Acute Medical Emergencies

**Acute Medical
Emergencies**

Useful website addresses

Advanced Life Support Group   http://www.alsg.org
Best Evidence in Emergency Medicine http://www.bestbets.org
Evidence based on-call   http://cebm.jr2.ox.ac.uk/eboc/eboc.html
Royal College of Physicians   http://www.rcplondon.ac.uk/

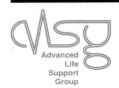

Acute Medical Emergencies
The Practical Approach

SECOND EDITION

Advanced Life Support Group

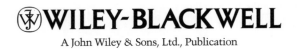

WILEY-BLACKWELL

A John Wiley & Sons, Ltd., Publication

BMJ | Books

Library of Congress Cataloging-in-Publication Data

Acute medical emergencies : the practical approach / Advanced Life Support Group. – 2nd ed.
    p. ; cm.
  Includes index.
  ISBN 978-0-7279-1854-3
  1. Medical emergencies–Handbooks, manuals, etc.   2. Emergency medicine–Handbooks, manuals, etc.   I. Advanced Life Support Group (Manchester, England)
  [DNLM: 1. Emergency Treatment–methods. 2. Emergencies. WB 105 A1895 2010]
  RC86.7.A282 2010
  616.02′5–dc22
                                     2009046382

ISBN: 9780727918543

A catalogue record for this book is available from the British Library.

Set in 10/13pt Meridien by Aptara® Inc., New Delhi, India
Printed and bound in Singapore by Markono Print Media Pte Ltd

1 2010

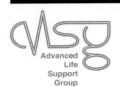

Contents

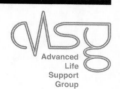

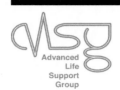

Working group

P Driscoll Emergency Medicine, *Manchester*
P Dyer General Medicine, *Birmingham*
C Duffy ALSG, *Manchester*
R Kishen Anaesthesia/ICU, *Manchester*
K Mackway-Jones Emergency Medicine, *Manchester*
G McCarthy Emergency Medicine, *Cork*
TD Wardle General Medicine, *Chester*
J Whitaker Care of the Elderly, *Harrogate*
S Wieteska ALSG, *Manchester*

REVIEWERS

P Driscoll Emergency Medicine, *Manchester*
M Emons Emergency Medicine, Rijen, *Netherlands*
A Eriksson Medicine, Stockholm, *Sweden*
R Kishen Anaesthesia/ICU, *Manchester*
D MacKechnie Emergency Medicine, *Rochdale*
G McCarthy Emergency Medicine, *Cork*
T D Wardle General Medicine, *Chester*

EDITORIAL GROUP

P Driscoll Emergency Medicine, *Manchester*
TD Wardle General Medicine, *Chester*
S Wieteska CEO, ALSG, *Manchester*

Contributors to first edition

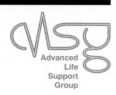

M Bhushan Dermatology, *Manchester*

P Davies Emergency Medicine, *Bristol*

P Driscoll Emergency Medicine, *Manchester*

CEM Griffiths Dermatology, *Manchester*

C Gwinnutt Anaesthesia, *Manchester*

J Hanson Emergency Medicine, *Preston*

R Kishen Anaesthesia/ICU, *Manchester*

K Mackway-Jones Emergency Medicine, *Manchester*

A McGowan Emergency Medicine, *Leeds*

G McMahon Emergency Medicine, *Manchester*

F Morris Emergency Medicine, *Sheffield*

C Moulton Emergency Medicine, *Bolton*

K Reynard Emergency Medicine, *Manchester*

P Sammy General Practice, *Manchester*

P Terry Emergency Medicine, *Manchester*

D Wallis Emergency Medicine, *London*

TD Wardle General Medicine, *Chester*

B Waters Anaesthesia/ICU, *North Wales*

J Whitaker Care of the Elderly, *Harrogate*

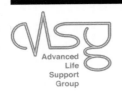

Contributors to second edition

Z L Borrill General Medicine, *Manchester*
P Davies Emergency Medicine, *Bristol*
P Driscoll Emergency Medicine, *Manchester*
P Dyer General Medicine, *Birmingham*
R Dowdle General Medicine, *Glamorgan*
J Hanson Emergency Medicine, *Preston*
R Hardern Emergency Medicine, *Durham*
P Hormbrey Emergency Medicine, *Oxford*
S J Hutchison Cardiology, *Abergavenny*
K Jones Respiratory Medicine, *Bolton*
T Jordan Respiratory Medicine, *Liverpool*
R Kishen Intensive Care, *Manchester*
G Lloyd Emergency Medicine, *Exeter*
A MacNab Emergency Medicine, *Swansea*
G McCarthy Emergency Medicine, *Cork*
D Wallis Emergency Medicine, *London*
T D Wardle General Medicine, *Chester*
J Whitaker Care of the Elderly, *Harrogate*
D W Wrathall Intensive Care, *Dumfries*

Preface to second edition

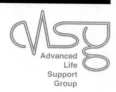

Since its first publication in 2001, this text has been a key component of an educational package that has trained in excess of 600 providers in the management of acute medical emergencies. The course is now running in the UK, Eire, the Netherlands and Sweden.

Over this time, new guidelines and changes in practice have provided impetus to produce the second edition. The challenge of updating this with ever evolving guidelines has now been met. However, despite evidence-based developments and improvement in medical practice, the foundation of MedicALS – the structured approach – remains unchanged, reassuringly.

The second edition will continue to promote the essence of MedicALS, which is to ensure that the candidate leaves the course equipped with a 'Practical Approach' that is safe to patients with any kind of acute medical emergency.

As new or updated guidelines become available, we will provide those on the ALSG website www.alsg.org to ensure that your Acute Medical Emergencies text remains current.

Over the years, an increasing number of experts have contributed to the work and we extend our thanks both to them and to our instructors, who unceasingly provide helpful feedback. Consultation with instructors has greatly contributed to this new edition and to the revised course.

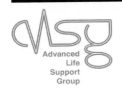

Preface to first edition

This book has been written to enable health care workers to understand the principles of managing an acute medical emergency safely and effectively. To achieve this aim it provides a structured approach to medical emergencies, describing relevant pathophysiology that will also help to explain physical signs and the rationale behind treatment. The first edition of this manual (written by Terry Wardle) has undergone significant modification directed by the working group and also, in particular, candidates from the first MedicALS courses. The requirements of these contributing doctors have meant that the contents and associated information may initially appear skewed – but this is evidence based.

Most textbooks are out of date by the time they are published – this manual is different in that it is both pragmatic and dynamic. Medicine is a rapidly evolving discipline and in order to ensure that this manual remains dynamic and up to date, reference web sites are available to ensure that the reader has constant access to relevant information. This will facilitate continual professional development that is the responsibility of the individual.

The book provides a structured approach that is applicable to all aspects of acute medicine, ensures the early recognition of signs of critical illness and will empower the individual to take immediate and appropriate action.

The text alone cannot provide all the necessary knowledge and skills to manage an acute medical emergency; therefore, readers are encouraged to attend the MedicALS course to further their theoretical and practical knowledge.

This book will continue to change to include new evidence-based practices and protocols to ensure a solid and safe foundation of knowledge and skills in this era of clinical governance.

Continued professional development is mandatory for all medical practitioners. This manual and the associated course will ensure both new knowledge acquisition and revision – and stimulate further learning.

Acknowledgments

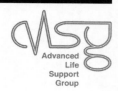

We would like to thank members of faculty and candidates who have completed the MedicALS course for their constructive comments that have shaped both the text and the course.

We would also like to thank Dr. Iomhar O'Sullivan for the use of Fig. 10.1.

We would also like to thank the Resuscitation Council (UK) and the British Thoracic Society for their permission to reproduce some of their algorithms and guidelines.

We would also like to thank Helen Carruthers, MMAA and Kate Wieteska for their work on some of the figures within the text.

Finally, our thanks to Clare Duffy of ALSG and the staff at the Wiley-Blackwell for their ongoing support and invaluable assistance in the production of this text.

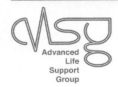

Advanced
Life
Support
Group

PART I
Introduction

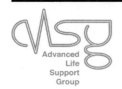

CHAPTER 1

Introduction

INTRODUCTION

After reading this chapter you will understand:
- the current problems in the assessment of acute medical emergencies
- the need for a structured approach to the medical patient.

THE PROBLEM

A medical emergency can arise in any patient, under a variety of circumstances, e.g.:
- previously fit
- acute on chronic illness
- post-surgical
- precipitating or modifying the response to trauma.

The acute problem can be directly or indirectly related to the presenting condition, an associated complication, any treatment and/or the result of inappropriate action.

Key point

Inappropriate action costs lives

Furthermore, with the increase in the elderly population there is a corresponding increase in the number and complexity of medical problems. The management of such patients is compromised by conflicting demands such as financial constraints, limited bed availability, workforce availability and increased medical specialisation.

For the last few years there has been an annual increase of emergency admissions in excess of 5%. These account for over 40% of all acute National Health Service beds. In the UK the mean hospital bed complement is 641, but only 186 are allocated for medical patients, with an average of 95% of these housing patients admitted as emergencies.

The common acute conditions can be broadly classified according to the body system affected (Table 1.1).

This information may be broken down further to reveal the common reasons for admission:
- myocardial infarction
- stroke
- cardiac failure
- acute exacerbation of asthma

Acute Medical Emergencies; The Practical Approach, 2nd edition.
Edited by Terence Wardle, Peter Driscoll, and Sue Wieteska.
© 2010 Blackwell Publishing Ltd.

Table 1.1 Classification of medical emergencies

Type	%
Cardiac	29
Respiratory	26
Neurological	21
Gastrointestinal	13

- acute exacerbation of chronic obstructive pulmonary disease
- deliberate self-harm.

Despite the fact that these are common conditions, frequent management errors and inappropriate action result in preventable morbidity and mortality.

A recent risk management study examined the care of medical emergencies. One or more avoidable serious adverse clinical incidents were reported. Common mistakes are listed in the box below.

Common mistakes

Failure to recognise and treat serious infection
Error in investigating – acute headache
– acute breathlessness
– epilepsy
Misinterpretation of investigations
Inadequate assessment of abdominal symptoms

This was only a small study but of the 29 patients who died, 20 would have had a good chance of long-term survival with appropriate management. In addition, out of the 11 patients who survived, 3 were left with serious neurological defects, 3 had avoidable intestinal resection and 4 patients suffered unnecessarily prolonged hospital admission.

The overall problems were identified as follows:
- Medical emergencies were not assessed by sufficiently experienced staff.
- A second opinion was not obtained.
- Assessment was inadequately performed before discharge.
- X-rays were not discussed with radiologists.
- Protocols were not used for standard conditions.

Diagnostic errors were made in 80% of patients because of inadequate interpretation of the clinical picture and initial investigations. Errors in patient assessment are listed in the box below.

Errors in patient assessment

Available clinical evidence incorrectly interpreted
Failure to identify and focus on very sick patients
Investigations misread or ignored
Radiological evidence missed
Standard procedures not followed
Inadequate assessment and/or treatment
Discharge from hospital without proper assessment

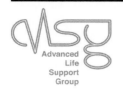

Furthermore, the assessment of medical patients requiring intensive care was either incomplete, inappropriate or too late to prevent increased morbidity and mortality.

Therefore, there are problems in the **fundamental** areas of medical patient care, i.e. clinical examination, requesting and interpreting appropriate investigations and communication. However, probably most important of all is knowing when and who to ask for help. One answer to this important problem is to provide a structured approach to patient assessment that will facilitate problem identification and prioritise management.

All that is required to manage medical emergencies is the application of focused knowledge and basic skills. These will ensure prompt accurate assessment and improve patient outcome. Avoidable deaths are due to inappropriate management, indecision or delays in assessment and/or treatment. In the study the average time for initial review after admission is 30 minutes, with a further 130 minutes passing before definitive management occurs.

In the UK, numerous studies have shown that specialist care is better than that provided by a generalist; e.g. prompt review by a respiratory physician has been shown to reduce both morbidity and mortality from asthma. The mortality from gastrointestinal haemorrhage falls from 40% to approximately 5% if the management is provided by a specialist in gastroenterology. Further, supportive evidence has been provided by studies in the US, where mortality from myocardial infarction or unstable angina was greater in patients managed by generalists.

However there are insufficient numbers of 'specialists' to manage all of these conditions. Besides, patients with sudden deterioration in their condition often present as 'undifferentiated medical emergencies', without a clear 'label' identifying which particular specialist is required. Some will require review by a general physician, whilst others will be managed at least initially by colleagues in the rapidly expanding, exciting discipline of acute medicine.

Thus, physicians need to know how to manage medical emergencies. This course will teach a structured approach for assessment that will enable you to deliver safe, effective and appropriate care.

Traditional medical teaching dictates that a history should always be taken from the patient before the clinical examination. This will subsequently allow a diagnosis or differential diagnosis to be postulated and dictate the investigations required. Unfortunately this approach is not always possible; e.g. trying to obtain a history from a patient who presents with breathlessness may not only exacerbate the condition but also delay crucial therapy.

This course has been developed by observing how experienced physicians manage medical emergencies. The results have shown quite an interesting cultural shift. Most of us, as we approach the patient, quickly scan for any obvious physical signs, e.g. breathlessness, and then focus our attention on the symptoms until the diagnosis is identified. Only when the patient's symptoms have been improved can a history be taken and the remainder of the examination performed. This process has been refined and formalised to produce a structured approach to patient assessment so that the most immediately life-threatening problems are identified early and treated promptly. Thus, this structured approach considers the conditions that are most likely to kill the patient.

All other problems will be identified subsequently as part of the overall classical approach to the medical patient, i.e. taking a comprehensive history and examining the patient fully. Being aware at all time that should the patient deteriorate a reassessment should start at the beginning.

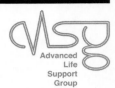

The key principles of MedicALS are shown in the box.

Key principles of MedicALS

Do no further harm

Focused knowledge and basic skills are essential for doctors dealing with acute emergencies

A structured approach will identify key problems and prioritise management

Prompt accurate assessment and treatment improves patient outcome

---

SUMMARY

The number and complexity of acute medical emergencies are increasing along with the potential for medical mishaps. Typically these result from a failure to assess acutely ill patients, interpret relevant investigations and provide appropriate management. This manual, and the associated course, will equip you with a structured approach to deal with these patients.

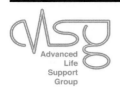

CHAPTER 2

Recognition of the medical emergency

OBJECTIVES

After reading this chapter you will be able to:
- understand the clinical features of potential respiratory, cardiac and neurological failure
- describe these clinical features and use them to form the basis of the primary assessment.

Irrespective of the underlying pathology, the acutely ill medical patient who dies does so from failures of the respiratory, circulatory or central neurological systems separately or in combination. It is of paramount importance that the physician can recognise potential failure of these systems, as early intervention will reduce morbidity and mortality. The ultimate failure, a cardiorespiratory arrest, can often be predicted in the hospital setting as it is generally preceded by a period of physiological deterioration.

This chapter will provide an overview of the clinical assessment of patients with potential respiratory, circulatory and neurological failure. The chapters in Part II will then use this format to develop an in-depth assessment that produces a structured approach to the patient with a medical emergency. An underlying principle of the assessment system described below is that it is physiologically based rather than using the more classical format of history taking, examination and investigation.

Time Out 2.1

Think about a patient you have treated recently who was critically ill, and reflect on the good and/or bad aspects of their treatment. List the staff involved and assessments that took place during the management of this patient.

Draw a timeline and place the information from your lists on the line. At the end of the line, write down the outcome of the episode.

RECOGNITION OF POTENTIAL RESPIRATORY FAILURE

This can be assessed by examining the respiratory rate, effort of respiration and effectiveness of ventilation, as well as the effects of respiratory inadequacy.

Acute Medical Emergencies; The Practical Approach, 2nd edition.
Edited by Terence Wardle, Peter Driscoll, and Sue Wieteska.
© 2010 Blackwell Publishing Ltd.

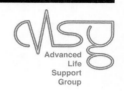

Respiratory rate

The normal adult respiratory rate is 14–20 breaths/min. Variation outside this range is an indication of potential respiratory failure. Tachypnoea (greater than 30 breaths/min at rest) generally indicates that increased ventilation is needed because of hypoxaemia associated with disease affecting the airway, breathing or circulation. It can also indicate compensatory hyperventilation due to a metabolic acidosis associated with a non-respiratory problem. Similarly, a respiratory rate of less than 10 breaths/min is an indication of respiratory fatigue or loss of central respiratory drive, both potentially requiring ventilatory support.

Effort of respiration

Assessment of effort gives an indication of how hard a patient is working to breathe. If the patient can count to 10 in one breath, there is usually no significant underlying respiratory problem. Features which suggest increased respiratory effort are tachypnoea, intercostal and subcostal recession and accessory muscle use.

Effectiveness of ventilation

Effectiveness of ventilation is assessed by measurement of chest expansion, percussion and auscultation. Chest expansion indicates the volume of air being moved during the respiratory cycle.

The presence or absence of breath sounds allows assessment of airflow to specific areas of both lung fields. Any asymmetry should be noted. Pathology is generally on the side of abnormal signs.

Any added sounds should be noted. Stridor is a loud inspiratory noise and is indicative of laryngeal/tracheal narrowing or obstruction. During auscultation you may hear wheezing and/or a prolonged expiratory phase due to lower airway narrowing.

Key point

A silent chest is an extremely worrying sign

Oxygen saturation

Pulse oximetry is used to measure the arterial oxygen saturation (SpO_2). It is inaccurate in the following circumstances:

- $SpO_2 < 70\%$
- poor peripheral perfusion
- in the presence of methaemoglobin or carboxyhaemoglobin.

Effects of respiratory inadequacy on other organs

Heart rate

Hypoxaemia initially produces a tachycardia. These changes are non-specific as other causes such as anxiety, fever or shock may coexist. However, severe or prolonged hypoxaemia will eventually lead to a bradycardia – a preterminal sign.

Skin colour

Hypoxaemia, via catecholamine release, produces vasoconstriction and hence skin pallor. Decreased oxygen concentration will lead to cyanosis as haemoglobin becomes deoxygenated. Central cyanosis in acute respiratory disease is indicative of imminent respiratory arrest. In the anaemic patient, cyanosis may be

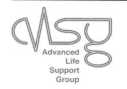

difficult to detect despite profound hypoxaemia, because the reduced total amount of haemoglobin may mean there is not enough deoxygenated haemoglobin to produce the cyanotic colour.

Mental status

The hypoxaemic patient will initially appear agitated and eventually will become drowsy. Similar features will also occur with hypercapnoea; in this situation the patient will be vasodilated and have a flapping tremor (asterixis).

RECOGNITION OF POTENTIAL CIRCULATORY FAILURE

Acute circulatory failure can also be defined as shock. Although this has multiple causes, during the initial assessment the overriding priority is to identify shock, rather than find a specific cause.

Circulatory failure is assessed by examining the heart rate, effectiveness of circulation and the effects of shock on other organs.

Heart rate

This increases in the shocked patient due to catecholamine release, generally secondary to a decreased circulatory volume in an effort to increase cardiac output. There are many reasons why a normal adult may experience a tachycardia (pulse rate > 100/minute) and other signs should be sought to confirm the clinical suspicion of circulatory failure.

Be aware that certain drugs (e.g β blockers) can prevent a compensatory tachycardia and very fit patients, in whom a pulse rate of 100/minute may be twice their resting pulse rate.

Effectiveness of circulation
Blood pressure

Compensatory mechanisms will try to maintain blood pressure. Consequently, during the early stages of shock it may be normal or even elevated. For this reason, blood pressure should not be used as the sole indicator of circulatory status. Hypotension in circulatory failure is an indicator of increased mortality. As the Blood pressure is such an important parameter always ensure that an appropriate cuff size is used when it is measured.

Pulses – central and peripheral; pulse volume

Although blood pressure is generally maintained until shock is very severe (loss of at least one third of the circulating volume), a rapid assessment of perfusion can be gained by examining peripheral and central pulses. The combination of absent peripheral pulses and weak central pulses is a sinister sign indicating advanced shock and profound hypotension.

Perfusion

Pressure on a central area (e.g sternum) for 5 s should normally produce a capillary refill within 2 s. A prolonged refill time indicates poor skin perfusion, a sign of shock. This sign is unreliable in hypothermic patients.

Effects of circulatory inadequacy on other organs
Respiratory system

A rapid respiratory rate with an increased tidal volume, without signs of increased respiratory effort, is predominantly caused by a metabolic acidosis associated with circulatory failure.

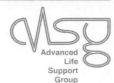

Skin

Mottled, cold and pale skin especially at the peripheries is an indicator of poor perfusion.

Mental status

Agitation, confusion, drowsiness and unconsciousness are the progressive stages of mental dysfunction associated with circulatory failure due to poor cerebral perfusion.

Urinary output

A urine output of less than 0.5 ml/kg/h indicates inadequate renal perfusion.

RECOGNITION OF POTENTIAL CENTRAL NEUROLOGICAL FAILURE

Maintaining adequate central neurological function is a priority during resuscitation of a critically ill patient. Both respiratory and circulatory failure will affect the assessment of neurological function, and must therefore be addressed before central neurological assessment.

Initial assessment is directed at global rather than specific function. Conscious level, posture, asymmetrical motor signs and pupillary response should be evaluated.

Conscious level

A rapid assessment of the patient's conscious level can be made by assigning the patient to one of the categories shown in the box.

AVPU grading of consciousness

A = Alert
V = response to Voice
P = response to Pain
U = Unresponsive

A painful stimulus should be applied by pressure over the supraorbital ridge on the superior orbital nerve. An adult who either responds only to pain (P) or is unresponsive (U) has a significant degree of coma equivalent to 8 or less on the Glasgow Coma Scale. These patients are at risk of losing control of their airway.

Posture

Abnormal posturing such as decorticate (flexed arms, extended legs) or decerebrate (extended arms, extended legs) is a sinister sign of brain dysfunction. A painful stimulus may be necessary to elicit these signs. Determine also if there is a difference in motor response between the right and left sides as this indicates a localised neurological disorder.

Pupils

The most important pupillary signs to seek are dilation, unreactivity and inequality. These indicate possible serious brain disorders. Many drugs and cerebral lesions have effects on pupil size and reaction.

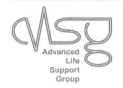

Respiratory effects of central neurological failure on other systems

There are several recognisable breathing patterns associated with raised intracranial pressure. However, they are often changeable and may vary from hyperventilation to periodic breathing and apnoea. The presence of any abnormal respiratory pattern in a patient with coma suggests brain stem dysfunction.

Circulatory effects of central neurological failure

Systemic hypertension with sinus bradycardia and erratic respiration (Cushing's triad) indicates compression of the medulla oblongata caused by herniation of the cerebellar tonsils through the foramen magnum. This is a late and preterminal sign.

Time Out 2.2

Refer back to the timeline you drew in Time Out 2.1.

Using the system described in this chapter, draw out an ideal timeline for your patient's assessment.

Do you think that this system would have any benefits to the patient's care you charted and particularly to the outcome you wrote at the end of the line?

On your ideal timeline, highlight the number of features that assess more than one system.

Finally, check that your list of clinical features is in a logical order to produce a rapid system for assessment of a critically ill patient.

SUMMARY

In the acutely ill medical patient a rapid examination will detect potential respiratory, circulatory and neurological failure. The clinical features are:
- respiratory – rate, effort and effectiveness of respiration
- circulatory – heart rate and effectiveness of circulation
- neurological – conscious level, posture and pupils.

These features will form the framework of the primary assessment. The components will be discussed in detail in Part II.

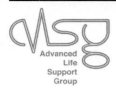

PART II
Structured Approach

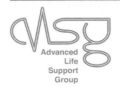

CHAPTER 3

A structured approach to medical emergencies

OBJECTIVES

After reading this chapter you will be able to describe the:
- correct sequence of priorities to be followed when assessing an acutely ill medical patient
- primary and secondary phases of assessment
- key components of a patient's history
- techniques used in the initial resuscitation, investigation and definitive care of a medical emergency.

INTRODUCTION

The management of a patient with a medical emergency requires a rapid assessment with appropriate treatment of life-threatening conditions as and when they are found. This can best be achieved using a structured approach. This chapter will give an overview of this approach and each component will be examined in greater detail in subsequent chapters.

Structured approach

Primary assessment and resuscitation
Secondary assessment and emergency treatment
Reassessment
Definitive care

Key point

The aim of the primary assessment is **to identify and treat any immediately life-threatening conditions with minimum delay and in a prioritised fashion.** Most acutely ill medical patients (75%) do not have an immediately life-threatening problem. However, a rapid primary assessment is still required.

The primary assessment should be repeated immediately in the event of any deterioration in the patient's condition. This allows early appropriate resuscitation to reverse the deterioration. Be prepared to act on a strong clinical suspicion as your intervention will be likely to reverse or halt a deterioration.

Acute Medical Emergencies; The Practical Approach, 2nd edition.
Edited by Terence Wardle, Peter Driscoll, and Sue Wieteska.
© 2010 Blackwell Publishing Ltd.

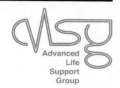

Remember that certain classical signs taught in medical school may be difficult to confirm in a noisy resuscitation area (e.g. quiet heart sounds in life-threatening cardiac tamponade).

Once any immediately life-threatening conditions have been either identified and treated, or excluded (i.e. primary assessment and resuscitation), you can then take a comprehensive history and complete a thorough examination (i.e. secondary assessment and emergency treatment). Following any emergency treatment the patient should be reassessed. Definitive care can then be planned including transportation to the appropriate ward and further investigation.

PRIMARY ASSESSMENT AND RESUSCITATION

Key point

The aim of the primary assessment is to **identify** and **treat** all (there may be more than one) **immediately life-threatening conditions**

Key point

Always use universal precautions before assessing an acutely ill patient

---

Key components of the primary assessment (ABCDE) are assessment and management of:

A – Airway
B – Breathing
C – Circulation
D – Disability
E – Exposure

A – Airway

Aims = assess patency and identify any imminent threat, e.g. mucosal oedema in anaphylaxis. If necessary, clear and secure the airway
    = administer high concentrations of inspired oxygen
    = appreciate the potential for cervical spine injury

Assessment

Assess airway patency by talking to the patient. An appropriate response to 'Are you okay?' indicates that the airway is clear, the patient is breathing and has adequate cerebral perfusion. If no answer is forthcoming, then open the airway with a chin lift or jaw thrust and reassess patency by:

* looking – for chest movement
* listening – for the sounds of breathing
* feeling – for expired air.

A check for upper airway obstruction should include inspection for foreign bodies, including dentures, and macroglossia.

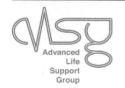

Resuscitation

If a chin lift or jaw thrust is needed, then an airway adjunct may be required to maintain patency. A nasopharyngeal airway is useful in the conscious patient. In contrast an oropharyngeal (Guedel) airway is typically used as a temporary adjunct in the unconscious patient before airway protection is achieved by endotracheal intubation.

Whilst gaining definitive control of the airway, supplemental oxygen should be given to all patients who are breathless, shocked, bleeding or suspected to be acutely ill from any cause. If the patient is not intubated, oxygen should be given using a non-rebreathing mask and reservoir. This enables the fractional inspired oxygen (FiO_2) concentration to reach a level of up to 0.85. All critically ill patients should receive high concentrations of inspired oxygen. For the purposes of this text and course, critically ill is defined as a patient with an early warning score of 3 or above (see Table 3.3). Even critically ill patients who have chronic obstructive pulmonary disease should receive high concentrations of inspired oxygen initially; this can subsequently be reduced according to its clinical effect and arterial blood gas results. You therefore need to maintain close observation of these patients until the optimum FiO_2 is determined.

Cervical spine problems are very rare in medical patients – except in those with rheumatoid disease, ankylosing spondylitis and Down's syndrome. The clinical features of these conditions are usually easily identifiable. However, be wary of the elderly patient found collapsed at the bottom of the stairs after an apparent 'stroke'. If you suspect cervical spine injury, ask for immediate help to provide in-line immobilisation.

Key point

Hypoxaemia kills

Hypercarbia is not a killer, provided the patient is receiving supplemental oxygen in a high dependency setting

---

Monitoring

Arterial oxygen saturation (SpO_2) monitoring is essential. End tidal carbon dioxide ($ETCO_2$) should be measured after endotracheal intubation, to check correct tube placement and alert you in the event of subsequent tube displacement.

See Chapter 4 for further details.

B – Breathing

Aim = detect and treat:
- life-threatening bronchospasm
- pulmonary oedema
- tension pneumothorax
- the presence of critical oxygen desaturation

Assessment

A patent airway does not ensure adequate ventilation. The latter requires an intact respiratory centre, adequate pulmonary function and the coordinated movement of the diaphragm and chest wall.

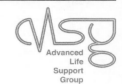

Chest inspection

Colour/marks/rash
Rate
Effort
Symmetry

Look for cyanosis, respiratory rate and effort, and symmetry of movement. Feel for tracheal tug or deviation. Tracheal deviation (in a distressed or unconscious patient) indicates mediastinal shift (consider tension pneumothorax and decompress immediately if suspected). Percuss the anterior chest wall in the upper, middle and lower zones, assessing the difference between the left and right hemithoraces. Repeat this on the posterior chest wall and axillae to detect areas of hyper-resonance (air), dullness (interstitial fluid) or stony dullness (pleural fluid). Listen to the chest to establish whether breath sounds are absent, present or masked by added sounds. Further information regarding oxygen saturation of blood will be provided by a pulse oximeter.

Key point

Some physical signs will be elicited that suggest a non-breathing cause for respiratory difficulty. Thus corroborative evidence must be sought to confirm a clinical diagnosis of, e.g., left ventricular failure.

Key point

Remember that if your patient is lying down:
The physical signs might be harder to elicit, e.g. dullness to percussion from an effusion will be posterior
Back examination must occur at some stage!

Resuscitation

Treat life-threatening bronchospasm as soon as it is identified, with nebulised salbutamol (β_2-agonist) and ipratropium bromide (muscarinic antagonist).

A tension pneumothorax requires urgent decompression with a needle thoracocentesis, followed by intravenous access and chest drain insertion.

Further clues to the cause of apparent respiratory difficulty may be found on examination of the patient's circulation.

Monitoring

Arterial oxygen saturation (SpO_2) should be monitored continuously.
Respiratory rate
See Chapter 5 for more comprehensive details.

C – Circulation

Aim = detect and treat shock

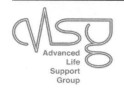

Assessment

Measure cardiovascular indices and level of consciousness. Examine a central pulse (ideally the carotid), for rate, rhythm and character. Compare both carotid pulses, but not simultaneously. A reduction or absence in one pulse may reflect focal atheroma or a dissecting aneurysm. Measure the blood pressure and assess peripheral perfusion using the capillary refill time. Assess the height (and character) of the JVP (Jugular Venous Pulse), the apex beat and listen to the heart sounds and for any extra sounds.

Hypotension indicates established decompensation, requiring prompt action to prevent shock becoming irreversible. A normal blood pressure in the young and previously healthy can be maintained despite well-established shock. Look for narrowing of the pulse pressure. This occurs when the systolic blood pressure is 'propped up' by the neuroadrenergic (catecholamine) response to a reduced stroke volume raising the diastolic blood pressure (increased tone/resistance).

Reduced blood volume can impair consciousness due to reduced cerebral perfusion.

Some causes of shock require specific treatment, e.g. adrenaline for anaphylaxis

Resuscitation

Intravenous access is needed in all acutely ill patients. If there is a suspicion of hypovolaemic shock, two large-bore cannulae should be inserted. The antecubital fossa is usually the easiest and most convenient site. Take blood for baseline haematological and biochemical values (including a serum glucose) and, in appropriate cases, a cross-match. You should strongly consider taking arterial blood gases to look for ventilatory inadequacy and metabolic acidosis in particular.

> **Key point**
>
> Fluid, antibiotics, glucose, adrenaline, inotropes, antidotes and electricity are crucial in the management of different types of shock

Hypovolaemic

If you suspect hypovolaemia (depletion of intravascular volume), give a fluid challenge of 2 litres of Ringer's lactate in 500 ml boluses. Further fluid requirements will be determined by the patient's response. If, after 2 litres of fluid, the patient remains hypotensive and haemorrhage is suspected, then blood and a **surgeon** are needed urgently.

Cardiogenic

A similar pale, cold and clammy picture will be found in cardiogenic shock. The presence of pulmonary oedema is a useful differentiating factor. Non-invasive positive pressure ventilation and/or inotropes will be required in this case. Consider emergency primary coronary intervention if myocardial infarction is the cause.

Cardiac rhythm

Cardiac rhythm disturbance causing haemodynamic instability should be treated according to UK and European resuscitation guidelines. This patient will almost certainly require sedation and cardioversion.

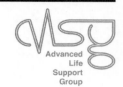

Septic

The hypotensive, warm, vasodilated and pyrexial patient is 'septic' until proven otherwise. Look for the non-blanching purpuric rash of meningococcal septicaemia. This condition, if suspected, requires immediate treatment with intravenous benzyl penicillin 2.4 g and ceftriaxone 1 g. Investigations should include blood cultures, C-reactive protein and blood for meningococcal polymerase chain reaction after initial resuscitation.

Diabetic keto acidosis (DKA)

Look (and smell) for diabetic ketoacidosis (raised blood glucose, ketonuria and acidaemia) in the tachypnoeic, dehydrated and hypotensive patient.Following confirmation of the diagnosis, treatment should be started as described in chapter 20.

Anaphylactic

Shock due to anaphylaxis is treated according to the UK and European resuscitation guidelines (see Chapter 9).

Occasionally, shock may have more than one cause. Dehydration is common in acute medical emergencies. If there is no evidence of either ventricular failure or a dysrhythmia, all patients should receive a fluid challenge (200–300 ml immediately). Subsequent management will depend on the patient's response and blood test results.

Monitoring

Continuous monitoring of oxygen saturation (pulse oximetry), pulse, blood pressure and ECG provides valuable baseline information about the patient and the response to treatment (reassessment). Consider a urinary catheter to monitor urinary output, in the shocked patient as this provides a useful indicator as to the adequacy of resuscitation.

See Chapter 6 for more comprehensive details.

D – Disability (neurological examination)

Aim = to detect and treat any immediately life-threatening neurological condition (e.g. prolonged fit, hypoglycaemia, opioid overdose, infection or suspected cerebral ischaemia).

Assessment

Measure pupillary size and reaction to light. Evaluate the conscious level, using either the AVPU system (see Chapter 2) or more commonly the Glasgow Coma Score (Table 3.1). Check the patient's posture and for the presence of lateralising signs in the limbs. Examine for signs of meningeal irritation. Remember FAST; **F**ace, **A**rms, **S**peech, **T**ime as pre-hospital indicators of a potential stroke.

Check serum glucose with either a glucometer or a BM stix in the presence of any neurological dysfunction. Hypoglycaemia is common, readily detectable, easily treatable and has serious implications if therapy is delayed. Hypoglycaemia should be treated immediately, once a venous blood sample has been taken for definitive glucose measurement.

Resuscitation

In the unconscious patient, it is vital to clear and secure the airway. Give supplemental oxygen until further clinical information and the results of investigations

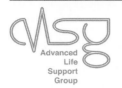

Table 3.1 The Glasgow Coma Scale

Eye Opening	
Spontaneous	4
To speech	3
To painful stimuli	2
Nil	1
Best Verbal Response	
Orientated	5
Confused	4
Inappropriate words	3
Incomprehensible sounds	2
Nil	1
Best Motor Response	
Obeys commands	6
Localises pain	5
Withdraws from pain	4
Abnormal flexion	3
Abnormal extension	2
Nil	1

Note: If there is focal limb weakness, the best motor response should be recorded.

are available. Prevent secondary brain injury by ensuring optimum management of A, B and C.

'Tonic–clonic' seizures usually resolve spontaneously within a minute or so. Ensure that the patient has a patent airway, is receiving supplemental oxygen and that vital signs are monitored regularly. Place the patient in the recovery position to prevent aspiration and injury on any adjacent objects. It is not uncommon to misinterpret reduction of tonic–clonic movements as the cessation of seizures. If you think the patient has stopped convulsing, check for ease of passive eye opening and absence of abnormal eye movements. Remember to check for hypoglycaemia.

If the fit is prolonged (longer than 2–5 min, depending on the patient's condition), give intravenous benzodiazepines, e.g. lorazepam 4 mg over 2 min (repeat after 10 min if the patient is still fitting), or increments of 2.5 mg of diazemuls (to a maximum of 20 mg). If benzodiazepines fail to control the fit, start intravenous phenytoin at 15 mg/kg over 30 min with ECG monitoring. This drug does not impair the conscious level and will facilitate early neurological assessment. An alternative is fosphenytoin (18 mg/kg phenytoin equivalent IV up to 150 mg/min). If this combination fails to control fitting, request urgent assistance from an anaesthetist regarding rapid sequence induction.

In hypoglycaemia, an infusion of 10% dextrose and/or intravenous glucagon (1 mg) is immediately necessary to prevent recurrence. If underlying alcohol use is suspected, give intravenous thiamine as well.

The unconscious patient showing signs of opioid excess (small and unreactive pupils) should be treated with intravenous naloxone 0.2 mg.

The unconscious or confused patient will need a CT brain scan. However, this must not delay antibiotic and/or antiviral treatment for suspected meningitis/encephalitis, or any other necessary resuscitation (including intubation to

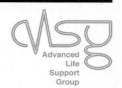

protect the airway, if necessary). As a general rule, unstable and/or inadequately resuscitated patients should not be moved to places of lesser safety (such as CT scan area), without the consultant in charge of the resuscitation agreeing that it is necessary and appropriate.

Patients with suspected cerebral ischaemia should have an early CT and, if indicated, should receive thrombolysis within 4 h.

Monitoring

Glasgow Coma Score, pupillary response and serum glucose.

See Chapter 7 for more comprehensive details.

E – Exposure

Aim = examine the entire patient and prevent hypothermia.

Severe life-threatening skin conditions are associated with problems in 'C', but also occasionally in A, B and D. These include hypovolaemia, vasodilatation, loss of temperature control and risk of infection. Hence you should have already treated these by the time you treat E.

Assessment

Examine for three important rashes (the non-blanching purpura of meningococcal septicaemia, erythroderma and blistering eruptions). Other physical signs may include bleeding or bruising (coagulopathy), injury, swelling and infection. Do not forget to look for needle marks.

Resuscitation

Patients should have received intravenous fluids and antibiotics, if indicated, earlier in the primary assessment. Urgent referral to a dermatologist may be necessary to guide further management and investigation.

Monitoring

• Temperature

It is impossible to do a comprehensive examination unless the patient is fully undressed. However, care must be taken to prevent hypothermia, especially in elderly patients. Therefore, adequately cover patients between examinations and ensure all intravenous fluids are warmed.

MONITORING

The effectiveness of resuscitation is measured by an improvement in the patient's clinical status. It is therefore important that repeat observations are measured and recorded frequently. Table 3.2 shows the minimum level of monitoring required by the end of the primary assessment in an acutely unwell patient.

It is important to reassess the patient regularly, especially after treatment has been started. This will ensure that the patient has responded appropriately, and not deteriorated.

Key point

The most important assessment is the reassessment

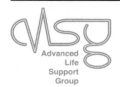

Table 3.2 Minimum patient monitoring in an acutely unwell patient

Pulse oximetry
Respiratory rate
Blood pressure
Continuous ECG monitoring, augmented by a 12-lead ECG
Chest X-ray when appropriate
Arterial blood gases when appropriate
Core temperature
Central venous pressure when appropriate
Glasgow Coma Score, lateralising signs and pupillary response
Urinary output

The majority of medical patients will only require a brief primary assessment, to establish that there is no need for aggressive resuscitation. In clinical practice, the usual patient–doctor introduction will provide a rapid assessment of the A, B, Cs. A patient who is sitting up and talking has a patent airway and sufficient cardiorespiratory function to provide oxygenation and cerebral perfusion.

A variety of scoring systems can be used to assess the acutely ill patient rapidly as a measure of 'how at risk the patient is'. These are based on the B, C, D and E components:

- Respiratory rate
- Pulse rate
- Systolic blood pressure
- Mental response
- Temperature

One such system, the Early Warning Score, is shown in Table 3.3. Scores may trigger actions at different levels in different settings.

In addition, the urine output can be included in patients who are catheterised. Each component is scored between 0 and 3. A patient who has a score of 3 for one component or 4 or more for a combination of components needs a more detailed assessment before physiological deterioration becomes too profound. Local protocols will dictate who does this detailed assessment, e.g. junior doctor, member of the outreach team or critical care team.

Where the early warning score is lower than that described above, one can skip quickly to the traditional style of history taking followed by a physical examination. This is referred to as the secondary assessment.

Table 3.3 Example early warning scoring system

Score	3	2	1	0	1	2	3
Respiratory rate		≤9		10–14	15–20	21–30	>30
Heart rate		<40	40–50	51–100	101–110	111–130	>130
Blood pressure (systolic)	≤70	71–80	81–100	101–199		≥200	
Central nervous system			SC	A	V	P	U
Temperature		<35		35–38		>38	
Urine output (ml/h)	Nil	<30	30–39	40–99	100–150	151–199	≥200

SC = sudden confusion; A = alert; V = responds to voice; P = responds to pain; U = unresponsive

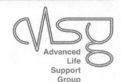

Advanced
Life
Support
Group

Time Out 3.1

After reading the case history, answer the following question:

A 54-year-old man is referred to the medical assessment unit because of an acute onset of confusion.

Briefly describe your primary assessment of this patient.

SECONDARY ASSESSMENT

> **The aims of the secondary assessment are to identify and treat all conditions not detected in the primary assessment, seek corroborative evidence to formulate a provisional diagnosis and prioritise the patient's management.**

The secondary assessment starts once vital functions have been stabilised and immediately life-threatening conditions have been identified and treated.

History

Nearly all medical diagnoses are made after a good history has been obtained from the patient. Occasionally, for a variety of reasons this may not be possible. Therefore information should be sought from relatives, the patient's medical notes, the general practitioner, friends or the police and ambulance service. A well-'phrased' history is required, and also serves as a useful mnemonic to remember the key features.

> **A well-'phrased' history**
>
> **P** Problem
> **H** History of presenting problem
> **R** Relevant medical history
> **A** Allergies
> **S** Systems review
> **E** Essential family and social history
> **D** Drugs

The history of the presenting problem is of paramount importance. A comprehensive systems review will ensure that significant, relevant information is not excluded. In addition, it will ensure that the secondary assessment focuses on the relevant systems.

Examination

Aims = find new features – often related to clues in the history
       = comprehensively reassess conditions identified in the primary assessment
       = seek corroborative evidence to support findings from the primary assessment and to formulate a diagnosis

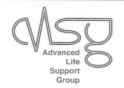

The examination should be directed by the history and primary assessment findings. It is a methodical, structured approach comprising a general overview and the detection of specific features.

General

A clinical overview of the patient's overall appearance 'from the end of the bed' can give clues to underlying pathology.

Clinical overview

Posture
Pigmentation
Pallor
Pattern of respiration
Pronunciation
Pulsations

Specific features include the following.

Hands

Inspect the hands for stigmata of infective endocarditis, chronic liver disease, thyrotoxicosis, carbon dioxide retention, polyarthropathy and multisystem disease. Palpate the radial pulse for rate, rhythm, character and symmetry, comparing it to the contralateral radial pulse and the femoral pulse.

Face

Examine for facial asymmetry, cyanosis, and the presence of any pigmentation, stigmata of hyperlipidaemia, titubation, and cutaneous features of internal pathology. Inspect the mouth, tongue and pharynx for the presence of ulcers, blisters, vesicles and erythema. Pigmentation of the buccal mucosa should be specifically sought (Addison's disease is an uncommon cause of collapse often associated with a delay in making the diagnosis).

Neck

Assess the height, waveform and characteristics of the internal jugular venous pulse. Palpate both internal carotid arteries in turn to compare and determine the pulse character. Check the position of the trachea and the distance between the suprasternal notch and the inferior aspect of the thyroid cartilage. A distance of less than 3 finger breadths indicates hyperexpansion of the chest. Feel for lymphadenopathy.

Chest

Assess the shape of the chest and breathing pattern. Recheck the rate, effort and symmetry of respiration. Look for surgical scars. Palpate the precordium to determine the site and character of the apex beat, the presence of a left and/or right ventricular heave, and the presence of thrills. Listen for the first, second and any additional heart sounds; and murmurs. Percuss the anterior and posterior chest walls bilaterally in upper, middle and lower zones comparing the note from the left and right hemithoraces. Auscultate these areas to determine the presence, type and quality of breath sounds as well as any added sounds. Check for evidence of peripheral oedema.

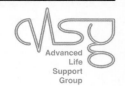

Abdomen

Systematically examine the abdomen according to the nine anatomical divisions. Specific features that should be sought include hepatosplenomegaly, peritonism/itis, abdominal masses, lymphadenopathy, ascites as well as renal angle tenderness. In appropriate cases examine the hernial orifices, external genitalia and rectum.

Locomotor

Inspect all joints and examine for the presence of tenderness, deformity, restricted movement, synovial thickening and inflammation. The patient's history, however, will indicate the joints that are affected. Although inflammatory polyarthropathies may present suddenly, acute monoarthropathies are potentially more sinister (see Chapter 17). Septic arthritis is an emergency that quickly destroys a joint if not diagnosed and treated.

Neurological

A comprehensive neurological examination is rarely required in the acutely ill patient. A screening examination of the nervous system can be accomplished as follows:

1 Assess the conscious state using the Glasgow Coma Scale.
2 A Mini Mental State Examination (see next box).
3 Examine the external ocular movements for diplopia, nystagmus or fatiguability. Elicit the pupillary response to light and accommodation (PERLA, i.e. pupils equally react to light and accommodation). Examine the fundi. The absence of dolls eye movement (oculocephalic reflex) indicates a brain stem problem. This is obviously only relevant in the unconscious patient and should not be elicited if there is a suspicion of cervical spine instability. Assess muscles of mastication and facial movement followed by palatal movement, gag reflex and tongue protrusion. When appropriate check the corneal reflex and visual fields (see Chapter 7).
4 Test the tone of all four limbs, the power of muscle groups, reflexes (including the Plantar/Babinski response) and coordination.
5 Sensory testing, although subjective, is useful in the acute medical setting, especially when a cord lesion is suspected.
6 Further neurological examination will be dictated by the patient's history and the examination findings, especially from the screening neurological assessment.

Skin

The skin and the buccal mucosa must be thoroughly inspected. Lesions may be a manifestation of internal pathology (e.g. buccal pigmentation in Addison's disease).

REASSESSMENT

The patient's condition should be monitored to detect any changes and assess the effect of treatment. If there is any evidence of deterioration, re-evaluate by returning to A in the primary assessment.

Some patients presenting with an apparent medical problem may require urgent specialist intervention to save their life, e.g. an early surgical opinion when treating patients with upper gastrointestinal haemorrhage.

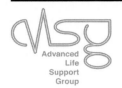

No.	Question	Assessment	Rating
1	How old are you?	Score for exact age only	
2	What is your date of birth?	Only date and month needed	
3	What is the year now?	Score for exact year only	
4	What is the time of the day?	Score if within 1 h of correct time	
5	Where are we? What is this building?	Score for exact place name, e.g. 'hospital' insufficient	
	Now ask subject to remember an address: 42, West Street		
6	Who is the current monarch?	Score only current monarch	
7	What was the date of the First World War?	Score for year of start or finish	
8	Can you count down backwards from 20 to 1?	Score if no mistakes or any mistakes corrected spontaneously	
9	Can you tell me what those 2 people do for a living?	Score if recognises role of 2 people correctly, e.g. doctor, nurse	
10	Can you remember the address I gave you?	Score for exact recall only	
		TOTAL	/10

Key point

Remember to examine the back of the patient either during the primary or secondary assessment

---

DOCUMENTATION

Always document the findings of the primary and secondary assessments. This record, along with subsequent entries into the patient's notes, should be dated, timed and signed. The patient's records must also contain a management plan, a list of investigations requested and the related results, as well as details of any treatment and its effect. This will not only provide an aide-mémoire but will also enable the patient's condition to be monitored and provide colleagues with an accurate account of a patient's hospital admission. This is assuming greater importance as patient care becomes more fragmented with increasing shift working and more patient movement between wards. Excellent written notes, and hence communication, are essential for good patient management.

DEFINITIVE CARE

Management plan

This should comprise a list of further investigations and treatment required for the particular patient. This is a dynamic plan that may change according to the clinical condition and test results. It needs to be reviewed regularly and updated.

Investigations

These will be dictated by the findings from the initial assessment and liaison with colleagues. Tests are not without risks; they should only be done if they directly benefit patient care.

Transport

All patients will be transferred sometime during their hospital stay. Irrespective of the transfer distance, appropriate numbers and grades of staff are required along with relevant equipment. Any period of transport is a period of potential patient instability. See Chapter 22 for further details.

Time Out 3.2

Your primary assessment of the confused 54-year-old man has revealed the following:

A	Assessment	Patent
	Resuscitation	$FiO_2 = 0.85$
	Monitor	Pulse oximetry ($SpO_2 = 99\%$)
B	Assessment	Rate 30/min
		No accessory muscle use
		Symmetrical expansion
		No focal features
	Resuscitation	Not required, as yet
	Monitor	Respiration rate
C	Assessment	Pulse – radial 140 beats/min
		Apex – 160 beats/min – atrial fibrillation
		Blood pressure 90/60
		Jugular venous pulse only visible when patient is lying flat
		Remainder of examination was normal
	Resuscitation	Following sedation cardioversion ($\times 3$) failed to convert patient to sinus rhythm therefore intravenous β blocker or amiodarone should be started
	Monitor	Radial pulse and apical rate
		Blood pressure
		Blood glucose, haemoglobin, urea and electrolytes
D	Assessment	PERLA
		Glasgow Coma Score 14/15: E = 4; V = 4; M = 6

a. What would be your next action?
b. What is the problem with this patient?
c. What is your management plan?

A WORD (OR TWO) OF COMMON SENSE

The structured approach is a safe comprehensive method of assessing any acutely ill patient. It should be regarded as the 'default method' in that it will prevent any further harm and cater for all medical problems. However, as most patients do not have an immediately life-threatening problem, a rapid primary assessment and/or an early warning score is all that is needed. Many patients do not require high

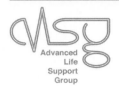

concentrations of inspired oxygen, intravenous access (×2) and a fluid challenge. Clinical judgement is still needed, combined with a modicum of common sense. If in doubt, revert to A.

SUMMARY

The acutely ill patient must be evaluated quickly and accurately. Thus, you must develop a structured method for assessment and treatment. In most acutely ill medical patients, the primary assessment is rapid and resuscitation is not required. Diagnosis is based on a well-'phrased' medical history obtained from the patient. However, if this is not possible then further information must be sought from medical records, relatives, general practitioners or colleagues from the emergency services.

Assessment and treatment are divided into two key assessment phases.

Primary assessment and resuscitation

The aim of the primary assessment is to identify and treat immediately life-threatening conditions.

- In most medical patients this can be done rapidly.
- Do not proceed to the secondary assessment until the patient's vital signs are normal or are moving towards normality.
- The most important assessment is the reassessment.

Assessment of:

A – Airway
B – Breathing
C – Circulation
D – Disability
E – Exposure

Resuscitation by:

- clearing and securing the airway and oxygenation
- ventilation
- intravenous access and shock therapy, including fluids, antibiotics, glucose, inotropes, dysrhythmia management
- exclude/correct hypoglycaemia
- consider anti-epileptic drugs, specific antidotes.

Monitoring to include oxygen saturation, respiration rate, pulse, blood pressure, cardiac rhythm, urinary output, pupillary response and Glasgow Coma Score; glucose and blood gases (if indicated).

Secondary assessment and emergency treatment

To gain corroborative evidence for primary diagnosis; to identify and treat new conditions.

Comprehensive physical examination including:

- general overview
- hands and radial pulse
- facial appearance
- neck – jugular venous pulse, carotid pulse, trachea
- chest – precordium and both lungs
- abdomen and genitalia
- locomotor system
- nervous system
- skin.

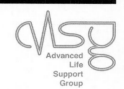

Reassessment

Now or if patient deteriorates at any stage.

Definitive care

- management plan
- investigations
- transport.

AIDE MEMOIRE

The flow diagrams depicted in Figs 3.1–3.6 are designed to aid your revision and provide an overview of the structured approach.

Note: *'BIG RED FLAGS' are findings that should alert you to an immediate life-threat and the need for urgent corrective action. The list is intended to be helpful, but not exhaustive.

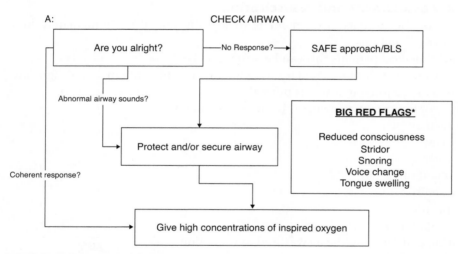

Fig. 3.1 Summary of airway assessment.

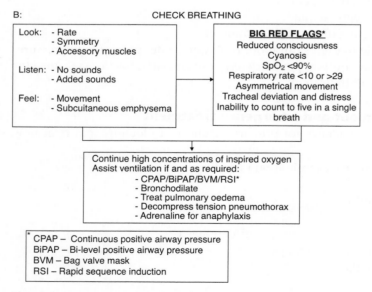

Fig. 3.2 Summary of breathing assessment.

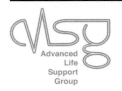

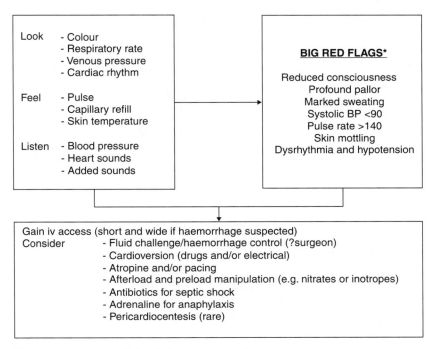

Fig. 3.3 Summary of circulation assessment.

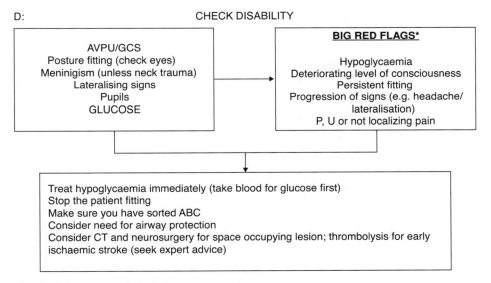

Fig. 3.4 Summary of disability assessment.

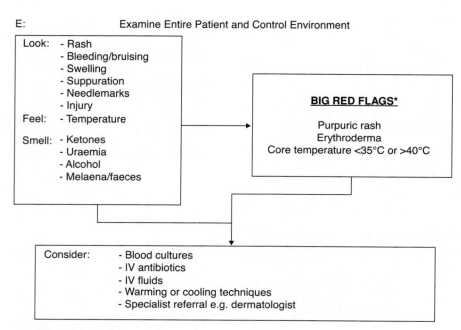

Fig. 3.5 Examine entire patient and control environment.

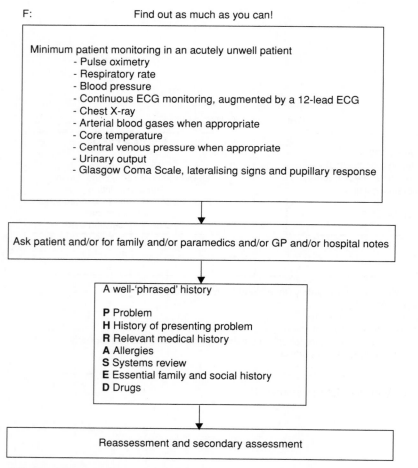

Fig. 3.6 Find out as much as you can.

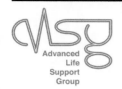

CHAPTER 4

Airway assessment

OBJECTIVES

After reading this chapter you will be able to:
- recognise the signs of airway obstruction
- understand how to use simple airway adjuncts
- describe advanced airway control and ventilation.

INTRODUCTION

- Airway problems are common in acute medical emergencies.
- Airway obstruction is the immediately life-threatening problem.

In the unconscious patient, it is essential to rapidly assess and control the airway; these simple manoeuvres can be life-saving. Therefore, in both basic and advanced life support, management of the airway is the first priority – the A of 'ABC'.

An obstructed airway can result in, or be caused by, a loss of consciousness. The obstruction can occur at many levels.

Immediately life-threatening causes of airway obstruction	
Pharynx	Tongue swelling
	Swelling of the epiglottis or soft tissues
Larynx	Oedema
	Spasm of the vocal cords (laryngospasm)
	Foreign body
	Trauma
Subglottic	Secretions or foreign body
	Swelling
Bronchial	Aspiration
	Tension pneumothorax
	Foreign body

In the unconscious patient, the most common level of obstruction is the pharynx due to:
- a reduction in muscle tone, allowing the tongue to fall backwards (Fig. 4.1)
- abnormal muscle activity in the pharynx, larynx and neck. This explains why obstruction may still occur when the patient is prone.

This situation can be rectified and an airway provided by using manoeuvres described in this chapter.

Acute Medical Emergencies; The Practical Approach, 2nd edition.
Edited by Terence Wardle, Peter Driscoll, and Sue Wieteska.
© 2010 Blackwell Publishing Ltd.

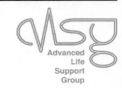

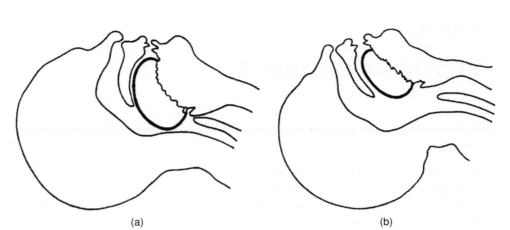

Fig. 4.1 (a) Obstruction of the airway by the tongue. (b) Head tilt, chin lift to clear the airway.

PRIMARY ASSESSMENT AND RESUSCITATION

This comprises:

Look at the chest for rate, depth and symmetry of movement. In complete airway obstruction, paradoxical movement of the chest and abdomen (see-sawing) will occur as a result of the increased respiratory effort. In addition, there may be use of accessory muscles; intercostal and supraclavicular recession may be visible and a tracheal tug may be palpable. Look in the mouth for blood, gastric contents, frothy sputum (pulmonary oedema) and foreign bodies.

Listen for breath sounds. Partial obstruction may be accompanied by the following:

- Inspiratory noises (stridor) commonly indicate upper airway obstruction.
- Expiratory noises, particularly wheezing, usually occur in obstruction of the lower airways as they collapse during expiration.
- 'Crowing' signifies laryngeal spasm.
- 'Gurgling' indicates the presence of liquid or semisolid material.
- 'Snoring' indicates that the pharynx is still partially occluded by the tongue.

Feel for:

- expired air against the side of your cheek
- chest movement, comparing one side with the other
- the position and 'tugging' of the trachea
- any subcutaneous emphysema.

Remove broken and very loose dentures, but leave well-fitting ones as they help to maintain the contour of the mouth and make using a bag–mask system easier (see later).

The possibility of an injury to the cervical spine must always be considered. However, medical patients are more likely to die from hypoxaemia than be rendered quadriplegic as a consequence of carefully conducted airway opening manoeuvres.

Airway adjuncts

These are often helpful to improve and maintain airway patency either during resuscitation or in a spontaneously breathing patient. Both oropharyngeal and nasopharyngeal airways are designed to overcome backward tongue displacement in the unconscious patient. In both cases, either the head tilt or jaw thrust techniques usually need to be maintained.

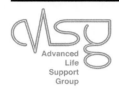

Oropharyngeal (Guedel) airways

These are curved, rigid, plastic tubes, flanged at the oral end and flattened in cross section to fit between the tongue and the hard palate. They are available in a variety of sizes which are suitable for all patients, from newborn babies to large adults. An estimate of the size required can be obtained by comparing the airway with the vertical distance from the centre of the incisors to the angle of the jaw (see Chapter 31 for further details).

The oropharyngeal airway is inserted either upside down and rotated through 180° or under direct vision with the aid of a tongue depressor or laryngoscope (see Chapter 31 for further details).

Incorrect insertion can push the tongue further back into the pharynx and produce airway obstruction, trauma, bleeding and force unrecognised foreign bodies further into the larynx. An oral airway may irritate the pharynx and larynx and cause vomiting and laryngospasm, respectively, especially in patients who are not deeply unconscious.

Nasopharyngeal airways

This airway is made from malleable plastic that is bevelled at one end and flanged at the other, and is round in cross section to aid insertion through the nose. Nasopharyngeal airways are sized according to the diameter of the patient's nares or the size of their little finger.

Nasopharyngeal airways are often better tolerated than oropharyngeal airways. They may be life-saving in a patient whose mouth cannot be opened, e.g. with trismus or in the presence of maxillary injuries. They should, however, be used with extreme caution in patients with a suspected base of skull fracture (very rare in the acutely ill medical patient).

Even with careful insertion, bleeding can occur from tissues in the nasopharynx. If the airway is too long, both vomiting and laryngospasm can be induced in patients who are not deeply unconscious.

A further problem with both of these types of airway is that air may be directed into the oesophagus during assisted ventilation. This results in inefficient ventilation of the lungs and gastric dilatation, which splints the diaphragm, making ventilation difficult and increasing the risk of regurgitation. This commonly occurs when high inflation pressures are used to try and ventilate a patient. In these circumstances, carefully check that ventilation is adequate and gastric distension is minimised.

If adequate spontaneous ventilation follows these airway opening manoeuvres, place the patient in an appropriate recovery position – provided there are no contraindications. This will reduce the risk of further obstruction.

Ventilatory support

If spontaneous ventilation is inadequate or absent, start artificial ventilation.

Exhaled air resuscitation

If no equipment is available, expired air ventilation will provide 16% oxygen. This can be made more pleasant, and the risks of cross-infection reduced, by the use of simple adjuncts to avoid direct person-to-person contact; an example of this is the Laerdal pocket mask. This device has a unidirectional valve to allow the rescuer's expired air to pass to the patient while the patient's expired air is directed away from the rescuer. The masks are transparent to allow detection of vomit or blood; one version has an additional attachment for supplemental oxygen.

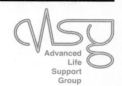

Oxygen

Oxygen should be given to all patients during resuscitation, with the aim of increasing the inspired concentration to greater than 95%. However, this concentration will depend on the system used and the flow available. In spontaneously breathing patients, a Venturi mask will deliver a fixed concentration (24–60%), depending on the mask chosen. A standard concentration mask will deliver up to 60%, provided the flow of oxygen is high enough (12–15 l/min). Some patients are more tolerant of nasal cannulae, but these only raise the inspired concentration to approximately 44%. The most effective system is a mask with a non-rebreathing reservoir in which the inspired concentration can be raised to 85% with an oxygen flow of 12–15 l/min. This is the most desirable method in spontaneously breathing patients.

Advanced airway control and ventilation

Airway control

In the deeply unconscious patient, airway control is best achieved by tracheal intubation. However, the technique requires a greater degree of skill and more equipment than the methods already described.

Tracheal intubation may be indicated for several reasons:

- to protect the airway against contamination from regurgitated stomach contents or blood
- to protect the airway and ensure ventilation when an investigation has to be done, e.g. CT scan
- when an airway cannot be secured by another route
- to allow safe transport of a patient
- to facilitate ventilation without leaks, even when airway resistance is high (e.g. in pulmonary oedema and bronchospasm)
- to achieve a safe environment for the patients (e.g. in drug overdosage)
- to facilitate mechanical ventilation for other reasons (e.g. exhaustion).

Tracheal intubation

This is the preferred method for airway control during cardiopulmonary resuscitation, for the reasons already outlined. Considerable training and practice are required to acquire and maintain the skill of intubation. Repeated attempts by the inexperienced are likely to be unsuccessful and traumatic, compromise oxygenation and delay resuscitation. Orotracheal intubation is the preferred route. Nasotracheal is rarely required and much more difficult than orotracheal intubation.

The technique of orotracheal intubation is described in Chapter 31. Nevertheless this is not intended as a substitute for practice using a manikin or, better still, an anaesthetised patient under the direction of a skilled anaesthetist.

Tracheal intubation may be difficult to perform during cardiac arrest. The patient may be in an awkward position on the floor, equipment may be unfamiliar, assistance limited, cardiopulmonary resuscitation obstructive and vomit copious. In these circumstances, it is all too easy to persist with the 'almost there' attitude. This must be strongly resisted. If intubation is not successfully accomplished in approximately 30–40 s (about the time one can breath-hold during the attempt), it should be abandoned. Ventilation with 12–15 l/min (95%) oxygen using a bag–valve–mask should be recommended before, and in between, any further attempts at intubation. Ideally, the tube should be seen to pass through the cords and then the circuit should be attached to a carbon dioxide monitor (end tidal or colorimetric) to ensure correct placement.

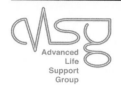

In certain circumstances such as acute epiglottitis, laryngoscopy and attempted intubation are contraindicated because they could lead to deterioration in the patient's condition. Specialist skills will be required, including the use of anaesthetic drugs or fibre-optic laryngoscopy.

Key point

It is not appropriate to learn and practice endotracheal intubation during resuscitation

---

Currently endotracheal intubation is the optimum method of managing the airway in an unconscious patient. For most people, acquiring this skill is time-consuming; continuous training is unavailable; and skill retention is poor. The laryngeal mask airway is an acceptable alternative.

The laryngeal mask airway

This comprises a 'mask' with an inflatable cuff around its edge that sits over the laryngeal opening. Attached to the mask is a tube that protrudes from the mouth and through which the patient either breathes or is ventilated (Fig. 4.2). This was originally designed for spontaneously breathing anaesthetised patients. However, supported ventilation is possible, provided that inflation pressures are not excessive. The main advantage of the laryngeal mask airway (LMA) is that it is inserted blindly, the technique may be mastered more easily than tracheal intubation and skill retention in the occasional practitioner is better. However, if either the seal around the larynx is poor or the mask is malpositioned, ventilation will be reduced and gastric inflation may occur. Furthermore, there is no guarantee against aspiration. Whenever possible, insertion of an LMA must be preceded by a period of preoxygenation. Any attempt at insertion must be limited to 30–40 s, after which ventilation with 12–15 l/min oxygen using a bag–valve–mask should be recommended before further attempts.

The LMA can be used as a conduit to allow the insertion of a tracheal tube to secure the airway in cases of difficult tracheal intubation. This technique is described in Chapter 31.

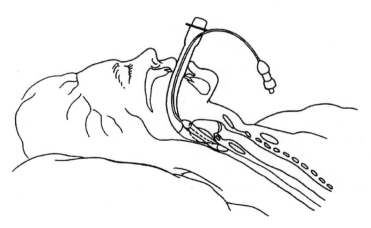

Fig. 4.2 Laryngeal mask *in situ*.

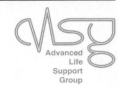

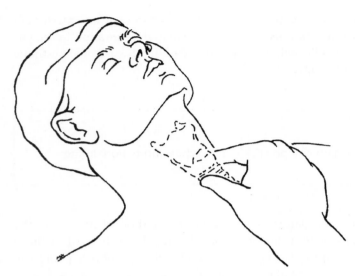

Fig. 4.3 Technique for cricoid pressure.

Cricoid pressure

This is a manoeuvre used by anaesthetists to prevent regurgitation and aspiration of gastric contents during induction of anaesthesia – often in acutely ill patients and/or those with a full stomach.

The cricoid cartilage forms a complete ring immediately below the thyroid cartilage. Pressure is applied on the cricoid by an assistant forcing the ring backwards, occluding the oesophagus against the body of the sixth cervical vertebra (Fig. 4.3), thus preventing the flow of any gastric contents beyond this point. This manoeuvre is maintained until:

- the tracheal tube is inserted into the larynx
- the cuff is inflated
- the person intubating indicates that pressure can be released.

Incorrectly applied pressure will make intubation more difficult. If the patient vomits, cricoid pressure must be released immediately because of the slight risk of oesophageal rupture. In such circumstances the patient needs to be turned onto their side, the trolley tipped head down and the airway cleared with suction.

In contrast to cricoid pressure, pressure on the thyroid cartilage by a trained assistant can facilitate endotracheal intubation. This is known as the BURP (Backward Upward Right Pressure) technique.

Ventilation

The ultimate aim is to achieve an inspired oxygen concentration of greater than 95%. The most common device used is the self-inflating bag with a one-way valve that can be connected to either a facemask or a tracheal tube (Fig. 4.4).

Squeezing the bag delivers its contents to the patient via the one-way valve. On release the bag re-inflates, refilling via the inlet valve at the opposite end. At the same time, the one-way valve diverts the expired gas from the patient to the atmosphere. Using the bag-valve alone (attached to mask or tracheal tube), the patient is ventilated with 21% oxygen as the bag refills with ambient air. This can (and should) be increased during resuscitation to around 50% by connecting an oxygen supply at 12–15 l/min directly to the bag adjacent to the air intake. This can be further increased to 95% by attaching a reservoir bag.

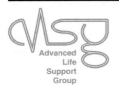

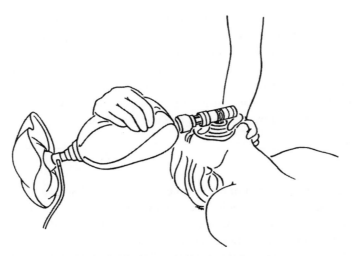

Fig. 4.4 Self-inflating bag–mask and reservoir.

Although the self-inflating bag–valve–mask will allow ventilation with higher concentrations of oxygen, it is associated with several problems.

- It requires considerable skill for one person to maintain a gas-tight seal between the mask and the patient's face, whilst at the same time lifting the jaw with one hand and squeezing the bag with the other.
- Any air leak will result in hypoventilation, no matter how energetically the bag is compressed.
- Excessive compression of the bag when attached to a facemask results in gas passing into the stomach. This further reduces effective ventilation and increases the risk of regurgitation and aspiration.
- The valve mechanism may 'stick' if it becomes blocked with secretions, vomit or heavy moisture contamination.

As a result of some of these problems, a two-person technique is recommended during ventilation of a patient with a bag–valve–mask. One person holds the facemask in place using both hands and an assistant squeezes the bag. Thus a better seal is achieved, the jaw thrust manoeuvre is easier to maintain and the patient can be ventilated more easily.

Clearly these problems can be overcome by tracheal intubation, which eliminates leaks and ensures that oxygen is delivered directly and only into the lungs (always assuming the tube is in the trachea!).

Patients requiring prolonged ventilation can be placed on a mechanical ventilator. When using these devices, the most important feature to remember is that they are good servants, but poor masters. Ventilators will only do what they are set to do, and will not automatically compensate for changes in the patient's condition during resuscitation. Therefore, it is imperative that they are set correctly and checked regularly.

A variety of small portable ventilators are used during resuscitation and are generally gas powered. If an oxygen cylinder is used as both the supply of respiratory gas for the patient and the power for the ventilator, its contents will be used more rapidly. This is particularly important if patients are being transported over long distances because adequate oxygen supplies must be taken.

Gas-powered portable ventilators are classified as time cycled and often have a fixed inspiratory/expiratory ratio. They provide a constant flow of gas to the patient during inspiration; expiration occurs passively to the atmosphere. The volume delivered depends on the inspiratory time (i.e. longer times and larger

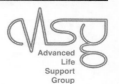

breaths) with the pressure in the airway rising during inspiration. As a safety feature, these devices can often be 'pressure limited' by a relief valve opening to protect the lungs against excessive pressures (barotrauma).

A ventilator should initially be set to deliver 7–10 ml/kg tidal volume at a rate of 12 breaths/min with 100% oxygen. Some ventilators have coordinated markings on the controls for rapid initial setting for different-sized patients. The correct setting will ultimately be determined by analysis of arterial blood gases.

Key point

Care should be taken when using ventilators which have relief valves fixed to open at relatively low pressures. These may be exceeded during cardiopulmonary resuscitation if a chest compression coincides with a breath from the ventilator, resulting in inadequate ventilation. Furthermore, by the same mechanism, ventilators with adjustable pressure relief valves, if set too high, may subject patients to excessively high pressures. These risks can be reduced by decreasing the rate of ventilation (breaths/min) to allow coordination of breaths and compressions.

If there is any doubt about the performance of the ventilator, the safest option is to temporarily disconnect it and continue by using a self-inflating bag–valve assembly with oxygen and reservoir, until skilled help is available.

Suction (endotracheal)

Once the trachea has been intubated, suction is performed to remove secretions, vomit or blood. To avoid making the patient hypoxaemic and bradycardic, this must be done carefully in the following way:

- Wear gloves.
- Ventilate the patient with 100% oxygen.
- Introduce a sterile catheter through the airway into the trachea without suction applied.
- The diameter of the catheter should be less than half that of the tracheal tube.
- Intermittent suction and withdraw the catheter using a rotating motion over 10–15 s.
- Irrespective of the amount of blood/mucus removed, do not reintroduce the catheter without a further period of oxygenation.
- Loosen tenacious secretions by instilling 10 ml of sterile saline, followed by five vigorous manual ventilations. Suction as described earlier.

Key point

Suction must not be applied directly to the tracheal tube as this will result in life-threatening hypoxaemia and dysrhythmias

---

Time Out 4.1

Take a break and list the clinical features of airway obstruction

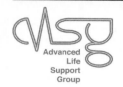

SUMMARY

Airway control and ventilation are essential prerequisites for successful management of the acutely ill patient. Airway obstruction should be recognised and managed immediately. Endotracheal intubation remains the best method of securing and controlling the airway, but requires additional equipment, skill and practice.

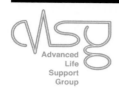

CHAPTER 5

Breathing assessment

OBJECTIVES

After reading this chapter you will be able to:
- understand the physiology of oxygen delivery
- describe a structured approach to breathing assessment
- identify immediately life-threatening causes of breathlessness
- describe the immediate management of these patients.

INTRODUCTION

The acutely breathless patient is a common medical emergency that is distressing for both the patient and the clinician. Often the effort required for breathing makes it virtually impossible for the patient to provide any form of medical history and questioning may only make the situation worse. Information should be sought from any available source. The clinician's skills will help to determine the underlying cause and dictate appropriate management.

Key point

Breathlessness can result from a problem in airway (A), breathing (B), circulation (C) and disability (D)

Immediately life-threatening causes of breathlessness

Airway
- Obstruction (see full list in box 1 in Chapter 4)

Breathing
- Acute severe asthma
- Acute exacerbation of chronic obstructive pulmonary disease (COPD)
- Pulmonary oedema
- Tension pneumothorax
- Critical oxygen desaturation

Circulation
- Shock

Disruption of oxygen delivery is a fundamental problem in these conditions. Therefore it is important to understand the mechanisms that maintain oxygen delivery in health.

Acute Medical Emergencies; The Practical Approach, 2nd edition.
Edited by Terence Wardle, Peter Driscoll, and Sue Wieteska.
© 2010 Blackwell Publishing Ltd.

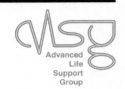

RELEVANT PHYSIOLOGY

Oxygen delivery

The normal respiratory rate is 14–20 breaths/min. With each breath, 500 ml of air (7–10 l/min) is inhaled and exhaled. This air mixes with alveolar gas and, by diffusion, oxygen enters the pulmonary circulation to combine mainly with haemoglobin in the red cells. The erythrocyte-bound oxygen is transported via the systemic circulation to the tissues, where it is taken up and used by the cells.

The delivery of oxygen (DO_2) to the tissues depends on:

- concentration of oxygen reaching the alveoli
- pulmonary perfusion
- adequacy of pulmonary gas exchange
- capacity of blood to carry oxygen
- blood flow to the tissues.

Concentration of oxygen reaching the alveoli

The two most important factors determining the amount of oxygen reaching the alveoli are:

- the fraction of inspired oxygen (FiO_2)
- ventilation.

Providing supplementary oxygen to a person increases the number of oxygen molecules getting to the alveoli. A variety of oxygen masks can be used to increase the **fraction of inspired oxygen**.

The effectiveness of this procedure depends on the lungs' ability to draw the inspired gas into the alveoli. The mechanism for transporting inspired air to, and expired gas from, the alveoli is called **ventilation** (V). Ventilation is subject to several regulatory processes which are summarised in the box below.

Key components in ventilation

Brain stem	Central respiratory chemoreceptors in medulla oblongata
Peripheral chemoreceptors	Carotid and aortic bodies for CO_2, O_2 and H^+
Vagus, phrenic and intercostal nerves	Ventilatory drive
Respiratory muscles	Intercostal muscles and diaphragm
Mechanics and compliance	Airways, lungs and chest wall

The normal ventilatory volumes and rates are summarised in Figs 5.1 and 5.2.

The **normal resting respiratory rate** is 15 (range 14–20) breaths/min. The amount of air inspired per breath is called the **tidal volume** and is equivalent to 7–8 ml/kg body weight (or 500 ml for the 70 kg patient). Therefore the amount of air inspired each minute, the **minute volume**, can be calculated by multiplying the **respiratory rate** by the **tidal volume** (15 × 500 ml) to produce a value of 7.5 l/min.

The tidal volume (500 ml) is distributed throughout the respiratory system but only 350 ml (70%) mixes with alveolar air. The remainder (150 ml) occupies the airways that are not involved in gas transfer. This volume is referred to as the **anatomical dead space**. In addition, there are certain areas within the lungs which are not involved with gas transfer because they are ventilated but not

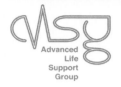

perfused. The volume produced by the combination of these areas and the anatomical dead space is called the **total or physiological dead space**. In healthy individuals, these two dead spaces are virtually identical because ventilation and perfusion are well matched.

It follows that the amount of air reaching the alveoli, i.e. **alveolar ventilation**, can be calculated from:

respiratory rate × (tidal volume − anatomical dead space)

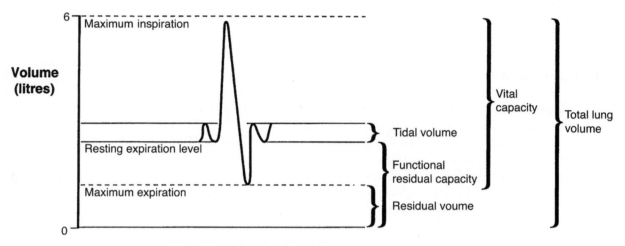

Fig. 5.1 Normal ventilatory volumes.

Using data from Fig. 5.2, this corresponds to 15 × (500 − 150) = 5250 ml/min.

Rapid shallow respiration causes a marked reduction in alveolar ventilation because the anatomical dead space is fixed, i.e. 30 × (200 − 150) = 1500. This is demonstrated further in Table 5.1, where the effect of different respiratory rates can be seen.

Finally, it is important to be aware of a crucial volume known as the **functional residual capacity** (FRC) (2.5–3.01). This is the amount of air remaining in the lungs at the end of a normal expiration. As 350 ml of each tidal volume is

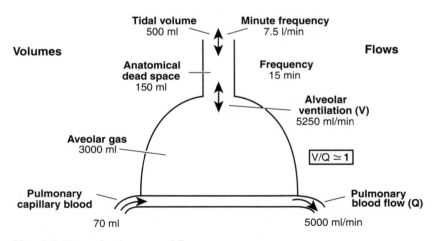

Fig. 5.2 Normal volumes and flows.

available for gas transfer, fresh alveolar air will only replace 12–14% of the functional residual capacity. The FRC therefore acts as a large reservoir, preventing sudden changes in blood oxygen and carbon dioxide concentration.

Table 5.1 The effect of respiratory rate on alveolar ventilation

Respiratory rate (breaths/min)	10	20	30
Tidal volume (ml)	600	400	200
Anatomical dead space (ml)	150	150	150
Alveolar ventilation (ml/min)	4500	5000	1500

Pulmonary perfusion

At rest, the cardiac output from the right ventricle is delivered to the pulmonary circulation at approximately 5.5 l/min. As alveolar ventilation is 5.25 l/min, the ventilation/pulmonary perfusion ratio is equal to 0.95 (5.25/5.5).

The pressures in the pulmonary vascular bed are low (around 20/9 mm Hg) and therefore affected by posture. As a result, there are differences in blood flow to different lung regions, contributing to the physiological dead space. In the upright position, basal alveoli are well perfused but relatively poorly ventilated. Consequently, in these areas, venous blood comes into contact with alveoli filled with low concentrations of oxygen and so less oxygen can be taken up. This effect is minimised in healthy individuals by pulmonary vasoconstriction which diverts blood to areas of the lungs that have better ventilation. In the apical regions of the lungs, there is ventilation but relatively poor perfusion.

There are also direct links between the right and left sides of the heart (mainly from blood supplying lung parenchymal tissue). These normally allow 2% of the right ventricle's output to bypass the lungs completely and are collectively known as the **physiological shunt**. As the blood in this shunt has had no contact with the alveoli, its oxygen and carbon dioxide concentrations will remain the same as those found in the right ventricle.

Pulmonary gas exchange

Oxygen continuously diffuses out of the alveolar gas into the pulmonary capillaries, with carbon dioxide going in the opposite direction. The rate of diffusion is governed by the following factors:
- partial pressure gradient of the gas
- solubility of the gas
- alveolar surface area
- alveolar capillary wall thickness.

The lungs are ideally suited for diffusion as they have both a large alveolar surface area (approximately 50 m^2) and a thin alveolar capillary wall. It is easy to understand why gas exchange would be compromised by a reduction in the former (e.g. pneumothorax) or an increase in the latter (e.g. interstitial pulmonary oedema).

Gases move passively down gradients from areas of high to low partial pressure. The partial pressure of oxygen in the alveoli (PaO$_2$) is approximately 13.4 kPa (100 mm Hg), whereas that in the pulmonary artery is 5.3 kPa (40 mm Hg). In contrast, the gradient for carbon dioxide is only small, with the alveolar partial pressure being 5.3 kPa (40 mm Hg), compared with 6.0 kPa (46 mm Hg) in the

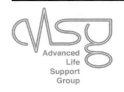

pulmonary artery. However, carbon dioxide passes through biological membranes 20 times more easily than oxygen. In health, the net effect is that the time taken for exchange of oxygen and carbon dioxide is virtually identical.

Although alveolar ventilation, diffusion and pulmonary perfusion will all affect the alveolar PO_2 (PaO_2) and hence the arterial PO_2 (PaO_2), the most important factor in determining the PaO_2 is the ratio of ventilation to perfusion.

Ventilation/perfusion ratio

To understand this concept, it is helpful to consider the normal situation and divide each lung into three functional areas: apical (a), middle (b) and basal (c) (Fig. 5.3).

The apical segment is well ventilated, but relatively poorly perfused. Therefore, not enough blood is available to accept all the alveolar oxygen. However, the red cells that are available are fully laden (saturated) with oxygen with the extra oxygen dissolved in plasma.

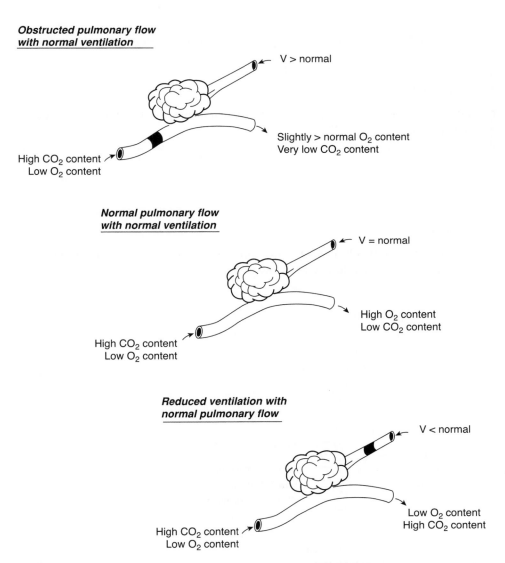

Fig. 5.3 Three different ventilation (V)/perfusion (Q) ratios: (a) normal ventilation with reduced perfusion; (b) normal ventilation with normal perfusion; (c) reduced ventilation with normal perfusion.

> **Key point**
>
> In the apical segment, there is more ventilation than perfusion, i.e. the V/Q ratio > 1

The middle segment has ventilation and perfusion perfectly matched. Alveolar oxygen diffuses into – and is correctly balanced by – the pulmonary capillary blood, ensuring that the red cells are fully saturated. There is relatively little oxygen left to dissolve in plasma.

> **Key point**
>
> In the middle segment, ventilation and perfusion are matched, i.e. the V/Q ratio = 1

The basal segment alveoli are well perfused, but poorly ventilated.

> **Key point**
>
> In the basal segment, ventilation is reduced when compared with perfusion, i.e. the V/Q ratio < 1

Remember that the overall ratio of ventilation to perfusion is nearly one (0.95).

> **Key point**
>
> An area of lung with a high V/Q ratio cannot offset the fall in oxygen content produced by an area of lung with a low V/Q ratio

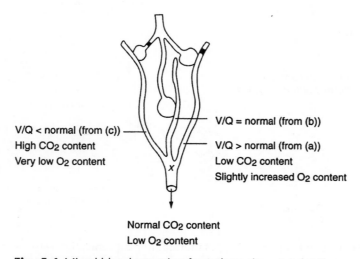

V/Q < normal (from (c))
High CO_2 content
Very low O_2 content

V/Q = normal (from (b))

V/Q > normal (from (a))
Low CO_2 content
Slightly increased O_2 content

Normal CO_2 content
Low O_2 content

Fig. 5.4 Mixed blood returning from three sites at point X.
To understand this point we need to consider how oxygen is carried in the blood.

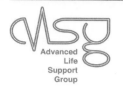

Oxygen content of arterial blood

The oxygen content of haemoglobin (Hb) going to tissues depends on the:

- saturation of haemoglobin with oxygen
- haemoglobin concentration
- oxygen-carrying capacity
- oxygen dissolved in plasma.

Haemoglobin is a protein comprising four subunits, each of which contains a haem molecule attached to a polypeptide chain. The haem molecule contains iron which reversibly binds oxygen; hence it is oxygenated but **not** oxidised (it carries oxygen, but does not react with it, i.e. it is not rust!). Each haemoglobin molecule can carry up to four oxygen molecules. Blood has a haemoglobin concentration of approximately 15 g/100 ml. Under normal conditions, each gram of haemoglobin can carry 1.34 ml of oxygen if it is fully saturated. Therefore, the **oxygen carrying capacity** of blood is:

$$Hb \times 1.34 \times 1$$
$$15 \times 1.34 \times 1 = 20.1 \text{ ml } O_2/100 \text{ ml of blood}$$
(A value of 1 indicates that Hb is fully saturated.)

This is approximately 60 times greater than the amount of oxygen dissolved in plasma.

Key point

Nearly all of the oxygen carried in the blood is taken up by haemoglobin, with only a small amount dissolved in the plasma

---

The relationship between the PaO_2 and oxygen uptake by haemoglobin is not linear, because the addition of each O_2 molecule facilitates the uptake of the next O_2 molecule. This produces a sigmoid-shaped oxygen dissociation curve (Fig. 5.5). Furthermore, because haemoglobin is 97.5% saturated at a PaO_2 of 13.4 kPa (100 mm Hg) (i.e. that found in the normal healthy state), increasing the PaO_2 further has little effect on oxygen transport.

The affinity of haemoglobin for oxygen at a particular PO_2 (commonly known as the O_2–Hb association) is also affected by other factors. A decreased affinity

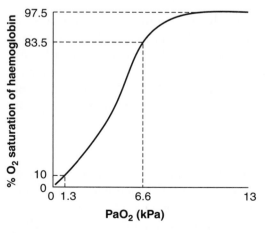

Fig. 5.5 The haemoglobin–oxygen dissociation curve.

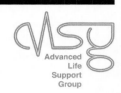

means that oxygen is more readily released. Thus the oxygen dissociation curve is shifted to the right.

Factors that decrease the affinity of haemoglobin for oxygen:

- hydrogen ion concentration (i.e. a fall in pH)
- $PaCO_2$
- concentration of red cell 2,3-diphosphoglycerate (2, 3-DPG)
- temperature.

(The opposite of these factors increases the affinity and moves the curve to the left. These will be discussed later.)

The normal haemoglobin concentration is usually just above the point at which the oxygen transportation is optimal. Consequently, a slight fall in haemoglobin concentration will actually increase oxygen transportation by decreasing blood viscosity.

In addition to the oxygen combined with haemoglobin, there is a smaller amount dissolved in plasma. This amount is directly proportional to the PaO_2 and is approximately 0.23 ml/l blood/kPa PaO_2 (0.003 ml/100 ml blood/mm Hg of PaO_2).

It follows from the description above that the total content of oxygen in blood is equal to the oxygen associated with haemoglobin (per litre) and that dissolved in plasma.

$$\text{Oxygen blood content} = (Hb \times 1.34 \times \text{saturation}) + (0.23 \times PaO_2) \text{ ml/l}$$

For example, in arterial blood with a haemoglobin content of 150 g/l and a PaO_2 of 15 kPa the oxygen content would be:

$$\text{Oxygen blood concentration} = (150 \times 1.34 \times 0.975) + (0.23 \times 15) = 199 \text{ ml/l}$$

Alternatively, in venous blood with a haemoglobin content of 150 g/l and a PaO_2 of 5 kPa the oxygen content would be:

$$\text{Oxygen blood concentration} = (150 \times 1.34 \times 0.75) + (0.23 \times 5) = 151 \text{ ml/l}$$

PRIMARY ASSESSMENT AND RESUSCITATION

Airway

This has been described in detail in Chapter 4. The following summary contains the relevant facts relating to the breathless patient.

Assessment

Most breathless patients will have a patent airway. The number of words said with each breath is a useful indicator of illness severity and the effects of treatment. If the patient can count to 10 in one breath, then the underlying condition is unlikely to warrant immediate intervention. Occasionally, however, the patient will be severely distressed with stridor, possibly coughing and making enormous but ineffectual respiratory efforts. Stridor is a sinister sign and should be regarded as indicating impending airway obstruction.

Resuscitation

If established or impending airway obstruction is suspected, immediate review by an anaesthetically competent person is required. If foreign body inhalation is suspected, then a Heimlich (or modified Heimlich in pregnant and obese patients) manoeuvre should be attempted. If the patient has a respiratory arrest, perform laryngoscopy and remove any identifiable foreign body. If this is unsuccessful,

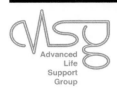

proceed to needle cricothyroidotomy and jet insufflation, followed by surgical referral for a surgical cricothyroidotomy.

Breathing

Assessment

This is summarised in the box.

Summary of breathing assessment	
Look	Colour, sweating
	Posture
	Respiratory rate, effort
	Symmetry
Feel	Tracheal position
	Tracheal tug
	Chest expansion
Percuss	Anterior and posterior aspects of both lungs in
Listen	the upper, middle and lower zones

The immediately life-threatening conditions need to be identified and treated during the primary assessment of breathing.

Specific clinical features

By the time 'B' is assessed, all critically ill patients should be receiving high concentrations of inspired oxygen (FiO_2 = 0.85 at 15 l/min) (Fig. 5.6). Do not be concerned about patients who retain CO_2. Provided that FiO_2 equals 0.85, a rise in $PaCO_2$ will not increase mortality – but untreated hypoxaemia will!

After the primary assessment has been completed, the FiO_2 can be titrated according to either the arterial blood gas results or the pulse oximeter reading.

A hyperinflated chest is indicative of asthma or COPD. **In an acute exacerbation** of these conditions, the trachea moves downwards during inspiration. This is referred to as tracheal tug and implies airway obstruction or increased respiratory effort. In addition, the internal jugular pressure may be elevated and accessory muscle use will be prominent, as will intercostal recession over the lower part of the chest during inspiration. Patients often adopt a seated or standing posture to aid breathing.

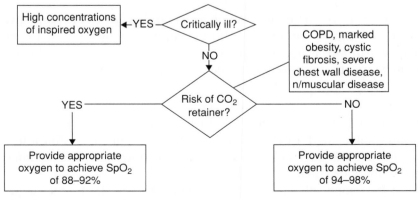

Fig. 5.6 Oxygen requirements.

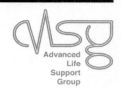

Bronchospasm is common to both asthma and COPD. In acute asthma, the inspiratory phase is snatched and expiration is prolonged. With COPD, however, the clinical picture ranges widely from a patient with preserved respiratory drive with pursed-lip breathing to one who is cyanosed, lethargic and mildly dyspnoeic. Wheezes may be heard on inspiration, but especially on expiration.

Acute pulmonary oedema can mimic or coexist with either of these conditions. However, the commonest cause of pulmonary oedema is left ventricular failure associated with ischaemic heart disease. Although there are many other causes, these will be seen only occasionally in most hospitals (see box below).

An idea of the 'chance' of meeting such a condition is displayed on an arbitrary scale in the box.

Causes of acute pulmonary oedema and 'chance' of meeting the condition*

Cause	Chance
Ischaemic heart disease	Daily
Myocardial infarction	
Cardiac dysrhythmias	
Fluid overload	Weekly
Severe hypertension	
Aortic stenosis/regurgitation	Monthly
Mitral stenosis/regurgitation	
Cardiomyopathy	
Non-cardiac	
Pulmonary oedema (ARDS, pneumonia)	
Left ventricular aneurysm	Annually
Infective endocarditis	
Cardiac tamponade	
Left atrial myxoma	Only in examinations

*Patients with some of the more common causes of pulmonary oedema may also feature in examinations.

Features that would support a diagnosis of pulmonary oedema include poor peripheral perfusion, absence of both neck vein distension and chest hyperexpansion. In addition, the percussion note is often dull, particularly at the lung bases. There are usually fine inspiratory crackles on auscultation and occasionally signs of a pleural effusion.

A deviated trachea (a very late sign) should alert the clinician to the possibility of a tension pneumothorax. Other signs, in particular tachypnoea, raised neck veins, reduced expansion, a hyperresonant percussion note and absent breath sounds, should be sought on the opposite side to the tracheal deviation.

Resuscitation

Irrespective of the underlying cause of the bronchospasm, treat the patients with nebulised bronchodilators whilst clues to the cause are sought. The clinical features described above will have helped distinguish bronchospasm due to asthma, COPD and pulmonary oedema.

Immediate management of a tension pneumothorax is needle thoracentesis, followed by intravenous access and then chest drain insertion.

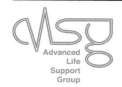

More comprehensive details of these conditions including pathophysiology, assessment and management can be found in Chapter 8.

Time Out 5.1

a Define: (i) tidal volume; (ii) minute volume
b How does the respiratory rate affect alveolar ventilation?
c Sketch a graph showing the relationship between PaO_2 and $\%SpO_2$.
d List the immediately life-threatening conditions that affect 'B'.

SUMMARY

Breathing is rapidly assessed using the look, feel, percuss and listen sequence to identify life-threatening:

- bronchospasm
- pulmonary oedema
- tension pneumothorax
- critical oxygen desaturation.

Life-threatening bronchospasm is common and treated initially with oxygen-driven bronchodilators. Tension pneumothorax is rare but, when present, requires immediate decompression with a needle thoracocentesis.

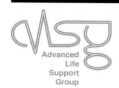

Advanced
Life
Support
Group

CHAPTER 6

Circulation assessment

OBJECTIVES

After reading this chapter you will be able to:
• understand the physiology of tissue perfusion
• describe a structured approach to circulatory assessment
• identify the immediately life-threatening causes of shock
• identify the anatomy for peripheral and central venous cannulation.

INTRODUCTION

The specific aim in 'C' is to identify and treat shock. The related immediately life-threatening conditions are shown in the box.

Immediately life-threatening conditions

Airway
• Obstruction (see full list in box 1 in Chapter 4)
Breathing
• Acute severe asthma
• Acute exacerbation of chronic obstructive pulmonary disease (COPD)
• Pulmonary oedema
• Tension pneumothorax
• Critical oxygen desaturation
Circulation
• Shock

It is important to understand the mechanisms that maintain tissue perfusion in health before considering the effects of disrupting the circulation.

RELEVANT PHYSIOLOGY

Blood flow to the tissues

The amount of blood reaching a particular organ depends on several factors:
• venous system
• cardiac output
• arterial system
• organ autoregulation.

Acute Medical Emergencies; The Practical Approach, 2nd edition.
Edited by Terence Wardle, Peter Driscoll, and Sue Wieteska.
© 2010 Blackwell Publishing Ltd.

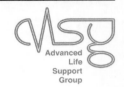

Venous system

This acts as a reservoir for over 70% of the circulating blood volume and is therefore often referred to as a **capacitance system**. The volume of blood stored at any one time depends on the size of the vessel lumen. This is controlled by sympathetic innervation and local factors (see later), which can alter the tone of the vessel walls. If the veins dilate, more blood remains in the venous system and less returns to the heart. Should there be a need to increase venous return, sympathetic stimulation reduces the diameter of the veins and hence the capacity of the venous system. A change from minimal to maximal tone can increase the venous return by approximately 1 litre in an adult.

Cardiac output

This is defined as the volume of blood ejected by each ventricle per minute. Clearly, over a period of time, the output of the two ventricles must be the same (or else all the circulating volume would eventually end up in either the systemic or pulmonary circulation). The cardiac output equates to the volume of blood ejected with each beat (stroke volume in ml) multiplied by the heart rate (beats per minute) and is expressed in litres per minute.

Cardiac output = stroke volume × heart rate = 4 − 6 l/min (normal adult)

To allow a comparison between patients of different sizes, the term cardiac index is used. This is the cardiac output divided by the surface area of the person and hence is measured in litres per square metre.

Cardiac index = cardiac output/body surface area
$$= 2.8 - 4.2 \; l/min/m^2 \; (normal \; adult)$$

The cardiac output can be affected by:
- preload
- myocardial contractility
- afterload
- heart rate.

Preload

This is the volume of blood in the ventricle at the end of diastole. The left ventricular end diastolic volume is about 140 ml and the stroke volume (SV) is 90 ml. Therefore, the end systolic volume is approximately 50 ml and the left ventricular ejection fraction (SV/EDV) ranges from 50 to 70%.

During diastole, the cardiac muscle fibres are progressively stretched as the ventricular volume increases in proportion to the venous return. Remember that **the more the myocardial fibres are stretched during diastole, the more forcibly they contract during systole; hence more blood will be expelled** (Starling's law). Therefore, the greater the preload, the greater the stroke volume. However, this phenomenon has an upper limit (due to the internal molecular structure of muscle cells) so that if the muscle is stretched beyond this point then a smaller contraction is produced (a situation that exists in ventricular failure).

Thus, the end diastolic fibre length is proportional to the end diastolic volume or force distending the ventricle. A clinical estimate of this volume, or force, is the end diastolic pressure (EDP). As the ventricular end diastolic pressure increases so does the stroke volume. If the end diastolic pressure exceeds a critical level then the force of contraction declines and eventually ventricular failure ensues (Fig. 6.1).

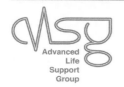

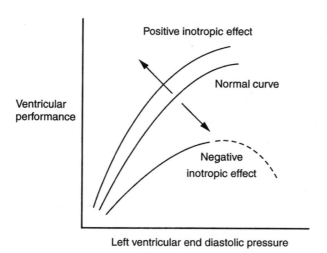

Fig. 6.1 Ventricular performance.

Current haemodynamic monitoring is based on measurements from a pulmonary artery flotation catheter. A commonly used recording is the pulmonary artery occlusion pressure because it is a useful estimate of the left ventricular end diastolic pressure.

Myocardial contractility

This is the rate at which the myocardial fibres contract for a given degree of stretch. Substances affecting myocardial contractility are termed inotropes, and they can be positive or negative in their actions. A positive inotrope produces a greater contraction for a given length (or end diastolic pressure (EDP)) (Fig. 6.1). Adrenaline and dopamine are naturally produced substances which have this effect. Dobutamine is a synthetic catecholamine with positive inotropic activity (however, it also has a potent vasodilator effect and must be used with caution). Therefore, depending on where you work, you may find some (or all) of these agents are used as part of the treatment of cardiogenic and septic shock.

Negative inotropes reduce contractility for a given muscle length (Fig. 6.1). These substances are often drugs, e.g. antiarrhythmics and anaesthetic agents. Rapid sequence induction of intravenous anaesthesia can precipitate circulatory collapse, if consideration has not been given to adequate fluid resuscitation and adjustment of dosage of induction agent (e.g. propofol or thiopentone) in the shocked patient. Many pathological states will also depress contractility, e.g. hypoxaemia, acidosis and sepsis. Myocardial damage also has a negative inotropic effect.

Afterload

As the left and right ventricular muscle contracts, pressures within the chambers increase until they exceed those in the aorta and pulmonary artery, respectively. The aortic and pulmonary valves open and the blood is ejected. The resistance faced by the ventricular myocardium during ejection is termed the afterload. In the left ventricle, this is mainly due to the resistance offered by the aortic valve and the compliance (stiffness) of the arterial tree. Usually this latter component is the most important and is estimated by calculating the **systemic vascular resistance**.

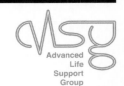

Using Ohm's law, where resistance equals pressure divided by flow, the systemic vascular resistance is defined as the mean arterial and venous pressure difference divided by the cardiac output.

(mean arterial pressure − central venous pressure) × 80/cardiac output =
770 − 1500 dyn/s/cm^5 (normal adult)

The value of 80 comes from converting mm Hg to SI units.

Key point

Reducing the afterload for a given preload will allow the myocardial fibres to shorten more quickly and by a greater amount. It therefore increases the stroke volume and cardiac output

---

Heart rate

An increase in heart rate is mediated via β_1 adrenoreceptors. These can be stimulated by the sympathetic nervous system, the release of catecholamines from the adrenal medulla and drugs (e.g. isoprenaline). This is termed a **positive chronotropic effect**. Conversely, the parasympathetic nervous system (PSNS) supplies the sinoatrial node and atrioventricular node via the vagus nerve. Stimulation of the PSNS decreases heart rate; i.e. it has a **negative chronotropic effect**. This effect can also be produced by drugs that inhibit the sympathetic nervous system, such as β blockers. In contrast, an increased heart rate may follow inhibition of the parasympathetic nervous system muscarinic receptors, e.g. atropine.

An increase in the heart rate can lead to an increase in cardiac output (see equation earlier). However, ventricular filling occurs during diastole and this phase of the cardiac cycle is shortened as the heart rate increases. A sinus tachycardia, above 160 beats/m in the young adult, drastically reduces the time during diastole for ventricular filling. This leads to a progressively smaller stroke volume and a fall in cardiac output. The critical heart rate also depends on the age of the patient and the condition of the heart; e.g. rates over 120 beats/min may cause inadequate filling in the elderly.

Key point

Increasing the heart rate will only lead to rise in the cardiac output if the rate is below a critical level (which differs in different individuals depending on age and the condition of the myocardium)

The main factors affecting the cardiac output are summarised in the box.

Main factors affecting cardiac output (of the left ventricle)

Preload, or left ventricular end diastolic volume
Myocardial contractility
Afterload, or systemic vascular resistance
Heart rate

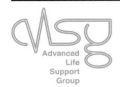

The arterial system

The walls of the aorta and other large arteries contain relatively large amounts of elastic tissue that stretches during systole and recoils during diastole. In contrast, the walls of arterioles contain relatively more smooth muscle. This is innervated by the sympathetic nervous system that maintains vasomotor tone. Stimulation of α adrenoreceptors causes vasoconstriction. A total loss of arterial tone would increase the capacity of the circulatory system so much that the total blood volume would be insufficient to fill it. As a consequence, the blood pressure would fall and the flow through organs would depend on their resistance. Some organs would receive more than normal amounts of oxygenated blood (e.g. skin) at the expense of others which would receive less (e.g. brain). To prevent this, the arterial system is under constant control by the sympathetic nervous system and local factors, to ensure that blood goes where it is needed most. This is exemplified in the shocked patient, where differential vasoconstriction is aimed at maintaining supply to the vital circuit of heart, lungs and brain at the expense of others (e.g. skin). Hence the skin is cold and looks pale in some states of shock (e.g. hypovolaemic shock).

> **Blood volume**
>
> Adult male = 70 ml/kg ideal body weight
> Adult female = 60 ml/kg ideal body weight

Systemic arterial blood pressure

This is the pressure exerted on the walls of the arteries. Systolic is the maximum and diastolic is the minimum pressure generated in the large arteries during the cardiac cycle. The difference between them is the pulse pressure. The **mean arterial pressure** is the average pressure during the cardiac cycle and is approximately equal to the diastolic pressure plus one third of the pulse pressure. As the mean arterial pressure is the product of the cardiac output and the systemic vascular resistance, it is affected by all the factors already discussed.

Autoregulation

Organs have a limited ability to regulate their own blood supply so that perfusion is maintained as blood pressure varies. This process, known as autoregulation, depends on the physiological control of smooth muscle tone in arteriolar walls. By altering the calibre of the vessels, flow to the organ is maintained over a wide range of arterial pressures. Other local factors, such as products of anaerobic metabolism, acidosis and a rise in temperature, all cause the local vascular tree to dilate. These local factors also shift the oxygen/haemoglobin dissociation curve to the right (see page 49).

Such effects enable active tissues to receive increased quantities of oxygenated blood and nutrients, and for this blood to 'give up' its oxygen more easily. Thus, the body attempts to halt the transition from reversible (where appropriate resuscitation will succeed) to irreversible shock. In the latter, the local tissue circulation has become so disrupted with large amounts of toxins from anaerobic metabolism, that the body becomes overwhelmed by negative inotropes, prothrombotic and procoagulant substances.

Remember that autoregulation may not work under pathological conditions.

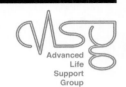

PRIMARY ASSESSMENT AND RESUSCITATION

A summary of the circulatory assessment is shown in the box.

Summary of circulatory assessment

Look	Pallor, sweating, venous pressure
Feel	Pulse – rate, rhythm and character
	Capillary refill time
	Blood pressure
	Apex beat
Listen	Blood pressure, heart sounds, extra sounds, lung bases

---

The aim of this brief assessment is to identify the patient who is shocked. This is a clinical syndrome resulting from inadequate delivery, or use, of essential substrates (e.g. oxygen) by vital organs. The causes of shock are described in detail in Chapter 9 and summarised in the next box.

Causes of shock

Preload reduction	Hypovolaemia	Haemorrhage
		Diarrhoea
		Excessive vomiting
		High fistulae loss
		Reduced intake
		Endothelial leak
	Impaired venous return	Pregnancy
		Pulmonary embolus
		Severe asthma
		Tension pneumothorax
Pump failure	Endocardial	Acute valve lesion
	Myocardial	Infarction
		Inflammation
		Dysrhythmia
	Epicardial	Tamponade
After load reduction	Vasodilation	Sepsis
		Anaphylaxis
		Toxic

SPECIFIC CLINICAL FEATURES

All patients with respiratory distress will have a tachycardia as described in the previous chapter. With severe airways obstruction, however, **pulsus paradoxus** may be present. Normally there is a reduction in systolic blood pressure of up to 10 mm Hg on inspiration. This is attributed to a fall in intrathoracic pressure (i.e. it becomes more negative on inspiration), which enlarges the pulmonary vascular bed and reduces return of blood to the left ventricle.

There is partial compensation by a simultaneous increase in right ventricular output. In severe asthma and COPD there is a more substantial fall in intrathoracic pressure on inspiration. This greatly increases the capacity of the pulmonary

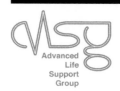

vascular bed that in turn reduces output from the left ventricle, resulting in pulsus paradoxus. This is an exaggeration of the **normal** systolic fall on inspiration and not a paradoxical change in the pulse as the name would imply. The abnormality is the extent by which the arterial pressure falls. If severe, the pulse may disappear on inspiration and this can easily be palpated at the radial artery. In contrast, if the fall in systolic pressure is not so marked, it can be detected using the sphygmomanometer. This physical sign indicates critical circulatory volume deficiency and can also occur in patients with cardiac tamponade.

Another pulse abnormality is **pulsus alternans** where evenly spaced beats (in time) are alternately large and small in volume. As this can indicate left ventricular failure, the clinician should check for corroborative signs such as a displaced apex beat, a **third heart sound** and a pansystolic murmur of mitral regurgitation. A third heart sound in patients over 40 years usually indicates elevated ventricular end diastolic pressure. This is because with increasing age, the myocardium and associated valvular structures become less compliant, i.e. stiffer. Thus, an increase in end diastolic pressure is needed to ensure adequate ventricular filling, during which sudden tension in these structures generates vibrations which correspond to the third heart sound.

Hypovolaemia

Hypovolaemia, commonly due to blood loss, can present with tachypnoea (an early sign, resulting from metabolic acidaemia) and a variety of other physical signs including tachycardia, hypotension (often a late sign of decompensation) and reduced urine output. Bradycardia occurs in advanced/preterminal shock (see Chapter 9 for further details).

Pulmonary embolus

The size and position of the pulmonary embolus will determine its haemodynamic effects. Non-fatal emboli blocking the major branches of the pulmonary artery (PA) provoke a rise in PA pressure due to hypoxaemia and vasoconstriction. In addition, tachypnoea follows stimulation of alveolar and capillary receptors. An acute increase in pulmonary vascular resistance and hence right ventricular afterload causes a sudden rise in end diastolic pressure and dilatation of the right ventricle. This produces a raised jugular venous pressure, a fall in systemic arterial pressure and a compensatory tachycardia (see Chapter 9 on Shock for further details).

Dysrhythmia

Shock resulting from a dysrhythmia is due to either pulmonary oedema or hypotension or a combination of these conditions. Under these circumstances tachydysrhythmias, irrespective of the QRS complex width, will require cardioversion. Unfortunately, atrial fibrillation may either fail to cardiovert (especially when chronic) or only transiently return to sinus rhythm. Remember to anticoagulate the patient with chronic atrial fibrillation (>48 h) before cardioversion.

The remaining options include:
- chemical cardioversion. Of the many drugs available, intravenous amiodarone is well tolerated. Flecainide is an excellent alternative, but has been shown to increase mortality in patients with ischaemic heart disease
- control the ventricular response with intravenous digoxin or β blockers.

In contrast, a patient with a bradydysrhythmia may require temporary support with either atropine and an inotrope (e.g. adrenaline) or external pacing whilst preparations are made for transvenous pacing (see Chapter 9 on Shock for further details).

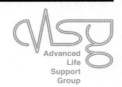

Cardiac tamponade

The signs of cardiac tamponade include pulsus paradoxus, raised internal jugular venous pressure that increases on inspiration (the opposite of normal; known as Kussmaul's sign) and an impalpable apex beat. As fluid accumulates, the elevated pressure in the pericardial sac is raised further during inspiration (this may be related to the downward displacement of the diaphragm). A corresponding increase is seen in the right atrial and central venous pressures. In contrast, pressures on the left side of the heart may be lower than that in the pericardium. As a consequence, filling of the left ventricle is compromised, stroke volume is reduced and the interventricular septum bulges into the left ventricular cavity. Thus, the stroke volume of the right ventricle is maintained at the expense of the left ventricle, which collapses on inspiration. With further increases in pericardial pressure there is diastolic collapse of the right atrium and ventricle. The venous pressure is always raised and is due to abnormal right heart filling. Kussmaul's sign can also be seen in right ventricular disease and pulmonary hypertension.

TREATMENT

All critically ill patients should receive high concentrations of inspired oxygen and have their oxygen saturation, pulse, blood pressure and cardiac rhythm monitored. Intravenous access is needed and at least one large cannula (12–14 gauge) is required.

Hypovolaemia

In acute hypovolaemia a fluid challenge should be given whilst the cause, usually haemorrhage, is sought (see Chapter 9). Chronic fluid depletion often presents as dehydration with features of acute renal impairment. Oxygen and careful fluid replacement are required, especially in patients with pre-existing cardiac conditions. Diuretics and angiotensin-converting enzyme inhibitors are a common cause of this problem in patients with a history of left ventricular failure. These drugs should be stopped and fluid replacement titrated against the patient's clinical condition and central venous pressure.

Acute severe left ventricular failure

The blood pressure is probably the most important feature in determining treatment. The combination of acute pulmonary oedema and hypotension requires inotropic support. Any patient who has a systolic pressure of less than 90 mm Hg should not be given diuretics, nitrates or opiates as their immediate action is to cause venodilatation. This, in turn, will reduce the cardiac preload and potentially exacerbate hypotension. However, once an inotrope has been started and the patient's condition is improving, a diuretic may be used to 'clear' pulmonary oedema.

Dysrhythmia – tachycardia

The acutely ill patient can develop a tachydysrhythmia in response to a variety of non-cardiac conditions:
- Hypoxaemia
- Hypovolaemia
- Hypokalaemia
- Hypomagnesaemia
- Acidosis
- Hypercarbia.

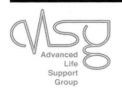

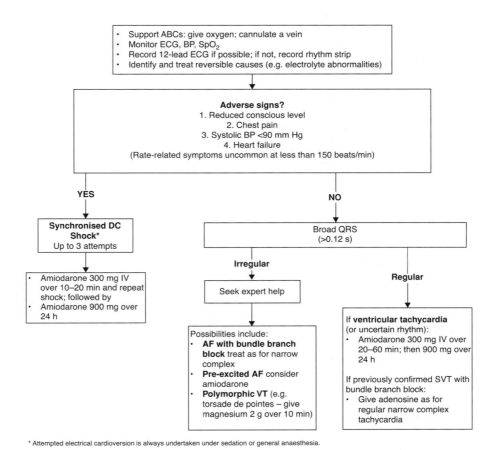

Fig. 6.2 Management of a broad complex tachycardia (UK and European guidelines). [Reproduced with permission from the Resuscitation Council (UK) and extracted from the Adult Tachycardia Algorithm.]

A tachydysrhythmia in the shocked or haemodynamically compromised patient necessitates electrical cardioversion (see Chapter 32). This is more likely to be successful if non-cardiac conditions have been treated. If cardio-version fails then drug treatment according to UK and European resuscitation committee guidelines is advocated (Figs 6.2 and 6.3). Remember that a sinus tachycardia can be the response of a failing ventricle or any other cause of shock. However, if the patient has another baseline rhythm such as atrial fibrillation, the increased sympathetic drive would result in atrial fibrillation with a rapid ventricular response. It can be difficult to decide whether a dysrhythmia is the cause of shock or vice versa. Previous ECGs are invaluable in this circumstance. If no such information is available, the treatment is dictated by the clinician's judgement. The following key points can help in this dilemma:

- A supraventricular tachycardia with a ventricular response of less than 150 is unlikely to cause failure.
- A broad complex tachycardia is almost always ventricular in a patient with ischaemic heart disease (>90%).

Time Out 6.1

Ensure that you have a sound understanding of this protocol (Fig. 6.2). If necessary take five minutes and copy the tachydysrhythmia management flow diagram to reinforce your knowledge.

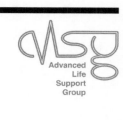

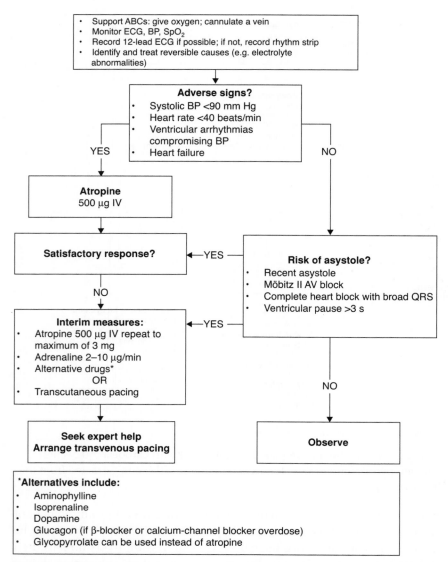

Fig. 6.3 Management of a bradydysrhythmia (UK and European guidelines). (Reproduced with permission from Resuscitation Council (UK).)

Dysrhythmia – bradycardia

This is treated according to UK and European resuscitation committee guidelines (Fig. 6.3).

Time Out 6.2

In a patient with a bradycardia, what are the risk factors for asystole? If you cannot answer this question, copy the bradycardia management flow diagram (Fig. 6.3) to reinforce your knowledge.

Pulmonary embolus

The minimum immediate management comprises high inspired concentrations of oxygen and anticoagulation. More comprehensive treatment details are provided in Chapters 8–10.

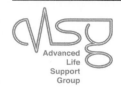

Cardiac tamponade

If this diagnosis is suspected clinically, then intravenous fluid should be given to raise the end diastolic pressure and volume to maintain the cardiac output. This is only a temporising procedure and immediate cardiological referral is required for echocardiography and pericardiocentesis (see Chapter 10).

INVESTIGATIONS

Appropriate investigations include:

- a full blood count to exclude anaemia (possibly exacerbating left ventricular failure)
- urea and electrolytes for baseline values particularly in patients who are being treated with vasodilators, diuretics or inotropes
- markers of myocardial injury troponin I or T, cardiac enzymes
- arterial blood gases
- 12-lead ECG
- portable chest X-ray
- echocardiography in selected cases.

Key point

If the patient is still breathless and the cause remains in doubt, a rapid re-evaluation of A, B and C is required

It is important to remember that hypovolaemia is an important cause of breathlessness

---

Once the patient's condition is stabilised, further information can be obtained from the secondary assessment.

Time Out 6.3

List the major causes of shock.

SUMMARY

- Tissue perfusion relies on venous return, myocardial contractility, afterload and autoregulation.
- Failure of one or more of these components will result in shock.
- In the primary assessment, the immediately life-threatening problems are:

– Airway	Obstruction
– Breathing	Acute severe asthma
	Acute exacerbation of COPD
	Pulmonary oedema
	Tension pneumothorax
	Critical oxygen desaturation
– Circulation	Shock

  These conditions can be identified and differentiated clinically.
- All shocked patients require oxygen and intravenous access.

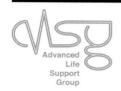

CHAPTER 7

Disability assessment

OBJECTIVES

After reading this chapter you will be able to:
- describe the neurological examination in both the primary and secondary assessment phases.

PRIMARY NEUROLOGICAL ASSESSMENT

This is the D component as described in Chapter 3. This brief examination comprises:
- pupil size and response to light
- Glasgow Coma Score
- lateralising signs
- signs of meningeal irritation
- glucose

SECONDARY NEUROLOGICAL ASSESSMENT

The most important component of the neurological examination is the history and this will follow the normal 'phrased' format (see Chapter 3). Particular attention should be directed at the key features shown in the box.

Key neurological features

Define the problem	
Describe the deficit	
Determine the	Onset
	Pattern
	Extent and duration
Associated symptoms	Neurological
	Other

A comprehensive neurological assessment is not required and so a screening examination will suffice. The components are listed in the box below.

Acute Medical Emergencies; The Practical Approach, 2nd edition.
Edited by Terence Wardle, Peter Driscoll, and Sue Wieteska.
© 2010 Blackwell Publishing Ltd.

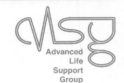

Advanced
Life
Support
Group

Components of the screening examination

Higher mental function

Speech

Pupil response

Visual fields

Fundoscopy

Eye movement

Facial sensation

Facial movement

Movement of mouth, tongue and palate

Motor

   Look for wasting and fasciculation

   Test tone

   Power

   Reflexes

Sensation

   Light touch and pinprick test

   Joint position sense (proprioception)

Coordination

Often higher function and speech are assessed whilst taking the patient's history.

Higher mental function tests

Whilst the clinical assessment of higher mental function is necessary for a comprehensive neurological examination, a full examination is rarely done in the first 24 h of admission. A brief assessment of cognition can be carried out using the AMTS (abbreviated mental test score; see Table 7.1). To allow comparison with scores obtained in the past it is important that the correct questions are asked and that they are scored consistently.

Table 7.1 Abbreviated mental test score

	Question	Assessment	Rating
1	How old are you?	Score for exact age only	
2	What is your date of birth?	Only date and month needed	
3	What is the year now?	Score for exact year only	
4	What is the time of the day?	Score if within 1 h of correct time	
5	Where are we? What is this building?	Score for exact place name, e.g. 'hospital' insufficient	
Now ask subject to remember an address: 42, West Street			
6	Who is the current monarch?	Score only current monarch	
7	What was the date of the first world war?	Score for year of start or finish	
8	Can you count down backwards from 20 to 1?	Score if no mistakes or any mistakes corrected spontaneously	
9	Can you tell me what those 2 people do for a living?	Score if recognises role of 2 people correctly, e.g. docor nurse	
10	Can you remember the address I gave you?	Score for exact recall only	
		TOTAL	/10

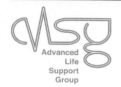

When to test higher mental function?

Usually when a doctor is suspicious that there is an underlying abnormality or occasionally if a concern is expressed by the patient or, more particularly, the family. Since delirium is frequently missed, there is an argument for assessing the AMTS in all patients who are admitted as an emergency (Table 7.1).

How to test?

Explain that you are going to ask a few questions that might seem strange.

A correct answer scores 1 mark. No half-marks are given. A score of 6 or below is abnormal.

Speech

Particular abnormalities that influence speech are shown in the box.

Important abnormalities affecting speech

Deafness
Dysphasia
Dysarthria
Dysphonia

The 'four D's' of speech can be easily assessed by remembering the following four questions.

Can the patient hear, understand, articulate and vocalise?

Lack of comprehension as well as failure of thought or word generation implies a dysphasia, of which there are two major types. Expressive or motor aphasia is where the patient can understand either verbal or written information but has aphasia or non-fluent speech. In contrast, poor comprehension and occasionally meaningless speech indicates receptive or sensory aphasia. These conditions are often referred to as Broca's or Wernicke's dysphasia respectively and occur predominantly in the dominant hemisphere.

Broca's dysphasia is usually a lesion in Broca's area in the inferior frontal gyrus that can be associated with a hemiplegia. In contrast, Wernicke's area (upper part of the temporal lobe and supramarginal gyrus of the parietal lobe) is often associated with a visual field defect. Total aphasia is a lesion of the dominant hemisphere that affects both Broca's and Wernicke's areas.

Key points in assessing aphasia

Establish whether the patient is right or left handed
Discover the first language
Ask the patient simple questions initially, requiring 'yes/no' answers
Increase complexity of questions starting with simple commands such as 'put out your tongue', followed by 'touch your right ear with your left index finger'
Always ensure that the patient has understood your instructions

---

Dysarthria is a failure of articulation that normally requires the coordination of breathing with movement of the vocal cords, larynx, tongue, palate and lips.

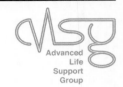

When taking the history, listen for slurring and the rhythm of speech along with the words or sounds which cause the greatest difficulty.

Types of dysarthria

Spastic – slurred, like 'Donald Duck' speech (also called pseudobulbar palsy)

Extrapyramidal – slurred and monotonous, e.g. in Parkinson's disease

Cerebellar – slurred, disjointed, scanning or staccato (equal emphasis on each syllable) seen in alcohol intoxication and disseminated sclerosis

---

Lower motor neurone lesions affecting speech include:
- facial (VII) – difficulty with the letters B, P, M and W
- palate (IX) – nasal speech (like nasal congestion)
- tongue (XII) – distorted speech with difficulty with T, S and D (bilateral lower motor neurone lesions of XII cause bulbar palsy).
  KLM is an easier way of remembering (X, XII, VII):
- X – affects the soft palate so impairs the sound, 'kuh, kuh, kuh . . .'
- XII – affects the tongue so impairs the sound, 'la, la, la . . .'
- VII – affects the lips so impairs the sound, 'mi, mi, mi . . .'

Dysphonia is a disturbance of voice production that may indicate laryngopharyngeal pathology or an abnormality of the vagus. Dysphonia is not formally assessed unless the patient is unable to produce a normal volume of sound or speaks in a whisper.

Pupil response

Check the pupils for:
- symmetry
- reaction to both light and accommodation
- both direct and consensual reflexes.

Be careful to shine the light obliquely; a torch shone directly in front of the eye may produce an accommodation response. Remember that the afferent pathway for light reaction is the optic nerve whilst the efferent pathway is the parasympathetic component of the third nerve. In contrast, the accommodation reaction afferent pathway arises in the occipital cortex but the efferent pathway remains the parasympathetic component of the third nerve bilaterally (see Fig. 7.1).

Examination should include assessment of a relative afferent pupillary defect (RAPD) by moving the light from eye to eye. If there is a RAPD, the pupil in the affected side will dilate when the light moves to it (as the direct stimulus is less intense than the consensual one). RAPD may occur with prechiasmal pathology such as optic neuritis.

A summary of pupillary abnormalities is given in Table 7.2.

Visual acuity

Some effort should always be made to assess acuity. If there is any doubt that visual acuity may be reduced formal assessment using a Snellen chart is needed.

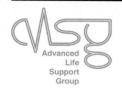

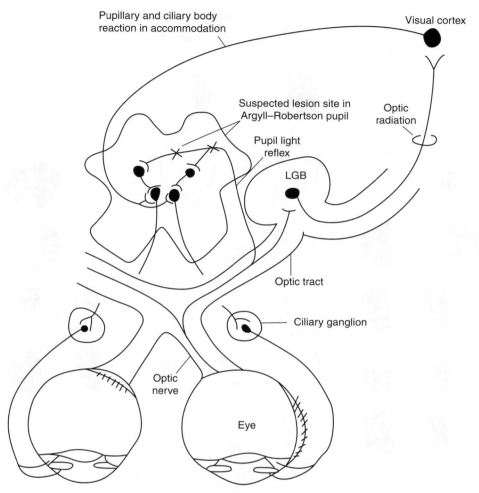

Fig. 7.1 Pathways for pupillary light reflex and accommodation.

Table 7.2 Pupillary abnormalities

	Pupillary response	Cause
Equal pupils	Small + reactive	Metabolic encephalopathy
		Midbrain herniation
		Senile miosis
	Pinpoint + fixed	Pontine lesion
		Opioids, organophosphates
	Dilated + reactive	Metabolic cause
		Midbrain lesion
		Ecstacy, amphetamines
	Dilated + fixed	Peri ictal
		Hypoxaemia
		Hypothermia
		Anticholinergics
Unequal pupils	Small + reactive	Horner's syndrome
	Small + 'non reactive'	Argyll Robertson (tertiary syphilis)
	Dilated + fixed	Uncal herniation
		IIIrd nerve palsy

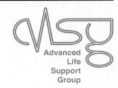

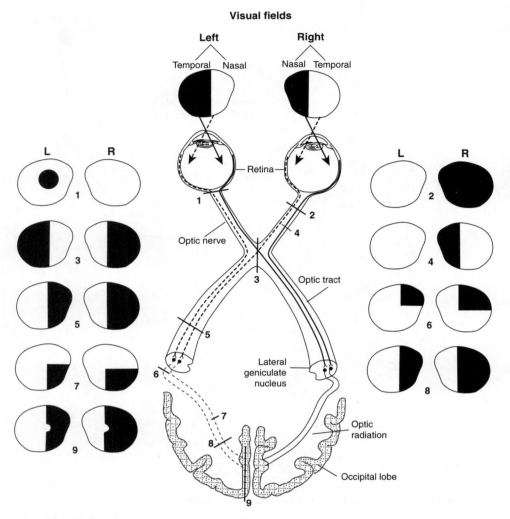

Fig. 7.2 Visual pathway with associated lesions.

Visual fields

These should be tested by confrontation which will identify any gross field defects. This way of assessing visual fields is quick, accurate and easy for patients to understand. To use this method:

- face the patient, who should cover one eye
- ask the patient to look at your corresponding pupil (i.e. their left to your right)
- hold up both hands with one or two fingers extended on each hand and ask the patient how many fingers there are in total.

All four quadrants should be covered. If an error is made, repeat changing the number of fingers in one hand to determine where the patient is not seeing well.

The visual pathway, with associated lesions, is demonstrated in Figs 7.2 and 7.3.

Interpretation

Monocular defects

These usually indicate ocular, retinal or optic nerve pathology.

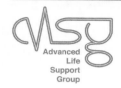

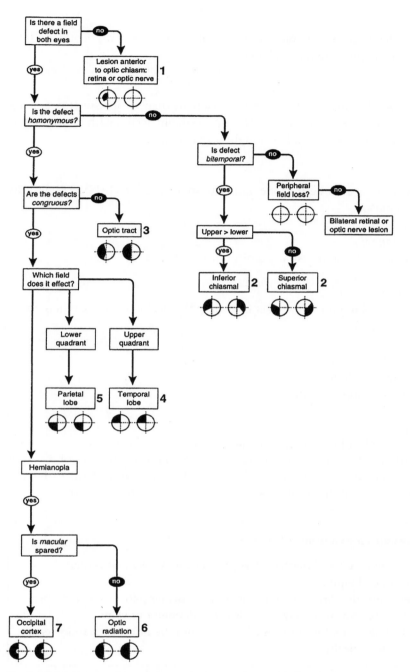

Fig. 7.3 Decision tree to determine the cause of visual field defects.

Key point

In monocular blindness due to a complete lesion of the optic nerve, the direct pupillary response to light is lost but the consensual response is retained

---

Tunnel vision

The size of the constricted field remains the same irrespective of the distance of the test object from the eye – usually functional.

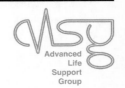

Constricted field
The field is reduced but is less marked as the object moves away from the eye; seen with chronic papilloedema or glaucoma.

Scotoma
A hole in the visual field, e.g. disseminated sclerosis or neuropathy (toxic or ischaemic), retinal haemorrhage/infarct. This occasionally occurs with migraine but other, more serious causes should be sought and excluded.

Binocular defects
These indicate a lesion at or behind the optic chiasm or very rarely bilateral lesions in front of the chiasm.

Bitemporal hemianopia
It indicates a chiasmal lesion, usually a pituitary adenoma.

Homonymous hemianopia
A lesion anywhere along the optic tract including the occipital cortex where macular sparing may be evident.

Homonymous quandrantanopia
   – upper = temporal lobe lesion
   – lower = parietal lobe lesion.

Fundoscopy

Many people make fundoscopy harder than it need be. For a successful examination, darken the room to allow the pupils to dilate. Stand to the side of a seated patient rather than in front and check the red reflex. It is important to have a system when examining the fundus. Key features are shown in the box.

Key features when examining the eye

Optic disc – colour, cup and margins; the presence or absence of venous pulsation can be helpful

Blood vessels – arteries, arteriovenous junctions, vascular patterns. Remember that arteries are approximately two thirds the diameter of veins

Background – follow the four groups of vessels from the disc and examine each quadrant systematically

---

Papilloedema is often sought. Usually the patient will retain normal vision but the optic disc will appear pink with indistinct margins. It is important to remember that papilloedema can be absent even with raised intracranial pressure.

Causes of papilloedema

Raised intracranial pressure
Arterial hypertension
Raised venous pressure due to obstruction of cerebral venous drainage
Others including hypercarbia and severe anaemia

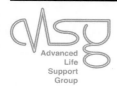

Eye movement

There are three control centres for eye movement.

Control centres for eye movement
Frontal lobe – command **Occipital lobe – pursuit** **Cerebellar/vestibular nuclei – positional**

The pathways from these three key centres are integrated in the brain stem to ensure that the eyes move together. In addition, the centre for lateral gaze is within the pons. The medial longitudinal fasciculus links the third, fourth and sixth nerve nuclei and these in turn control the external ocular muscles (see Fig. 7.4).

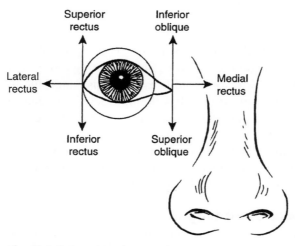

Fig. 7.4 External ocular muscles.

Nystagmus must also be actively sought. To avoid spurious nystagmus, the target should not be moved too quickly and/or too far away from the visual axis.

The commonest form of nystagmus is horizontal; vertical and rotary are rare. Specific examples include:

- Ataxic nystagmus, which is greater in the abducting than the adducting eye; caused by multiple sclerosis and cerebro-vascular disease.
- Multidirectional gaze evoked nystagmus which occurs in the direction of gaze, occurring in more than one direction. This is often seen in cerebellar syndromes, associated with drugs, alcohol or disseminated sclerosis.
- Unidirectional nystagmus, second or third degree horizontal nystagmus usually implies a cerebellar syndrome or central vestibular syndrome.
- Contrasting vertical horizontal nystagmus may be central or peripheral. The latter is usually associated with fatigue and vertigo.
- Downbeat nystagmus normally indicates a lesion at the level of the foramen magnum.

Third nerve palsies

Oculomotor nerve lesions can affect movement of the eye, the pupil and the upper eyelid. In complete third nerve palsy, there is ptosis, paralysis of the eye (except in abduction and intorsion, in which the eye is rotated 'down and out') and a

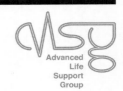

pupil that is dilated and paralysed to all stimuli. Sometimes the palsy is complete except pupil reaction remains; this indicates a 'medical' problem (e.g. diabetes) rather than compression. This 'pupil sparing rule' should be applied only in isolated third nerve palsies.

Facial sensation

Test for gross deficit using the finger tip in all three divisions of the trigeminal nerve. The corneal reflex should be tested since an abnormal response may be the first sign of trigeminal pathology. It is vital that the cornea rather than the conjunctiva is touched with a fine wisp of cotton wool and that the stimulus is brought in from the side.

Jaw jerk

This can be useful in patients with upper motor neurone signs in all limbs to help determine if the pathology is above or below the fifth nerve nucleus. If above, a pathologically brisk jaw jerk may be found.

Facial movement

After checking for symmetry, ask the patient to screw up their eyes tightly. Asymmetric power will result in the eyelids on the weaker side protruding more than on the stronger side. There are two points to remember: (1) ptosis is not due to a seventh nerve lesion; (2) corneal reflex usually has the ophthalmic branch of the trigeminal nerve as the afferent pathway whilst the efferent pathway uses the seventh nerve.

Seventh nerve palsies can be either upper motor neurone where only movements of the forehead and orbicularis oculi are preserved or lower motor neurone lesions when latter all movements on the affected side are involved.

Movement of the mouth, palate and tongue

Clues to problems in these three areas may have been elicited when testing the integrity of the fifth nerve and the patient's speech.

Abnormalities are shown in the box.

Abnormalities when examining the mouth

Small tongue with fasciculation – lower motor neurone lesion

Reduced range of tongue movement – bilateral upper motor neurone lesion often associated with labile emotions and pseudobulbar palsy

Tongue deviates to one side (with normal bulk) – unilateral upper motor neurone weakness associated with a stroke (common)

Unilateral wasting or fasciculation of tongue – unilateral lower motor neurone lesion (rare)

Uvula does not move on saying 'ah' or gag – bilateral palatal muscle paresis

Uvula moves to one side – contralateral upper or lower motor neurone lesion of the vagus nerve

---

Risk of aspiration after stroke

The best bedside way to assess the risk of aspiration in patients who have had a stroke is the water swallow test. Testing the gag reflex is much less helpful in this setting. The ability to swallow a small amount of water normally is associated with a low risk of aspiration; inability to do so is associated with a high risk and

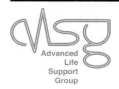

such patients should normally be kept nil by mouth until expert assessment (such as by a speech and language therapist) has been made.

Table 7.3 Classification of muscular weakness

Type of weakness	Clinical features
Upper motor neurone lesion	Increased tone, increased reflexes, pyramidal pattern of weakness, i.e. weak arm extensors and leg flexors
Lower motor neurone lesion	Wasting, fasciculation, decreased tone, absent reflexes
Neuromuscular junction	Fatiguable weakness, normal or decreased tone, normal reflexes
Muscle disease	Wasting, decreased tone, impaired or absent reflexes
Functional weakness	No wasting, normal tone, normal reflexes, variable and inconsistent power

Motor system

Examination of the motor system is designed to detect muscular weakness. The five categories are given in Table 7.3.

Thus the sequence of your examination should include the following.

Observation
Look for wasting, fasciculation, posture and gait.

Tone
Ensure that the patient is either relaxed or distracted by conversation but remember that telling the patient to relax often has the opposite effect. Tone in the upper limb is assessed by passive movement of the wrist and elbow joints. Tone in the lower limbs is assessed by rolling the legs (with the hands on the patella) and observing movement at the ankle, and by lifting the knee quickly and observing if the heel slides along the surface (normal) or is lifted in the air (indicates increased tone). Common abnormalities in tone are listed in the box.

Common abnormalities in tone

Increased spasticity – upper motor neurone lesion (the tone will be greater in flexors in upper limb and extensors in lower limb). This is sometimes called 'clasp knife' rigidity

Increased rigidity – this is sometimes called 'lead pipe' rigidity as the resistance to movement is increased in all directions. The combination of increased rigidity and a tremor e.g. extrapyramidal syndromes like Parkinson's disease produces a cogwheel effect.

Reduced tone – lower motor neurone lesion

Power
When assessing any component of the nervous system, patient cooperation is vital. Instructions such as 'pull your foot towards your bottom' can seem complex and difficult to understand, especially when the patient is anxious. It is, therefore, recommended that you not only explain to the patient what you are going to do and what you would like them to do, but also show them. This demonstration can save a lot of time and frustration.

Before formally testing power, ask the patient to hold their arms out in front of their chest with palms uppermost and close their eyes. Watch the position of the arms as this will give you a clue as to underlying abnormalities. For example, pyramidal weakness will cause the arm to pronate and drift downwards. Muscular weakness, which can occur bilaterally, may make the arms drift downwards irrespective of whether the patient's eyes are open or closed. With cerebellar disease the arm may rise spontaneously; or a sharp tap on the back of the hand will cause exaggerated displacement, excessive compensatory return and overshoot. Disorders of joint position sense are manifested by the fingers moving up or down or the arm drifting, particularly when the eyes are closed.

If you suspect the patient's apparent weakness is factitious, ask the patient to lift one leg while you palpate under the other heel. If the patient is trying to lift one leg, there will be downwards pressure from the other side (unless there is bilateral paralysis of the lower limbs).

The key movements to be tested are listed in Table 7.4, along with the muscle, root value, and associated nerve.

The radial nerve supplies all the extensors in the arm. The ulnar nerve supplies all the intrinsic hand muscles except for the lateral two lumbricals, opponens pollicis, abductor pollicis brevis and flexor pollicis brevis. These muscles are supplied by the median nerve and can often be remembered by the acronym LOAF.

Once the muscles in the arms have been tested, it is easier to assess power in the legs rather than sensation in the arms. The reason for that will become apparent. The key movements and the appropriate muscles, nerves and root values for the lower limbs are listed in Table 7.5.

Table 7.4 Key movements of the arm

Movement	Muscle	Nerve	Root value
Shoulder abduction	Deltoid	Axillary	C5
Elbow flexion (with forearm supinated)	Biceps brachialis	Musculocutaneous	C5 C6
Elbow extension	Triceps	Radial	C6 C7
Finger extension	Extensor digitorum	Posterior interosseous	C7
Finger flexion	Flexor digitorum superficials and profundus	Median and ulnar	C8
Thumb abduction	Abductor pollicis brevis	Median	T1
Index finger abduction	First dorsal interosseous	Ulnar	T1
Index finger adduction	Second palmar interosseous	Ulnar	T1

Table 7.5 Key movements of the leg

Movement	Muscle	Nerve	Root
Hip flexion	Iliopsoas	Lumbar plexus	L1, 2
Knee extension	Quadriceps femoris	Femoral	L3, 4
Knee flexion	Hamstrings	Sciatic	L5, S1
Foot dorsiflexion	Tibialis anterior	Deep peroneal	L4/5
Foot plantarflexion	Gastrocnemius	Posterior tibial	S1
Big toe extension	Extensor digitorum longus	Deep peroneal	L5
Hip extension	Gluteus maximus	Inferior gluteal	L5, S1

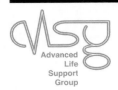

When testing muscle power, always:
- ensure the joint is pain-free
- allow the patient to move the joint through the full range before testing power
- compare the strength of right side with left side
- grade your findings according to the MRC scale.

Power grading – MRC scale

5 = normal power
4 = moderate movement against resistance
3 = movement against gravity but not resistance
2 = movement with gravity eliminated
1 = flicker
0 = no movement

Reflexes

Remember that tendon reflexes are increased in upper motor neurone lesions and decreased with abnormalities in lower motor neurones and muscles. Reflexes are graded (see Table 7.6 below).

Table 7.6 Grading reflexes

4 = clonus
3 = increased
2 = normal
1 = diminished
0 = absent

When eliciting a tendon reflex:
- first palpate to ensure that the tendon is present and not tender
- make sure that the patient is relaxed
- use the whole length of the patella hammer and let it fall through a gentle arc – the force should come from gravity alone not from your arm muscles
- watch the belly of the muscle you are testing
- use reinforcement if a reflex is unobtainable directly. A way of doing this that patients find easy to understand is to ask them to clench a fist. Remember, reinforcement does not last for long, so ask the patient to clench the fist just as you are about to let the tendon hammer fall.

It may be easier to elicit the triceps reflex if the patient sits forward while their shoulder is passively extended. The triceps will now be on the upper surface of the upper arm and is easily accessible.

Striking the sole of the foot with the tendon hammer rather than striking the Achilles tendon elicits the ankle jerk more easily, comfortably and accurately.

The major reflexes are listed in Table 7.7 (see page 80).

In the presence of increased reflexes, check for ankle and patella clonus and for increased tone. Reflex abnormalities are listed in Table 7.8 (see page 80).

Reflexes can be absent in the early stages of a severe upper motor neurone lesion. This is often, inappropriately, referred to as spinal shock. There is no evidence of shock but the nerves have been in effect stunned. The classic features of an upper motor neurone lesion will develop subsequently.

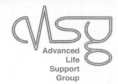

Table 7.7 Major reflexes

Muscle	Nerve	Root
Triceps	Radial	C7
Brachioradialis (supinator)	Radial	C6
Biceps	Musculocutaneous	C5
Knee	Femoral	L3, 4
Ankle	Tibial	S1, 2

Table 7.8 Reflex abnormalities

Reflex response	Interpretation
Increased, clonus	Upper motor neurone lesion
Absent, generalized	Peripheral neuropathy
Absent, isolated	Lesion of either peripheral nerve or nerve root
Pendular	Cerebellar disease
Slow relaxing	Hypothyroidism
Inverted supinator – no elbow flexion on striking brachioradialis but finger flexion occurs	C6 myelopathy

The plantar or Babinski response completes the assessment of the major reflexes. It is important to be aware of the following:

- A positive Babinski response is manifested by extension of the big toe and spreading of the adjacent toes.
- A negative Babinski response may be found in an upper motor neurone lesion.
- A positive Babinski response that does not fit in with other neurological features should be interpreted with caution.

There are a number of other eponymous manoeuvres that supply the same information as the Babinski. Details do not need to be remembered, but it is useful to know that if the patient is unable to tolerate stimulus applied to the sole of the foot they will usually be able to tolerate the same stimulus applied to the tibial border.

A summary of the common motor abnormalities is shown in Table 7.4.

Sensation

The five basic types of sensation are shown in a cross section of the spinal cord in Fig. 7.5. It is important to remember that on entry to the cord, the spinothalamic tract (pain and temperature) will cross within one or two segments. In contrast, the posterior columns (joint position sense) remain ipsilateral until they cross in the medulla. Pinprick and light touch are rarely lost without discernible symptoms. As the different sensory modalities are carried predominantly in two tracts, the preliminary sensory examination should focus on pinprick and joint position sense.

The sensory examination is used:

- as a screening test
- for assessment of symptomatic patients
- to confirm signs detected on examination of the motor system.

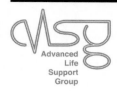

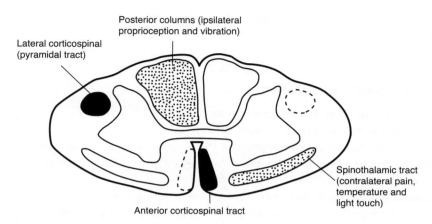

Lateral corticospinal
(pyramidal tract)

Posterior columns (ipsilateral
proprioception and vibration)

Anterior corticospinal tract

Spinothalamic tract
(contralateral pain,
temperature and
light touch)

Fig. 7.5 Cross section of the spinal cord.

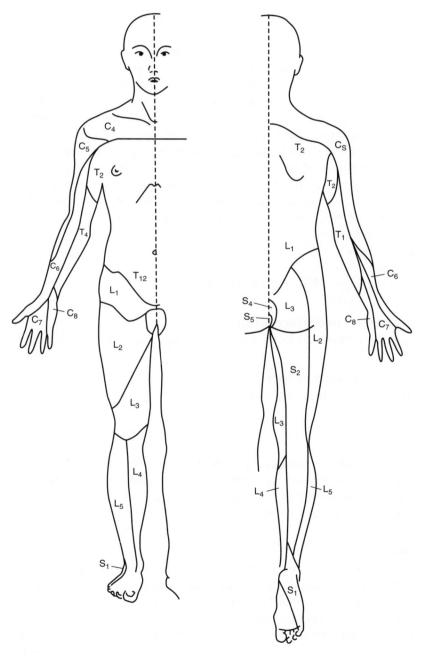

Fig. 7.6 Dermatomes.

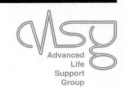

There are several key points to consider when examining sensation. These are listed in the next box.

Key points for sensory examination

Explain to the patient what you are going to do

Demonstrate to the patient what you want them to do

Always ensure that the patient can appreciate the sensory modality to be tested

Assess dermatomes in a sequential fashion. The relevant dermatomes are shown in Fig. 7.6

Ask the patient to keep their eyes open but look away during the test. Patients usually find it easier to concentrate when their eyes are open than when closed

---

Pinprick

Use a 'neuro tip' not a hypodermic needle. Check intermittently using a blunt stimulus that the patient has recognised the 'pin' appropriately. During sensory assessment, test the integrity of each dermatome and whether there is any difference when comparing left and right sides of the body. It is also convenient at this time to test whether the patient can distinguish between two stimuli applied simultaneously to the left and right sides. Failure to do this indicates sensory inattention and therefore a parietal lobe lesion (most commonly non-dominant). Do not forget to test sacral sensation. Whilst this is not part of the screening test, it must be done in patients who have any of the following features (and should be accompanied in each of these cases by assessment of anal tone):

- urinary or bowel symptoms
- bilateral leg weakness
- sensory loss in both legs
- suspicion of a conus medullaris or cauda equina lesion.

Joint position sense (proprioception)

It is important to remember that Romberg's test assesses joint position sense.

Types and causes of sensory loss

Patterns of sensory loss fall into three broad categories:

- peripheral nerves
- spinal cord
- brain.

The major abnormalities for each category are listed in Tables 7.9 and 7.10.

A bizarre distribution of sensory loss which does not conform to an anatomical distribution is suggestive of a functional disorder. This, however, is a difficult diagnosis to make (and a dangerous one to rush into).

Coordination

This requires integration of sensory feedback and motor output. Thus it is logical to assess coordination after any sensory motor abnormalities have been identified. The cerebellum is responsible for integrating information related to coordination. A clue to an underlying abnormality is often present during examination of the motor system. Watch for the exaggerated response when the patient

Table 7.9 Peripheral nerve abnormalities

Lesion	Sensory loss	Cause
Single nerve lesions	Within the distribution of a single nerve	Entrapment neuropathy, diabetes mellitus, rheumatoid disease
Multiple single nerve lesions	Distribution of relevant nerves	Vasculitis or more diffuse neuropathy
Root lesion	Confined to single root or number of roots in close proximity	Prolapsed intervertebral disc
Peripheral nerves	Glove and stocking distribution	Diabetes mellitus, alcohol, thiamine deficiency

Table 7.10 Spinal cord and brain sensory loss

Lesion	Sensory loss	Cause
Complete transverse lesion	Loss of all modalities a few segments below the lesion	Trauma, spinal cord compression by tumour, transverse myelitis
Hemisection	Ipsilateral loss of joint position sense, contralateral loss of pain and temperature a few segments below the lesion	As with complete transection plus subacute combined degeneration of the cord and tabes dorsalis
Posterior column loss	Loss of joint position sense and vibration only	
Central cord syndrome	Loss of pain and temperature sensation at the level of the lesion	Syringomyelia
Anterior spinal syndrome	Loss of pain and temperature below the level of the lesion	Anterior spinal artery lesions
Brain stem	Loss of pain and temperature sensation in the face (ipsilateral) and body (contralateral)	Demyelination, lateral medullary syndrome
Thalamic	Hemicentral loss of all modalities	Stroke, tumour or disseminated sclerosis
Cortical parietal lobe dysfunction	The patient recognises all sensory modalities but localises them poorly. In addition, there is loss of sensory attention, two-point discrimination and astereognosis	Stroke, cerebral tumour, disseminated sclerosis

has outstretched arms and you tap the back of their hands. Tests for demonstrating coordination are complex activities. It is therefore important to tell the patient what you are going to do as well as demonstrate the movement required. Assess the finger–nose test (ensuring they have to extend the elbow to touch your finger), and the heel-shin test (ensuring the heel is slid down to the hallux as poor coordination may be evident only when the heel is moved this far) as well as the presence of truncal ataxia (if the patient is mobile assess their heel-toe walking).

Other signs indicating cerebellar dysfunction are shown in the box.

Signs of cerebellar dysfunction

Speech abnormalities: slurred, scanning, staccato
Nystagmus
Pendular reflexes
Truncal ataxia
Intention tremor
Hypotonia
Dysdiadochokinesis

Interpretation

The presence of unilateral incoordination suggests ipsilateral cerebellar disease, such as demyelination or vascular disease. In contrast bilateral signs usually reflect alcohol, drugs or demyelination. The presence of truncal ataxia and/or gait ataxia without limb coordination indicates a midline (vermis) lesion.

Time Out 7.1

Draw an outline of a man and label the appropriate dermatomes.

SUMMARY

This chapter has provided an overview of the key components of a screening neurological examination. Although there are many other tests that may be relevant to comprehensive neurological assessment, the framework provided in this chapter will enable detection of neurological signs.

The primary neurological assessment (D) comprises:

- pupil size and response to light
- Glasgow Coma Score
- lateralising signs
- signs of meningeal irritation.

The secondary neurological assessment comprises:

- the history, which is the most important component. It is important to develop a simple common personalised structure to neurological assessment. A screening neurological examination is the minimum that should be done
- examine the motor components in a logical, systematic fashion followed by sensory assessment. An isolated abnormality should be interpreted with caution. Neurological problems are associated with a well-described pattern of clinical features
- test coordination after motor and sensory assessment. Clues to the presence of cerebellar disease are obtained from other parts of the examination before coordination is assessed.

Unlike other components of the physical examination, the nervous system is often not examined as there are no clinical indications. It is therefore important to take every opportunity to hone your clinical neurological skills.

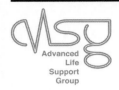

Advanced
Life
Support
Group

PART III
Presenting Complaints

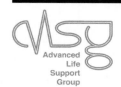
Advanced
Life
Support
Group

CHAPTER 8

The patient with breathing difficulties

OBJECTIVES

After reading this chapter you will be able to:
- describe a structured approach to the breathless patient
- understand why a structured approach is important in the management of such patients
- differentiate between the immediately life-threatening and potentially life-threatening causes of breathlessness
- describe the immediate management of these patients and appropriate definitive care.

INTRODUCTION

Acute breathlessness is a common emergency condition. The effort required for breathing often makes it virtually impossible for the patient to provide any form of medical history and questioning may only make the situation worse. The clinician's skills will help to determine the underlying cause and dictate appropriate management.

Immediately life-threatening causes and signs of breathlessness

Airway
- Obstruction (see full list in box 1 in Chapter 4)

Breathing
- Acute severe asthma
- Acute exacerbation of chronic obstructive pulmonary disease (COPD)
- Pulmonary oedema
- Tension pneumothorax
- Critical oxygen desaturation

Circulation
- Acute severe left ventricular failure
- Dysrhythmia
- Hypovolaemia
- Pulmonary embolus (PE)
- Cardiac tamponade

Key point

It is important to remember that the breathless patient does not always have pathology arising primarily from the respiratory or cardiovascular systems

---

Acute Medical Emergencies; The Practical Approach, 2nd edition.
Edited by Terence Wardle, Peter Driscoll, and Sue Wieteska.
© 2010 Blackwell Publishing Ltd.

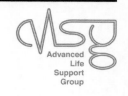

PRIMARY ASSESSMENT AND RESUSCITATION

Airway
Assessment
This has been described in Chapter 4 and is summarised in the box below.

Summary of airway assessment

Look	Respiratory	Rate
		Effort
		Symmetry
Feel	Expired air	
	Trachea	
Listen	Count to 10'	
	Breath sounds	
	Added noises	

Resuscitation
High concentrations of inspired oxygen ($FiO_2 = 0.85$) may relieve some of the patient's distress. If airway obstruction is suspected, request **immediate** review by a specialist. If a foreign body has been inhaled, attempt a Heimlich or modified Heimlich manoeuvre.

Breathing
Assessment
This has been discussed in Chapter 5 and is summarised in the box.

Summary of breathing assessment

Look	Colour, sweating
	Posture
	Respiratory – rate
	– effort
	– symmetry
Feel	Tracheal position
	Tracheal tug
	Chest expansion
Percuss	Anterior and posterior aspects of both lungs in
Listen	the upper, middle and lower zones

Resuscitation
If bronchospasm is suspected, treat patients with oxygen-driven nebulised bronchodilators irrespective of the underlying cause, whilst clues to the cause are sought.

Immediate management of a tension pneumothorax is needle thoracocentesis followed by intravenous access and then chest drain insertion.

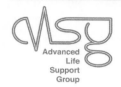

Time Out 8.1
Take 30 s to mentally rehearse the key components of your assessment.

Circulation

Assessment

This has been described in Chapter 6 and is summarised in the box.

Summary of circulatory assessment	
Look	Pallor, sweating, venous pressure
Feel	Pulse – rate, rhythm and character
	Capillary refill time
	Blood pressure
	Apex beat
Listen	Blood pressure, heart sounds, extra sounds, lung bases

Resuscitation

All patients should receive high concentrations of inspired oxygen, be treated in a 'seated' position (if level of consciousness permits) and have their oxygen saturation, pulse, blood pressure and cardiac rhythm monitored. Intravenous access is necessary and at least one large cannula (12–14 gauge) is required.

The management of the 'shocked' patient will depend on the underlying cause. Treatment options are summarised in the box.

Treatment of shock	
Cause	**Treatment**
Acute, severe, left ventricular failure	Inotropes
Dysrhythmia – Tachycardia	Cardioversion
– Bradycardia	Atropine
	Inotropes
	Pacing
Hypovolaemia	Fluids
Pulmonary embolus	Anticoagulation
	Thrombolysis
	Fluids
Sepsis	Fluids
	Antibiotics
	Inotropes
Anaphylaxis	Adrenaline
	Fluids
	Chlorpheniramine
	Hydrocortisone
Cardiac tamponade	Fluids
	Pericardiocentesis

Once the patient's condition is stabilised and the primary assessment completed, further information can be obtained from the secondary assessment.

Summary

In the breathless patient, the immediately life-threatening problems are:

- Airway   Obstruction
- Breathing   Acute severe asthma
                       Acute exacerbation of COPD
                       Pulmonary oedema
                       Tension pneumothorax
                       Critical oxygen desaturation
- Circulation   Acute severe left ventricular failure
                       Dysrhythmia
                       Hypovolaemia
                       Pulmonary embolus
                       Cardiac tamponade

These conditions can be identified and differentiated clinically.
All patients require oxygen and intravenous access.

Time Out 8.2

Mentally rehearse your approach to the patient with breathing difficulties. Then list the major components of the primary assessment. Armed with this structure read the following information and then answer the associated questions.

A old man with known ischaemic heart disease was admitted to the coronary care unit after becoming acutely breathless. He denied any chest pain or cough. The following physical signs were elicited:

- respiratory rate 26/min
- fine inspiratory crackles were heard at both bases
- pulse rate 140/min and regular
- blood pressure 80/50
- peripherally shut down
- no other relevant features

a What would be your immediate management?
b What investigations would you request?

SECONDARY ASSESSMENT

Many patients with breathlessness will be able to give a history, albeit fragmented. The conditions diagnosed in this assessment phase are shown in the box.

Potentially life-threatening causes of breathlessness

Respiratory
- Asthma
- Acute on chronic respiratory failure
- Pulmonary oedema

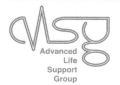

- Simple pneumothorax
- Pneumonia
- Pleural effusion
- Pulmonary embolus

Non-respiratory
- Metabolic acidosis e.g. diabetic ketoacidosis, salicylate overdose
- Pontine haemorrhage

SPECIFIC CONDITIONS

Asthma

Asthma is a chronic inflammatory condition resulting in reversible narrowing of the airways. It affects approximately 5% of the population and can occur for the first time at any age with a male predominance in childhood and females in later life. Asthma in children is usually associated with atopy, whilst in adults it is more commonly non-atopic. Both, however, have an inherited component.

Although there are many potential triggers, asthma is characterised by wheezing due to widespread narrowing of the peripheral airways. There may be an associated increase in sputum volume and viscosity. Occasionally a nocturnal cough will be a prominent symptom and patients may describe tightness in the chest or a sensation of choking rather than wheezing. Furthermore, exposure to external stimuli such as viruses, cold air, cigarette smoke and paint fumes may induce an acute 'asthmatic' attack. This does not indicate an allergic response but demonstrates that the airways are hyperreactive and produce an exaggerated response to non-specific irritants.

Pathophysiology

Acute attacks of bronchospasm may be precipitated by IgE mediated mast cell degranulation. In contrast, when exposed to environmental factors, e.g. allergens and pollutants, the airways of known asthmatics are susceptible to chronic inflammation characterised by eosinophil and T lymphocyte infiltration. These cells are responsible for liberating inflammatory mediators that evoke a variety of responses (see next box) culminating in airways narrowing and hence increased airflow resistance. Since resistance is inversely proportional to the fourth power of the radius (Poiseulle's law) a small increase in airways thickness will have a marked effect on airways resistance and therefore reduce airflow. The change in airway radius is usually due to bronchial muscle contraction, but in the asthmatic this is exacerbated by mucosal oedema, increased mucus production and epithelial cell damage. In addition, the chronic inflammatory response reduces elastic recoil of the airways, further exacerbating the narrowing (Fig. 8.1).

Inflammatory mediator induced changes in asthma

- Disrupt the functional and structural integrity of the epithelium
- Stimulate   mucus secretion
                      oedema formation
                      smooth muscle contraction
- Induce collagen deposition under the basement membrane.

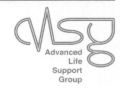

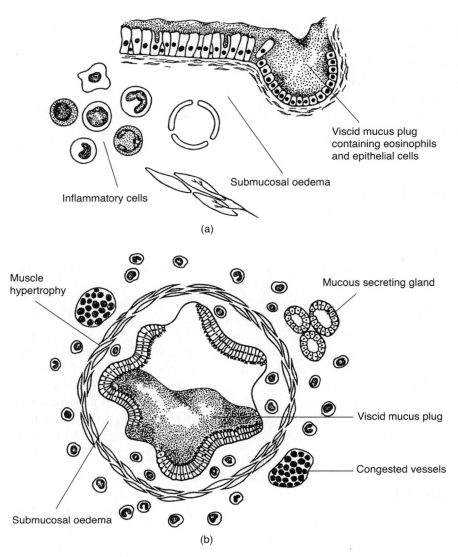

Fig. 8.1 Diagrammatic representation of the pathophysiology of asthma:
(a) longitudinal section and (b) cross section.

This disturbed and decreased airflow is manifest clinically as audible wheeze, reduced forced expiratory volume in one second and peak expiratory flow rate, along with increased functional residual capacity due to air trapping. Thus, because of increased airways resistance the work of breathing is increased and the patient feels breathless.

In an acute asthmatic attack some of the airways become blocked by mucus plugs resulting in hypoxaemia due to ventilation perfusion (V/Q) mismatch. This further increases the work of breathing, causing hyperventilation in an attempt to reverse the hypoxaemia.

Key point

Failure to sustain this increased respiratory effort, usually in a severe exacerbation, will be manifest by a silent chest, hypoxaemia and a rising PaCO$_2$

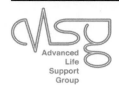

Management

> **Key point**
>
> Preventable deaths from acute asthma still occur due to treatment delay

The management summarised in Fig. 8.2 is from the British Thoracic Society guidelines.

Life-threatening asthma

Assessment

This is characterised by:

- airway – normally patent but can be compromised by exhaustion
- breathing – cyanosed, exhausted, minimal respiratory effort and a silent chest
- circulation – tachycardia greater than 130 beats per minute or bradycardia, hypotension.

In addition, the peak expiratory flow is less than 33% of the predicted or the patient's best.

> **Key point**
>
> A silent chest is a life-threatening sign as it means there is insufficient air being moved (in and out of the chest) to generate a wheeze

Immediate treatment

All patients need high concentrations of inspired oxygen ($FiO_2 = 0.85$); oxygen should also be used to drive nebulised bronchodilators. See Fig. 8.2. It is important to remember that acute breathlessness in an asthmatic is usually due to bronchospasm. However, because of 'gas trapping' there is an increase in positive end expiratory pressure. This increases the potential to develop a pneumothorax that can further inhibit the respiratory and cardiovascular systems. Always be alert to this possibility in asthmatics who either fail to respond to treatment or become acutely breathless. Regular reassessment and an urgent chest X-ray are required.

Role/action management

Intravenous fluids should be given as most patients have coexisting dehydration (increased insensible losses, the possibility of an underlying chest infection and reduced intake). Adequate hydration also helps to render the sputum less tenacious. In addition, hypokalaemia can occur as a consequence of either asthma or coexistent β_2 agonist therapy. Thus, careful monitoring and appropriate replacement therapy are required.

The patient's clinical response to treatment (as described earlier) should be monitored continuously along with frequent arterial blood gases.

If the patient either becomes exhausted, retains CO_2 or adequate oxygenation is not possible then intermittent positive pressure ventilation will be required (see box). Early liaison with the anaesthetist/intensivist is vital. Patients who have previously required intubation and ventilation have an increased risk of requiring this again during an acute severe attack.

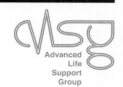

Indications for intensive care

Hypoxaemia ($PaO_2 < 8$ kPa despite $FiO_2 > 0.6$)

Hypercapnia ($PaCO_2 > 6$ kPa)

Acidaemia

Exhaustion

Altered conscious level (confused, drowsy, unconscious)

Respiratory arrest

MANAGEMENT OF ACUTE ASTHMA IN ADULTS ASSESSMENT OF SEVERE ASTHMA	
B	Health care professionals must be aware that patients with severe asthma and one or more adverse psychosocial factors are at risk of death
☑	• Keep patients who have had near fatal asthma or brittle asthma under specialist supervision indefinitely • A respiratory specialist should follow up patients admitted with severe asthma for at least one year after admission

INITIAL ASSESSMENT	
MODERATE EXACERBATION	**LIFE THREATENING**
• Increasing symptoms • PEF >50-75% best or predicted • No features of acute severe asthma	In a patient with severe asthma any one of: • PEF <33% best or predicted • SpO_2 <92% • PaO_2 <8 kPa • normal $PaCO_2$ (4.6-6.0 kPa) • silent chest • cyanosis • poor respiratory effort • arrhythmia • exhaustion, altered conscious level
ACUTE SEVERE	**NEAR FATAL**
Any one of: • PEF 33-50% best or predicted • respiratory rate ≥ 25/min heart rate ≥ 110/min • inability to complete sentences in one breath	Raised $PaCO_2$ and/or requiring mechanical ventilation with raised inflation pressures

Clinical features	Severe breathlessness (including too breathless to compete sentences in one breath), tachypnoea, tachycardia, silent chest, cyanosis or collapse *None of these singly or together is specific and their absence does not exclude a severe attack*
PEF or FEV_1	PEF or FEV_1 are useful and valid measures of airway calibre. PEF expressed as a % of the patient's previous best value is most useful clinically. In the absence of this, PEF as a % of predicted is a rough guide
Pulse oximetry	Oxygen saturation (SpO_2) measured by pulse oximetry determines the adequacy of oxygen therapy and the need for arterial blood gas (ABG). The aim of oxygen therapy is to maintain SpO_2 94-98%
Blood gases (ABG)	Patients with SpO_2 <92% or other features of life threatening asthma require ABG measurement
Chest X-ray	Chest X-ray is not routinely recommended in the absence of: - suspected pneumomediastinum or pneumothorax - suspected consolidation - life threatening asthma - failure to respond to treatment satisfactorily - requirement for ventilation

Taken from The British Thoracic Society – British Guidelines on the Management of Asthma – Revised June 2009

Fig. 8.2 The British Thoracic Society guidelines for asthma assessment [Reproduced with permission from the British Thoracic Society].

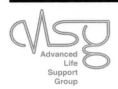

	MANAGEMENT OF ACUTE ASTHMA IN ADULTS CRITERIA FOR ADMISSION
B	Admit patients with any feature of a life threatening or near fatal attack
B	Admit patients with any feature of a severe attack persisting after initial treatment
C	Patients whose peak flow is greater than 75% best or predicted one hour after initial treatment may be discharged from ED, unless there are other reasons why admission may be appropriate

TREATMENT OF ACUTE ASTHMA

OXYGEN		β₂ AGONIST BRONCHODILATORS	
C	• Give supplementary oxygen to all hypoxaemic patients with acute asthma to maintain an SpO₂ level of 94-98%. Lack of pulse oximetry should not prevent the use of oxygen.	A	Use high dose inhaled β₂ agonists as first line agents in acute asthma and administer as early as possible. Reserve intravenous β₂ agonists for those patients in whom inhaled therapy cannot be used reliably.
A	• In hospital, ambulance and primary care, nebulised β₂ agonist bronchodilators should be driven by oxygen	☑	In acute asthma with life threatening features the nebulised route (oxygen-driven) is recommended.
C	• The absence of supplemental oxygen should not prevent nebulised therapy being given if indicated	A	In patients with severe asthma that is poorly responsive to an initial bolus dose of β2 agonist, consider continuous nebulisation with an appropriate nebuliser.

STEROID THERAPY		IPRATROPIUM BROMIDE	
A	Give steroids in adequate doses in all cases of acute asthma	B	Add nebulised ipratropium bromide (0.5 mg 4-6 hourly) to β2 agonist treatment for patients with acute severe or life threatening asthma or those with a poor initial response to β2 agonist therapy.
☑	Continue prednisolone 40-50 mg daily for at least five days or until recovery		

OTHER THERAPIES		REFERRAL TO INTENSIVE CARE
B	Consider giving a single dose of IV magnesium sulphate for patients with: • Acute severe asthma who have not had a good initial response to inhaled bronchodilator therapy • Life threatening or near fatal asthma.	Refer any patient: • Requiring ventilatory support • With acute severe or life threatening asthma, failing to respond to therapy, evidenced by: - deteriorating PEF - persisting or worsening hypoxia - hypercapnoea - ABG analysis showing ⇓ pH or ⇑ H⁺ - exhaustion, feeble respiration - drowsiness, confusion, altered conscious state - respiratory arrest
☑	IV magnesium sulphate (1.2-2g IV infusion over 20 minutes) should only be used following consultation with senior medical staff	
B	Routine prescription of antibiotics is not indicated for patients with acute asthma.	

Taken from The British Thoracic Society – British Guidelines on the Management of Asthma – Revised June 2009

Fig. 8.3 British Thoracic Society's Guidelines for Treatment of Asthma in hospital [Reproduced with permission from the British Thoracic Society].

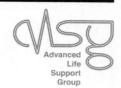

Please also see Fig. 8.3 for the assessment and management of patients with acute asthma that is not immediately life-threatening.

Time Out 8.3

Have a five-minute break, then answer the following questions.
a What type of condition is asthma?
b List the major components of this response.
c What is the overall effect of this process?
d How does this affect pulmonary physiology?
e Describe how you would manage life-threatening asthma
f What are the indications for ventilation?

Acute on chronic respiratory failure
This is an important cause of breathlessness and is considered in detail in Chapter 20 on organ failure.

Pulmonary oedema
This is an important cause of breathlessness and is considered in detail in Chapter 20.

Pneumothorax
A pneumothorax results from gas entering the potential space between the visceral pleura and the parietal pleura. This may arise spontaneously from the rupture of a bulla or cyst on the lung surface, or as a consequence of underlying lung disease. However, there are a number of invasive procedures such as subclavian vein cannulation that can also be responsible (see box).

Iatrogenic pneumothoraces

Attempted internal jugular/subclavian vein access
Pleural aspiration/biopsy
Percutaneous lung/liver biopsy
Transbronchial biopsy
Intermittent positive pressure ventilation

Pathophysiology
The outward recoil of the chest and inward elastic retraction of the lung produces negative pressure in the potential space between the visceral pleura and parietal pleura. This pressure, with respect to atmosphere, becomes more negative during inspiration. Following a breach of the visceral pleura, air preferentially moves from the alveolus into the pleural space until these pressures equilibrate – hence the lung collapses, resulting in a simple pneumothorax. If, however, the breach in the pleura acts as a one-way valve then air will preferentially enter the pleural space during inspiration and not return during expiration. Thus the pressure in the intrapleural space rises above atmospheric pressure. The

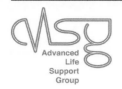

resulting hypoxaemia acts as a respiratory stimulus causing deeper inspiratory efforts, which in turn further increase the intrapleural pressure. This produces a tension pneumothorax, which can impair venous return. If untreated, mediastinal shift occurs, distorting the great vessels, further impairing venous return, and compressing the opposite lung. This process exacerbates hypoxaemia and eventually causes pulseless electrical activity (electromechanical dissociation).

Key point

Tension pneumothorax is a clinical diagnosis. Needle thoracocentesis is the immediate management

---

Primary pneumothorax
This condition is relatively uncommon (affecting about 9/100,000 patients with a male to female ratio of approximately 4:1). It occurs in previously normal lungs and is attributed to rupture of a surface bulla or cyst, which is often at the apex. About 20% of patients will have recurrent pneumothoraces on both the ipsilateral and the contralateral sides.

Secondary pneumothorax
This condition is associated with pre-existing lung disease (see next box) and medical procedures (see previous box on page 96).

Pre-existing lung conditions associated with pneumothoraces

Emphysema
Chronic obstructive pulmonary disease
Acute exacerbations of asthma
Infections: Empyema
                 Staphylococcal pneumonia
                 Tuberculosis
Malignancy
Pulmonary fibrosis
Cystic fibrosis

Assessment
Simple pneumothorax
Symptoms and signs may be absent but commonly the patient will present with breathlessness and pleuritic chest pain localised to the affected side. Breathlessness may be related to pain, size of pneumothorax and pre-existing lung disease.

Key point

In a patient with pre-existing lung disease even a small pneumothorax can produce acute respiratory failure

---

Clinical signs are difficult to detect when the pneumothorax is small or when there is coexistent emphysema. Often there is reduced chest expansion on the affected side (usually due to pain) and the percussion note is typically resonant. Hyperresonance is very difficult to detect even when comparing with the non-affected side. The most consistent sign is a reduction in breath sounds over the pneumothorax. However, a large bulla can easily be misdiagnosed as a pneumothorax. Review of the previous chest X-rays and CT scans will often solve the dilemma and prevent inappropriate chest drain insertion.

Tension pneumothorax

Presenting complaints for this condition differs depending on whether the patient is spontaneously breathing or is receiving Positive Pressure Ventilation (PPV).

Spontaneous
- More gradual onset
- Presents with mainly respiratory symptoms – tachypnoea, increase in effort, chest pain, tachycardia, falling SpO_2, agitation
- Early – contralateral HYPER mobility and Ipsilateral HYPO mobility
- Late – classic physical findings of condition
- Pre-terminal signs are a low SpO_2, fall in blood pressure, decreasing consciousness

Receiving PPV
- Onset quickly
- Fall in SpO_2 (immediate), blood pressure, tachycardia
- Late – pressure alarm (excessive pressure on inspiration)
- Other physical signs include hyperesonance, hyper-expanded chest, chest hypomobility

Radiological features of a tension pneumothorax
- Splayed ribs
- Depressed hemi-diaphragm
- Mediastinal displacement

Key point

Tension pneumothorax is a clinical diagnosis in the non-ventilated patient.

Management

Simple pneumothorax

Spontaneous resolution will occur in an asymptomatic patient with only partial lung collapse (and no deterioration for 24 h) at approximately 1.25% of the volume of the hemithorax per day. Under these circumstances no intervention will be required. Occasionally pain relief is required with non-steroidal anti-inflammatory drugs. Do not forget to reassure the patient!

The management of pneumothorax, however, depends on the size of the collapse and the presence of underlying lung disease. It is summarised in Figs 8.4 and 8.5.

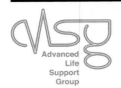

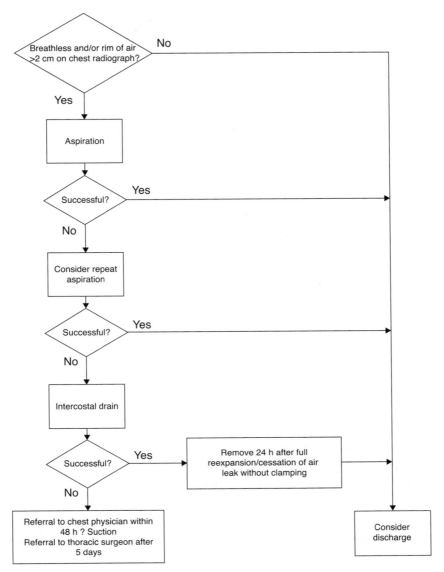

Fig. 8.4 Recommended treatment of a primary pneumothorax.

Aspiration is a simple technique with negligible morbidity. If successful it produces rapid resolution of breathlessness and chest discomfort.

Early drainage and early surgical referral are needed if the patient has either cystic fibrosis or AIDS:

AIDS patients
2–5% of AIDS patients will develop a pneumothorax. Pneumocystis Jiroveci is the most likely cause which produces necrotising alveolitis that impairs healing. This infection leads to a high risk of bilateral and recurrent pneumothorax.

Tension pneumothorax
Immediate needle thoracocentesis is needed. This will relieve the tension and the acute problems, but the residual pneumothorax will need chest drain insertion after securing intravenous access (see Chapter 31). This is a precaution because

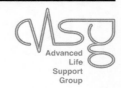

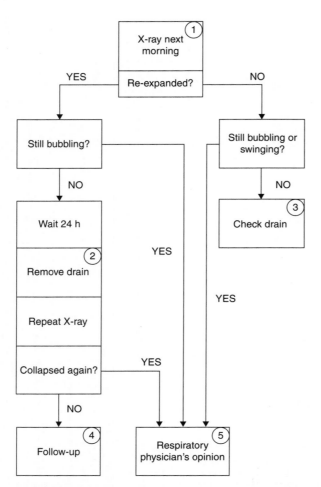

Fig. 8.5 Guidance for removing a chest drain inserted for a pneumothorax.

occasionally a pneumothorax can be complicated by a haemothorax, possibly due to tearing of a pleural lesion or from an adjacent necrotic tumour.

Investigation
Radiological confirmation of a simple pneumothorax is important and will guide appropriate therapy. In contrast, tension pneumothorax is a clinical diagnosis and an X-ray is only needed after chest drain insertion.

Discharge
- Avoid air travel until the pneumothorax has resolved radiologically. Airlines recommend 6 weeks between treatment and flying. If no intervention is necessary then there is a risk of recurrence for up to 1 year. A patient with a secondary pneumothorax without any intervention should therefore avoid flying for up to 1 year.
- Diving should be avoided permanently unless the patient has had a bilateral surgical pleurectomy
- After aspirating a primary pneumothorax – observe the patient to ensure that the signs and symptoms resolve before discharge. After aspiration for a secondary pneumothorax admit the patient for 24 h to ensure that there is no recurrence.

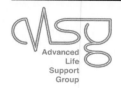

Potential problems

- Lung fails to re-expand after intercostal drain insertion – liaise with respiratory physician regarding use of low pressure suction.
- Recurrent pneumothoraces – liaise with a cardiothoracic surgeon regarding either additional chest drains, chemical endoscopic (VATS – video assisted thorascopic surgery) or formal surgical pleurodesis. Surgical advice should also be sought if there are bilateral pneumothoraces.

Explanatory notes for Fig. 8.5

1 Chest X-ray

If the underwater seal is always kept below the level of the chest, clamping is unnecessary and potentially dangerous. As far as possible, an X-ray film should be taken in the department, rather than on the ward with a portable machine; an expiration film is unnecessary.

2 Removal of chest drain

Bubbling should have stopped for at least 24 h. Some patients find tube removal unpleasant, consider sedation as above. Remove the suture holding the chest drain in place, withdraw the tube while the patient holds their breath in full inspiration. Use the two remaining sutures to seal the wound.

3 Check chest drain

If the lung has not re-inflated and there is no bubbling in the bottle, then the tube is either kinked which can be corrected or blocked. A replacement must be inserted through a clean incision.

4 Follow-up

Arrange for a chest clinic appointment in 7–10 days after discharge. The patient must be given a discharge letter and told to attend again immediately in the event of deterioration. Air travel should be avoided until changes seen on radiographs have resolved.

5 Respiratory physician's opinion

Should advice from a specialist be required, transfer of continuing care is advisable. Important considerations in management are:

- Assessing why re-expansion has not been achieved (e.g. air leaking around the drain site, tube displaced or blocked, large persistent leak/bronchopleural fistula);
- The use of suction to re-expand the lung (this can be lengthy, requires appropriate equipment and pressure settings, influences how and where confirmatory radiographs are taken and involves care from experienced nursing staff);
- is a second drain required?
- Whether early thoracic surgery would be appropriate (e.g. failure of conservative measures, need to prevent recurrence);
- Consideration of chemical pleurodesis in certain cases;
- Management of subcutaneous emphysema.

Time Out 8.4

A 72-year-old lady, who has COPD presents with acute breathlessness. She has a respiratory rate of 28/min, a hyperexpanded chest with scattered wheezes and a prolonged expiratory phase. Her SpO$_2$ is 72% on 28% oxygen. What is your immediate management?

Pneumonia

Pneumonia is a general term used to describe a respiratory infection with new chest radiographic shadowing. Traditionally pneumonia has been classified according to its radiological appearance, i.e. lobar, lobular or broncho pneumonia. Unfortunately these do not help in either the diagnosis or the management. In contrast, the circumstances of the illness and the clinical background of the patient, as described in the box, provide helpful clues to aid investigation, management and treatment.

Classification of pneumonia

Community acquired
Hospital acquired (nosocomial)
Aspiration and anaerobic
Recurrent
Immunosuppression associated
Travel related

Management principles – checklist
Diagnosis

- History
- Examination
- Investigations

	Chest X-ray	PA
	Pulse oximetry	
	Arterial blood gases	
	Venous blood	Cultures
		Full blood count and film
		Electrolytes, glucose and liver profile
		C-reactive protein
		Initial serology: Mycoplasma, Legionella, Chlamydia
	Sputum	Culture and sensitivity
		Microscopy
		Acid and alcohol fast bacilli
	Urine	Legionella antigen
		Pneumococcal antigen

Treatment
- Oxygen – unless blood gases are normal
- Antibiotic – choice depends on severity, likely cause, test results and local policies (Fig. 8.6)
- Fluid replacement, either oral or intravenous according to clinical picture
- Analgesia if required
- Consider early liaison with clinical microbiologist, respiratory physician or intensivist.

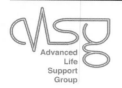

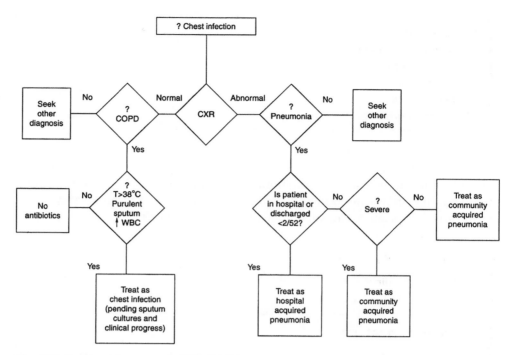

Fig. 8.6 Pneumonia management algorithm.

> **Key point**
>
> Early use of antibiotics in patients with pneumonia reduces morbidity and mortality

Community acquired pneumonia

This is a common cause of acute hospital admission and often occurs in the winter months. Community acquired pneumonia can affect previously healthy individuals or patients with coexisting lung disease. The age of the patient is likely to influence the pathogen involved.

> **Modes of infection transmission**
>
> Extension of bacteria colonising respiratory tract
> Droplet, e.g. respiratory viruses from infected individuals
> Birds, e.g. *Chlamydia psittaci*
> Water droplet, e.g. *Legionella pneumophila*

The organisms likely to cause community acquired pneumonia in the UK are shown in the box.

> **Organisms causing community acquired pneumonia**
>
> *Streptococcus pneumoniae*
> *Haemophilus influenzae*
> *Staphylococcus aureus*

Advanced
Life
Support
Group

Influenza virus
Mycoplasma pneumoniae
Chlamydia psittaci
Coxiella burnetti
Legionella species
Moraxella catarrhalis

Streptococcus pneumoniae (pneumococcal pneumonia) is the major pathogen involved, whilst influenza is the commonest viral infection. It is important to realise that viral infections caused by influenza, parainfluenza and respiratory syncytial virus can be associated with superadded bacterial infections.

Assessment
The clinical features are very variable.

Respiratory symptoms

Clinical:	Cough	Prodromal:	Pyrexia
	Sputum production		Malaise
	Breathlessness		Anorexia
	Pleuritic pain		Sweating
	Haemoptysis		Myalgia
			Arthralgia
			Headache

On examination most patients appear flushed and unwell with tachypnoea and/or tachycardia. The temperature can exceed 39.5°C and rigors are not uncommon in young people. In contrast, elderly patients may remain afebrile. Herpes simplex labialis is present in approximately one third of patients with pneumococcal pneumonia. Often chest movement is reduced on the affected side, especially if pleuritic pain is present. Inspiratory crackles are the commonest sign and bronchial breathing is infrequent. A pleural rub can be heard even when pleuritic pain is absent. **Occasionally the physical examination is entirely normal;** therefore a chest X-ray is necessary.

It is important to realise that non-respiratory symptoms may predominate; e.g. a patient with lower lobe pneumonia may present with abdominal pain and peritonism. Confusion may be due to hypoxaemia and/or metabolic derangement. In addition, *Legionella pneumophila* is associated with severe headache, cerebellar dysfunction, and amnesia. Vomiting and diarrhoea may occur as a direct manifestation of the illness or related to antibiotic therapy.

Moraxella catarrhalis causes bronchitis or pneumonia in children and adults with underlying chronic lung disease and is occasionally a cause of bacteraemia or meningitis, especially in patients who are immunocompromised.

Unfortunately the mortality from severe pneumonia remains high. Clinical features associated with severe pneumonia are listed in the box and their presence indicates a poor prognosis. Early liaison with an anaesthetist/intensivist is needed if **two** or more are present.

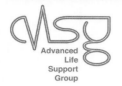

These features have been modified to form the 'CURB 65' score for community acquired pneumonia (Table 8.1). The risk of death from pneumonia ranges from 3% with a score of 1 to 57% with a score of 5.

Table 8.1 The Curb 65 score

Clinical factor	Score
Confusion	1
Urea > 7 mmol/l	1
Respiratory rate > 30/min	1
Systolic blood pressure < 90 or diastolic blood pressure < 60	1
Age > 65 years	1

High risk features in patients with severe pneumonia

Clinical	Investigations
Confusion	Blood urea > 7 mmol/l
Respiratory rate > 30/min	White cell count $< 4 \times 10^9$ or $> 20 \times 10^9$
Systolic < 90 mm Hg, diastolic < 60 mm Hg	PaO_2 < 8 kPa (60 mm Hg) (on room air)
	Serum albumin < 25 g/l
Old age and coexistent illness	Multilobe involvement on chest radiograph

Treatment

Patients with scores of 1 or less may not require admission to hospital. Manage all patients in bed; treat fever and pleuritic pain with appropriate non-steroidal anti-inflammatory drugs.

Correction of hypoxaemia and fluid balance is very important as described above. Chest physiotherapy is rarely helpful in the acute phase.

Specific treatment: When the patient presents acutely the microorganism responsible for the pneumonia is not usually known. Therefore, the choice of antibiotic is made according to the limited number of organisms that cause community acquired pneumonia. Most hospitals have devised specific antibiotic policies based on an assessment of the severity of the pneumonia – Fig. 8.6 (page 103). This should be started within 1 h of the diagnosis being made.

- *Severe pneumonia* (CURB 65 ≥4). This can affect even previously fit individuals. As the mortality is high parenteral antibiotics must be given immediately. Considering the potential organisms that may be responsible (see earlier) potential treatments include either IV Tazocin (4.5 g tds) or a combination of cefotaxime 1 g tds combined with Clarithromycin 250 mg qds is advised. Rifampicin should be added if legionella is suspected. The duration of intravenous therapy is based on the patient's clinical response.
- *Mild pneumonia* (CURB 65 ≤ 1). In most previously fit people the likely organism is *Streptococcus pneumoniae* or occasionally *Mycoplasma pneumoniae*, *Chlamydia* species, *Legionella* species or *Coxiella burnetii*. The combination of amoxycillin and erythromycin is both cheap and effective. Erythromycin alone is appropriate for patients who are allergic to penicillin or if an atypical organism is suspected, e.g. *Mycoplasma, Chlamydia, Legionella*. If the patient fails to respond to this combination, then levofloxacin should be used.

Time Out 8.5

Factual overload? Take a five-minute break and then answer the following questions.
a What is the major pathogen responsible for community acquired pneumonia?
b What are the clinical features?
c How would you manage a patient with severe community acquired pneumonia?
d List the high risk features in patients with severe pneumonia that indicate the need for critical care.

Hospital acquired pneumonia (nosocomial)

This is defined as pneumonia developing more than 48 h after hospital admission, irrespective of the reason.

Pathophysiology

Bacterial colonisation of the nasopharynx changes markedly in hospital patients, particularly those who receive broad spectrum antibiotics and are severely ill. These bacteria arise either from the hospital environment or the patient's gastrointestinal tract. Such pathogens are likely to be aspirated in patients who are ill, bed bound or who have impaired consciousness for whatever reason. This may be exacerbated by an inability to clear bronchial secretions after a general anaesthetic or where coughing is impaired due to thoracic or abdominal surgery. The risk of postoperative pneumonia is associated with increasing age, smoking, obesity, underlying chronic illness and prolonged anaesthesia. Pathogens may also be spread from contaminated equipment such as nebulisers, ventilators, suction equipment and even from the hospital staff.

A large number of pathogens are responsible for hospital acquired pneumonia (see box). Gram negative bacilli are commonly implicated and to a lesser extent, Gram positive bacteria, especially *Staphylococcus aureus*, except if the patient is immunocompromised.

Hospital acquired pneumonia in specific circumstances

Streptococcus pneumoniae	
Haemophilus influenzae	Early post—elective surgery, especially if chronic chest pathology
Pseudomonas	
Klebsiella	Contaminated respiratory equipment
Pseudomonas	
Klebsiella	
Bacteroides	Aspiration
Clostridium	
Legionella	Contaminated water (cooling towers, heating and showers

---

Specific treatment

As there are a wide range of potential organisms responsible for hospital acquired pneumonia, initial therapy is usually Tazocin (Pipparicillin and Tazobactum). If a pseudomonal infection is suspected then an appropriate penicillin derivative such as ticarcillin should be used. Early liaison with a clinical microbiologist is recommended.

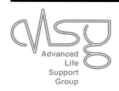

Antibiotic therapy can be tailored according to the results of investigations.

Ideally, treatment should be proactive in preventing such infections by scrupulous hygiene practices, appropriate infection control and preoperative advice for the patient.

Time Out 8.6

a Define the term hospital acquired pneumonia.
b List those patients at risk.
c How would you manage a patient with hospital acquired pneumonia?

Aspiration and anaerobic pneumonia

This is commonly associated with impaired consciousness and/or dysphagia. Infection is usually with either *Pseudomonas aeruginosa* or an *Enterobacter* species in the hospital environment. Treatment with Tazocin is advised as true anaerobes do not survive the oxygen rich environment in the lung.

Recurrent pneumonia

If a patient experiences two or more pneumonic episodes, consider the following:
- localised bronchiectasis
- bronchial obstruction, e.g. foreign body, carcinoma or external compression
- a generalised respiratory disorder if the pneumonia recurs in different sites
- COPD with or without bronchiectasis
- aspiration of oesophago-gastric contents in patients with, e.g. motor neurone disease, disseminated sclerosis, achalasia, epilepsy, alcoholism, drug/substance use and oesophagotracheal fistula.
- chronic organising pneumonia (bronchiolitis obliterans organising pneumonia)
- recurrent pulmonary infarction
- immunosuppression/deficiency.

Immunosuppression associated pneumonia

An in-depth discussion on this topic is well beyond the scope of this book. However, the following practical guidelines are suggested.

Pneumonia of acute onset and rapid progression suggests bacterial origin. Therefore, initial treatment should include a combination of cefotaxime and gentamicin to ensure adequate cover against *Streptococcus pneumoniae*, *Haemophilus influenzae*, *Staphylococcus aureus* and many other Gram negative species. If the patient fails to respond or the pace of the illness is less acute then specialist help should be sought early.

Travel related pneumonia

With the increase in worldwide travel, a variety of unexpected respiratory infections may be seen and/or enter into the differential diagnosis of pneumonia. This subject is too extensive to be covered here, but do not forget to:
- take a full:
  - travel history
  - drug history
  - sexual history
- consider bacterial, viral and fungal infections
- consider tuberculosis

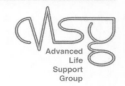

- consider an esoteric infection if the patient fails to respond appropriately, but remember that rare manifestations of common infections occur more frequently than common manifestations of rare infections
- liaise early with a consultant in infectious diseases/clinical microbiology/ respiratory medicine.

Key point

Antibiotics can cause side effects, and *Clostridium difficile* is a major concern. Thus change from broad spectrum to specific antibiotics as soon as possible

---

Time Out 8.7

Pneumonia is a common condition. You have already boosted your knowledge by reading this section and answering the associated questions. To complete your understanding review the management of pneumonia as shown in Fig. 8.5

PLEURAL EFFUSION

Pathophysiology

The pleural surfaces are lubricated by a thin layer of fluid that allows the lung and chest wall to move with minimum energy loss. The volume of pleural fluid is a balance between production by the parietal pleura and absorption by the visceral pleura. The increase in hydrostatic pressure within the capillaries of the parietal pleura ensures that fluid passes into the pleural space. Thus, the parietal pleura acts like a plasma ultrafiltrator. In comparison, the pressure within the capillaries of the visceral pleura is lower ensuring that fluid is absorbed. Lymphatic drainage also facilitates removal of fluid and protein from the pleural space.

A pleural effusion results from an excessive accumulation of fluid within the pleural space. Considering the normal production of pleural fluid, as described earlier, the potential factors involved in the production of excess fluid are summarised in the box.

Factors involved in the production of excess pleural fluid

An imbalance between the hydrostatic and oncotic pressures
Alteration in pleural capillary permeability
Impaired lymphatic drainage
Disruption of structural integrity
Transdiaphragmatic passage of fluid

More than one of these factors may be involved in the production of pleural fluid according to the underlying disease process as described below.

Causes of pleural effusion

Some of the reasons why a patient may develop a pleural effusion are listed in the next box. The estimated 'chance' of meeting these causes is given in brackets.

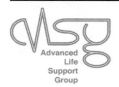

Specific pleural effusions

Transudate

These are characterised by low protein concentrations (<30 g/l). Excess fluid forms when there is an increase in pleural hydrostatic pressure, e.g. in congestive cardiac failure, or when there is a reduction in colloidal osmotic pressure, e.g. with hypoalbuminaemia associated with nephrotic syndrome or liver disease.

Small effusions can be associated with failure of either the left or right or both ventricles.

Elevated left heart pressures will be transmitted to the pulmonary circulation and hence result in reduced fluid absorption from the visceral pleura. In contrast, increased pressure from the right heart is transmitted to the systemic capillaries and this leads to increased production of fluid from the parietal pleura. Resolution occurs with treatment of heart failure, but unilateral effusions that fail to respond to this treatment require further investigation.

Hypoalbuminaemia, as listed earlier, is a major contributory factor in the development of generalised oedema. Thus, both pleural effusions and ascites are common. Formation of pleural fluid is due to a reduction in colloidal osmotic pressure combined with the transdiaphragmatic passage of fluid.

Causes of pleural effusion

(a) Transudate	**Cardiac failure**	**Daily**
Hypoalbuminaemia	**Nephrotic syndrome**	**Weekly**
	Cirrhosis	**Daily**
	Malabsorptions	**Annually**
	Peritoneal dialysis	**Monthly**
	Myxoedema	**Only in exams**
(b) Exudate		
Infective	**Pneumonia**	**Daily**
	Empyema	**Monthly**
	Subphrenic abscess	**Monthly**
	Tuberculosis	**Annually**
Inflammatory	**Pancreatitis**	**Weekly**
	Connective tissue disease	**Monthly**
	Dressler's syndrome	**Annually**
Neoplastic	**Metastatic carcinoma**	**Daily**
	Lymphoma	**Annually**
	Mesothelioma	**Annually**
	Meig's syndrome	**Only in exams**
Haemothorax	**Pulmonary emboli**	**Monthly**
	Trauma	**Monthly**
	Spontaneous bleeding disorders	**Annually**
Chylothorax	**Trauma**	**Annually**
	Carcinoma	**Annually**
	Lymphoma	**Annually**

Key point

In patients with cardiac failure the nature of the pleural effusion can change from transudate to exudate following treatment with diuretics

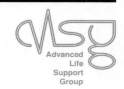

Exudate
Malignancy The commonest cause of a large pleural effusion is malignant involvement of the pleura. This can occur as:
• direct spread from an adjacent bronchogenic carcinoma
• metastatic spread via the lymphatics, e.g. from breast malignancy
• haematogenous spread from the gastrointestinal tract.
In contrast, primary pleural tumours (mesotheliomas) are rare.
   Excess pleural fluid is formed by a combination of mechanisms, including:
• disruption of the integrity of the pleura
• an associated adjacent inflammatory response
• the tumour secreting fluid
• infiltrating malignancy causing haemorrhage
• interference with lymphatic drainage.
   Initial treatment is symptomatic and referral to an oncology specialist is recommended.

Connective tissue diseases Pleural involvement is common in patients with systemic lupus erythematosus but to a much lesser extent in those who have rheumatoid disease.

Haemothorax As an acute medical emergency this is rare because most cases occur in association with penetrating or non-penetrating trauma. However, it can occur after:
• attempts at central venous access due to disruption of associated arteries or veins
• secondary to intercostal vessel damage during the course of percutaneous liver or pleural biopsy.
   Haemothorax is a rare sequel to bleeding diatheses, overanticoagulation or following a dissection/rupture of the thoracic aorta.

Chylothorax This is rare. It is associated with trauma to, or malignant invasion of, the thoracic duct. This structure can also be damaged during an oesophageal resection or mobilisation of the aortic arch. It is important to differentiate a chylothorax from a pyothorax. A chest drain is the initial management of choice.

Assessment
Symptoms
Pain and breathlessness are the cardinal symptoms of pleural disease. Their presence will, however, vary according to the underlying pathology. Pleuritic pain, which is worse on deep inspiration or coughing, is typical of dry pleurisy. As fluid accumulates, however, the pain spontaneously improves. Breathlessness, as described earlier, only becomes apparent if the pleural effusion is either large or rapidly expanding or there is significant underlying pulmonary pathology.

Signs
Physical signs are often absent unless the effusion is large. Tachypnoea and tachycardia may be present. Chest wall movement and expansion are often reduced on the affected side. The percussion note is 'stoney dull' and both vocal resonance (or tactile vocal fremitus) and breath sounds will be diminished or absent. Above the effusion, however, the lung may collapse with signs of consolidation, i.e. bronchial breathing and increased vocal resonance. Remember that consolidated lung tends to filter out low frequency sounds; thus high pitched bronchial

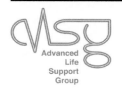

breathing is prominent. Furthermore, vocal sounds, i.e. '99' or '11' are transmitted by normal lung and, in particular, solid lung but not by air space or fluid.

Investigation of pleural effusion

Radiology

Chest radiographs are of limited value in identifying the cause of a pleural effusion. Ultrasound can help confirm the site and presence of an effusion. It is especially useful when a drain has to be placed into loculated fluid.

Examination of pleural fluid

Macroscopic appearance

- Straw coloured fluid, which does not clot on standing, typifies a transudate.
- Turbid fluid is usually due to the increased protein content, which often reflects an exudate.
- Bloodstained fluid is likely to be associated with an underlying malignancy or pulmonary embolus.
- Chyle is odourless and milky in appearance.
- Empyema fluid is often very viscous, yellow and frequently foul smelling.

Microscopic and cytological examination

- Transudate cell count less than $100/mm^3$
  - often mixed cells, i.e. lymphocytes, neutrophils and mesothelial cells.
- Exudate has high white cell count
  - neutrophil leucocytosis often indicative of bacterial infection
  - lymphocytosis suggests tuberculosis or lymphoma.

The presence of malignant cells is likely to be diagnostic though on occasion the precise cell of origin may be difficult to determine.

Microbiology Fluid should be sent for Gram stain, culture and identification of acid and alcohol-fast bacilli.

Biochemistry Pleural fluid has been described as either a transudate or an exudate based on the protein concentration of less than or greater than 30 g/l, respectively. Unfortunately this is only a rough guide. A better assessment can be obtained by comparing the pleural fluid concentrations of protein and lactate dehydrogenase with those of blood as shown in the box.

Criteria for identifying an exudate

Total protein pleural fluid to serum ratio greater than 0.5

Lactate dehydrogenase concentration in pleural fluid more than two-thirds the upper limit of normal serum LDH

Lactate dehydrogenase pleural fluid to serum ratio greater than 0.6

Other important investigations include:

- glucose – which is consistently low in rheumatoid associated effusions as well as malignancy, empyema and tuberculosis
- amylase – as pancreatitis can result in a pleural effusion which is most frequently on the left
- pleural fluid pH – pH $<$ 7.2 suggests infection and requires tube drainage

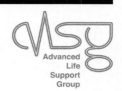

Pleural biopsy
This is only indicated when pleural fluid analysis fails to establish a diagnosis and ideally should be done at thoracoscopy, which is usually video assisted.

Specific management
Frequently all that is required, initially, is a sample of pleural fluid for laboratory investigations.

Immediate drainage of pleural fluid is only required if the patient is breathless. This usually occurs if pleural effusion is massive, rapidly accumulating or there is underlying pulmonary disease. The symptoms usually resolve rapidly if 1.5 litres of fluid are aspirated. Chest drains are rarely required, except for empyema, complicated parapneumonic effusions and pleurodesis.

Transudates rarely require direct treatment as they usually resolve with improvement in the underlying condition. In contrast, the management of an **exudate** is governed by the results of investigations. A chest drain may be required for the reasons listed earlier and in the presence of an empyema or pyopneumothorax. The latter should alert the clinician to the presence of either necrotic lung tissue or oesophageal rupture. Antibiotic treatment with intravenous cefotaxime and metronidazole is advocated.

PULMONARY EMBOLISM

Pulmonary embolism is an important condition because it is potentially fatal, often preventable and sometimes treatable. The majority of pulmonary emboli originate in the deep veins of the legs and pelvis. Occasionally, however the right side of the heart can be the source of emboli, e.g. atrial fibrillation, right ventricular infarction or a dilated right ventricle. Major risk factors of pulmonary embolism are shown in the box.

Risk factors for pulmonary embolism and the 'chance' of meeting this factor

Recent surgery	Daily
Immobility for greater than four days	Daily
Age over 40 years	Daily
Previous venous thrombosis/embolism	Daily
Malignant disease	Daily
Lower limb fractures	Daily
Obesity	Daily
Varicose veins	Daily
Pregnancy/oral contraceptive pill	Daily
Nephrotic syndrome*	Weekly
Diabetic ketoacidosis*	Weekly
Resistance to activated protein C*	Annually
Deficiency of antithrombin III*	Annually
Deficiency of protein C and S*	Annually
Prothrombin Gene	Annually
Paroxysmal nocturnal haemoglobinuria*	Only in examinations
Behçet's disease*	Only in examinations

* Risk factors for recurrent thromboembolic disease.

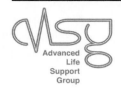

Prothrombin gene mutation

Prothrombin gives rise to thrombin in the coagulation cascade. The mutation leads to an increased amount of thrombin circulating in the blood which leads, by unclear reasons, to a thrombophilic state.

This condition is common in the Caucasian population. About 1–2% of the general population are heterozygous (one copy) for the prothrombin gene mutation.

Risks of the prothrombin gene mutation

Thrombophilic status	Relative risk of venous thrombosis
Normal	1
Oral contraceptive (OCP) use	4
Factor V Leiden, heterozygous	5–7
Factor V Leiden, heterozygous + OCP	30–35
Factor V Leiden, homozygous	80
Factor V Leiden, homozygous + OCP	??? >100
Prothrombin Gene Mutation, heterozygous	3
Prothrombin Gene Mutation, homozygous	??? possible risk of arterial thrombosis
Prothrombin Gene Mutation, heterozygous + OCP	16
Protein C deficiency, heterozygous	7
Protein C deficiency, homozygous	Severe thrombosis at birth
Protein S deficiency, heterozygous	6
Protein S deficiency, homozygous	Severe thrombosis at birth
Antithrombin deficiency, heterozygous	5
Antithrombin deficiency, homozygous	Thought to be lethal prior to birth
Hyperhomocysteinemia	2–4
Hyperhomocysteinemia combined with Factor V Leiden, heterozygous	20

Pathophysiology

One of the normal functions of the lungs is to filter out small blood clots. This process occurs without any symptoms. However, emboli blocking larger branches of the pulmonary artery provoke a rise in pulmonary arterial pressure causing rapid shallow respiration. The rise in pressure is believed to be due, in part, to reflex vasoconstriction via the sympathetic nerve fibres and also hypoxaemia. Tachypnoea is a reflex response to the activation of vagal innervated luminal stretch receptors and interstitial J receptors within the alveolar and capillary network.

Furthermore, vasoactive substances such as 5-hydroxytryptamine and thromboxane released from activated platelets may enhance vasoconstriction and neurotransmission.

Key point

The effect on haemodynamics will be related to the size of the pulmonary embolus

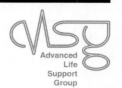

To explain the variations in pathophysiology and management of pulmonary emboli they will be classified as massive, moderate and minor.

Massive pulmonary embolism
This usually follows an acute obstruction of at least 50% of the pulmonary circulation. An embolus in the main pulmonary trunk or at the bifurcation of the pulmonary artery (saddle embolus) can produce circulatory collapse, i.e. pulseless electrical activity (PEA or electromechanical dissociation) and death. However, an identical clinical picture may arise with lesser degrees of obstruction when there has been previous cardiorespiratory dysfunction. An acute massive pulmonary embolus, without immediate death, elicits the haemodynamic response as described earlier. The acute increase in pulmonary vascular resistance and thus right ventricular afterload causes a sudden rise in end diastolic pressure and hence dilatation of the right ventricle. This may be manifest clinically as an elevated jugular venous pressure and tricuspid regurgitation. The dilated right ventricle and rise in pulmonary arterial pressure cause a marked fall in systemic arterial pressure by the following mechanisms.
- A fall in left ventricular stroke volume. Dilatation of the right ventricle and increased pulmonary artery pressure ensures that the right ventricular stroke work is depressed. This results in delayed emptying of the right ventricle, and hence a fall in left ventricular stroke volume.
- Interventricular septum displacement. The dilated right ventricle and associated increased pressure cause displacement of the interventricular septum into the left ventricular cavity (the reverse Bernheim effect) reducing left ventricular volume.

These processes culminate in a fall in systemic stroke volume, which to some extent is offset by the sympathetic mediated increase in systemic (peripheral) vascular resistance. Thus, the patient with a massive pulmonary embolus can present with the features of 'shock' (see Chapter 9).

Moderate pulmonary emboli
Whilst the pathophysiology is identical to that described above, the effect on pulmonary arterial resistance and hence right ventricular function is minimal. The mechanisms underlying breathlessness have already been described. Infarction of the pulmonary parenchyma and associated pleura induces inflammation, both processes culminating in haemoptysis and pleuritic pain.

Minor emboli
These will often go unnoticed but repeated attacks can result in progressive breathlessness, hyperventilation and possibly effort-induced syncope. If this problem remains undiagnosed pulmonary hypertension will develop leading to hypertrophy and subsequently failure of the right ventricle.

Assessment
The different sites of pulmonary emboli are shown in Fig. 8.7.

Differential diagnosis
Acute circulatory collapse is a cardinal feature of massive pulmonary embolism. The differential diagnosis of this shocked state is considered in detail in Chapter 9. However, specific conditions that warrant mention here in the context of acute breathlessness, hypotension, central chest pain and unconsciousness are acute

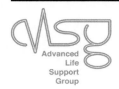

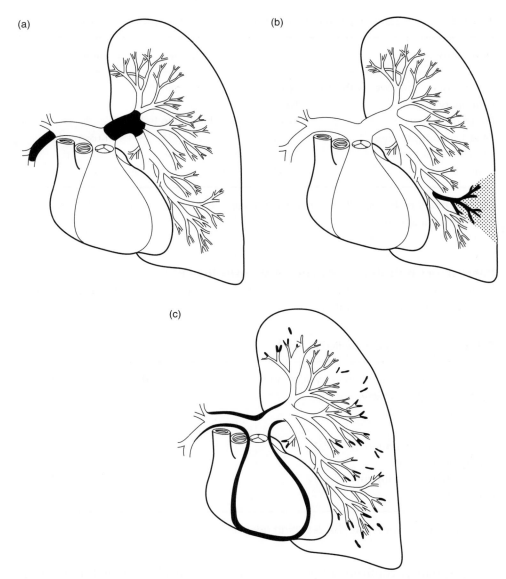

Fig. 8.7 The different sites of pulmonary emboli: (a) main trunk (massive), (b) third division vessels (moderate) and (c) multiple peripheral (minor).

ventricular failure, myocardial infarction and cardiac tamponade. All of these major features are related to diminished cardiac output and hence hypoxaemia and relative hypovolaemia in the acutely ill patient. The differential diagnosis of these conditions can be difficult but there are several key features that can help (Table 8.2).

As with all shocked patients high concentration of inspired oxygen (FiO_2 = 0.85) are required. More comprehensive details regarding the management of the shocked patient are provided in Chapter 9.

Investigations can also help differentiate between these conditions, of which left ventricular failure is the commonest.

Assess the Well's score (page 116) and request D-dimer.

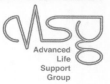

Table 8.2 Key features in the differential diagnosis of breathlessness

Symptoms/signs	PE	LVF	RVF	MI	Tamponade
Breathlessness improves with sitting	No	Yes	No	No	No
Pulmonary oedema	No	Yes	No	No	No
Pulsus paradoxus	Yes	No	No	No	Yes
Raised venous pressure	+++	+	+++	No	+++ (Kussmaul's)
Palpable apex beat	Yes	Yes	Yes	Yes	No
Heart sounds	+ S3/S4	+ S3	+ S3	+ S4	Quiet

PE, pulmonary embolus; LVF, left ventricular failure; RVF, right ventricular failure; MI, myocardial infarction.

Pretest probability of Pulmonary embolus (PE)

Wells score, modified by the Manchester group to include intravenous drug users, provides a pre-test probability:

Table 8.3 Wells score, modified by the Manchester group

Clinical signs of DVT – minimal swelling and pain on palpation of the deep veins	3.0
Other diagnosis less likely	3.0
Intravenous drug user	3.0
HR > 100	1.5
Stasis ≥ 3/7 or operation in <4/52	1.5
History of DVT or PE	1.5
Active cancer or treatment in <6/12	1.0
Haemoptysis	1.0

Low risk 2 or less; moderate risk 2–6; high risk >6.

In pregnancy, confirming the diagnosis can be difficult. Although there is an increased risk of PE the D-dimer is of limited use unless it is negative. Usually, the D-dimer is raised from 6/52 gestation to 3/12 post partum. If a PE is considered obtain a Chest X-ray (less radiation than CT angiography). A perfusion (Q) scan is safe. It is important to balance the risks of delayed treatment (which can be fatal to mother and child) against the risks of the investigations.

This protocol results in <1% missed venous thromboembolic events during follow-up.

Investigations in pregnancy

Objective scoring and D-dimer are less reliable.
- If critically ill arrange a portable echocardiogram otherwise:
  - Chest X-ray to exclude infection and pneumothorax
  - Consider ultrasound Doppler of the legs – no risk to fetus and if positive can treat
  - Consider half dose VQ if normal lungs and Chest X-ray
  - CT pulmonary angiogram if abnormal Chest X-ray or lung disease
  - Discuss with mother and specialist

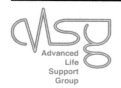

Investigations

- **ECG** changes will occur in approximately 75% of all patients after a massive pulmonary embolus. However, these are often non-specific and T wave inversion in the chest leads (V1 – V3) is the most frequent abnormality. In addition, rhythm disturbances, usually a sinus tachycardia or atrial fibrillation, can occur along with manifestations of acute right heart strain ranging from the classic S1, QIII, TIII pattern to right bundle branch block and voltage criteria of right ventricular hypertrophy. Small complexes, possibly with electrical alternans, can occur in cardiac tamponade.

Key point

A normal ECG does not exclude either an acute pulmonary embolus or a myocardial infarction

---

- **Chest X-ray**. It is usually unhelpful in the diagnosis of acute pulmonary embolus. Occasionally the affected main pulmonary artery may be prominent or there may be loss of lung volume or rarely a 'wedge' shaped defect. However, the chest radiograph will be helpful in the diagnosis of both pulmonary oedema and, to a lesser extent, cardiac tamponade.
- **Arterial blood gases**. Hypoxaemia and acidosis are common after massive or moderate pulmonary emboli. In contrast, a respiratory alkalosis/alkalaemia secondary to hyperventilation is compatible with recurrent small emboli.
- **Plasma D-dimer**. This is a breakdown product of cross-linked fibrin, which is released in thromboembolism. This investigation has become widely used. There are many causes of false positive test results including sepsis. It is generally used to exclude a diagnosis of thromboembolism. The only useful D-dimer is a negative one!
- **Ventilation/perfusion** scans. These can be used to detect pulmonary emboli in patients with normal chest X-rays. They can exclude pulmonary embolism if completely normal but the majority of scans are non-diagnostic. The clinician then has to proceed to further imaging or treat on the basis of clinical suspicion.
- **Echocardiography**. This will show right ventricular abnormalities in 40% of patients and also raised pulmonary arterial pressure.
- **Pulmonary angiography**. This remains the gold standard but very few hospitals have the facilities (Fig. 8.8)
- **Lower limb doppler** studies. They may show a DVT if V/Q scanning is inconclusive.
- **CTPA** (computed tomographic pulmonary angiography). **It is now the recommended imaging modality**.

Specific treatment for acute pulmonary embolism

Most patients with a definitive or suspected diagnosis of pulmonary embolus are treated with a low molecular weight heparin (LMWH) (stops propagation of the embolus/clot and further embolisation from the source thrombus) given subcutaneously. If unfractionated heparin is used, check the activated partial thromboplastin time 6 h after either starting or changing the dose, but be wary of the increased risk of heparin induced thrombocytopenia. Other advantages of LMWH are that there is only one injection per day and there is no loss monitoring unless the patient has renal impairment.

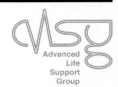

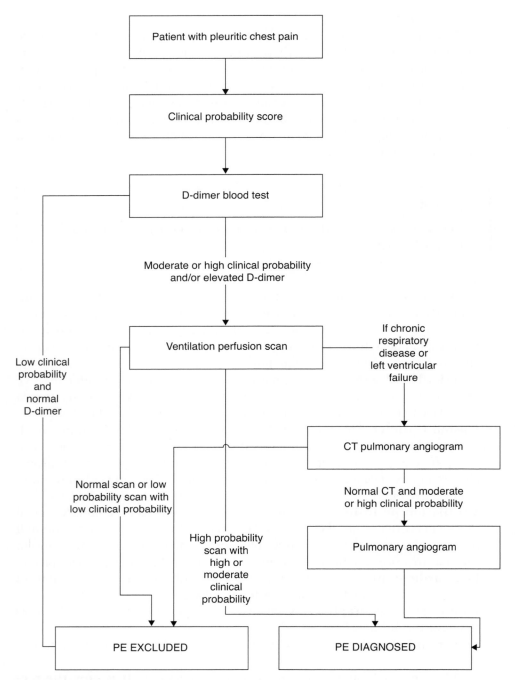

Fig. 8.8 Diagnosis of pulmonary embolism.

Irrespective of the results of investigations, if the clinical suspicion of a pulmonary embolus remains high then the patient should be treated appropriately. If pulseless electrical activity (electromechanical dissociation) results from a massive pulmonary embolus then resuscitation should follow the European and UK guidelines. With the patient who is hypoxaemic and hypotensive, then immediate resuscitation should reduce hypoxaemia and maintain cardiac output. The major decision is medical versus surgical therapy. This will depend primarily on:
• whether the patient has any contraindications to thrombolysis
• local surgical expertise.

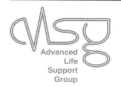

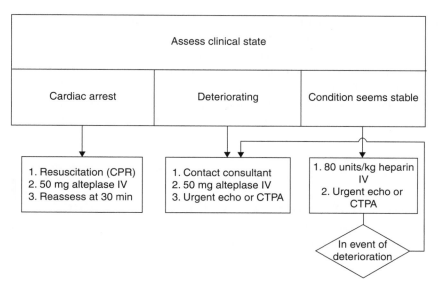

Fig. 8.9 British Thoracic Society protocol for PE thrombolysis.

Comments on Fig. 8.9

In stable patients massive PE is highly likely if:
1 Collapse/hypotension, and
  • Unexplained hypoxaemia and
  • Engorged neck veins, and
  • Right ventricular gallop (often)
2 In patients without haemodynamic compromise where massive PE has been confirmed, IV dose of alteplase is 100 mg in 90 min (i.e. accelerated myocardial infarction regimen)
3 Thrombolysis is followed by unfractionated heparin after 3 h, preferably weight adjusted
4 A few units have facilities for clot fragmentation via pulmonary artery catheter. Elsewhere, contraindications to thrombolysis should be ignored in life-threatening PE (see next box)
5 'Blue light' patients with out-of-hospital cardiac arrest due to PE rarely recover.

Contraindications to thrombolysis are shown in the box.

Contraindications to thrombolysis

Previous haemorrhagic stroke
Any stroke in previous 6 months
Active internal bleeding / active peptic ulceration
Known or suspected aortic dissection
Recent major surgery / head injury / arterial surgery
Pregnancy
Prolonged CPR
Hypertension BP > 180/110
Previous allergic reaction to the thrombolytic agent

Thrombolysis (embolus dissolution), usually in the form of alteplase can be given intravenously as a bolus of 50 mg. This should only be used in a patient who has a massive PE and can be given on clinical grounds alone if cardiac arrest is imminent. Urgent echocardiography, if **immediately** available, can be very useful in confirming your clinical suspicion, by showing a relatively full right ventricle and relatively empty left ventricle). Invasive approaches such as clot fragmentation and 'open heart surgery' can be used if facilities are immediately available.

Time Out 8.8

Take a 5-min break and reflect on the previous section whilst you drink your tea or coffee, and answer the following question.
   Why do patients with pulmonary emboli become breathless?

Non-cardiopulmonary causes of breathlessness

The respiratory centre is under the influence of both chemical and neurogenic stimuli. Hypoxaemia, e.g. at high altitude or acidaemia due to diabetic ketoacidosis or salicylate overdose may, therefore, stimulate the respiratory centre in an attempt to provide more oxygen or promote carbon dioxide excretion. Disruption of the integrity of this centre, e.g. by a brain stem haemorrhage, will also result in breathlessness. Other non-pulmonary causes of breathlessness are: any critical illness, shock from any cause especially hypovolaemic, septic or cardiogenic or severe sepsis.

Key point

Be wary of labelling people as 'hysterical hyperventilators' unless underlying pathology has been excluded

---

SUMMARY

- Breathlessness is a common medical emergency.
- The structured approach will ensure that the immediately life-threatening causes are identified and treated.
- Immediately life-threatening causes of breathlessness are:
  - Airway Obstruction
  - Breathing   Acute severe asthma
                Acute exacerbation of COPD
                Acute pulmonary oedema
                Tension pneumothorax
  - Circulation   Acute severe left ventricular failure
                Dysrhythmia
                Hypovolaemia
                Pulmonary embolus
                Cardiac tamponade.
- The pathophysiology of these conditions has been linked to their diagnosis, investigation and management.
- A similar framework has been applied to non-immediately life-threatening conditions, in particular pneumonia and pleural effusion.

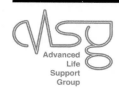

CHAPTER 9

The patient with shock

OBJECTIVES

After reading this chapter you will be able to understand the:
- definition and causes of shock
- underlying pathophysiology of shock
- importance of oxygen delivery
- structured approach to the shocked patient.

INTRODUCTION

Shock is the result of a series of pathophysiological processes that differ according to the underlying cause. Nevertheless, they culminate in a final common pathway that prevents tissues having enough oxygen to meet their metabolic needs.

Shock can therefore be defined as a clinical syndrome resulting from inadequate delivery, or use, of oxygen by vital organs.

It has many causes, but this chapter will concentrate on those giving rise to inadequate delivery of oxygen to the tissues. The other causes will be mentioned only briefly, but with cross-references to more detailed descriptions elsewhere in this manual.

PATHOPHYSIOLOGY

The amount of oxygen delivered to a particular organ depends on how much blood the heart is pumping out each minute (i.e. the cardiac output) and how much oxygen the blood is carrying:

The oxygen content of blood

Although the majority of oxygen carried in blood is by haemoglobin, we have also mentioned that an additional small volume is physically dissolved in plasma. Therefore, the total volume of oxygen carried in blood at any time is the sum of that carried by the haemoglobin plus that dissolved in the plasma. This total is termed as the **oxygen content**.

The volume of oxygen dissolved in plasma from arterial blood is directly proportional to the PaO_2 and is approximately:

$$0.003 \text{ ml per 100 ml blood per mm Hg } PaO_2$$
$$\text{or}$$
$$0.023 \text{ ml per 100 ml blood per kPa } PaO_2$$

Acute Medical Emergencies; The Practical Approach, 2nd edition.
Edited by Terence Wardle, Peter Driscoll, and Sue Wieteska.
© 2010 Blackwell Publishing Ltd.

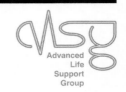

It follows that the oxygen content per 100 ml of arterial blood (i.e. the amount associated with the haemoglobin molecule as well as that dissolved in the plasma) is equal to[1]:

(Hb conc × oxygen carrying capacity of Hb
× saturation of Hb)   +(0.003 × PaO$_2$)
Oxygen content of haemoglobin   **Oxygen content of the plasma**

When the SpO$_2$ = 100%, each gram of haemoglobin in the arterial system carries 1.34 ml oxygen – a figure known as the **oxygen carrying capacity of haemoglobin.**

Therefore, the oxygen content per 100 ml of arterial blood is:

(Hb conc × 1.34 × saturation of Hb)   +(0.003 × PaO$_2$)
Oxygen content of haemoglobin   **Oxygen content of the plasma**

Consider now a normal person who has a PaO$_2$ of 100 mm Hg with a haemoglobin concentration of 15 g per 100 ml which is 97% saturated with oxygen. In this person, the oxygen content per 100 ml of arterial blood would be equal to:

$$(15 \times 1.34 \times 97\%) + (0.003 \times 100) = 19.5 + 0.3$$
$$= \textbf{19.8 ml oxygen per 100 ml blood}$$

OXYGEN DELIVERY TO THE TISSUES

So far, we have considered only the volume of oxygen in terms of how much oxygen is contained in aliquots of 100 ml of blood, when exposed to varying partial pressures of oxygen. Under normal circumstances, the heart pumps out 5000 ml blood per minute (the cardiac output). Therefore, the total volume of oxygen delivered to the tissues per minute is the product of the cardiac output and the oxygen content:

Oxygen delivery (DO$_2$) = cardiac output × oxygen content
In normal circumstances, DO$_2$ = 5000 ml/min × 19.8 ml/100 ml
= **approximately 1000 ml oxygen per minute**

Compensatory mechanisms

When a body is under stress it does not immediately fail as several compensatory mechanisms attempt to maintain adequate oxygen delivery to the essential organs.

Oxygen uptake

One mechanism is to increase the respiratory rate in an attempt to take up more oxygen. This is mediated by the sympathetic nervous system. Unfortunately, this does not produce any significant increase in oxygen uptake, because the haemoglobin in blood passing ventilated alveoli is already 97.5% saturated. However, the clinician can help by increasing the inspired concentration of oxygen and ensuring there is adequate ventilation. The slight rise in alveolar oxygen due to the hypocapnia from hyperventilation increases this value by around 1%.

---

[1] For simplicity, we have just used the values for PaO$_2$ measured in mm Hg. For those using kPa, you will need to alter the equation in the way indicated above.

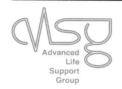

Circulatory control

A more effective method of ensuring oxygen delivery to the vital organs is seen with changes in the cardiovascular system. Pressure receptors in the heart and baroreceptors in both the carotid sinus and aortic arch respond to hypovolaemia by triggering a reflex sympathetic response, via control centres in the brain stem. The sympathetic discharge stimulates many tissues in the body, including the adrenal medulla, increasing the release of systemic catecholamines. These combine with the direct sympathetic discharge to prevent, or limit, the fall in cardiac output by positive inotropic and chronotropic effects on the heart and by increasing venous return secondary to venoconstriction.

Furthermore, selective arteriolar and pre-capillary sphincter constriction of non-essential organs (e.g. skin and gut) maintains perfusion of vital organs (e.g. brain and heart). Selective perfusion also leads to a lowering of the hydrostatic pressure in those capillaries serving non-essential organs. This reduces the diffusion of fluid across the capillary membrane into the interstitial space. It also has the effect of increasing the diastolic pressure and thereby reducing the pulse pressure.

Key point

Sympathetic stimulation can give rise to the commonly recognised cardiovascular clinical presentation of patients in advanced shock:
Sweaty and tachycardic – direct sympathetic stimulation
Pale and cool – reduced skin perfusion
Thready pulse – reduced pulse pressure
Ileus – reduced gut perfusion

Any reduction in renal blood flow is detected by the juxtaglomerular apparatus. The resulting increase in renin secretion leads to the formation of angiotensin II and aldosterone. These, together with antidiuretic hormone released from the pituitary, increase the reabsorption of sodium and water by the kidney and reduce urine volume. In addition, the thirst centre of the hypothalamus is stimulated. The overall result is that the circulating volume is increased. Renin, angiotensin II and antidiuretic hormone can also produce generalised vasoconstriction and so help increase the venous return. The body also attempts to enhance the circulating volume by releasing osmotically active substances from the liver. These increase plasma osmotic pressure and so cause interstitial fluid to be drawn into the intravascular space.

Key point

A fall in blood pressure will only take place when no further compensation is possible. It is therefore a **late** sign in shock. Shock should be identified and resuscitation begun before this point is reached

---

Autoregulation

Most organs have some capacity to regulate their own blood flow by a process known as autoregulation (see page 59). This enables tissues to compensate for moderate changes in perfusion pressure, by altering local vascular resistance.

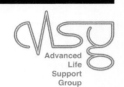

However, as the 'shock' state develops, there is paralysis of the smooth muscle in the small blood vessel walls. This allows flow to become pressure dependent and vessels, such as skin arterioles, will begin to distend. This can lead to blood going to non-vital areas at the expense of more clinically important tissues. Autoregulation is further compromised when the vessels become rigid, e.g. with atheroma. As a result, tissue flow will begin to fall at a higher perfusing pressure than normal.

Microcirculatory changes in the late stages of shock lead to stagnation of blood flow, sludging of red cells and a further impairment of tissue perfusion. In addition, the hydrostatic pressure within the capillaries increases, because blood can still perfuse the capillaries but cannot escape. Consequently, further intravascular fluid is lost as it diffuses through the capillary wall into the interstitial space.

Tissue oxygen extraction

At the tissue level, the partial pressure gradient of oxygen is opposite to that found at the alveolar/capillary interface. The capillary PO_2 is approximately 20 mm Hg (2.6 kPa) and cellular PO_2 is only 2–3 mm Hg (<0.4 kPa). Furthermore, local factors also decrease the affinity of haemoglobin for oxygen (shifting the oxygen dissociation curve to the right), allowing O_2 to be released more readily. As mentioned earlier (see Chapter 5), this occurs with an increase in:

- hydrogen ion concentration (i.e. fall in pH)
- $PaCO_2$
- 2,3-DPG
- temperature.

Key point

To help remember these effects, think of the athlete during a race. Active muscles require more oxygen than when they are at rest. With increased metabolism lactic acid, CO_2 and heat are generated. All of these facilitate the release of oxygen from haemoglobin

---

The total consumption of oxygen per minute (VO_2) for a resting healthy male is 100–160 ml/min/m². As the delivery of oxygen (DO_2) is 500–720 ml/min/m², the tissues use only 20–25% of the oxygen that is available. This percentage is referred to as the **oxygen extraction ratio**. This low value indicates that body tissues have a tremendous potential to extract more oxygen from the circulating blood.

The total consumption of oxygen per minute is constant throughout a wide range of oxygen delivery in a healthy subject (Fig. 9.1). Under normal circumstances, an increase in oxygen demand is met by increasing the oxygen delivery, usually from a rise in the cardiac output. However, should this not be possible, or inadequate, then VO_2 can be maintained to a limited extent by increasing the oxygen extraction ratio. Should this also fail, then VO_2 will begin to fall, because it is now directly dependent on the delivery of oxygen (Fig. 9.1).

Increasing the oxygen extraction ratio leads to a fall in the venous oxygen saturation. This is difficult to detect clinically early on and its actual value varies from organ to organ. However, it can be measured from a mixed venous sample directly usually by a pulmonary artery catheter (superior venacaval oxygen saturation – $ScVO_2$ is used now as it is easier to obtain and serves similar purpose (normal $ScVO_2$ should be >70%)). Under normal circumstances, this is approximately 75%, with values below 70% indicating that global delivery of oxygen is becoming inadequate.

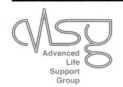

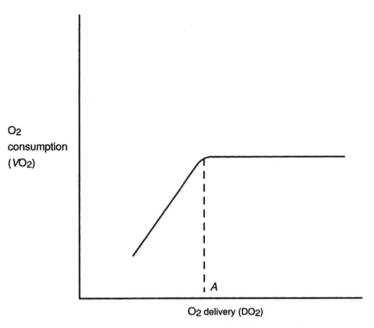

Fig. 9.1 The relationship between oxygen delivery and consumption A is the critical level for DO_2. VO_2 below A depends directly on DO_2.

The amount of anaerobic metabolism increases as the oxygen debt increases. As a result, the plasma lactate level rises in the shocked patient. These levels not only correlate with the severity of the shock, but also allow the body's response to therapy to be assessed.

Resuscitation is completed when tissues return to normal aerobic metabolism and any oxygen debt has been repaid. This is manifested by correction of any metabolic acidosis. Beware that patients may appear adequately resuscitated when simply using clinical vital signs as a measure. Unfortunately, these may not indicate that the body is still trying to compensate for an ongoing lack of tissue oxygenation. If not corrected, this can lead to organ dysfunction and even death in compromised patients. The use of a series of endpoints to measure the shock state, including plasma lactate, is therefore recommended (see later).

Key point

There is a chain of events that delivers oxygen to tissues, where it is used by the cells. Each part has a finite capacity to compensate when one or more links in the chain are defective. When the compensatory capacity is exceeded, shock will develop

---

Time Out 9.1

a Take a moment to list the five factors that influence the delivery of oxygen to tissues.

b How does the sympathetic nervous system help to compensate for a defect in oxygen delivery?

CAUSES OF SHOCK

Many conditions can lead to an inadequate delivery of oxygen to vital structures of the body (Table 9.1, Fig. 9.2).

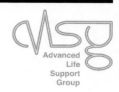

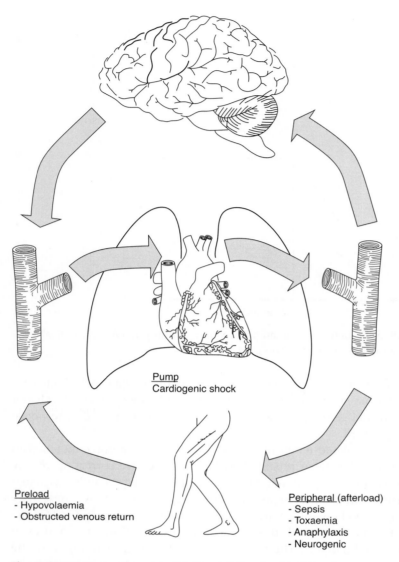

Pump
Cardiogenic shock

Preload
- Hypovolaemia
- Obstructed venous return

Peripheral (afterload)
- Sepsis
- Toxaemia
- Anaphylaxis
- Neurogenic

Fig. 9.2 Diagrammatic representations of the causes of shock.

Table 9.1 Mechanisms and causes of inadequate oxygen delivery

Mechanism	Cause
Decrease in oxygen uptake by the lungs	Pneumonia, massive pulmonary embolus, tension pneumothorax, sepsis, anaemia
Reduced venous return	Hypovolaemia, obstructed venous return, sepsis
Impaired cardiac function	Ischaemic heart disease, cardiomyopathy, dysrhythmia, pulmonary emboli, valvular disease (especially severe aortic stenosis and regurgitation), sepsis
Reduced arterial tone	Anaphylaxis, neurogenic shock, sepsis
Impaired organ autoregulation	Sepsis
Decrease oxygen uptake and use by tissues	Poisoning with carbon monoxide, cyanide, sepsis

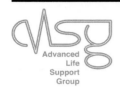

Decrease in oxygen uptake by the lungs

The airway and pulmonary conditions leading to a fall in oxygen uptake are described in detail in Chapters 5, 8 and 20.

Reduced venous return

Hypovolaemia

True hypovolaemia is associated with loss of either blood or plasma (see next box). Upper gastrointestinal haemorrhage is a common cause in medical patients. In contrast, excessive plasma loss is often seen at the extremes of age with gastroenteritis. However, there may be more than one mechanism involved, e.g. in diabetic ketoacidosis; the fluid loss is related to a combination of hyperventilation, osmotic diuresis, decreased body sodium, vomiting and possibly the precipitating condition.

Causes of hypovolaemic shock

True loss	Common examples
Blood loss	Gastrointestinal haemorrhage
	Ruptured aortic aneurysm
Plasma loss	Diarrhoea and vomiting
	Diabetic ketoacidosis
	Osmotic diuresis
	Pancreatitis
	Hyponatraemia and mineralocorticoid deficiency
	Fistula and ostomies
	Burns

Apparent loss	Common examples
Venodilators	Nitrates, opiates, intravenous loop diuretics
Hyponatraemia	Glucocorticoid deficiency

Many drugs cause hypotension by reducing preload. Although this effect may be beneficial to patients with left ventricular failure, it can lead to a marked fall in blood pressure, particularly in patients with low blood volumes. The true hypovolaemia and hyponatraemia associated with Addison's adrenal insufficiency are attributed to the deficiency of both mineralo- and gluco-corticoid hormones.

Estimating volume loss and grading shock

The compensatory mechanisms evoked by 'shock' are related to the decline in function of various organs. Respiratory rate, capillary refill (see later), heart rate, blood pressure, urine output and conscious level can be readily measured and so are important indicators of both the grade of shock and the response to treatment. As an approximation, these physiological changes can be used to divide hypovolaemic shock into four categories, depending on the percentage blood loss (Table 9.2). The important features are as given:

- A tachycardia often occurs early due to the sympathetic response.
- In grade II shock, the diastolic blood pressure rises, without any fall in the systolic component, leading to a narrowed pulse pressure. This is due to the compensatory sympathetic nervous system mediated vasoconstriction. Consequently, a narrow pulse pressure with a normal systolic blood pressure is an early sign of shock.

Table 9.2 Categories of hypovolaemic shock

	Category			
	I	II	III	IV
Blood loss (litres)	<0.75	0.75–1.5	1.5–2.0	>2.0
Blood loss (%BV)*	<15%	15–30%	30–40%	>40%
Respiratory rate	14–20	20–30	30–40	>35 or low
Heart rate	<100	>100	>120	140 or low
Systolic BP	Normal	Normal	Decreased	Decreased ++
Diastolic BP	Normal	Raised	Decreased	Decreased ++
Pulse pressure	Normal	Decreased	Decreased	Decreased
Capillary refill	Normal	Delayed	Delayed	Delayed
Skin	Normal	Pale	Pale	Pale/cold
Urine output (ml/h)	>30	20–30	5–15	Negligible
Mental state	Normal	Anxious	Anxious/confused	Confused/drowsy

*% B/V = % of blood volume.

- Tachypnoea can indicate shock as well as underlying respiratory or metabolic pathology.
- Hypotension indicates a loss of at least 30% of the circulating volume.

Limitations to estimations of hypovolaemia

Blindly following the signs in Table 9.2 will lead to gross errors in blood loss estimation – particularly in certain patient types (see box). It is therefore important that management is based on the overall condition of the patient and not isolated physiological parameters.

Pitfalls in assessing blood loss

Elderly
Drugs
Pacemaker
Athlete
Pregnancy
Hypothermia
Compensation
Tissue damage

The **elderly patient** is less able to compensate for acute hypovolaemia as their sympathetic drive is reduced. Consequently the loss of smaller volumes can produce a fall in blood pressure. Reliance only on the blood pressure could therefore lead to an overestimation of blood loss (see Chapter 21).

A variety of **drugs** that are commonly taken can alter the physiological response to blood loss. For example, β blockers will prevent tachycardia and also inhibit the normal sympathetic positive inotropic response. Therefore, after a 15% circulating volume loss, compensatory tachycardia is unlikely to occur in a β-blocked patient. This could lead to an underestimation of the blood loss. It is also

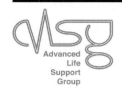

important to remember that the blood pressure falls at lower volumes of blood loss in these patients, by the same mechanisms.

An increasing number of patients have **pacemakers** fitted each year. These devices may only allow the heart to beat at a particular rate, irrespective of the volume loss or sympathetic drive. Therefore they will give rise to the same errors in estimation as β blockers.

The physiological response to training will mean that the **athlete** will have a larger blood volume and a resting bradycardia (about 50 beats/min). The blood volume can increase by 15–20%; thus, it is possible to underestimate blood loss, especially as a compensatory increase in heart rate can mean that the pulse is less than 100 beats/min.

During **pregnancy**, the heart rate progressively increases so that by the third trimester it is 15–20 beats faster than normal. Blood pressure falls by 5–15 mm Hg in the second trimester and returns to normal during the third, as the blood volume increases by 40–50%. Supine hypotension, due to uterine compression of the inferior vena cava, has been discussed earlier (also see Chapter 23).

Hypothermia will reduce the respiratory rate, pulse and blood pressure irrespective of any other cause of shock. Depending on the temperature, hypothermic patients are often resistant to cardiovascular drugs, cardioversion or fluid replacement. The estimation of the fluid requirements of these patients can therefore be very difficult and often invasive monitoring is required (see Chapter 21).

Delays in resuscitation, especially in the young increases the action of the normal **compensatory mechanisms**. This can lead to improvements in respiratory rate, heart rate and blood pressure, thus the clinician may possibly underestimate the volume of blood lost.

The degree of **tissue damage** can have a profound effect on the patient's physiological response. The initial tachycardia can deteriorate into a bradycardia when there is a significant haemorrhage with little tissue damage (e.g. a gastrointestinal bleed). At this stage, the blood pressure also begins to fall. Conversely, when there is marked tissue damage even with a significant haemorrhage, the blood pressure and tachycardia are maintained. Consequently, the degree of blood loss can be over- or underestimated depending on the absence or presence of significant tissue damage.

Obstructed venous return

Blood returning to the heart depends on the pressure gradient created by the high hydrostatic pressure in the peripheral veins and low hydrostatic pressure in the right atrium of the heart. Any reduction in this gradient, e.g. by increasing right atrial pressure, will lead to a fall in venous return to the heart. External compression on the thorax or abdomen can have a similar action in obstructing the venous return. Consequently in the supine position, the gravid uterus can compress the inferior vena cava and impair venous return.

The common causes of obstructed venous return, reducing preload, are shown in the box.

Causes of obstructed venous return

High mean airway pressure (e.g. high PPV)	Daily
Acute asthma	Daily
Pregnancy	Weekly
Massive pulmonary embolus, tension pneumothorax	Monthly
Cardiac tamponade	Annually

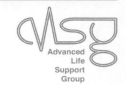

Impaired cardiac function

A variety of conditions can adversely influence ventricular function and lead to shock (see next box).

It is important to remember that antiarrhythmic drugs may have a significant negative inotropic effect. The same effect is seen with certain drugs taken as an overdose, e.g. tricyclic antidepressants. Myocardial function can also be impaired by infection (myocarditis), an underlying cardiomyopathy or toxins associated with the systemic inflammatory response syndrome (see later). Cardiac tamponade, in addition to its effect on venous return, impedes ventricular filling.

Cardiogenic shock occurs when around 40% or more of the left ventricle has infarcted. Clinically, it is defined as Class IV on the Killip classification – i.e. a systolic blood pressure of 90 mm Hg or lower, peripheral vasoconstriction, oliguria and pulmonary vascular congestion.

Summary of the cardiac causes of shock

Myocardial	Ventricular failure/ conduction problems	Ischaemia/infarction
		Myocarditis
		Drugs
		Toxins
		Cardiomyopathy
Endocardial	Acute valve lesion	Infective endocarditis
		Papillary muscle rupture
		Aortic root dissection
Epicardial	Acute tamponade	Ventricular wall rupture
		Malignancy
		Post-surgery
	Constrictive pericarditis	Viral
		Tuberculosis
		Radiotherapy

Key point

In cardiogenic shock, the compensatory sympathetic and catecholamine response, i.e. increased heart rate and systemic vascular resistance, only serve to raise the myocardial oxygen demand and exacerbate the degree of myocardial ischaemia

---

Reduced arterial tone
Anaphylactic shock

Anaphylaxis is an acute reaction to a foreign substance to which the patient has already been sensitised. This leads to an IgE-triggered rapid degranulation of mast cells and basophils (see box). Anaphylactoid reactions have an identical clinical presentation but are not triggered by IgE and do not necessarily require previous exposure. Furthermore, they may not produce a reaction every time.

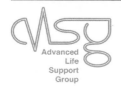

Common causes of anaphylaxis/anaphylactoid reactions

Anaphylaxis	Drugs (protein and non-protein) – commonly penicillin or other β lactam drugs, blood products and immunoglobulins
	Vaccines
	Food – especially nuts, shellfish
	Venoms – especially bees, wasps and hornets
	Parasites
	Chemicals
	Latex
Anaphylactoid	Complement activation
	Coagulation/fibrinolysis system activation
	Direct pharmacological release of mediators
	Exercise induced
	Radiological contrast
	Idiopathic

Key point

The most common causes of anaphylactic fatalities are parenteral drugs, bee stings and food-related reactions. Radio-contrast and non-steroidal anti-inflammatory medications are the most common anaphylactoid fatalities

---

The body's response to these stimuli is to release a collection of mediators from mast cells and basophils that have inflammatory, spasmogenic and chemotactic actions. The inflammatory activators induce vasodilatation and oedema. This leads to a reduction in tissue perfusion as a result of the fall in arterial tone and venous return. The spasmogens cause bronchial smooth muscle contraction, increased mucus production and mucosal oedema. The chemotactic agents attract platelets and white blood cells to the affected area.

In addition, the variety of chemical mediators released cause cardiovascular collapse from one, or more, of the following:

- arrhythmia
- hypovolaemia
- decreased myocardial function
- pulmonary hypertension.

Arrhythmias may result from direct mediator effects, as well as hypoxaemia, hypotension, acidosis, pre-existing cardiac disease and adrenaline given during resuscitation. Hypovolaemia can occur very quickly, with up to 50% of the circulating plasma volume being lost within 10–15 min in severe cases. This is due to a combination of increased vascular permeability, vasodilatation and decreased venous return from raised intrathoracic pressure secondary to bronchospasm and positive pressure ventilation.

The vast majority of serious anaphylactic reactions occur unexpectedly. Over 50% of fatalities occur within the first hour. Seventy five percent of these deaths are due to asphyxia from upper airway obstruction or bronchospasm. The remaining cases die from circulatory failure and hypotension.

Key point

The diagnosis is not difficult when a patient presents with generalised urticaria, wheeze and hypotension following a known stimulus. However, circulatory collapse can occur without preceding warning signs

SEPTICAEMIA, SEPSIS, SEVERE SEPSIS, SEPTIC SHOCK

Septicaemia is an ambiguous term, does not explain the various syndromes associated with infection or the body's response to infection and should, therefore, not be used in clinical practice. This term is also often confused with *bacteraemia*, which refers to the presence or detection of bacteria in blood where they normally do not exist.

Sepsis, caused by invading microorganisms, is a well-known clinical entity, usually known by its common name: infection. Generally, such patients are not systemically severely ill. Confusion is caused by either not recognising systemic illness consequent upon severe infections or erroneously diagnosing severe sepsis where widespread systemic inflammatory response does not accompany infective illness. There are internationally recognised definitions of sepsis, severe sepsis and septic shock. Sepsis must be distinguished from severe sepsis and septic shock, which in turn must also be distinguished from systemic inflammatory response syndrome as the therapeutic priorities are different in different conditions.

Systemic inflammatory response syndrome (SIRS) is the systemic response to severe inflammation (e.g. pancreatitis) or major trauma. Two or more of the following criteria define SIRS when such inflammation is present:
- respiratory rate of $\geq$20 breaths/min or $PaCO_2$ of ≤ 4.25 kPa
- heart rate $\geq$90 beats/min
- core temperature $\geq$38.0°C or $\leq$36.0°C
- white cell count of $\geq$12,000/mm^3 or $\leq$4,000/mm^3.

Sepsis is defined as evidence of SIRS with a known or suspected source of infection. In clinical practice, it is sometimes difficult to distinguish between SIRS and sepsis. It is, therefore, very important that a diligent search is made for the source of infection in these patients. Aggressive treatment with antibiotics and/or drainage (radiological, endocopic, surgical) of the source will help to prevent patients slipping into severe sepsis and/or septic shock and progress to multiple organ dysfunction syndrome (MODS), thus reducing mortality.

Severe sepsis is sepsis accompanied by hypoperfusion and organ dysfunction. Any one of the following organ dysfunctions may be present:
- Cardiovascular: Systolic blood pressure $\leq$90 mm Hg or mean arterial pressure $\leq$70 mm Hg for at least 1 h despite **adequate** volume resuscitation
- Renal: Urine output $\leq$0.5 ml/kg body weight/h (despite **adequate** fluid loading) or acute renal failure (now called *acute renal injury*)
- Pulmonary: PaO_2/FiO_2 ratio of $\leq$33.3–26.5 (kPa) depending on the presence or absence of other organ dysfunction (Normal PaO_2/FiO_2 ratio is $\approx$63.4 for a healthy adult breathing room air.)
- CNS: Acute alteration in mental status, e.g. delirium or a Glasgow Coma Score < 14
- Haematological: Platelet count of $\leq$80,000/mm or a decrease of 50% over 3 days or disseminated intravascular coagulation

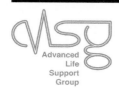

- Gastrointestinal: Paralytic ileus, delayed gastric emptying, abnormal liver function tests
- Metabolic: pH $\leq$7.30 or a base deficit >5.0 mmol/l and/or a plasma lactate >1.5 times the upper limit of normal (usually 2.8–3.0 mmol/l).

Septic shock is severe sepsis with persistent hypoperfusion, despite aggressive and adequate fluid resuscitation. This is usually, but not always, manifested as hypotension. The hypotension of septic shock always requires vasopressors (e.g. norepinephrine) and/or inotropes (dopamine, dobutamine, epinephrine depending on the patients' condition, disease severity and comorbidities).

Mortality increases proportionately from sepsis to severe sepsis to septic shock. Many conditions may mimic sepsis and, in an emergency, any of the following conditions may be mistaken for sepsis:
- acute myocardial infarction
- acute pulmonary embolism
- acute pancreatitis
- fat embolism syndrome
- acute adrenal insufficiency
- acute decompensation of chronic liver disease; mild infections in patients with liver disease
- acute gastrointestinal haemorrhage
- 'overzealous' diuresis or unnecessary and inappropriate use of diuretics
- adverse drug reactions
- transfusion reactions
- procedure-related transient bacteraemia (e.g. urethral instrumentation, removal of an infected central line)
- amniotic fluid embolism
- last stages of malignant diseases, carcinomatosis and mild infections in patients with advanced malignancy.

With sepsis, the circulating endotoxins (inflammatory mediators such as prostaglandins, cytokines and nitric oxide) have a negative inotropic effect, cause vasodilatation and impair energy use at a cellular level; the source is usually Gram negative bacteria. Occasionally, Gram positive bacteria release toxins causing the **toxic shock syndrome**. *Staphylococcus aureus* is the usual organism, although some severe streptococcal infections can have a similar presentation. Much less commonly in the UK, viruses, fungi and protozoa are the sources of the sepsis.

Causes of toxic shock syndrome
Retained tampon
Abscess
Empyema
Surgical wound infection
Osteomyelitis
Cellulitis
Infected burns
Septic abortion

Eventually, septic shock will affect all parts of the circulatory system. Venous return is reduced as pro-inflammatory cytokines increase capillary permeability. Further cellular damage by endotoxins causes the release of proteolytic enzymes. These paralyse precapillary sphincters, enhance capillary leakage and increase

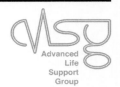

hypovolaemia. The resultant loss of fluid and protein causes hypovolaemia which, combined with venodilatation, produces a fall in preload. The reduction in tissue blood flow resulting from decreased perfusion, and the increased viscosity, leads to platelet aggregation and clot formation. At the same time, thromboplastins are activated. Consequently, disseminated intravascular coagulation can result and lead to further falls in tissue perfusion.

Myocardial depression occurs, especially in severe sepsis. This is due to multiple factors including hypoxaemia, acidosis, myocardial oedema and circulating negative inotropes. Tissue autoregulation is disrupted and there is marked peripheral arterial dilatation. Arteriovenous shunts also develop, resulting in maldistribution of blood flow. This either increases the chances of, or exacerbates, tissue ischaemia. In addition to all of these changes, tissue oxygen demand increases, but uptake is impaired. It will not, therefore, be surprising to find that septic shock has an extremely high mortality rate (>50%).

The diagnosis of septic shock can be difficult. In contrast with other causes of shock (except anaphylactic), the physiological features are usually (but not always) high cardiac output and low systemic vascular resistance (Table 9.3). The classic signs are a wide pulse pressure and warm skin (due to the dilated peripheral vessels), agitation, pyrexia and an increased respiratory rate (due to hypoxaemia). The classic features of hypovolaemic shock are manifested later, with peripheral vasoconstriction and a low or normal core temperature. There may also be evidence of disseminated intravascular coagulation. This abnormality often manifests as blood oozing around wounds and cannula sites.

Table 9.3 Haemodynamic variables in shock (adult mean values)

	Left atrial pressure (mm Hg)	Cardiac output (l/min)	Systemic vascular resistance (dyn/s/cm^2)
Normal	10	5	1200
Left ventricular failure	25	2	3000
Haemorrhage	0	3	3000
Sepsis and anaphylaxis	2	12	300

Key points

Maintain a high index of suspicion, because diagnosing septic shock can be difficult

Always check for the non-blanching purpuric rash of meningococcal septicaemia

Consider the diagnosis in any ill patient with an altered conscious level and haemodynamic abnormalities

---

As described before, the type of septic shock known as the toxic shock syndrome has many potential causes. However, the clinical presentation remains the same:

- temperature 39°C or above
- macular, blanching rash
- hypotension
- evidence of involvement of at least three systems.

The rash can be localised or general and tends to lead to desquamation after one or two weeks in survivors. Common systems that are involved are gastrointestinal

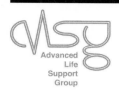

(diarrhoea and vomiting); neurological (confusion, drowsiness); renal (impaired function); muscle (myalgia, high creatine phosphokinase); haematological (leucocytosis, disseminated intravascular coagulation, thrombocytopenia).

Multiorgan dysfunction

Organ dysfunction of more than one organ is called multiple organ dysfunction syndrome (MODS; previously called multiple organ failure). Severe sepsis and septic shock are the commonest causes of MODS in the critically ill.

Neurogenic shock

Neurogenic shock is caused by disruption of the sympathetic nervous system outflow following spinal injures above T6. The higher the lesion, the greater the impairment and the more marked the effect.

In the context of acute medical emergencies, neurogenic shock is rare. Patients who are susceptible to spontaneous cervical vertebral subluxation include those with:

- rheumatoid disease
- Down's syndrome
- ankylosing spondylitis (an inflexible cervical spine that fractures following minimal trauma).

The lack of sympathetic activity results in generalised vasodilatation, bradycardia, loss of temperature control and lack of both the reflex tachycardia and vasoconstriction responses to hypovolaemia. As neurogenic shock leads to a reduction in blood supply to the spinal column, it also gives rise to additional nervous tissue damage.

Clinically, the patient with a high spinal lesion often has a systolic blood pressure of approximately 90 mm Hg, with a heart rate of around 50/min. In addition, the patient has warm and pink skin due to vasodilatation. However, due to an initial pressor response releasing catecholamines into the circulation, the onset of these signs can take from a few minutes to 24 h to develop.

During the initial neurological assessment using the AVPU scale or Glasgow Coma Scale, an asymmetrical weakness may become apparent by a lack of response to peripheral stimulation. These should be noted and a definitive neurological examination performed in the secondary assessment (see Chapter 7). However, these are difficult in the unconscious patient. If in doubt, immobilise the cervical spine and request a neurosurgical/orthopaedic review. Appropriate imaging can then be chosen and interpreted.

Key points

Be wary of the unconscious patient who is admitted following a fall downstairs. The initial neurological features are often falsely attributed to an underlying stroke

Spinal immobilisation must be maintained until specialist advice is obtained if a spinal injury is suspected, from either the mechanism of the injury or the physical signs

---

PRIMARY ASSESSMENT AND RESUSCITATION

Patients cannot remain permanently in a state of shock; they either improve or die. Shock could be viewed as a momentary pause on the way to death. Its detection depends on certain physical signs that are produced as a result of poor

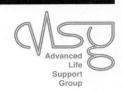

oxygen delivery. Thus, the treatment of shock necessitates restoring adequate delivery of oxygen, and not simply restoring a normal blood pressure.

Airway

The first priority in any shocked patient is to clear and, if necessary, secure the airway so that high concentrations of inspired oxygen can be given (see Chapter 4). The patient should also be attached to a pulse oximeter and, if intubated, a capnograph.

Breathing

Once the airway has been cleared, adequate ventilation with a high inspired oxygen concentration is required. This is often difficult (e.g. in patients with active haematemesis); therefore, early liaison with an anaesthetist is necessary. Record the respiratory rate and examine for signs of bronchospasm, pulmonary oedema, and tension pneumothorax, and treat as appropriate.

Circulation

Look at the patient noting colour, sweating and distress. Assess the height and character of the jugular venous pulse. Then **feel** the arterial pulse for either a brady or a tachycardia. Is the patient vasodilated with a bounding pulse? Then check the position and character of the apex beat if it is palpable. Finish by **listening** for the presence of extra heart sounds and/or heart murmurs.

Connect the patient to an ECG and blood pressure monitor. Obtain peripheral intravenous access with the largest cannula possible (ideally a 14 or 16 gauge) and take 20 ml of blood for laboratory tests. These include full blood count, urea and electrolytes, glucose, lactate and an arterial blood gas sample. If clinically appropriate, blood should also be taken for cross-match, markers of myocardial damage, amylase, blood cultures and toxicology.

Plasma lactate is a useful measure, particularly in hypovolaemia where it is related to the degree of hypovolaemic shock and risk of death. The time to normalise the plasma lactate level is also a predictor of survival.

> **Key point**
>
> All shocked patients will have a metabolic acidosis. It should be treated by correcting any A, B and C problems and NOT by giving sodium bicarbonate

---

If a peripheral site is not available in adults, central venous access is advocated. This procedure should **only** be done by experienced staff, because of the potential for damaging the vein and neighbouring structures. Ultrasound guidance is increasingly being used to locate the central veins and facilitate cannulation.

By the end of this assessment, the answers to the following questions should have been ascertained:

- Is shock present?
- If present, what is its likely cause?

Further information from a well-'phrased' history will help in deciding the answers to these questions.

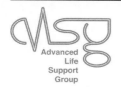

SPECIFIC TYPES OF SHOCK

Hypovolaemia

In the majority of 'medical patients' with hypovolaemic shock, the primary aim is to restore fluid loss from, e.g. vomiting and diarrhoea. Occasionally, however, the primary aim of treatment is to prevent further bleeding if at all possible. Examples of this include the use of a Sengstaken tube for a variceal bleed (see cautionary comments below) or urgent surgery for a ruptured ectopic pregnancy. Often there is no definite source for blood or fluid loss. In these cases, the clinician should devise a management plan based on the likely cause of fluid loss, or the bleeding source, the degree of hypovolaemia and the patients pre-existing medical condition.

General

In grade I shock, a litre of crystalloid is infused and the response monitored. If hypovolaemia is estimated to be grade II or higher, 500 ml intravenous colloid, or another litre of crystalloid, is required. The aim should be to maintain the haematocrit (packed cell volume) at 30–35%, so that oxygen delivery is optimised. Red cell replacement is secondary, becoming more important with progressively larger blood losses.

All fluids need to be warmed before they are given to patients to prevent iatrogenically induced hypothermia. A simple way of achieving this is to store a supply of crystalloids and colloids in a warming cupboard. However, if this method is used, care must be taken to push the fluids rapidly through a wide-bore short cannula (Poiseuille's law) to prevent the fluids cooling down in the giving set. This eliminates the need for warming coils, which increase resistance to flow and thereby slow the rate of fluid administration. 'Level One' rapid fluid infusors, if available, allow rapid infusion of large volumes of warm fluid.

The above management should be modified in hypotensive patients where there is a definite bleeding source that has not been controlled. In these cases, vigorous fluid resuscitation will lead to further bleeding and a worse prognosis. These patients require the source of the bleeding controlled urgently. In the meantime fluid needs to be administered so that the blood pressure is maintained at 20 mm Hg below the baseline. This is known as **hypotensive resuscitation**.

Specific

The source of bleeding in the acutely ill medical patient is often the upper gastrointestinal tract and, as a group, accounts for 1–2% of medical admissions. The specific causes are listed in the box.

Upper gastrointestinal haemorrrhage: causes and frequency	
34%	Duodenal ulcer
19%	Gastric ulcer
15%	No lesion identified
11%	Oesophagitis
8%	Gastroduodenitis
5%	Malignancy (upper gastrointestinal tract)
4%	Varices
4%	Others

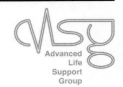

In addition to the general management principles described earlier, the clinician should ensure **early** liaison with surgical colleagues. Immediately after resuscitation has started, inform the surgical gastroenterology team of the clinical problem and request a review. Combined medical and surgical management is the ideal. The decision to operate is usually based on continuing haemorrhage and the patient's transfusion needs.

Need for surgery with upper gastrointestinal tract bleed

Six units of blood in patients aged less than 65 years, unless there is a history of non-steroidal anti-inflammatory drugs (NSAIDs) use or comorbid pathology
Four units of blood in patients greater than 65 years of age or those less than 65 years with a history of NSAID use or comorbid pathology

---

If oesophageal varices are suspected, based on the presence of chronic liver disease stigmata or from the history, give terlipressin (2 mg bolus IV over 1 min, then 20 mg/kg (1 mg) every 4–8 h, max 120 µg/kg/day). Early liaison with a gastroenterologist is important for endoscopic intervention. Tamponade devices are rarely required and should only be introduced by an appropriately trained individual.

Key point

Bleeding from varices is rare when compared with gastroduodenal inflammation/ulceration, even in alcohol users

---

Obstructed venous return

Severe bronchospasm and a gravid uterus are common causes of obstructed venous return. Please read pages 90 and 372.

Other causes include cardiac tamponade where the symptoms (see Chapter 6) can be transiently improved by a fluid challenge to assist ventricular filling pressures. If, however, this presents as a pulseless electrical activity, then resuscitation according to the UK and European protocol is required, including pericardiocentesis. Ideally, echocardiography should be used to facilitate pericardiocentesis. If the equipment/skill is unavailable and the patient is deteriorating, then drainage of the pericardium should be done blindly, using ECG control, to gain time, allowing the subsequent insertion of a pericardial drain under more controlled conditions.

Both pulmonary emboli and tension pneumothorax are described in detail in Chapter 8.

Impaired cardiac function

Shock resulting from heart failure is common. The signs are described in detail in Chapter 20 and summarised in the box. When the signs of shock are resulting solely from myocardial damage, there is an 80% mortality. There are often other, more treatable, causes adding to the shock state. It is therefore essential that hypovolaemia, vasovagal reactions, arrhythmias and drug reactions are identified and treated.

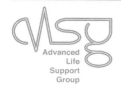

Signs of cardiogenic shock

Breathlessness and central cyanosis
Fine bi-basal crackles
Tachycardia
Hypotension
Raised JVP
Third heart sound
Murmurs, e.g. mitral valve regurgitation (due to ventricular dilatation)

The first management priority is to correct hypoxaemia. The use of non-invasive ventilation (CPAP or NIPPV) is increasing. However, there is still debate on which is the optimum method of non-invasive ventilation for these patients. Occasionally, the patient may require intubation so that optimal oxygenation can be achieved. The high cardiac filling pressures also need to be reduced in a controlled fashion. Intravenous nitrates are often used, but with caution, because of the risk of aggravating hypotension, as they lower the systemic vascular resistance. Dopamine and dobutamine may also be required to provide inotropic support and improve the cardiac output. Any dysrhythmia causing haemodynamic compromise must also be treated.

When cardiogenic shock is due to right heart failure, give a fluid challenge of 200 ml of colloid and assess the effect, and repeat according to the clinical response.

It is not unusual to find that a combination of mechanical ventilation, vasodilators, inotropes and fluids is required to increase the cardiac index and the delivery of oxygen. Clearly, these procedures require the facilities available in either coronary care or high dependency or intensive treatment units.

Patients with heart failure are less able to compensate for hypovolaemia, should that coexist. This problem is compounded by the fact that measurement of the central venous pressure (CVP) does not provide an accurate estimate of the left ventricular end diastolic pressure (see the box below). These patients are therefore best managed using a pulmonary artery catheter. This enables both the filling pressure of the left side of the heart and the cardiac output to be estimated and accurate fluid resuscitation provided. Many non-invasive haemodynamic monitoring devices are now also available but need specialist training to use them (as does the pulmonary artery catheter).

CVP monitoring in heart failure

Measures right ventricular pressure affected by:
- Intravascular volume
- Intrathoracic pressure
- Right ventricular function
- Venous tone

As a result, the CVP can be raised in:
- Pulmonary pathology
- Positive pressure ventilation
- Malposition causing false elevations

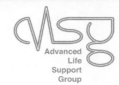

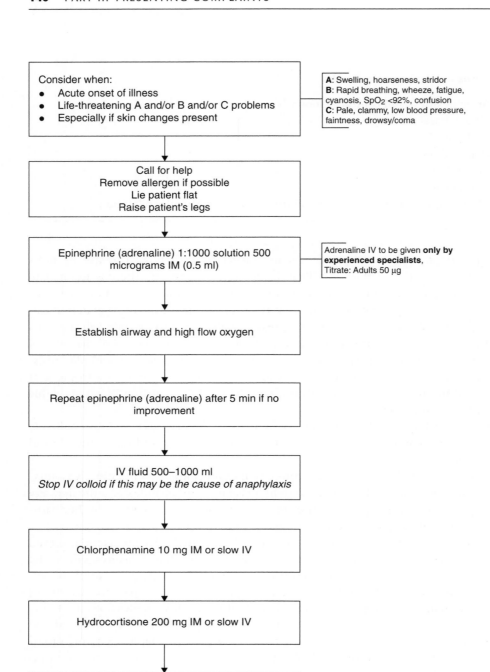

Fig. 9.3 Management of anaphylactic shock (RCUK guidelines 2008) [Reproduced with permission from the Resuscitation Council (UK)].

Anaphylactic shock

The management of anaphylactic shock is dependent on a rapid ABC assessment and resuscitation, considering the diagnosis and preventing any further absorption of the suspected causative agent (Fig. 9.3). Always be wary because airway obstruction, bronchospasm and hypotension can have a delayed, but ultimately sudden, presentation.

If profound shock is judged immediately life-threatening, give cardiopulmonary resuscitation/advanced life support as necessary. Consider slow intravenous (IV) adrenaline (epinephrine) 1:10,000 (i.e. very dilute) solution. This is hazardous

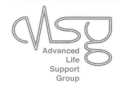

and is recommended only for an experienced practitioner who can also obtain IV access without delay. Note the different strength of adrenaline (epinephrine) that is required for IV use. A crystalloid may be safer than colloid.

Following resuscitation, the patient should be admitted for 8–12 h of monitoring to detect those cases that develop a protracted or biphasic response. The latter is more likely following oral antigen ingestion, or when symptoms started over 30 min after exposure.

Septic shock

Therapeutic priorities are different in different 'stages' of sepsis. Hypotension constitutes a medical emergency. This is a sign of advanced decompensation and will lead to rapid worsening of tissue hypoxaemia, organ dysfunction, organ failure and increase in mortality. A first priority in severe sepsis and/or septic shock, therefore, is to improve tissue oxygenation by supportive measures. These include high concentrations of inspired oxygen, aggressive fluid resuscitation with balanced salt solutions (Hartmann's preferred to 0.9% saline), vasopressors/inotropes as necessary and assessment and management according to the familiar steps of ABC. Some of the supportive measures may not be available in general medical or surgical wards. However, as stated above, severe sepsis and septic shock are emergencies and the resuscitative measures should be started immediately while an appropriate place (a bed in HDU, ICU) for the patient's further care is identified. On no account should the patient be left alone.

Once resuscitative measures have been started, appropriate help should be sought, e.g. an intensivist's opinion either a radiologists or, a surgical opinion for percutaneous or surgically accessible sources of infection or help from microbiologists etc. Initially, after taking appropriate cultures, broad spectrum antibiotics (including those for gram negative bacteria, e.g. aminoglycosides; cover for anaerobes is usually not required) may be started empirically; these should later be changed when microbiological culture results are available. If meningitis is suspected, antibiotics should not be withheld or delayed because appropriate cultures (e.g. cerebrospinal fluid) have not been taken. Blood cultures can usually be taken when gaining venous access.

If septic patients are to survive, the source of infection needs to be identified, treated and removed. When there is a collection of pus, drainage will be required by either surgery or percutaneously under imaging control.

Repeated blood cultures may be required to determine the causative organism. In the meantime, antibiotic therapy should be aimed at the most likely organism. Often a combination of a penicillin, aminoglycoside and metronidazole is used according to the hospital antibiotic policy. If meningococcal septicaemia is suspected, give benzyl penicillin 2.4 g and ceftriaxone 2 g intravenously **immediately**.

The patient will require cardiovascular and respiratory support, as well as intensive monitoring of their fluid and antibiotic regimes. The former aims to maintain a high cardiac index (over 4.5 l/min/m^2), high oxygen delivery (above 600 ml/min/m^2) and tissue perfusion pressure. This usually entails intubating and ventilating the patient with supplemental oxygen, correction of hypovolaemia and the use of inotropes. The response to all vasoactive drugs is unpredictable. It is therefore advisable to start with a low dose and titrate further amounts until the cardiac index is sufficient to allow acceptable tissue perfusion. In adults, this is usually at a level greater than 4.5 l/min/m^2.

The indications for ventilation are no different from those routinely used:
- inability to maintain an airway
- inability to maintain normal PaO_2 and $PaCO_2$

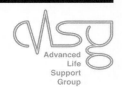

- persistant tachypnoea despite adequate oxygenation and volume replacement
- persistant metabolic acidaemia
- elevated serum lactate.

Noradrenaline is frequently needed for its α-agonist activity that helps counteract some of the profound vasodilatation.

Clinical objectives in treating sepsis

Maximise oxygenation
Improve haemodynamic function
Correct any metabolic derangement
Remove source

These patients are very ill. It should not be assumed that starting resuscitation and antibiotics is the end of their care. Many of these patients deteriorate despite best therapy and care. They need constant monitoring and evaluation. Many will need multiple organ support. These patients behave differently from 'standard' patients on the wards and their needs and priorities are different. They are best cared for in critical care units where their needs will be adequately met. Mortality is high and early recognition and aggressive therapy cannot be overemphasised. Although the survivors of MODS may recover from their critical illness and be discharged from ICU and finally from hospital, their physical and psychological recovery is often slow and prolonged and may take up to 18–24 months after an episode of severe sepsis and MODS (Fig. 9.4).

SSC 'treatment bundles'

Sepsis resuscitation bundle (to be started immediately and completed within 6 h)

Serum lactate measured
Blood cultures obtained prior to antibiotic administration
From the time of presentation, broad-spectrum antibiotics administered within
    3 h for admissions to the emergency department and within 1 h for
    non-emergency department admissions to the intensive care unit (ICU).
In the event of hypotension and/or lactate levels >4 mmol/l (36 mg/dl):
deliver an initial minimum of 20 ml/kg crystalloid (or colloid equivalent)
give vasopressors for hypotension not responding to initial fluid resuscitation to
    maintain mean arterial pressure ≥65 mm Hg
In the event of persistent arterial hypotension despite volume resuscitation
    (septic shock) and/or initial lactate >4 mmol/l (36 mg/dl):
achieve central venous pressure of ≥8 mm Hg
achieve central venous oxygen saturation ≥70%*

Sepsis management bundle (to be started immediately and completed within 24 h)

Low-dose steroids administered for septic shock in accordance with a standard
    ICU policy
Drotrecogin alfa (activated) administered in accordance with a standard ICU
    policy

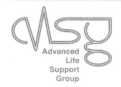

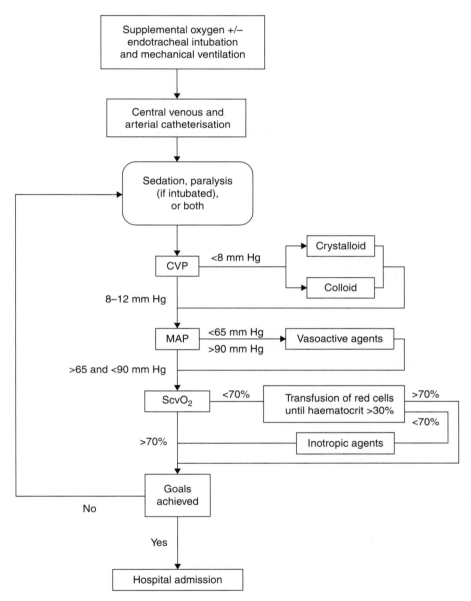

> Glucose control maintained ≥lower limit of normal but <150 mg/dl (8.3 mmol/l)
> For mechanically ventilated patients, inspiratory plateau pressures maintained
> <30 cm H_2O
>
> *Achieving a mixed venous oxygen saturation of 65% is an acceptable alternative.

Fig. 9.4 Management of septic shock.

Neurogenic shock

These patients usually require intubation, as the risks of regurgitation and aspiration are increased due to paralytic ileus, a full stomach and an incompetent gastro-oesophageal sphincter.

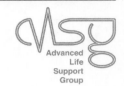

As close to 100% oxygen as is possible should be given, not least because the damaged spinal cord is very sensitive to hypoxaemia. Always maintain in-line cervical spine immobilisation, by an assistant holding the head during intubation, or by the use of commercially available apparatus.

Be aware that the lack of sympathetic tone decreases the patient's compensatory response to other types of shock. It also enhances the vagal effect produced by stimulation of the pharynx, e.g. during laryngoscopy. This can lead to profound bradycardia, requiring treatment with glycopyrrolate. Atropine can be used, but it produces dry, thick secretions that increase the lung dysfunction. Finally, remember to keep the patient covered by warm sheets and blankets. This not only avoids embarrassment but also prevents heat loss from vasodilatation that occurs after high spinal injuries.

Key point

Intubation is not contraindicated in the presence of cervical spine instability, as long as in-line immobilisation is maintained

---

Persistent signs or symptoms of shock must not be attributed to the presence of spinal cord injury, particularly if there is evidence of haemorrhage or trauma. Identification and control of any bleeding source is equally relevant in cases of spinal injury, because of the risks of hypoperfusion of the spinal cord. In the presence of an isolated spinal cord injury, a systolic blood pressure of 80–90 mm Hg is initially acceptable and usually achieved with a fluid challenge of 0.5–1 litre. Patients with a bradycardia of less than 50 beats/min should be given atropine 0.5–1 mg intravenously, repeated as necessary until the heart rate is acceptable. If this fails, inotropes and/or pacing may be required. It is important that these patients are neither under- nor overtransfused. The former leads to further spinal injury, the latter leads to pulmonary oedema. A central line is an important way of monitoring the patient's condition.

Early insertion of an arterial line is necessary to provide continuous, accurate blood pressure recordings as well as facilitating repeated arterial blood gas sampling. High doses of methyl prednisolone in the first 24 h after blunt spinal injury are beneficial (see box below). The reason for this improvement is not known, but workers have postulated that it could be due to a decrease in lipid peroxidation, protein degradation, catabolic activity or an increase in impulse conduction by activation of ion pumps.

The early use of methyl prednisolone following blunt spinal injury

30 mg/kg IV over 15 min immediately
Then 5.4 mg/kg/h for 23 h

MONITORING AND ONGOING CARE

The shocked patient's vital signs should be continuously monitored (see next box). Be aware, however, that despite this monitoring it is still possible to miss ongoing tissue hypoxaemia. Consequently, a number of other devices of varying complexity and invasiveness are available (pulmonary capillary wedge

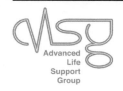

pressure, gastric tonometry, right ventricular diastolic volume index, subcutaneous and muscle oxygenation). However, the risks and practical problems associated with using some of these devices need to be weighed against their potential benefits.

In the shocked patient, coexistent pathology can be present and for those with ischaemic heart disease, the increase in cardiac work and oxygen demand may be critical. Often these patients will require more invasive monitoring and the care of at least a high dependency environment.

Monitored vital signs in hypovolaemic patients

Respiratory rate
Peripheral oxygen saturation
Heart rate
Blood pressure
Pulse pressure
Capillary refill
Chest leads (ECG rhythm and wave form)
Temperature (core and peripheral)
Urinary output
Glasgow Coma score

Time Out 9.2

Take a moment to write down how you would manage a 60-year-old man who presents after a haematemesis. Initial vital signs recorded by the nurse are:

Respiratory rate	28/min
SpO$_2$	92% (air)
Pulse rate	120/min
Blood pressure	90/60
Pale, sweating and anxious	

SUMMARY

There are many causes of shock, but all lead to inadequate delivery of oxygen to vital tissues. The management goal is to treat hypoxaemia and hypovolaemia, whilst excluding the immediately life-threatening conditions. It is also important to realise that resuscitation, though crucial, only plays a preliminary part in the patient's long-term management. It is therefore important that shocked patients receive multispecialty input from the beginning.

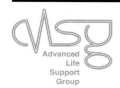

CHAPTER 10

The patient with chest pain

OBJECTIVES

After reading this chapter you will be able to:
- identify and treat immediate life-threatening causes of chest pain
- formulate a differential diagnosis for non-immediately life-threatening causes of chest pain
- discuss the investigation and management of other causes of chest pain.

INTRODUCTION

Chest pain has many underlying causes and these range from the immediately life-threatening to the trivial. The nature of the pain (site, severity, radiation and associations) varies with the actual cause, but in clinical practice immediately life-threatening causes (next box) can be difficult to identify rapidly. Therefore, a structured approach to care is advocated, starting with a primary assessment and resuscitation followed by secondary assessment and emergency treatments.

Life-threatening causes of chest pain

Myocardial infarction
Dissecting aortic aneurysm
Massive pulmonary embolus
Tension pneumothorax
Oesophageal rupture

PRIMARY ASSESSMENT AND RESUSCITATION

This concentrates on evaluating and maintaining the ABCs. If the patient is conscious, it is usually also possible to gain key information about their chest pain at the same time.

Airway

Airway patency must be assessed and secured where necessary. If the patient's conscious level is fluctuating, then simple airway adjuncts may be needed. If the airway cannot be maintained despite these measures, then endotracheal intubation may be needed. Tolerance of a Guedel airway suggests the patient's airway is

Acute Medical Emergencies; The Practical Approach, 2nd edition.
Edited by Terence Wardle, Peter Driscoll, and Sue Wieteska.
© 2010 Blackwell Publishing Ltd.

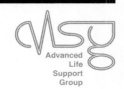

currently unprotected from the risk of gastric aspiration (although prompt resuscitation may improve this situation).

Breathing

All patients will require high concentrations of inspired oxygen at 12–15 l/min, via a non-rebreathing mask with reservoir.

The rate, symmetry and effort of respiration should be noted. Palpation in the sternal notch will determine if there is tracheal deviation or tug. After percussing the anterior chest wall for areas of hyper-resonance or dullness, breath sounds should be auscultated and any additional sounds, such as a pleural rub, identified.

Inadequate breathing should be supported – initially by bag–valve–mask ventilation and then by intubation and mechanical ventilation. Pulmonary emboli producing pleuritic chest pain are, in themselves, rarely life-threatening. However, such a symptom should raise the clinician's suspicion of the potential for a larger embolus that may have a significant haemodynamic effect, including pulseless electrical activity (PEA, or previously electromechanical dissociation).

Tension pneumothoraces are a rare cause of chest pain, but are rapidly fatal if ignored. You must be alert to this problem, in particular in patients with pre-existing lung disease. Once the diagnosis has been made, time should not be wasted getting X-rays. An immediate needle thoracocentesis is required. This converts the tension into a simple pneumothorax and allows time for chest drain insertion.

Circulation

Check for the presence of an arterial pulse and assess the rate. The carotid artery is the first choice but radial, carotid and femoral arteries should be palpated to determine their pressure, volume and radio-radial or radio-femoral delay. Check the precordium for the position and character of the apex beat, plus any thrills or heaves. Listen for the presence of normal, altered and added heart sounds, as well as murmurs.

Ideally, all patients should have IV access – the antecubital fossa is usually the easiest site. Monitoring should include SpO_2, pulse, blood pressure and ECG.

Immediate investigations

All patients with non-traumatic chest pain will require an immediate 12-lead ECG, as it can help in differentiating the causes of chest pain (next box).

Key point
A normal ECG does not exclude an acute coronary syndrome of any sort

A diagnosis of myocardial infarct made on ECG should lead to rapid emergency treatment. A 12-lead ECG may be normal during the evolution of myocardial infarct. If pericarditis is present, then the classic concave ST elevation occurs in the leads that lie over the affected area.

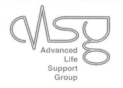

ECG features of immediately life-threatening causes of chest pain	
Myocardial infarction	Normal
	1 mm (01 mV) ST elevation in two of the inferior leads (II, III and aVF)
	1 mm (01 mV) ST elevation in leads 1 and aVL
	2 mm (02 mV) ST elevation in two contiguous anterior chest leads
	New left bundle branch block
	True posterior infarct
Pulmonary emboli	Normal
	Sinus tachycardia
	Atrial fibrillation or tachycardia
	Right axis deviation
	Symmetrical T wave inversion in the anterior chest leads
	Right ventricular strain
	Right bundle branch block
Dissecting aortic aneurysm	Normal
	Signs of left ventricular hypertrophy and strain due to hypertension
	Acute ischaemic changes, including changes of classical myocardial infarction, when coronary ostia are involved (very rare)

Once intravenous access has been secured, blood should be taken for full blood count, markers of myocardial damage (e.g. troponin I or T), electrolytes and blood glucose. If a dissecting aneurysm is suspected, blood transfusion may be required and, therefore, a sample should be taken for cross-match. Arterial blood gas measurement is also ideally required to exclude any underlying acid–base disturbance, ventilation–perfusion mismatch and inadequate ventilation.

SECONDARY ASSESSMENT

Immediately life-threatening conditions are rare, but it is important that they have been excluded or treated. Attention can then be directed to the secondary assessment, where the crucial exclusions are myocardial infarction, pulmonary embolus, oesophageal rupture, pneumonia and pneumothorax. These last two conditions are usually easily diagnosed radiologically; therefore, the essential management plan is to rule out myocardial infarction and pulmonary embolus. If neither myocardial infarction nor pulmonary embolism seems likely, oesophageal rupture should be considered. Other minor conditions can be investigated, often as an outpatient.

History
Clinical diagnoses are frequently made on the basis of a medical history. The features of chest pain should be assessed in a regular and orderly sequence, paying particular attention to the site, character, radiation, precipitation and relieving factors as well as any other associated symptoms.

A pertinent history can provide invaluable clues as to the differential diagnosis of conditions giving rise to chest pain.

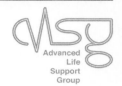

A patient with an acute myocardial infarct and associated ECG changes should be identified immediately and treated appropriately. The remaining patients will have diagnoses ranging from acute coronary syndrome to musculoskeletal pain. While the particular diagnosis in individual patients may take some time to establish, the risks of either myocardial infarction or of later complications can be rapidly assessed by repeating and reviewing the ECGs, taking a focused history and examining the patient. This will allow appropriate decisions about further care to be made.

The most important finding is a history of cardiac-type chest pain, and any patient presenting with such a history requires continuous ECG monitoring in an area where cardiopulmonary resuscitation – especially defibrillation – can be provided immediately. Subsequent investigations by assay of chemical markers of cardiac damage, particularly cardiac troponins, will both help identify patients with cardiac ischaemia presenting with normal ECGs and will help risk stratify all patients, as does pre-discharge exercise testing or nuclear perfusion imaging. Both ECG and clinical findings can predict a high risk of subsequent myocardial infarction and its complications. Dynamic ECG changes, elevation of troponin levels or clinical evidence of left ventricular dysfunction are adverse findings and should prompt consideration of early – pre-discharge – coronary angiography. The approach to clinical risk assessment is shown in Fig. 10.1.

The pain from a dissecting thoracic aortic aneurysm may be severe and poorly responsive to opiates. It usually starts in the centre of the chest, radiates through to the back between the scapulae and may involve the upper limbs. It is often described as tearing, but the nature of the pain may change as the dissection progresses. Dilatation of the aortic root caused by aortic dissection can lead to aortic valve incompetence and regurgitation. Any patient who has evidence of both myocardial infarction and aortic regurgitation should be screened for aortic dissection. Risk factors need to be sought, in particular a family history of ischaemic heart disease, hyperlipidaemia, hypertension, diabetes mellitus, Marfan's syndrome, homocystinuria, procoagulant disorder and a history of cigarette smoking. Oral contraceptive pill use or pregnancy may influence the differential diagnosis, as may the patient's occupation.

Tension pneumothorax can present with progressive dyspnoea, occasionally pleuritic pain, and in extreme cases, a cardiorespiratory arrest. A similar range of presentations may be encountered in patients with pulmonary emboli. It is therefore important to enquire about the history of breathlessness and haemoptysis, as this may help in establishing the correct diagnosis (see Chapter 8).

Oesophageal rupture is a rare cause of severe chest pain, but carries a poor prognosis if not recognised early. Whereas myocardial infarction often has chest pain associated with vomiting, oesophageal rupture has vomiting as an initial symptom, followed by chest pain caused by mediastinitis. The pain is severe and often there are no clinical signs. Be wary of diagnosing a 'functional disorder'.

The clinician should ascertain additional information, so that a well-'phrased' history has been obtained by the end of the secondary assessment.

Examination

The secondary assessment ensures that the physical examination started in the primary assessment is completed in a comprehensive fashion. The blood pressure, pulse pressure and the height and character of the jugular venous pulse should also be recorded. Assessment of the site and character of the apex beat, as well as the presence of normal and additional heart sounds can then be done.

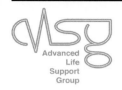

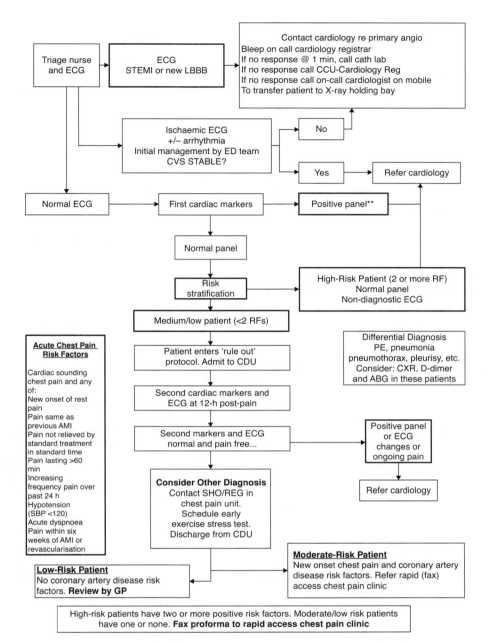

Fig. 10.1 Chest pain assessment.

Occasionally, a blowing early diastolic murmur may be heard when a dissecting thoracic aortic aneurysm has involved the aortic valve. This may be the only initial physical sign.

The clinician should then consider and integrate the facts from the history with the examination findings to pinpoint the cause of the chest pain. The commonest causes of chest pain are listed in Tables 10.1–10.5. For clarity, these are divided into body systems:

- Cardiac chest pain
- Chest pain caused by respiratory disease and oesophageal rupture
- Chest pain caused by gastrointestinal disease
- Chest wall pain
- Functional chest pain

Table 10.1 Clinical features of cardiac chest pain

	Ischaemia	Pericarditis
Site	Retrosternal Deep Arms alone (infrequently)	Surface – according to site of pericarditis
Character	Constricting, band like, heavy	Sharp
Radiation	Left arm > right arm Throat/jaw/teeth (rare)	Left arm > right arm Throat (very rare)
Precipitation (**Stable angina only**)	Exertion Cold winds Anxiety Heavy meals	Deep inspiration Coughing Postural variation – according to site of pericarditis
Relief (**Stable angina only**)	Rest Nitrates (within 1–2 min)	Postural variation
Associated symptoms	Strangling sensation in the throat	Occasionally pleuritic pain (on respiration)
Clinical examination	Limited value Occasionally signs of hyperlipidaemia or atherosclerosis	Pericardial rub

Table 10.2 Clinical features of chest pain caused by respiratory disease and oesophageal rupture

	Pleuritic	Spontaneous pneumothorax	Mediastinitis
Site	Anterior/lateral/posterior	Anterior/lateral/posterior or none	Mid-line Retrosternal
Character	Sharp, stabbing, catching	Sharp, stabbing, catching	Usually stabbing, but may mimic cardiac pain if severe
Radiation	Shoulder tip if basal pleuritis		Neck, back
Precipitation	Coughing Deep inspiration	Coughing Deep inspiration	Coughing Deep inspiration Postural variation
Relief	Shallow breathing Postural variation	Shallow breathing	Postural variation
Associated symptoms	(a) Infective 　　Cough 　　Purulent sputum 　　Prodromal symptoms (b) Embolic 　　Cough 　　Breathless 　　Haemoptysis (see earlier)	Breathless Cough (see earlier re: Tension pneumothorax)	Cough Neck and facial subcutaneous emphysema
Clinical examination	Pleural rub ± signs of consolidation	Hyper-resonant percussion note Reduced breath sounds	Mediastinal friction rub Subcutaneous emphysema

Table 10.3 Clinical features of chest pain caused by gastrointestinal disease

	Peptic ulcer disease	Gastro-oesophageal reflux disease – GORD	Diffuse oesophageal spasm
Site	Epigastric Right hypochondrium	Retrosternal Epigastric	Retrosternal Deep
Character	Postprandial constant/gnawing	Burning	Squeezing Constricting
Radiation	Posteriorly (posterior duodenal ulcer)	Retrosternal Throat	Throat Arms (rare)
Precipitation	Eating Alcohol	Drinking Eating Lying/bending	–
Relief	Acid suppressants Antacids	Standing Antacids Acid suppressants	Antispasmodics Nitrates
Associated symptoms	Nausea Vomiting Waterbrash	Nausea Waterbrash Bronchospasm	Dysphagia
Clinical examination	Epigastric tenderness	Often overweight	Often associated with GORD

Table 10.4 Clinical features of chest wall pain

	Muscular	Cervical spondylosis	Costochondritis	Herpes zoster (shingles)
Site	Intercostal, periscapular, localised	Upper chest, arms (corresponding to nerve root involved)	Costochondral junctions	Chest wall dermatomes
Character	Sharp, stabbing ache	Ache Constant	Ache Sharp	Severe lancing
Radiation	Shoulder	Arms Inframammary	–	Affected nerve root(s)
Precipitation	Coughing Deep inspiration Physical effort involving upper limbs	Movement Physical effort involving upper limbs	Deep inspiration Lying on anterior chest wall	Previous varicella zoster
Relief	Rest Analgesia (NSAIDs) Heat	Rest Analgesia (NSAIDs) Immobilisation	Anti-inflammatory drugs (NSAIDs)	Analgesia Aciclovir Carbamazepine
Associated symptoms	Focal tenderness over muscle mimicked by compression of thoracic cage, movement of muscle group	Paraesthesia (nerve root distribution)	Focal erythema/swelling Tenderness over joint	Erythematous vesicular rash (pain precedes rash)
Clinical examination	Focal tenderness	Restricted neck movement Nerve root signs	Focal erythema/tenderness	Rash

Table 10.5 Clinical features of functional chest pain

Site	Anywhere
	Often left inframammary
Character	Often sharp and stabbing, but may be dull
	Often unrelenting, lasting many hours or even days
Radiation	None, usually
	Arms, infrequently
Precipitation	Anxiety
	Tension
Relief	Reassurance
	Treat underlying cause
Associated symptoms	Palpitations
	Breathless
	Headaches
	Other somatic symptoms
Clinical examination	Unremarkable

EMERGENCY TREATMENT

ST elevation myocardial infarction

In the presence of myocardial infarction, aspirin and vasodilators, i.e. sublingual or intravenous nitrates, will be required. If this combination fails to relieve pain, then opiates should be used. Direct reperfusion with percutaneous coronary intervention is the treatment of choice, if available within 90 min. Pre-treatment with clopidogrel 600 mg and heparin 5000 IE IV can be given, depending on local protocols, along with the aspirin and nitrates.

If coronary intervention is not available, thrombolysis should be started as soon as possible, provided there are no contraindications (next box). Clinical trials have shown that the beneficial effect of thrombolysis is significantly reduced with time, particularly if it is started over 12 h after the onset of chest pain.

Contraindications to thrombolysis

History of gastrointestinal or genitourinary bleeding in the previous two months
Recent major surgery (including dental extraction), trauma, biopsy or head injury
History of intracranial or spinal cord haemorrhage, aneurysm or neoplasm
History of cerebrovascular disease, especially recent events or with any residual disability
Reduced level of consciousness
History of bleeding disorder
Pregnancy or heavy vaginal bleeding (normal menstrual period is not a contraindication)
Traumatic cardiopulmonary resuscitation within the previous 10 days
Non-compressible intra-arterial diagnostic procedures within previous 14 days
Aortic dissection
Acute pancreatitis
Severe liver disease, oesophageal varices

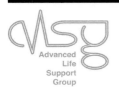

Systolic blood pressure greater than 200 mm Hg or diastolic greater than 110 mm Hg (Thrombolysis may be given if treatment successfully lowers BP to acceptable levels)

The benefits of thrombolysis can be expected to be:

Greatest in patients presenting early – within 4 h, with extensive ST segment changes in many leads, with marked ST segment elevation – more than 5 mm and involving the anterior chest leads – V1 to V6

Least in patients presenting late – approaching 12 h, with limited ST segment changes – in few leads with minor ST segment elevation – 1 or 2 mm and involving the inferior leads – II, III and aVF

The risks of thrombolysis are not time dependant and there is, in particular, a risk of intracerebral haemorrhage of 1%, with half of these patients dying and half of the survivors being disabled. In the elderly, this risk increases to 2.4% in those over 75 years of age. Those at greatest risk are older patients, with hypertension (systolic BP >140 mm Hg or diastolic BP >100 mm Hg) lighter body weight (<67 kg), female and black. Clinical judgements need to be made in each case to optimise patient care. If thrombolytic therapy is contraindicated, aspirin can still be given and affords equal benefit.

Unstable angina and non-ST elevation myocardial infarction (NSTEMI)

In common with all patients with possible cardiac chest pain, patients with unstable angina and NSTEMI should receive aspirin and appropriate analgesia. Antithrombotic therapy should be given to all patients with unstable angina or NSTEMI. Low molecular weight heparin is more effective than unfractionated heparin at reducing the incidence of ischaemic events and the need for revascularisation procedures. The incidence of major bleeding complications is the same for both forms of heparin. Thus, all patients who have chest pain of probable cardiac origin and who are not eligible for fibrinolytic drugs should receive low molecular weight heparin. Patients who have high risk features such as dynamic ECG changes or elevated cardiac troponin levels, are also candidates for additional antiplatelet therapy with glycoprotein IIb/IIIa receptor inhibitors depending on local protocols

Pulmonary embolus

If the diagnosis is suspected, start treatment with heparin (either unfractionated or low molecular weight) immediately, after which embolic, pleuritic pain often melts away within 2–6 h. Thrombolysis is a useful therapeutic adjunct in severe disease (see Chapter 8 and 9).

Dissecting aortic aneurysm

This condition is rare, but be alert to the patient with classical myocardial infarction and aortic regurgitation who may have aortic dissection. When a dissecting aortic aneurysm is discovered, the optimum systolic blood pressure is considered to be 100 mm Hg. This may be achieved by either pharmacological reduction of hypertension or titrated fluid replacement with hypotension. Cardiothoracic advice must be sought urgently.

Tension Pneumothorax

This is considered in detail in Chapter 8.

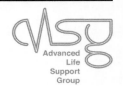

Oesophageal Rupture

This condition is also rare, and like dissecting aortic aneurysm rarity leads to difficulties in diagnosis which, if delayed, can significantly increase mortality due to the development of mediastinitis. Oesophageal rupture occurs when vomiting takes place against a closed glottis and is often associated with alcohol excess. The sequence of events is that of vomiting then chest pain, rather than the opposite order, which may occur in myocardial infarction. Other causes include therapeutic, and occasionally diagnostic, upper gastrointestinal endoscopy. The patients suffer severe pain that seems out of proportion to other symptoms and signs, especially when initial tests are negative. Hence such patients may be diagnosed as 'functional pain'. Beware! The diagnosis is usually made from the history. The key finding is the presence of air in the mediastinum on chest X-ray, or clinically as surgical emphysema in the subcutaneous tissues of the neck. Arrange for urgent assessment by an intensivist and either an upper gastrointestinal or cardiothoracic surgeon.

DEFINITIVE CARE

After taking a history and examining the patient, the clinician will have either established a diagnosis or postulated a differential diagnosis. The patient with a suspected acute coronary syndrome will be transferred to coronary care, whilst patients with other causes of chest pain will be managed – at least initially – either in another critical care area or on a medical ward. Appropriate investigations will then be required to confirm or refute these conclusions. The choice will depend on which body system(s) is involved.

Investigations

ECG

All patients with chest pain need 12-lead ECGs. Those with possible acute coronary syndromes should have continuous electrocardiograph monitoring, during their initial assessment. Exercise stress testing is a useful tool for risk stratification, both after myocardial infarction and other acute coronary syndromes, where it is used to identify potential candidates for coronary angiography. In addition, it is used to identify patients with ischaemic heart disease who have not shown any other markers following their presentation with chest pain

Imaging

Chest X-ray

A chest X-ray is of limited diagnostic use in patients with angina and myocardial infarction, unless the latter is complicated by heart failure and/or aneurysm of the left ventricle. Similarly, it is usually unremarkable in patients with pericarditis unless there is a coexisting pericardial effusion. A plain chest radiograph may be normal in uncomplicated pleuritis and even with pulmonary emboli. It may, however, show evidence of pulmonary parenchymal infection and either a wedge shaped peripheral defect or hyperlucency associated with pulmonary embolus. Atelectasis is also a manifestation of both of these conditions. A chest X-ray is essential for diagnosing spontaneous, simple pneumothorax, especially when the film is taken in expiration.

In the case of dissecting aneurysm, a chest X-ray may show widening of the mediastinum, deviation of trachea to the right, elevation of right main bronchus and depression of left main bronchus, a pleural cap, the obliteration of the aorticopulmonary window and, more obviously, the aortic knuckle.

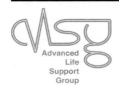

The chest X-ray may be normal in a patient with an oesophageal rupture. Other features include air in the mediastinum and/or soft tissues of the neck, and a pleural effusion.

VQ scans

Ventilation perfusion (VQ) scans are rarely used for the immediate diagnosis of pulmonary emboli.

CT Pulmonary Angiography

This is the investigation of choice in patients with suspected pulmonary embolic disease (see Chapter 8).

Echocardiogram

Transthoracic echocardiography is helpful in the diagnosis of pericardial effusion and dissecting aneurysm. However, in the latter, a trans-oesophageal echocardiogram is preferred. CT aortography is an alternative, which may be more readily available, and magnetic resonance imaging has also been used. Transthoracic echocardiography may also help in assessing valvular pathology, pulmonary artery pressures and the presence of thrombus as well as function of the left and right ventricles and atria.

Markers of myocardial damage

These should be requested in all patients with chest pain.

The traditional markers of creatine phosphokinase, aspartate transaminase and lactate dehydrogenase are being superceded by newer tests. Other markers such as the cardiac troponins, Troponin I and T, are used in routine clinical practice. It is important to be aware of your local laboratory protocols and reference ranges.

Endoscopy

Endoscopy is essential for investigating peptic ulcer as well as gastro-oesophageal reflux disease. A normal endoscopy, however, does not exclude this disease and formal pH manometry and a semisolid phase barium swallow may be required to confirm the diagnosis – similarly for diffuse spasm.

Either a barium swallow and/or a CT scan are needed in order to investigate suspected oesophageal perforation. Endoscopy should be avoided unless it is done by the surgeon who is contemplating an operation.

DIAGNOSTIC PITFALLS

- Treat all patients with a good history of cardiac type chest pain as having an acute cardiac syndrome until proven otherwise.
- Remember that elderly patients may have atypical presentations of acute cardiac ischaemia and have fewer ECG changes.
- Diabetic patients may have 'silent ischaemia' as may elderly patients.
- Patients with chest pain, irrespective of the cause, will manifest clinical features of anxiety.
- Always reassess every episode of chest pain as though it were the first, even in frequent attenders.
- The absence of deep vein thrombosis does not rule out a diagnosis of pulmonary embolus.
- If the patient's history suggests a pneumothorax but there is no radiological evidence, re-evaluate the X-ray for evidence of pneumomediastinum.

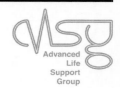

- A normal chest X-ray and white cell count does not exclude the diagnosis of pulmonary infection.
- Rapid pain relief with nitrates does not point to a diagnosis of angina – diffuse oesophageal spasm responds in an identical fashion.
- Gastro-oesophageal reflux is a common problem and does not indicate that chest pain is due to this cause.

SUMMARY

- Chest pain is a common presentation requiring acute medical admission.
- Most causes of chest pain are not immediately life-threatening.
- Rule out myocardial infarction and pulmonary embolus in patients with a compatible history.

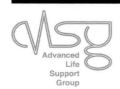
Advanced
Life
Support
Group

CHAPTER 11

The patient with altered conscious level

OBJECTIVES

After reading this chapter you should be able to:
- understand the physiology of the conscious state and how this may be disturbed
- understand how the structured approach can be applied to the unconscious patient
- discuss the initial management of such a patient
- discuss how clinical signs detected in the secondary assessment will influence your diagnosis and subsequent management.

INTRODUCTION

The care of the unconscious patient is a common medical emergency. To understand why patients become unconscious, it is necessary to review briefly the physiology of consciousness, by considering:
- neurophysiology
- cerebral metabolism
- cerebral perfusion
- intracranial pressure.

Neurophysiology

There are two interlinked areas that are of paramount importance in maintaining the conscious state:
- the reticular formation
- the cerebral cortex.

The reticular formation arises in the brain stem, in the midst of a host of neural pathways communicating between the brain and spinal cord and vice versa. It contains the primary centres for cardiovascular and respiratory control, as well as a distinct area called the reticular activating system (RAS). This is crucial for maintaining the conscious state. Neurones in the RAS system pass via the thalamus to synapse in the cortex. There is no specific individual area in the cortex that is responsible for the conscious state, but the coordinated interaction of many cortical areas is required.

It is important to note that the cerebral cortex and the interconnections (including thalamus and hypothalamus) have to be affected bilaterally to affect consciousness. Metabolic disorders, toxins, hypoxaemia and a postictal state are more

Acute Medical Emergencies; The Practical Approach, 2nd edition.
Edited by Terence Wardle, Peter Driscoll, and Sue Wieteska.
© 2010 Blackwell Publishing Ltd.

likely to affect conscious level by affecting the cerebral cortices, whereas the RAS is affected by supratentorial pressure, infratentorial pressure or intrinsic brainstem lesions.

Cerebral metabolism

Glucose and oxygen are the essential fuels for cerebral metabolism. The brain, however, only has a small store of glucose and thus its supply is critically dependent on adequate cerebral blood flow. In practice, the brain can only function for approximately 2–3 min in the absence of glucose. If the brain is deprived of both glucose and oxygen, as in cardiorespiratory arrest, then normal energy metabolism can only continue for about 15 s.

Cerebral perfusion

Adequate ventilation and cerebral perfusion are necessary to ensure that the brain is provided with oxygen and glucose. Under normal resting conditions, the brain receives approximately 15–20% of the resting cardiac output. Cerebral blood flow is autoregulated to ensure a constant supply of blood with a mean arterial pressure of 60–160 mm Hg. Within this range, a rise in blood pressure is balanced by intracranial vasoconstriction and, conversely, a fall by vasodilatation. Cerebral blood flow depends not only on the mean arterial pressure, but also on the resistance to blood flow due to intracranial pressure and, to a lesser extent, the central venous pressure.

Cerebral perfusion pressure (CPP) = mean arterial pressure − intracranial pressure

Autoregulation is impaired in conditions like infection and trauma, and, in particular, chronic hypertension. However, under normal circumstances, if cerebral blood flow falls (mean arterial pressure drops below 60 mm Hg) then cerebral ischaemia occurs. In contrast, cerebral oedema and hypertensive encephalopathy may ensue if the mean arterial pressure exceeds 160 mm Hg.

Intracranial pressure

In the adult the volume of the intracranial contents, comprising the brain, cerebrospinal fluid, blood and blood vessels, is fixed by the surrounding rigid skull. These contents produce an intracranial pressure of 6–13 mm Hg. To maintain this normal range, any increase in volume of one of the contents must be balanced by a corresponding decrease in one or more of the others.

The brain is a compliant organ that will mould to accommodate an increase in pressures. Furthermore, cerebrospinal fluid can be displaced into the spinal system and the volume of cerebral venous fluid, in particular within the dural sinuses, can be displaced into the systemic venous circulation. These mechanisms will initially offset any rise in intracranial pressure.

Once these normal compensatory measures are exhausted, any further small increase in intracranial volume will lead to large increases in intracranial pressure, which, in turn, will reduce cerebral perfusion pressure.

Therefore, disruption of one or more of these four mechanisms will result in loss of consciousness.

CAUSES OF COMA

The causes of coma are listed in Tables 11.1–11.3 according to the presence of neck stiffness and/or lateralising signs.

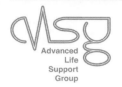

Table 11.1 Causes of coma: no menigism: no focal/lateralising signs

Drug overdose	Daily
Ischaemia/hypoxaemia*	Daily
Hypoglycaemia*	Daily
Cardiac failure	Daily
Respiratory failure	Daily
Alcohol*	Daily
Renal failure	Weekly
Diabetic ketoacidosis	Weekly
Hepatic failure*	Monthly
Hyponatraemia	Monthly
Sepsis	Monthly
Wernicke's encephalopathy	Monthly
Carbon monoxide poisoning	Annually
Hypernatraemia	Annually
Hypothermia	Annually

*These rarely present with focal signs.

Table 11.2 Causes of coma and neck stiffness: no focal/lateralising signs

Bacterial meningitis	Daily
Encephalitis	Weekly
Subarachnoid haemorrhage	Weekly
Cerebral/Cerebellar haemorrhage with extension into subarachnoid space	Monthly
Cerebral malaria	Only in exams

Table 11.3 Causes of coma with focal/lateralising signs

Intracerebral tumour	Daily
Intracerebral haemorrhage	Daily
Intracerebral infarction	Daily
Intracerebral abscess	Monthly

PRIMARY ASSESSMENT AND RESUSCITATION

In the primary assessment, airway, breathing and circulation need to be assessed and managed appropriately. Irrespective of the underlying pathology, every effort should be made to prevent secondary brain damage by identifying and treating hypoxaemia, hypercapnia, hypotension, hypoglycaemia and raised intracranial pressure.

Senior help including an anaesthetist should be sought immediately for all comatose patients, who should be managed – initially – in the resuscitation area.

A – airway and cervical spine

In the patient with altered consciousness, the potential for airway obstruction is high.

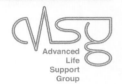

Clear and control the airway using the techniques described in Chapter 4. If a patient is comatose (a Glasgow Coma Score of eight or less), the risk of aspiration is increased if the gag reflex is absent, swallowing (even saliva) is uncoordinated and the airway is unprotected. In such cases, the insertion of a cuffed endotracheal tube, by means of rapid sequence induction of anaesthesia should be considered. All patients require high concentrations of inspired oxygen using an appropriate delivery system.

Acute cervical spine problems are rare in acute medicine, but be wary of the patient found unconscious/confused at the bottom of the stairs. Consider a potential cervical spine/cord injury if there is no clear history, and especially if there are external signs of trauma above the clavicle. Seek specialist help to immobilise the cervical spine if you are concerned.

B – breathing

Unconscious patients often have low respiratory rates and if less than 10/min, may need assisted ventilation. Ensure the patient is connected to a pulse oximeter.

Patients in respiratory distress (i.e. respiratory rate greater than 30) may have a life-threatening chest problem. Examination of the chest during the primary assessment is designed specifically to pick up any such chest problems. Give naloxone (100 µg/min IV or 400 µg IM if IV access is not possible) to any patient with signs of opioid toxicity. Intubation and ventilation should be considered if the respiratory rate is less than 10/min and there is inadequate or no response to naloxone.

C – circulation

Shock has to be treated appropriately to prevent secondary brain injury. Once intravenous access is established, blood should be taken for immediate glucose estimation, using a glucometer. Unless hypoglycaemia (<4 mmol/l) can be excluded rapidly and reliably, 50 ml of 50% dextrose should be given intravenously. If intravenous access is difficult, glucagon 1 mg intramuscularly should be given instead.

Thiamine deficiency can occur in any acutely ill patient, especially those with chronic liver disease, folate deficiency, malnutrition, anorexia nervosa and high alcohol intake. Thiamine should be given intravenously (for at least 3 days) especially in patients with Wernicke's encephalopathy.

In addition to the 'routine' blood tests, arterial blood gases must be measured. Patients should be connected to the cardiac monitor and a urinary catheter inserted if the unconsciousness is not quickly reversed.

D – disability

The initial neurological assessment should be a rapid evaluation of the Glasgow Coma Score and pupil size, equality and reaction to light. Check for meningeal irritation – if there are no contraindications. Remember, at this stage, you are looking for conditions which are immediately life-threatening! Consider:
- hypoglycaemia
- antidotes, e.g. naloxone if pinpoint pupils/needle track marks
- antibiotics
- aciclovir
- antiepileptic drugs.

E – exposure

The patient must be fully exposed to allow complete assessment. The temperature must be taken, with a low reading rectal thermometer if necessary. Do not forget

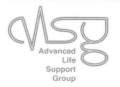

that hypothermia is an important cause of coma and should not be missed. Be wary of inducing hypothermia by fully exposing the patient. The patient's clothes should be searched for useful information such as medical cards, drugs and details of next of kin.

SECONDARY ASSESSMENT

The secondary assessment should only be done once the immediately life-threatening conditions have been treated. A well-'phrased' history should be sought, followed by a complete examination. Further appropriate investigations can be requested.

History

The history is particularly important in this context and must be sought from attending relatives, friends, paramedics and other witnesses. Additional and useful information may be obtained from the hospital notes or the general practitioner.

Examination

A thorough head-to-toe examination of the patient should then take place, looking for evidence of precipitating factors such as head injury, infection, drug use and vascular pathology. In the unconscious patient, particular attention should be paid to the following:
- level of consciousness
- assessment of brain stem function
- focal neurological signs.

Level of consciousness

The Glasgow Coma Scale (GCS, range 3–15) gives a qualitative measurement of the patient's conscious level. The Glasgow Coma Score is the sum of scores in three areas of assessment.
E – best eye opening
V – best verbal response
M – best motor response

Eye opening response

Response	Score
Spontaneous	4
To speech	3
To painful stimuli	2
Nil	1

Verbal response

Response	Score
Orientated	5
Confused	4
Inappropriate words	3
Incomprehensible sounds	2
Nil	1

Motor response

Response	Score
Obeys commands	6
Localises pain	5
Withdraws from pain	4
Abnormal flexion (decorticate)	3
Abnormal extension (decerebrate)	2
Nil	1

If the patient does not respond to commands, then a painful stimulus is applied by pressure on the supraorbital ridge. If assessment of a verbal response is not possible, e.g.due to an *in situ* endotracheal tube, then this fact should be documented in the patient's notes. The best response of any limb is recorded. If there are differences between limbs, this may suggest a potential neurological lesion. Patients who have a GCS of eight or less are by definition comatose. It is important to recheck the GCS every 15 min.

Assessment of brain stem function

The initial brain stem assessment comprises:

- pupillary response
- eye movements
- corneal response
- respiratory pattern.

Pupillary response

The size, shape and response to light of both pupils should be assessed. An understanding of the common changes in pupillary reflexes is important as this will help to localise lesions (see Table 11.4).

Table 11.4 Pupillary abnormalities

	Pupillary response	Cause
Equal pupils	Small + reactive	Metabolic encephalopathy
		Midbrain herniation
		Senile miosis
	Pinpoint + fixed	Pontine lesion
		Opioids, organophosphates
	Dilated + reactive	Metabolic cause
		Midbrain lesion
		Ecstacy, amphetamines
	Dilated + fixed	Peri ictal
		Hypoxaemia
		Hypothermia
		Anticholinergics
Unequal pupils	Small + reactive	Horner's syndrome
	Small + 'non reactive'	Argyll Robertson (tertiary syphilis)
	Dilated + fixed	Uncal herniation
		IIIrd nerve palsy

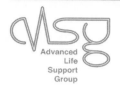

Eye movements

Many comatose patients have roving or dysconjugate eye movements; these are common and are of no particular significance.

The oculocephalic response (doll's head/eye movement) provides useful information about the oculomotor and vestibular components of brain stem function. Hold the eyelids open and observe eye movements. Illicit the response by quickly turning the head to the right and then to the left.

- Eyes move in opposite direction to head turn – normal
- Eyes move to one side but not the other – unilateral brain stem lesion – lateral gaze palsy
- Eyes fail to move in any direction – bilateral brain stem lesions

---

Key point

Do not attempt to elicit the oculocephalic response if cervical spine pathology is suspected

---

The oculovestibular (caloric) test is a much more potent stimulus to brain stem function than the oculocephalic reflex. It is more time consuming to perform and often unsuitable for emergency assessments. However, it is particularly useful in differentiating psychogenic unresponsiveness from coma.

Having first ensured that the ear drums are intact, the head is inclined at 30° to the trunk and the external auditory canal of one ear is irrigated with ice cold water while the eyes are held open. The following responses may occur:

- Tonic deviation of the eyes towards the irrigated ear in those comatose patients with an intact vestibular component.
- Nystagmus (the quick phase is away from the irrigated side) and vomiting in patients not in coma.
- No movement of the eyes when brain stem function is lost.
- Asymmetry of the oculovestibular response is characteristic of focal brain stem lesion.
- A fixed conjugate gaze due the absence of the fast component indicates cortical damage with an intact brainstem.

Corneal reflexes

They are usually preserved in coma. In the absence of drugs, the loss of this reflex is a very poor prognostic sign.

Respiratory pattern

Alterations in brain stem function produce a variety of respiratory patterns, which may help to localise the lesion. In practice, however, they are of limited value.

- Normal breathing (eupnoeic), e.g. postictal, metabolic coma
- Periodic breathing (Cheyne–Stokes), e.g. lesions in the thalamus and hypothalamus, though there are many non-cerebral causes, including heart failure
- Central neurogenic hyperventilation, e.g. lesions in the midbrain or upper pons
- Slow and irregular breathing (apneustic) lesions in the medulla
- Deep sighing respiration (Kussmaul's) associated with a metabolic acidosis.

Focal neurological signs

The motor system must be assessed for asymmetry of tone, response to pain and deep tendon reflexes. Focal signs with intact brain stem reflexes occur with a focal

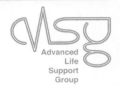

hemispheric lesion, whereas focal signs with absent brain stem reflexes are signs of a lesion in the posterior fossa. Assessment of the brain stem reflexes can be very valuable in localising the lesion and selecting patients for immediate further investigation, e.g. CT or MR scanning.

Key point

The absence of papilloedema does not exclude raised intracranial pressure

---

The fundi must always be examined. The presence of papilloedema indicates raised intracranial pressure. Subhyaloid haemorrhage should be sought as this may indicate subarachnoid haemorrhage or basal skull fracture. Furthermore, changes associated with diabetes mellitus and hypertension also need to be noted.

It cannot be overemphasised that the initial neurological examination is only the beginning. The initial findings are a 'baseline' for comparison with repeated neurological examinations.

Do not forget that specific evidence should also be sought of meningeal irritation (usually neck stiffness, Kernig's sign and Brudzinski's sign). Neck stiffness should not be elicited if cervical spine instability is suspected. It is important to realise that neck stiffness is often absent if the patient's conscious level is depressed.

Investigations
Neuroradiology
Computerised tomography (CT) of the brain is the primary investigation in coma. It is relatively quick and will identify 99% of supratentorial masses, especially when the non-contrast scan is supplemented with one using intravenous contrast. It is important to maintain adequate resuscitation during the scan. Restless or uncooperative patients will need to be electively anaesthetised, intubated and ventilated to get good quality images, avoiding movement artefact.

In comparison with CT scanning, cranial magnetic resonance imaging (MRI) is a more sensitive imaging modality. It not only will demonstrate most cerebral disease processes, but is also the ideal method for imaging posterior fossa lesions. These cannot be seen on CT imaging, because of obtrusive artefacts (e.g. the dense bone of the skull base). CT is the investigation of choice for subarachnoid haemorrhage as it is more sensitive for fresh blood. MRI is, however, highly sensitive for infective/inflammatory changes to cerebral tissue enabling identification of encephalitic disorders at an earlier stage when the CT scan will be normal. A further advantage is that magnetic resonance angiography can be done as a non-invasive, radiation-free technique for the investigation of intra- and extracerebral vascular structures. Unfortunately MRI is a very lengthy process when compared with CT scanning. Furthermore, it is extremely difficult to continue resuscitation in the MRI scanning area, as metal components are not allowed within the area of the 'magnet'. Therefore, for practical reasons, CT is still the initial modality of choice. It is important to realise that the scan must not delay the diagnosis and treatment of conditions like meningitis and encephalitis. These should be treated early with appropriate antibiotics and/or antiviral agents based on a clinical diagnosis before scanning.

Lumbar puncture
A lumbar puncture should not be done in the unconscious patient until a CT scan has excluded a mass lesion. Failure to do this may precipitate central/uncal

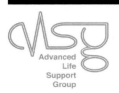

herniation as cerebrospinal fluid is drained via the lumbar puncture needle. Furthermore, a diagnosis of subarachnoid haemorrhage on CT will negate the need for lumbar puncture. However, CT scans can miss a small subarachnoid bleed and as this often heralds subsequent catastrophic haemorrhage, a lumbar puncture must be done in any patient who has a clinical history suggestive of subarachnoid haemorrhage and a negative CT scan. Other conditions which may cause coma and neck stiffness are shown in Table 11.2. See further details on lumbar puncture in Chapter 33.

It is important to remember that meningeal irritation may be absent when conscious levels are depressed. The pyrexial unconscious patient without evidence of mass lesion on CT scan will warrant a lumbar puncture. The prognosis is extremely poor for patients with meningitis who are unconscious before treatment is started.

Emergency management

The aims of emergency management are to maintain adequate cerebral metabolism and prevent and/or treat intracranial hypertension whilst a specific diagnosis is made and treatment started.

Maintain cerebral metabolism

The principal metabolic requirements of the brain are oxygen and glucose. Delivery of adequate levels of these substrates must be ensured. The oxygen content of the blood depends on the haemoglobin level and arterial oxygen concentration. The arterial oxygen concentration can be assessed using blood gas analysis and pulse oximetry. Low arterial oxygen tension also has profound effects on cerebral blood flow. When it falls below 50 mm Hg (6.7 kPa), there is a rapid increase in CBF and intracranial blood volume. Supplementary oxygen must be given to prevent this threshold being reached.

The concentration of glucose in the blood must be considered early and the brain must be protected from hypo- or hyperglycaemia. Close control of blood sugar concentrations between 4 and 8 mmol/l offers better preservation of cerebral function in hypoxaemia, cerebral haemorrhage and traumatic brain injury.

Maintain cerebral blood flow

The cerebral blood flow depends on the difference between systemic arterial pressure and intracranial pressure.

Systemic arterial pressure

The aim is to maintain a normal blood pressure, considering the nature of the intracranial pathology and pre-existing medical conditions, e.g. hypertension.

Although autoregulation will endeavour to preserve cerebral perfusion, causes of hypotension, e.g. hypovolaemia and sepsis, must be identified and treated immediately. Conversely, hypertension is often a compensatory response to maintain cerebral perfusion in patients with raised intracranial pressure. Therefore, treat the underlying condition and not the hypertension in patient with raised intracranial pressure. Any reduction in blood pressure will reduce cerebral perfusion pressure resulting in global cerebral infarction.

Intracranial pressure

Several approaches can be taken to keep pressure to acceptable levels:
- $PaCO_2$ should be kept within the normal range. Elevations in $PaCO_2$ will be associated with cerebral vasodilatation and exacerbate the raised intracranial

pressure. In contrast, hyperventilation will not only reduce the arterial carbon dioxide tension and hence reduce cerebral oedema, but also reduce cerebral blood flow, resulting in ischaemia. Keeping the $PaCO_2$ within the range 4.0–4.5 kPa should therefore be the goal. Seek an early liaison with an intensivist/neurosurgeon, maintain a normal $PaCO_2$ and monitor the $PaCO_2$ and intracranial pressure as required.

- Overhydration must be avoided as this may increase cerebral oedema.
- Hyperosmolar fluids must be avoided.
- Diuretics, either loop or osmotic, can be used in certain situations. Cerebral oedema formation is reduced as right atrial pressure is lowered. As the diuresis will produce a negative fluid balance, it is important to avoid jeopardising the circulation. Therefore, they should only be used in consultation with a neurosurgeon, intensivist or neurologist. Mannitol 0.5–1 g/kg is given to patients with signs of cerebral oedema and raised ICP. It is thought to exert its effects initially by increasing circulating blood volume and reducing blood viscosity (improving microcirculatory flow and oxygen delivery) and then reducing brain water by its osmotic action.
- *Corticosteroids*: These are commonly used in less urgent situations. Dexamethasone 4 mg 6 hourly may produce symptomatic relief by reducing tumour associated oedema. They have not been shown to be of benefit in any other situations except in pneumococcal meningitis where dexamethasone (give before the antibiotics) improved outcome. However, beware that dexamethasone reduces the concentration of vancomycin (the antibiotic of choice for penicillin resistant pneumococci).
- *Seizures*: Prolonged seizures are associated with brain damage. Therefore, they should be controlled rapidly. Lorazepam 4 mg intravenously should be used, as it has better ability to control seizures than diazepam. The dose can be repeated. If this is unsuccessful, then phenytoin, 15 mg/kg diluted in 0.9% saline, should be infused over 30 min. Fosphenytoin is a water-soluble pro-drug that is converted into phenytoin by non-specific phosphatases. In comparison with phenytoin, it can be infused faster, causes phlebitis and is soluble in dextrose. The patient should have ECG monitoring, as too rapid an infusion of phenytoin can cause hypotension, bradycardia and asystole. If phenytoin fails to control the seizures, an anaesthetic induction agent should be used and the patient anaesthetised and ventilated as necessary.
- *Temperature control*: Hyperthermia is detrimental to patients with intracerebral pathology. An elevated temperature increases metabolism and therefore substrate requirements, i.e. oxygen and glucose.

Time Out 11.1

Take a 15-min break from reading.
a. List the mechanisms that maintain consciousness.
b. Describe briefly how you would assess brain stem function.

SPECIFIC CONDITIONS

Subarachnoid haemorrhage
Pathophysiology

The causes of subarachnoid haemorrhage are shown in the next box.

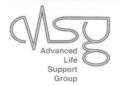

Causes of subarachnoid haemorrhage

Intracranial saccular aneurysm
Arteriovenous malformation
Others:
- extension from intracranial haemorrhage
- intracranial venous thrombosis
- haemostatic failure
- vascular tumour
- drug use

Conditions associated with intracranial saccular aneurysms

Polycystic kidney disease
Aortic stenosis
Infective endocarditis
Coarctation of the aorta
Thyromuscular dysplasia
Others:
- Marfan's syndrome
- Ehler–Danlos syndrome
- Pseudoxanthoma elasticum

The commonest cause is rupture of an intracranial saccular aneurysm. In contrast, only about 5% of patients bleed from arteriovenous malformations. Intracranial saccular aneurysms develop on medium-sized arteries at the base of the brain. The commonest sites are the distal internal carotid/posterior communicating artery and the anterior communicating artery complex. Multiple aneurysms are present in approximately 25% of patients. Aneurysms vary in size from a few millimetres to several centimetres in diameter. Whilst some are undoubtedly congenital, others develop during adult life, possibly as a consequence of atherosclerosis and hypertension. Conditions associated with intracranial saccular aneurysms are shown in the box above. The prevalence of unruptured aneurysms, as derived from prospective autopsy series, is in the region of 3/100 patients.

Assessment

Clinical features

The clinical picture is usually, but not always, dominated by an acute severe occipital headache. There may be a preceding history (usually over 1–2 weeks) of an acute transient severe headache, indicating a sentinel bleed. This can radiate over the head and, around, down into the neck, sometimes as far as the back or legs as blood tracks down the spinal cord. If the haemorrhage is extensive, the patient may become comatosed. If not, consciousness may be either lost transiently or impaired. Vomiting is common. Chemical meningitis (induced by blood) may take several hours to develop and focal signs are rare unless blood has extended into, or emanated from, the cerebral parenchyma. Occasionally, there is an oculomotor nerve palsy from a posterior communicating artery aneurysm. Arteriovenous

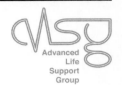

malformations may be diagnosed from the history because of recurrent unilateral migrainous headaches or very rarely on examination when an intracranial bruit is heard.

The patients are often irritable, confused and drowsy for several days. Headache may persist for weeks. Fundoscopy may reveal subhyaloid haemorrhages, which are believed to follow a rapid rise in intracranial pressure at the onset of intracranial haemorrhage.

Diagnosis

The diagnosis of subarachnoid haemorrhage is usually made on CT brain scan. However, a negative head CT does not exclude a subarachnoid haemorrhage. In these circumstances, a lumbar puncture (LP) is required. The three-tube test (i.e. a decreasing CSF red blood cell count in three consecutive tubes being indicative of a bloody tap) is unreliable. Only the absence of xanthrochromia, formally assessed by spectrophotometry, can be relied on to exclude subarachnoid haemorrhage following an LP. Xanthochromia refers to the yellowish discolouration of CSF supernatant from breakdown products of haemoglobin (oxyhaemoglobin and bilirubin). After a subarachnoid haemorrhage, red cells are gradually lysed within the CSF.

Released haemoglobin is metabolised to oxyhaemoglobin and bilirubin.. Oxyhaemoglobin can be detected within hours, but bilirubin requires up to 12 h to appear. Timing of an LP is therefore crucial and should be delayed until at least 12 h after the onset of symptoms. However, some neurosurgeons advocate immediate lumbar puncture irrespective of the time of the headache onset as blood may be detected. Thus, timing of the initial LP depends on local policy.

The CSF should be centrifuged and examined promptly so that red cells from a bloody tap do not undergo lysis *in vitro*. Xanthochromia is found in the CSF of all patients with subarachnoid haemorrhages from 12 h to 2 weeks after the haemorrhage, gradually disappearing thereafter.

The reliability of CT and lumbar puncture in the diagnosis of subarachnoid haemorrhage vary with time after the onset of headache as shown:

CT – detection of SAH		LP – presence of bilirubin	
<24 h	98%	1–12 h	Variable
24–48 h	86%	12 h–2 weeks	100%
2–5 days	76%	3 weeks	70%
5 days	58%	4 weeks	40%

The complications of subarachnoid haemorrhage are shown in the next box:
Occasionally, organised blood clot within the subarachnoid space may obstruct cerebrospinal fluid flow, causing acute hydrocephalus. This may lead to a deterioration in the patient's conscious level days or weeks after the haemorrhage. Other causes of neurological deterioration correspond to the complications of subarachnoid haemorrhage shown in the next box. Any change in neurological status is likely to warrant a CT scan to assess the presence of any treatable complication, e.g. hydrocephalus.

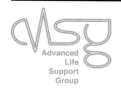

Complications of subarachnoid haemorrhage

Local recurrent haemorrhage
Cerebral oedema
Haemorrhage into brain parenchyma
Hydrocephalus
Secondary cerebral infarction due to vasospasm
Epileptic seizures
Hyponatraemia (inappropriate antidiuretic hormone production)
Central/uncal herniation
General hypoxaemia
Pulmonary embolus
Hypertension
Dehydration
Pneumonia/septicaemia
Hyperglycaemia

Management

The aim is to prevent secondary brain injury by following the structured approach. In addition, severe vasospasm may occur and this can be reduced by nimodipine (60 mg orally or NG every 4 h for 3 weeks). Other conditions that can arise include hypertension, cardiac dysrhythmias and neurogenic pulmonary oedema.

Do not forget that haemorrhage into the 4th ventricle can cause a transient rise in blood sugar. This is believed to be due to rapid autonomic nervous system discharge. The blood sugar will rapidly return to normal. Treatment with insulin could be fatal in precipitating hypoglycaemia.

Definitive management

Aneurysms detected on angiography may be treated either by endovascular coiling of the aneurysm with platinum wire coils, craniotomy and clipping of the neck of the aneurysm or, rarely, by stereotactic radiotherapy. The choice depends on individual expertise, the size, position and shape of the aneurysm. Coiling has become increasingly popular, due to its lower morbidity compared with craniotomy.

Outcome

Approximately 25% of patients die within 24 h of their subarachnoid haemorrhage. A further 25% die within the first month as a consequence of either recurrent haemorrhage or vasospasm induced infarction. The remainder survive for longer, but with an increased risk of rebleeding of approximately 2% per year.

Bacterial meningitis

Meningitis is an inflammatory condition of the lining of the brain and the ventricles. Causative organisms will influence the clinical presentation, management and outcome. Bacteria may reach the leptomeninges and produce meningitis in several ways:

• Bacterial seedlings by haematogenous spread.
• Local extension from contiguous extracerebral infections.
• Direct implantation of bacteria into the meninges.

Haematogenous spread

This type of meningitis is usually community acquired. The majority of cases are caused by *Streptococcus pneumoniae* or *meningococcus*. Of the remainder

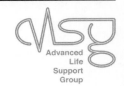

(approximately 20%), *Listeria monocytogenes*, anaerobic gram negative bacilli (e.g. *Escherichia coli*), *Haemophilus influenzae* and *Staphylococcus aureus* are responsible. Risk factors for *Strep. pneumoniae* meningitis are shown in the box below.

Risk factors for *Strep. pneumoniae* meningitis

Hypogammaglobulinaemia (primary or secondary, e.g. chronic lymphatic
  leukaemia)
Sickle cell disease
Previous skull trauma with dural fistula

Listeria tends to affect people at the extremes of age, pregnant women and those patients who have prolonged immunosuppression from steroids or alkalating agents, e.g. azathioprine. Contaminated foods, in particular unpasteurised soft cheeses, pâté and poorly refrigerated precooked chicken have been implicated.

Local extension
Local extension from contiguous extracerebral infection (e.g. otitis media or sinusitis). Possible pathways for migration of pathogens from the middle ear to the meninges can be (1) via systemic route in the bloodstream (2) along fascial planes (e.g. posterior fossa) (3) via temporal bone fractures (4) through the oval or round window membranes (e.g. the labyrinths).

Direct implantation
Post-traumatic meningitis can follow trauma to the skull or spine. It often occurs early in the post-traumatic period due to a breach in the meninges; however, it may occur years later. If the infective organism is acquired in the community, then *Strep. pneumoniae* or *H. influenzae* are the likely responsible organisms. In contrast, hospital acquired infections are usually caused by the anaerobic gram negative bacilli (*E. coli, Klebsiella, Enterobacter* and *Pseudomonas* species).

Post-surgical meningitis may follow an operation on the head, neck or spine, or the insertion of cerebrospinal fluid drains and shunts. The majority of the post-surgical meningitides are caused by anaerobic gram negative bacilli (as described earlier).

Key point

It is important to remember that:
• approximately 2% of meningitides will be culture negative
• with recurrent meningitis, cerebrospinal fluid leak, hypogammaglobulinaemia
  and complement deficiencies should be excluded

Most infections affecting cerebrospinal fluid drains and shunts are hospital acquired, predominantly caused by coagulase negative staphylococci and *Staph. aureus*. Whilst it is easy to understand how organisms may contaminate the cerebrospinal fluid as a result of trauma or surgery, the precise mode of invasion in spontaneous meningitis is currently unknown.

All organisms induce inflammatory injury to the meninges. This increases the permeability of the blood–brain barrier and raises intracranial pressure due to cerebral oedema. This is due to a combination of:
• interstitial fluid accumulation

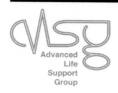

- communicating hydrocephalus due to decreased cerebrospinal fluid reabsorption
- cellular swelling
- vasculitis affecting the large vessels traversing the subarachnoid space.

A major consequence of increased intracranial pressure and vascular inflammation is decreased cerebral perfusion and therefore impaired delivery of oxygen and substrates. As the acute inflammatory response affects the pia and arachnoid mater, the cerebrospinal fluid contains numerous neutrophils and fibrin. Therefore, pus accumulates over the surface of the brain, in particular around its base, and can extend over the associated cranial nerves and spinal cord.

The early diagnosis of meningitis is difficult as many of the symptoms are non-specific and include malaise, fever, headache, myalgia and vomiting. As the disease progresses, the picture is dominated by irritability, severe headache and vomiting with the exception of meningococcal infection where diarrhoea is common. The classic non-blanching purpuric rash is common with meningococcal septicaemia, but occurs in only approximately 50% of those with meningococcal meningitis. The precise reason why some patients will develop meningococcal septicaemia rather than meningitis or vice versa is unknown.

Assessment
Clinical signs
The classic triad of fever, headaches and neck stiffness is usually present in 85% of cases. Limitation of neck movement is obvious, but meningitis is unlikely if the patient can shake their head or place their chin on their chest. Meningism is best elicited by passive flexion of the neck when the patient is supine. Confirmatory evidence may be obtained from Kernig's test, where the lower limb is flexed at the hip and the knee gradually extended. Resistance to this manoeuvre by contraction of the hamstrings is indicative of meningeal irritation. In contrast, Brudzinski's test is performed with the patient seated with their legs straight. Flexion of the neck in the presence of meningeal irritation will be associated with flexion of the hips and knees. Marked meningeal irritation can manifest as opisthotonus, i.e. the neck and back fully extended. **Meningism may be absent in patients who are either immunosuppressed or deeply comatosed.** Herpes labialis is commonly seen in **all** forms of bacterial meningitis.

Physical examination must exclude primary sites of infection, in particular otitis media, sinusitis, mastoiditis and pneumonia. Watery rhinorrhoea or otorrhoea should be collected and tested for glucose. Rhinorrhea or otorrhea fluid can also be tested for beta-transferrin, but the results will probably not be available in a useful timeframe, depending on local laboratory resources. Beta-transferrin is a protein that is produced by neuraminidase activity in the brain and is unique to CSF and perilymph fluid. Under these circumstances, a basal skull fracture must be excluded. The other clinical signs in the box below are not always present.

Clinical signs of a basal skull fracture

Bruising over mastoid process – Battle's sign
Otorrhoea – CSF ± blood
Rhinorrhoea – CSF ± blood
Periorbital bruising (panda or racoon eyes)
Subhyaloid haemorrhage

As the disease progresses, cranial nerves may become involved as they cross the inflamed basal meninges – commonly II, III, VI, VII and VIII. Papilloedema means that either cerebral oedema, hydrocephalus, a subdural effusion or empyema is contributing to the development of intracranial hypertension. Headache, vomiting, fever and decreasing level of consciousness usually dominate the clinical picture. Patients with infected shunts may present as described earlier. These devices can become infected in the cranium, the venous circulation or the peritoneal cavity, where they may produce symptoms akin to meningitis, right-sided infective endocarditis and peritonitis, respectively.

Diagnosis

The diagnosis is made clinically and often confirmed by lumbar puncture, provided there are no contraindications. In the majority of patients, the cerebrospinal fluid features of bacterial meningitis, are:

- raised white cell count (>100 white blood cells/ml), the majority of which are neutrophils
- cerebrospinal fluid glucose less than 40 mg/dl
- cerebrospinal fluid protein elevated
- gram staining of the cerebrospinal fluid will reveal organisms in over 50% of cases (see box below).

Gram staining of cerebrospinal fluid in pyogenic bacterial meningitis

Appearance	Probable organism
Gram positive cocci	Strep. pneumoniae, Staph. aureus
Gram negative cocci	N. meningitidis
Gram positive rods	L. monocytogenes
Gram negative rods	H. influenzae, Enterobacter

The causes of a predominant lymphocyte count are listed in the box below:

Meningitis with high cerebrospinal fluid lymphocyte count

Early or partially treated cryogenic bacterial infection
Tuberculosis, leptospirosis, brucellosis, syphilis, *Listeria*
Viral infection
Fungal infection, e.g. *Cryptococcus*
Parameningeal infection – intracerebral abscess or subdural empyema
Neoplastic infiltration

Specific treatment

Antibiotic therapy must be started immediately, as bacterial meningitis progresses rapidly and has a high mortality. The following are appropriate antibiotic agents. You should always refer to local hospital antibiotic policies.

Suspected meningococcal meningitis/septicaemia.
The patient should be given an immediate dose of ceftriaxone 2 g IV or benzylpenicillin 2.4 g qds IV.

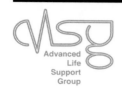

Suspected meningitis

In adults, spontaneous meningitis is usually caused by *Strep. pneumoniae* or *Neisseria meningitidis*.

There is an increased risk of *L. monocytogenes* and infections caused by anaerobic gram negative bacilli, e.g. Eschericia coli in patients with hospital acquired meningitis. The recommended first line management is cefotaxime 2 g tds IV.

Remember the benefits of IV dexamethasone (10 mg qds for 4 days) in patients with pneumococcal meningitis (see page 168)

Postsurgical meningitis

This is usually caused by hospital acquired, multiresistant organisms. Often, specific hospital antibiotic policies exist; if not, an initial choice is ceftazidine 2 g every 8 h as this will also provide antipseudomonal cover. Either ceftazidine or ceftriaxone is a good first line antibiotic for patients who have acute infections of either shunts or drains, before they are removed.

Outcome

Mortality rates vary considerably depending on the study and type of organism. The overall mortality ranges from approximately 10% for *N. meningitidis* and *H. influenzae* to over 20% for *L. monocytogenes* and *Strep. pneumoniae meningitis*.

Mortality is much greater in the very young; the elderly, and patients with pre-existing debilitating illnesses. Furthermore, progression from consciousness through to confusion and then coma is associated with an increased mortality. Complications are not uncommon and are listed in the box below.

Complications of meningitis

Raised intracranial pressure
Seizures
Hyponatraemia
Venous sinus thrombosis
Cranial nerve deficit
Hydrocephalus
Cerebral infarcts
Cerebritis and abscess
Subdural effusions and empyema
Ventriculitis
Cerebral oedema

Tuberculous meningitis

There has been an increased incidence of tuberculosis in many parts of the world, related to the human immunodeficiency viral infection. These patients have a high risk of meningeal involvement. Other high risk groups include immigrants from Pakistan, India, Africa and the West Indies, alcoholics, intravenous drug users, immunocompromised patients and those with previous pulmonary tuberculosis.

Pathophysiology

Infection spreads from the primary lesion, or site of chronic infection, through the blood stream to the brain and meninges, where microtubercles are formed.

These rupture and discharge tubercular protein and mycobacteria into the sub-arachnoid space, inciting an inflammatory response. Many patients develop miliary tuberculosis at this stage because of haematogenous spread. As with bacterial meningitis, the base of brain and associated cranial nerves can be affected. Tuberculous meningitis is also associated with endarteritis. This can produce ischaemia/infarction of superficial cortical areas, internal capsule, basal ganglia and brain stem.

Assessment
Symptoms
The onset is usually subacute with two to eight weeks of non-specific prodromal symptoms, including malaise, irritability, lethargy, headache and vomiting.

Clinical signs
Meningeal irritation and cranial nerve damage (most often involving VI, but also II, IV and VII) are common, as is papilloedema. Raised intracranial pressure usually occurs because of obstruction of cerebrospinal fluid circulation, in particular, through the basal cisterns. The neurological features associated with raised intracranial pressure and hydrocephalus have been described earlier. The development of focal neurological signs, however, does not always imply raised intracranial pressure as these patients are prone to arteritis and hence cerebral infarction. Inappropriate antidiuretic hormone secretion is also common and may precipitate or exacerbate unconsciousness.

British Medical Research Council staging for disease severity is:

Stage I – early non-specific features, including apathy, irritability, headache, fever, anorexia and vomiting without alteration of conscious level.

Stage II – altered conscious level, without delirium or coma, but with minor neurological signs. Signs of meningism are present, with cranial nerve palsies or involuntary movements.

Stage III – advanced state with stupor or coma, severe neurological deficits, seizures, abnormal posturing and/or abnormal movements.

The prognosis is related directly to the clinical stage at diagnosis.

Diagnosis
The cerebrospinal fluid is clear or slightly turbid, with a white cell count less than 500 cells/ml. This is composed of both lymphocytes and neutrophils, in varying proportions. The cerebrospinal fluid glucose is low and the protein concentration is elevated. Tubercle bacilli are rarely seen on cerebrospinal fluid microscopy; however, centrifugation of the sample can increase the diagnostic yield. The most sensitive and specific test uses the polymerase chain reaction (PCR) to detect the *Mycobacterium tuberculosis* genome.

Treatment
This comprises combination chemotherapy with isoniazid (300 mg), rifampicin (600 mg) and pyrazinamide (1500 mg) for 12 months. Streptomycin can also be added for the first two months. Para-aminosalicylic acid should not be used, because it does not enter the cerebrospinal fluid. In view of the numerous complications and morbidity and mortality, specialist advice should be sought early.

Outcome
Prognosis is related to the clinical state at diagnosis. Mortality is still high, at approximately 25%, irrespective of whether patients have coexistent human

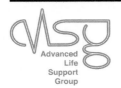

immunodeficiency virus. Permanent sequelae occur in approximately 25% of survivors, ranging from cranial nerve deficit (including blindness) to hemiparesis and intellectual impairment.

Summary of the CSF findings in meningitis are shown in Table 11.5.

Encephalitis and viral meningitis

There is considerable geographical variation in the type of virus causing encephalitis. In the UK, however, the commonest diagnosed cause of encephalitis is mumps. Other causes are shown in the box below.

Causes of viral encephalitis

Mumps
Echo virus
Coxsackie virus
Herpes simplex
Herpes zoster
Epstein – Barr virus
Adenovirus
Enterovirus

Many of these infections occur in seasonal peaks or epidemics; e.g. mumps encephalitis is common in the late winter or early spring whilst enterovirus infections occur in summer and early autumn. Other viral infections, in particular herpes simplex encephalitis, are sporadic. Although viral infections affect all age groups, they are most frequent and severe in children, the elderly and those who

Table 11.5 Summary of CSF findings in meningitis

Agent	Opening pressure (mm H$_2$O)	WBC count (cells/mm^3)	Glucose (mmol/l)	Protein (g/l)	Microbiology
Normal values	80–200	0–5; lymphocytes	60% of blood glucose	0.15–0.40	Negative
Bacterial meningitis	200–300	100–105; >80% PMNs	Very low	< 3	Specific pathogen demonstrated in 60% of gram stains and 80% of cultures
Viral meningitis	90–200	10–2000; lymphocytes	Normal, reduced mumps	< 1.5	Viral isolation, PCR
Tuberculous meningitis	180–300	Up to 4000; lymphocytes	Reduced, 1–4	1–6	Acid-fast bacillus stain, culture, PCR
Aseptic meningitis	90–200	10–300; lymphocytes	Normal	Normal but may be slightly elevated	Negative

PMN, polymorphonuclear lymphocyte; PCR, polymerase chain reaction.

have decreased T-cell immunity, e.g. Hodgkin's disease. Whilst herpes simplex encephalitis affects all age groups, it shows distinct peaks in those patients aged either between 5 and 30 years or greater than 50 years.

Pathophysiology

Most viral infections reach the central nervous system from the primary site of infection, via the blood stream. Nervous system damage is a consequence of direct invasion and immunological reaction. These processes culminate in:

- destruction and phagocytosis of neurones
- inflammatory oedema
- vascular lesions
- demyelination.

Characteristically, viral encephalitides cause lymphocytic infiltration of the meninges. Other features include perivascular cuffing of lymphocytes, plasma cells and histiocytes within the cortex and white matter as well as proliferation of microglia. This results in Neuronal degeneration and demyelination.

Herpes simplex encephalitis has characteristic features, in particular gross oedema, severe haemorrhage and necrotising encephalitis. These features are often asymmetrical and localised to the temporal lobe or, to a lesser extent, the frontal lobe. Demyelination is rare. The unique localisation of herpes simplex encephalitis has not been satisfactorily explained as yet.

Assessment

Clinical features

The symptom profile is similar to that of meningitis, dominated by headache, vomiting, fever and malaise.

Clinical signs

A wide spectrum of clinical signs includes confusion, convulsions, coma, focal neurological signs, features of raised intracranial pressure and psychiatric manifestations.

However, specific symptoms may arise as herpes simplex encephalitis involves primarily the temporal and frontal cortex. These include gustatory and olfactory hallucinations, amnesia, expressive dysphasia, temporal lobe seizures, anosmia and behavioural abnormalities. Cerebral oedema is common with herpes simplex encephalitis and untreated patients usually lapse into coma towards the end of the first week.

Diagnosis

The aim is to demonstrate a specific viral agent, especially herpes simplex, or exclude potentially treatable causes. Provided there are no contraindications, as described earlier, a lumbar puncture is needed. The cerebrospinal fluid pressure is usually increased, especially in herpes simplex encephalitis (related to the intense cerebral oedema) unless it is early in the evolution of the illness. There is often a marked increase in white cells, with lymphocytes and other mononuclear cells predominating. Furthermore, the cerebrospinal fluid may contain erythrocytes or be xanthochromic if there is a haemorrhagic element to the encephalitis, as with herpes simplex. Protein concentration is usually increased in excess of 50 mg/dl, with an increase in the proportion of immunoglobulin G (IgG). A prominent monoclonal IgG band will be seen in the cerebrospinal fluid due to *de novo* synthesis of IgG combined with leakage of IgG from the serum. The cerebrospinal fluid glucose is usually normal.

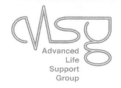

A specific virus can be found in the majority of patients, from either a throat swab or samples of stool, cerebrospinal fluid and blood. CSF PCR for Herpes Simplex viral DNA is 100% specific and 75–98% sensitive within the first 24–45 h. Magnetic resonance imaging has provided greater detail about the structural damage in patients who have encephalitis. Further supporting evidence may be provided by an EEG that shows irregular activity over the affected area.

Specific treatment

Aciclovir (10 mg/kg every 8 h for 14–21 days), a nucleoside analogue, is an effective treatment for herpes simplex encephalitis. It has the advantage that it is only taken up by infected cells and is therefore non-toxic to normal uninfected cells. If the diagnosis is suspected clinically, then treatment should be started immediately as untreated HSE has a mortality rate of 50–75%. Corticosteroids can be used in an attempt to combat cerebral oedema, but there is no convincing evidence of any benefit.

Often, however, the precise initial diagnosis is in doubt hence patients are treated with both aciclovir and antibiotics until definitive results are available.

Outcome

Neurological sequelae are common in patients following herpes simplex encephalitis and include mental retardation, amnesia, expressive aphasia, hemiparesis, ataxia and recurrent seizures, along with various behavioural and personality disturbances.

Aseptic meningitis

This is a common, rarely fatal condition usually caused by certain viruses. Less commonly it results from nonviral infections (e.g. partially treated bacterial meningitis; TB; fungi and parasites) and many noninfectious causes (e.g. drug reactions; CT disease). It occurs in individuals of all ages, although it is more common in children, especially during summer.

Clinical symptoms vary – typically there is headache and fever which are mild and go without treatment. However some develop full-blown life-threatening meningitis.

Treatment

As encephalitis. Subsequent changes depend on confirmation of the cause.

Cerebral malaria

Malaria remains the most important human parasitic disease globally. *Plasmodium falciparum* is the only malarial parasite that causes cerebral pathology but this is the predominant species in the highly endemic areas of Africa, New Guinea and Haiti.

Infection in man is acquired from either the female anopheles mosquito, which inoculates parasites into the human blood stream, or by transfusion of blood containing the parasite. The parasite, at this stage referred to as a sporozoite, enters hepatic parenchymal cells. *Plasmodium falciparum* does not have a dormant phase within the liver so relapses do not occur. After a period of 6–8 days, mature forms (merozoites) are liberated into the blood stream. Here they attach to and invade circulating erythrocytes. Parasites undergo many morphological changes in the erythrocytes to eventually produce shizonts containing daughter erythrocytic merozoites.

These are liberated by red cell lysis and immediately invade uninfected erythrocytes, resulting in a cycle of invasion and multiplication. The intraerythrocytic division is relatively regular, as is red cell lysis and merozoite release. These processes and the inflammatory components they provoke (e.g. cytokines) are responsible for the regular attacks of fever that occur at approximately the same time of day for the duration of the infection.

Pathophysiology

Plasmodium falciparum, in contrast to the other three forms of human malaria (*P. ovale, P. malariae, P. vivax*), affects the brain as well as other tissues. This unique difference is attributed to the fact the mature parasites adhere to specific endothelial receptors, in particular, on the venule. As a consequence, partial occlusion of small vessels occurs, which reduces perfusion. The resulting tissue anoxia and damage is exacerbated by red cells impacting on the parasites adhering to the vascular endothelium. Consequently areas of the brain will be deprived of oxygen and appropriate substrates, in particular glucose.

Assessment

Clinical features

Prodromal symptoms often predominate and include malaise, headache, myalgia, anorexia and mild fever. These are present for several days before the first rigor. This typically starts with the patient feeling cold and apprehensive. Shivering rapidly evolves into a rigor lasting for 1 h associated with vomiting, throbbing headache, palpitations, breathlessness and fainting. Culminating in a drenching sweat. The whole episode lasts for approximately 8–12 h, after which the exhausted patient sleeps. A high irregular continuous fever is not uncommon in a patient with falciparum malaria. In addition, generalised seizures, confusion, delirium, irritability and loss of consciousness may occur. Mild meningism can be present but neck stiffness, photophobia and papilloedema are rare. A conjugate gaze palsy is common, but pupillary, corneal and oculocephalic reflexes are normal. Muscle tone is increased symmetrically, knee reflexes are generally brisk and both plantar responses are extensor. Furthermore, extensor posturing is common and can be associated with sustained gaze. Other clinical features are shown in the box.

Non-neurological features associated with cerebral malaria

Anaemia
Spontaneous bleeding from the gastrointestinal tract
Jaundice
Hypoglycaemia
Shock
Oliguria
Acute renal failure
Pulmonary oedema

Diagnosis

Malaria should be considered in the differential diagnosis of any acute febrile illness until it can be excluded by definite lack of exposure, repeated examination of blood smears or following a therapeutic trial of antimalarial chemotherapy.

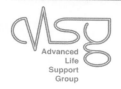

Examination of at least three thick and thin blood films is required to exclude the diagnosis.

Other techniques include:

- rapid diagnosis tests which use a finger prick blood sample to give results within 15 min. These tests are ideal in areas where microscope facilities and/or diagnostic expertise are limited.
- polymerase chain reaction which detects either DNA or mRNA from particular plasmodium species.

These tests have lower specificities and sensitivities. The gold standard remains thick and thin film examination.

Key point

Do not dismiss the possibility of malaria in patients who have taken prophylactic drugs, as protection is never complete

---

Absence of parasites in peripheral blood smears may indicate partial antimalarial treatment or sequestration in deep vascular beds. Treatment must be started and the diagnosis may be made on bone marrow aspirate.

If there are no contraindications, lumbar puncture must be done because it is important to exclude other treatable encephalopathies. The cerebrospinal fluid will show approximately 15 lymphocytes/ml, with increased protein and normal glucose, unless the patient is hypoglycaemic.

Specific therapy

Quinine is the drug of choice. This should be given by an intravenous infusion to patients who are seriously ill or unable to swallow tablets.

- Loading dose 20 mg/kg of quinine salt diluted in 5% dextrose over 4 h.
- Maintenance dose 10 mg/kg of quinine salt given over 4 h by intravenous infusion every 8–12 h until the patient can swallow tablets to complete a 7-day course. If patients require more than 48 h of parenteral therapy, the maintenance dose should be halved to 5 mg/kg.

Note that quinine can induce hypoglycaemia as a result of islet cell stimulation. This may be combined with hypoglycaemia due to extensive hyperparasitaemia. Thus, regular monitoring of blood glucose is necessary. Contraindications to quinine therapy are shown in the box below.

Contraindications to quinine therapy

Hypersensitivity to quinine
Concurrent use of cimetidine, amiodarone or digoxin
Therapeutic administration of mefloquine within the previous 14 days
Resistant *Plasmodium falciparum*

Side effects from quinine are rare and usually follow rapid intravenous injection (see box below). Thus, careful monitoring of the infusion speed is required.

Side effects following quinine administration	
Cardiovascular	Sinus arrest, junctional rhythms, arteriovenous block, ventricular tachycardia/fibrillation, sudden death, prolongation of QT interval
Neurological	Visual disturbances, partial deafness, headache, tinnitus, myopathy
Haematological	Thrombocytopenia, haemolytic anaemia
Endocrine	Hypoglycaemia

Any of the following regimes are appropriate for patients who are not seriously ill and can swallow tablets:

- quinine 600 mg three times a day for 7 days
- fansidar–three tablets as a single dose
- doxycycline 200 mg daily for at least 7 days.

Key point

Tetracyclines, sulfadoxine and pyrimethamine are contraindicated in pregnancy

The first line treatment for uncomplicated chloraquine resistant falciparum malaria (WHO recommended) is artemether combination regime (artemisinin 10–12 mg/kg total does over 3–5 days) with e.g. mefloquine. Avoid combinations with drugs that have a reduced effect due to resistance such as chloraquine or sulfadoxine-pyrimethamine.

Outcome

Mortality is approximately 10%, but varies according to the medical facilities available. Severe falciparum malaria can occur with the following conditions:

- impaired acquired immunity
- post splenectomy
- pregnancy
- immunosuppression.

Complications such as retinal haemorrhage, renal failure, hypoglycaemia, haemoglobinuria, metabolic acidaemia and pulmonary oedema carry a poor prognosis.

Intracranial abscess

These can be extradural, subdural or intracerebral. Occasionally, subdural and intracerebral abscesses may rupture into the subarachnoid space, resulting in meningitis.

Pathophysiology

Intracerebral abscess

These occur as a consequence of middle ear infection, frontal sinusitis and penetrating trauma to the head. Other causes include sepsis related to infective endocarditis, lung abscess and bronchiectasis. As most abscesses are related to disease affecting either the middle ear or sinuses, they tend to be found in the temporal lobes, cerebellum or frontal lobes. Not surprisingly, sepsis can be associated with multiple intracerebral abscesses.

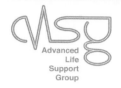

Large intracerebral abscesses may rupture into the ventricular system producing ventriculitis.

Many of the organisms involved are described earlier and also under the section entitled subdural abscess/empyema.

Subdural abscess

This is often a sequel to an infection in the paranasal sinuses or middle ear. Other causes include meningitis and sepsis related to cyanotic congenital heart disease and lung abscesses. Penetrating trauma and intracranial surgery can also be implicated. Subdural abscesses may be extensive with pus extending over the surface of the brain. The most common organisms include *Strep. pneumoniae*, *Strept. milleri*, *Strept. pyogenes*, *Staph. aureus* and *Bacteroides* species along with *H. influenzae*.

Extradural abscess

As the dura mater is tightly adherent to the periosteum of the skull, epidural collections of pus are usually localised. They are related to either infections within the mastoid and nasal sinuses or focal osteomyelitis of the skull. Occasionally, infection may spread intracranially as described previously. This is more likely to occur in penetrating trauma to the skull or rarely following craniotomy. Common organisms include *Streptococcus*, *Staph. aureus*, Enterobacteriaceae, *Bacteroides* and many anaerobic species.

Assessment

Clinical features

The clinical features will depend on the number, site and extent of the lesions, as well as the impact on surrounding structures.

- *Intracerebral* abscess can present as headache, vomiting, impaired consciousness, hemiparesis and seizures. There may also be features to suggest either a pulmonary or cardiac primary focus of infection.
- *Subdural* abscess is often associated with severe headache, pyrexia, confusion, seizures and coma. A contralateral hemiparesis can be present. There may be evidence of either mastoiditis, frontal sinusitis or a scalp infection.
- *Extradural* abscess is often difficult to diagnose clinically, but may present with a localised headache in association with mastoiditis and sinusitis.

Diagnosis

This is usually made on either CT scan or magnetic resonance imaging. Lumbar puncture is rarely needed and is contraindicated when raised intracranial pressure is present. Usually the results are non-specific, consisting of an elevated protein level, pleocytosis with variable neutrophil count, a normal glucose level and sterile cultures. A lumbar puncture is mostly of value to rule out other disease processes, especially bacterial meningitis

Specific management

Neurosurgical opinion is necessary. Most supratentorial abscesses can be aspirated via a burr hole but subdural collections usually require evacuation through a craniotomy. Small abscesses are usually treated with antibiotics.

Outcome

The mortality is 10–20%. However, one third of survivors will have persistent epilepsy, in particular, as a sequel to temporal lobe or subdural abscesses.

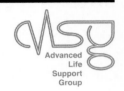

Intracranial haematoma

Classification is identical to 'intracranial abscess', i.e. extradural, subdural and intracerebral.

Intracerebral haematoma

Occasionally, spontaneous haemorrhage can produce a haematoma within the substance of the brain. This is the result of rupture of small arteries affected by lipohyaline degeneration (Charcot–Bouchard aneurysm). It typically occurs in patients with hypertension and occurs at well-defined sites – basal ganglia, pons, cerebellum and subcortical white matter. The site and extent of the lesion will determine the clinical findings. One such condition which deserves mention is a cerebellar haematoma, because surgical treatment can be life saving. The patient presents with acute occipital headache, dizziness, truncal ataxia and rapid reduction in consciousness.

Subdural haematoma

This may be acute in patients who are overanticoagulated or chronic in the elderly, epileptic or alcoholic. A chronic subdural haematoma is usually associated with a trivial injury that may go unnoticed by the patient. Haemorrhage is due to rupture of the small veins crossing the subdural space with blood forming a localised collection between the dura and arachnoid mater.

Absorption of fluid from the adjacent arachnoid space causes expansion of the blood clot. The onset of symptoms is insidious, with headache, often mental changes, drowsiness and vomiting. There may be mild hemiplegia, but raised intracranial pressure is not initially prominent.

Extradural haematoma

This usually follows a tear to the middle meningeal artery following a fracture in the temporoparietal region. In a third of cases there is a triad of symptoms: unconscious for a short time recovery (the lucid interval, where confusion is common) and then comat, minutes or hours later as the extradural haematoma raises the intracranial pressure. The other two thirds of patients are either unconscious from the initial impact or do not have an initial period of unconsciousness.

Diagnosis

In all cases, the diagnosis is confirmed by either a CT scan or magnetic resonance imaging. An extradural haematoma is 'egg-shaped' and a subdural haematoma is 'saucer-shaped' on CT scan.

Specific management

For all of these conditions, urgent neurosurgical consultation is required. It is important to realise that patients with such lesions can deteriorate very quickly. Regular monitoring is necessary, as is prevention of secondary brain injury.

Prognosis

The outcome for extradural haematoma is good provided there is no underlying brain damage and the haematoma is evacuated rapidly (less than 4 hours).

For subdural haematoma and intracranial haematoma the prognosis is worse as there is invariably primary brain damage. Factors affecting survival are:
- Age ≥ 60 years
- Presenting GCS ≤ 6 (poor conscious level), significant comorbidity on coagulation/antiplatelet therapy

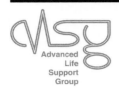

- Dominant hemisphere, deep-seated clot
- Clot >50 cm^3

Intracranial tumours

These may be benign or malignant, primary or secondary. The clinical effects are related to the site and extent of the lesion(s) as well as the impact on neighbouring structures. An in-depth discussion on the different types of tumour is beyond the scope of this text. Furthermore, this will not influence the initial management.

Pathophysiology

The effect of any intracranial neoplastic lesion depends on the following:
- type of tumour
- growth rate
- site
- extent
- capacity to incite oedema formation in the adjacent brain tissue
- effect on neighbouring structures
- potential to obstruct flow of cerebrospinal fluid and blood.

The precise effects that these will have on intracranial pressure have been explained earlier.

Assessment

Clinical features

Patients with intracerebral tumours tend to present with either epilepsy, or focal neurological signs, or raised intracranial pressure or a combination of these features. Late onset epilepsy (patients over 25 years) should always raise the suspicion of an intracranial tumour. Focal neurological deficits will obviously be related to the site and extent of the tumour, as well as its effect on adjacent structures. The effects of raised intracranial pressure have been discussed earlier. The progressive development of clinical signs is the most significant factor in the diagnosis of intracerebral tumours.

Investigations

Imaging, either CT scan or MRI, is the investigation of choice.

Specific management

Dexamethasone (4 mg tds) can reduce oedema surrounding the tumour(s). Neurosurgical consultation is required.

Time Out 11.2

Check your knowledge acquisition by answering the following questions.
a. What is the commonest site for a saccular aneurysm?
b. List the two common causes of subarachnoid haemorrhage.
c. How long does it take for xanthochromia to develop?
d. What is the mortality in the first 24 h after a subarachnoid haemorrhage?
e. List the two common bacteria that cause spontaneous meningitis.
f. Which categories of patients are 'high risk' for TB meningitis (a clue – six major groups)?
g. List the characteristic features of herpes simplex encephalitis.
h. In which patients would you consider a diagnosis of cerebral malaria?
i. List the non-neurological features of *Plasmodium falciparum* infection.

j. List any differences between abscesses in the extradural, subdural and intracerebral locations

k. List any differences between haematomata in the extradural, subdural and intracerebral locations.

SUMMARY

- The patient with altered conscious level is a common medical problem.
- Prevent secondary brain injury by ensuring appropriate provision of supplemental oxygen and glucose.
- It is important that CT scanning is the critical first investigation providing all immediately life-threatening problems have been treated and hypoglycaemia excluded. If either meningitis or encephalitis is suspected treatment should be given before investigations are done.
- Late onset epilepsy may indicate an intracranial tumour.
- Early liaison with specialist colleagues in microbiology, neurology or neurosurgery is important.

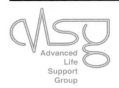

CHAPTER 12

The 'collapsed' patient

OBJECTIVES

After reading this chapter you will be able to:
- describe the structured approach to the collapsed patient
- understand the pathophysiology of collapse
- discuss the causes and initial investigation of transient loss of consciousness
- describe some of the common conditions that present as 'collapse'.

INTRODUCTION

A wide variety of medical conditions present to hospital as 'collapse'. This term has different meaning to different groups of medical professionals and patients. To some it refers to any patient who has been found on the floor, or less responsive than normal. To others it refers to a transient loss of consciousness with return to pre-existing neurological function (more correctly called syncope). To yet others it may include near-syncope or dizziness. Regardless of the cause – which may not be known even after investigation – the same structured approach is applicable.

PRIMARY ASSESSMENT AND RESUSCITATION

An overview of this has been described in Chapter 3. Specific details relating to the collapsed patient will now be considered.

A – airway (and cervical spine)

Assess and clear the airway as described in Chapter 4. Patients with syncope are unlikely to have airway problems. Those with other causes of collapse especially stroke and epilepsy have significant potential for airway compromise due to position, loss of or increase in muscle tone, loss of protective reflexes and inability to swallow.

Trauma due to the collapse may compromise the airway due to bleeding or loose teeth. Although cervical spine injury is unusual in patients falling to the floor from their own height, it does occur, especially in the elderly and those with rheumatoid arthritis and ankylosing spondylitis. Remember the potential for this condition in patients found collapsed at the bottom of the stairs. Consider and treat for potential cervical spine injury if there is no clear history, especially in patients with signs of injury above the clavicles. Give supplementary oxygen (12–15 l/min via non-rebreathing mask with reservoir bag) titrated to oxygen saturation in all acutely ill patients (see Chapter 3).

B – breathing

Examine for evidence of a condition that may have either caused the collapse (e.g. pulmonary oedema) or more likely be a consequence (e.g. aspiration pneumonia in an unconscious patient).

Acute Medical Emergencies; The Practical Approach, 2nd edition.
Edited by Terence Wardle, Peter Driscoll, and Sue Wieteska.
© 2010 Blackwell Publishing Ltd.

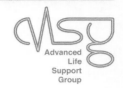

C – circulation

Seek features of shock and treat with intra-venous fluids for hypovolaemia. Institute cardiac rhythm monitoring and treat life-threatening arrhythmias according to UK and European resuscitation council guidelines. Other causes of shock and collapse, e.g. anaphylaxis are considered in Chapter 9.

D – disability

The aim of this brief examination is to identify and begin treatment for immediately life-threatening conditions such as hypoglycaemia, status epilepticus and meningitis. Assess:

- pupil size and reaction
- conscious level using Glasgow Coma Scale (GCS)
- for evidence of meningism
- for signs of seizure activity
- bedside glucose.

As neurological signs may develop and change, monitor GCS, pupillary response and glucose.

E – exposure

Quickly identify signs that may point to a life-threatening cause of collapse. Look for non-blanching purpuric rash, cutaneous opioid patches, evidence of illicit drug use, recent surgical scars, signs of deliberate self harm. Check the temperature. Remember that a patient who has collapsed may have spent several hours on the floor. Hence also consider the risk of rhabdomyolysis and pressure sores.

STROKE/TIA

Introduction

Stroke is a syndrome characterised by an acute onset of focal (at times global) loss of neurological function lasting more than 24 h (or causing earlier death) due to cerebrovascular disease. Therefore, it is a clinical diagnosis. Traditionally, a transient ischaemic attack (TIA) has been defined as a neurological deficit caused by focal brain ischaemia that completely resolves within 24 h. Most have a much shorter duration than this, and with increased use of magnetic resonance imaging (MRI) it has become clear that over half of the patients who present with TIA have evidence of infarction in the corresponding territory.

TRANSIENT ISCHAEMIC ATTACK

> **Score to predict of early stroke within 7 days (after TIA):**
>
> A – Age ≥ 60 years = 1 point
> B – BP (SBP ≥ 140; DBP ≥ 90; Both) all = 1 point
> C – Clinical sign – unilateral weakness 2 pts; speech 1 pt; other 0 pt
> D2 – Duration ≥ 1 h = 2 pt; 10–59 min = 1 pt; < 10 min 0 pt
> –Diabetes mellitus (1 point)

With TIA, it is important to assess the patient's risk of a subsequent stroke. One way is the National Institute of Health scoring system described in the next box. Those with a score of 3 or less can be referred to the TIA clinic within 2 weeks.

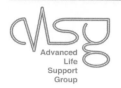

Patients scoring 4 or more or those in atrial fibrillation should be admitted for specialist assessment. This score can then be used to predict the risk of stroke.

A–D2 score	Risk of stroke within 2 days
6–7	8 fold
4–5	4 fold
<4	1 fold

Treatment includes one or more of the following:
- anti-platelet therapy
- anticoagulation
- endarterectomy.

If a vascular stenosis is detected and treated early (<2/7 ideally) – the chance of stroke is reduced by 30%.

If the patient is already on aspirin give dipyridamole. This combined tablet is called asasantin. Remember that dipyridamole cannot be used if the patient has either severe coronary artery disease or contra indications for aspirin use.

Stroke

Acute stroke affects about 2/1000 population per annum. This incidence increases steeply with increasing age (20/1000 in those over 85). Stroke is more common in men.

Mortality is high (20% within 30 days after a first stroke), as is prevalence of disability in survivors (about one third are dependent on others at one year). The risk of stroke after a first TIA is approximately 10% in the first 3 months – half of such strokes occurring in the first 48 h. The risk factors that make stroke more likely within a short interval are:
- age over 60
- diabetes mellitus
- weakness or speech impairment during the episode
- duration longer than 10 min
- occurrence despite aspirin
- probable cardiac embolic source.

Pathophysiology

The types of stroke are listed in the box

Types and causes of stroke	
Cerebral infarction	**80%**
(large vessel disease 50%)	
(small vessel disease [lacunar] 25%)	
(cardiogenic embolism 20%)	
Primary intracerebral haemorrhage	**10%**
(hypertension 50%)	
Subarachnoid haemorrhage	**5%**
Unknown	**5%**

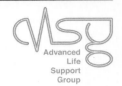

Atherosclerosis of the major vessels supplying the brain can precipitate a stroke by causing either embolisation from atherosclerotic plaques or major vessel occlusion. Small vessel disease, with occlusion of small penetrating arterioles, leads to small infarcts in the subcortical white matter, internal capsule and basal ganglia (lacunar infarcts). Atrial fibrillation, valvular heart disease, recent myocardial infarction and ventricular aneurysm can cause embolic strokes.

Intracerebral haemorrhage usually follows the sudden rupture of microaneurysms caused by hypertensive vascular disease, characteristically in the basal ganglia, brain stem and cerebellum.

Subarachnoid haemorrhage is commonly caused by a rupture of an aneurysm arising on one of the arteries at the base of the brain, but it may arise from an arteriovenous malformation. (See Chapters 11 and 14 for further details.)

The distinction between strokes in the internal carotid (anterior circulation) territory and those in the vertebrobasilar (posterior circulation) territory is not always easy on clinical grounds. Dysphasia or visual spatial apraxia indicates definite carotid distribution. In contrast, simultaneous bilateral weakness or sensory loss, cortical blindness, diplopia, vertigo, ataxia and dysphagia suggest vertebrobasilar distribution.

Lacunar strokes tend not to affect conscious level or cognitive function. They may cause pure motor stroke, pure sensory stroke, sensorimotor stroke, ataxic hemiparesis and, rarely, movement disorders such as hemiballismus or hemichorea.

Primary assessment and immediate treatment

In a patient presenting with stroke, it is essential to follow the structured approach previously described to optimise oxygenation and cerebral perfusion, and to limit secondary cerebral damage. Specific problems in the stroke patient include:

A – Airway may not be maintained. Clear and secure if necessary.

B – Respiratory drive may be depressed.

C – Cardiovascular compromise may have precipitated the stroke. Treat hypotension and tachycardias/bradycardias appropriately.

D – Check glucose. Hypoglycaemia may present with focal signs or depressed conscious level. Look for evidence of seizure activity.

E – Check temperature. Both hypothermia and hyperthermia may complicate stroke.

Secondary assessment and emergency treatment
Phrased history

An account of the onset of symptoms must be obtained from the patient or relative. A rapid onset of a focal neurological deficit is characteristic of a stroke (minutes or hours). A history of sudden onset of a severe headache associated with neck stiffness suggests subarachnoid haemorrhage. In contrast, a slower onset of symptoms is more likely to indicate other diagnoses, e.g. intracranial tumour or chronic subdural haematoma.

Note any vascular risk factors including history of transient ischaemic attacks, hypertension, atrial fibrillation, ischaemic heart disease, cigarette smoking, diabetes mellitus, hyperlipidaemia and family history.

Examination

A full neurological assessment will help localise the lesion and record the degree of disability.

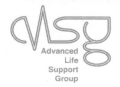

One way of recognising stroke in the emergency room is shown in the next box:

ROSIER (Recognition of stroke in the ER) score

History
LOC   −1
Convulsion   −1

Examination
Face, arm, leg   +1 for each affected
Speech defect   +1
Visual field defect   +1

Negative score – consider stroke mimic
For scores over zero: PPV for stroke – 90%; NPV for stroke 88%

Examination of the fundi may reveal changes of raised intracranial pressure or show evidence of previously undiagnosed hypertension or diabetes mellitus.

The cardiovascular examination should assess:
- heart rhythm (in particular atrial fibrillation)
- blood pressure, taken in both arms (subclavian steal, aortic dissection)
- the presence of any valvular heart disease
- reduced carotid blood flow (pulse pressure/bruit)
- peripheral pulses.

Listen carefully at the lung bases. Patients with swallowing difficulty are at risk of aspiration.

Look for evidence of development of pressure sores or rhabdomyolysis in patients who may have been on the floor for some time.

Investigations

CT scan

This is essential to establish whether the underlying pathology is infarction or haemorrhage and to exclude possible cerebral tumour or subdural haematoma.

Key point

It is not possible to distinguish cerebral infarction from cerebral haemorrhage on clinical grounds

---

CT scanning has several advantages over MRI in the acute stage and is the current method of choice as it is:
- more widely available
- cheaper
- more sensitive at identifying haemorrhage in the early stages
- easier to monitor the patient during a CT scan.

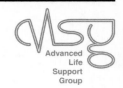

However, there are disadvantages to CT scanning.

- It will not identify an infarction in the first few (possibly up to 48) hours after the onset of symptoms.
- It has limited ability to show vascular lesions in the brain stem and cerebellum and small ischaemic infarcts deep in the cerebral hemispheres.

MRI modalities such as diffusion weighted imaging can detect ischaemia within minutes of onset.

Other investigations

- ECG is essential to demonstrate rhythm disturbance, particularly atrial fibrillation, and evidence of ischaemic, hypertensive or valvular heart disease.
- Chest X-ray may reveal features consistent with a potential cardiogenic source of emboli as well as evidence of aspiration.
- Full blood count and clotting will exclude polycythaemia, thrombocytosis and clotting disorders.
- Plasma viscosity/ erythrocyte sedimentation rate as a screen for infection, vasculitis.
- Blood glucose, to exclude hypoglycaemia and diabetes mellitus.
- Urea and electrolytes, to identify:
  - electrolyte disturbances in patients on diuretics
  - evidence of renal impairment in patients with hypertension
  - hyponatraemia (a rare cause of focal neurological deficit).
- Fasting lipids, in all but the very elderly (although levels in acute phase of a stroke may not reflect premorbid profile).
- Syphilis serology, to identify meningovascular syphilis as a treatable, but rare, cause of cerebral ischaemia.

Management

The immediately life-threatening problems will have been identified and treated as part of the primary assessment. As soon as the CT has shown that it is not intracranial haemorrhage the stroke team should be informed and thrombolysis started.

Other important considerations at this stage include the following:

Antiplatelet therapy: In acute stroke, aspirin should be started as soon as the CT scan confirms there is no cerebral bleed. A starting dose of 150–300 mg daily should be given and continued until decisions have been made about secondary prevention. Depending on local policy other agents such as clopidogrel may be used instead, especially in patients where there are contraindications to aspirin.

Anticoagulant therapy: There is no evidence at present to support the use of anticoagulants in **acute** stroke, even for patients in atrial fibrillation. However, all patients in atrial fibrillation will require anticoagulation, provided there are no contraindications.

Thrombolysis: Intravenous thrombolytic therapy is a potentially effective treatment of acute thrombotic stroke, to provide early reperfusion of ischaemic cerebral tissue and limitation of infarct size. However, all thrombolytic drugs need to be given early after the onset of symptoms (probably within 3 h) and involve a risk of cerebral haemorrhage. Results of trials so far suggest an increase in the proportion of patients making a good recovery by six months, but a substantial increase in cerebral haemorrhage within the first two weeks.

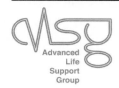

The National Institute for Neurological Disorders (NINDS) has set down time goals for the management of acute stroke in the context of thrombolysis as follows:

- Clinical assessment within 10 min of Emergency Department (ED) arrival.
- CT scan performed within 25 min of ED arrival.
- CT scan interpreted within 45 min of ED arrival.
- Initiation of fibrinolytic therapy (if indicated) within 1 h of ED arrival and 3 h of onset.
- Door-to-admission time of 3 h.

In view of the potential risks and service implications, the most recent advice from the Intercollegiate Stroke Working Party (Royal College of Physicians, 2006) is that hospitals offering thrombolysis for acute stroke, outside a clinical trial, should have registered with the UK Safe Implementation of Thrombolysis in Stroke Monitoring Study programme. The recommendations on the use of thrombolysis in acute stroke have been produced by the National Institute of Clinical Excellence in July 2008.

Cardiovascular: Hypotension must be corrected (hypovolaemic hypotension may occur due to inadequate oral fluid intake). Hypertension must be managed cautiously. Some elevation in blood pressure is often seen with an acute stroke. Too drastic a reduction in blood pressure may reduce cerebral blood flow in the area around the infarct, causing extension of the stroke. Mild to moderate elevations in blood pressure do not require treatment unless they are maintained for several days after the acute event. If the diastolic blood pressure is persistently above 120 mm Hg, the blood pressure must be lowered cautiously, using oral agents, e.g. sublingual nifedipine. Avoid intramuscular preparations which may cause precipitous falls in blood pressure.

Respiratory: Patients with swallowing difficulty are at risk of bronchopulmonary aspiration. Monitor carefully for evidence of aspiration in the early stages and treat accordingly. An early review by the speech and language therapy team is beneficial.

Metabolic: Blood sugar must be maintained within normal limits. Hyperglycaemia is harmful. Monitor fluid and electrolyte balance, in view of probable inadequate oral intake in the early stages.

Surgery: Neurosurgery may need to be considered for some cases of intracerebral haemorrhage. Evacuation of a cerebellar haematoma may be life saving and result in good long-term recovery. Evacuation of supratentorial haematomas may also be life saving but survivors usually have greater disability.

Other investigations and treatments will need to be considered later to reduce the risk of recurrent stroke, but these are beyond the scope of this text.

Summary

- Stroke is common.
- Mortality is high.
- Prevalence of dependency in survivors is high.
- The history and clinical assessment provide the diagnosis in the majority of patients, but a CT brain scan is necessary to exclude other pathology and to distinguish between thrombosis and haemorrhage.
- In the acute phase, the main aim is to optimise cerebral oxygen supply and ensure normal glucose, fluid and electrolyte balance.

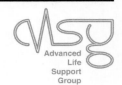

- Aspirin is of benefit and should be started once cerebral thrombosis has been confirmed.
- Early thrombolysis in appropriate cases is essential to minimise further brain injury.

TRANSIENT COLLAPSE

Collapse is common. It accounts for about 3% of visits to the emergency department and between 1 and 6% of general medical admissions. Collapse may be an isolated episode or a recurrent problem.

Recurrent collapse is important because it:
- is common
- is disabling
- may cause serious injury to the patient or to others
- can indicate life-threatening underlying pathology.

Certain factors increase the likelihood of a serious cause for syncope, warranting hospital admission. These include abnormal ECG, shortness of breath in the history of the presenting complaint, systolic blood pressure less than 90 mm Hg and haematocrit less than 30%.

Cerebral function can be disturbed by interruption of blood supply, epilepsy or metabolic factors. Some causes are listed in the next box. Whatever the cause, the initial approach to the patient should be a primary assessment and appropriate resuscitation before moving on to the secondary assessment and a more detailed history.

The prevalence of the various causes depends on the population studied. Some recently published pooled data are summarised in the box. However, carotid sinus hypersensitivity may cause up to 47% of syncope in the elderly.

Causes of recurrent collapse – prevalence

Vasovagal syncope	18%
Arrhythmia	14%
Epilepsy	10%
Postural hypotension	8%
Situational syncope	5%
Organic heart disease	4%
Medications	3%
Psychiatric	2%
Carotid sinus hypersensitivity	1%
Unknown	35%

Pathophysiology

The causes and associated reasons for a transient disturbance of consciousness are summarised in the following box.

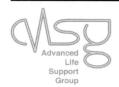

Causes of transient disturbances of consciousness

Reduction in cerebral blood flow:
  Generalised cerebral hypoperfusion (syncope)
    (i) Cardiac:

Reduced cardiac output	Myocardial ischaemia	Daily
	Hypovolaemia	Daily
	Aortic stenosis	Monthly
	Hypertrophic obstructive cardiomyopathy (HOCM)	Annually
	Pulmonary hypertension	Annually
Reduced ventricular filling	Arrhythmia	Daily
	Pulmonary embolism	Weekly
	Atrial myxoma	Only in exams

    (ii) Reflex mediated:

Vasovagal	Daily
Situational (micturition, cough)	Weekly
Carotid sinus hypersensitivity	Weekly

    (iii) Postural hypotension — Daily
  Localised vascular disease

Vertebrobasilar	Weekly
Transient ischaemic attack	Annually
Basilar artery migraine	Daily

Epilepsy
Metabolic disturbances/drugs:

Hypoxaemia	Daily
Hypoglycaemia	Daily
Hyperventilation	Only in exams

Syncope

Syncope is defined as a transient loss of consciousness associated with an acute reduction in cerebral blood flow. Although cerebral autoregulation compensates for minor changes in blood pressure, more severe reductions will cause a fall in cerebral perfusion pressure. This will lead to a loss of consciousness.

Syncope is the most common cause of recurrent loss of consciousness. The other main differential diagnosis to consider is epilepsy. The distinction is usually clear from the history. However, seizures can sometimes be precipitated by cerebral hypoperfusion due to a primary cardiac problem. It is not unusual to see abnormal jerking movements at the onset of loss of conciousness due to an arrhythymia that causes decreased cerebral perfusion (especially VT) and at the start of a witnessed cardiac arrest.

Postural hypotension is common – especially in the elderly – due to a combination of reduced baroreceptor sensitivity, excessive venous pooling and autonomic dysfunction. It is often exacerbated by drugs and dehydration.

In vasovagal syncope, venous pooling in the upright posture reduces venous return resulting in increased sympathetic activity. In response to the vigorous

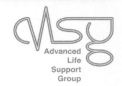

contraction of the underfilled ventricles, stimulation of ventricular mechanoreceptors initiates a brain stem reflex. This causes profound hypotension due to a combination of vagal stimulation (causing bradycardia) and withdrawal of sympathetic stimulation (causing vasodilatation) – the Bezold–Jarisch reflex.

Situational syncope occurs when the parasympathetic nervous system is activated by a trigger such as micturition or coughing.

It is important to remember ectopic pregnancy as a cause of syncope in women of child bearing age. A normal pregnancy can also cause syncope (see Chapter 23 for further details). In UK emergency medicine practice it is considered negligent not to exclude this diagnosis.

Localised vascular disease

Any disorder of the cerebral blood vessels can result in reduced cerebral perfusion. Syncope in isolation is not typically a feature of transient ischaemic episodes. Loss of consciousness does not usually occur with a stroke in the carotid artery territory. A brain stem vascular episode may result in impaired consciousness but other symptoms usually occur, e.g. vertigo, diplopia and ataxia.

Metabolic causes

Metabolic causes of transient loss of consciousness are uncommon. Hypoglycaemia must not be forgotten. It is usually due to overtreatment of diabetes mellitus but may occur in other situations, e.g. cirrhosis, Addison's disease (adrenocortical failure), postgastrectomy and insulinoma.

Hyperventilation can cause a respiratory alkalosis, which rarely predisposes to syncope.

Chronic catecholamine oversecretion with phaeochromocytoma can be associated with postural hypotension.

Drugs

Drugs can cause collapse by:
- interfering with cardiac conduction (e.g. digoxin, β blockers, calcium channel blockers, amiodarone)
- causing postural hypotension (e.g. diuretics, antihypertensives, antidepressants, levodopa preparations).
- altering conscious level – alcohol
- disturbing electrolyte balance (diuretics, B2 agonists, glucocorticoids).

Assessment

The paroxysmal nature of the problem means that you are likely to see the patient between episodes of collapse, when primary assessment is likely to reveal no major problems. Secondary assessment with a careful history and physical examination will provide the diagnosis in the majority of patients.

History

It is important to obtain a history from the patient, and also a witness if available. The circumstances of the collapse may be relevant, e.g. cough or micturition syncope.

Vasovagal syncope is usually associated with a hot environment or stressful, emotional situations. Collapse associated with head turning may indicate carotid sinus hypersensitivity. Episodes associated with exertion suggest

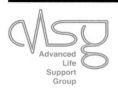

mechanical limitation of cardiac output (aortic stenosis, Hypertrophic Obstructive Cardiomyopathy (HOCM)) or an exercise induced arrhythmia. Symptoms on prolonged standing suggest postural hypotension or vasovagal syncope.

Ask specifically about cardiovascular symptoms (palpitations, chest pain, breathlessness) and neurological symptoms (headache, weakness/parasthesiae, autonomic dysfunction). **The importance of an accurate drug history cannot be over-emphasised**. A family history of syncope or sudden death may be relevant. It is also important to establish the occupation, hobbies and driving status of the patient to enable you to advise them appropriately prior to discharge. Be aware of the DVLA guidelines on driving after episodes of collapse.

The distinction between epilepsy and syncope can be difficult. A witnessed tonic–clonic convulsion associated with tongue biting and incontinence is obviously helpful in making a diagnosis, but the story may not always be so clear.

- A patient with syncope usually reports symptoms of light-headedness, nausea, sweating or blurring of vision before consciousness is lost. In contrast, a generalised tonic–clonic seizure usually has minimal prodromal symptoms.
- In syncope the duration of unconsciousness is shorter than epilepsy (seconds versus minutes) and recovery is more rapid without the usual drowsy confused postictal period.
- Brief twitching may be seen with an episode of syncope but this is usually very transient.
- Pallor may be seen before the collapse. This is common with syncope, although it may be seen with epilepsy.

Key point

The distinction between epilepsy and syncope is important. A careful history from the patient and witnesses will clarify the situation in the majority of cases

---

Examination

Assess the pulse rate, rhythm and character. Measure the lying and standing blood pressure. A fall in systolic blood pressure of 20 mm Hg after 2 min standing is significant. Remember that postural hypotension may indicate serious pathology – it is found in hypovolaemia and in some patients with peritoneal irritation. Examine the precordium for evidence of structural heart disease, especially aortic stenosis or other causes of outflow obstruction. Listen for carotid bruits.

A thorough neurological assessment is essential. Look for patterns of signs including upper motor neurone features extrapyramidal pathology, cerebellar features, brain stem signs and evidence of peripheral neuropathy.

Remember to look for injuries relating to the collapse. If the skin is broken check the tetanus status.

Actively seek evidence of tongue biting and incontinence (patients may deny the latter).

Many physicians only examine the patient on the bed. After collapse it is important to ensure the patient is still able to walk: fractured pubic rami often do not cause symptoms until the patient is weight bearing.

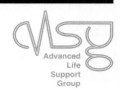

Investigations

Further investigations will be guided by the history and clinical findings.

(a) Cardiological

○ 12-lead ECG is needed for all patients with recurrent collapse looking for evidence of ischaemia, left ventricular hypertrophy or conduction abnormalities.

○ 24-h ECG monitoring may be useful if there is a suspicion of paroxysmal rhythm disturbances, even though 12-lead ECG may be normal.

○ Echocardiography is invaluable if either left ventricular outflow obstruction is suspected or left ventricular function is impaired and in patients with pulmonary hypertension.

○ Exercise testing may be useful when collapse is associated with exertion (providing left ventricular outflow obstruction has been excluded), as it may reveal ischaemia, hypotension, an arrhythmia and also hypoxaemia.

○ Specialist referral for either left and/or right heart catheterisation.

(b) Neurological

○ CT/MRI scanning is rarely required unless there are focal neurological signs or there has been a witnessed seizure.

○ Electroencephalogram is of little value in the assessment of patients with recurrent collapse. It may be helpful in confirming a diagnosis of epilepsy, when this is suspected clinically, but it is not indicated routinely in the assessment of syncope.

○ Carotid or transcranial doppler ultrasonography is rarely helpful. It should only be considered in the presence of bruits, a palpaple discrepancy between carotid pulses or when the history suggests either carotid or vertebrobasilar insufficiency.

(c) Laboratory tests

○ Laboratory tests have a poor yield unless there is clinical suspicion of an abnormality. However, it is worth checking glucose, urea and electrolytes, and haemoglobin.

○ Rarely the clinical features may indicate either Addison's disease (adrenocortical failure) or phaeochromocytoma; therefore, a short Synacthen® test or 24-h urine collection for catecholamines, respectively, may be needed.

(d) Other investigations

○ Carotid sinus massage. This is contraindicated:

(i) in the presence of carotid bruits or cerebrovascular disease

(ii) if there is a history of ventricular arrhythmias or recent myocardial infarction.

Providing there are no contraindications, place the patient in the supine position and monitor ECG and blood pressure. The right carotid artery is massaged longitudinally, with the neck slightly extended, for a maximum of 5 s. If the response is negative there should be a 30-s interval before the left carotid artery is massaged (maximum 5 s).

Key point

Bilateral carotid massage must never be attempted at the same time.

A positive cardioinhibitory response is defined as a sinus pause of 3 s or more. A positive vasodepressor response is defined as a fall in systolic blood pressure of more than 50 mm Hg.

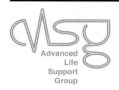

○ Tilt testing is useful in the further assessment of unexplained recurrent syncope after exclusion of other cardiac causes including arrhythmias. Briefly:

(i) Baseline pulse and blood pressure recordings are measured with the patient lying supine for 30 min.

(ii) The patient is tilted to 60–75° for up to 45 min and asked to report any symptoms.

(iii) A positive result is a cardioinhibitory response and/or a vasodepressor response in association with symptoms.

(iv) If a positive response occurs, the patient is immediately returned to the horizontal position.

Other measures may be used to increase the sensitivity of the test.

Key point

With both carotid sinus massage and tilt testing full resuscitation facilities must be available immediately

---

SPECIFIC CONDITIONS

Status epilepticus

Status epilepticus is defined as either a single seizure lasting for 30 min or repeated seizures between which there is incomplete recovery of consciousness. However, seizures lasting more than 5 min can indicate impending status epilepticus. This may be prevented by immediate treatment.

Key point

Generalised convulsive status epilepticus is a common and serious medical emergency. There is a significant risk of permanent brain damage and death from cardiorespiratory failure (5–10% mortality in those admitted to intensive care units)

Primary assessment and resuscitation – specific summary for epilepsy management

A – Maintain patency/initially with nasopharyngeal airway

Give oxygen ($FiO_2 = 0.85$)

Do not attempt to insert oral airway/intubate while jaw is clenched

Early liaison with anaesthetist

B – Pulse oximeter. Respiratory rate. Occasionally respiration may need to be assisted

C – Establish IV access

Monitor ECG

D – IV benzodiazepine to terminate seizure. Lorazepam is probably better than diazepam as it lasts longer, has a lower incidence of cardio-respiratory side effects and has the same speed of onset

In the absence of IV benzodiazepine access, rectal diazepam may be used.

Check glucose-immediate bedside test and laboratory test

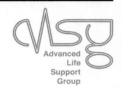

IV thiamine (250 mg over 10 min) especially if there is a history of chronic alcohol abuse

Look for evidence of head injury

E – Check temperature

Look for purpura (meningococcal septicaemia)

Respiratory depression and hypotension may occur after IV diazemuls or lorazepam. The dose of lorazepam is 0.1 mg/kg, max 4 mg by slow IV injection (2 mg/min), that of diazepam 10 mg at a rate of 2.5 mg/30 s. Both can be repeated if necessary. If control is not achieved, phenytoin 15 mg/kg IV should be given with ECG monitoring (reduce dose if patient is previously on phenytoin). The infusion rate should not exceed 50 mg/min because of the risk of cardiac arrhythmias. Further doses up to a total of 30 mg/kg may be given if seizures persist. Then maintenance doses of 100 mg IV should be given every 6–8 h. Phenytoin has the advantage of suppressing seizures without causing cortical or respiratory depression. An alternative is fosphenytoin (18 mg/kg phenytoin equivalent IV up to 150 mg/min). If seizures continue, the patient should be anaesthetised and ventilated.

Cerebral function monitoring is very useful in this situation. Anaesthesia and ventilation should continue until 12–24 h after the last seizure.

Secondary assessment

A history from a relative is important. Are there any symptoms to suggest tumour, meningitis or head injury? Ask about alcohol consumption. If the patient is a known epileptic, ask about current drug regime, compliance or any recent changes in drug therapy.

Physical examination includes a careful neurological assessment, looking particularly for evidence of meningeal irritation, raised intracranial pressure and focal neurological deficits.

Arrhythmia

Bradycardia

Bradycardia may be diagnosed on 24-h ECG monitoring but it is important to document associated symptoms. Review the patient's medications and stop those which may cause bradycardia.

In the presence of sino-atrial node disease, pacing may be considered if pauses greater than 3 s are documented.

With atrioventicular node dysfunction, pacing should be considered for second-degree or third-degree heart block, in the absence of a reversible cause (drugs or ischaemia).

Tachycardia

Supraventricular tachycardias, including atrial fibrillation, often cause palpitations and dizziness but rarely present with syncope. Ventricular tachycardia is more likely to cause syncope. The Wolff–Parkinson–White syndrome and the prolonged QT syndrome should be considered in patients with recurrent syncope. The type of tachycardia will determine the treatment. This comprises anti-arrhythmic drug therapy, occasionally an anti-tachycardia pacemaker/defibrillator or radio-ablation. Transient rhythm abnormalities are increasingly common with increasing age, e.g. short runs of atrial fibrillation and sinus bradycardia occur at night. Do not treat unless there is clear evidence that these arrhythmias are associated with symptoms or predispose to further pathology, e.g. paroxysmal atrial fibrillation and stroke.

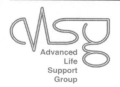

Vasovagal syncope

The mechanism of collapse in vasovagal syncope and the assessment of patients by tilt testing has been described. Treatment is not always satisfactory. β blockers may be used to inhibit the initial sympathetic activation in vasovagal syncope. With a positive cardioinhibitory response to tilt testing, disopyramide may be useful (to block the vagal outflow) or dual chamber pacing may be necessary. With a predominant vasodepressor response, ephedrine, dihydroergotamine or fludrocortisone have been tried with variable success.

Carotid sinus hypersensitivity

Hypersensitivity of the carotid artery baroreceptors can cause bradycardia and/or vasodilatation due to vagal activation. The patient complains of dizziness or syncope associated with head turning or the wearing of a tight collar. Diagnosis is by carotid sinus massage as described previously. A positive cardioinhibitory response to this technique responds well to cardiac pacing. As with vasovagal syncope, a vasodepressor response is more difficult to treat.

Postural hypotension

Postural hypotension is associated with:
- hypovolaemia (dehydration, haemorrhage, diuretics)
- drugs (nitrates, levodopa preparations)
- autonomic failure (diabetes mellitus, Parkinson's disease, old age).

It is difficult to treat patients who have postural hypotension. Attempt to correct intravascular volume and rationalise the drug therapy as much as possible. Patients should be advised to stand up slowly and to avoid prolonged standing. Graduated elastic stockings may reduce venous pooling. Fludrocortisone increases salt and water retention and is occasionally helpful. Midadrine, an alpha agonist, can be used orally to increase systemic vascular resistance, but should only be used on the advice of a cardiologist.

Left ventricular outflow obstruction

Advanced aortic stenosis may cause exertional dizziness and syncope because cardiac output is reduced. Such symptoms indicate urgent assessment with a view to aortic valve replacement.

HOCM is associated with restricted cardiac output during stress. Treatment is with negatively inotropic drugs (β blockers, verapamil) to reduce the outflow tract gradient. Dual chamber pacing or surgery may be needed in more advanced cases.

Time Out 12.1

a Define 'stroke'.
b Describe your immediate management of a patient with a suspected transient ischaemic attack.

SUMMARY

Recurrent collapse is common.
- It can be associated with life-threatening underlying pathology and can cause serious injury.

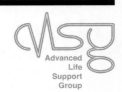

- History and physical examination provide a likely diagnosis in the majority of patients.
- Further investigation will be guided by clinical judgment and by the frequency and severity of the symptoms.

Following stroke:

- Early CT scanning will identify patients suitable for thrombolysis.
- A normal CT brain scan excludes a cerebral bleed.

In transient collapse:

- loss of consciousness is an uncommon feature of transient ischaemic attack
- prodromal symptoms of light headedness, nausea and sweating suggest syncope rather than epilepsy as a cause of collapse
- a sinus pause of 3 s or more with carotid sinus massage is significant.

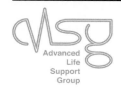
Advanced
Life
Support
Group

CHAPTER 13

The overdose patient

OBJECTIVES

After reading this chapter you will be able to:
- describe how the structured approach can be applied to patients who have taken an overdose
- discuss the diagnostic clues that may be available in the primary assessment
- understand the indications and contraindications of measures to minimise drug absorption
- describe specific treatment strategies for drugs commonly taken as an overdose

---

INTRODUCTION

The management of overdose patients is a challenging aspect of emergency medicine. The diagnosis can be difficult in the absence of a clear history, so medical staff should have a high index of suspicion when assessing patients who may have taken a drug overdose. This is especially important in patients presenting with reduced conscious level. Furthermore, many patients are reluctant to cooperate during their initial assessment. The potentially significant effects of substances taken may not be immediately obvious, but may require emergency intervention to limit morbidity and mortality.

The majority of cases are a result of deliberate self-harm. Remember that 'overdose' is a description of an action, not a definitive diagnosis. Overdoses with multiple different medications is no longer a rarity. Be aware of those drugs with high lethality in overdose and narrow therapeutic windows (see below) and be sure to enquire by proper, forensic history taking about the likelihood of the patient having taken any other medications, as well as the apparent one.

Accidental overdose is also fairly common, especially in children and in recreational drug users. Accidental chronic overdose can also occur in elderly patients on multiple medications and in patients with long-standing health problems such as chronic renal failure. The presentation of these patients is variable and may include unusual behaviour, decreased conscious level, fits or cardiac arrhythmias.

Whatever the presentation, medical care should follow the structured approach described in Chapter 3 – with primary assessment and resuscitation preceding secondary assessment, emergency treatment and definitive care. Psychiatric assessment is often necessary in this group of patients and should take place as soon as is reasonably possible.

Acute Medical Emergencies; The Practical Approach, 2nd edition.
Edited by Terence Wardle, Peter Driscoll, and Sue Wieteska.
© 2010 Blackwell Publishing Ltd.

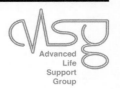

PRIMARY ASSESSMENT AND RESUSCITATION

A – airway

An appropriate answer to the question, 'Are you all right?' will allow the examining doctor to establish that the patient has a patent airway with reasonable laryngeal function, is conscious with adequate cerebral perfusion, and has sufficient respiratory function to speak. A patient who fails to respond to this question should prompt more detailed airway assessment as to the need for supporting airway adjuncts, as described in Chapter 3. Remember that a patient with a reduced conscious level is likely to have impaired protective airway reflexes and is therefore at risk of regurgitation and aspiration. As always with the unconscious patient, consider the risk of spinal column injury, avoid unnecessary movement of the neck and consider formal cervical spine immobilisation if you feel it is indicated.

B – breathing

Since a number of agents taken in overdose can produce respiratory depression, it is very important to look for adequate breathing. The rate, depth and work of breathing should be assessed. If there are any signs of ventilatory inadequacy, breathing should be supported by the use of a bag–valve–mask device attached to high concentrations of inspired oxygen; consider reversing the cause of the inadequate ventilation (e.g. naloxone in opiate overdose). Even in the patient who appears to be breathing adequately, high concentrations of inspired oxygen should be given until it is deemed unnecessary. Remember that adequate oxygen saturation on pulse oximetry does not guarantee adequate ventilation and carbon dioxide retention may be present with normal oxygen saturation. Arterial blood gases should be measured if there is any concern about the patient's ventilation.

Remember that unexplained tachypnoea may reflect a metabolic acidosis resulting from the overdose, e.g. following salicylates.

C – circulation

Pulse rate, adequacy of peripheral perfusion, cardiac rhythm and blood pressure should be assessed. Inadequate circulation in the overdose patient is generally caused by hypotension or cardiac arrhythmia.

Hypotension is usually caused by a relative hypovolaemia secondary to peripheral vasodilation, often compounded by poor intake during a period of reduced consciousness or the diuretic effect of alcohol taken in association with the overdose. This responds well to fluid resuscitation.

The cause of cardiac arrhythmias differs from those seen in ischaemic heart disease, as they are likely to be due to drug toxicity, and therefore require a different approach in their management. Arrhythmias are often surprisingly well tolerated in the overdose patient and specific anti-arrhythmic drug treatment should be avoided, if possible. Treatment should initially be directed at minimising the effects of the drug likely to be provoking the arrhythmia, in particular correcting abnormalities in electrolytes, calcium and magnesium in the bloodstream. If anti-arrhythmic treatment becomes necessary, cardioversion should be considered as an alternative to medical treatment to avoid potential drug interactions and side effects.

Intravenous access should be established at this stage, providing a route for fluid resuscitation, emergency medication and an opportunity to take blood samples for relevant investigations.

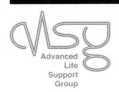

D – disability

Assess conscious level using either the AVPU or Glasgow Coma Scale (see Chapter 3) and measure the pupillary size and response to light. These latter observations can be helpful in establishing a diagnosis if the agent that has been taken is unknown. Although the Glasgow Coma Scale has not been validated for poisoned patients, it remains the most useful objective measure of conscious level.

Many drugs, such as paracetamol and alcohol, can cause rapid hypoglycaemia, so a bedside glucose level should be measured, followed by a formal laboratory sample.

E – exposure

Full exposure is necessary, looking for signs of injury, rashes and possible needle track marks. It is very important to assess temperature at this stage, since a number of drugs can alter thermoregulatory mechanisms, e.g. phenothiazines. Once patients have been fully exposed and the required examination has been completed, cover immediately, as many will lose heat rapidly in this situation.

By the end of the primary assessment, the minimum essential monitoring should include pulse oximetry and ECG monitoring. The respiratory rate, pulse, blood pressure, Glasgow Coma Score, temperature and glucose concentration should have been documented. These observations need to be repeated on a regular basis, to monitor the patient's condition and response to treatment.

Diagnostic clues from the primary assessment may provide a pointer towards the specific drug or drugs ingested and therefore guide specific management. These are listed in Table 13.1.

LETHALITY ASSESSMENT

At the end of the primary assessment, it is important to assess the potential lethality of the overdose. This requires knowledge of the substance, the time it was taken and the dose. Corroborative evidence may need to be sought from other sources, such as family members, friends or paramedic staff. If the nature of the overdose is unknown then a high potential lethality should be assumed.

The UK National Poisons Information Service (NPIS) provides the online TOXBASE database, which provides evidenced-based advice on diagnosis, treatment and management of patients who have been poisoned. This is supported by a second tier consultant-led information service for more complex clinical advice. TOXBASE is available to all health care workers, usually via a registered hospital department or general practice and should be the first point of contact for poisons information. The NPIS has six regional poisons centres which can also be accessed by phone 24 h a day for advice consistent with that available on TOXBASE.

IMMEDIATE MANAGEMENT

Problems identified in the primary assessment should be treated in the standard way. In addition, there are techniques available to reduce absorption of ingested drugs from the gastrointestinal tract and to increase elimination of drugs that have already been absorbed.

Table 13.1 Diagnostic clues from the primary assessment

	Sign	Drug
B	Tachypnoea	Aspirin, ethylene glycol
	Bradypnoea	Opioids
		CNS depressants
C	Tachycardia	Antidepressants
		Sympathomimetics
		Amphetamines
		Cocaine
	Bradycardia	β blockers
		Digoxin
		Clonidine
	Hypertension	Amphetamines
		Cocaine
D	Small pupils	Opioids
		Cholinesterase inhibitors
	Large pupils	Tricyclic antidepressants
		Anticholinergics
		Antihistamines
		Ephedrine
		Amphetamines
		Cocaine
	Coma	Barbiturates
		Tricyclic antidepressants
		Opioids
		Benzodiazepines
		Ethanol
E	Hypothermia	Tricyclic antidepressants
		Barbiturates
		Phenothiazines
	Hyperthermia	Amphetamines
		Cocaine

Reducing absorption

Methods to minimise drug absorption have been used liberally in the past. Recent evidence shows that such techniques are of limited value and only have a role in a minority of patients. It should be noted that they should never be used as a punitive measure, as their use does not deter patients from further episodes of overdose and they expose the patient to the risk of side effects without likely therapeutic benefit. These measures should be used on the advice of Toxbase or NPIS.

Activated charcoal

Charcoal works by absorbing ingested drugs onto its large surface area. It is the treatment of choice when efforts to decrease the systemic absorption of drugs in the overdose patient are indicated. Its dose is 50 g (1 g/kg in children). However, it is usually limited to patients presenting within 1 h of taking a life-threatening overdose. This time period may be increased for certain drugs which prolong gastric emptying, most commonly aspirin and tricyclic antidepressants (Table 13.2).

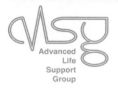

Table 13.2 Drugs which delay gastric emptying

Drug	Minimum dose	Maximum time since ingestion
Paracetamol	12 g	4 h
Theophyllines	>2.5 g	4 h
Tricyclic antidepressants	>750 mg	8 h
Aspirin	15 g	12 h

Charcoal will only absorb 10% of its own weight of a drug, so in large overdose repeated doses of charcoal can be considered. Compliance with taking charcoal is generally low, due to its unpleasant black appearance and taste. The use of a naso-gastric or oro-gastric tube may help those patients unwilling to drink charcoal. Consider endotracheal intubation, to prevent aspiration either in unconscious patients, or in those who have recently taken an overdose that will render them unconscious.

Certain agents are not absorbed by charcoal; these include metal salts (iron, lithium), alcohols, acids/alkalis, solvents, hydrocarbons, cyanide and fluoride.

Whole bowel irrigation

Polyethylene glycol (e.g. Kleen Prep) is given either orally or via a naso-gastric tube, at a rate of 2 l/h, until the resulting watery diarrhoea becomes clear. It should not be used in the presence of a paralytic ileus or suspected mechanical obstruction. It is indicated after ingestion of large volumes of agents not absorbed by charcoal, body packers and significant ingestion of sustained release or enteric coated formulations.

Gastric lavage

Gastric lavage has largely been superceded by the use of activated charcoal. Delayed gastric lavage has little value and may propel drugs further along the gastrointestinal tract. It may be considered for those drugs not absorbed by charcoal, such as iron and lithium. It is absolutely contraindicated after ingestion of caustic agents (Table 13.3). If the patient's airway is compromised and gastric lavage is thought to be of value, the airway should be managed by a doctor with anaesthetic training and will usually require insertion of a cuffed endotracheal tube.

Table 13.3 Contraindications to gastric lavage

Corrosive agents	Acid
	Alkali
	Bleach
Petroleum derivatives	Petrol
	Paraffin
	White spirits
	Turpentine substitute
	Kerosene

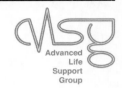

Therapeutic emesis

Centrally acting emetics such as ipecacuanha have been used historically to promote active vomiting. The symptoms produced can often cloud an already complicated clinical picture. There is no evidence that it decreases absorption and its use in emergency practice is now obsolete.

Increasing elimination

Adequate cardiovascular and fluid resuscitation of the patient in the primary assessment will maximise the body's normal routes for excretion of toxins via the liver and kidneys. Measures to increase elimination of life-threatening overdoses are specific to the drugs ingested and include therapeutic diuresis, alkalinisation, chelation, haemoperfusion and haemodialysis. Such treatments should only be used on the advice of specialists.

Multiple dose activated charcoal

Fifty grams can be given every 4 h for large ingestions of drugs that have a significant entero-hepatic circulation, such as carbamazepine, theophylline, phenobarbitone, quinine, dapsone, digoxin and salicylate.

Urinary alkalinisation

This can be used for large ingestions of aspirin, phenobarbitone, chlorpropramide, mecoprop and phenoxyacetate herbicides. Urinary alkalinisation can be achieved by giving intravenous sodium bicarbonate (1 litre of 1.26% over 3 h). Renal function and plasma potassium must be checked first, as it is difficult to produce alkaline urine in the presence of hypokalaemia. Potassium levels may fall during the diuresis, so they should be checked regularly and replaced with 20–40 mmol of potassium in each litre of sodium bicarbonate if needed. The therapeutic goal is a blood gas base excess reading of +8 and urinary pH > 7.5.

Extracorporeal methods

These include charcoal haemoperfusion, haemofiltration and haemodialysis. They are only indicated in a limited number of situations and are usually done in an HDU or ITU setting. However, when clearly indicated/advised by the Poisons Information Centre, these treatments are life-saving and should be started immediately.

SECONDARY ASSESSMENT

As in all other emergency presentations, the secondary assessment involves taking as full a history as possible. A full examination is also necessary, and should include examining for physical evidence of self-harm and injury such as cutting, needle marks and signs of head injury. Some symptoms and signs elicited in the secondary assessment may provide clues to specific types of overdose. These are listed in Table 13.4.

Appropriate investigations should be ordered, based on the findings in the secondary assessment. A 12-lead ECG should be recorded in all patients with any kind of rhythm disturbance or with potential cardiac sequelae from their overdose, in particular looking carefully for signs of conduction abnormalities that may precede frank rhythm disturbance. A chest X-ray is necessary in unconscious patients, those with possible aspiration and those with abnormal findings on respiratory examination.

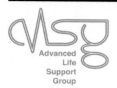

Table 13.4 Clues to possible overdose from secondary assessment

Pulmonary oedema	Salicylate
	Ethylene glycol
	Opiate
	Organophosphates
	Paraquat
Hypoglycaemia	Insulin
	Oral hypoglycaemic
	Ethanol
	Paracetamol
	Salicylate
Hyperglycaemia	Salbutamol
	Theophylline
Hypokalaemia	Salbutamol
	Theophylline
	Salicylates
Metabolic acidosis	Salicylates
	Paracetamol
	Ethanol
	Ethylene glycol
	Tricyclics
Raised osmolality	Ethanol
	Methanol
	Ethylene glycol
Prolonged prothrombin time	Salicylates
	Paracetamol

Blood investigations depend on the drugs ingested. They are likely to include full blood count, glucose, urea and electrolytes, renal and liver function, coagulation screen and serum osmolality. Arterial blood gases will help to quantify any respiratory compromise and also indicate an acid–base disturbance. Toxicology screening is generally limited by local resources to paracetamol and salicylate estimation, but blood and urine may be saved for further testing, depending on the services available.

Commercially available urinary dip tests can be used to indicate the presence of certain drugs used recreationally such as benzodiazepines, opioids, cocaine, amphetamines and cannabinoids. It is worth remembering that some of these chemicals remain present in the urine for several weeks. 'Recreational' drug use is common. As with all investigations, treat the patient, not the result. If the patient's condition does not clearly fit the 'toxidrome/toxic drug syndrome' produced by the drug that has been shown to be present search for another cause of the patient's medical emergency. In particular, for example the patient with altered consciousness may have head trauma, stroke or intracranial infection.

EMERGENCY TREATMENT OF SPECIFIC OVERDOSES

In addition to the general management described previously, certain poisons require specific antidotes. Some of the more commonly used antidotes are listed in Table 13.5.

Table 13.5 Specific measures in overdose

Drug	Treatment
Paracetamol	*N*-Acetyl cysteine
Opioids	Naloxone
Tricyclic antidepressants	Sodium bicarbonate
Digoxin	Specific Fab antibodies
Ethylene glycol	Ethanol, fomepizol, haemodialysis
Iron	Desferrioxamine
Methanol	Ethanol
Cyanide	100% oxygen, amyl nitrite, sodium thiosulphate, high dose vitamin B_{12}
Organophosphates	Atropine, pralidoxime
β blockers	Glucagon, dobutamine, atropine, isoprenaline, temporary pacing
Aspirin	Dose dependent: diuresis, alkaline diuresis, haemodialysis

Paracetamol, tricyclic antidepressant and opioid overdoses are common. These drugs will be discussed in more detail, due to their, risk of high morbidity and mortality and because of the potential benefit from correct management.

Paracetamol

Paracetamol overdose is very common in the UK, with a risk of high morbidity and mortality. With correct treatment, most patients will make a full recovery with no long-term sequelae.

Paracetamol is normally metabolised in the liver to form non-toxic metabolites which are excreted in the urine. If the normal pathways of metabolism are saturated, the excess paracetamol will form toxic metabolites which are rapidly conjugated with glutathione and excreted. Accumulation of the toxic metabolites results in hepatocellular damage and liver necrosis.

The antidote to paracetamol overdose is *N*-acetylcysteine (NAC), which works by preventing toxic metabolite formation, increasing availability of glutathione and acting as a glutathione analogue. It also has vasodilatory, anti-inflammatory and anti-oxidant effects, which limit morbidity and mortality once hepatotoxicty is established.

Certain patient groups are at greater risk of morbidity in paracetamol overdose, either from glutathione deficiency (alcoholism, AIDS, anorexia nervosa, malnutrition) or enhanced enzyme activity, which increases toxic metabolite formation (patients on rifampicin, barbiturates, anti-convulsants).

Important factors in the assessment of the patient are: amount taken, time taken and whether the overdose was staggered over a period of time. Significant overdose is considered to occur if the patient has ingested a total of at least 12 g or 150 mg/kg of paracetamol. This level is reduced to 75 mg/kg in the at-risk patient groups described above.

The serum paracetamol level is valuable to diagnosis and management, as the patient may exhibit non-specific symptoms or be asymptomatic for up to 24 h following ingestion. The level should be taken 4 h after single ingestion and plotted on the paracetamol treatment graph to determine need for NAC therapy. The level should not be taken until 4 h have elapsed from ingestion, as the result is likely to

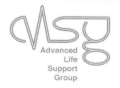

be inaccurate and can lead to under-treatment of the patient. Paracetamol levels are also extremely difficult to interpret in cases of staggered overdose or when 24 h have elapsed since the time of ingestion. In these cases, markers of hepatic and renal damage such as prothrombin time, creatinine and electrolytes, venous bicarbonate and arterial blood gases (and, of course, expert advice), should guide management.

In situations where there is strong clinical suspicion of significant overdose or the paracetamol level will not be available within 8 h of ingestion, start NAC therapy until either paracetamol levels are available or other markers of toxicity are available to guide further management. Although NAC is most effective if started early, it should not be started without clear clinical indication as it can cause an anaphylactoid reaction in susceptible patients. The safe management of patients with paracetamol overdose can be complicated and is beyond the scope of this chapter. Detailed advice relating to individual patients, in particular those who have taken a staggered overdose over a period of time, should be obtained from the NPIS phone lines or from TOXBASE.

Tricyclic antidepressant drugs

The toxicity of tricyclic antidepressant (TCA) drugs is mainly due to anticholinergic effects and a quinidine-like effect on the myocardium (blocking of fast sodium channels). The majority of life-threatening problems occur in the first 6 h following ingestion and are principally due to seizures and arrhythmias. The patient may show signs of agitation, tachycardia, dilated pupils and ataxia. This may progress rapidly to drowsiness or coma, increased tone, hyperreflexia, hypotension, and respiratory depression. The ECG may show tachycardia and, in severe poisoning, bizarre rhythms may be present. Widening of the QRS complex indicates a greater risk of seizures and arrhythmias.

These patients are often under-resuscitated and may need intensive care. Assisted ventilation may be needed to correct hypoxaemia and hypercapnia. Blood should be taken for urea and electrolytes, glucose and arterial blood gases. A 12-lead ECG is needed to look for conduction disturbance and the patient must be monitored for a rhythm disturbance.

If the patient has possibly taken a significant overdose ($>$1 g of TCA in an adult), they must be placed in a high dependency treatment area on a cardiac monitor until at least 6 h have passed from the latest possible time of ingestion, even if their initial ECG and physical examination signs are normal. If the initial ECG or GCS is abnormal, they should remain on a cardiac monitor for at least 12 h after their ECG has returned to normal.

Cardiac arrhythmias should be treated by correction of hypoxaemia, electrolyte disturbance and acidosis, rather than by drugs wherever possible. The exception to this, however, is sodium bicarbonate which is of particular value in these patients. Alkalinisation alters the binding of TCAs to the myocardium and the sodium load counteracts the sodium channel blockade, both of which are cardioprotective. Even in the absence of acidosis, treat adults with arrhythmias or ECG abnormalities with 50 mmol sodium bicarbonate intravenously. (500 ml of 1.26% contains 75 mmol sodium bicarbonate and 50 ml of 8.4% contains 50 mmol sodium bicarbonate), but remember the stronger concentration as it is very irritant to veins and can cause skin necrosis if extravasation occurs. Further doses may be required depending on the clinical response. The patient with significant physiological disturbance should have their pH maintained above the upper range of normal, at 7.5–7.55, by means of manipulation of hyperventilation, where possible, and further doses of sodium bicarbonate.

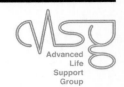

Convulsions should be treated in the usual fashion with intravenous benzodiazepines. If seizures persist, the patient may need to be intubated, paralysed and ventilated. Further anti-convulsants need to be administered. **Phenytoin should not be given** in TCA overdose as it blocks sodium channels and can increase the risk of arrhythmias.

If the patient is thought to have taken a combined TCA and benzodiazepine overdose, **flumazenil should not be used** to reverse the benzodiazepine component. In combined overdose, the benzodiazepine is protective and reversal may precipitate seizures or cardiac arrest, which may be refractory to treatment.

Opioids

Acute opioid poisoning is commonly accidental in intravenous drug users, either from diamorphine (heroin) or from methadone. These patients often present with pinpoint pupils and profound respiratory depression, or even respiratory arrest. Fresh and old venepuncture marks, track marks and thrombosed superficial veins may give a clue to the diagnosis.

Immediate management should be aimed to ensure a patent airway and oxygenation. This can usually be achieved on a short-term basis with bag valve mask ventilation and high concentrations of inspired oxygen. Endotracheal intubation may be required. Be careful not to fall into the trap of letting an apnoeic patient become more and more cyanosed while hunting for venous access to give naloxone. Ensure adequate oxygenation and ventilation first.

Naloxone is a specific opioid antagonist and should be given intravenously as a therapeutic trial as soon as safely possible in suspected opioid poisoning. The naloxone should be titrated in small aliquots against the patient's response, as a large bolus runs the risk of rapid complete reversal. In chronic users, this will precipitate an acute withdrawal syndrome (AWS) or 'cold turkey' characterised by profound agitation, nausea, abdominal pain and diarrhoea. This can result in an angry, uncooperative, potentially violent and often slightly confused patient taking their own discharge from the resuscitation room. The therapeutic effect of naloxone is much shorter than most of the opioids taken recreationally, due to more rapid redistribution of naloxone away from the receptor sites. Therefore, the patient is at considerable risk of relapsing into life-threatening respiratory depression shortly after leaving the hospital.

To avoid precipitating AWS, titrate naloxone at a rate of 0.1 mg/min, aiming for a respiratory rate of greater than 10 and a GCS of 13–14/15. The patient may still be drowsy at this level of reversal, but should maintain their own airway and self ventilate adequately. An infusion of naloxone may be indicated in some patients, usually at a dose of 2/3 of the initial dose per hour. The patient should be carefully monitored until the opioid is fully reversed. Avoid using subcutaneous and intra muscular routes if possible as absorption from these sites is unpredictable. However, if intravenous access is impossible and the patient is collapsed, doses of 0.8 mg subcutaneously or 0.4 mg intramuscularly can be given and the patient observed carefully for at least 2 h.

MENTAL HEALTH ASSESSMENT

It is essential that all patients who have taken an intentional drug overdose undergo mental health assessment. This is important for two reasons. Firstly, it is important to make a risk assessment as soon as reasonably possible to determine the patient's risk of immediate further self-harm. This risk assessment can help to direct the care each patient requires. This may include the need for one-to-one

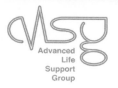

psychiatric nursing for those patients at risk of further suicide attempts. A number of factors can help to indicate the seriousness of the individual's intent for self-harm and some of these are summarised in the next box. Secondly, the patient's need for ongoing psychiatric support needs to be decided.

Factors defining intent in deliberate self-harm

Patient's perception of lethality
Evidence of premeditation
Measures to prevent discovery
Social circumstances
Evidence of depression
Evidence of psychosis

A common error in the management of deliberate self-harming patients is to delay mental health assessment until all medical treatment is completed. This can put vulnerable patients at considerable risk, by delaying recognition and appropriate management of severe mental illness. In most cases, the medical and psychiatric care can be conducted in parallel, e.g. the psychiatric liaison nurse can perform a risk assessment while medics await blood results. Similarly, moderate alcohol consumption is not a contraindication to mental health assessment. The exceptions to this are grossly intoxicated patients, those who are critically ill or have reduced conscious level.

All doctors involved in the medical management of overdose patients should be trained in basic mental health risk assessment and be able to recognise when psychiatric referral is appropriate. Many emergency departments have a mental health liaison team, consisting of specially trained psychiatric nurses who work as independent practitioners and are able to assess, manage and discharge patients with mental health problems. These practitioners' skill and experience can lend invaluable support to emergency medical teams.

DEFINITIVE CARE

Some patients may require admission to the medical wards or to an emergency department short stay ward, either for active management or for a short period of observation. However, a large number will be fit for medical discharge after immediate assessment. It should be remembered that many of the effects of drug overdose are delayed, e.g. nephrotoxic renal failure due to either paracetamol or aspirin. It is important to anticipate such complications and where possible take measures to prevent them. Unfortunately this is not always possible if there is a prolonged time between ingestion and presentation to hospital.

SUMMARY

- The structured approach to the seriously ill patient should be used when dealing with patients who have taken overdoses.
- The potential lethality of the overdose must be assessed at the end of the primary assessment.

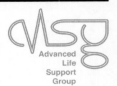

- If indicated, measures should be taken to stop absorption and increase excretion of the ingested compound.
- Specific treatment may be indicated once the substance ingested has been identified.
- A mental health assessment must be made in all patients to determine the risk of further self-harm and need for psychiatric support.

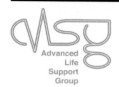

CHAPTER 14

The patient with a headache

OBJECTIVES

After reading this chapter you should be able to:
- understand the causes of headache
- describe a classification of headache that will be useful in clinical practice
- discuss the initial management of a patient with headache
- describe how clinical signs detected in the secondary assessment influence diagnosis and subsequent management.

INTRODUCTION

Patients presenting with a headache of acute onset account for less than 2.5% of new emergency attendances. Of these, only 15% will have a serious cause for their headache. Therefore, the aim is to identify the relatively small group of high risk patients.

PATHOPHYSIOLOGY

Pain sensitive structures that can cause a headache include:
- dura
- arteries
- venous sinuses
- paranasal sinuses
- eyes
- tympanic membranes
- cervical spine.

These are innervated by somatic afferents from the V, VII, IX and X cranial nerves (linked via the spinal tract of the trigeminal nerve) and the upper three cervical nerve roots. Pain will occur if there is traction, inflammation or distension of these structures, in particular, the dura, blood vessels and nerves. A throbbing headache is non-specific because it is common to many intracranial conditions. Similarly the site of pain is non-specific, but it can provide clues to underlying pathology as outlined below.

• Frontal	Ipsilateral forehead and eye pain, referred via the trigeminal nerve, can indicate a lesion in the anterior or middle cranial fossa.
	Bifrontal headache can be a presenting feature of acute hydrocephalus secondary, e.g. to either a supra- or infratentorial lesion. The pain is attributed to vascular distortion following dilatation of the lateral ventricles.

Acute Medical Emergencies; The Practical Approach, 2nd edition.
Edited by Terence Wardle, Peter Driscoll, and Sue Wieteska.
© 2010 Blackwell Publishing Ltd.

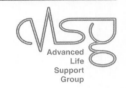

- Frontotemporal Unilateral pain is common with sinusitis and dental problems. In addition, orbital cellulitis, glaucoma, and cavernous sinus thrombosis have a similar presentation.

- Occipital Posterior fossa or upper cervical spine pathology (referred via the upper three cervical nerve roots) can present with occipital pain.

In contrast, the distribution of pain can be more specific.

- Trigeminal Neuralgia is restricted to the distribution of the trigeminal nerve. The searing paroxysms of intense pain are usually unilateral and confined to one division. Occasionally, two or all three divisions are involved. This specific distribution of pain is attributed to distortion of the blood vessels supplying the trigeminal nerve.

- Somatic afferent Postherpetic neuralgia is secondary to inflammation and will occur in the distribution of the affected nerve, i.e. the V, VII, IX and X cranial nerves.

CLINICAL ASSESSMENT

A useful way to categorise patients presenting with a headache is shown in the next box.

Clinical classification of headache

Headache with **altered Glasgow Coma Score** and/or **focal neurological signs**
Headache with **papilloedema** but no focal neurological signs
Headache with **fever** but no focal neurological signs
Headache with **extracranial** signs
Headache with **no** abnormal signs

This classification will form the framework of the remaining sections in this chapter. It is important to note that some conditions occur in more than one category – reflecting their diverse manifestations. The structure of the initial assessment and the above classification is designed to ensure early detection and management of an immediately life-threatening problem, i.e. headache with **altered Glasgow Coma Score** and/or **focal neurological signs**. The remaining, non-immediately life-threatening causes will be identified in the secondary assessment.

HEADACHE WITH ALTERED GLASGOW COMA SCORE AND/OR FOCAL NEUROLOGICAL SIGNS

After assessing 'D' the following will have been identified:
- a reduction in the Glasgow Coma Score
- the presence of lateralising signs
- pupillary abnormalities
- meningeal irritation.

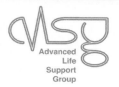

Table 14.1 Causes of headache with altered Glasgow Coma Score and/or focal neurological signs

Vascular	Stroke	Daily
	Subarachnoid haemorrhage	Weekly
	Chronic subdural haematoma	Monthly
Infective	Meningitis	Daily
	Encephalitis	Monthly
	Cerebral abscess	Monthly
	Subdural empyema	Annually
	Cerebral malaria	Annually
Neoplastic	Secondary intracerebral tumour	Weekly
	Primary intracerebral tumour	Monthly

Although the specific diagnosis is often unknown at this stage, the patient should receive optimum oxygenation and appropriate control of both blood pressure and serum glucose.

An immediately life-threatening event either causing or following a headache will be identified in the **primary assessment**. Such conditions are listed in Table 14.1.

Key point

Remember that the goal of initial management is to prevent secondary brain injury

---

Key management issues
- The mode of onset of symptoms will help distinguish different conditions, e.g.:
  - acute onset = vascular
  - subacute onset = infective
  - chronic onset = neoplastic.
- If the patient is febrile, take blood cultures and start appropriate antibiotic therapy to cover bacterial meningitis. If there is a history of foreign travel to relevant areas, request thick and thin films to exclude malaria. Subsequent investigations will include imaging, either CT or MR. This should precede lumbar puncture (see Chapter 11).
- Further management should be discussed with appropriate clinicians, i.e. neurologist, microbiologist, neurosurgeon and/or infectious disease physician.

Specific management of the conditions shown in Table 14.1 is considered in the unconscious patient (Chapter 11).

Key point

Emphasis should be placed on seeking meningeal irritation, fever, reduced conscious level, focal neurological features and skin rash

---

The primary assessment will detect any changes in the Glasgow Coma Score, pupillary response and lateralising signs. However, physical signs can change.

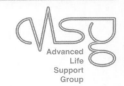

Table 14.2 Key features of the assessment of a patient with a headache

Characteristics	New onset
	Acute onset
	Progressive
	Wakens from sleep
	Worst ever
Associated symptoms	Photophobia
	Neck stiffness
	Fever
	Altered mental state
	Neurological dysfunction
Examination findings	Temperature
	Meningeal irritation
	Abnormal neurological signs
	Rash

Thus, the secondary assessment facilitates re-evaluation, combined with obtaining further information and a more comprehensive examination. The relevant secondary assessment features are summarised in Table 14.2.

Most patients presenting with a headache will not have an immediately life-threatening condition. Thus, in the **secondary assessment** the doctor has time to take a full history. A new headache, or one different from normal, can indicate intracranial pathology.

Key point

Over one third of patients with major subarachnoid haemorrhage will have suffered a minor (sentinel) bleed in the preceding hours or days

---

It is important to elicit the frequency of headache and what the patient was doing at the onset of the pain, e.g. a headache that wakes a patient from sleep suggests significant pathology. Furthermore, headaches that become progressively more severe, or chronic ones that are different from usual, may be caused by raised intracranial pressure.

An important part of this assessment is to exclude raised intracranial pressure. Features that would indicate this diagnosis are listed in the box below.

Headache with features suggestive of raised intracranial pressure

Worse on waking
Aggravated by coughing, vomiting, straining, standing and sitting
Relieved by lying down
Papilloedema and neurological signs (these are late signs)

Key point

It is important to realise that the classic early morning headache of raised intracranial pressure is uncommon

---

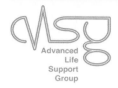

Headache exacerbated by changes in posture or associated with nausea, vomiting or ataxia requires further investigation, especially cranial imaging, when neurological signs are detected.

Specific information should also be sought regarding photophobia, neck stiffness, altered mental function, neurological dysfunction and the presence of a fever or skin rash. These features may be transient.

HEADACHE WITH PAPILLOEDEMA BUT NO FOCAL NEUROLOGICAL SIGNS

The mechanism of cerebrospinal fluid production and the relationship to intracranial pressure is discussed in Chapter 11.

It is also important to remember the pathophysiology of raised intracranial pressure. The brain is contained within a rigid skull with little room for expansion. There are four ways to disturb the normal cerebral homeostasis:
- increasing the pressure in the arteries
- adding to the intracranial contents, e.g. tumour or oedema
- obstructing cerebrospinal fluid drainage
- preventing venous drainage, e.g. congestion.

In the context of headache, the relevant causes are listed in Table 14.3.

Key point

Papilloedema:

is usually bilateral and causes minimal interference with vision

is associated with hypertension due to optic nerve vascular damage and cerebral oedema

---

Key management issues
- Antihypertensive therapy is required if the diastolic blood pressure is greater than 120 mm Hg and retinal haemorrhages are present.
- CT is warranted, especially if the blood pressure is normal.
- The CT scan result will guide further management, e.g. dexamethasone for tumour associated oedema and neurosurgical referral for evacuation of haematoma.
- Further management will follow discussion with appropriate clinicians, especially a neurologist or neurosurgeon.

Table 14.3 Causes of headache and papilloedema, but with no focal or neurological signs

Arterial	Accelerated hypertension/arterial dilatation
Intracranial	Mass lesions, e.g. tumour, haematoma
	Cerebrospinal fluid accumulation
	Cerebral oedema
	Benign intracranial hypertension
Venous	Obstruction to outflow, i.e. sinus thrombosis
	Congestion

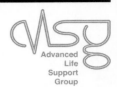

Table 14.4 Causes of headache with fever but no focal neurological signs

Intracranial		Meningitis	Daily
		Subarachnoid haemorrhage	Weekly
		Encephalitis	Monthly
Extracranial	– focal	Acute sinusitis	Daily
	– systemic	Viral illness	Daily
		Malaria	Annually
		Typhoid	Annually

- Although neurological signs may be absent at presentation, they can develop as the condition progresses. For example, hypertension can lead to a stroke; a host of focal features can be associated with either an intracerebral tumour (depending on the site and extent) or venous sinus thrombosis. In addition, they can all present as epilepsy.

HEADACHE WITH FEVER BUT NO FOCAL NEUROLOGICAL SIGNS

This is a common mode of presentation and the major conditions are listed in Table 14.4. However, headaches and fever are common to many infectious diseases. One particularly useful differentiating feature is the presence of neck stiffness.

Key point

Do **not** assess neck stiffness in patients with potential cervical spine instability, e.g. rheumatoid disease, ankylosing spondylitis, Down's syndrome and trauma

---

Neck stiffness is a non-specific sign that should be assessed with the patient flat, your hands supporting the occipital region and by feeling for increased tone while:
1 gently rotating the head (as if the patient is saying no)
2 slowly lifting the head off the bed. During this manoeuvre also watch for hip and knee flexion. This response, referred to as Brudzinski's sign, indicates meningeal irritation. The latter will also produce a positive Kernig's sign, i.e. whilst the patient is lying flat with one leg flexed at both the hip and knee, resistance is experienced when trying to extend the knee. Repeat on the other limb. A bilateral response indicates meningeal irritation., A positive Kernig's sign can occur with a radiculopathy but here other symptoms and signs of nerve root irritation will be found.
Neck stiffness can be elicited in the following conditions:
- Meningeal irritation
  ○ Infective – Commonly bacterial or viral
  ○ Chemical – Subarachnoid haemorrhage
- Cervical spondylosis
- Parkinsonism
- Myalgia, e.g. as a prodromal feature of a viral illness
- Pharyngitis
- Cervical lymphadenopathy.

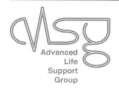

Other features from the history and examination will provide clues to the underlying diagnosis.

Key point

In a patient with neck stiffness:
Kernig's sign usually indicates meningeal irritation
discomfort only on forward flexion suggests pharyngitis and/or cervical
    lymphadenopathy

If meningeal irritation is present, a lumbar puncture is necessary after a CT scan, to exclude either meningitis or subarachnoid haemorrhage. Similarly, cerebrospinal fluid is required to establish a diagnosis of encephalitis. In contrast, if there is a history of foreign travel, further details and investigations are required to exclude relevant infectious diseases, especially malaria and typhoid.

Time Out 14.1

During your 5-min break answer the following questions.
a List the conditions that can present as 'headache with fever but no focal signs'.
b List the diagnostic signs of a radiculopathy.

HEADACHE WITH EXTRACRANIAL SIGNS

Many conditions can present with headache and extracranial signs; some examples are listed in Table 14.5.

Acute sinusitis

This acute infection commonly causes frontal and/or maxillary sinusitis. However, it may extend to involve the ethmoid and sphenoid sinuses. In contrast, isolated infection in these areas is rare. Sinusitis is usually secondary to either the common cold or influenza and both streptococci and staphylococci are involved. On occasions, anaerobes can be present when maxillary sinusitis is associated with a dental apical abscess.

Patients usually relate an initial history of an upper respiratory tract infection. This can be followed by headache and facial pain (which is often supraorbital (frontal sinusitis) and infraorbital (maxillary sinusitis)). The pain is often worse in the morning and exacerbated by head movements or stooping. Nasal obstruction is invariably present. The clinical signs are listed in the box.

Table 14.5 Causes of headache with pericranial signs

Acute sinusitis	Daily
Cervical spondylosis	Daily
Giant cell arteritis	Monthly
Acute glaucoma	Annually

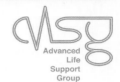

Clinical signs of sinusitis

Pyrexia
Tenderness over the affected sinus
Oedema of the upper eyelid

Key point

Swelling of the cheek:
is very rare in maxillary sinusitis
is commonly of dental origin
from antral pathology usually implies a carcinoma

The treatment comprises:

- analgesia
- antibiotics
- nasal decongestants.

Most patients with acute sinusitis will recover completely. However, liaison with an ear, nose, and throat (ENT) specialist is required when either chronic infection or complications may occur (see Table 14.6).

Further investigations are often needed and the results will dictate referral to the relevant specialist colleague.

Cervical spondylosis

This is a common condition caused by intervertebral disc degeneration producing two main effects:

- *Annulus bulging,* which elevates the periosteum from adjacent vertebral bodies, resulting in osteophyte formation.
- *Disc space narrowing* causes malalignment of posterior facet joints, which develop hypertrophic osteoarthritic changes, and ligament folding, and disruption as the vertebral bodies become closer.

These chronic degenerative changes are referred to as spondylosis and, in the cervical spine, occur commonly at the C4/5, C5/6 and C6/7 interspaces. The combination of disc space narrowing, posterior facet joint malalignment and ligament folding results in either anterior or posterior displacement of one vertebral body

Table 14.6 Indications for ENT referral in patients with acute sinusitis

Potential for chronic infection	Poor drainage
	Virulent infection
	Dental infection
	Immunocompromised patient
Complications	Laryngitis
	Pneumonia
	Orbital cellulitis/abscess
	Meningitis
	Cerebral abscess
	Osteomyelitis
	Cavernous sinus thrombosis

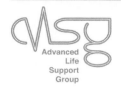

on another. Any of these effects, either individually or combined, can cause compression of the spinal cord (producing a myelopathy) or adjacent nerve roots (radiculopathy).

Another feature of this degenerative condition is headache. This is thought to arise not only from posterior facet joints and the associated ligaments, but also from osteophytes, which may irritate the C2 nerve root and branches of the greater occipital nerve. The pain classically involves one or both sides of the neck, extending to the occiput or even the temporal and frontal areas. It is often aggravated by movement and is worse in the morning after the neck has been inappropriately positioned on, or inadequately supported by, pillows.

Clinical examination usually reveals restriction of neck movements, especially lateral flexion and rotation.

> **Key point**
>
> **Always check for signs of a myelopathy or radiculopathy**

The headache will usually respond to antiinflammatory drugs, but local infiltration with lignocaine and hydrocortisone may be required. It is best to leave this type of treatment to the 'pain specialist'.

Despite the extensive degenerative changes and associated neurology, the cervical spine is usually stable and acute cord compression is rare (the exception is an acute disc prolapse). Assessment for spinal surgery is advocated, as it may be possible to prevent further neurological compromise.

Giant cell arteritis (cranial arteritis, temporal arteritis and granulomatous arteritis)

This condition predominantly affects large/medium sized arteries. It is rare before the age of 50 and commonly affects those aged between 65 and 75 years.

Giant cell arteritis classically involves the branches of the arteries originating from the aortic arch in a patchy distribution. Microscopically, the affected vessels show infiltration with lymphocytes, macrophages, histiocytes and multinucleate giant cells. These result in intimal fibrosis and thickening producing narrowing or occlusion of the vessel lumen.

Giant cell arteritis also affects the extracranial branches of the vertebral artery in 70–100% of cases. It commonly presents with neurological deficits due to vertebro-basilar insufficiency (VBI) which may present as abnormal gait, dizziness, vertigo, vomiting and slurred speech.

> **Tip: Beware VBI involvement can occur without the symptoms of temporal arteritis.**

The onset of arteritis may be acute, but the symptoms are often present for many months before the diagnosis is made. Thus, a high degree of suspicion is needed. Most patients have clinical features related to the arteries involved, i.e. mainly those originating from the aortic arch. Therefore, symptoms and signs related to the head and neck are common.

Presentation
- Usually > 50 year
- Female > male

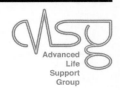

- Insidious onset over weeks
- Often associated with jaw claudication on chewing (very specific sign) and diplopia
- Risk of blindness if not treated.

Headache is a frequent presentation, localised to the superficial temporal or occipital arteries, and described as throbbing and worse at night. On examination, these vessels can be tender, red, firm and pulseless. In addition, increased scalp sensitivity may predominate with complaints like, 'It is painful to comb my hair'. Visual problems (see next box) are associated with involvement of the following:

- ciliary artery producing an ischaemic optic neuropathy
- posterior cerebral artery leading to hemianopia
- vessels supplying the III, IV and VI cranial nerves resulting in ophthalmoplegia.

Visual problems associated with giant cell arteritis

Blurred vision

Visual hallucinations

Amaurosis fugax

Loss of vision   – Transient

                 – Permanent

Hemianopia

Ophthalmoplegia

Although the head and neck vessels are commonly affected, arteritis can be widespread (see next box). However, these features are rare. In contrast, constitutional symptoms are common and include weight loss, fever, malaise and a low-grade anaemia (often a normocytic normochromic picture). Furthermore, polymyalgia rheumatica is present in approximately 50% of patients who have giant cell arteritis.

Other manifestations of giant cell arteritis

Intermittent claudication

Peripheral neuropathy

Myocardial ischaemia/infarction

Gut ischaemia/infarction

Stroke

Aortic arch syndrome

Diagnosis

The diagnosis is confirmed, in approximately 75% of cases, by biopsy of an affected vessel, usually the temporal artery. However, the histology changes may be patchy. Other laboratory investigations yield non-specific results, which reflect the inflammatory response, e.g. elevated ESR and CRP. The vessels can be imaged by Colour flow Doppler or MR angiography which can distinguish VBI from giant cell arteritis from atherosclerotic disease.

Key point

A normal ESR and CRP do not exclude the diagnosis of giant cell arteritis

---

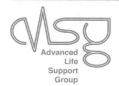

Treatment

The lack of readily available supportive laboratory data means that the diagnosis relies on the clinician's skills. Despite the many potential modes of presentation, treatment should be started as soon as the condition is suspected, because of the profound morbidity and mortality. Do not wait for a biopsy to confirm the diagnosis. This can be done at a later stage, if required, as the histological changes persist for approximately 14 days. Prednisolone 60 mg daily, in divided doses, is an effective treatment. This is reduced slowly, according to the patient's response, to achieve a maintenance dose of 10 mg after one year. Occasionally, 'pulse' intravenous methylprednisolone is used to treat ocular involvement. Early liaison with specialist colleagues is necessary when patients present with clinical signs or when giant cell arteritis has entered into the differential diagnosis. This is very important as correct diagnosis and treatment will reduce morbidity and prevent inappropriate chronic therapy with corticosteroids (and their related side effects).

Acute glaucoma

Acute closed angle glaucoma results from raised intraocular pressure. It commonly occurs in patients who are over 50 years. Under normal circumstances, aqueous humour circulates from the capillaries of the iris and ciliary muscle in the posterior chamber (between the iris and the lens) to reach the anterior chamber (between the iris and the cornea) (Fig. 14.1).

With raised intraocular pressure, the iris root protrudes into the back of the cornea and closes the canal of Schlemm preventing drainage of aqueous (Fig. 14.2). The precise cause of glaucoma is unknown, but patients who have diabetes mellitus or an affected first-degree relative are at increased risk. Furthermore, it is more common in individuals who are long sighted (hypermetropia). The shorter eyeball has a shallow anterior chamber, hence a very narrow drainage angle, which is more readily obstructed. The sudden rise in intraocular pressure causes vascular insufficiency, which can lead to ischaemia of the optic nerve and retina, if left untreated.

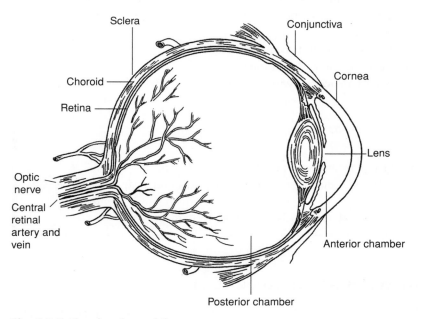

Fig. 14.1 The chambers of the eye.

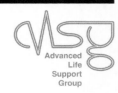

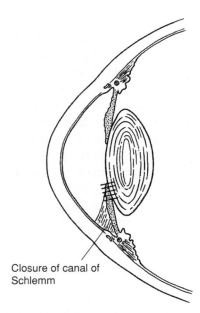

Closure of canal of
Schlemm

Fig. 14.2 The mechanism of acute closed angle glaucoma.

Acute glaucoma usually presents with severe pain in, and around, the eye. Visual changes include blurring, photophobia and marked impairment of acuity to such an extent that only light can be perceived. In addition, the patient experiences either nausea or vomiting.

The affected eye is red (ciliary congestion) with a cloudy cornea (oedema) and a mid-dilated, oval pupil that is unreactive to light. Urgent referral to an ophthalmologist is required.

Key points

Subacute glaucoma occurs with mild, transient episodes of intraocular hypertension. The patient may describe 'coloured haloes around lights' especially at night. This should be regarded as a danger signal indicating an imminent acute attack

Coloured haloes around lights can also occur as:
- light diffuses through an early cataract
- a scintillating aura associated with migraine

Time Out 14.2

Assess your knowledge by answering the following questions.

a What is the differential diagnosis in a patient presenting with a headache with extracranial signs?

b List the major complications associated with each condition.

HEADACHE WITH NO ABNORMAL SIGNS

In most patients presenting with an acute headache, no abnormal signs are detected (Table 14.7).

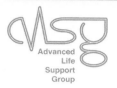

Table 14.7 Causes of headache with no abnormal signs

Tension	Daily
Migraine	Daily
Drugs	Daily
Toxins	Daily
Subarachnoid haemorrhage	Weekly
Giant cell arteritis	Monthly
Cluster headache	Annually
Coital migraine/cephalgia	Annually
Hyponatraemia	Annually

Tension type headache

This is common and also referred to as muscle contraction headache. Patients are usually aged 20–40 years, predominantly female (female/male = 3:1) and may describe either an acute or chronic history.

Acute

After an acute onset, the pain rapidly increases in severity over a few hours. The patient often appears pale and anxious with tachycardia, photophobia and neck stiffness (attributed to muscle spasm). These latter two clinical features mandate lumbar puncture to exclude meningitis. The main treatment is to reassure the patient, provide adequate analgesia and help to sort the emotional problems that are invariably associated.

Chronic

This common problem is the classic presentation of a tension type headache. The features are listed in Table 14.8. Patients can seek medical advice at any stage. Therefore, a comprehensive history is important to exclude other conditions, identify patient concerns (usually a brain tumour) and possible therapeutic avenues. Clinical examination provides some reassurance, but referral for

Table 14.8 Features of tension type headache

Site	Diffuse, but commonly at the vertex
	Often starts at forehead or neck
	Frequently bilateral
Character	Pressure sensation or pain
	Tight band, vice or clamp like, squeezing
	'As if my head is going to explode'
	'On fire or stabbing from knives or needles'
	Daily, increasing throughout the day
Radiation	Forehead to occiput or neck – vice versa
	Over the vertex or around the side – band like
Precipitation	Stress, anxiety
Relief	Nothing
Associated symptoms	Nausea, tiredness
Clinical examination	Often unremarkable

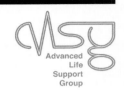

psychological advice may be necessary. Drug therapy has little to offer. The shorter the history, the better the chance for effective treatment.

Key points

Important discriminating factors in a patient with a tension headache:
headache starts each morning and increases in severity throughout the day
vomiting does not occur
visual disturbance does not occur

Migraine

This common condition affects approximately 20% of women and 15% of men, who usually present with paroxysmal headaches before the age of 30 years. There is often a family history, but the genetic basis remains unknown. Many patients will identify specific things that will precipitate an attack of migraine.

Common migraine precipitants

Dietary	Fasting
	Alcohol
	Specific foods
Drugs	Oral contraceptives
Affective	Anxiety/stress
	Post stress relaxation
Physiological	Exercise
	Menstruation
Visual	Bright light

Migraine appears to be of neural/cerebral origin. This primary event somehow triggers the release of substances that influence vasomotor tone and neuronal activity. The resultant distension of arteries in the scalp and dura causes pain, whilst decreased neuronal activity is responsible for the aura.

Migraine is often described as common, classic or variant. As its name suggests, most patients (75%) have the common variety and only 20% experience classic symptoms. However, all of these people will have prodromal features and paroxysmal headaches.

Prodromal features occur in the 24 h before the headache and comprise changes in mood, ranging from excess energy and euphoria to depression and lethargy. In addition there can be craving or distaste for specific foods.

Paroxysmal headaches can be either unilateral, bilateral or unilateral progressing to bilateral. They occur on wakening or during the day and are described as throbbing or pounding.

Patients with classic migraine can also have other presenting symptoms.

- **Visual aura** described as, e.g. flashing lights, fragmented images and micropsia. The aura lasts for 30 min and is followed by headache.
- **Sensory disturbances** can signify the onset of an attack, with numbness and tingling of one or both hands or the face, lips and tongue.
- **Motor disturbances** include weakness, hemiparesis and dysphasia.

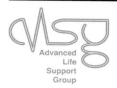

- Most patients experience nausea, prostration and vomiting. Other somatic symptoms include shivering, pallor, diarrhoea, fainting and fluid retention.
  The attacks gradually subside after 48 h. Some relief is gained from rest in a dark room, but either vomiting or sleep usually relieves the pain.

Immediate treatment
- Rest in a dark, quiet environment
- Analgesia – usually aspirin, paracetamol or a non-steroidal anti-inflammatory drug, such as diclofenac or piroxicam melt.
- Antiemetics, e.g. metoclopramide or domperidone, can be given as either suppository or intravenous preparations.
- Sumatriptan (or other triptan), a selective 5HT1 antagonist, can be used (oral, subcutaneous, intranasal) if the patient either has failed to respond to analgesia and/or is vomiting. A 6 mg subcutaneous injection of sumatriptan provides prompt, effective relief in nearly 70% of patients. Only one dose should be given for each attack. However, if a second attack occurs, a further 6 mg can be given, provided at least 1 h has elapsed following the first dose (maximum: 12 mg in 24 h).

Key points

Sumatriptan is contraindicated in patients with ischaemic heart disease

---

Prophylactic treatment
- Seek and exclude known precipitants.
- Treat precipitants appropriately, e.g. amitriptyline if anxiety/stress related; atenolol for the tense patient.
- Oral pizotifen (1.5 g at night) is useful if a specific precipitant cannot be identified.

Key points

Migraine should not be:
diagnosed in anyone presenting for the first time over the age of 40 years, until other conditions have been excluded
confused with tension headache (non-paroxysmal, no vomiting or visual features)

Drugs
A variety of drugs can cause headache because of their effect on vascular muscle tone, e.g. nitrates and calcium channel antagonists. A medical history will establish the link and provocation tests are rarely required.

Key points

Caffeine is often added to analgesic preparations to enhance their effect.
Remember that the addition or withdrawal of caffeine can also cause headache

---

Toxins
Alcohol: Both alcohol excess and withdrawal can cause headache.

Subarachnoid haemorrhage
Always consider this condition for any patient with an unexplained headache of acute onset. Please see Chapter 11 for further information.

Giant cell arteritis
The differential diagnosis of a sudden headache, in any patient over the age of 50 years, includes giant cell arteritis as described earlier in this chapter.

Cluster headache
This distinctive condition comprises:
- unilateral headache with ipsilateral:
  - corneal injection and epiphora (90%)
  - nasal congestion or rhinorrhoea (90%)
  - transient Horner's syndrome (25%).

It can be present at any age, commonly between 20 and 50 years, and predominantly affects men (male: female = 10:1). The headache is centred around the orbit and is described as severe, boring or stabbing with radiation to the forehead, temple or cheek and jaw. Brief bouts of this unilateral pain last 30–120 min each day for between four and 16 weeks. Characteristically, the pain occurs shortly after the onset of sleep, although it can occur during the day. During attacks the patient is usually crying, restless and prefers walking. The cause remains unknown, but alcohol can precipitate an attack as can other vasodilators.

Oxygen delivered through a face mask at a dose of 8 l/min for 10 min, early on during an attack, often terminates or diminishes the intensity of the attack. This is postulated to be the result of oxygen being a vasoconstrictor leading to increased production of serotonin in the CNS.

Prophylactic ergotamine should be given approximately 1 h before an attack. Suppositories are the most useful preparation and should be continued for one week. If the headache recurs, treatment should be restarted on a weekly basis until the cluster ends. Oral sumatriptan and verapamil are alternatives if the patient does not respond to ergotamine.

Coital migraine/cephalgia
This is a severe headache that begins suddenly during sexual intercourse or immediately following orgasm. It is more common in males and nearly 50% will have a previous history of migraine. Some patients require propranolol 40–80 mg before intercourse. This drug can be stopped once the patient has remained asymptomatic for one month.

Key points

Subarachnoid haemorrhage must be excluded in patients who present with coital migraine

---

Hyponatraemia
This can be associated with headache, nausea, vomiting and weakness. The diagnosis and management are considered in detail in Chapter 26.

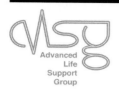

Advanced
Life
Support
Group

Time Out 14.3

a List the features that would differentiate between tension headache, migraine and cluster headache.

b In a patient presenting with headache and no abnormal signs, under what circumstances would you consider doing a lumbar puncture?

SUMMARY

Headache of acute onset accounts for less than 2.5% of new emergency attendances. Of these, 15% will have an immediately life-threatening condition. These need to be identified and treated in the primary assessment. Some of the remaining patients will have sinister pathology. The characteristics of headache that suggest a serious underlying cause are:

- new onset
- acute onset
- progressive
- wakens from sleep
- worst ever.

Important associated signs that should be sought include:

- photophobia
- meningeal irritation
- fever
- altered mental state
- neurological dysfunction.

Physical examination should be thorough, with particular emphasis on:

- meningeal irritation
- papilloedema
- pyrexia
- pericranial signs
- focal neurological features
- rash.

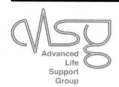
Advanced
Life
Support
Group

CHAPTER 15

The patient with abdominal pain

OBJECTIVES

After reading this chapter you should be able to describe:
- the different mechanisms of abdominal pain
- the primary assessment and resuscitation of the patient with abdominal pain
- the associated secondary assessment
- emergency treatment and definitive care.

INTRODUCTION

Abdominal pain is a common complaint and can be the presenting symptom of a wide range of conditions which have their origin both inside and/or outside the abdomen. Making an accurate diagnosis and starting appropriate treatment for the patient with abdominal pain may be difficult. Although the majority do not have an immediately life-threatening problem, identification of those who require urgent investigation and treatment is essential to avoid preventable morbidity and mortality. The structured approach gives priority to life-threatening conditions and initial resuscitation, and a PHRASED history and examination are particularly important in the patient with abdominal pain.

ANATOMY AND PATHOPHYSIOLOGY

The basic pathological processes in intra-abdominal causes of abdominal pain are:
- inflammation (e.g. gastroenteritis, appendicitis, pancreatitis, pyelonephritis)
- perforation (e.g. peptic ulcer, carcinoma of the colon)
- obstruction (e.g. intestine, bile duct, ureter)
- haemorrhage (e.g. leaking aortic aneurysm, bleeding ulcer, ectopic pregnancy)
- infarction (e.g. bowel, spleen).

An alternative classification is based on the system affected (see the next four boxes):
- Gastrointestinal causes
- Vascular causes
- Urological causes
- Gynaecological/obstetric causes

Acute Medical Emergencies; The Practical Approach, 2nd edition.
Edited by Terence Wardle, Peter Driscoll, and Sue Wieteska.
© 2010 Blackwell Publishing Ltd.

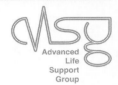

Gastrointestinal causes of abdominal pain

Non-specific abdominal pain	Daily
Gastroenteritis	Daily
Acute appendicitis	Daily
Gall stone disease and acute cholecystitis	Weekly
Peptic ulcer disease	Weekly
Intestinal obstruction	Weekly
Diverticular disease	Weekly
Pseudoobstruction	Monthly
Acute pancreatitis	Monthly
Perforated viscus	Monthly
Hernia (incarcerated/strangulated)	Monthly
Hepatitis	Monthly
Malignancy (carcinoma, lymphoma)	Monthly

Vascular causes of abdominal pain

Leaking abdominal aortic aneurysm	Monthly
Infarction of bowel, kidney or spleen	Monthly
Inflammatory bowel disease	Monthly
Primary infective peritonitis	Only in exams

Urological causes of abdominal pain

Lower urinary tract infection/pyelonephritis	Daily
Ureteric/renal colic	Daily
Acute urinary retention	Daily
Testicular torsion	Monthly

Gynaecological/obstetric causes of abdominal pain

Miscarriage	Daily
Pelvic inflammatory disease	Daily
Ovarian cyst	Monthly
Ectopic pregnancy	Monthly
Labour	Monthly
Retained products of conception	Annually
Placental abruption	Annually
Red degeneration of a uterine fibroid	Only in exams

Abdominal pain may also arise from the retroperitoneum, the pelvis and, occasionally, outside the abdomen (see box below).

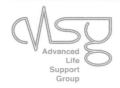

Extraabdominal causes		
Psychosomatic (including drug seeking behaviour)		Monthly
Chest (myocardial infarction, basal pneumonia, pulmonary embolus)		Monthly
Haematological (sickle cell crisis, haemophilia)		Annually
Metabolic (diabetic ketoacidosis, Addisonian crisis, uraemia, porphyria, drug withdrawal symptoms)		Annually
Neurological	– spine/disc disease	Weekly
	– radiculopathy	Monthly
	– herpes zoster	Annually
Vasculitis (e.g. polyarteritis nodosa, systemic lupus erythematosus)		

This classification of abdominal pain by system is neither comprehensive nor user friendly in clinical practice. An alternative classification – which may be clinically more useful – is to consider three mechanisms by which abdominal pain may occur:

- visceral pain
- parietal pain
- referred pain.

Visceral pain

Visceral pain is characteristically caused by inflammation, ischaemia, neoplasia and distension of either the wall of a hollow viscus or the capsule of a solid intraabdominal organ. Most gastrointestinal organs are served by afferent nerves from both sides of the spinal cord. Visceral pain is usually perceived in the midline, transmitted via autonomic nerve fibres in the wall or capsule of the organ; and the site of pain is characteristically poorly demarcated and may not correspond to the site of tenderness on examination. Pain is often described as cramp-like, colicky, dull, burning or gnawing, and associated with autonomic features such as nausea, vomiting, pallor and sweating.

The pain is usually localised to one of three regions according to the embryological origin of the organ involved.

- Foregut structures – stomach, proximal duodenum, liver, gall bladder and pancreas – characteristically produce pain in the epigastrium.
- Midgut structures – distal duodenum, small intestine, appendix and ascending and proximal part of the transverse colon – produce periumbilical pain.
- Hindgut structures – descending colon, kidneys, bladder, ureter and pelvic organs – produce pain that is characteristically felt in the hypogastrium and/or lower back.

Parietal pain

Parietal or somatic pain is characteristically caused by inflammation (bacterial or chemical) of the parietal peritoneum. It is mediated by segmental spinal nerves associated with specific dermatomes. Consequently the pain is more precisely localised to the structure from which the pain originates. This corresponds to the site at which tenderness and guarding develop. The pain is also characteristically sharper and is aggravated by movement, coughing and sometimes breathing.

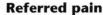

Referred pain

Referred pain is localised to a site distant from the organ that is the source of pain. The organ involved and the site at which the pain is felt share a common embryological origin and associated peripheral nerves share a common segmental origin. A classical example is pain felt in the shoulder tip, supraclavicular area and side of the neck due to irritation (by blood or pus) of the diaphragm that is derived from the fourth cervical segment. Pain may be referred to the abdomen from the chest (e.g. inferior myocardial infarction, basal pneumonia), the back and external genitalia.

PRIMARY ASSESSMENT AND RESUSCITATION

The presence of a rapidly life-threatening condition presenting with abdominal pain should be recognised by the end of the primary assessment (see box).

Life-threatening conditions in the patient with abdominal pain

Hypovolaemic shock:

• gastrointestinal bleeding	Daily
• leaking abdominal aortic aneurysm/aortic dissection	Monthly
• ectopic pregnancy	Monthly
• splenic rupture (usually traumatic but may be spontaneous)	Annually
Acute pancreatitis	Monthly
Small bowel infarction	Monthly
Sepsis (e.g. following perforation of colon)	Monthly
Acute myocardial infarction/acute right heart failure	Monthly
Diabetic ketoacidosis	Monthly

Patients with abdominal pain generally have a patent **airway**. It is important to be aware of the risk of aspiration with profuse vomiting, particularly if the conscious level is reduced. A nasogastric tube should be passed early in patients with small bowel obstruction to drain fluid and air and reduce the risk of aspiration.

In the patient with abdominal pain, abnormalities on **breathing** assessment such as tachypnoea and signs of hypoxaemia (including low oxygen saturation) may occur for a variety of reasons. Severe abdominal pain may cause splinting of chest movement. There may be symptoms and signs of pathology within the chest (causing pain localised to the upper abdomen), such as basal pneumonia. Other clinical abnormalities (e.g. tachypnoea) may be a manifestation of shock (due to intra-abdominal or retroperitoneal haemorrhage) or sepsis. Deep sighing respiration (Kussmaul's respiration) suggests metabolic acidosis (e.g. diabetic ketoacidosis or sepsis).

Initial treatment is with high concentrations of inspired oxygen via a facemask with a non-rebreathing reservoir bag. However, intubation and ventilation may be required if oxygenation is inadequate despite supplemental oxygen, e.g. in patients with severe acute pancreatitis who develop acute respiratory distress syndrome or in patients with septic shock.

An immediately life-threatening condition in the patient with abdominal pain most commonly becomes apparent when assessing circulation (see next box and Chapter 6).

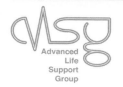

Assessment of circulation: signs of circulatory failure

Pulse: tachycardia, low volume

Blood pressure: hypotension (but remember systolic blood pressure may be normal in a patient who has lost up to 30% of circulating volume);

Pulse pressure is narrow in hypovolaemic shock (>Grade II)

Cerebral perfusion: agitation, confusion

Peripheral perfusion: pallor, cool extremities, sweating, prolonged capillary refill time

---

Occult bleeding can occur in the gut lumen, peritoneal cavity or retroperitoneum. While signs of hypovolaemia occurring early after the onset of pain suggest haemorrhage, hypovolaemia may occur later due to loss of extracellular fluid:

- with diarrhoea and vomiting
- into obstructed bowel
- into inflamed retroperitoneum or peritoneal cavity.

Patients with septic shock are classically vasodilated and warm with hypotension and a fever, but many (particularly if presenting late) are peripherally vasoconstricted and have a normal or even low body temperature. Atrial fibrillation is a risk factor for mesenteric artery embolism.

Key point

If a patient over 50 years has a clinical presentation of 'ureteric colic', always consider the possibility of aortic aneurysm or dissection, particularly if there is any sign of circulatory failure

---

Insert two large-bore (14-gauge) peripheral intravenous cannulae. Take blood for baseline full blood count, biochemistry (including glucose stick test and amylase), blood crossmatch or save, coagulation screen, blood cultures and, when appropriate, sickle screen and pregnancy test.

If hypovolaemia due to blood loss is suspected, start fluid resuscitation with 2 litres of warmed crystalloid, followed by blood; if there is evidence of anaemia as well as circulatory failure, it may be preferable to substitute blood for crystalloid earlier.

A portable ultrasound scan (if available) may confirm the cause of hypovolaemic shock (e.g. a leaking aortic aneurysm or an ectopic pregnancy). This should not delay urgent referral to a surgeon or gynaecologist when prompt surgery may be life saving (see next two boxes).

Indications for urgent referral to a surgeon

Abdominal pain or tenderness plus a pulsatile mass and/or a history of aortic aneurysm, or a leaking aortic aneurysm suspected for any other reason

Gastrointestinal bleeding in a patient of 60 years or over or in a patient of any age with signs of shock, haemoglobin less than 10 g/dl, significant coexistent disease or varices

Any evidence of free intraperitoneal fluid in the patient with abdominal pain and signs of circulatory failure

Suspected pancreatitis

Suspected mesenteric ischaemia

Suspected testicular torsion

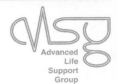

Indications for urgent referral to a gynaecologist

Suspected ectopic pregnancy
Suspected torsion or rupture of an ovarian cyst

Key point

Urgent surgical (or gynaecological) referral of the patient with abdominal pain and shock may be life saving; do not wait for the results of investigations

---

If a diagnosis of either myocardial infarction or pulmonary embolism is possible, investigate and start specific treatment (see Chapters 8 and 10). If septic shock (see Chapter 9) is suspected, treat with intravenous broad-spectrum antibiotics before the result of cultures is known.

If there is any depression of conscious level in the patient with abdominal pain, check that hypoxaemia and shock are being adequately treated, and consider hypoglycaemia, diabetic ketoacidosis and sepsis.

Time Out 15.1

a What is the differential diagnosis of abdominal pain and shock in (i) a 75-year-old man and (ii) a 25-year-old woman?
b What are the management priorities?

SECONDARY ASSESSMENT

A PHRASED history and careful examination are important for making a diagnosis in the patient with abdominal pain. An improvement in diagnostic and decision making skills has been attributed to the use of computer-assisted diagnosis based on a proforma (Fig. 15.1). This ensures more effective collection of information from the patient's history and examination findings.

'Phrased' History
The well-'phrased' history may be applied to the patient with abdominal pain.

Problem
It is important to establish the patient's main complaints, particularly as abdominal pain may be a presenting symptom of such a wide variety of conditions.

History of presenting problem
The **site**, any change in location and **radiation** of pain are important. Inquire about the site of pain at onset in particular: pain which is lateralised from the outset is consistent with pain from a paired structure (e.g. kidney, ureter, gonad), whereas pain which is felt centrally (or bilaterally) is consistent with a gastrointestinal cause. The level of early pain – epigastric, periumbilical or hypogastric – may suggest the affected viscus, pain being referred to the segment corresponding to the root level of the afferent nerves to the organ involved. Ill-defined pain may indicate visceral pain early in the disease process, referred pain or a metabolic,

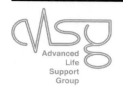

Abdominal Pain Chart

NAME		REG NUMBER	
MALE FEMALE AGE		FORM FILLED BY	
PRESENTATION (999, GP. etc)		DATE	TIME

PAIN

SITE	AGGRAVATING FACTORS	PROGRESS
ONSET	movement	better
	coughing	same
	respiration	worse
	food	DURATION
	other	
	none	
		TYPE
	RELIEVING FACTORS	intermittent
	lying still	steady
PRESENT	vomiting	colicky
	antacids	
	food	SEVERITY
	other	moderate
RADIATION	none	severe

HISTORY

NAUSEA	BOWELS	PREV SIMILAR PAIN
yes no	normal	yes no
	constipation	
VOMITING	diarrhoea	PREV ABDO SURGERY
yes no	blood	yes no
	mucus	
ANOREXIA		DRUGS FOR ABDO PAIN
yes no		yes no
	MICTURITION	
PREV INDIGESTION	normal	♀ LMP
yes no	frequency	
	dysuria	pregnant
JAUNDICE	dark	vag. discharge
yes no	haematuria	dizzy/faint

EXAMINATION

MOOD	TENDERNESS	INITIAL DIAGNOSIS & PLAN
normal		
distressed	REBOUND	
anxious	yes no	
SHOCKED	GUARDING	RESULTS
yes no	yes no	amylase
COLOUR	RIGIDITY	blood count (WBC)
normal	yes no	computer
pale		urine
flushed	MASS	X-ray
cyanosed	yes no	other
TEMP PULSE	MURPHY'S	DIAG & PLAN AFTER INVEST
	+ve −ve	
SP	BOWEL SOUNDS	
ABDO MOVEMENT	normal absent + + +	(time)
normal		
poor nil	RECTAL – VAGINAL TENDERNESS	DISCHARGE DIAGNOSIS
peristalsis	left	
	right	
SCAR	general	
yes no	mass	
	none	
DISTENSION		
yes no		

History and examination of other systems on separate case notes

Fig. 15.1 Abdominal pain chart.

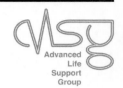

toxic or psychological cause. Migration of pain is characteristic of an inflamed viscus; e.g. pain migration from the periumbilical region to the right lower quadrant in acute appendicitis or from the epigastrium to the right upper quadrant in cholecystitis.

Pain arising from the stomach or duodenum is characteristically localised to the epigastrium in the midline. Pain from the gall bladder is also felt in the epigastrium and/or right upper quadrant, sometimes radiating to the area below the inferior angle of the right scapula (dorsal segmental radiation). Pain from pancreatitis is generally felt in the upper abdomen, with radiation through to the back. Other important conditions to consider in the patient who reports pain radiating to the back are leaking aortic aneurysm and renal or ureteric disease. Small bowel pain is characteristically felt symmetrically, centrally and may radiate to the back, while pain from the large bowel is felt in the hypogastrium and may radiate to the back and thighs.

Sudden **onset** of severe pain is characteristic of either a vascular problem such as a leaking abdominal aortic aneurysm, torsion of a gonad or a perforated viscus. The pain of acute pancreatitis may come on relatively rapidly, but over minutes rather than seconds. Whereas pain due to an inflammatory condition, such as diverticulitis or appendicitis, progresses more gradually, over hours or days. Collapse associated with the onset of pain suggests leaking aortic aneurysm, acute pancreatitis, perforated ulcer or (in females) ruptured ectopic pregnancy.

Note the **duration** of pain and whether it can be characterised as steady (present all the time at a similar intensity – e.g. bowel infarction), *intermittent* (pain resolves for periods of time – e.g. pain from gastroenteritis) or *colicky* (present all the time with fluctuating intensity). Determine whether the pain is improving, worsening or remaining much the same over a period of 1–2 h or more.

Somatic pain is characteristically described as sharp, whereas vague terms are used for visceral pain. Otherwise, it is difficult to draw diagnostic inferences from the description of the **character** of abdominal pain by patients who may use a variety of terms in different ways. The **severity** of pain may be assessed by the patient's own account and by observation of the patient who may appear distressed, sweating or crying out. Although conditions such as a perforated viscus, bowel infarction or acute pancreatitis often cause severe pain, this does not reliably distinguish them from non-specific abdominal pain.

Ask about the main **exacerbating/relieving** factors – *movement* (particularly movements which cause the patient to tense the anterior abdominal wall muscles and movement of inflamed peritoneal surfaces), *coughing and deep inspiration*. The effect on pain of vomiting (which may provide transient relief in small intestinal obstruction), food and antacids should also be noted. Also inquire about any relationship to position and to micturition.

Other gastrointestinal symptoms including anorexia, nausea and vomiting are common and relatively non-specific. The frequency of vomiting and its relationship to the onset of pain may be significant; pain before nausea and vomiting suggests a surgical cause (such as peritonitis and obstruction), whereas nausea and vomiting followed by pain is more characteristic of gastroenteritis. Ask about blood or bile in the vomit; faeculent vomiting indicates intestinal obstruction. Pre-existing indigestion may lead to a diagnosis of a perforated or bleeding peptic ulcer and previous symptoms of cholelithiasis suggest a cause for acute pancreatitis.

Diarrhoea and constipation may also be non-specific (either may occur in patients with appendicitis). In common with vomiting, diarrhoea from the beginning of an illness is characteristic of gastroenteritis, whereas onset after several hours may occur in appendicitis and peritonitis. Ask about blood or mucus in

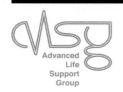

diarrhoea (inflammatory bowel disease, ischaemic bowel or malignancy). Change in bowel habit over a period of time raises the possibility of malignancy especially in a patient aged 55 years or over.

Abdominal pain, vomiting and absolute constipation are virtually pathognomonic of intestinal obstruction. Early vomiting and more frequent episodes of colicky abdominal pain are features of more proximal small bowel obstruction; on arrival at hospital the patient may not yet be aware of constipation. By contrast, constipation will be prominent in the patient with large bowel obstruction.

Relevant medical history

The past history should include details of:

- similar episodes of pain, investigation (leading to a diagnosis of inflammatory bowel disease, for example), treatment and outcome
- previous abdominal surgery (with possible subsequent adhesions, the leading cause of small bowel obstruction)
- other conditions – including diabetes mellitus; cardiac, cerebrovascular and respiratory disease; and psychiatric illness – may be relevant to the cause of abdominal pain or complicate its treatment.

Allergies

Note any previous allergies and adverse reaction to drugs, particularly antibiotics, analgesics and, if surgery is a possibility, topical antiseptics, dressings and anaesthetic agents.

Systems review

- Burning dysuria, frequency and urgency, with or without haematuria, are characteristic of urinary tract infection, but an inflamed appendix or diverticulum adjacent to the ureter or bladder may cause urinary symptoms and pyuria. Establish whether dysuria is an exacerbation of the patient's abdominal pain or a different pain.
- A gynaecological history should be taken from women with abdominal pain, to include information about pregnancies, menstrual pattern, contraception, abnormal vaginal discharge, and – if pelvic inflammatory disease is suspected – new or multiple sexual partners.
- Ask patients with upper abdominal pain in particular about chest pain, shortness of breath, cough and haemoptysis. Coexistent cardiovascular disease may be a clue to the diagnosis of intra-abdominal vascular pathology.

Essential family and social history

A family history of intra-abdominal conditions (such as inflammatory bowel disease or carcinoma) or of an inherited condition (Marfan's, sickle cell disease, acute intermittent porphyria, haemophilia) and ethnic origin may be relevant to diagnosis and treatment. A group of people affected by vomiting, diarrhoea and abdominal pain suggests an infectious agent or carbon monoxide poisoning.

Drugs

This part of the history should include medicines taken either for the present problem or other conditions (particularly corticosteroids, non-steroidal anti-inflammatory drugs, anticoagulants and antibiotics), alcohol consumption and drug use.

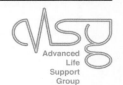

Examination

Objectives of examination include:

- assessment of the patient's general condition – the ABCDEs should be re-assessed
- localisation of an intra-abdominal source of pain (generally related to the area of maximum tenderness)
- detection of any extra-abdominal cause of pain.

General examination

Pallor, sweating and signs of distress in a patient with abdominal pain suggest (but are not diagnostic of) a more serious cause for abdominal pain, such as a vascular event, perforated viscus or acute pancreatitis. Classically, patients with visceral pain (e.g. ureteric colic) roll around. In contrast, those with peritonitis lie immobile, showing signs of pain if the bed on which they are lying is inadvertently knocked. The lethargic patient may be septic.

Mucous membrane pallor may indicate anaemia due to chronic blood loss. Look at the sclerae for jaundice. Stigmata of chronic liver disease (spider naevi, palmar erythema, Dupuytren's contracture, leuconychia and clubbing, abnormal veins around the umbilicus, loss of body hair, gynaecomastia and testicular atrophy, ascites and signs of encephalopathy) may provide useful clues to the cause of either upper gastrointestinal bleeding or abdominal distension. Features of uraemia in patients with abdominal pain are rare. The pigmentation of Addison's disease, seen in scars, the flexor creases of the palm, over pressure areas and on the buccal mucosa opposite the molar teeth, may be missed if not actively sought. Purpura in characteristic distribution over the lower limbs will suggest the possibility of Henoch–Schönlein purpura, but abdominal pain can precede the rash; petechiae can represent an underlying haematological abnormality; both mandate consideration of meningococcal septicaemia. Erythema nodosum is one of the extra-intestinal manifestations of inflammatory bowel disease and photosensitivity is a feature of porphyria.

Pyrexia is significant. A normal temperature, particularly in the elderly, does not exclude conditions such as cholecystitis and appendicitis; although perforation of the appendix is usually associated with a temperature greater than 38°C. A temperature above 38.5°C, especially with a history of rigors, is a common feature of bacterial infections, such as pyelonephritis, acute salpingitis or ascending cholangitis. A furred tongue and foetor are common and non-specific; the smell of acetone, if detected, may facilitate the rapid diagnosis of diabetic ketoacidosis. Signs of dehydration imply extracellular fluid loss due to gastroenteritis, diabetic ketoacidosis or intestinal obstruction.

Rapid shallow respiration may be a feature of either peritonitis or pneumonia. Look also for the deep (Kussmaul's) sighing respiration of diabetic ketoacidosis or other metabolic acidoses. Signs of circulatory failure due to hypovolaemia would usually have been detected in the primary assessment; other causes of tachycardia include sepsis, untreated pain and anxiety.

A brief systematic examination of the cardiovascular system (including peripheral pulses), the chest and back is important to identify any extra-abdominal cause of pain and to assess the patient's general condition.

Abdominal examination

Adequate exposure is vital if subtle but important signs (such as a small incarcerated femoral hernia) are not to be missed.

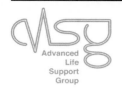

On **inspection** look for:

- the contour of the abdomen (particularly distension) and any gross deformity
- visible peristalsis (suggesting intestinal obstruction) or the abdominal wall held immobile in peritonitis; get the patient to move the anterior abdominal wall by coughing and watch the patient's facial expression. (If there is peritonitis, coughing or any movement of the bed is likely to cause sharp pain due to the movement being transmitted to the inflamed peritoneum.)
- scars from previous surgery (which may be the clue to adhesions as the cause of small bowel obstruction)
- visible pulsation of an aneurysm
- discolouration or bruising around the umbilicus (Cullen's sign) or in the flank (Grey Turner's sign) which are rare but important features of haemorrhagic pancreatitis; retroperitoneal haemorrhage from an aortic aneurysm may also produce flank bruising.

Palpation (with a warm hand) should be gentle and start in an area of the abdomen away from the site of pain. Distinguish between the symptom of pain and the sign of tenderness on examination, and the site of each. Localised tenderness suggests the site of an inflammatory source of the patient's pain. However, it may be absent in appendicitis, either because the pain is visceral early in the inflammatory process or because the appendix is retrocaecal. Conversely, abdominal tenderness may be present in biliary colic, small bowel obstruction or gastroenteritis. A particular pitfall for the unwary is the elderly patient with bowel infarction due to mesenteric artery thrombosis or embolism: characteristically these patients present with pain of sudden onset which is steady and severe, apparently out of proportion to the limited tenderness on examination. If the diagnosis is not suspected there may be a dangerous delay in arranging surgery.

The presence of guarding (reflex contraction of the abdominal wall muscles in response to palpation) and rebound tenderness suggest local peritonitis and rigidity is a sign of generalised peritonitis.

Palpate for any masses and/or organomegaly. A distended bladder may be identified on palpation or percussion.

Percussion may give information about the size of solid organs and distinguish between gas and fluid as the cause of abdominal distension (shifting dullness in ascites). Percussion tenderness may identify signs of localised or generalised peritonitis, in which case subsequent examination should be modified to avoid unnecessary painful palpation.

On **auscultation**, loud high pitched (tinkling) bowel sounds suggest obstruction and absent bowel indicate peritonitis (e.g. perforated viscus) or ileus; neither sign is sensitive and normal bowel sounds do not exclude serious intra-abdominal pathology.

Listen for bruits over the upper quadrants of the abdomen and costovertebral angles (for renal artery stenosis or aneurysm).

Inflammation close to the psoas muscle may be confirmed by stretching the psoas muscle. Lie the patient on the unaffected side and then passively extend the thigh at the hip on the affected side. In a different manoeuvre, passive rotation of the flexed thigh to the limit of internal rotation. This may produce pain in the hypogastric region, if there is a perforated appendix, abscess or other collection overlying the fascia of obturator internus in the pelvis.

Examination of the abdomen should include examination of the flanks, the external genitalia (in particular the scrotum and testes) and the inguinal and femoral canals for herniae; an incarcerated hernia is the second most common cause of small bowel obstruction. **Vaginal examination** – when indicated – may

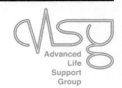

provide information about gynaecological causes of abdominal pain or an inflamed appendix palpable in the pelvis.

On **rectal examination**, assess for perianal disease (in inflammatory bowel disease), pelvic tenderness, abnormal masses, blood or melaena, sphincter tone and, where relevant, the prostate.

Investigations

All patients with abdominal pain should have a **blood glucose stick test** (to exclude diabetes) and **urinalysis**. Microscopic haematuria can occur with either ureteric colic or urinary tract infection (but remember also the possibility of infective endocarditis, symptoms of which include abdominal pain). Pyuria (more than 5–10 white cells/cubic mm) is commonly due to urinary tract infection but it may also be due to inflammation of an adjacent organ, such as appendicitis or diverticulitis. In the presence of jaundice or suspected biliary tract disease test the urine for urobilinogen and bilirubin. A **urine pregnancy test** (for the β subunit of human chorionic gonadotrophin) should be done in all women of childbearing age, regardless of the history.

On the **full blood count,** a raised white cell count supports the diagnosis of a significant cause for abdominal pain but is neither sensitive nor specific for a surgical condition. For example, a patient with an acute appendicitis may have a normal white cell count, while a raised white cell count may be due to pyelonephritis or other bacterial infection. Nevertheless, a white cell count of greater than 15×10^9/l in a patient with acute pancreatitis is one factor associated with increased mortality (see box of adverse prognostic factors in the section on acute pancreatitis). The haemoglobin concentration does not reflect acute blood loss but may indicate chronic bleeding where serial values may be useful.

A **serum amylase** of greater than five times the upper limit of normal, suggests acute pancreatitis, but a normal amylase does not exclude pancreatitis and a lesser rise may be seen in a variety of conditions which cause abdominal pain (including cholecystitis and peptic ulcer). A raised serum lipase may be a better test, but is not always available. Estimation of urea and electrolytes does not usually contribute to the diagnosis of the patient with abdominal pain, but forms part of the assessment of the general condition of any patient who is haemodynamically unstable or dehydrated, e.g. due to vomiting or diarrhoea. A **liver enzyme profile and prothrombin time** are required for patients who are jaundiced. Baseline coagulation studies are indicated in the patient who is bleeding, has a suspected coagulopathy or requires blood transfusion.

An **arterial blood gas** sample will assess oxygenation and acid–base status in the patients with hypovolaemia, pancreatitis or a suspected pulmonary problem.

An **electrocardiogram** is recommended in patients over the age of 40 (or younger if there is a specific indication), as either acute myocardial infarction or pulmonary embolism can cause abdominal pain. In addition, an ECG may identify coexistent cardiac disease which predisposes to an intra-abdominal vascular event (e.g. atrial fibrillation leading to mesenteric artery embolism) or complicates treatment.

The role of **radiology** is primarily to confirm or refute a diagnosis suspected on clinical assessment and is not a substitute for an effective history and clinical examination.

Plain X-rays

The principal indications for plain X-rays in patients with abdominal pain are suspicions of one of the following:

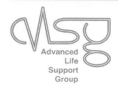

- intestinal obstruction
- perforated viscus
- toxic megacolon
- foreign body
- ureteric/renal colic
- chest pathology.

The abdominal film may also yield useful information in peritonitis and/or suspected mesenteric ischaemia, but should not be used indiscriminately in patients with abdominal pain.

Standard views are the erect chest X-ray (CXR) and the supine abdominal film. The erect CXR should be taken after the patient has been sitting upright for 5–10 min (after which as little as 1–2 ml of free air may be shown); it may also show pneumonia or other pathology in the chest. If the patient is unable to stand or sit, the left lateral decubitus view of the abdomen is an alternative when looking for 'free gas'. An unsuspected abdominal aortic aneurysm may be outlined by a calcified vessel wall. The erect abdominal view does not generally add useful information. An unprepared barium enema may be required urgently to elucidate the cause of suspected large bowel obstruction and to exclude pseudo-obstruction.

A KUB (kidney, ureter, bladder) X-ray is the initial imaging for patients with ureteric colic. Although more than 80% of ureteric calculi are radiopaque, they are often missed on plain X-ray. This film should be followed by either an intravenous urogram (IVU), ultrasound scan or more commonly computed tomography (CT) to demonstrate the size and location of a stone and the extent of obstruction to the ureter and kidney.

Ultrasound

Urgent ultrasound scan is indicated in the following situations:
- suspected abdominal aortic aneurysm
- right upper quadrant pain, jaundice or suspected cholelithiasis
- acute renal failure
- suspected urinary tract colic or obstruction, particularly if there is any contraindication to an intravenous urogram
- lower abdominal pain in women of childbearing age
- suspected intra-abdominal abscess/bleeding.

Visualisation of a normal appendix may be useful in ruling out appendicitis.

Computed tomography

This is an important urgent investigation, but the patient must be well enough to be moved to the CT suite. It is particularly useful:
- as an alternative for imaging suspected urinary tract obstruction
- in suspected perforation of a viscus
- to visualise retroperitoneal structures, including the pancreas and aorta
- in the subsequent investigation of selected patients with acute abdominal pain, to help with making a definitive diagnosis and planning treatment.

In many countries non-contrast CT (CT urogram) is now the initial radiological investigation of choice for suspected urolithiasis. It is quicker than IVU, avoids the use of contrast and can identify other pathologies, e.g. abdominal aortic aneurysm.

Angiography and labelled red cell scans

These have a beneficial role in evaluating intestinal ischaemia and gastrointestinal haemorrhage (after negative endoscopy of the upper and lower tracts). The choice

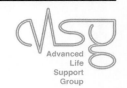

of investigation may be influenced by the rate of bleeding as labelled red cell scans are more sensitive.

Potential pitfalls in the assessment of patients with abdominal pain

Elderly patients with acute abdominal pain have a higher mortality. Several factors may contribute to this, some of which put the elderly at risk of delayed diagnosis:

- Different spectrum of disease: a greater proportion have a malignancy or a vascular cause for pain (which may not initially be recognised).
- General peritonitis may be due to a perforated colon rather than a perforated ulcer or appendix.
- A different presentation of intra-abdominal disorders: in comparison with younger patients, the pain is often not as marked. Fever, tachycardia and leucocytosis are uncommon with inflammatory conditions such as appendicitis. These factors can lead to a delay in diagnosis and an increased risk of perforation.
- Delayed presentation is more common.
- Coexistent illness is likely to make the elderly more vulnerable to complications.

Key point

Glucocorticoids can mask both clinical and laboratory responses to inflammation or perforation of a viscus in the abdomen, including the degree of pain and tenderness and fever

---

Similarly other immunosuppressive drugs, coexistent diabetes mellitus and immunodeficiency can influence the patient's response to inflammatory conditions. These patients may display minimal clinical signs and normal laboratory tests, despite a serious intra-abdominal disorder.

Finally, the clinical features of surgical conditions may be unexpectedly non-specific in late pregnancy.

EMERGENCY TREATMENT

After the primary assessment, a well-'phrased' history and examination of the patient, a differential diagnosis can be formulated and appropriate investigations requested. Treatment should be initiated simultaneously with assessment and investigation. Consider:

- analgesia
- review of fluid resuscitation
- antiemesis and nasogastric suction
- antibiotics
- urethral catheter.

Analgesia

Early judicious analgesia is advocated for any patient with acute abdominal pain, including those who require referral for a surgical opinion. If opioid analgesia is given as a dilute solution by slow intravenous injection, the dose can be titrated against the patient's pain.

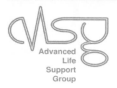

Key point

Acute abdominal pain is **not** a contraindication to opioid analgesia

---

Adequate analgesia reduces suffering with no evidence that appropriate analgesia makes diagnosis of a surgical condition more difficult, providing the patient's condition is reviewed regularly and that necessary investigations are done. A patient who is not distressed is more likely to give a clearer coherent history and cooperate with an examination.

Review fluid resuscitation

Reassess the patient for signs of intravascular volume depletion and the response to fluid resuscitation.

Dehydration in patients with acute abdominal pain may be due to a combination of factors including vomiting and diarrhoea, inadequate oral intake and 'third space' loss (including loss into the bowel lumen or retroperitoneum). Pathology affecting the small bowel mucosa and intestinal obstruction can produce profound electrolyte disturbances. Replace fluid and electrolytes with an appropriate crystalloid solution; this may be either definitive treatment for gastroenteritis or preparation for urgent surgery in patients with intestinal obstruction.

Central venous pressure monitoring is often required in the elderly or those with cardiac disease. Careful fluid balance is necessary in any patient who is seriously ill.

Antiemesis and nasogastric suction

An antiemetic is often needed for the patient with acute abdominal pain, especially if opioid analgesia has been used, although effective analgesia may also relieve vomiting. A nasogastric tube should be passed to decompress the stomach in patients with small bowel obstruction, pancreatitis and persistent vomiting despite the use of an antiemetic.

Antibiotics

Antibiotics are needed for either localised infection such as pyelonephritis or where clinical sepsis is thought to have an intra-abdominal source (e.g. perforation of the colon in an elderly patient). In patients who are septic and/or in whom perforation is suspected, broad-spectrum intravenous antibiotics should be started as soon as possible without waiting for the result of blood cultures (according to local protocols).

Urinary catheter

Measurement of urine output (via a urethral catheter) is needed in any patient who is seriously ill.

DEFINITIVE CARE

After secondary assessment and emergency treatment, some patients with abdominal pain will require referral to a surgeon (see next box). This is likely if the pain:
- has preceded other symptoms
- has persisted for more than 6 h

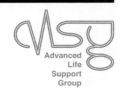

- is asymmetrical and distant from the umbilicus and accompanied by distension, bile stained or faeculent vomiting or significant abdominal tenderness.

Indications for surgical referral

Suspected generalised peritonitis
- significant diffuse tenderness, with or without a rigid silent abdomen

Suspected localised peritoneal inflammation
- significant localised tenderness with or without other signs of peritoneal irritation
- tenderness and a mass
- tenderness and a fever

Suspected bowel obstruction
- pain and bile stained or faeculent vomiting

Tenderness plus uncontrolled vomiting

Suspected pancreatitis

Suspected aortic aneurysm

Suspected bowel infarction/ischaemia

Gastrointestinal bleeding
- upper gastrointestinal bleeding in a high risk patient
- lower gastrointestinal bleeding

Age greater than 65 years

Patients with ureteric colic should be referred to the urology team (or general surgeons depending on local arrangements). Gynaecological assessment is required for women with suspected ectopic pregnancy, miscarriage, pelvic inflammatory disease or complications of an ovarian cyst. Other patients, including those with gastroenteritis, gastrointestinal haemorrhage or pyelonephritis will be admitted under the medical team. Diverticulitis and acute pancreatitis can be treated 'medically', but the ideal situation is combined management by physicians and surgeons on a high dependency unit.

Some patients may be discharged (with or without arrangements for outpatient follow-up) if they have uncomplicated cholelithiasis, ureteric colic or gastroenteritis or where a diagnosis has not been made but the patient appears clinically well and no serious condition is suspected. Advice should be given to these patients to return to hospital without delay if their symptoms deteriorate or new symptoms develop. A proportion may have presented at an early stage of an intra-abdominal problem such as appendicitis. However, if in doubt or the patient is unable to cope at home, admit for observation.

SPECIFIC CONDITIONS

Acute gastroenteritis

Gastrointestinal infection is one of the commonest abdominal disorders, and symptoms commonly include abdominal pain. Worldwide, intestinal infections account for significant morbidity and mortality. The elderly are particularly vulnerable to the effects of dehydration and electrolyte imbalance and may present with life-threatening cardiovascular collapse.

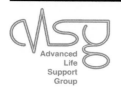

Pathophysiology

There are three different pathophysiological mechanisms that can be used to explain the clinical features and treatment rationale.

Inflammatory diarrhoea (dysentery) can follow bacterial invasion of the mucosa of the colon and distal small intestine. This leads to both impairment of absorptive function and to loss of blood, protein and mucus which contribute to diarrhoea.

Bacterial infections, which produce inflammatory diarrhoea, include *Salmonella enteritidis*, *Shigella* and *Campylobacter jejuni*. Cytopathic toxins are produced by *Clostridium difficile* which is the commonest cause of antibiotic associated colitis and by verotoxin producing *Escherichia coli*, one type of which (O157:H7) is associated with haemolytic uraemic syndrome. *Entamoeba histolytica* also produces dysentery of varying severity.

The patient may report blood and pus in the diarrhoea (which characteristically contains faecal leucocytes). Severity varies from mild self-limiting diarrhoea to severe colitis which may be complicated by toxic megacolon, perforation and sepsis.

Non-inflammatory (secretory) diarrhoea is classically due to enterotoxin of *Vibrio cholerae* in the small bowel. The toxin blocks passive absorption of sodium (and water) and stimulates active sodium (and water) excretion. This leads to an outpouring of isotonic sodium and water into the bowel lumen, which exceeds the absorptive capacity of the small intestine and colon. Active sodium absorption by a glucose dependent mechanism is, however, generally unaffected; hence rehydration may be achieved by oral glucose solutions which contain both sodium *and* carbohydrate.

Characteristically the patient has profuse watery diarrhoea (and vomiting), which may lead to severe dehydration, shock and death.

Viruses (e.g. rotavirus), *Giardia lamblia* and *Cryptosporidium*, toxins of *Staphylococcus aureus* and *Bacillus cereus* (in food poisoning) and *enterotoxogenic E. coli* (a major cause of traveller's diarrhoea) may also produce secretory diarrhoea.

Systemic infection results from infection that penetrates the mucosa of the distal small bowel, invades lymphatic structures and causes a bacteraemia. Invasive organisms include *Salmonella typhi* (typhoid or enteric fever), *Salmonella paratyphi* and *Yersinia enterocolitica*.

Although about 50% of patients with typhoid may develop diarrhoea and fever, other features are prominent (including headache, cough, malaise, myalgia, abdominal tenderness and hepatosplenomegaly, relative bradycardia and 'rose spots' on the trunk). Complications include small bowel ulceration and occasionally perforation.

Diagnosis and assessment of severity

The diagnosis is essentially clinical, supported by the result of investigations in some cases.

Clinical features

Diarrhoea, nausea and vomiting, abdominal pain, tenesmus and fever occur in various combinations. Pain may be cramp-like and transiently relieved by the passage of diarrhoea, but (with *Salmonella* or *Campylobacter infection*) may mimic a surgical acute intra-abdominal emergency.

To make the diagnosis of gastroenteritis there should be a history of diarrhoea and vomiting, although this will not always be the case. A history of affected family or other contacts supports a diagnosis of gastroenteritis; foreign travel,

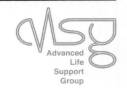

ingestion of suspect food and/or immune compromised state may be risk factor(s) for infection.

Antibiotic therapy may suggest *C. difficile* colitis. The elderly and patients who are immune compromised are at increased risk from complications of infection with *Salmonella*. Patients with enteric fever may be constipated rather than have diarrhoea at the time of presentation. The diagnosis will depend on evaluation of systemic symptoms and signs in a patient who has potentially been exposed to infection (recent travel to the tropics).

On the secondary assessment examine for signs of dehydration which – particularly in the elderly – may be accompanied by circulatory failure, fever, systemic signs of bacteraemia and abdominal signs. Record the patient's weight and stool output.

Key point

Do not diagnose gastroenteritis in patients with abdominal pain and vomiting, without diarrhoea. Consider other conditions, e.g. acute pancreatitis, appendicitis

---

Investigations

Stool specimens (at least three on consecutive days) should be sent to microbiology (to reach the laboratory immediately) for microscopy (leucocytes, red blood cells, ova, cysts and parasites) and culture (particularly for *Salmonella, Shigella, Campylobacter* and *E. coli* O157). If amoebiasis is suspected, a 'hot stool' specimen should be sent directly to the laboratory (and the laboratory forewarned) to enable detection of trophozoites. Suspicion of *Clostridium difficile* should prompt specific examination for the associated toxin.

Check the electrolytes, urea and creatinine in any patient with signs of dehydration or requiring intravenous therapy. Request the following additional investigations in any patient who is febrile or systemically unwell:
- full blood count
- C-reactive protein
- blood cultures
- chest X-ray
- serum lactate (a useful marker of the severity of *C. difficile* infection)
- thick and thin blood films for malaria (if history indicates possible infection)

Treatment

Most patients require only supportive therapy as acute gastroenteritis is a self-limiting disease irrespective of the causative organism and most patients require only supportive therapy for self-limiting disease.

If there are signs of volume depletion, treat initially with 1–2 litres of 0.9% saline and reassess. Volume and rate of replacement may be determined clinically (by signs of peripheral perfusion, jugularvenous pulse, auscultation over lung bases and urine output) or, in the critically ill patient, by central venous pressure measurement. Add potassium, if appropriate, once the serum result is known and there is evidence of urine output.

After restoring the circulating volume, correct dehydration gradually, replacing deficit and maintenance requirements for water and electrolytes. The majority of patients with gastroenteritis can be managed with oral rehydration alone, taking

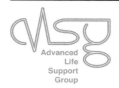

advantage of the active glucose dependent mechanism for absorption of sodium. Proprietary rehydration powders for reconstitution are available.

Antibiotics should be used for the following specific indications:

- cholera
- typhoid
- occasionally those with non-typhoid *Salmonella* or Campylobacter (associated bacteraemia and systemic symptoms, immune compromise, significant coexistent medical problem, e.g. malignancy, sickle cell disease, prosthetic device)
- *C. difficile* colitis, particularly if antecedent antibiotic therapy cannot be stopped (according to local policy). If *Clostridium difficile* is suspected (especially the elderly, patients with prior antibiotic use, patients who are immunocompromised or have a raised WBC) start treatment with metronidozole. Early liaison with a microbiologist/gastroenterologist is advised.
- specific parasitic infections (amoebiasis, giardiasis)
- Antibiotic medication neither prolongs nor increases illness complications. An antiemetic (e.g. prochlorperazine by IM injection) may be helpful.

Infection control staff should be involved in the in-patient management of gastroenteritis, especially in relation to isolation, barrier nursing and cohorting of outbreaks.

The need for surgical intervention is rare, except for complications such as perforation. Inform the local Public Health Department of notifiable diseases. Those whose occupation involves handling food require appropriate advice regarding time away from work.

Acute pancreatitis

The majority of patients with acute pancreatitis have a self-limiting illness and recover with supportive treatment on a general ward. About 20–25% will develop severe acute pancreatitis, requiring vigorous resuscitation and multidisciplinary care on the intensive treatment unit. These patients are likely to be severely hypovolaemic due to retroperitoneal fluid loss, generalised extravasation of fluid through leaky capillaries and loss of extracellular fluid from profuse vomiting. They have a mortality of 25–30%.

Cause

The common causes are gall stones and alcohol, accounting for about 80% of cases. Others include metabolic conditions (hyperlipidaemia, hypercalcaemia), drugs, trauma, infection, ischaemia, autoimmune, genetic, post-ERCP and hypothermia. In about 10% of patients no cause is found.

Clinical features

Characteristically, patients with acute pancreatitis report an acute onset of pain in the upper half of the abdomen. The initial pain may be felt in the epigastrium, right or left upper quadrant or rather vaguely in the centre of the abdomen; the pain may radiate to the back or encircle the upper abdomen. A small proportion of patients describe pain that is either overwhelming generalised pain or localised to the chest. The pain is often severe, aggravated by movement or inspiration and may be colicky. Nausea is common. During the first 12 h, most patients vomit; this may be profuse and repeated.

Most patients with acute pancreatitis are shocked; tachypnoea and tachycardia may reflect hypoxaemia, hypovolaemia and pain. Cyanosis may occur early but is less common than in patients who have suffered an intra-abdominal vascular problem or myocardial infarction. Jaundice occurs in about one quarter of

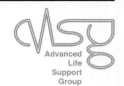

patients, particularly those who have either gall stone pancreatitis or an alcohol related illness.

The abdomen looks normal, moves with respiration and can be distended in the upper half of the abdomen, where there may be a mass. The majority of patients have tenderness over the upper half of the abdomen and occasionally this is restricted to the right upper quadrant. About half of patients have guarding, but rebound tenderness and rigidity are less common. Bowel sounds are reduced or absent in about one third of patients (and duration of ileus is an indicator of severity).

Gall stone pancreatitis presents with jaundice, pain and tenderness localised to or maximal in the right upper quadrant and a positive Murphy's sign. Seriously ill patients with acute pancreatitis may be pyrexial, tachypnoeic and hypotensive (but sometimes peripherally vasodilated) and have pleural effusions, ascites, Cullen's and/or Grey Turner's sign and/or a prolonged paralytic ileus.

Investigations

A serum amylase level greater than 3–4 times the upper limit of normal confirms the clinical diagnosis. However the serum amylase is not always raised in acute pancreatitis. Patients with alcoholic pancreatitis often have a normal amylase as may those presenting late. The amylase level returns to normal soon after the onset of an episode of acute pancreatitis, and the urinary amylase should be checked. Conversely a raised amylase is not specific. A significantly raised (greater than two times normal) serum lipase is considered more specific, but is less commonly available.

A plain abdominal X-ray is generally not diagnostic but may show an elevated diaphragm, localised gastroduodenal ileus or a sentinel loop of small bowel, or pancreatic calcification indicative of previous disease. In patients where the diagnosis is not clear, ultrasound scan or contrast enhanced CT may be helpful. Both may show a swollen pancreas or fluid in the lesser sac; CT may show non-perfused necrotic areas of pancreas and give information about severity and pseudocyst formation.

> **Key point**
>
> **A normal amylase does not exclude acute pancreatitis**

Early complications

The most significant early complication is multiple organ failure.

- Cardiovascular collapse: hypovolaemia and myocardial depression
- Respiratory failure: pleural effusions, atelectasis, pulmonary infiltrates, intrapulmonary shunting, acute respiratory distress syndrome
- Acute renal failure
- Coagulopathy
- Metabolic: hypocalcaemia, hyperglycaemia.

Severity and prognosis

Complications, including multiple organ failure, may develop rapidly and unpredictably. Identify patients at increased risk of developing severe acute pancreatitis. This will ensure that they receive high dependency or intensive care and may help avoid potentially unnecessary hazardous interventions. Evidence of three or more factors in the modified Glasgow Scoring System (next box) is associated with

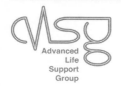

increased morbidity and mortality; the greater the number of factors present, the worse the prognosis.

Adverse prognostic factors in acute pancreatitis

On admission:
Age > 55 years
White blood cell count > 15 × 10⁹/l
Blood glucose > 10 mmol/l (no diabetic history)
Serum urea > 16 mmol/l (no response to IV fluids)
PaO₂ < 8 kPa

Within 48 hours
Serum calcium < 2.0 mmol/l
Serum albumin < 32 g/l
Lactate dehydrogenase > 600 IU/l

Management

Baseline investigations should include electrolytes, calcium, glucose, renal function, liver enzymes, coagulation screen, full blood count, arterial blood gases, chest X-ray and ECG.

Treatment
The priorities are to correct/prevent hypoxaemia and restore circulating volume. This limits ischaemic damage to the pancreas and reduces the risk of multiple organ failure. Those with severe disease may have a clinical picture similar to that of acute respiratory distress syndrome; if adequate oxygenation cannot be achieved with supplemental oxygen ($FiO_2 = 0.85$), the patient should be intubated and ventilated.

Rapid infusion of high volumes of crystalloid and synthetic colloid (up to 4–5 litres or more during the first 24 h) may be required. Monitoring in patients with severe disease should include a urinary catheter and central venous pressure measurement, to guide fluid resuscitation. Blood transfusion may be required for a falling haemoglobin level (due to haemorrhagic pancreatitis). Patients with persistent circulatory failure despite adequate fluid replacement may require inotropic support; those with renal impairment may need either haemofiltration or dialysis.

Pain should be treated with intravenous opioid, titrated to effect, possibly followed by patient controlled analgesia. A nasogastric tube will reduce nausea and vomiting in those with severe vomiting or an ileus. Address the cause where possible, e.g. discontinuation of drug or alcohol. Arrange ultrasound of the gall bladder and if gall stones are demonstrated in the bile duct, request an opinion on early endoscopic retrograde cholangiography and either stenting or sphincterotomy with stone extraction.

Antibiotics are given:
- for suspected cholangitis (cholestatic jaundice and fever)
- in severe acute pancreatitis as prophylaxis against infection of necrotic pancreatic tissue from bacterial translocation
- to cover endoscopic retrograde cholangiography.

Early surgery may be needed:
- to debride infected necrotic pancreatic tissue
- to exclude other treatable intra-abdominal pathology
- to remove gall stones after acute pancreatitis has subsided.

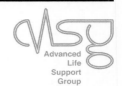

> **Time Out 15.2**
>
> List eight adverse prognostic factors in patients with acute pancreatitis.

Acute upper gastrointestinal bleeding
Cause and clinical presentation
Melaena, haematemesis and symptoms of hypovolaemia and/or anaemia are the common presenting features of acute upper gastrointestinal bleeding. However, there may be a history of abdominal pain due to inflammation and/or ulceration in the oesophagus, stomach or duodenum. Ingestion of non-steroidal antiinflammatory drugs (NSAIDs) is an important contributory factor in patients with peptic ulcer disease. Other causes of upper gastrointestinal bleeding include varices, Mallory–Weiss tear, oesophagitis and tumour.

Haematemesis and/or melaena suggest bleeding from the oesophagus, stomach or duodenum, although black stools may occasionally be due to bleeding into the distal small bowel or 'right' colon. Vomiting of fresh blood, compared with altered blood, suggests more serious bleeding. Rapid upper gastrointestinal bleeding can present with dark red blood per rectum, although (particularly in the absence of hypotension) this is more likely to originate in the lower gastrointestinal tract.

Primary assessment and resuscitation
The airway should be managed as described in Chapters 3 and 4. Patients with a reduced level of consciousness (e.g. those with hepatic encephalopathy) are at risk of aspiration, and may require endotracheal intubation. Restore intravascular volume, initially with warmed crystalloid (0.9% sodium chloride) and subsequently blood (see Chapter 9 for further details). Packed cells may be preferable in patients with anaemia. Vitamin K and fresh frozen plasma may be required for patients with liver disease, or for those on warfarin prothrombin complex concentrate can also be used. A central venous pressure line should be inserted in patients with evidence of shock, particularly if there is a history of cardiovascular disease, sign(s) of rebleeding or if the patient is on a β blocker. Emergency surgery (preceded by endoscopy) may be required for those with bleeding and hypovolaemia, unresponsive to fluid resuscitation and treatment of any coagulopathy. Early surgical consultation is therefore necessary.

Secondary assessment
The history should include details of the duration and severity of bleeding, recent dyspepsia, vomiting, alcohol or drugs (NSAIDs, bisphosphonates, SSRIs, anticoagulants, β blockers), jaundice, previous gastrointestinal haemorrhage and other medical problems. Look for signs of chronic liver disease and splenomegaly or malignancy. Melaena may only be apparent on rectal examination. Ensure that the important early investigations have been done including a full blood count, crossmatch, coagulation screen, biochemistry including liver enzyme profile, hepatitis serology, chest X-ray and a 12-lead ECG if appropriate.

Evidence of rebleeding includes:

- signs of hypovolaemia (fall in central venous pressure, rise in heart rate, fall in systolic blood pressure)
- fresh haematemesis or melaena
- fall in haemoglobin (3 g/dl over 48 h).

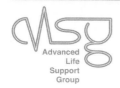

Definitive care

After resuscitation, early endoscopy (within 12–24 h) will identify the source of bleeding, provide prognostic information on the risk of rebleeding and offer an opportunity for haemostatic therapy. Emergency endoscopy should be done in patients with severe, continued or recurrent bleeding, persistent or recurrent signs of hypovolaemia, haemoglobin less than 8 g/dl or suspected varices.

Patients with an increased mortality risk (see next box) should be admitted to a high dependency area.

Adverse prognostic features in patients with gastrointestinal haemorrhage

Age $\geq$ 60 years
Signs of hypovolaemia/shock (systolic blood pressure < 100 mm Hg)
Haemoglobin concentration < 10 g/dl
Severe coexistent disease
Continued bleeding or rebleeding
Varices

The need for surgery for a bleeding peptic ulcer is determined by the severity, persistence or recurrence of bleeding and patient risk factors. A surgical team should be informed of all patients, especially those at increased risk (see previous box). In general, surgery should be considered for patients:
- with severe, continuing gastrointestinal bleeding
- aged > 60 years, or younger with other risk factor(s), who have either persistent bleeding requiring four units of blood or one rebleed
- aged < 60 years old with no risk factor(s), who have either persistent bleeding requiring six to eight units of blood or two rebleeds.

Key point

Patients with an increased risk of death from a gastrointestinal bleed (e.g. the elderly with persistent or recurrent bleeding) may benefit most from prompt surgery

---

Vascular causes of acute abdominal pain

Vascular causes of abdominal pain are important because they include conditions which are life-threatening but treatable if recognised early. Early recognition may be difficult because:
- these conditions are relatively uncommon
- initial symptoms – though severe – may be non-specific
- 'surgical' signs of an acute abdomen may be lacking
- affected patients are often elderly and have coexistent medical problems

Delay in diagnosis and referral for surgery when appropriate may result in increased mortality and morbidity. The possibility of a vascular cause for abdominal pain should always be considered in patients over the age of 50 and particularly above the age of 70. The three most common vascular causes of abdominal pain are abdominal aortic aneurysm, acute mesenteric ischaemia and myocardial infarction presenting with abdominal pain.

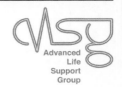

Abdominal aortic aneurysm

A leaking abdominal aortic aneurysm is the commonest intra-abdominal vascular emergency and may present as:

- vague abdominal pain
- a preceding history of back pain for hours or days, with or without a previously diagnosed aneurysm
- shock with a distended tender abdomen (if the patient has not exsanguinated before reaching hospital)
- atypical abdominal pain
- severe pain of sudden onset in the abdomen radiating to the flank and back, with a pulsatile mass, an abdominal bruit and reduced pulses in one or both lower limbs (due to emboli or shock), accompanied by signs of hypovolaemia.

Key point

In the patient previously known to have an abdominal aortic aneurysm, beware of attributing pain to another cause, however well the patient may appear

---

However, a majority of these patients will not be known to have an aneurysm, pain may not be severe, a mass may be difficult to detect and signs of hypovolaemia may be minimal. Pain in the abdomen, flank or back in these patients may be misdiagnosed as ureteric colic or acute pancreatitis. Others present with collapse, with neurological symptoms (spinal cord affected) or pain in the lower limbs (distal emboli). Risk factors include age over 65 years, male, hypertension, smoking, known vascular disease, as well as conditions such as Marfan's syndrome. If the diagnosis is not to be missed, the possibility of an aortic aneurysm must be actively considered in any middle aged or elderly patient with a history of abdominal pain, back pain or collapse, even though there is no evidence of haemodynamic compromise.

If abdominal aortic aneurysm is suspected, the principles of management are:

- resuscitation aiming for a systolic blood pressure of about 90 mm Hg (if the patient is conscious)
- carefully titrated IV opioid analgesia
- immediate surgical referral
- crossmatch blood and warn blood transfusion staff
- portable ultrasound (the aneurysm may also be outlined by calcification on an abdominal X-ray)
- rapid transfer to the operating theatre once the diagnosis has been made (because of the possibility of sudden decompensation).

Key point

Always consider the possibility of an aortoenteric fistula in a patient who presents with upper gastrointestinal haemorrhage and has an abdominal aortic aneurysm especially if it has been repaired

---

Acute mesenteric infarction

Acute intestinal ischaemia commonly affects the superior mesenteric artery. If diagnosis and treatment are delayed, complications include necrosis of the small

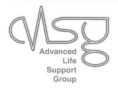

bowel, ascending colon and proximal transverse colon. Diagnosis depends on a high index of suspicion, particularly in patients at increased risk (see next box), and appropriate history and examination.

Risk factors for acute mesenteric ischaemia

Elderly (older than 50 years, greater risk with increasing age)
Known atheromatous vascular disease
Source of embolus (atrial fibrillation and other arrhythmias, myocardial
    infarction, ventricular aneurysm, valvular heart disease, infective endocarditis)
Prolonged hypoperfusion
Procoagulant disorders

Characteristically the pain is acute, severe out of proportion to physical signs and poorly localised in the periumbilical region or below. There may be a short preceding history of abdominal pain after eating. An alternative presentation is of pain with an insidious onset over 24–48 h, initially poorly localised and becoming generalised throughout the abdomen. The pain is colicky initially, becoming steady and unrelenting. Vomiting is common, sometimes with haematemesis.

The patient is pale, distressed and usually has diarrhoea with blood. As bowel infarction develops the abdomen becomes distended with worsening tenderness, guarding and rebound, and absent bowel sounds. Fever and shock due to bacteraemia often occur.

The key to management is clinical suspicion at an early stage when abdominal signs are minimal. An abdominal X-ray may show dilatation of the intestine with multiple fluid levels; the appearance of gas in the portal vein indicates intestinal necrosis.

Treatment includes vigorous fluid resuscitation, opioid analgesia, antibiotics and urgent surgical referral with a view to laparotomy once the patient has been resuscitated.

Myocardial infarction

An acute inferior myocardial infarction may present with upper abdominal pain. If nausea and vomiting are prominent features, a primary intra-abdominal problem may be suspected. In acute cardiac failure, distension of the liver capsule causes right upper quadrant pain mimicking a biliary or upper gastrointestinal tract problem.

Complete heart block complicating inferior myocardial infarction and causing collapse can be mistaken for intra-abdominal bleeding. All patients with abdominal pain over 40 (and younger if there is any reason to suspect the diagnosis) should have an ECG.

Inflammatory bowel disease
Ulcerative colitis

Ulcerative colitis is an inflammatory disease of uncertain cause affecting the rectum and colon. Many patients experience a gradually progressive illness in which symptoms related to bowel habit are prominent. However, some present with an acute illness characterised by fever, abdominal pain, diarrhoea with blood and mucus and tenesmus. A proportion of these patients develop fulminant colitis (associated with pancolitis).

> **Key point**
>
> Abdominal signs and leucocytosis may be masked if the patient is on steroids. However, remember that steroids can cause a leucocytosis

> **Features of severe colitis**
>
> Severe diarrhoea (more than six stools a day) with blood
> Systemic features: tachycardia, signs of hypovolaemia, fever and drowsiness, weight loss
> Progressive abdominal pain, distension and tenderness over the colon
> Raised ESR, CRP and white cell count, low haemoglobin and albumin, electrolyte disturbance

Toxic megacolon is a medical emergency and the possibility of this complication should be considered in all patients with severe colitis. In addition to the features of severe colitis (see box above), abdominal X-ray shows dilatation of the colon with a diameter greater than 6 cm and loss of haustrations. Bowel perforation occurs in patients with fulminant colitis, with or without toxic megacolon. Symptoms and signs of perforation may be obvious, but if the patient is on steroids these may be masked, and a deterioration in the patient's condition may be the only clue to this complication. Free air may be seen on X-ray.

> **Key point**
>
> The patient may be 'toxic' without any evidence of colonic dilatation

The patient with severe colitis/toxic megacolon should be managed by both medical and surgical gastroenterologists. The initial treatment includes resuscitation with fluid and electrolyte replacement, intravenous steroids and antibiotics. Parenteral nutrition is frequently required, as is blood transfusion. If surgery is delayed until after the colon has perforated, mortality is significantly increased. In the acutely ill patient colectomy is needed for:

- perforation
- features of severe colitis (with or without toxic megacolon) which deteriorate or do not improve after 24–48 h on medical treatment
- massive continuing haemorrhage.

Crohn's disease

Crohn's disease is a chronic granulomatous inflammatory disease of undetermined cause. Any part of the gastrointestinal tract may be involved often with 'skip lesions', but the ileum is affected in most patients.

The clinical presentation of Crohn's disease is variable. Abdominal pain, diarrhoea, anorexia, weight loss and fever are common features. Although a chronic illness with recurrent symptoms over years is common, patients with terminal ileitis can present acutely and be misdiagnosed as acute appendicitis. Think of Crohn's disease (as opposed to appendicitis) if the pain is poorly localised to the right lower quadrant and of more than 48-h duration, or there is a history of

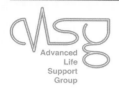

previous surgery (remember the possibility of a retrocaecal inflamed appendix). Other findings include a palpable mass, perianal signs (more frequently than in ulcerative colitis), sepsis and extraintestinal features. Crohn's colitis can also present with a clinical picture similar to that of ulcerative colitis.

Initial investigations include stool samples for microbiology to exclude infectious diarrhoea, abdominal X-ray, haematology and biochemistry, followed by specialist investigation. Treatment includes fluid and electrolyte replacement as required and nutritional supplements, medical treatment and surgery for complications.

SUMMARY

Abdominal pain may be due to any one of a wide variety of conditions, both intra- and extra-abdominal.

Primary assessment and resuscitation

A minority of patients will have life-threatening conditions. Rapid diagnosis and immediate treatment are required. Consider the following:

- Is the patient's airway at risk (recurrent vomiting with a depressed level of consciousness)?
- Is oxygenation and ventilation adequate (often impaired with chest pathology, severe acute pancreatitis and sepsis)?
- Are there signs of circulatory failure (when abdominal pain is due to a condition causing life-threatening hypovolaemia or sepsis)?

Urgent surgical (or gynaecological) referral is required, as part of resuscitation, for haemorrhagic shock. Septic shock due to an intra-abdominal cause is a multidisciplinary emergency; treatment includes vigorous fluid resuscitation, IV broad-spectrum antibiotics and early specialist consultation.

Secondary assessment and emergency treatment

- A detailed history and careful examination are the most important elements in making a diagnosis.
- Selective imaging and investigation may confirm the diagnosis and/or provide useful supplementary information.
- Careful attention to fluid and electrolyte replacement, analgesia, antibiotics and nasogastric drainage are important, particularly when the patient needs surgery.

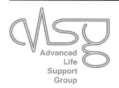

CHAPTER 16

The patient with hot red legs or cold white legs

OBJECTIVES

After reading this chapter you will be able to describe:
- the assessment and initial management of common medical problems which arise in the lower limb
- the complications that may arise from limb pathology.

INTRODUCTION

Trauma is the most common condition to affect the lower limb. In addition:
- systemic diseases and dermatological problems often lead to symptoms in the legs
- degenerative diseases may cause pain in the hip and the knee
- oedema usually gravitates to the legs
- chronic venous disease is common in older people.

However, a variety of acute medical problems may also arise in the lower limb. This chapter describes the assessment and initial management of the most common of these conditions (see next box).

Common acute medical problems in the lower limb	
Venous thrombosis	Daily
Phlebitis	Daily
Venous problems in IV drug users	Daily
Cellulitis	Daily
Arterial embolism	Weekly
Intraarterial injection	Monthly
Compartment syndrome	Monthly
Rupture of a Baker's cyst	Monthly

GENERAL PRINCIPLES OF ASSESSMENT OF THE LOWER LIMB

Key point

Always look at the 'whole patient' before examining their legs

---

Acute Medical Emergencies; The Practical Approach, 2nd edition.
Edited by Terence Wardle, Peter Driscoll, and Sue Wieteska.
© 2010 Blackwell Publishing Ltd.

For a full initial assessment, see Chapter 3.

The history of a condition that affects the legs takes the same format as any other history. Pain, swelling and loss of function (i.e. inability to weight bear) are usually the most important features. Always consider:

- recent injury/surgery
- smoking
- recent infections
- diabetes
- venous or other vascular disease
- pregnancy or use of oral contraception
- known malignancy (may cause coagulopathy)
- drug use
- long distance travel (venous stasis)
- family history.

The examination of the lower limb should follow the sequence of 4 four-letter words:

LOOK
FEEL
MOVE
X-RAY

Look for: site, spread, symmetry, systemic effects, swelling, bruising and redness

Feel for: temperature, tenderness, oedema and pulses

Move for: passive and active range of movements, function (including weight bearing)

X-ray for: suspected traumatic conditions.

Investigations should usually include blood glucose, full blood count and plasma chemistry. Special imaging may be appropriate (see later).

VASCULAR CONDITIONS OF THE LOWER LIMB

Venous thrombosis

Facts and figures about deep vein thrombosis (DVT):

- Around 2–5% of the population have a venous thrombosis at some time during their lives (see later box on incidence).
- DVT occurs in up to 40% of postoperative patients and increases in incidence with age. Three per cent of such patients progress to pulmonary embolism.
- DVT is estimated to occur in nearly one in every thousand pregnancies and 15–20% of these women will have pulmonary embolis if left untreated. Pulmonary embolism is the commonest cause of maternal death in the UK and similar developed countries.

Factors predisposing to thrombosis in pregnancy

- Increased concentrations of clotting factors and fibrinogen
- Production of inhibitors of fibrinolysis by the placenta
- Venous stasis
- Changes in blood vessels and patterns of blood flow
- Relative immobility

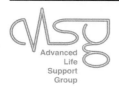

> **Time Out 16.1**
>
> Make a list of some types of patients who are at a high risk of DVT.

Thrombosis of the deep veins of the lower limb or pelvis may be caused by changes in:
- blood coagulation (smoking, oral contraceptive, procoagulant conditions)
- blood vessels (pregnancy)
- blood flow (immobility, plaster casts).
  There is:
- swelling and oedema distal to the occlusion
- warmth, redness and deep tenderness of the thigh or calf
- dilated superficial veins.

> **Key points on clinical findings in suspected DVT**
>
> The classic signs depend on venous occlusion. In contrast, there may be no signs in the presence of an extensive, non-occlusive but potentially lethal thrombus. Moreover, there is some evidence that non-occlusive thrombi float in the middle of the vein and break free very easily
>
> Homan's sign cannot be relied on – it is non-specific and may cause a pulmonary embolus and should not be done
>
> Calf muscle tear, ruptured Baker's cyst and superficial phlebitis may all be mistaken for DVT; oedema may occur with ischaemia
>
> DVT may be the first sign of occult malignancy – hence the need for abdominal and pelvic examination and investigation

Diagnosis

The first step in diagnosis of DVT involves assigning a clinical probabilty of DVT to the patient. On the basis of Well's criteria (see Table 16.1 below) patients can be classified as being 'likely' or 'unlikely' to have DVT. Patients deemed 'likely' to have DVT require diagnostic imaging.

Table 16.1 Incidence of venous thromboembolic disease in women

Characteristics	Cases per 100,000 women per year
Healthy, non-pregnant, not taking oral contraceptive	5
Using a second-generation pill (i.e. containing levonorgestrel)	15
Using a third-generation pill (i.e. containing desogestrel or gestodene)	25
	100,000 pregnancies
Pregnant	60

All of the above numbers increase with age and other known risk factors such as obesity

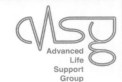

Clinical prediction rule to rank DVT risk

Ask about:	Score
Active cancer (ongoing treatment, diagnosed in last 6 months or having palliative care)	+1
Paralysis, paresis or plaster immobilisation of a leg	+1
Recently bedridden >3 days or major surgery within past 4 weeks	+1

Look for:	
Localised tenderness over distribution of the deep veins	+1
Entire leg swollen	+1
Calf circumference 10 cm below tibial tuberosity >3 cm greater than other calf	+1
Pitting oedema only in the symptomatic leg	+1
Collateral dilated (but not varicose) veins	+1
An alternative diagnosis as/or more likely than DVT	−2

Match the patient's score to the risk

Score	Risk of DVT
2 or more	Likely
1 or less	Unlikely

If a DVT is suspected, the patient should have a D-dimer assay. This test measures the breakdown products of cross-linked fibrin and is thus more specific for thrombosis than measurement of fibrin degradation products which arise from the breakdown of fibrinogen and fibrin monomer. A positive D-dimer mandates further diagnostic imaging, as above. A negative D-dimer in an 'unlikely' patient excludes the diagnosis.

The subsequent tests depend on local availability. Plethysmography, and its various modifications, can be used – often for screening. Doppler ultrasound studies are replacing the traditional venogram in many centres. If neither investigation is immediately available, the patient must be treated on clinical suspicion alone.

Management
Once the diagnosis is confirmed, treatment depends on local protocol. Anticoagulation is required with either an intravenous infusion of standard unfractionated heparin or, more commonly nowadays, with low molecular weight heparins given subcutaneously (e.g. enoxaparin 1.5 mg/kg every 24 h). The availability of subcutaneous treatment has increasingly led to patients with DVT being treated at home by community nurses. Heparin is discontinued when adequate oral anticoagulation is established. This is continued for a minimum of 3 months.

Thrombosis of veins distal to the popliteal vein (below-knee DVT) is common because of the venous sinuses present in the soleus muscle of the calf. Clinicians treat below-knee DVT with anticoagulation, but the condition is increasingly managed conservatively with:
- elastic stockings
- non-steroidal anti-inflammatory drugs
- rest and elevation
- clinic review.

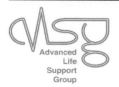

> **Key point**
>
> At least 5% of below-knee deep vein thromboses spread to the proximal veins and 50% of all above-knee venous thromboses embolise to the lungs

For diagnosis and management of suspected pulmonary embolism, see Chapter 8.

Phlebitis

Inflammation of the long or short saphenous vein usually occurs in patients with varicose veins. Phlebitis (usually in the arm) can also follow intravenous therapy. The vein is red, hot and tender.

Management

Phlebitis usually settles with topical therapy and oral non-steroidal anti-inflammatory drugs. If the patient is pyrexial, an antibiotic can be added. Superficial thrombophlebitis affecting varicose veins is treated with non-steroidal anti-inflammatory drugs.

Venous disease in intravenous drug abusers

Repeated injection into any vein causes chronic venous obstruction. There is swelling and oedema of the whole lower limb and dilatation of the superficial vessels; sinuses are often found in the groin. Acute thrombosis may occur, in which case the limb becomes hot, red and painful.

Management

This DVT is potentially life-threatening and should be treated with heparin as described earlier.

Arterial embolism

Thrombi which embolise to peripheral arteries may arise from several sites:
- the left atrial appendage (usually in the presence of atrial fibrillation)
- the left ventricle (invariably on an area damaged by a recent myocardial infarction or dilated ventricle or an aneurysm)
- an atheromatous plaque
- an aortic aneurysm
- a thrombosis in a deep vein in a patient with a patent foramen ovale (paradoxical embolism).

All of these possibilities should be considered although the first two are by far the most common. Emboli tend to lodge at the sites of bifurcation of arteries. Their effects depend on the extent of the occlusion of the circulation and on the degree of collateral circulation that exists. Common sites that involve the lower limb include:
- the aortic bifurcation (bilateral ischaemia to the level of the knees)
- the origin of the deep femoral artery (ischaemia to the mid-calf)
- the bifurcation of the popliteal artery (ischaemia of the foot).

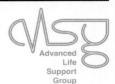

Sudden occlusion of the femoral artery causes the six 'P's:

Findings in arterial occlusion of the lower limb

- Pain
- Pallor
- Pulselessness
- Paraesthesiae
- Paralysis
- Perishing cold

Management

Embolism must be treated within 6 hours of the onset of symptoms or else propagation of thrombus distal to the embolus will greatly worsen prognosis.

Treatment includes:

- oral aspirin (300 mg)
- intravenous analgesia
- intravenous fluids
- referral to a vascular surgeon for embolectomy and/or fibrinolytic therapy.

Intraarterial injection

Irritant substances may cause critical ischaemia if injected into an artery. Intravenous drug users are the commonest sufferers from this problem; temazepam is the drug most usually involved. The ischaemia results from a mixture of vasospasm and multiple small emboli. Severe pain is the prominent symptom but the other signs described above (six 'P's) may be absent.

Management

This is similar to that described earlier for arterial embolism. Drugs that cause arterial dilatation may be considered.

Acute compartment syndrome

Closed compartment syndrome is caused by swollen, contused muscle or bleeding inside a rigid fascial envelope. The onset may be delayed after injury and insidious. Early symptoms are pain – particularly on muscle stretching – and paraesthesia. The affected part may also (but not invariably) be pale and cool with a slow capillary refill. Ischaemia results from compression of small blood vessels and so the presence of distal pulses is of no help in excluding the diagnosis.

Compartment syndrome can easily develop unseen under a plaster cast or below an eschar from a burn. The most common site to be affected is the lower leg, which has four anatomical compartments, but the syndrome is also seen in the forearm (three fascial compartments), buttock, thigh, foot and the hand.

Key point

In compartment syndrome, the limb may not be broken, distal pulses may be present and pulse oximetry may be normal

---

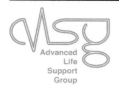

Management

Suspicion of compartment syndrome is an indication for immediate orthopaedic referral. Manometry is useful, particularly in patients with a depressed level of consciousness. There are four compartments in the lower leg and all may require extensive fasciotomy.

> **Key point**
>
> Arteriography will reveal arterial lesions but will not demonstrate compartment syndrome

OTHER MEDICAL CONDITIONS OF THE LOWER LIMB

Rupture of a Baker's cyst

Bursae in the popliteal fossa occur either spontaneously or may be connected to the knee joint. An enlarged and isolated popliteal bursa (a Baker's cyst) can be associated with rheumatoid arthritis. If this cyst bursts, it causes pain in the upper calf as the synovial fluid is squeezed between the calf muscles. The condition is often misdiagnosed as either a muscle injury or a DVT.

> **Key point**
>
> A popliteal aneurysm may also present as an extra-articular swelling behind the knee

Management

Ultrasound is the initial investigation. Arthrography is diagnostic. The patient should be referred to an orthopaedic surgeon or a rheumatologist.

Cellulitis of the lower limb

Infection of the skin may arise around a wound or without any obvious port of entry. The skin is red, swollen and tender, although the degree of pain is very variable. A cause for the infection should be sought but is not usually found. Without treatment, cellulitis can progress rapidly, leading to lymphangitis, lymphadenopathy and sepsis.

Management

Analgesics and antibiotics should be prescribed. The infection may be streptococcal and/or staphylococcal and so a combination of penicillin V and flucloxacillin is usually appropriate.

Admission for observation, elevation and intravenous therapy is indicated for extensive or rapidly progressing lesions. Lesser cases can be treated with oral antibiotics at home but should be reviewed within 36 hours. The limits of the infection should be marked on the skin with a pen so that changes are obvious at review.

Athlete's foot is a fungal infection which gives rise to an itchy whitish area between the toes (usually in the web space between the third and the fourth toes). It may be the cause of an ascending cellulitis and so the toes should always

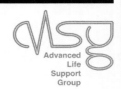

be examined in patients with cellulitis of the leg. If found, athlete's foot is treated with a topical cream, such as clotrimazole.

Time Out 16.2

Make a list of signs that differentiate arterial embolism from compartment syndrome.

SUMMARY

A number of serious medical and surgical problems are commonly seen in the lower limb.

- The assessment and management of these conditions follows a logical sequence.
- Trauma is the commonest problem to affect the leg but medical (especially vascular) conditions must always be considered.
- If untreated, some of these conditions can present a threat to life or limb.

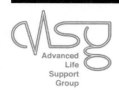

CHAPTER 17

The patient with hot and/or swollen joints

OBJECTIVES

After reading this chapter you should be able to:
• discuss the general principles of recognising, assessing and managing patients presenting with hot and/or swollen joints.

INTRODUCTION

A systematic approach will help in the diagnosis and management of these patients. This entails:
• recognition of the condition
• assessment of the patient
• determining the cause
• organising appropriate investigation relevant to the suspected diagnosis
• providing appropriate treatment.

Key point

The aim is to immediately identify and treat those patients with septic arthritis

---

GENERAL PRINCIPLES OF MANAGING PATIENTS WITH HOT AND/OR SWOLLEN JOINTS

Recognition (the history)

This is usually the easy part. The patient presents with any, or all, of the following symptoms and signs related to their joints:
• red joints
• swollen joints
• hot joints
• tender joints
• painful joints
• decreased function.

Together, these signs and symptoms represent manifestations of inflammation. Swelling indicates organic disease and may be due to intra-articular fluid, synovitis, bone hypertrophy or a swollen periarticular structure.

Acute Medical Emergencies; The Practical Approach, 2nd edition.
Edited by Terence Wardle, Peter Driscoll, and Sue Wieteska.
© 2010 Blackwell Publishing Ltd.

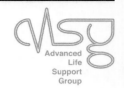

The nature of the pain provides clues to the cause of the condition. Pain at the end of the day implies a mechanical cause and is therefore often found in patients with osteoarthritis. In contrast, pain due to inflammatory disease tends to be worse in the morning and after rest, and may improve with exercise.

Loss of function is usually due to the joint being painful and stiff. The latter is most marked in the morning in inflammatory disease. In addition, with chronic joint problems, tendon and articular damage can exacerbate both neurological impairment and muscle weakness.

Assessment

There are many causes for a 'hot and/or swollen joint'. As treatment varies with the cause, the clinician needs to try to identify the likely causes as soon as possible. Differentiation can be helped greatly in this task by assessing the six 'S's (see box below).

The six 'S's of hot joint assessment

Single or several joints involved
Site(s)/symmetry
Sequence of symptoms
Systemic effects
Supplementary features
Specific findings on joint examination

Systemic effects include pyrexia and gastrointestinal upset. Supplementary features include the signs of other organ involvement.

The social impact of the condition needs to be considered when developing a management plan. This includes assessment of the patient's current occupational, social and domestic situation and how this has been affected following the onset of arthritis.

Causes

One of the most important clues is the number of joints involved. There are four causes which can potentially manifest as either mono- or polyarthropathies.

Potential causes of both mono- and polyarthropathy

O – Osteoarthritis	Daily
R – Rheumatoid arthritis	Weekly
C – Connective tissue disease	Annually
S – Spondyloarthritis	Annually

Once these have been excluded, you can divide the remaining causes into those which affect either a **single** joint or **several** joints.

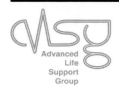

Causes of monoarthropathy (Common)

S – Sepsis	Weekly
I – Injury	Weekly
N – Neoplasm	Annually
G – Gout/pseudogout	Daily
L – Loose body	Weekly
E – Erythrocytes	Monthly

Causes of polyarthropathy (Rare)

S – Sexually transmitted disease	Annually
E – Endocrine/metabolic*	Annually
V – Viral	Monthly
E – Endocarditis	Only in examinations
R – Rheumatic fever	Only in examinations
A – Allergies/drug associated	Only in examinations
L – Lyme disease	Only in examinations

*E.g. Wilson's disease, alkaptonuria.

Investigations

Appropriate investigations should be requested to confirm or refute your suspected diagnosis. These consist of:

- blood tests
- radiography
- joint aspiration.

Blood tests

Although many blood tests can be requested, it is best initially to concentrate on the baseline measurements given in Table 17.1.

Non specific markers of active inflammation are:

- normocytic normochromic anaemia
- raised platelet count
- elevated erythrocyte sedimentation rate and C-reactive protein
- low albumin.

Table 17.1 Blood tests

Test	Condition
Uric acid	Gout
Rheumatoid factor	Present in 50–75% of rheumatoid arthritis and 30% of collagen/vascular disease
Antinuclear antibodies	Common in connective tissue disorders
Full blood count	Anaemia common in chronic conditions
Erythrocyte sedimentation rate	Reflects severity of inflammation
C-reactive protein	Reflects severity of inflammation

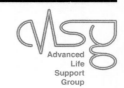

Radiography

During the development of the arthritis, the radiological features may vary from nothing to complete joint disruption (see next box). In addition, particular conditions have specific radiological features.

Radiological features of a hot joint (each finding can be present in isolation or in combination with others)

Normal
Soft tissue swelling
Joint space widening
Underlying bone lucency
Joint space narrowing
Bone destruction
Crystal deposition
Subluxation/dislocation
Loose body

Joint aspiration

See practical procedure in Chapter 33. The aspirate should be tested for the following:

- Gram stain
- Culture – bacterial and viral
- Crystals – with polarising microscope
- Red blood cells
- White blood cells
- Glucose
- Protein

Treatment

In the acute phase, all inflamed joints benefit from analgesia and splintage. However, appropriate treatment for the specific cause must also be started.

SPECIFIC TYPES OF HOT JOINTS

Septic arthritis
Causes

Staphylococcus aureus is the causative organism in 80% of cases, often spreading via the bloodstream, rarely from adjacent local osteomyelitis. It is more common in patients with one or more of the following risk factors:

- chronic disease
- rheumatoid arthritis
- intravenous drug use
- immunocompromise
- prosthetic joint.

The six 'S's

- **Single/multiple joint involved?** – Single
- **Site(s)?** – Any, but commonly around the knee in teenagers

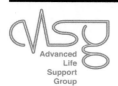

- **Sequence of symptoms?** – Develops gradually over a matter of hours to days. In addition to the signs of a hot joint, there is usually little or no movement and it is very tender
- **Systemic effects?** – Pyrexia and other signs of bacteraemia. Look carefully for potential portals of entry of infection.
- **Supplementary features?** – Related to the risk factors.
- **Specific findings on joint examination?** – There is usually a hot, tense joint effusion and marked pain on any compression/movement.

Investigation

Blood culture may show the causative organism. The joint aspirate may show pus, but a gram stain is necessary to help decide on an immediate antibiotic. This may be modified after the culture results are known.

Septic arthritis and pseudogout both give rise to pus in the aspirate and positive birefringent crystals in plane polarised light.

Treatment

Key point

Sepsis can destroy a joint in under 24 h!

Intravenous antibiotics must be started immediately the diagnosis is suspected. The choice will depend on local hospital policy but, using the gram stain, a good initial 'blind' combination is given in the next box.

Gram positive cocci   1 g flucloxacillin – 6 hourly – IV
Gram negative cocci   1.2 g benzylpenicillin – 6 hourly – IV
Gram negative rods   Gentamicin – dose according to body weight and renal function

---

Orthopaedic referral should be made without delay as urgent surgical drainage is probably required.

Gout
Cause

Normally nucleic acids in cells are metabolised into purines, which in turn are converted into uric acid. This is eliminated predominantly by the kidneys (67%) and the remainder by the gut. In gout, sodium monourate accumulates and crystals precipitate into joints, inducing an inflammatory reaction.

It follows from this metabolic pathway that uric acid can accumulate following reduced renal excretion of uric acid or increased production (see box below).

Causes of gout

Causes of reduced renal excretion of uric acid:
   Intrinsic kidney disease
   Diuretics (thiazide & loop)

Continued

Causes of gout (Continued)

Diabetic ketoacidosis
Lactic acidosis
Starvation
Causes of increased uric acid production:
Foods high in purines: – all meats
– meat extracts and gravy
– seafood
– yeast
– beer
– beans and lentils

Increased cell destruction:
Leukaemia
Polycythaemia
Some cancer therapies

The six 'S's
- **Single/multiple joint involved?** – Single initially
- **Site(s)?** – Classically the metatarsophalangeal joint of the hallux (other joints can be involved)
- **Sequence of symptoms?** – Comes on abruptly, typically at night
- **Systemic effects?** – Usually none
- **Supplementary features?** – Chronic tophaceous gout: tophi (urate deposits) develop in avascular areas after repeated attacks. Sites include pinna, tendons and the elbows. Urate nephropathy. Uric acid stones
- **Specific findings on joint examination?** – Gout is usually very painful on palpation of the synovial or perisynovial tissues, but not very painful on axial compression of the joint or minor passive movement.

Investigations
Aspirate – Negative birefringent needle shaped crystals

Key point

The serum urate may be normal even in acute gout

Treatment
Remove the precipitating cause. Patients should cut down on these foods, but dietary purines only contribute 1 mg/dl to the serum urate level so dieting only helps a small amount.

Analgesia: A non-steroidal anti-inflammatory drug will usually provide good symptomatic relief. Be wary of gastrointestinal complications, particularly in the elderly. It is therefore advisable to co-prescribe a proton pump inhibitor for gastromucosal protection. In patients unable to use non-steroidal anti-inflammatory drugs, colchicine can be helpful.

After three weeks, consider using allopurinol. This reduces the plasma urate level by blocking the production of uric acid, via inhibition of the enzyme xanthine oxidase (see next box).

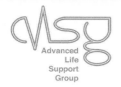

Advanced
Life
Support
Group

> **Indications for allopurinol therapy**
>
> Recurrent attacks of gout
> Chronic tophaceous gout
> Polyarticular gout
> Clinical or X-ray signs of gouty arthritis
> Recurrent uric acid renal stones
> Prophylaxis before cytotoxic chemotherapy for haematological malignancy

> **Key point**
>
> Aspirin in high doses (300 mg tds) can be used to treat gout, although seldom used today. In contrast, low doses (<150 mg daily) can cause gout

Pseudogout
Causes
Pseudogout results from the precipitation of calcium pyrophosphate crystals in joints. This is more likely when any of the following risk factors are present: old age, dehydration, illness, hypothyroidism, diabetes mellitus, any arthritis, high serum calcium and low serum magnesium or phosphate.

> **Tip**
>
> Pseudogout is the commonest cause of an acute monoarthropathy in the elderly

The six 'S's
- **Single/multiple joint involved?** – Single
- **Site(s)/symmetry?** – Mainly the knee
- **Sequence of symptoms?** – Less severe and longer lasting than gout. In chronic form it leads to destructive changes like osteoarthritis
- **Systemic effects?** – Usually none, unless associated with a metabolic condition, e.g. haemochromatosis
- **Supplementary features?** – Usually none
- **Specific findings on joint examination?** – Pseudogout is usually very painful on palpation of the synovial or perisynovial tissues, but not very painful on axial compression of the joint or minor passive movement.

Investigations
Aspirate the joint and check the fluid for weakly positive birefringent rod shaped crystals in plane polarised light. Calcium pyrophosphate deposits in cartilage, ligaments and joint capsules may also be seen on X-ray. This can occur in any cartilaginous joint but the knee is classically involved. There may also be joint destruction.

Treatment
Correct any cause and provide analgesia. As this analgesia is usually a nonsteroidal anti-inflammatory drug, the same precautions need to be applied as described for gout.

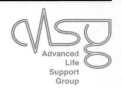

Rheumatoid arthritis (disease)

Cause

For reasons that are unclear, patients with this condition develop a systemic, autoimmune inflammatory disease which acts mainly on the synovial linings. Often this leads to irreversible destruction of joints and, in some cases, systemic complications. This type of arthritis is common, affecting approximately 1% of the adult population, particularly females (ratio 3:1) and peaks in the fourth decade.

As part of the inflammatory process, B lymphocytes secrete autoantibodies, known as rheumatoid factors, which act on the synovium as well as extra-articular sites. The latter explains the systemic symptoms which are present in these patients.

The six 'S's

- **Single/multiple joint involved?** – Usually more than three joints are involved but rarely it affects a single joint. When it does, it is typically a large joint, such as the knee, ankle, shoulder or wrist.
- **Site(s)?** – Hands and feet initially. Symmetrical.
- **Sequence of symptoms?** – Initially, it tends to affect the hands and feet. In the elderly, it can present as an acute hot joint. With time, larger joints become involved while previously affected joints remain painful, stiff and fusiform in shape. In keeping with its inflammatory aetiology, the stiffness is most noticeable in the morning and typically lasts over 30–60 min. When the patient moves about, the nocturnal accumulation of soft tissue fluid disperses and the stiffness eases. In contrast, the presence of erythema extending beyond the joint margin can indicate septic arthritis or cellulitis.

  In addition, the onset may be acute self-limiting attacks (palindromic), rapid with severe polyarticular involvement (explosive), non-articular features (systemic) or limited to one joint (mono).

  As the disease process progresses, ulnar deviation and volar subluxation of the metacarpophalangeal joints occur, along with swan neck and *boutonnière* deformities of the fingers, and Z-deformities of the thumbs. Some changes in the feet, especially subluxation of the metatarsophalangeal joints, are common. In addition, there can be extensor tendon rupture and intrinsic muscle wasting of the hands and feet. It is important to remember that the atlantoaxial joint can also be involved. This, along with other changes in the cervical spine, can lead to subluxation and potential spinal cord compression during airway maneouvres. Rheumatoid arthritis can also complicate airway management through reduced range of movement in the neck and temporomandibular joints.
- **Systemic effects?** – Anaemia, weight loss
- **Supplementary features?** – In addition to rheumatoid nodules (hence seropositive), these include:
  ○ respiratory system – pulmonary fibrosis, pleuritis, bronchiolitis obliterans, cricoarytenoid involvement
  ○ cardiovascular system – valvulitis, vasculitis, pericarditis
  ○ liver – hepatitis
  ○ central nervous system – carpal tunnel, multifocal neuropathies
  ○ eyes – episcleritis, scleritis, dry eyes, scleromalacia
  ○ kidney – amyloid
  ○ reticuloendothelial – lymphadenopathy, splenomegaly
  ○ skin – rash, nodules.

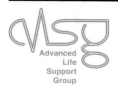

- **Specific findings on joint examination**? – There is joint swelling and tenderness along the joint line. Pain on compression of metacarpophalangeal or metatarsophalangeal joints is an early feature of rheumatoid arthritis. Ulnar deviation and volar subluxation of the metacarpophalangeal joints, swan neck and *boutonnière* deformities of the fingers, and Z-deformities of the thumbs as outlined above, are found at various stages of the disease. There are some changes in the feet, especially subluxation of the metatarsophalangeal joints.

> **Key point**
>
> Rheumatoid disease affects multiple systems. Early referral to a rheumatologist is essential

Investigation

Laboratory investigations help only to support the diagnosis of rheumatoid arthritis or to exclude alternative diagnoses. They do not help to confirm or exclude rheumatoid arthritis. Investigation results can all be negative at the onset of the disease.

Rheumatoid factor can be detected in about 50–70% of patients with rheumatoid arthritis, but can be absent in up to 60% of patients with early disease. Therefore, negative rheumatoid factor should not be taken as evidence against rheumatoid arthritis. A positive result should also be interpreted with caution, as it occurs in several conditions (e.g. TB, hepatitis C, SLE) as well as occurring in 5% of healthy individuals.

> **Key point**
>
> Rheumatoid factor should never be used on its own to diagnose rheumatoid arthritis. Results can all be negative at the onset of the disease

A chest X-ray may show pulmonary fibrosis, nodules and rarely pleural effusions

Plain radiographs of hands and feet are normal or show only soft tissue changes in up to 70% of patients with early rheumatoid arthritis.

Treatment

Cases of suspected rheumatoid arthritis should be referred to a rheumatologist, to confirm the diagnosis and take over the long-term care of these patients. In the meantime, analgesia must be provided. Start treatment with paracetamol and add a non-steroidal anti-inflammatory drug.

Disease-modifying drugs (e.g. methotrexate, sulphasalazine and monoclonal antibodies such as infliximab) are used if there is no response to the non-steroidal antiflammatory or synovitis has persisted for more than six months. The difficulty for the clinician is that many patients with early undifferentiated inflammatory arthritis have self-limiting disease such as postviral arthritis. It is important not to expose such patients to potentially toxic therapy with these drugs.

Other potential therapies include:

Non-specific

- Regular exercise
- Household aids

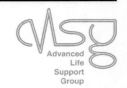

Specific
- Intra-articular injection
- Surgery

Gonococcal arthritis (*Neisseria gonorrhoeae*)
Cause
This occurs most frequently in young people. A purulent effusion is uncommon (<30%).

The six 'S's
- **Single/several joints involved?** – Multiple
- **Site(s)/symmetry?** – Involves midsized joints such as knee, wrist and elbow
- **Sequence of symptoms?** – Usually migratory arthralgia
- **Systemic effects?** – Skin rash and other symptoms associated with gonococcal infection
- **Supplementary features?** – Associated with red rash/vesicles over the distal part of the limbs. May also get tenosynovitis of the wrist and hands
- **Specific findings on joint examination?** – The signs are those of an acutely inflamed joint, without any specific to gonococcal arthritis.

Investigations
- Aspirate – send for GCFT (gonococcal fixation test)
- Serum for GCFT
- Urethral or high vaginal swab

Treatment
- Antibiotics
- Refer to genitourinary medicine for treatment, contact tracing and screening for other sexually transmitted diseases

Viral
Arthralgia is a common symptom of viral infection along with malaise, fatigue, fever, myalgia, headache and sore throat. These features will occur before any arthritis.

The six 'S's
- **Single/several joints involved?** – Multiple
- **Site(s)/symmetry?** – Symmetrical, small joints, of the hands, wrists, knees (parvovirus, rubella)
- **Sequence of symptoms?** – Self limiting (usually), stiffness is most marked in the morning
- **Systemic effects?** – As above
                                    – Morbilliform rash and lymphadenopathy with rubella
- **Supplementary features?** – As above
- **Specific findings on joint examination?** – Painful, tender, swollen joints.

Investigations
Positive viral serology, Interestingly rheumatoid factor may be positive in rubella.

Treatment
This is symptomatic with analgesia and NSAIDs (for further detail on NSAIDs, see Chapter 9).

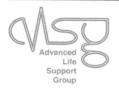

Spondyloarthritis

This represents a collection of conditions that are seronegative (for rheumatoid factor) and have several common symptoms. The types you are most likely to see can be remembered by the acronym 'PEAR'.

P – Psoriatic arthritis
E – Enteropathic arthritis
A – Ankylosing spondylitis
R – Reactive arthritis (Reiter's syndrome)

The six 'S's

- **Single/several joint involved?** – Multiple or monoarthritis of large joints (small joints involved in psoriatic arthritis); characterised by enthesopathy, i.e. develop inflammation at the site of ligamentous insertion into bone
- **Site(s)/symmetry?** – Spine and sacroiliac joints; asymmetrical when involves several joints
- **Sequence of symptoms?** – Depends on the specific type of spondyloarthritis (see later)
- **Systemic effects?** – Can include uveitis
- **Supplementary features?** – Depends on the specific type of spondyloarthritis, but can include calcification of tendon insertions, uveitis, aortic regurgitation, upper zone pulmonary fibrosis, and amyloidosis
- **Specific features on joint examination?** – Asymmetrical, dactylitis, oligoarticular, sacroiliitis.

Psoriatic arthritis

Commonly, this involves the terminal interphalangeal joints asymmetrically, but there are other different presentations. The patient usually also has the skin and nail manifestations of psoriasis.

Enteropathic arthritis

Usually involves the knees and ankles. Typically this person has associated inflammatory bowel disease.

Ankylosing spondylitis

Typically seen in young males presenting with back stiffness and pain, especially in the morning. Although rare, they may eventually get the 'question mark' spinal posture (kyphotic spine with hyperextended neck) due to progressive spinal fusion, a fixed spinocranial ankylosis and restricted respiration. In 50% of cases, the hip is involved and in 25%, the knee and ankle are affected. Associated with anterior uveitis and aortic regurgitation.

Reactive arthritis (Reiter's syndrome)

This comprises a triad of urethritis, conjunctivitis and seronegative arthritis. In the UK this typically presents in young male patients with lower limb involvement including enthesitis (heels) dactylitis, asymmetrical oligoarticular changes. Asymmetrical with extra-articular features including oral ulceration, circinate balanitis and keratoderma blennorrhagicum. A recent history of non-specific urethritis or diarrhoea can occasionally be elicited.

Investigations

HLA B-27 is present in 88–96% of patients with ankylosing spondylitis, but only 20% of the HLA B-27 population develops ankylosing spondylitis. The spinal

X-ray may also show 'bamboo spine' as well as squaring of the vertebra and erosions of the apophyseal joints. Obliteration of the sacroiliac joint is also commonly visible in established cases. Bilateral sacroiliitis is the characteristic radiological feature.

Treatment

Early rheumatological referral is necessary. Exercise must be started early to maintain as much mobility and posture as possible. In the other types of spondyloarthritis, exercise should be started once the acute symptoms have settled. Treat the underlying condition.

Time Out 17.1

Construct an algorithm to include the important steps in the diagnosis and management of a hot swollen joint.

Key point

Do **not** leave a septic joint until the next day – infection can destroy a joint in under 24 h

---

SUMMARY

A hot joint is easy to recognise, but has many causes. A systematic approach is therefore needed. This includes a well-'phrased' history followed by a six 'S' assessment and appropriate investigations.

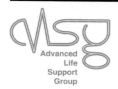

CHAPTER 18

The patient with a rash

OBJECTIVES

After reading this chapter you will be able to:
- understand the common terms used in dermatology
- discuss cutaneous manifestations of life-threatening illness
- apply a structured approach to the assessment and management of the patient with a rash.

INTRODUCTION

The skin is a large organ which may be affected by a primary disorder or manifest signs of systemic illness. It may also provide the signs required to diagnose immediately life-threatening illnesses. Careful assessment using a structured approach is necessary to distinguish the serious from a coincidental or innocuous rash. Early recognition of these signs will allow prompt, potentially lifesaving, disease specific therapy to be initiated.

This chapter will provide you with a structured approach to common dermatological problems – some of which are life-threatening.

USEFUL TERMINOLOGY

- **Angio-oedema:** Similar to urticaria but involves the subcutaneous tissues, especially the face, lips and tongue. Presents with swelling rather than wheals. It is rarely life-threatening, but be wary of laryngeal compromise. Hypotension/anaphylaxis can occur (uncommonly), as can bronchospasm and gastrointestinal disturbance. ABC treatment should include intramuscular adrenaline, intravenous hydrocortisone and antihistamines.
- **Bulla:** A fluid-filled blister greater than 1 cm in diameter, e.g. as in pemphigoid.
- **Ecchymoses:** Bruises (i.e. confluent petechiae).
- **Erosion:** Partial epidermal loss (no scar usually).
- **Erythema:** Redness that blanches on pressure, indicating dilated capillaries. It should be distinguished from purpura, which can be red, orange, purple or brown but do not fade on firm pressure.
- **Erythroderma:** Widespread erythema (i.e. greater than 90% body surface area affected).
- **Macule:** Flat lesions, any colour, e.g. a freckle, and less than 5 mm in diameter.
- **Nikolsky's sign:** Gentle rubbing of the skin causes the epidermis to separate from the underlying dermis with subsequent erosions.
- **Nodule:** A raised rounded lesion greater than 1 cm in diameter.

Acute Medical Emergencies; The Practical Approach, 2nd edition.
Edited by Terence Wardle, Peter Driscoll, and Sue Wieteska.
© 2010 Blackwell Publishing Ltd.

- **Papule:** A raised rounded lesion less than 1 cm in diameter, e.g. a mole. Therefore a maculopapular rash consists of raised and flat lesions. These are often less than 1 cm diameter, e.g. as seen in a penicillin rash.
- **Patch:** Larger version of a macule (greater than 5 mm in diameter).
- **Petechiae:** Pinpoint haemorrhage.
- **Plaque:** A raised patch, e.g. a plaque of psoriasis on an elbow.
- **Purpura:** A condition that can be red, orange, purple or brown but does not fade on firm pressure (unlike erythema).
- **Pustule:** A pus filled blister, usually less than 1 cm in diameter, e.g. as in a furuncle (i.e. boil).
- **Ulcer:** Full loss of epidermis and some dermis (scar possible).
- **Urticaria:** Formation of pruritic, transient (<24 h) wheals (like nettle rash). These are collections of dermal oedema surrounded by erythema. Systemic symptoms are extremely rare.
- **Vesicle:** A fluid-filled blister less than 1 cm diameter, e.g. as in herpes labialis.

IMMEDIATELY LIFE-THREATENING EMERGENCIES

Life-threatening illnesses involving the skin may present with signs relating to airway, breathing or circulation.

Immediately life-threatening illnesses with signs in the skin		
Airway	Obstruction	Anaphylaxis
		Angio oedema
Breathing	Bronchospasm	Anaphylaxis
Circulation	Shock	*Meningococcal sepsis*
		Gonococcal sepsis
		Cellulitis
		Anaphylaxis
		Erythroderma

These conditions can be usefully grouped into four different areas by the type of rash associated with the underlying condition. These are:
- urticaria
- erythema
- purpura and vasculitis
- blistering disorders.

Urticaria

This is a common presentation and 15–20% of the population will present to the emergency department with varying degrees of severity. Urticaria can present in many different ways with many associated features, e.g., with:
- anaphylaxis
- angio oedema or
- urticaria alone.

Anaphylaxis

This may present with predominantly dermatological features including pruritus and urticaria. These features are usually florid but may be subtle.

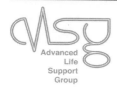

A – Airway

Anaphylaxis can present with upper airway obstruction.

B – Breathing

This can be affected with anything from mild to severe bronchospasm.

C – Circulation

The patients are often hypotensive and can have complete cardiovascular collapse, which is due to a combination of increased vascular permability and vasodilatation.

Specific features

Anaphylaxis can present with gastrointenstinal disturbance. The specific management of this condition is considered in detail in Chapter 9.

Angio oedema

This is a condition that may present with some features similar to anaphylaxis. It is characterised by swelling of the subcutaneous tissues, predominantly affecting the face. Notably these lesions are rarely itchy in contrast to the intense pruritus often associated with urticaria.

A – Airway

Involvement of mucous membranes or the tongue, larynx or pharynx may result in airway obstruction. Angio oedema may herald the onset of anaphylaxis.

Specific features

Frequently no cause is apparent and attacks may be recurrent. Angio oedema should be treated in the same manner as anaphylaxis. Rarely patients may have angio oedema resulting from C1 esterase inhibitor deficiency. This should be treated similarly to other causes of angio oedema but may require specific treatment with either fresh frozen plasma or C1 esterase inhibitor concentrate where available.

Urticaria specific features

Dermographism

This is produced by firm stroking of the skin and leads to the development of an urticarial 'wheal' within 30 min.

Solar and heat urticaria

This is rare and solar urticaria settles once the light stimulus has been removed.

Cholinergic urticaria

This is produced by exercise, heat or emotional stress and is associated with itching, headaches and nausea.

Cold urticaria

This is usually familial or acquired and can be associated with underlying illnesses, e.g. connective tissue disorders. This can be treated with cypoheptadine 2–4 mg twice a day, although there are side effects, specifically drowsiness and increased appetite.

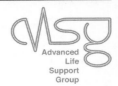

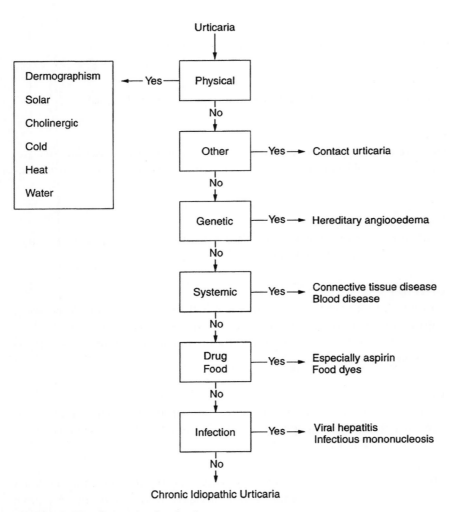

Fig. 18.1 The diagnosis of urticaria.

Contact urticaria
This is produced by foods, textiles, animal dander, plants, tropical medicines and cosmetics. Foods that are commonly involved are fish, eggs and nuts. The most important thing is to remove the causative agent and treat with antihistamines (Fig. 18.1).

Erythema
The patient with red skin (erythema). This is defined as **redness that blanches on pressure** and indicates dilated capillaries. It should be distinguished from purpura which can be red, orange, purple or brown but does not fade on firm pressure. Erythroderma means widespread erythema (i.e. greater than 90% of the body surface area affected).

Erythroderma and Exfoliation
They may result from a number of causes (see next box) although the common feature is marked vasodilatation. Shock may occur from a number of mechanisms including vasodilatation, fluid loss and endotoxin related. A striking clinical feature is the heat radiated by these patients, which may result in problems with thermoregulation.

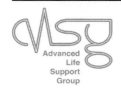

Causes of erythroderma and exfoliation

Psoriasis
Toxic epidermal necrolysis
Drug eruptions
Staphylococcal scalded skin syndrome
Toxic shock syndrome
Lymphoma
Seborrhoeic dermatitis
Contact dermatitis
Idiopathic
Necrotising Fasciitis

Primary assessment

A–B – Airway and breathing

In view of the widespread erythema, the oxygen consumption is greatly increased, thus high concentrations of inspired oxygen are required.

C – Circulation

Patients with erythroderma, especially where the skin has peeled leaving a large moist area, will continue to lose large amounts of fluid. This fluid should be replaced. The amount of fluid required can be calculated with standard formulae used for burn injuries. Hypovolaemia should be corrected with crystalloid as described in Chapter 9. Inotropic support or vasoconstrictor drugs may occasionally be required to treat the shock after adequate fluid resuscitation. This step should be undertaken in conjunction with specialist advice from Intensive Care. Vascular access preferably in unaffected skin.

D – Disability

Do not forget confusion as a sign of untreated shock

E – Exposure

Distribution of eruption – reassess frequently (necrotising fasciitis, cellulitis) if it grows rapidly it is more urgent. Thermoregulation – prevent heat loss.

Secondary assessment

This will often reveal the underlying cause for erythroderma. A well-'phrased' history may help to identify specific diseases.

Psoriasis, seborrhoeic/contact dermatitis

It is important to obtain a history of previous skin diseases and an enquiry should be made about the recent use of the systemic or topical steroids as abrupt withdrawal may precipitate an acute flare up. There may be other precipitating factors in the history which has caused an acute flare up, of which the patient will be aware.

Toxic epidermal necrolysis

See blistering eruptions.

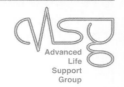

Drug eruptions

A full drug history must be obtained, including all topical medications. This enquiry must not be limited to prescribed medications but should include over the counter medications, herbal remedies and cosmetic use. The reaction to topical applications may be local or systemic.

Staphylococcal scalded skin syndrome

This commonly occurs in children and there will be history of recent or current infection, e.g. conjunctivitis or otitis media. The patient will be irritable and have a fever, with an orange red macular rash, which is tender. There is a positive Niklosky's sign and within 48 h there is a blistering eruption. Sheets of the epidermis are lost and healing is complete in 5–7 days.

Toxic shock syndrome

This has menstrual and non-menstrual forms and there is also a streptococcal variety – all show similar features. The mortality rate is 1–5% in toxic shock syndrome and 25–75% in streptococcal toxic shock syndrome. The history may include recent tampon use. There is usually an infection with *staphococcal aureus* in the non menstruating toxic shock syndrome and the predisposing factors include influenza, sinusitis, tracheitis, IVDA, HIV, burns, infected contact dermatitis, gynecological infection, post partum and post operative infections. There is usually a fever of greater than 38.9°C, diffuse macular erythroderma with hypotension, nausea, diarrhoea, myalgia and headache. This may lead to acute kidney injury and septic shock. Commonly there is desquamation in 1–2 weeks.

Lymphoma

Erythroderma can occur in patients with Hodgkin's lymphoma and presents with severe pruritus, weight loss and night sweats. Erythroderma is also seen in lymphocytic leukaemia.

Necrotising fasciitis

This usually presents after an insect bite, wound or abscess or following infection of needle tracts (in an IV drug user) or surgical wounds. Mortality rate can be as high as 25% and in some cases there is no associated initial wound. It is characterised by fever, vesicle formations with serious fluid drainage and the erythema rapidly spreads and may become violet in colour. There may be pain, crepitus or painless ulcers. It is caused by synergism between the streptococcal and anaerobic bacterii causing a rapid spread.

Specific treatment of causes of erythroderma

Specific treatment can be started after resuscitation, which includes providing oxygen and IV fluids and a working diagnosis. These may include:

- Covering weeping or open lesions with saline soaked dressings. This may reduce contamination and secondary infection. If large areas are to be dressed, dry sterile dressings should be used to reduce heat loss in the early stages. It may be useful to photograph the rash before covering it.
- Intravenous flucloxacillin should be given (unless contraindicated) if staphylococcal infection is suspected. Topical and prophylactic antibiotics are of no benefit and may cause later complications.
- Intravenous opioid analgesia may be required.
- If necrotising fasciitis is suspected, immediate surgical referral and antibiotics should be arranged.

  Disease specific treatment should be initiated on the basis of specialist advice.

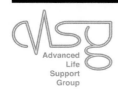

Summary

The assessment and management of the erythematous patient is shown in Fig. 18.2.

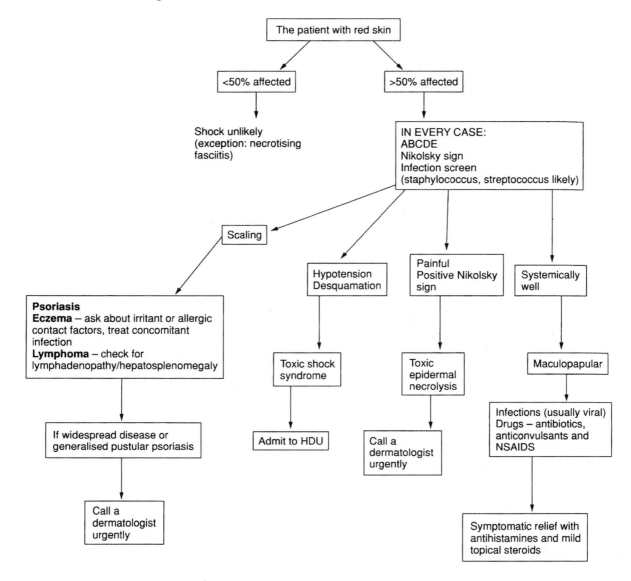

Fig. 18.2 Assessment and management of the erythematous patient.

> **Key point**
>
> Nikolsky's sign – shearing stress on epidermis causes new blisters

Purpura and vasculitis

Purpura are caused by red cells leaking out of blood vessels into the dermis. Although the main cause is inflammation of these blood vessels, i.e. vasculitis (see later), other conditions have to be considered.

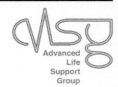

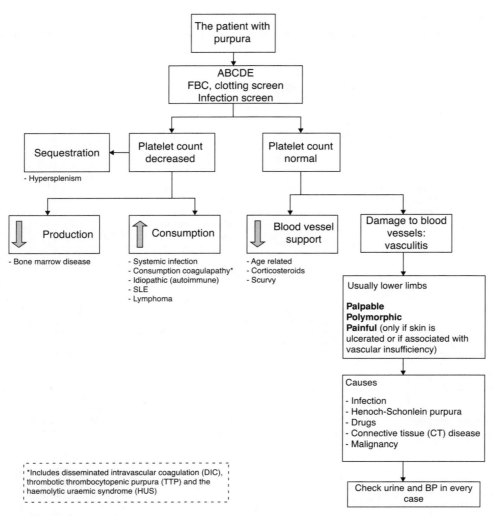

Fig. 18.3 The patient with purpura: an algorithm to aid differential diagnosis.

Key point

Unlike erythema, purpura does not blanch on firm pressure

Purpura may be part of either a rapidly progressive – often septic – illness or, in contrast, a component of a longstanding stable vasculitis. The hallmark of a purpuric rash is the failure to blanch with pressure. This is best seen by pressing on the rash with a microscope slide or a clear drinking glass.

Purpura may be caused by an abnormality of the blood or the vessels. These points are summarised in Fig. 18.3.

Key point

The presence of a purpuric rash in an ill patient is due to overwhelming sepsis until proven otherwise

---

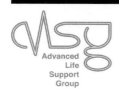

Primary assessment

There are a number of infections that produce a characteristic clinical picture of a purpuric rash associated with shock.

Infections associated with shock and purpura

Meningococcus (*Neisseria meningitidis*)
Gonococcus (*Neisseria gonorrhoeae*)
Staphylococcus aureus
Rickettsia
Arbovirus

The most common cause is *meningococcal septicaemia*. It is important to remember that this can occur without any symptoms or signs of meningitis. Its management is discussed fully in Chapters 9, 11 and 14 but remember that cefotaxime or ceftriaxone IV (80 mg/kg) should be given immediately. A third-generation cephalosporin is used as penicillin resistant strains of *Neisseria meningitidis* have been isolated. If possible blood cultures should be taken before the first dose of antibiotics.

Key point

If in doubt, treat with ceftriaxone/cefotaxime IV (80 mg/kg) first and investigate for alternative causes later

---

Secondary assessment

The well-'phrased' history may reveal the presence of systemic symptoms, e.g. urinary symptoms, and abdominal pain combined with fever or joint symptoms may suggest a systemic vasculitis such as Henoch–Schönlein purpura, or polyarteritis, or a systemic infection. A detailed drug history must be obtained. Further investigations should include urine analysis for blood and protein, full blood count, and urea and electrolytes.

The comprehensive physical examination should seek specific clues as to the underlying cause of purpura or vasculitis. Changes to the mental state may be present but may be subtle. This can occur with meningitis, connective tissue diseases or with intracranial bleeding or thrombosis (e.g. in thrombotic thrombocytopenia).

Definitive care of the underlying problem will frequently involve the input of a number of specialties including haematology, immunology, rheumatology, general medicine and intensive care. Do not delay resuscitative treatment for a specialist opinion.

Blistering disorders

- Blisters are accumulations of fluid that occur in two common sites.
- Within the epidermis (intraepidermal) – often having a thin roof and therefore burst early, like herpes, pemphigus.
- Under the epidermis (subepidermal) – often thick walled, like pemphigoid.
- Any may contain blood.

Although there are more comprehensive classifications, the differential diagnosis of blistering eruptions is based on whether they are painless (Fig. 18.4) or painful (Fig. 18.5).

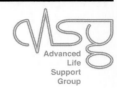

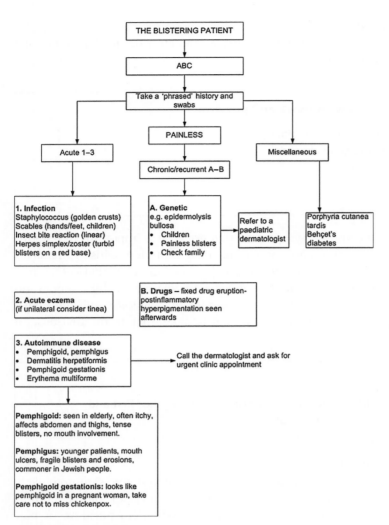

Fig. 18.4 Painless blistering eruptions.

IS THIS STEVENS–JOHNSON SYNDROME (SJS) OR TOXIC EPIDERMAL NECROLYSIS (TEN)?

Terminology in these conditions can be confusing. Stevens–Johnson syndrome is considered to be erythema multiforme characterised by purpuric macules and 'target lesions' in association with mucous membrane (ocular, oral, genital) involvement. However, erythema multiforme is often maculopapular rather than the classic target appearance. To help differentiate it from the usual maculopapular eruptions, there is mucosal involvement, pain and possible progression to toxic epidermal necrolysis. This is heralded by the development of the Nikolsky sign.

Toxic epidermal necrolysis, with full thickness loss of the epidermis, presents with tenderness and widespread red macules and target lesions of the skin followed by exfoliation (like a scald). It may follow Stevens–Johnson syndrome or appear *de novo* and often starts in the flexures. This is a dermatological emergency, which requires swift recognition and treatment. The mortality rate is 30–35%, which increases in the elderly (who are usually on the most medication). Management needs to be on a high dependency unit.

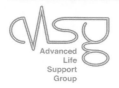

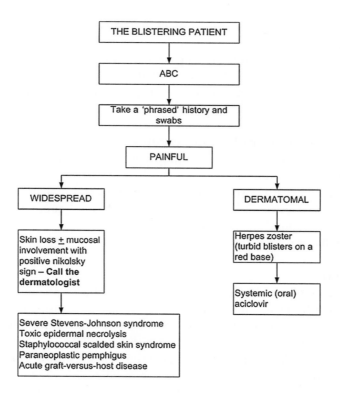

Fig. 18.5 Painful blistering eruptions.

Causes of Stevens–Johnson syndrome
- Sulphonamides and NSAIDs
- Herpes simplex, streptococcus, mycoplasma

Causes of toxic epidermal necrolysis
- Drugs are the commonest cause of toxic epidermal necrolysis (TENs) including anticonvulsants, antibiotics (especially sulphonamides) and NSAIDs
- Infection (bacterial, viral, fungal)
- Idiopathic
- As a sequel to Stevens–Johnson syndrome
- Rarely as a paraneoplastic phenomenon
- Human Immunodeficiency Virus (HIV)

If you suspect Stevens–Johnson syndrome/toxic epidermal necrolysis
ABCDE (IVI should be peripherally placed in uninvolved skin; oral intake of fluids may be impossible). Admission to critical care must be considered.

pain relief is crucial

take a detailed drug history and stop any offending drugs

an infection screen is needed as sepsis is the main cause of death

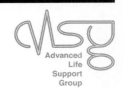

do not use flamazine (crossreacts with sulphonamides and causes neutropenia)
do not give steroids
call the dermatologist urgently to confirm the diagnosis and supervise treatment
keep the environmental temperature 30–32°C to prevent heat loss.
a prompt referral decreases the risk of infection, mortality rate and length of hospital stay.

Differential diagnosis of toxic epidermal necrolysis

Staphylococcal scalded skin – seen in children, may see evidence of impetigo, especially around the mouth and nose.
Paraneoplastic pemphigus – usually associated with haematological malignancy; may look very similar to Stevens–Johnson syndrome with subsequent toxic epidermal necrolysis but responds to steroids; characteristic histology.
Acute graft-versus-host disease.

Infection and the skin

The skin may be directly involved in an infective process. Cellulitis is a common problem that can occasionally become life- or limb threatening if necrotising fasciitis develops or sepsis ensues. The infecting organism causing cellulitis is usually a group A streptococcus. First-line treatment should be with penicillin.

Primary herpes zoster (varicella or chicken pox) is an unpleasant illness. However, it may become life-threatening in immunocompromised patients (e.g. post transplant, high dose steroids, acquired immunodeficiency syndrome). The rash is characterised by the simultaneous presence of vesicles, pustules and crusted lesions. It is important in the immunocompromised patient to recognise the illness as early as possible, when only a handful of vesicles may be present. The illness may be complicated by pneumonitis. Immunocompromised patients with primary herpes zoster should be treated with an intravenous antiviral agent, such as aciclovir.

Time Out 18.1

a List the four categories of dermatological conditions that can be immediately life-threatening.

b Draw the algorithm for each condition.

SUMMARY

- Life-threatening skin conditions are rare but may be rapidly fatal.
- Resuscitation may involve specific treatments including adrenaline for anaphylaxis and benzyl penicillin for *meningococcal septicaemia*.
- A careful history and examination may be required to elicit subtle features in the early stages of life-threatening illness.
- Seek specialist advice early.
- Most dermatological conditions presenting as an emergency are not life-threatening.

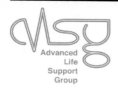
Advanced
Life
Support
Group

CHAPTER 19

The patient with acute confusion

OBJECTIVES

After reading this chapter you will understand:
- why acute confusional states occur
- the underlying cause
- the immediate management.

INTRODUCTION

Acute confusional state is a common condition. These medical emergencies can occur at home or arise in any hospital patient, usually as an unexplained behavioural change. The particular role of the reticular formation in the brain stem and the cerebral cortex in maintaining consciousness has been discussed in chapter 11 on the unconscious patient. This interlink to neurological activity is often suppressed in the acute confusional state, commonly caused by an acute illness (usually an infection, or the adverse effect of a drug).

Key point

Always consider an acute confusional state in any patient who is difficult, uncooperative or unable to give a reliable, accurate, history

---

CAUSES OF ACUTE CONFUSION

There are many causes of confusion; some of the common ones are listed in Table 19.1.

INITIAL ASSESSMENT

This should follow the standard format. Rather than describe a complete assessment, this will be tailored to specific features relevant to the patient with an acute confusional state.

Primary assessment

Ensure airway patency.

Exclude hypoxaemia.

Exclude shock; check glucose.

Exclude meningeal irritation, reduction in Glasgow Coma Score and lateralising signs. Make sure pupil response is appropriate.

Check temperature. Examine for a rash.

Acute Medical Emergencies; The Practical Approach, 2nd edition.
Edited by Terence Wardle, Peter Driscoll, and Sue Wieteska.
© 2010 Blackwell Publishing Ltd.

Table 19.1 Common causes of confusion

Systemic illness	Infection	Urinary or respiratory
	Organ failure	Hypoxaemia
		Hypoglycaemia
		Uraemia
		Liver failure
	Metabolic	Hypoglycaemia
		Electrolyte imbalance
		Hypercalcaemia
Primary neurological Disease		Status epilepticus
		Postictal state
		Non-dominant parietal lobe stroke
		Subarachnoid haemorrhage
		Subdural haematoma
		Raised intracranial pressure
		Viral encephalitis
Drugs		Recreational opioids
		Benzediazepines
		Tricyclics
		Antiparkinsonian treatment
Alcohol		Intoxication
		Withdrawal

SECONDARY ASSESSMENT – PHRASED HISTORY

This is only available from relatives or carers – or may not be available at all. However if present, the history usually describes impairment of consciousness over hours or days and typically worse at night. Confusion can manifest as global impairment of cognitive processes or impairment of thought, perception and memory. The patient is usually disorientated as assessed by the Abbreviated Mental State Score (see Chapters 3 and 7). There are often wild changes in behaviour which are out of character, and range from inactivity to irritability, hyperactivity and noisiness.

Thought processes are often slow, with delusion. Visual hallucinations classically dominate but perceptual defects can also include auditory and tactile hallucinations.

During the secondary assessment, it is important to repeat the primary assessment observations and check for any focal signs of infection.

Key point

Core temperature is more reliable than peripheral in the confused patient

---

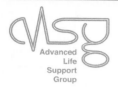

Request a urine dipstick. Check for clinical features of uraemia or hepatic encephalopathy, including flapping tremor (asterixis) and stigmata of chronic liver disease. A comprehensive neurological examination is required, but this may be limited by lack of cooperation from the confused patient. Recheck the Glasgow Coma Score to ensure that there has been no deterioration and reassess the pupils.

Look for lateralising signs and features that may suggest drug use, in particular nystagmus and ataxia of Wernicke's encephalopathy. Exclude urinary retention and faecal impaction – which occasionally, in the elderly, may be responsible for a change in conscious level.

By the end of the secondary assessment, a series of investigations will have been requested, to either support the clinical diagnosis or find the underlying cause of confusion. The minimum list of immediate investigations is shown in the next box.

List of immediate investigations in the confused patient

Glucometer and formal blood glucose
Sodium, potassium, urea and creatinine
Plasma calcium
Full blood count
Prothrombin time
C reactive protein/ESR
Blood cultures, urine dipstick test, microscopy and culture, chest X-ray
Arterial gases
ECG

Management

Specific management is directed at the underlying cause. Sedation should not routinely be required. If, however, the patient is aggressive or is at risk of self-injury, then sedation should be given; ideally with the patient being fully monitored on a high dependency unit. Remember the risk of sudden collapse or paradoxical agitation with some of the commonly used sedating agents in these circumstances.

Most patients with an acute confusional state have an underlying organic cause, especially if there is no previous psychiatric history. Always check the drug chart in hospital patients who become confused. Consider status epilepticus if there are myoclonic movements of the eyelids, face or hands. Demented patients are often diagnosed as confused and vice versa. Remember that patients with dementia often deteriorate and become confused, in response to an acute illness. Features differentiating acute confusional state, dementia and acute function psychosis are given in Table 19.2.

Table 19.2 Clinical features of acute confusional state, dementia and acute functional psychosis

Characteristic	Acute confusional state	Dementia	Acute functional psychosis
Onset	Sudden	Insidious	Sudden
Course over 24 h	Fluctuating, nocturnal exacerbation	Stable	Stable
Consciousness	Reduced	Clear	Clear
Attention	Globally disordered	Normal, except in severe cases	May be disordered
Orientation	Usually impaired	Often impaired	May be impaired
Cognition	Globally impaired	Globally impaired	May be selectively impaired
Hallucinations	Usually visual, or visual and auditory	Often absent	Predominantly auditory
Delusions	Fleeting, poorly systematised	Often absent	Sustained, systematised
Psychomotor activity	Increased, reduced or shifting unpredictably	Often normal	Varies from psychomotor retardation to severe hyperactivity
Speech	Often incoherent, slow or rapid	Difficulty finding words, perseveration	Normal, slow or rapid
Involuntary movements	Often asterixis or coarse tremor	Often absent	Usually absent
Physical illness or drug toxicity	One or both present	Often absent	Usually absent

SPECIFIC CONDITIONS

Alcohol

There are many causes of confusion related to alcohol use (see the next box).

Causes of a confusional state associated with alcohol abuse

Hypoglycaemia
Acute intoxication
Alcohol withdrawal
Wernicke's encephalopathy
Head injury
Chronic subdural haematoma
Alcoholic hepatitis
Hepatic encephalopathy
Acute pancreatitis
Alcoholic ketoacidosis
Lactic acidosis
Other illnesses, particularly pneumonia

If a history is available, then it is possible to exclude some of the above causes – in particular eliminating features of alcohol withdrawal (Table 19.3).

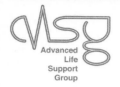

Table 19.3 Clinical features that may occur with alcohol withdrawal

Last drink	Features
Within 6–12 h	Tremor, sweating, anorexia, nausea, insomnia, anxiety ('morning shakes')
	Mild confusional state with agitation
Within 48 h	'Rum fits' – one to six tonic-clonic fits, without focal features, occurring within a 6 h period
After 72 h	Delirium tremens (DT) with tremor, severe confusional state, agitation, visual and auditory hallucinations and paranoid ideation
	Tachycardia, sweating and fever

MANAGEMENT OF ALCOHOL WITHDRAWAL

Exclude hypoglycaemia. If treating hypoglycaemia with IV glucose, it is essential to also give high dose parenteral B vitamins to minimise the risk of precipitating Wernicke's encephalopathy. Rehydration is often required, as is treatment of any intercurrent illness. Vitamin supplements are also required. Thiamine is best given parenterally for at least 72 h (followed by oral thiamine 250 mg/day and vitamin B strong compound, 2 tablets daily). If however, Wernicke's encephalopathy is present, parenteral thiamine should be continued for one week.

The presence of delirium tremens or severe agitation is managed according to local policy and will probably include the use of chlorpromazine (contraindicated in the presence of liver disease), chlordiazepoxide or another benzodiazepine. Any patient who needs intravenous sedation must be managed on a high dependency unit.

ELECTROLYTE DISTURBANCES

Physiology

A 70-kg man has a: total fluid volume of 42 litres (60% body weight). This comprises: Intracellular fluid = 28 litres (67% body fluid), extracellular fluid = 14 litres (33% body fluid) of which the intravascular component = 3 litres plasma (5 litres of blood).

The distribution between intra- and extravascular compartments is determined by osmotic equilibrium, and the 'oncotic pressure' exerted by non-diffusible proteins.

Over 24 h the fluid balance is roughly:

Input (l ml water)	Output (1 ml water)
Drink; 1500	Urine 1500
Food: 800	Insensible loss: 800
Metabolism of food: 200	Stool: 200
Total: **2500**	Total: **2500**

Osmolarity is the number of osmoles per litre of solution.
Osmolality is the number of osmoles per kg of solvent (normally 280–300).

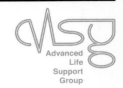

A mole is the molecular weight expressed in grams.

To estimate plasma osmolality calculate $2[Na^+ + K^+] + Urea + glucose$. If the measured osmolality is greater than this (i.e. an osmolar gap of >10 mmol/l), consider diabetes mellitus, high blood ethanol, methanol or ethylene glycol.

SODIUM

Sodium control

Renin is produced by the juxtaglomerular apparatus in response to decreased renal blood flow and catalyses the formation of angiotensin 1 from angiotensinogen. This is then converted by angiotensin-converting enzyme to angiotensin 11. The latter has several important actions including efferent renal arteriolar constriction (so increasing perfusion pressure); peripheral vasoconstriction and stimulation of the adrenal cortex to produce aldosterone. This activates the sodium pump in the distal renal tubule, leading to reabsorption of sodium, in exchange for potassium and hydrogen ions (excreted in urine).

A *high glomerular filtration rate* results in high sodium loss, where as *high renal tubular blood flow* and haemodilution decrease sodium reabsorption in the proximal tubule.

Water control

Water is controlled mainly by sodium concentration. An increased plasma osmolality causes thirst and the release of antidiuretic hormone (ADH) from the posterior pituitary. This, in turn, increases the passive water reabsorption from the renal collecting duct, by opening water channels to allow water to flow from the hypotonic luminal fluid into the hypertonic renal interstitium.

Abnormalities

Hyponatraemia

The assessment of a patient with hyponotraemia is based on the history and the fluid balance status, i.e. whether there is evidence of:

- dehydration
- normal volume
- peripheral oedema.

Do not base treatment on the plasma sodium concentration alone.

There may be symptoms and signs of water excess such as confusion, fits, hypertension, cardiac failure, oedema, anorexia, nausea and, muscle weakness.

Diagnosis

The key decision is whether the patient is either dehydrated or overloaded with fluid. History, clinical examination and serum urine analyses are your guides.

Causes of hyponatraemia

- Diuretics, especially thiazides
- Water excess, either orally, or IV as excess 5% dextrose
- Others – see Fig. 19.1.

If the patient is not dehydrated, renal function good, and if Na >125 mmol/l, treatment rarely needed. If Na <125 mmol/l, restrict water to 0.5–1 l/day if tolerated. Consider frusemide (furosemide) 40–80 mg/24 h IV slowly/PO for a few days only. SIADH (below) is occasionally treated by producing nephrogenic diabetes insipidus with demeclocycline.

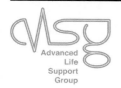

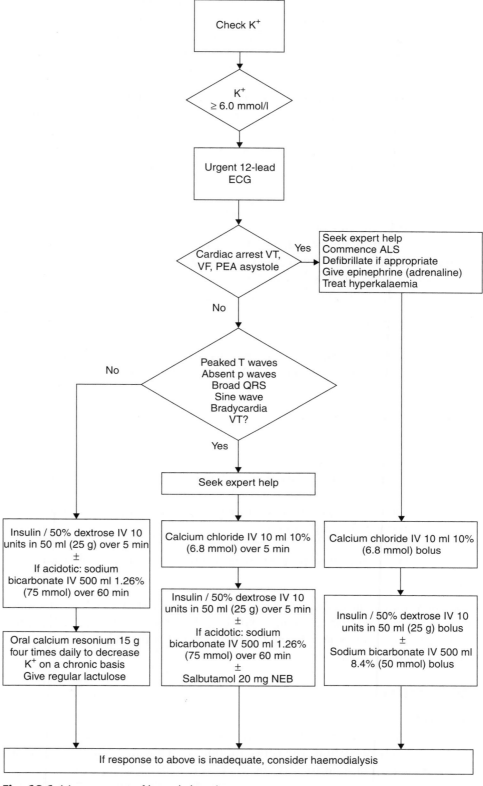

Fig. 19.1 Management of hyperkalaemia.

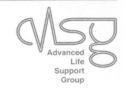

If the patient is dehydrated and kidney function good, 0.9% saline can be given. In emergency (seizures, coma) consider rapid IVI infusion of 0.9% saline or hypertonic saline (e.g. 1.8% saline) at 70 mmol Na^+/h. Aim for a gradual increase in plasma sodium by 1 mmol/h to about 125 mmol/l. Watch out for heart failure, and central pontine myelinolysis. Seek expert help.

Syndrome of inappropriate ADH secretion (SIADH)

This is an important cause of hyponatraemia, but is over-diagnosed. The diagnosis is made by finding a concentrated urine sodium (>20 mmol/l) in the presence of hyponatraemia (<125 mmol/l) and an inappropriately low plasma osmolality (<260 mmol/kg), with no evidence of hypovolaemia, oedema or diuretics.

Causes
- Malignancy (lung small-cell, pancreas, prostate, lymphoma).
- CNS disorders (meningoencephalitis, abscess, stroke, subarachnoid, subdural haemorrhage, head injury, Guillain–Barré, vasculitis (e.g. SLE).
- Chest disease (TB, pneumonia, abscess, aspergillosis)
- Metabolic disease (porphyria, trauma)
- Drugs (opiates, chlorpropramide, psychotropics, cytotoxics).

Hypernatraemia

Symptoms and signs
Thirst, confusion, coma and fits – with signs of dehydration: dry skin, reduced skin turgor, postural hypotension and oliguria if water deficient.

Laboratory features
Elevated PCV, albumin and urate.

Causes
- Usually due to water loss in excess of sodium loss.
- Fluid loss without water replacement (e.g. diarrhoea, vomiting, burns).
- Incorrect IV fluid replacement
- Diabetes insipidus. Suspect if large urine volume. This may follow head injury, or CNS surgery, especially pituitary
- Osmotic diuresis
- Primary aldosteronism: suspect if hypertension, hypokalaemia and alkalosis.

Management
Give water orally if possible. Otherwise, dextrose 5% IV slowly (4 l/24 h), guided by urine output and plasma sodium. Some authorities recommend giving 0.9% saline, since this causes less marked fluid shifts and is hypotonic in a hypernatraemic patient.

POTASSIUM

Physiology

Most potassium is intracellular, and thus serum potassium levels are a poor reflection of total body potassium. The concentrations of potassium and hydrogen ions in extracellular fluid tend to vary together. This is because these ions compete with each other as they are exchanged with sodium across most cell membranes (sodium is pumped out of the cell) and in the distal tubule of the kidney (sodium is reabsorbed from the urine). Electrical neutrality has to be maintained thus, if the hydrogen ion concentration is high, fewer potassium ions will be excreted into the urine. Similarly K^+ will compete with H^+ for exchange across cell membranes and extracellular K^+ will accumulate.

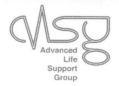

ABNORMALITIES

Hypokalaemia

If <2.5 mmol/l needs urgent treatment. Note that hypokalaemia exacerbates digoxin toxicity.

Symptoms and signs
Muscle weakness, hypotonia, cardiac arrhythmias, cramps and tetany.

ECG
Small or inverted T waves, prominent U waves, prolonged P-R interval, depressed ST segment.

Causes
- Diuretics
- Vomiting
- Pyloric stenosis
- Alkalosis
- Villous adenoma of the rectum
- Intestinal fistulae
- Cushing's syndrome/steroids/ACTH
- Conn's syndrome
- Purgative and liquorice use
- Renal tubular failure.

If the patient is using diuretics, a raised bicarbonate is the best indication that the hypokalaemia is likely to have been long-standing. The magnesium level may also be low, and hypokalaemia is often difficult to correct until magnesium levels are restored to normal. In hypokalaemic periodic paralysis, intermittent weakness lasting up to 72 h appears to be caused by potassium shifting from the extracellular to the intracellular fluid. Suspect Conn's syndrome if hypertensive, hypokalaemic alkalosis in someone not taking diuretics.

Treatment
mild: (>2.5 mmol/l, no symptoms) give oral potassium supplement (at least 80 mmol/24 h, e.g. Sando-K® 2 tablets bd). If the patient is taking a thiazide diuretic, hypokalaemia >3.0 mmol/l rarely needs treating.
severe: (<2.5 mmol/l, dangerous symptoms) give IV potassium cautiously, not more than 20 mmol/h, not more than 40 mmol/l. Do not give potassium if the patient is oliguric.

> **Key point**
>
> Never give potassium as a fast 'stat' bolus dose

Hyperkalaemia

A plasma potassium >6.5 mmol/l needs urgent treatment, but first ensure that this is not an artefact (e.g. due to haemolysis during or after venesection).

Symptoms and signs
Muscle weakness/paralysis and cardiac arrhythmias, sudden death.

ECG
Tall tented T waves, small flat P waves, wide QRS complex becoming sinusoidal, VF.

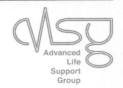

Causes
- Oliguric renal failure
- Potassium sparing diuretics
- Angiotensin converting enzyme inhibitors (especially if the patient has type IV renal tubular acidosis)
- Rhabdomyolysis
- Metabolic acidosis
- Excess K^+ therapy
- Artefact. Haemolysis of blood sample; delay in analysis – potassium leaks out of RBCs; thrombocythaemia – platelets leak potassium as sample clots in tube
- Addison's disease (see page XXX)
- Massive blood transfusion

Treatment
Ensure correct fluid balance. Treat or remove the underlying cause. Then consider:
- Check K^+ and other electrolytes (1–4 hourly) and monitor ECG
- $K^+ > 6.0$ – Give 100 ml 50% glucose solution with 10 units regular (rapid-acting) insulin IVI.
- $K^+ > 6.5$ – Treat as for (a), but infuse calcium gluconate, 10 ml 10% solution over 10–15 min (stabilizes cardiac cell membranes) until ECG changes revert to normal.
- $K^+ > 7.0$ – as for (a) and (b) above, and infuse 50–100 ml 8.5% sodium bicarbonate over 30 min (unless patient in respiratory failure). Repeat glucose and insulin 2–4 hourly prn
- Rectal calcium resonium 30 mg once daily to decrease K^+ on a chronic basis.

If response to above is inadequate, consider nebulised salbutamol, furosemide and haemodialysis.

CALCIUM

Physiology
About 40% of plasma calcium is bound to albumin. Usually it is the total plasma calcium which is measured. The unbound, ionised portion is important. Therefore, *adjust calcium level for albumin as follows*: Add 0.1 mmol/l to calcium concentration for every 4 g/l that albumin is below 40 g/l, but subtract 0.1 mmol from calcium contraction for every 4 g/l that is raised above 40 g/l albumin. However, many factors affect binding (e.g. other proteins in myeloma, cirrhosis, individual variation) so be cautious in your interpretation. If in doubt over a high Ca^{2+}, take a blood sample with the limb uncuffed and the patient fasted.

Calcium metabolism is controlled by:
- Parathyroid hormone (PTH): PTH secretion is controlled by ionised plasma calcium levels. A rise in PTH causes a rise in plasma calcium and a decrease in plasma phosphate: This is due to an increased calcium and phosphate: reabsorption from bone; and increased calcium but reduced phosphate reabsorption from the kidney. PTH secretion enhances active vitamin D formation.
- Vitamin D: Calciferol (vitamin D_3) and ergocalciferol (vitamin D_2) are biologically identical in their actions. Serum vitamin D is converted in the liver to 25-hydroxy Vitamin D (25-(OH)D). In the kidney a second hydroxyl group is added to form the biologically active 1.25-dihydroxy vitamin D (1.25-(OH)2-D), also called calcitriol, or the much less active 24.25-(OH)2-D. Calcitriol production is stimulated by reduced calcium reduced phosphate and PTH. Its

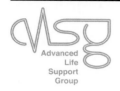

actions include increased absorption of calcium and phosphate from the gut; increased reabsorption of calcium and phosphate by the kidney; enhanced bone turnover; and inhibition of PTH release. Disordered regulation of 1.25-(OH)2-D underlies familial normocalcaemic hypercalciuria which is a major cause of calcium oxalate renal stone formation.

- Calcitonin: From thyroid C cells, causes a decrease in plasma calcium and phosphate, but its physiological role is unclear. It is a marker for medullary carcinoma of the thyroid.
- Thyroxine: (=Levothyroxine) may increase plasma calcium, although this is rare.
- Hypomagnesaemia: Prevents PTH release, and may cause hypocalcaemia.

> **Key point**
>
> A low Mg is associated with either a low calcium, or a low potassium or both

Abnormalites
Hypocalcaemia
Apparent hypocalcaemia may be an artefact of hypoalbuminaemia (above).

Symptoms and signs
Tetany, depression, perioral paraesthesiae, carpo-pedal spasm (wrist flexion and fingers drawn together), especially if brachial artery occluded with blood pressure cuff (Trousseau's sign), neuromuscular excitability, e.g. tapping over parotid (facial nerve) causes facial muscles to twitch (Chvostek's sign). Cataract formation, if chronically reduced calcium.

ECG
Prolongation of Q-T interval.

Causes
It may be a consequence of thyroid or parathyroid surgery. If the phosphate level is raised, consider either chronic renal failure, hypoparathyroidism or pseudohypoparathyroidism. If the phosphate level is either normal or reduced suspect either osteomalacia (high alkaline phosphatase), overhydration or pancreatitis.

Treatment
- Mild symptoms, give calcium 5 mmol/6 h PO. Do daily plasma calcium levels. In chronic renal failure, if necessary, add alfacalcidol; start at 0.5—1 mg/24 h PO.
- Severe symptoms, give 10 ml (2.32 mmol) calcium gluconate 10% IVI over 30 min (bolus injections are only needed very rarely). Repeat as necessary.

Hypercalcaemia
Symptoms and signs
Abdominal pain, vomiting, constipation, polyuria, polydipsia, depression, anorexia, weight loss, tiredness, weakness, hypertension, confusion, pyrexia, renal stones, renal failure, corneal calcification, cardiac arrest.

ECG
Q-T interval reduced.

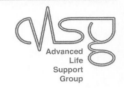

Causes and diagnosis
Bloods: Measure U&Es, magnesium, creatinine, calcium phosphate, ALK PHOS. Most commonly malignancy (myeloma, bone metastases, PTHrP increased and 10 hyperparathyroidism). Pointers to malignancy are: low plasma albumin, low-ish chloride, hypokalaemia, alkalosis, raised phosphate and raised alkaline phosphatase. Other investigations (e.g. isotope bone scan, CXR, FBC) may also be of diagnostic value.

Treatment
Treat the underlying cause. Patients who have a calcium >3.5 mmol/l, or with hypotension, severe abdominal pain, vomiting, pyrexia, confusion, aim to reduce calcium as follows:
- Fluids: Rehydrate with IVI 0.9% saline, e.g. 4–6 litres in 24 h as needed. Correct hypokalaemia and hypomagnesaemia (mild metabolic acidosis does not need treatment). This will reduce symptoms, and increase renal calcium loss. Monitor U&E during treatment.
- Diuretics: Frusemide 40 mg/12 h IV, once rehydrated. Avoid thiazides.
- Bisphosphonates: A single dose of pamidronate (30 mg IVI over 4 h in 0.9% saline) will lower calcium over 2–3 days. Maximum effect is at 1 week. Inhibit osteoclast activity, and so bone reabsorption.
- Steroids: Occasionally used, e.g. in sarcoidosis.
- Salmon calcitonin: Now rarely used. More side effects than bisphosphonates, but quicker onset. Again inhibits osteoclasts.
- Other: Chemotherapy may reduce calcium in malignant disease, e.g. myeloma.

Magnesium
Physiology
Magnesium is distributed 65% in bone and 35% in cells. Its level tends to follow those of Ca^{2+} and K^+. Magnesium excess is usually caused by renal failure, but rarely requires treatment in its own right.

Hypomagnesemia
Symptoms and signs
Paresthesiae, fits, tetany, arrhythmias. Digitalis toxicity may be exacerbated.

Causes
Severe diarrhoea, ketoacidosis, alcohol, total parenteral nutrition (monitor weekly), accompanying hypocalcaemia, accompanying hypokalaemia (especially with diuretics).

Treatment
If needed, give magnesium salts either orally or IV (dose example: 10 mmol $MgSO_4$ IVI over 3 min–2 h, depending on severity; monitor Mg^{2+}).

Hypermagnesaemia
Symptoms and signs
Neuromuscular depression, followed sequentially by hypotension, CNS depression and finally coma.

Causes
- Acute on chronic renal failure
- Metabolic acidosis

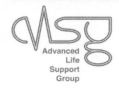

- Magnesium containing medications
- Adreno-cortisol insufficiency

Treatment

With cardiac conduction defects urgent treatment is needed, intravenous calcium may be given cautiously with ECG monitoring. Forced diuresis can also be used, although dialysis is the treatment of choice especially in renal failure.

SUMMARY

- Acute confusion is a common medical condition.
- An infection or an adverse effect of drugs is the usual cause.
- Most causes of confusion are not immediately life-threatening.

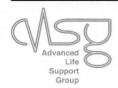
Advanced
Life
Support
Group

PART IV
Organ Failure

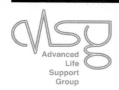

CHAPTER 20

Organ failure

OBJECTIVES

After reading this chapter you will be able to:
- understand the concept of organ failure and its impact on other body systems
- describe the structured approach to management.

INTRODUCTION

Organ failure is a common medical problem. It may be complete or partial; acute or chronic and single organ or multiple organs. However, it is not a diagnosis but the final stages of an underlying condition.

Patients with organ failures often require intensive medical and nursing management: the presence of organ failure thus has resource implications as well as prognostic implications.

This chapter will consider the management of individual failing organs and the diagnosis and management of some of the underlying conditions.

ACUTE ORGAN FAILURE

Acute organ failures are a medical emergency. The structured approach in Chapter 3 will ensure failing organs are detected and supported.

Primary assessment and resuscitation
- Support life-threatening organ dysfunction
- Limit further organ damage

Secondary assessment and emergency treatment
- Detect and support failing organ systems
- Diagnose underlying disease process

Definitive care
- Treat underlying disease processes
- Place patient in a critical care environment for ongoing organ support

Classification of the level of critical care will ensure that patients with organ dysfunction are managed in the correct environment.

Acute Medical Emergencies; The Practical Approach, 2nd edition.
Edited by Terence Wardle, Peter Driscoll, and Sue Wieteska.
© 2010 Blackwell Publishing Ltd.

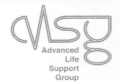

Level of critical care	Organ systems failing	Environment
Level 1	None (at risk)	Ward (with close observation)
Level 2	One (excluding respiratory failure requiring invasive ventilation)	High dependency unit
Level 3	More than one (or respiratory failure requiring invasive ventilation)	Intensive care unit

The severity of acute multiple organ dysfunction may be scored using the Sequential Organ Failure Assessment (SOFA). This is mainly a tool for audit and research purposes but it illustrates that organ failure is not an all-or-nothing process, and despite its simplicity the score has prognostic implications (Table 20.1).

Table 20.1 SOFA score

Respiratory system	
PaO_2/FiO_2	SOFA score
>400	0
<400	1
<300	2
<200	3
<100	4

Nervous system	
Glasgow Coma Score	SOFA score
15	0
13–14	1
10–12	2
6–9	3
<6	4

Cardiovascular system	
MAP/vasopressors	SOFA score
No hypotension	0
MAP <70 mm Hg	1
Dop ≤5, or dob, any dose*	2
Dop >5, or adr ≤0.1 or noradr ≤0.1	3
Dop >15, or adr >0.1 or noradr >0.1	4

Dop, dopamine; dob, dobutamine; adr, adrenaline; noradr, noradrenaline.
*Doses of inotropes in µg/kg/min for at least 1 h

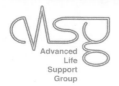

Liver	
Bilirubin (mg/dl)	SOFA score
<1.2	0
1.2–1.9	1
2.0–5.9	2
6.0–11.9	3
≥12.0	4

Coagulation	
Platelets	SOFA score
>150	0
≤150	1
≤100	2
≤50	3
≤20	4

Renal	
Creatinine (mg/dl) or urine output (u.o.)	SOFA score
<1.2	0
1.2–1.9	1
2.0–3.4	2
3.5–4.9 (or u.o. <500 ml/day)	3
>5.0 (or u.o. <200 ml/day)	4

Any patient with acute respiratory failure should be admitted to either a respiratory care unit or an other level 2–3 facility. Hypoxaemia is the most life-threatening facet of respiratory failure. The goal is to ensure adequate oxygen delivery to tissues, which is generally achieved with a PaO_2 above 8.0 kPa or SpO_2 of at least 92%. Apart from oxygen therapy, various types of respiratory support are used to treat respiratory failure. As well as treating the underlying cause (e.g. antibiotics for pneumonia), the ventilation can be supported in the following ways:

- through an invasive airway, e.g. by intubating the patient
- non-invasive respiratory support via a tight-fitting mask.

CHRONIC ORGAN FAILURE

Chronically dysfunctional organ systems may deteriorate acutely ('acute on chronic failure'). Chronic single organ failure typically produces abnormalities

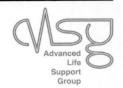

in multiple other physiological systems which may affect the way a patient copes with a new acute illness. Consider, e.g., the cardiovascular, nutritional and immunological implications of chronic renal failure.

The management of chronic organ failure is beyond the scope of this manual. The principles are given below.

Principles of management of chronic organ failure

- Support failing organ systems.
- Limit further deterioration in organ function.
- Prevent and aggressively treat intercurrent illness.
- Manage multi system consequences of chronic organ failure.

RESPIRATORY FAILURE

Respiratory failure may be defined as an inability of the lungs to maintain normal gaseous composition of the blood when breathing air and is usually classified as:

Type 1 respiratory failure is hypoxaemia without hypercapnia. This is usually due to ventilation/perfusion mismatch and/or shunt.

Type 2 respiratory failure is hypoxaemia and hypercapnia. This is due to reduced alveolar ventilation (reduced total ventilation and/or increased dead space ventilation)

Hypoxaemic respiratory failure is characterised by a low PaO_2 leading to an elevated alveolar-arterial gradient and a low $PaCO_2$ reflecting adequate ventilation but inadequate gas exchange. Hypoxaemia is most commonly due to mismatch of ventilation and perfusion or intrapulmonary right to left shunt. Hypercapnia (or, at least, the reason why $PaCO_2$ rises) is often misunderstood. CO_2 retention occurs with uncontrolled oxygen therapy in patients with chronic hypoxaemia (e.g. some patients with chronic obstructive pulmonary disease). Ventilatory capacity is the amount of spontaneous ventilation that can be maintained without the development of respiratory muscle fatigue. Normally, ventilatory capacity matches demand. Hypercapnic respiratory failure results from either a reduction in ventilatory capacity or an increase in ventilatory demand that cannot be met by the patient's own ventilatory capacity.

These definitions, however, do not recognise early compensated respiratory failure where blood gases may be normal at rest due to compensatory mechanisms, predominantly hyperventilation. Tissue hypoxaemia at rest and on exercise arises as the result of failure of multi-system compensatory mechanisms (see box)

Compensatory mechanisms in respiratory failure	
Respiratory	Tachypnoea increases alveolar PO_2
Cardiovascular	Tachycardia and increased cardiac output increase oxygen delivery to tissues
Haematological	Polycythaemia increases blood oxygen carrying capacity

There is inevitably a decrease in exercise ability. Thus, the diagnosis of respiratory failure is largely a clinical one based on symptoms and signs, supported by pulse oximetry and/or blood gas estimation.

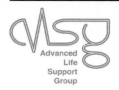

Acute respiratory failure

This is most often seen in patients with one of the following:

- a severe asthma attack
- tension pneumothorax
- pulmonary embolus
- severe pneumonia (see Chapter 8).

The management, irrespective of the cause (see the box below) is to ensure a patent airway and supply high concentrations of inspired oxygen via an appropriate mask, assisting ventilation when necessary. The decision to assist ventilation is a **clinical** one, aided by investigations such as blood gas estimation. Assisted ventilation is discussed with acute on chronic respiratory failure below.

Causes of acute respiratory failure

Pulmonary	Asthma, pneumonia, pulmonary embolus
Cardiac	Dysrhythmia, failure, arrest
Neurological	Unconsciousness, Status epilepticus, Guillain–Barré syndrome
Neuromuscular	Myasthenia gravis
Trauma	Head, neck, chest, spinal cord

Chronic respiratory failure

Acute exacerbations of chronic pulmonary disease are amongst the most common reasons for acute medical admission. The common underlying causes, along with an estimation of their frequency, are listed below.

Causes of chronic respiratory failure

Parenchymal disease	Chronic bronchitis	Daily
	Emphysema	Daily
	Pulmonary fibrosis	Weekly
	Bronchiectasis	Weekly
	Pulmonary vascular disease	Weekly
Obstructive sleep apnoea		Weekly
Chest wall problems	Kyphoscoliosis	Weekly
	Extreme obesity	Weekly
Neuromuscular disorders	Motor neurone disease	Annually
	Cervical cord lesion	Annually

The commonest causes are now considered in more detail.

Chronic obstructive pulmonary disease

This is a collective term referring to patients who have chronic bronchitis and/or emphysema. The major cause of both conditions is cigarette smoking.

Pathophysiology

In **chronic bronchitis**, there is an initial increase in mucous production and reduction of ciliary motility reducing sputum clearance. This is followed by airway oedema, inflammation, bronchoconstriction and subepithelial airway

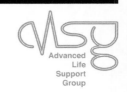

fibrosis. This has the greatest impact on small airways, causing fixed obstruction and leading to the well-known clinical consequences (see box below).

Pathophysiology	Clinical consequences
Increased mucus production, decreased mucus clearance	Cough and increased sputum volumes Susceptibility to infection
Airway inflammation and bronchocon-striction	Variability of symptoms, particularly wheeze
Airway narrowing	Ventilation perfusion mismatching with hypoxaemia Breathlessness, wheeze and decreased exercise ability Prolonged expiration, chest hyperinflation
Chronic hypoxaemia	Respiratory, cardiovascular and haematological compensatory changes (see box above) Hypoxaemia, pulmonary vasoconstriction and pulmonary hypertension leading to right heart failure

In **emphysema**, the alveolar walls are destroyed and, consequently, the alveolar spaces coalesce. This causes two main structural problems:
- Loss of elastic recoil, increasing lung size and compliance
- Loss of support for small airways, allowing dynamic airways collapse during expiration.

The net effect is to cause gross hyperinflation and **air trapping**, where exhalation cannot fully occur. Bronchodilators have limited clinical effect, because the pathology is at alveolar, rather than bronchiolar, level.

Chronic bronchitis and emphysema usually coexist in smoking related lung disease. The respiratory failure produced is typically type 1 (hypoxaemic), because of ventilation-perfusion mismatch. Chronic severe disease may lead to decreased alveolar ventilation and development of type 2 (hypercapnic/hypoxaemic) respiratory failure, as the patient cannot continue to meet the high work of breathing associated with the airway obstruction and 'wasted' dead space ventilation.

Pulmonary fibrosis

Diseases associated with diffuse pulmonary fibrosis are shown in the box.

Diseases associated with diffuse pulmonary fibrosis

Cryptogenic fibrosing alveolitis
Occupation, e.g. asbestosis/pneumoconiosis
Extrinsic allergic alveolitis (usually upper lobe and late in the disease)
Drug, e.g. busulphan, bleomycin, paraquat
Rheumatoid disease
Systemic sclerosis
Systemic lupus erythematosus
Sarcoid

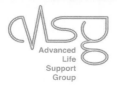

Hypoxaemia is often severe and present at rest, whilst the $PaCO_2$ is generally normal or low. The latter is attributed to hyperventilation increasing the elimination of carbon dioxide. Lung compliance is markedly reduced and, although there may be thickening of the alveolar wall reducing gas diffusion, the main cause of the hypoxaemia is ventilation-perfusion mismatch.

Bronchiectasis

This condition is characterised by chronic dilatation of at least some of the bronchi. The bronchial wall is irreversibly damaged as a consequence of early inflammation or infection of either the bronchus or adjacent lung parenchyma. The normal transport of mucus is impaired and chronic local suppuration ensues.

A variety of conditions are associated with bronchiectasis and they are shown in the box.

Conditions associated with bronchiectasis

Infection:	Measles pneumonia
	Whooping cough
	Tuberculosis
	Aspergillosis
Immune related:	Immunoglobulin deficiency
	Complement deficiency
Inhalation:	Gastric aspiration
	Ammonia inhalation
	Foreign body inhalation
Others:	$\alpha1$ antitrypsin deficiency
	Kartagener's syndrome
	Immotile cilia

The clinical hallmark of bronchiectasis is chronic copious sputum production, typically infected. The mainstay of chronic treatment is assisted sputum clearance with physiotherapy and postural drainage. Acute exacerbations require management of the respiratory failure as well as assisted sputum clearance and careful choice of antibiotics.

Management of acute exacerbations of chronic respiratory failure

The structured approach to medical emergencies (Chapter 3) is followed. In the **Primary Assessment and Resuscitation** phase, the priority is to:
- treat hypoxaemia with controlled oxygen therapy, with or without assisted ventilation (see below)
- assess the severity of the respiratory failure
- identify and treat the reason for the acute exacerbation
- monitor the response to treatment.

Controlled oxygen therapy

Hypoxaemia kills and must be treated. High concentrations of inspired oxygen should be given initially and then arterial oxygenation should be monitored with pulse oximetry and blood gas estimation. Titrate oxygen therapy to achieve an SpO_2 of 90–92% (PaO_2 of 8 kPa).

The major cause of hypoxaemia in a patient with COPD is impaired ventilation/perfusion matching. Patients will compensate by increasing the rate of

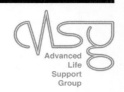

ventilation, but this increases the work of breathing (the pink puffer; type 1 respiratory failure).

In contrast, patients with severe COPD and hypercapnia usually have lower tidal volumes, due to a short inspiratory time and an increased respiratory rate ('blue bloater', type 2 respiratory failure). There is little evidence to support the theory that supplemental oxygen in COPD patients 'removes the hypoxaemic drive', causing alveolar hypoventilation and hypercapnia. The major effect is to increase dead space ventilation, probably secondary to worsening ventilation/perfusion mismatch due to a loss of hypoxaemic pulmonary vasoconstriction. Therefore, oxygen therapy should be given to ensure a saturation of 90–92% to reduce hypoxaemia and prevent further hypercapnia. However, in the acute situation, especially when the diagnosis remains in doubt, high concentrations of inspired oxygen should be given and adjusted according to arterial blood gas results. In patients who respond appropriately, it is only necessary to increase the flow to ensure a PaO_2 of 8 kPa. If life-threatening hypoxaemia persists, without increasing hypercapnia to an unacceptable level, the patient will require some form of assisted ventilation.

Key point

The presence of hypercarbia is not a reason to accept hypoxaemia

---

Hypercarbia is often present during acute exacerbations of chronic respiratory disease. The use of oxygen will usually cause a slight rise in $PaCO_2$, due to a small increase in alveolar dead space. This is usually well tolerated by the patient. On rare occasions, the rise in CO_2 is severe enough to cause obtundation and, ultimately, hypoventilation. These patients are best monitored clinically in a high dependency environment aided by blood gas estimation.

The reason for clinical deterioration is usually bronchospasm further impairing ventilation. Nebulised β_2 agonists will reduce this burden as will therapy with steroids and antibiotics. These will also help to reduce the luminal inflammatory response and infected secretions. Aminophylline is often beneficial in patients who have an acute exacerbation of COPD. This bronchodilator has other benefits, including inotropic stimulation, increased cardiac output and improved renal perfusion. This is of particular benefit in patients who have coexistent ventricular failure.

If the patient does not respond appropriately to treatment, reassessment is required to identify any of the possible causes listed in the next box.

Causes of treatment failure in respiratory failure

Untreated bacterial infection
Sputum retention
Coexistent pneumothorax
Inadequate bronchodilator therapy
Coexistent pulmonary oedema
Underlying dysrhythmia
Inappropriate sedation
Wrong diagnosis

If there is not a rapid improvement in the patient's condition after titrating oxygen therapy (see above) and treating the underlying condition, consider

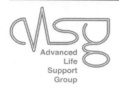

ventilation. Doxapram as a respiratory stimulant rarely leads to a sustained improvement and is not often used as assisted ventilation is more readily available. Hence, early liaison with an anaesthetist/intensivist is needed.

Assisted ventilation

Advances in technology and application of assisted ventilation have improved outcome in patients with acute-on-chronic respiratory failure. It may be 'non-invasive', delivered by face mask, or 'invasive', delivered via an endotracheal tube or tracheostomy. Non-invasive ventilation has the advantage of maintaining an awake, conversant patient and has a lower risk of hospital acquired pulmonary infection.

Unfortunately, not all suitable patients can tolerate the close fitting masks for long periods. Both types require specialist knowledge to deliver.

Non-invasive ventilation is increasingly available in emergency departments, respiratory wards and medical high dependency areas using simple portable equipment.

The indications and relative contraindictions are shown in the following boxes.

Indications for non-invasive ventilation (NIV)

Respiratory acidosis pH <7.35, PaCO$_2$ >6.5 kPa despite controlled oxygen therapy

Moderate to severe breathlessness with accessory muscle use and paradoxical abdominal motion

Respiratory rate >25/min

Relative contraindications to non-invasive ventilation

Respiratory acidosis pH <7.25

Confused

Somnolence, agitation, lack of cooperation

High risk of gastric aspiration

Glasgow Coma Score <8

Copious or viscous sputum

Facial or pharyngeal trauma, deformity or recent surgery

Recent gastro-oesophageal surgery

Untreated pneumothorax

Non-invasive ventilation in the form of BiPAP (bilevel positive airway pressure) provides the possibility of giving two levels of respiratory support:

- EPAP (expiratory positive airway pressure, similar to CPAP) maintains the airways in an open state, improves alveolar gas exchange, improves oxygenation and increases the functional residual capacity.
- IPAP (inspiratory positive airway pressure) supports the inspiratory effort, reducing the effort of breathing, improves tidal volume and improves CO$_2$ removal.

Intubation and ventilation may be indicated when hypoxaemia and respiratory acidosis persist despite NIV, or when contraindications for NIV exist. Modern ventilatory techniques and appropriate use of tracheostomy have improved outcome.

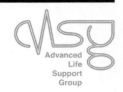

The need for invasive ventilation in acute on chronic respiratory failure is a poor prognostic indicator- only a minority of patients survive 12 months. The prognosis improves if there is a treatable cause for the exacerbation.

In the **Secondary Assessment and Emergency Management** phase the priority is to identify and treat the cause of the exacerbation. This is often not clear-cut and typically a combination of therapy is indicated (see box below).

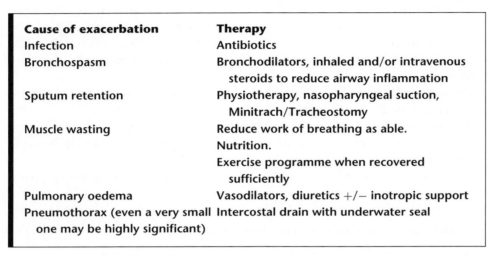

Cause of exacerbation	Therapy
Infection	Antibiotics
Bronchospasm	Bronchodilators, inhaled and/or intravenous steroids to reduce airway inflammation
Sputum retention	Physiotherapy, nasopharyngeal suction, Minitrach/Tracheostomy
Muscle wasting	Reduce work of breathing as able. Nutrition. Exercise programme when recovered sufficiently
Pulmonary oedema	Vasodilators, diuretics +/− inotropic support
Pneumothorax (even a very small one may be highly significant)	Intercostal drain with underwater seal

Summary

Acute on chronic respiratory failure is a common medical emergency. All patients should initially receive high concentrations of inspired oxygen and this should be titrated according to pulse oximetry and the results of blood gas analysis. Early intervention is required by either a respiratory physician or intensivist if the patient fails to respond to treatment with controlled oxygen therapy, bronchodilators, steroids and antibiotics.

Time Out 20.1

A 72-year-old lady, who has COPD presents with acute breathlessness. She has a respiratory rate of 28/min, a hyperexpanded chest with scattered wheezes and a prolonged expiratory phase. Her SpO_2 is 72% on 28% oxygen. What is your immediate management?

CARDIOVASCULAR FAILURE

Introduction

Cardiovascular failure may be defined as failure of the circulation to transport sufficient oxygenated blood to the tissues. In its most acute and severe form, this is **shock**, and is discussed in detail in Chapter 9.

In this section, another manifestation of cardiovascular dysfunction will be considered: cardiac failure leading to pulmonary oedema and/or right ventricular failure.

Acute pulmonary oedema

Pulmonary oedema occurs when there is excessive extravascular lung water, which interferes with pulmonary gas exchange. The factors influencing the accumulation of lung water are defined.

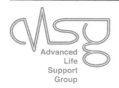

Factors increasing extravascular lung water	Disease process
Increased pulmonary capillary hydrostatic pressure	Cardiac failure Fluid overload (renal failure, iatrogenic) Neurogenic pulmonary oedema
Increased pulmonary capillary permeability	Sepsis Systemic inflammatory response syndrome Acute respiratory distress syndrome Neurogenic pulmonary oedema
Decreased plasma oncotic pressure	Hypoproteinaemia (rarely an isolated cause)
Negative pressure in alveoli	Airway obstruction with active inspiration ('Negative pressure pulmonary oedema')

The most common cause of pulmonary oedema is cardiac failure, which is now considered in detail.

Cardiogenic pulmonary oedema
Pathophysiology

In **acute cardiogenic pulmonary oedema**, there is an increase in left atrial pressure and consequent increase in pulmonary venous and pulmonary capillary pressure. The rise in left atrial pressure may be due to obstruction to the outflow from the left atrium (e.g. mitral stenosis) or a rise in left ventricular end diastolic pressure (e.g. left ventricular failure).

The distension of pulmonary vessels is sufficient to cause symptomatic breathlessness through vascular neural receptors. However, as the process progresses, fluid accumulates in the pulmonary interstitial spaces as lymphatic drainage is overwhelmed. Finally, fluid may accumulate in the alveolar space. By this stage the patient is fighting for breath and terrified, leading to sympathetic activation increasing left ventricular afterload and heart rate. This usually causes a further decrease in cardiac performance – hence the often explosive onset of pulmonary oedema.

As a consequence of this process, the following changes may occur.

- The lung becomes firm and less compliant producing **increased work of breathing.**
- Reflex **hyperventilation** is due to stimulation of vagal sensory 'J receptors' because of distortion of the lung tissue by oedema.
- Small airways become either narrowed by interstitial oedema or filled with oedema. When they open during inspiration they do so with a click which is represented clinically as **fine crackles**.
- During expiration, early airway closure occurs, producing **wheezing**.
- Reduced ventilation in less compliant areas leads to local **hypoxaemia** and reflex arteriolar constriction. This reduces perfusion and diverts blood to less affected areas. This improves the V/Q mismatch, but raises pulmonary artery pressures and increases right ventricular afterload.

In **acute on chronic heart failure**, there may be several other pathophysiological and compensatory mechanisms already active which influence the progression of the heart failure:

- Chronically reduced cardiac output leading to:

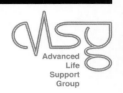

- renal retention of sodium (renin–angiotensin–aldosterone mechanism) and water (ADH), increasing ventricular preload
- sympathetic nervous system induced vasoconstriction, increasing ventricular afterload
- sympathetic nervous system mediated increased heart rate and force of contraction (positive chronotropy and inotropy)
- downregulation of myocardial β1 receptors reducing the positive inotropic effect of sympathetic stimulation (and exogenous adrenoceptor agonists such as dobutamine and dopamine)
- disordered calcium release and binding within the heart muscle cells further limiting the effectiveness of endogenous and exogenous positive inotropes.
- Decreased myocardial compliance reducing diastolic ventricular filling
- Ventricular dilatation due to chronically increased preload
  - Functional valvular regurgitation
  - For a given end-diastolic pressure, the dilated ventricle has a greater tension within the myocytes (Laplace's law). A further increase in preload is therefore produced.

Principles of therapy in cardiogenic pulmonary oedema

- Clear excessive lung water:
  - improve left ventricular performance (cardiac output)
  - optimise heart rate and rhythm
  - decrease total body sodium and water load.

Preload needs to be reduced, both to improve ventricular performance and reduce pulmonary venous pressures. Afterload is usually severely increased and needs reduction if the consequent reduced blood pressure can be tolerated. Contractility may need improving if the above measures are ineffective or cannot be tolerated (Fig. 20.1).

The optimum **heart rate** depends on the condition producing the heart failure. Slower heart rates (less than 60–80/min) may reduce cardiac output, but faster heart rates impair diastolic ventricular filling, particularly if the ventricle is hypertrophied and non-compliant. The onset of atrial fibrillation may precipitate heart failure in conditions of slow ventricular diastolic filling, e.g. mitral stenosis.

Decreasing total body sodium and water with diuresis takes more time than the previous measures and requires adequate cardiac output and blood

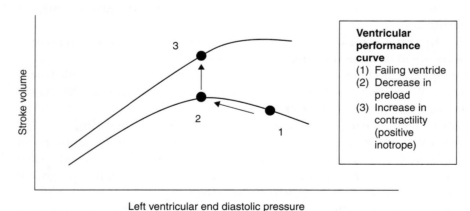

Ventricular performance curve
(1) Failing ventricle
(2) Decrease in preload
(3) Increase in contractility (positive inotrope)

Left ventricular end diastolic pressure

Fig. 20.1 Ventricular performance is improved by optimising preload, afterload and contractility. In cardiac failure, the ventricle is often on the unfavourable part of the performance curve (see Chapter 10).

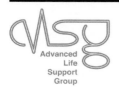

pressure for renal perfusion. Overly aggressive diuresis may reduce preload sufficiently to reduce cardiac output if there is not a concomitant reduction in afterload. Fortunately, frusemide has an arterial and venous dilator effect that precedes the diuresis.

Key point

Preload and afterload reduction has a more rapid effect on pulmonary oedema than diuresis

---

Causes of cardiogenic pulmonary oedema

Myocardial disease	**Myocardial infarction and ischaemia**
	Hypertensive cardiomyopathy
	Dilated cardiomyopathy
	Hypertrophic obstructive cardiomyopathy
Endocardial disease	**Valvular heart disease**
	Endocarditis
	Atrial myxoma
Pericardial disease	**Constrictive pericarditis**
	Pericardial tamponade
Rhythm disturbances	**Tachy- and bradydysrhythmias**

Myocardial diseases, especially ischaemia and hypertrophy (due to hypertension), are by far the most common.

Clinical presentation

Breathlessness is invariably present, often accompanied by much distress. There may be cough and, in severe cases, frothy blood-stained sputum. Examination reveals a distressed, tachypnoeic and tachycardic patient, pale, sweaty and perhaps cyanosed.

Fine crackles are usually heard at the lung bases, sometimes with an associated wheeze. Blood pressure is often elevated, and cardiac examination may reveal a third heart sound. There may be specific features present relating to the cause of the cardiac failure, e.g. signs of valvular heart disease and perhaps symptoms and signs of chronic heart failure (orthopnoea, paroxysmal nocturnal dyspnoea, ankle swelling).

Recognition of an episode of pulmonary oedema is not always easy. None of the symptoms or signs are specific. Fortunately, the generic approach to the breathless patient remains valid and the history and investigations in the secondary assessment will often reveal whether pulmonary oedema is the cause of breathlessness and if so, the cause of pulmonary oedema.

Management of acute pulmonary oedema
Primary assessment and resuscitation

Give high concentrations of inspired oxygen by face mask. Sit the patient upright, unless severely obtunded. Consider using CPAP by face mask at 5–10 cm H_2O, as it reduces preload, afterload and increases alveolar pressures.

Assess heart rate, rhythm, blood pressure and perfusion. Obtain venous access. Treat severe brady or tachydysrhythmias as appropriate (see Chapter 10).

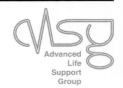

Drug therapy options

Intravenous diamorphine 2.5 mg is an excellent drug which reduces afterload, heart rate, distress and sympathetic overactivity: hypotension is a common side effect.

If the systolic BP>90 mm Hg give either GTN 200–400 µg sublingually to reduce preload and afterload or an intravenous GTN infusion, titrated up to 2 µg/kg/min (approximately 1–10 mg/h), may be added.

Alternatively, furosemide, 20–40 mg IV (more if on large doses already) may be given. This initially reduces preload through venodilation, then causes a diuresis.

If the systolic BP <90 mm Hg and the patient has pulmonary oedema and hypotension then outlook is poor unless a treatable cause is found. Positive inotropic support may 'buy time' until definitive treatment is established:

- Dobutamine may be used at 1–20 µg/kg/min. This inodilator increases heart rate and contractility and also reduces afterload by vasodilatation. Cardiac output increases, but blood pressure may either rise or fall and needs to be monitored carefully during therapy. Unfortunately, the tachycardia induced by Dobutamine may limit therapy.
- Dopamine 1–10 µg/kg/min. increases contractility, heart rate and blood pressure even in the low doses previously regarded as 'renal'. It is also a mild diuretic through Dopamine1 receptors in the renal tubules, but the renal vascular dilatation produced by dopamine in healthy subjects does not appear to improve outcome in renal failure in critically ill patients. It has the advantage over dobutamine that a rise in blood pressure is more reliably produced, but in higher doses it induces severe vasoconstriction, which is not beneficial to the failing heart.

Other inotropic agents are available and, as in many areas of medical practice, have produced conflicting results about outcomes in studies. There may be local protocols for their use. Noradrenaline is generally reserved for patients with profound hypotension (e.g. systolic BP <60 mm Hg).

Secondary assessment and emergency management

- A detailed history and examination should confirm the presence of pulmonary oedema and give a differential diagnosis for its cause.
- Investigations should always include 12-lead ECG, CXR, urea, electrolytes and full blood count.
- Elevated blood levels of brain natriuretic peptide shows promise as a relatively specific indicator of the presence of cardiogenic pulmonary oedema.
- More specific, investigations may be warranted, e.g. urgent echocardiogram if acute valvular dysfunction is suspected. An early echocardiogram is indicated in most cases of suspected cardiogenic pulmonary oedema.
- Thromboprophylaxis with low dose heparin is usually indicated.
- Emergency management may now be directed towards the underlying diagnosis. Thrombolysis angioplasty or urgent revascularisation may be indicated in myocardial infarction/ischaemia.
- Cardiac surgery may be indicated in acute valvular dysfunction. A senior opinion is always indicated if the management plan is not clear.

Reassessment

If the patient does not respond to the initial treatment, the following should be considered:

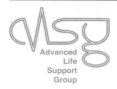

- Is the diagnosis correct?
- CPAP via face mask
- Optimise afterload reduction
- Inotropic support
- Monitor continuous pulse oximetry and ECG and hourly respiratory rate, pulse, blood pressure and urine output are always indicated. A central venous line to optimise inotropic delivery, intra-arterial monitoring (in shock or in aggressive vasodilatation therapy), cardiac output monitoring may all be useful.
- Intensive care opinion if there is ongoing hypoxaemia, shock or multiple organ failures.
- Urgent haemodialysis if there is fluid overload and no response to diuresis once shock has been corrected.
- Consider mechanical cardiac support, such as intra-aortic balloon pumping (IABP). This may 'buy time' if a treatable underlying cause of pulmonary oedema is present. Insertion (by an appropriately experienced practitioner) of an intra-aortic balloon pump may be a life-saving intervention in patients awaiting emergency surgery for acute mitral regurgitation secondary to papillary muscle rupture or those with ventricular septal defect as a complication of myocardial infarction. IABP reduces afterload and thereby reduces the severity of mitral regurgitation. It enhances forward cardiac output, reduces left atrial pressure and improves pulmonary oedema.

Definitive care

Placement will usually be dictated by the nature of the ongoing therapy and the extent and complexity of monitoring.

In addition to the specific therapeutic options mentioned above, consider long-term therapy after the acute event has been treated. This may include angiography, surgery, ACE inhibitors, β blockers, lifestyle changes and weight loss overseen by a specialist.

Causes of cardiogenic pulmonary oedema

- Left ventricular failure (see Chapters 8 and 9 for further details)
- Valvular heart disease
- Mitral stenosis

Pathophysiology

Chronic rheumatic heart disease is by far the most common cause. The mitral valve cusps are thickened and often fused, with associated thrombus on the atrial surface.

Calcification may also occur. The left atrium is characteristically enlarged and mural thrombus may be present proximal to the posterior mitral valve cusp.

Mitral stenosis reduces left ventricular filling. Consequently, cardiac output falls and pulmonary vascular resistance increases. Left ventricular cavity size usually remains normal. In contrast, the left atrium enlarges and chronic left atrial hypertension induces a rise in pulmonary capillary pressure and, hence, pulmonary oedema formation. Reactive pulmonary hypertension, repeated pulmonary emboli, frequent chest infections or even haemosiderosis, may occur.

Treatment

Pulmonary oedema associated with mitral stenosis responds well to diuretic therapy.

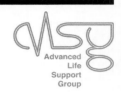

Heart rate and rhythm control is particularly important: tachycardia is not well tolerated. If the patient is in atrial fibrillation with a rapid ventricular response, then appropriate treatment is with digoxin. In addition, low molecular weight heparin should be started as a prelude to either cardioversion or formal anti-coagulation, because of the high incidence of arterial embolism from left atrial thrombus.

Rarely, left atrial myxomas (present in 2 per 100,000 of the population) may present as progressive breathlessness, orthopnoea, paroxysmal nocturnal dysp-noea or fluid retention. The acute management is described under mitral stenosis. As there is a significant risk of emboli, surgery is the definitive treatment.

Mitral regurgitation
Pathophysiology
Of the many causes of mitral regurgitation (Table 20.2), the most common is the floppy mitral valve. Irrespective of the cause, however, the main physiological disturbance is an increase in left ventricular output. The pressure within the aorta is significantly greater than that in the left atrium, so the majority of the left ventricular ejection fraction enters the left atrium. The left ventricular output is maintained, however, by a sinus tachycardia. If severe, mitral regurgitation can lead to pulmonary oedema and/or a low output state. Atrial fibrillation is common and, when present, the risk of thromboembolism is high.

During diastole there is a large flow of blood from the left atrium to the left ventricle, comprising blood received from the pulmonary circulation combined with that regurgitated during the preceding systole. This increased volume will lead to left ventricular failure, raised pulmonary capillary pressures and hence pulmonary venous hypertension.

Treatment
Medical treatment does not differ from that described for mitral stenosis. Vasodi-latation to reduce afterload is also helpful, especially in acute mitral regurgitation. The different mitral valve operations used currently for correction of mitral re-gurgitation are mitral valve repair (MVR) with preservation of part or all of the mitral apparatus, and MVR with removal of the mitral apparatus. Improved post-operative function occurs with repair.

Aortic stenosis
Pathophysiology
The causes of aortic stenosis are listed in the box.

Table 20.2 The causes of mitral regurgitation

Structure affected	Pathogenesis
Valve cusps	Floppy mitral valve, infective endocarditis, rheumatic heart disease
Chordae	Floppy mitral valve, connective tissue diseases, infective endocarditis
Papillary muscle	Acute myocardial infarction, cardiomyopathy
Valve ring	Left ventricular dilatation

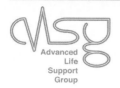

> **Causes of aortic stenosis**
>
> Congenital bicuspid (fused commissure)
> Rheumatic heart disease
> Calcified 'senile' valve
> Infective endocarditis

Aortic stenosis gives rise to left ventricular hypertrophy. This produces diastolic stiffness of the myocardium, higher end diastolic pressures and, eventually, pulmonary oedema. As the disease progresses, the left ventricular cavity becomes dilated, especially in severe cases.

Treatment

Aortic stenosis is a mechanical problem that will, in most cases, require surgical intervention. Acute pulmonary oedema, in this context, can be managed by diuretic therapy and bed rest before surgery. This, however, is only a temporary measure. Indications for surgery are:

- any symptoms attributable to aortic stenosis
- left ventricular failure
- critical stenosis (peak systolic gradient >50 mm Hg).

Aortic regurgitation

Pathophysiology

The causes of aortic regurgitation are listed in the box.

> **Causes of aortic regurgitation**
>
> Infective endocarditis
> Rheumatic heart disease
> Trauma
> Rheumatoid disease
> Marfan's syndrome
> Dissecting aneurysm
> Syphilis
> Ankylosing spondylitis

Aortic regurgitation is associated with an increase in left ventricular stroke volume. The regurgitant flow is greatest in early diastole, when the difference in pressure between the aorta and left ventricle is maximal. The volume of regurgitated blood is determined not only by the severity of the aortic valve disease, but also by the compliance of left ventricle and systemic vascular resistance. The left ventricular output may be more than double.

The end diastolic pressure in the aorta is low and the resistance to ejection of blood by the left ventricle is reduced. This reduction in resistance, allied to a large stroke volume, is responsible for the rapid upstroke and wide pulse pressure.

In acute aortic regurgitation the only physical sign may be the early blowing diastolic murmur.

Treatment

Acute aortic regurgitation is a surgical emergency. It is nearly always secondary to infective endocarditis in the presence of acute pulmonary oedema. Vasodilatation, as with acute mitral regurgitation, is the treatment of choice, whilst plans are being made for emergency aortic valve replacement.

> **Key point**
>
> All patients must receive appropriate advice and treatment, where relevant, for infective endocarditis – irrespective of the valvular problem

Acute hypertension

Pathophysiology

Increased left ventricular load, possibly augmented by increased sympathetic nerve activity, is responsible for left ventricular hypertrophy. The consequent increase in muscle mass may be responsible for the development of ischaemia and also ventricular dysfunction, both predisposing to left ventricular failure.

Treatment

Patients with malignant hypertension usually are admitted to a critical care unit for continuous cardiac monitoring and frequent assessment of neurologic status and urine output. An intravenous line is started for fluids and medications. Patients typically have altered blood pressure autoregulation, and overzealous reduction of blood pressure to reference range levels may result in organ hypoperfusion. The initial goal of therapy is to reduce the mean arterial pressure by approximately 25% over the first 24–48 h. An intra-arterial line is helpful for continuous titration of blood pressure.

Sodium and volume depletion may be severe, and volume expansion with isotonic sodium chloride solution must be considered.

Sodium nitroprusside is the agent of choice, as its action can be immediately reversed by stopping the infusion (50 mg of sodium nitroprusside added to 500 ml of 5% dextrose gives a solution of 100 µg/ml). Intra-arterial pressure monitoring is necessary. An infusion of sodium nitroprusside at 10 µg/min (6 ml/h) should be started with increments of 10 µg/min every 5 min, until a maximum dose of 75 µg/kg is reached.

Right ventricular failure

Pathophysiology

The commonest cause of right ventricular failure is inferior myocardial infarction. Failure of the ventricle to contract appropriately reduces forward flow into the pulmonary circulation and hence manifests as low output left ventricular failure. This may be the first clue to the underlying diagnosis. Further signs include tachycardia, hypotension, and a third heart sound. However, there is no pulmonary oedema. Right ventricular dilatation often produces tricuspid regurgitation with a systolic murmur and regurgitant V waves in the JVP. Features of systemic venous hypertension predominate. This clinical picture may initially be confused with a pericardial effusion or constrictive pericarditis, but Kussmaul's sign is negative and there is no pulsus paradoxus.

Treatment

This comprises a fluid challenge to increase the right ventricular filling pressure. Often, inotropes have to be added. Under ideal circumstances, these patients should be monitored on the coronary care unit and their treatment facilitated by readings from a pulmonary arterial flotation catheter.

> **Key point**
>
> Cardiac tamponade and constrictive pericarditis are rare

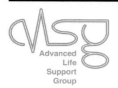

Summary

Cardiac failure is a common medical emergency. Knowledge of the pathophysiology of the conditions producing heart failure help apply the structured approach to the management of this condition. The underlying cause is usually ischaemic heart disease. A critical feature in the management of these patients is blood pressure. This will dictate whether vasodilatation and/or inotropic support is the management of choice.

BRAIN FAILURE

Introduction

Acute brain failure may be manifested as a decrease in consciousness, pupillary abnormalities or abnormal movements and posture, as described in Chapter 7. However this section will examine the more subtle types of brain failure manifested by intellectual dysfunction, loss of intelligence or loss of intellectual capacity. This condition must be differentiated from learning difficulties, where there is a subnormal intellectual capacity from the outset that is often caused by brain disease acquired during prenatal or early life.

In this context brain failure is not a medical emergency, but it is considered because the differential diagnosis often causes concern (see box).

Differential diagnosis of brain failure

Dementia
Pseudodementia   Acute confusional state
                             Inattention
                             Depression

All of these conditions will affect the mental state but, in the context of acute medicine, the important diagnosis to establish is that of an acute confusional state. This is the commonest condition that affects the mental state and the commonest form of pseudodementia.

Intellectual functions are best examined using a mental state examination, as described in Chapter 7. In both acute confusion and dementia, there is a **global** impairment in the mental state. However, there are some specific features which will help to distinguish one from the other.

Acute confusional state

In a patient who is acutely confused, the abnormality in mental state is due to reduced cerebral function, commonly secondary to a toxin, hypoxaemia or ischaemia; i.e. the patient has an encephalopathy. Diagnostic clues are the acute onset, a decrease in conscious level and an underlying disease process or exogenous toxin that has precipitated the acute confusion.

Key point

Acute confusional state is associated with a subtly decreased conscious level

---

The confused patient is unable to maintain a coherent stream of thought or action. This is best assessed by tests of mental attention such as the 'serial sevens'

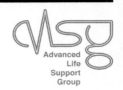

or '1 tap/ 2 tap' test. Explain to the patient that if you tap once the patient should respond by tapping twice; however, if you tap twice the patient should not tap. A similar test is to ask the patient to recite rapidly all the letters of the alphabet that rhyme with tree.

This ensures that they have to keep the task in mind whilst reciting the appropriate letters.

Dementia

Dementia is characterised by a chronic and often progressive onset of global intellectual dysfunction. Memory impairment is the most commonly found abnormality of cognitive function.

Key point

Do not focus on 'overlearned' knowledge, such as details of the family, as even the most demented patient may still be able to recollect some relevant details

---

The mini mental state examination is a 30 point score that is easily assessed (see Chapter 7). Search for **Global** impairment of the components (orientation, recent and remote memory, calculation, language). Scattered abnormal results should not be overinterpreted, as mistakes are common. Normal results in these tests are very useful in excluding a diagnosis of dementia.

Dementia is a chronic disabling disease and, therefore, before a firm diagnosis is made it is important not to miss a treatable condition. A full history and physical examination is performed and help should be sought from either a neurologist or a geriatrician.

Some causes of dementia

Common

Alzheimer's disease	Alcoholism
Cerebrovascular disease	Parkinson's disease

Uncommon

Vitamin B_1, B_{12} deficiency	Heavy metal poisoning
Hypothyroidism	Vasculitis
Syphilis	Sarcoidosis
HIV infection	SLE
Subdural haematoma	Huntington's chorea
Cerebral tumour	Multiple sclerosis
Hydrocephalus	

A computed tomography scan is usually necessary, as are some laboratory tests, but a battery of screening tests for rare diseases is unrewarding, especially for those that have other clinical manifestations detectable on examination.

Summary

Brain failure commonly presents as an acute confusional state. The differential diagnosis includes dementia, inattention and depression, and is facilitated by a comprehensive medical history and search for an underlying treatable cause. In

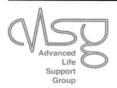

the context of acute confusional state, this is usually a toxin, hypoxaemia or ischaemia. In contrast, treatable causes for dementia include meningioma, chronic bilateral subdural haematomata, hydrocephalus and vitamin B_{12} deficiency.

ACUTE RENAL FAILURE/ACUTE KIDNEY INJURY

Introduction
Acute renal dysfunction is common in a sick patient with multiple organ dysfunction and is usually secondary to circulatory failure. As a single organ failure, it is usually due to a nephrotoxin, intrinsic renal disease or post-renal obstruction. Intrinsic renal disease is relatively rare. Approximately 5% of emergency admissions have transient disturbances in renal function.

Definition
The traditional definition of acute renal failure was the abrupt loss of kidney function resulting in the:
- Retention of urea and other nitrogenous waste products
- Dysregulation of electrolytes and extra cellular volume

There have been many problems with this and other definitions. To obviate these problems the term 'acute kidney injury' has been adapted to embrace the spectrum of acute renal failure. The diagnostic criteria are:
- abrupt onset (within 48 h)
- absolute increase in serum creatinine of 26.4 µmol/l above baseline
- an increase of >50% of serum creatinine
- oliguria of less than 0.5 ml/kg/h for more than 6 h.

The SOFA score criteria (see introduction) recognises that acute renal injury is not an all or nothing phenomena.

Causes
Although the causes are divided into three groups (see box) those grouped as prerenal are the commonest. Often, you will suspect that acute kidney injury is likely from either the clinical features or the history. Occasionally, however, it will come to light when laboratory results are examined.

Causes of acute renal failure	
Prerenal	Hypotension, e.g. following shock
	Hypovolaemia, e.g. gastrointestinal haemorrhage, persistent vomiting or diarrhoea, diuretic or hyperglycaemic states
	Selective renal ischaemia, e.g. hepatorenal syndrome
Intrinsic renal disease	Glomerular, e.g. primary part of a systemic disease
	Vascular, e.g. vasculitis, coagulopathy
	Tubular, e.g. acute tubular necrosis (often ischaemic)
	Interstitial, e.g. drug related acute interstitial nephritis
Postrenal	Urethral obstruction, e.g. prostatic pathology
	Ureteric obstruction, e.g. carcinoma of the bladder

Primary assessment and resuscitation
The priority in acute kidney injury is to treat life-threatening abnormalities in airway, breathing and circulation. Hypotension, shock and hypovolaemia must

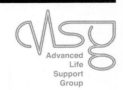

be aggressively corrected. Fluid replacement is usually indicated if pulmonary oedema is absent. If pulmonary oedema is present, it should initially be treated conventionally as detailed above, although diuretics will not usually be effective.

Principles of management of acute kidney injury

Resuscitate ABC to normal
Treat life-threatening pulmonary oedema and hyperkalaemia
Look for and treat other organ failures and infection
Make a diagnosis of the cause of renal failure and treat accordingly
    Exclude renal tract obstruction
    Exclude all potential renal toxins
    Examine the urine/urinary sediment
Consider timing of renal replacement therapy if indicated

Secondary assessment and emergency treatment

A full history should consider potential nephrotoxins (see the next box). Clinical examination should always include rectal and pelvic examinations to search for a pelvic tumour.

Common nephrotoxins

Non steroidal anti-inflammatory drugs	Radiocontrast media
ACE inhibitors angiotensin receptor	Amphotericin
antagonists	Aminoglycosides

The presenting features of renal disease are summarised in the next box. A urinary catheter must be inserted. Multiple organ dysfunction should be sought and managed appropriately.

Symptoms and signs of renal disease presentation

Altered function	Decreased/no urine output
	Flank pain
	Hypertension
	Discoloured urine
Failure	Weakness, lethargy
	Anorexia
	Vomiting
	Oedema
	Confusion, fits
Concurrent disease	Fever
	Arthralgia
	Breathless
Incidental findings (asymptomatic)	Abnormal creatinine
	Urine analysis
	Renal scan

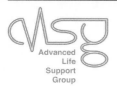

When acute renal injury is suspected, some urgent investigations are required (see the next box).

Urgent investigations in suspected acute renal failure

Plasma sodium, potassium, urea, creatinine and glucose
Urine stick test, microscopy, biochemistry and culture
Arterial blood gases
ECG
Renal ultrasound scan

Hyperkalaemia is a life-threatening emergency and should be carefully managed (see next box).

Emergency Management of hyperkalaemia

Ensure correct fluid balance. Treat or remove the underlying cause. Then consider:
   Check K^+ and other electrolytes (1–4 hourly) and monitor ECG:
a K^+ > 6.0 – 100 ml 50% glucose solution with 10 units regular (rapid-acting) insulin IVI
b K^+ > 6.5 – as for (a), but infuse calcium gluconate, 10 ml 10% solution over 10–15 min first (stabilises cardiac cell membranes) until ECG changes revert to normal
c K^+ > 7.0 – as for (a) and (b) above, and infuse 50–100 ml 8.5% sodium bicarbonate over 30 min (unless patient in respiratory failure). Repeat glucose and insulin 2–4 hourly prn
d Rectal calcium resonium 30 mg once daily to decrease K^+ on a chronic basis
e If response to above is inadequate, consider nebulised salbutamol furosemide and haemodialysis.

Urine analysis is useful in the differential diagnosis of acute renal injury. Urine biochemistry may be helpful, but the values in Table 20.3 are of limited use in the presence of pre-existing renal disease, diuretic therapy, liver disease and intrinsic glomerular disease.

With acute renal injury urine sodium measurement can help distinguish hypovolaemia (pre renal) from acute tubular necrosis. However, urine sodium is

Table 20.3 Urine biochemistry in acute renal injury

	Prerenal	Acute tubular necrosis
Urine sodium (mmol/l)	<20	>40

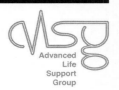

influenced by urine output. The effect of variations in urine volume can be determined by calculating the fractional excretion of sodium (Fe Na):

$$\text{Fe Na (\%)} = \frac{\text{Urine Na} \times \text{Plasma creatines} \times 100}{\text{Plasma Na} \times \text{Urine creatines}}$$

A value of below 1% = pre renal disease
Above 2% = acute tubular necrosis
(values below 1 and 2 = either disorder)

Urine stick testing and microscopy is more useful. The presence of dysmorphic red cells, red cell casts and proteinuria on urine microscopy is suggestive of acute glomerulonephritis. In contrast, a positive urine stick test for blood, but negative microscopy for red cells, is indicative of rhabdomyolysis. This may be confirmed by the laboratory detection of urine myoglobin and raised blood creatinine kinase. The presence of tubular cell casts, tubular cells and granular casts is highly suggestive of acute tubular necrosis.

It is vital to exclude urinary obstruction as a cause of acute renal failure. Dilation of the renal collecting system, ureters or bladder on renal ultrasound makes obstruction likely and this investigation should be performed urgently in oliguric acute renal failure. The ultrasound will also be useful to confirm number, site and shape of the kidneys including any cortical thinning and scarring, suggestive of pre-existing disease.

Monitoring is usually dictated by any associated multiple organ dysfunction but, as a minimum, should include:

- hourly — urine output and clinical examination
- 4 hourly — pulse, blood pressure
- twice daily — serum, urea, electrolytes and creatinine, arterial blood gases (more frequently if hyperkalaemia or rhabdomyolysis present)

Definitive management

Once resuscitation is complete and acute life-threatening complications have been managed successfully, the next decision is the timing and necessity for renal replacement therapy and the manner in which it is delivered. Low dose dopamine is not thought to be of benefit, on current evidence. There is little evidence for high dose frusemide (e.g. 250 mg over 1 h), but it is often prescribed.

Indications for early renal replacement therapy in acute renal injury

Hyperkalaemia
Pulmonary oedema
Severe metabolic acidosis
Uraemic encephalopathy or pericarditis

Intermittent haemodialysis is the usual renal replacement therapy used in isolated acute renal injury, often within a specialist medical area. The patient with multiple organ failures, especially haemodynamic instability, may benefit from continuous renal replacement therapy, usually in an intensive care unit. All renal replacement therapy will be under the guidance of a nephrologist and/or intensivist.

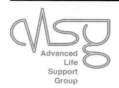

Summary

Acute renal injury is usually associated with other failing organs. The priorities are to:

- identify all failing organ systems
- treat life-threatening hyperkalaemia and pulmonary oedema
- recognise and treat the underlying cause
- organise dialysis when appropriate.

LIVER FAILURE

Introduction

The incidence of both acute and acute-on-chronic liver failure is increasing. The patient with acute on chronic liver failure is a frequent medical emergency. The immediate management of these two conditions is virtually identical.

Definition

Liver failure is a syndrome that follows severe impairment of hepatocyte function, hence it is also referred to as hepatocellular failure.

Clinical features

These usually develop over several days, but coma onset may occur over hours.

Cardinal signs of acute hepatocellular dysfunction

Jaundice

Hepatic encephalopathy

Ascites (particularly acute on chronic liver failure)

Coagulopathy

Jaundice indicates impaired release of conjugated bilirubin and its intensity is proportional to the extent and duration of hepatocellular necrosis.

Hepatic encephalopathy is manifested as a broad spectrum of neuropsychiatric features that are epitomised by impaired mental state and neuromuscular dysfunction. This form of neurological dysfunction occurs when blood is shunted from the portal venous system into the systemic circulation without hepatic extraction of substances such as ammonia, phenols and GABA (γ-aminobutyric acid)–like glycoprotein. These compounds are believed to act as inhibitory neurotransmitters, depressing both motor function and the conscious level. This may easily be assessed using the Glasgow Coma Score, but hepatologists in particular prefer to use Childs grading.

Childs grading of hepatic encephalopathy

Grade 1	Prodromal phase – euphoria or irritability
Grade 2	Impending coma – drowsiness, lethargy and confusion interspersed with agitated or aggressive behaviour
Grade 3	Stupor – somnolent but rousable
Grade 4	Coma

Patients with encephalopathy can present with a variety of neurological signs ranging from flexor, equivocal or extensor plantars (positive Babinski response)

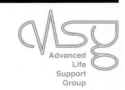

to extrapyramidal features. The classic sign is asterixis; a non-specific 'flapping' tremor associated with liver failure, carbon dioxide retention and uraemia. This is due, in part, to neuromuscular incoordination of the wrist flexors and extensors.

Differential diagnosis of hepatic encephalopathy: three 'H's *and* four 'I's

Hypoxaemia
Hypovolaemia
Hypoglycaemia
Alcohol
Neurodegenerative conditions
Drugs
Infection
Impaction of faeces
Intracranial haemorrhage
Imbalance of electrolytes

Ascites occur primarily due to a raised portal venous pressure, secondary to distortion and destruction of the sinusoids with superadded impaired venous drainage. It is uncommon as a presenting feature in acute liver failure, but common in acute on chronic.

Coagulopathy associated with liver failure is multifactorial. Bleeding tendency is primarily due to impaired synthesis of all coagulation factors (factor VIII is predominantly produced by the endothelium). This is often exacerbated by thrombocytopenia (e.g. secondary to hypersplenism) or platelet dysfunction. Therefore, it is advisable to check both the prothrombin and activated partial thromboplastin times. Occasionally, disseminated intravascular coagulation is present, but this is rarely severe and, if present, often has another cause, e.g. sepsis. Check a blood film and D-dimer or fibrin degradation products.

In addition, two other features worth mentioning are foetor hepaticus and immunocompromise. Foetor hepaticus is a characteristic smell of the patient's breath which is due to sulphur compounds. All patients with liver failure are relatively immunocompromised and severe infection may be present without coexistent pyrexia or leucocytosis.

Critical clinical features

Life-threatening features of acute liver failure

Hypoxaemia	Gastrointestinal haemorrhage
Hypovolaemia	Coma
Hypoglycaemia	Multiple organ failure

- *Hypoxaemia:* This is multifactorial in origin and is primarily related to widespread peripheral pulmonary vasodilatation. This results in approximately two thirds of patients becoming hypoxaemic, but the precise cause remains unknown. It is exacerbated by abnormalities in ventilation, perfusion and transfer factor. The hypoxaemia is usually readily reversible with high concentrations of inspired oxygen.
- *Hypotension:* This is a manifestation of systemic vasodilatation combined with a hyperdynamic circulation. Patients therefore exhibit a bounding pulse,

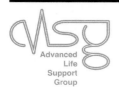

prominent left ventricular impulse and a flow murmur. Of interest is the fact that, whilst the systemic blood flow is increased, renal perfusion is reduced along with urine output. Hypotension associated with liver disease is therefore a combination of systemic vasodilatation and hypovolaemia. The situation can be compounded by the fact that patients can have a coexistent dysrhythmia

> **Key point**
>
> Fifty per cent of patients with acute liver disease will have coexistent gastrointestinal haemorrhage

- *Hypoglycaemia:* This is extremely important and easy to miss. Hepatic glucose synthesis and release is impaired and this process is exacerbated by raised levels of circulating insulin.

It is important to be aware of the potential for acute hypoglycaemia. Failure to prevent and recognise this condition can lead to irreversible brain damage – unlike the situation with hepatic encephalopathy.

> **Key point**
>
> Hypoglycaemia is common in patients with liver dysfunction and may mimic hepatic encephalopathy

Other key features include:
- *Cerebral oedema* is attributed to arterial vasodilatation and failure of cellular osmoregulation with reduction in cerebral oxygen consumption. The crucial factor is how to distinguish cerebral oedema from hepatic encephalopathy. Often this is impossible. However, in patients with grade 4 coma, both cerebral oedema and hepatic encephalopathy coexist. Thus, early discussion with a hepatologist and intensivist is required.
- *Renal failure* is very common in patients with liver failure, but only a minority are associated with true hypovolaemia. Most patients have a 'functional' renal failure.
- *Impaired water clearance,* sodium pump failure, intravenous fluids and diuretics can give rise to hyponatraemia. These may also contribute to hypokalaemia and the coexistent metabolic alkalosis. Other acid–base disturbances include centrally driven respiratory alkalosis associated with hypovolaemia and metabolic acidosis due to anaerobic metabolism from lactate accumulation and tissue destruction.

> **Key point**
>
> In patients with liver failure, remember that urea and creatinine are not reliable indicators of renal function as hepatic synthesis of urea is reduced and tubular excretion of creatinine is increased

Management of liver failure
Primary assessment and resuscitation
The priority is to treat the hypoxaemia, hypovolaemia and hypoglycaemia characteristic of the condition. These are all treated in a conventional manner as detailed

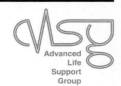

elsewhere in this manual. The presence of gastrointestinal haemorrhage must always be suspected and blood cross-matched urgently. A coagulation screen is requested urgently and this will guide blood product replacement if haemorrhage is present. Coma may require emergency airway management and, once hypoglycaemia is excluded, oral lactulose is started.

Management of liver failure

Universal precautions
High concentrations of inspired O_2
Secure IV access and treat hypovolaemia
Recognise and proactively treat the potential for:
   Hypoglycaemia
   Hepatic encephalopathy
   Thiamine deficiency
   Underlying infection

Secondary assessment and emergency management

This part of the assessment focuses on establishing the cause of hepatic failure and detecting treatable sequelae. A full history should include travel and contact with infectious diseases, drug ingestion (recreational and therapeutic, particularly ecstasy, alcohol and paracetamol) and a sexual history. The presence of encephalopathy may make taking a history difficult.

Urgent investigations in liver failure

Full blood count	Liver enzyme profile
Clotting times	Viral serology
Urea and electrolytes	Serum/Urine for toxicology
Glucose	Urine – Microscopy/Culture
Arterial blood gases	Ascites – Microscopy/Culture
Blood cultures	Protein/Amylase
Paracetamol level	Cytology
	Cell count

If gastrointestinal haemorrhage is present, this is assumed to be variceal until proven otherwise, particularly in acute on chronic liver failure. The mortality from variceal haemorrhage in these circumstances is around 30–50%, illustrating the need for early expert advice. Shock is treated conventionally, octreotide or vasopressin analogue commenced according to local protocol, and an urgent endoscopy arranged. If variceal bleeding cannot be controlled with endoscopy, a Sengstaken or Minnesota tube can be passed.

Definitive care

Early liaison with a specialist hepatology unit will be guided by the local gastroenterologist. The important issues in this final stage of management are listed in the box.

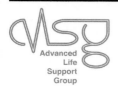

Important issues in the definitive care of liver failure

Treatment of vasodilatation and increasing oxygen uptake
Prevention or treatment of cerebral oedema
Treatment of coexistent renal failure with haemofiltration
Temporary hepatic support versus emergency transplant

Outcome measures

Many features will dictate the outcome.

- The shorter the interval between onset of jaundice and hepatic encephalopathy, the better the outcome.
- Severe hepatic encephalopathy is associated with a poor prognosis.

Summary

Irrespective of the cause of either acute or acute on chronic liver failure, the initial management is the same. Treat hypoxaemia, hypovolaemia and hypoglycaemia (the three Hs). Early liaison with a gastroenterologist/hepatologist is necessary.

ENDOCRINE FAILURE

Introduction

Of all conditions that are associated with endocrine failure, the two that cause most concern are related to hyperglycaemia and adrenocortical insufficiency. The latter may be related to either a primary adrenal problem or secondary to pituitary pathology.

Hyperglycaemic states: diabetic ketoacidosis

Clinical features of diabetic ketoacidosis

Hyperventilation
Dehydration and shock
Decreased conscious level
Smell of ketones on breath

Primary assessment and resuscitation

The structured approach will ensure that the patient is receiving oxygen and appropriate vigorous fluid therapy, especially if there are signs of either dehydration or shock. Coma will mean that the airway needs protecting. An initial high glucometer reading must be confirmed with a formal blood glucose. Plasma or urine testing for ketones is necessary.

Key points

Consider ketoacidosis in any ill diabetic, especially if there is vomiting and/or tachypnoea
Never diagnose primary hyperventilation until diabetic ketoacidosis has been excluded
Always exclude ketoacidosis in patients who are confused, comatosed or have a metabolic acidosis

---

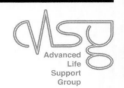

As soon as an elevated blood glucose is identified, the patient should receive 10 units of intravenous soluble insulin whilst an infusion is being prepared.

Treatment of shock is a priority. Hyperglycaemia and hypovolaemia are treated simultaneously and consequently the serum potassium may fall sharply. Regimes for fluid, insulin and potassium have reduced the morbidity and mortality from this condition; an example is given in the box below. This may slightly differ from your local policy; so note any changes. Thromboprophylaxis is usually indicated.

Insulin infusion
10 units IV bolus
6 units per hour
Reduce to 'sliding scale' when
　glucose <15 mmol/l
Subcutaneous regime when eating
　and ketones gone

Potassium
Urgent U & E

Fluids
Bolus 1 l normal (N.) saline
1st hour 1 l N. saline
2nd hour 500 ml N. saline
3rd hour 500 ml N. saline
Then 250 ml/h N. saline until rehydrated
Add 10% dextrose 62.5 ml/h (500 ml in 8 h)
　when glucose < 15 mmol/L
If severe hypernatraemia (Na>155 mmol/l),
　use 0.45% saline and monitor hourly

Serum K+	KCl added per litre
<3.5 mmol/l	40 mmol
3.5–5.5 mmol/l	20 mmol
>5.5 mmol/l	None

Secondary assessment and emergency treatment

Monitoring in an appropriate environment is essential to assess the response to treatment and the development of any complications. Shock, coma, glucose level, acidosis and ketosis should all steadily improve. If ketosis persists, it is important to ensure sufficient glucose is being given with insulin, appropriate to the blood glucose.

Monitoring progress in diabetic ketoacidosis

15 min checks: respiratory rate, pulse, blood pressure and Glasgow Coma score
1 hourly checks: glucometer, urine output
2 hourly checks: blood glucose (until less than 20 mmol/l), serum potassium and
　sodium

This is the minimum monitoring, along with continuous ECG and SpO_2, if the patient does not improve:

- A clinical search for infection is made and blood and urine cultures taken. The skin is examined thoroughly, including the perianal region and perineum, for signs of infection. If infection is suspected, a broad-spectrum antibiotic such as Tazocin is given.

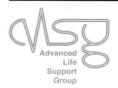

- Other causes of ketoacidosis should be considered, such as non-compliance with insulin, myocardial infarction.
- Sodium bicarbonate use in severe acidosis is controversial, but if pH <6.9, 50 mmol of sodium bicarbonate may be infused and rechecked, targeting a pH >6.9 (rather than normal levels).

> **Key point**
>
> Patients with ketoacidosis can have a neutrophil leucocytosis without any evidence of an infection. Do not treat with antibiotics

Definitive management

The patient with ketoacidosis will usually need either high dependency or intensive care.

The insulin infusion should be continued until either plasma urinary ketones are negative and the venous bicarbonate is normal. Most patients will be tolerating a normal diet by this stage and it is, therefore, safe to convert to subcutaneous insulin. However, the infusion should be continued for approximately 60 min after the first subcutaneous dose. In the newly diagnosed diabetic, start with short acting soluble insulin three times per day before meals. After 24 h, it should be possible to estimate the total daily insulin dose. This should then be given as two thirds of the daily dose before breakfast and the remainder before supper. Each dose should comprise half of soluble insulin and half of intermediate acting insulin. Glucometer readings should be taken before breakfast, lunch and dinner, and the insulin should be adjusted accordingly. Other long-term regimes may be recommended by a diabetologist.

In contrast, known diabetic patients can be restarted on their normal insulin regime; however, they should be monitored in case this has to be amended.

Hyperosmolar non-ketotic hyperglycaemia

> **Key points**
>
> This diagnosis should be considered in any patient with severe hyperglycaemia, dehydration and drowsiness
>
> Hyperosmolar non-ketotic coma is differentiated from diabetic ketoacidosis by:
> - blood glucose greater than 30 mmol/l, but only 1+ or absence of ketonuria
> - plasma osmolality greater than 350 mosmol/kg

The patient with hyperosmolar non-ketotic hyperglycaemia is usually elderly, but the management should follow the guidelines for diabetic ketoacidosis with the following exceptions:

- Half normal saline is used for fluid replacement if the plasma sodium is greater than 150 mmol/l. Frequent checks of serum sodium are important to ensure serum sodium does not fall too quickly. Insulin sensitivity is greater in the absence of severe acidosis, therefore, the infusion should be started at 3 ml/h.

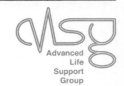

- The risk of thromboembolism is high; therefore, the patient should be fully anticoagulated with heparin according to local policy unless there are contraindications.
- Total potassium is low and plasma level is more variable.

Acute adrenal insufficiency

The causes of adrenal insufficiency are listed in the box.

Causes of acute adrenal insufficiency

Rapid withdrawal of corticosteroids after chronic therapy

Sepsis or surgical stress in patients with chronic adrenal dysfunction from:
    chronic corticosteroid therapy
    autoimmune adrenalitis

Rare causes such as tuberculosis, age related infection with cytomegalovirus and
    adrenal metastases

Bilateral adrenal haemorrhage (rare) secondary to fulminant meningococcal
    sepsis or anticoagulant therapy

Sepsis or surgical stress in patients with hypopituitarism

Septic shock may produce 'relative' adrenal insufficiency

Key point

This diagnosis should be considered in any patient with:
    unexplained hypotension
    mild hyponatraemia
    corticosteroid therapy
    pigmentation
    preceding anorexia, vomiting, diarrhoea and weight loss

Emergency management issues

The patient will be treated appropriately by the structured approach according to their presenting symptoms, especially if they are comatosed, hypotensive or confused. Remember that the patient may be hypoglycaemic. As soon as the diagnosis of acute adrenal insufficiency is suspected, draw blood for a random cortisol and adrenocorticotrophic hormone (ACTH) measurement. If the patient has an impaired conscious level or shock give hydrocortisone 100 mg immediately followed by 100 mg three times per day.

The urgent investigations will not differ from those normally requested in the primary assessment. The results of the cortisol and ACTH estimations above may provide supportive evidence of the clinical diagnosis. A short Synacthen® test should be done to confirm the diagnosis once the patient has improved begin treatment. Change hydrocortisone to an appropriate dose of dexamethasone before testing with using 250 μg of Synacthen® after baseline cortisol levels. The cortisol levels should be repeated after 30 min and then 1 h.

The typical biochemical findings in acute adrenal insufficiency are low sodium (120–130 mmol/l), raised potassium (5–7 mmol/l), raised urea (>6.5 mmol/l) and low glucose.

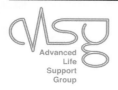

Intravenous fluid replacement, dextrose and hydrocortisone should continue until the patient is asymptomatic. Maintenance therapy usually comprises hydrocortisone 20 mg in the morning and 10 mg at night. Fludrocortisone is not always necessary and will be co-prescribed according to local policy or if the patient has postural hypotension.

> **Key point**
>
> **Patients with acute adrenal insufficiency do not always exhibit classic biochemical features**

Summary

Diabetic emergencies are common in medical practice. Consider hyperglycaemia in all patients who are hyperventilating, confused, comatosed or acidotic. Fluid replacement and intravenous insulin are the essential therapy.

Acute adrenal insufficiency should be suspected in any patient who has unexplained hypotension, mild hyponatraemia, corticosteroid therapy, pigmentation or preceding anorexia, nausea, vomiting and weight loss. The mainstay of therapy is to provide adequate inspired oxygenation and fluid replacement while increasing the serum glucose (if required) and providing intravenous hydrocortisone replacement.

> **Time Out 20.2**
>
> List the causes of:
> - **(i)** respiratory failure
> - **(ii)** cardiac failure
> - **(ii)** brain failure
> - **(iv)** renal failure
> - **(v)** liver failure
> - **(vi)** endocrine failure
>
> For each cause list the underlying problems, e.g. hypoxaemia, hypovolaemia.
> Note how common problems occur, irrespective of the cause, and how and when these problems will be treated in the initial assessment.

SUMMARY

Organ failure is a common medical emergency. Initial treatment is directed at the manifestations of failure, rather than at the underlying cause.

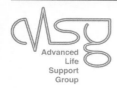
Advanced
Life
Support
Group

PART V
Special Circumstances

PART V

Special Circumstances

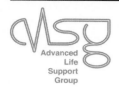
Advanced
Life
Support
Group

CHAPTER 21

The elderly patient

OBJECTIVES

After reading this chapter you will be able to understand:
- why age does not influence the structured approach to patient assessment
- how age influences homeostasis
- how age influences disease pathophysiology
- the special considerations that are needed when assessing and managing an acutely ill elderly patient.

INTRODUCTION

Defining 'elderly' is not easy. Some patients in their 60s are physiologically older than those in their 80s. In general, 'elderly' characteristics become more prevalent after the age of 75 years.

When the elderly become acutely unwell, assessment and treatment will follow the structured approach previously described. However, the elderly differ in a number of ways, which may affect presentation, assessment and treatment.

MULTIPLE CONDITIONS

The prevalence of most diseases increases with increasing age. The elderly, therefore, tend to have multiple conditions. In addition to any acute presenting problem, there are usually other coexisting chronic disorders. These make assessment more difficult and may influence prognosis and management.

> **Key point**
>
> Multiple pathology is the rule in the elderly

NON-SPECIFIC/ATYPICAL PRESENTATION

Illness in the elderly often presents with confusion, falls, immobility or incontinence, rather than the typical pattern seen in a younger population, e.g.:
- pneumonia is equally as likely to present with either confusion or pleuritic pain and breathlessness
- cardiac failure may present with confusion or falls rather than breathlessness.

Acute Medical Emergencies; The Practical Approach, 2nd edition.
Edited by Terence Wardle, Peter Driscoll, and Sue Wieteska.
© 2010 Blackwell Publishing Ltd.

The reasons for this are multiple. The physiological and pathological changes associated with ageing produce a reduction in physical and mental reserves. Under normal circumstances, the elderly person is able to function satisfactorily with these limited reserves, remaining mobile, continent and mentally clear. However, with the additional stress of an acute illness these abilities may be overcome. Consequently, confusion, falls, immobility and incontinence are common presenting features.

Acute myocardial infarction, pleurisy or acute abdominal emergencies may not present with pain in the elderly. Possible reasons for this include:
- reduced perception of visceral pain
- multiple pathology – diminished awareness of a symptom amongst a complex of symptoms
- associated mental impairment or communication difficulties.

Key point

Any acute medical problem in the elderly can present with confusion, falls, immobility or incontinence. An acute abdomen or acute myocardial infarction may be painless

---

POLYPHARMACY AND ALTERED DRUG HANDLING

Adverse drug reactions are an important cause of morbidity, even mortality, in older people.

Key point

Approximately one in ten older patients will experience an adverse drug reaction. This may either precipitate their admission to or follow treatment in hospital

---

Factors underlying adverse drug reactions are complex (see Fig. 21.1). Old people usually have multiple conditions which give more opportunity for prescribing and may lead to polypharmacy.

The elderly may have impaired hearing, eyesight, memory and manual dexterity which can affect their ability to follow a prescribed drug regime (reduced compliance).

Polypharmacy, especially if the drug regime is complex, is also associated with reduced compliance.

A number of changes in pharmacokinetics and pharmacodynamics occur with increasing age:
- Reduced renal clearance – increases the risk of toxicity for water-soluble drugs excreted by the kidney (especially digoxin, gentamicin).
- Reduced hepatic clearance – reduces first-pass metabolism for certain drugs, increasing the likelihood of adverse effects (important for propranolol and morphine). Reduced activity of hepatic mixed-function oxidase causes a decline in clearance of diazepam and chlordiazepoxide.

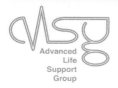

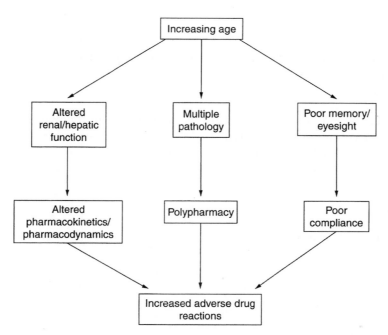

Fig. 21.1 Factors underlying adverse drug reactions in the elderly.

- Altered body composition – there is a relative increase in body fat and a reduction in body water (associated with a reduction in lean body mass) with increasing age. This results in a reduced volume of distribution for water-soluble drugs and an increased volume of distribution for lipid soluble drugs. Therefore, following a given dose of digoxin (based on body weight), a higher serum level is achieved in the elderly compared with the young. The increased volume of distribution for lipid soluble drugs (diazepam, chlordiazepoxide, thiopental) increases the amount of drug bound in body fat and increases the half-life of these drugs.
- Reduced protein levels – may be important with some drugs which bind to albumin.
- Increased sensitivity – has been demonstrated with opiates and benzodiazepines. The elderly require lower doses of warfarin to achieve anticoagulation, without any demonstrable changes in warfarin pharmacokinetics.

Some drugs which are commonly associated with adverse effects in the elderly include the following.

Digoxin

There is an age-related decline in renal function. Therefore, the body is less able to excrete digoxin and hence levels may rise. The levels required to produce both a therapeutic effect and toxicity are very close. Thus, there is a significant risk of toxicity with increasing age and any intercurrent illness.

The adverse effects of digoxin are multiple and may be life-threatening, e.g.:

- cardiac   arrhythmias
- gastrointestinal anorexia
                   nausea/vomiting
                   diarrhoea
- neurological   confusion/agitation
                   visual disturbance

> **Key point**
>
> Be suspicious of digoxin toxicity in any patient on digoxin who develops anorexia, vomiting or confusion

As a general rule, the elderly require a reduced loading dose of digoxin, because of the reduced volume of distribution (0.5 mg compared with 1.0 mg in younger patients). They also require a reduced maintenance dose (125 or 62.5 μg daily, compared with 250 μg in a younger patient), because of the reduced renal clearance. Estimation of serum digoxin levels is helpful.

Diuretics
Diuretics are commonly used in the elderly, often inappropriately (for leg oedema associated with venous stasis). Homeostatic mechanisms are less efficient (see later) than in younger patients. Thus, elderly patients taking diuretics are more prone to dehydration, metabolic disturbances and postural hypotension, especially when there is intercurrent illness.

Antihypertensives
The use of antihypertensives is increasing in the elderly. These drugs are more likely to cause adverse effects, particularly postural hypotension, because of impaired homeostasis.

Non-steroidal anti-inflammatory drugs
Non-steroidal anti-inflammatory drugs are responsible for a quarter to a third of hospital admissions for gastrointestinal bleeding in older people. They can cause renal failure, fluid retention and worsening of heart failure.

Sedatives and hypnotics
Drowsiness and falls are caused by sedatives and hypnotics. Their half-life tends to be prolonged (due to increased volume of distribution and reduced hepatic clearance of diazepam and chlordiazepoxide). The elderly are more sensitive to the effects of sedatives and hypnotics. Withdrawal reactions are common if these drugs are stopped abruptly. An acute confusional state a couple of days after admission may be the first indication that the patient had been taking sleeping tablets (or alcohol).

Antidepressants
Common side effects from tricyclic antidepressants include postural hypotension, confusion, dry mouth and urinary retention in males. The newer selective seretonin reuptake inhibitors antidepressants are less likely to cause side effects.

Major tranquillisers
Phenothiazines and haloperidol commonly cause side effects including drowsiness, unsteadiness, postural hypotension, constipation and drug-induced Parkinsonism.

Treatment for Parkinson's disease
Levodopa preparations are associated with a high prevalence of side effects, mainly postural hypotension, confusion and dyskinesia. Anticholinergic drugs are even more likely to cause confusion.

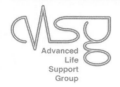

Advanced
Life
Support
Group

Key points

An accurate drug history is essential

Always be suspicious that any new problem may be a side effect of an existing medication, rather than an indication for additional drug therapy

The drug regime should be as simple as possible (in terms of the number and the frequency of dosing), to improve compliance and reduce the risk of adverse reactions

When introducing new drugs, start with a low dose and increase slowly. Review regularly. Always question whether a particular drug is needed. If it is, what would be the correct dose?

IMPAIRED HOMEOSTASIS

This is important in a number of ways. Postural hypotension due to impaired blood pressure control is mentioned in Chapter 12. Two other important areas are fluid and electrolyte imbalance and temperature homeostasis.

Fluid and electrolyte imbalance

A number of changes which affect sodium and water homeostasis occur with increasing age, increasing the risk of fluid and electrolyte disturbance. These changes include:

- a reduction in renal blood flow
- loss of nephrons
- impaired ability to:
  excrete an extreme sodium load
  conserve sodium and other electrolytes
  concentrate urine
  excrete a water load
- a decrease in total body water with age (associated with the reduction in lean body mass)
- decline in thirst with age
- reduction in the levels of plasma renin and aldosterone (although no changes in angiotensin II concentrations have been found). This probably contributes to the reduced ability to preserve sodium when necessary.

Fluid and electrolyte imbalance can be exacerbated by increased fluid loss (diarrhoea and/or vomiting) and reduced fluid intake (which is more likely to cause serious metabolic disturbance). Water replacement is less effective because of the reduced sensation of thirst. The elderly have impaired water conservation. In addition, the reduced total body water means the patient starts from a lower baseline and that dehydration occurs more readily.

Temperature homeostasis

Core body temperature is held within a narrow range around 37°C. Heat is generated in most tissues of the body and lost by radiation, convection, conduction and evaporation. The balance between heat production and heat loss is regulated by the hypothalamus.

If the core temperature rises, the hypothalamus is perfused by 'heated' blood and responds by causing cutaneous vasodilatation and sweating. This allows increased heat loss.

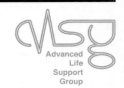

In contrast, if the core temperature falls, the hypothalamus increases core heat production (increased muscle tone with shivering) and reduces heat loss from the skin (cutaneous vasoconstriction). In the elderly, these processes are impaired because of:

- a delayed vasoconstrictor response to cold
- a smaller increase in metabolic heat production (probably due to the reduced muscle bulk)
- a decline in the perception of cold, which affects behavioural responses, e.g. wearing extra clothes, seeking shelter.

> **Key point**
>
> Homeostatic mechanisms are less efficient in the elderly. The stress of an acute illness or the effects of drugs are more likely to be associated with postural hypotension, fluid and electrolyte disturbance and disturbances of temperature control

The main clinical manifestation of impaired temperature homeostasis seen in the UK is hypothermia.

HYPOTHERMIA

Introduction

Hypothermia is defined as a core body temperature of 35°C or less. The true prevalence is unclear. Mortality is high, especially in the elderly, with estimates varying from 30 to 75%.

Multiple factors usually contribute to hypothermia. The elderly are at particular risk because of impaired temperature homeostasis. Other important factors include:

- physical – poor mobility, risk of falling
- social – living alone, inadequate heating
- medical conditions – affecting heat production, heat loss or temperature control
- drugs/alcohol – phenothiazines cause vasodilatation and act directly on the temperature control centre in the hypothalamus. Benzodiazepines, antidepressants and opioids act centrally and may increase the risk of falling
- Alcohol will predispose to hypothermia by inhibiting shivering, impairing hepatic gluconeogenesis and inducing peripheral vasodilatation.

The causes of hypothermia are listed in the next box.

Pathophysiology
Mild hypothermia (35–32°C)

The initial response to a fall in temperature is to increase the metabolic rate by shivering and to reduce heat loss by peripheral vasoconstriction. Even at this early stage, psychomotor function can be impaired especially in the elderly manifested by confusion, dysarthria and incoordination.

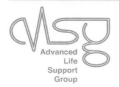

Causes of hypothermia

Excessive heat loss
  environmental exposure
  increased cutaneous blood flow
Inadequate heat production
  malnutrition
  hypoglycaemia
  hypothyroidism
  diabetic ketoacidosis
  adrenal insufficiency
  hepatic failure
  uraemia
Altered thermoregulation
  hypothalamic dysfunction
  spinal cord injury (T1 or above)
Drugs
  (i) Central effects
      alcohol
      phenothiazines
      barbiturates
      opioids
      benzodiazepines
  (ii) Peripheral vasodilatation
      alcohol
      phenothiazines

Moderate hypothermia (32–28°C)

As the core temperature falls below 32°C, cardiac conduction becomes impaired, heart rate falls and cardiac output decreases. Atrial fibrillation with a slow ventricular response is common. In addition, shivering stops and is replaced by hypertonia. Coma may develop.

Severe hypothermia (below 28°C)

There is a high risk of ventricular fibrillation. As the temperature continues to fall, hypotension results and eventually asystole occurs. In severe hypothermia, coma may be associated with a flat electroencephalogram, but this is not indicative of brain death and may be reversible.

In addition to these cardiovascular and neurological effects, hypothermia has other important effects.

Respiratory

Respiratory effects include tachypnoea in the early stages, followed by hypoventilation as hypothermia becomes more severe. Loss of cough and gag reflexes predispose to aspiration pneumonia.

Renal

A 'cold diuresis' occurs, due to increased central blood volume (peripheral vasoconstriction shunting blood from peripheral to central circulation). There may be additional sodium and water losses due to impaired function of epithelial transport mechanisms in the kidney. The result is severe volume depletion and hypotension.

Gastrointestinal

Hypomotility of the gastrointestinal tract is common. Gastric dilatation may occur, with increased risk of aspiration. Hypothermia may cause acute pancreatitis and acute peptic ulceration with haematemesis.

Haematological

The haemoconcentration associated with the reduced plasma volume may predispose to thrombotic complications. In addition, there may be bleeding problems. Clotting factors work less efficiently at lower temperatures and thrombocytopenia may occur due to sequestration of platelets.

Impaired oxygen delivery

As the temperature falls, the haemoglobin oxygen dissociation curve shifts to the left. Thus oxygen delivery to hypothermic tissues is impaired. However, hypothermia also reduces the tissues oxygen requirements.

Hyperglycaemia

Moderate to severe hypothermia inhibits the action of insulin. This leads to reduced glucose utilisation and hyperglycaemia.

Assessment

Primary assessment and resuscitation

Airway
- Airway may be obstructed due to depressed conscious level.

Breathing
- Respiratory rate is reduced with moderate/severe hypothermia.
- May be evidence of aspiration pneumonia (although slow shallow breathing may make clinical signs difficult to detect).

Circulation
- Check blood pressure. Treat hypotension due to hypovolaemia ('cold diuresis'). Fluid replacement has to be carefully controlled, as the cold myocardium does not tolerate excessive fluid loads.
- Check core temperature with a low reading thermometer or rectal thermocouple probe. Initiate rewarming measures.
- Check pulse for 60 s.
- ECG monitoring (risk of atrial fibrillation, ventricular fibrillation, asystole).

Disability
- Neurological dysfunction may be either the cause or the effect of hypothermia.
- Check glucose.

Rewarming

Rewarming techniques can be active or passive, and active rewarming can be external or internal. Which method is most appropriate will depend on a number of considerations including the degree of hypothermia, the rate of development of hypothermia, the age of the patient and the patient's cardiovascular status. A young person who is hypothermic due to cold exposure will usually tolerate rapid, active, surface rewarming. In contrast, this will lead to circulatory collapse in an elderly patient. An ideal rate of rewarming is 0.5°C/h. In the presence of

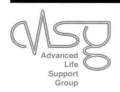

cardiac arrest, core temperature must be raised as rapidly as possible. However, if the patient does not have a life-threatening arrhythmia, interventions aimed at rapid rewarming should be used with caution to minimise the risk of precipitating arrhythmias.

> **Key point**
>
> **The hypothermic myocardium is very sensitive. Any physical manipulation of the patient (central lines, nasogastric tubes, endotracheal tubes, rapid rewarming techniques) increases the risk of developing ventricular fibrillation. This is resistant to defibrillation until the core temperature has risen to 32°C**

Passive rewarming

This uses the patient's own heat production to raise core temperature. Any wet clothing is removed and the patient is dried and then insulated with blankets. It is important to keep the head covered as up to 30% of body heat can be lost from this site. Warm humidified oxygen minimises respiratory heat loss.

Active external rewarming

Immersion in warm water (40°C) can be appropriate in conscious uninjured patients with a core temperature of greater than 30°C, where hypothermia has been of short duration and rapid onset. However, it is inappropriate and impractical for the majority of hypothermic patients. Circulating water blankets, electric blankets, warm air blankets and heating cradles are less efficient than warm water immersion but more practical. There are a number of potential dangers with active external rewarming.

When hypothermia has developed slowly and has been prolonged, there is hypovolaemia due to 'cold diuresis' and profound acidosis in the underperfused peripheral tissues. The vasodilatation caused by external heating may therefore cause hypotension and a metabolic acidosis. Active external rewarming also causes a significant 'afterdrop' in core temperature that can potentially trigger arrhythmias.

Active internal rewarming

Intravenous fluids should be heated to 40°C but their small volume means that they have a minimal effect on core temperature. Inspired humidified air heated to 42°C minimises respiratory heat loss but contributes little to active rewarming. Irrigation of hollow organs (stomach, bladder) and body cavities (pleura, peritoneum) with warm fluid (40°C) can be used in extreme conditions, such as cardiac arrest, but may need to be continued for several hours. Irrigation fluids should be isotonic and potassium free. Haemodialysis and cardiopulmonary bypass can bring about rapid rewarming but they require specialised skills and availability is limited.

Management of arrhythmias

Atrial arrhythmias are common and usually reversible with rewarming alone; specific antiarrhythmic therapy is rarely needed. Ventricular arrhythmias in the hypothermic patient are usually refractory to drugs and defibrillation. Antiarrhythmic drugs should not be used until the body temperature is normal. Below 32°C, defibrillation is unlikely to succeed. Therefore, the initial three cycles of shocks of the ventricular fibrillation algorithm should be given but, if

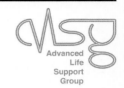

unsuccessful, further attempts should be withheld until the temperature is greater than 32°C. Repeated defibrillation in the hypothermic patient will simply cause myocardial damage.

It is difficult to distinguish reversible from irreversible hypothermia. Apnoea, asystole and absence of brain activity are usually signs of death but can also be present in severe reversible hypothermia. Patients should continue with cardiopulmonary resuscitation until a deep body temperature of at least 32°C has been achieved or the temperature has failed to rise despite effort. Only then can a definite diagnosis of death be made.

> **Key point**
>
> **The patient is not dead until both warm and dead**

Secondary assessment

In all hypothermic patients chest X-ray and 12-lead ECG are essential. ECG may show 'J' waves although they have no prognostic significance. Recheck urea and electrolytes, amylase and glucose, together with thyroid function, a drug screen and alcohol estimation. Arterial blood gases will need to be corrected for the low core temperature. Take blood cultures and start empirical broad-spectrum antibiotic therapy, as the usual signs of infection may be masked.

Once rewarming has been initiated and the patient stabilised, reassess for any underlying condition that may have precipitated the hypothermia.

> **Time Out 21.1**
>
> The percentage of elderly hospital admissions associated with drug side effects is:
> **a** 1%
> **b** 4%
> **c** 10%

> **Key points**
>
> **Hypothermia is a life-threatening condition**
> **Assessment and treatment follows the structured approach previously described**
> **The rate of rewarming needs to be adjusted according to the clinical situation**
> **Ventricular fibrillation or circulatory collapse can be precipitated by rapid**
>   **rewarming techniques**
> **The patient is not dead until both warm and dead**

SUMMARY

In the elderly patient:
- assessment follows the structured approach
- multiple conditions are common
- disturbances in mobility, mental function and continence are common presentations of many conditions.

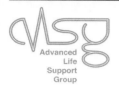

CHAPTER 22

Transportation of the seriously ill patient

OBJECTIVES

After reading this chapter you will be able to:
- discuss the principles necessary for the safe transfer and retrieval of critically ill patients
- describe the systematic 'ACCEPT' approach for managing such patients.

Key point

Transport is a potential period of instability

INTRODUCTION

There is an increasing need to transfer patients who are medically ill. Historically, patients are often transferred from home to hospital by ambulance and this will continue. However, with changes in the provision of health care more patients are being transferred because of the following:
- reduction in number of, and increased pressure on, hospital beds
- transfer for tertiary care, e.g. neurosurgery, cardiothoracic surgery
- the need for intensive care treatment, either supra-specialist care or because of a local shortage of beds.

Thus, it is common for patients to be transferred between hospitals, because of a bed shortage in one region or throughout the United Kingdom. It is important to remember that the transfer distance is irrelevant to the need for meticulous preparation before transfer. Movement from one ward to another is just as important, and can be associated with just as many problems as a transfer over 500 miles. Commonly reported problems are shown in the next box.

Most commonly reported adverse events

No capnography available (when clinically indicated, with potential for raised intracranial pressure)
Cardiovascular problems during transfer
    Tachyarrhythmias
    Bradycardias
    Hypotension
    Hypertension

Continued

Acute Medical Emergencies; The Practical Approach, 2nd edition.
Edited by Terence Wardle, Peter Driscoll, and Sue Wieteska.
© 2010 Blackwell Publishing Ltd.

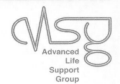

Most commonly reported adverse events (Continued)

Hospital equipment problems
   Monitor failure
   Pump failure
   Equipment not available
   Mechanical ventilator not available
Significant hypoxaemia
Ambulance breakdown/lost en route
Cardiac arrest in ambulance
Death during transfer

PRINCIPLES OF SAFE TRANSFER

The aim of a safe transfer policy is to ensure that there is continuing medical treatment for the patient without any detrimental effect. To achieve this, the **right** patient has to be taken at the **right** time, by the **right** people, to the **right** place by the **right** form of transport. This requires a systematic approach that incorporates a high level of planning and preparation before the patient is moved.

The systematic approach to patient transfer

A – assess the situation
C – control the situation
C – communication
E – evaluate the need for transfer
P – package and prepare
T – transportation

By following the ACCEPT approach, appropriate procedures are done in the correct order and are not forgotten. The acronym also emphasises the need for a great deal of preparation before the patient is transported.

ASSESSMENT

The initial clinician involved with patient management does not always accompany the patient during transfer. It is therefore important that the transportation procedure begins with assessing the situation. This is helped by answering several key questions.

Assessment questions

What are the patient's basic details?
What is the problem?
What has been done?
What was the effect?
What is needed now?

The clinician should also determine the lines of responsibility for the patient not only before transfer, but also during any future transportation. In practice,

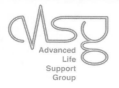

this responsibility is usually held jointly by the referring consultant clinician, the receiving consultant clinician and the transfer personnel. However, there should be a named person with overall responsibility to organise the transfer.

Conditions requiring transfer

There is an increasing need to transfer patients who require active resuscitation. Some of the more frequent medical conditions needing transfer between hospitals are listed in Table 22.1 (see over).

Potential problems during transfer

From the above list of conditions requiring transfer, one can predict potential problems that may arise – as in any clinical practice. For reference, these will be listed in the following seven boxes.

Potential respiration problems

Airway	Hypoxaemia
Breathing	Hypercarbia
	Severe bronchospasm
	Acute/chronic respiratory failure
	Respiratory arrest
Circulation	Cardiac arrest

Potential circulation problems

	Primary
Airway	Hypoxaemia
Breathing	Hypercarbia
Circulation	Myocardial infarction
	Dysrhythmia
	Cardiac failure (either left, right or biventricular)
	Rupture of papillary or ventricular muscle
	Cardiac tamponade
	Pulmonary embolus
Disability	Deterioration in Glasgow Coma Score
	Secondary
	Pain
	Peripheral embolus

Most cardiac patients requiring transfer will receive appropriate analgesia and anticoagulation or thrombolysis before transfer. The two most likely problems during transfer are either dysrhythmia, including cardiac arrest, or cardiac failure. Management of any dysrhythmia should follow the guidelines specified by the European and United Kingdom Resuscitation Councils (see Chapter 6). In contrast, the presence of cardiac failure would require treatment either with venodilators or inotropes (left or biventricular failure) or with a fluid challenge (right ventricular failure).

It is unusual for patients to develop these problems during transfer, as the potential for deterioration should have been recognised. Thus most patients at risk of these complications are sedated, paralysed and ventilated prior to transfer – but this is not always the case.

Table 22.1 Conditions requiring transfer

Respiration (AB)	Respiratory failure (to a respiratory physician, intensivist or *rarely* to an extracorporeal membrane oxygenation unit) • Acute severe asthma, chronic obstructive airways disease • Severe pneumonia • Adult respiratory distress syndrome
Circulation (C)	Critical ischaemic heart disease (to a cardiologist or cardiac surgeon) • Unstable angina, myocardial infarction • Heart failure, cardiogenic shock • Arrhythmia • Valvular or septal rupture Other cardiac disease (to a cardiologist) • Cardiomyopathy, myocarditis, pericarditis Critical vascular insufficiency (to a vascular surgeon) • Aortic aneurysm or dissection • Limb ischaemia
Nervous system (D)	Central nervous system failure (to a neurologist, neurosurgeon, spinal surgeon, stroke unit or psychiatric unit) • Intracerebral haemorrhage or infarction • Intracranial abscess, encephalitis or meningitis • Intracranial tumour or hydrocephalus • Spinal cord compression • Acute psychosis or suicidal behaviour Peripheral nervous system failure (to a neurologist) • Myasthenia gravis • Guillain-Barré syndrome (post-infectious polyneuropathy)
Metabolism/Excretion	Metabolic failure (to a renal, hepatic, gastrointestinal or endocrine unit) • Renal failure • Acute liver failure • Variceal or other gastrointestinal haemorrhage • Diabetic ketoacidosis or lactic acidosis • Thyrotoxicosis or other endocrine/metabolic derangement
Host defense	Infection (to an infectious diseases unit or ICU) • Septic shock including meningococcaemia • Specific infections Immune failure (to a specialist immunological unit, haematologist or oncologist) • Severe allergy or autoimmune process • Immune deficiency or marrow suppression Intoxication (to an ICU or specific poisons unit, e.g. hyperbaric unit) • Poisoning/Overdose • Carbon monoxide poisoning Immersion/Other environmental injury (to an ICU) • Near drowning • Hypothermia

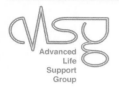

Patients with neurological conditions are commonly transferred to a tertiary referral centre, as most hospitals do not have the relevant facilities. The potential problems encountered are listed in the box.

Potential neurological problems

Airway	Hypoxaemia
Breathing	Hypercarbia
	Respiratory arrest
Circulation	Cardiac arrest
	Hypoglycaemia
	Hyponatraemia
Disability	Deterioration in Glasgow Coma Score
	Fit
	Subarachnoid haemorrhage

Similarly, most hospitals do not have facilities for managing patients with renal or hepatic disease. The relevant potential problems are listed in the next two boxes.

Potential renal problems

Airway	Hypoxaemia
Breathing	Hypoxaemia
Circulation	Hypovolaemia
	Fluid overload
	Hypertension
	Dysrhythmia
	Metabolic acidosis
	Hyperkalaemia
Disability	Deterioration in Glasgow Coma Score
	Fit

Potential hepatic problems

Airway	Hypoxaemia
Breathing	Hypercarbia
Circulation	Hypovolaemia: vasodilation
	Hyponatraemia
	Hypokalaemia
	Hypoglycaemia
	Lactic acidosis
	Dysrhythmia
	Haemorrhage
Disability	Deterioration in Glasgow Coma Score
	Fit

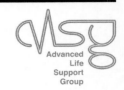

Two other groups of patients that often require transfer are those who have taken an overdose or who are septic and the associated problems are listed in the next two boxes.

Potential problems associated with a septic patient

Airway	Hypoxaemia
Breathing	Pulmonary oedema
Circulation	Hypovolaemia
	Haemorrhage
	Hypoglycaemia
	Disseminated intravascular coagulation
Disability	Reduced Glasgow Coma Score
	Fit

Potential problems associated with overdose

Airway	Hypoxaemia
Breathing	Hypercarbia
Circulation	Hypovolaemia
	Haemorrhage
	Hypokalaemia
	Hypotension
	Dysrhythmia
Disability	Reduced Glasgow Coma Score
	Fit

Although there is a broad spectrum of clinical conditions, there are clearly defined common potential problems, notably hypoxaemia, fluid balance, fitting, changes in Glasgow Coma Score and electrolyte disturbances. Thus, once the patient's condition has been stabilised, there are only a limited number of common complications. These will be prevented or reduced by ongoing treatment and monitoring. There are three major principles:

1 Do no further harm
2 Ensure ABCDE are maintained during transport
3 The most important assessment is the reassessment.

CONTROL

This comprises:
- identify the team leader
- identify the tasks to be done
- allocate tasks.

The person in charge needs to take control of the situation following the primary assessment (Chapter 3).

All immediately life-threatening conditions need to be identified and treated and the patient monitored. The responsible clinician should also decide the most appropriate place for further management, e.g. whether in the resuscitation room or ward, or whether to move the patient to an area in the hospital with greater resources.

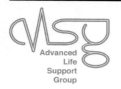

A common example of this is moving a patient from the ward to a high dependency unit.

The secondary assessment includes a head-to-toe survey, perusal of the medical notes and formulating a management plan by considering the clinical findings, response to treatment, and the results of any investigations. At the end of this phase, you should know whether transportation will be necessary and if so the ultimate destination.

COMMUNICATION

Moving critically ill patients from one place to another obviously requires the cooperation and involvement of several people. Therefore, key personnel need to be informed when transportation is being considered, as shown in the next box.

Communication

The patient's consultant
Your consultant (if different from above)
The intensive care unit consultant, where appropriate
The patient's relatives
The accepting consultant
Ambulance control
Special transportation controls (when appropriate)

It can be quite time consuming if all communication is delegated to one person. Therefore, delegate the tasks to appropriate people, taking into account their expertise and the local policies. In all cases, it is important that information is passed on clearly and unambiguously. This is particularly true when talking to people over the telephone. A useful tip is to plan what you wish to say before telephoning and use the systematic summary shown in the box.

Communication plan

Who you are
What is needed from the listener
What are the patient's basic details
What is the problem
What has been done
What was the response
What is needed

The second statement is repeated at the end to help summarise the situation and inform the listener what is required. The response to all these points should be documented in the patient's notes. The person in overall charge can then assimilate this information so that a proper evaluation of the patient's requirements for transportation can be made. In doing this, the clinician has to balance the risks involved in transfer against the risks of staying and the potential benefits of treatment from the receiving unit.

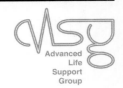

EVALUATION

Critically ill patients require transfer because of the need for:

- specialist treatment, such as haemodialysis
- specialist investigations unavailable in the referring hospital
- intensive care or high dependency unit facilities
- a bed.

Having identified the need for transfer, the responsible clinician has to triage the patient, considering their priority in relation to other patients on the intensive care or high dependency unit, the urgency of transfer and the nature of the medical support required. Following acute life-threatening illnesses or injuries, the patient may require urgent transfer after resuscitation, e.g. the movement of a patient with a subarachnoid haemorrhage to the neurosurgical centre. In contrast, patients with organ failure may require less urgent transfer to a tertiary hospital. Under these circumstances, it may be possible to use the transfer team from the specialist centre. On occasions, when empty beds are scarce, it is possible to transfer a less critically ill patient rather than the one currently being dealt with. This obviously requires formal triage of the patients involved and it needs to be done by the consultants in charge of their care.

Triage – categories of clinical urgency

Intensive
Time critical
Ill and unstable
Ill and stable
Unwell
Well

PREPARATION AND PACKAGING

Preparation: principles   stabilise patient
obtain and check all equipment
fully prepare transport personnel

Patient preparation

Key point

Inadequate resuscitation will result in problems during transfer

---

To avoid complications during any journey, meticulous resuscitation and stabilisation should be done **before** transfer. This may involve procedures requested by the receiving hospital or unit. The transferring team must also ensure that the patient's airway is assessed for patency and protection and appropriate respiratory support is being provided. In many cases, this will mean intubating the patient if it has not been done previously. Blood gases should be taken following this procedure, or after a change in ventilator setting, to make sure that the patient is maintaining an adequate PaO_2 (ideally more than 13 kPa) and $PaCO_2$ of 4.0–4.5 kPa.

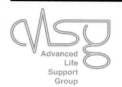

Advanced
Life
Support
Group

> **Key point**
>
> Remember a patient with pulmonary pathology may take up to 15–20 min to stabilise on a new ventilator or ventilator setting

The ventilator obviously needs to be portable. In addition, it must be able to provide the functions the patient requires. This includes variable FiO_2, inspiratory/expiratory ratio, respiratory rate, tidal volume and positive end expiratory pressure. For safety, there should also be a disconnect alarm and an ability to measure airway pressure. Those requiring intubation should be connected to an end tidal carbon dioxide monitor in addition to the basic monitoring equipment required for all critically ill patients.

> **Basic monitoring equipment**
>
> Pulse oximetry
> Suction
> ECG, defibrillator
> Blood pressure – preferably direct intra-arterial monitoring
> Thermometer
> Urinary catheter
> Naso/orogastric tube

Chest drains should be secured and unclamped with any underwater attachment replaced by a Portex drainage bag.

> **Key point**
>
> Before transfer, chest drains need to be inserted prophylactically if the patient has a simple pneumothorax or is at risk of developing one as a result of fractured ribs

Venous access is essential and preferably should be by two large bore cannulae. The patient must receive adequate fluid resuscitation to ensure optimal tissue oxygenation. Preferably, the haematocrit should be over 30%. In some patients inotropic support may also be necessary. Before transfer, invasive central monitoring may have been used to optimise volume replacement. During transfer, however, these lines become unreliable.

Appropriate drugs must be available to maintain the patient's airway, breathing and circulation. This may require infusion pumps (with a backup power source).

A urinary catheter is frequently necessary to monitor urinary output and for patient comfort.

The transfer team should confirm that all equipment is functioning, including battery charge status and oxygen availability, against what is calculated as necessary. The oxygen supply should be sufficient to last the maximum expected duration of the transfer, with a reserve of 1–2 h. There should also be a non-invasive blood pressure device and a self-reinflating bag (such as an Ambu Bag), so that resuscitation can be maintained in the event of either a power or gas failure. A member of the team should also be given the task of ensuring that all the patient's documents are taken.

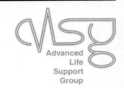

These include case notes, results of any investigations and the transfer form. All lines and drains should then be secured to the patient and the patient secured to the trolley. The trolley should then be secured to the ambulance and positioned such that all monitors are visible and lines are accessible.

Transport – time/mode

The choice of transport needs to take into account several factors.

Factors involved with transport

Nature of illness
Urgency of transfer
Mobilisation time
Geographical factors
Weather
Traffic conditions
Cost

Road ambulances are by far the most common means used in the United Kingdom. They have a low overall cost, rapid mobilisation time and are less affected by weather conditions. They also give rise to less physiological disturbance. Air transfer is used for journeys over 50 miles or 2 h in duration, or if road access is difficult.

Although this mode of transport is fast, this has to be balanced against the organisational delays and the inter-vehicle transfer at the beginning and end of the journey. Helicopters are used for distances of approximately 50–150 miles and are particularly useful when road or fixed winged air ambulances are not possible. They are, however, often cramped, noisy and uncomfortable. Fixed winged aircraft should ideally be pressurised and are used for transfers of distances greater than 150 miles.

Depending on the geographical location, other forms of transport are used, particularly outside the UK. These include anything from a boat to horseback.

Personnel

In addition to the ambulance crew, a minimum of two attendants should accompany a critically ill patient. One attendant should be an experienced medical practitioner who is competent in resuscitation and organ support. Ideally this doctor should have received training in intensive care and transportation medicine. The Intensive Care Society (ICS) recommend at least 2 years' experience in anaesthesia, intensive care medicine or other equivalent specialties. The clinician must be accompanied by another experienced attendant, who is usually a nurse. This person should be qualified with, ideally, 2 years' intensive care experience. All personnel should be competent in the transfer procedure and familiar with the patient's clinical condition. They should have adequate insurance to cover both death and disability occurring during transfer.

Personal equipment

In addition to the medical equipment described previously, the transfer team needs their own personal equipment.

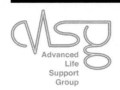

> **Personal equipment**
>
> P – phone
> E – enquiry number and name
> R – revenue
> S – safe clothing
> O – organised route
> N – nutrition
> A – A–Z
> L – lift home

This equipment will ensure that the journey is more comfortable and that a number of contingencies are available should problems occur. The telephone will enable direct communication with both the receiving and home unit. However, they should be given contact names and numbers before leaving. All personnel require appropriate clothing to ensure safety and enough money to enable them to get home should the ambulance be re-diverted to other duties. They also require a planned route and food if a long journey is envisaged.

TRANSPORTATION

Physiological problems during transfer can arise from both the patient's condition as well as the effects of movement. The latter include tipping, vibration, acceleration and deceleration forces, as well as barometric pressure and temperature changes seen with air transport. Adequate preparation can minimise many of these effects.

The standard of care and monitoring before transfer needs to continue. This will include SpO_2, ECG and arterial pressure monitoring. The end tidal carbon dioxide recording needs to be maintained in all patients who are intubated. Non-invasive arterial pressure monitor is sensitive to motion artefacts and, therefore, the intraarterial route is recommended. As mentioned previously, many of the central monitoring devices, such as central venous pressure or pulmonary artery wedge pressure, may be inaccurate due to movement of the ambulance.

The patient should be well covered and kept warm during the transfer. With ground transfer, road speed decisions depend both on clinical urgency and the availability of limited resources, such as oxygen (although the oxygen requirement should have been calculated as outlined above). Ambulance staff should therefore be advised whether a particularly smooth ride is required or a short journey time is important.

With adequate preparation, the transportation phase is usually incident free. Occasionally, untoward events occur; thus, the patient must be reassessed using the structured approach. Appropriate corrective measures should then be taken. This reassessment has to be thorough and cannot be done when faced with excessive vehicular motion. Therefore, in the case of land vehicles, ask the driver to stop at the first available place. Following such events, it is important to communicate with the receiving unit. They can then be adequately prepared and may be able to provide ongoing advice. Again this communication should follow the systematic summary described previously. A continuous record of the patient's condition during the transfer should be made. This can be helped by having monitors with memory functions, which can be accessed later.

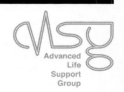

At the end of the transfer, the team should make direct contact with the receiving team. A verbal, succinct, systematic summary of the patient can then be provided. This must be accompanied by a written record of the patient's history, vital signs, treatment and significant clinical events during transfer. All the other documents which have been taken with the patient should also be handed over. Whilst this is going on, the rest of the transferring team can help move the patient from the ambulance trolley to the receiving unit's bed. A copy of the transfer sheet should then be handed over, with one copy retained by the transfer team who can then retrieve all their equipment and personnel for the return journey.

The data collection sheets should be subjected to regular audit by a designated consultant in each hospital. This will ensure transfers are appropriate and to the correct standards. Problems can also be addressed and corrected.

Time Out 22.1

A 27-year-old mechanic presented with an occipital headache. A clinical diagnosis of subarachnoid haemorrhage is confirmed by CT scan and lumbar puncture. The local neurosurgical centre is 30 miles away by road. The patient's vital signs are:

A – patent (FiO_2 0.85)
B – rate 14/min – no focal signs
C – sinus tachycardia 110/min BP 120/70
    (IV access secured)
D – GCS 15/15; PERLA, no lateralising signs glucose 7.0 mmol/l

Write down an outline of how you, as the doctor in charge, would arrange this patient's transfer to the neurosurgical centre.

SUMMARY

The safe transfer and retrieval of a patient requires a systematic approach. By following the ACCEPT method, important activities can be done at the appropriate time (see the STaR Transfer Master below).

STaR Transfer Master

Assessment	Problem (Sound bite)	
	Action	
	Effect	
	Next	
Control	Team members	Task
	1	Team leader
	2	Look after patient
	3	Communications
	4	Equipment collection
	5	Additional tasks

(*Continued*)

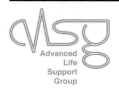

(Continued)

Communicate	Who are you	
	What is needed	
	Basic details	
	The problem (Sound bite)	
	Action (what has been done)	
	Effect (is it effective)	
	What is needed (repeated)	
Evaluate	Is the need agreed?	
	Triage = when (how soon) + mode + who (competencies)	

	MINT	
	M & N	**I** = (Equipment)
Preparation and package	PERSONAL	A
	Phone	
	Enquiry number	B
	Revenue	
	Safe clothing	C
	Organised route	
	Nutrition	D
	A to Z	
	Lift home	E
Transport	min...**T**	Handover (CLEAR)
		Case notes
		Laboratory
		Evaluation
		Audit
		Return equipment

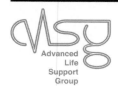
Advanced
Life
Support
Group

CHAPTER 23

The pregnant patient

OBJECTIVES

After reading this chapter you will be able to understand:
- the anatomical and physiological changes that occur during pregnancy
- how these changes may influence your initial assessment.

INTRODUCTION

Acute medical problems in the pregnant patient are rare. For that reason, the physician may feel apprehensive about the management of the acutely ill pregnant patient. This chapter will demonstrate that whilst there are significant physiological changes occurring in virtually every system of the body, pregnancy does not alter the initial assessment of the mother. These anatomical and physiological changes will be described and how these changes may influence the presentation, clinical features and detection of underlying conditions. A thorough understanding of the relationship between the mother and her fetus is essential.

Key point

Optimum treatment of the mother provides the optimum treatment for the fetus

---

ANATOMICAL AND PHYSIOLOGICAL CHANGES DURING PREGNANCY

These changes will be described and linked to the stages of the initial assessment.

Primary assessment
Airway–

The airway may be difficult to control due to neck obesity, breast enlargement and possible supraglottic oedema. There is an increased risk of aspiration, because of:
- increased incidence of gastro-oesophageal reflux
- delayed gastric emptying
- the pressure on the stomach from the gravid uterus.

Breathing–

Oxygen consumption is increased due to the metabolic demands of pregnancy. There is a physiological tachypnoea. As a result, hypocapnia is common. In particular in late pregnancy, diaphragmatic elevation results in a reduced functional residual capacity. This is offset by an increase in inspiratory capacity.

Acute Medical Emergencies; The Practical Approach, 2nd edition.
Edited by Terence Wardle, Peter Driscoll, and Sue Wieteska.
© 2010 Blackwell Publishing Ltd.

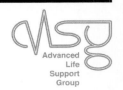

Circulation–
The heart rate increases gradually throughout pregnancy by approximately 10–15 beats/min, reaching a maximum in the third trimester. In contrast, the blood pressure falls by 10–15 mm Hg during the second trimester, returning to normal levels preterm.

Supine hypotension can occur as described above aggravated by the gravid uterus causing reduced venous return by compression of the vena cava. By the end of the first trimester, the cardiac output has increased by approximately 1.5 l/min, due to:
- an increase in plasma volume
- decreased vascular resistance of the uteroplacental unit.

Cardiac output may be significantly reduced in the supine position for reasons described earlier.

The effects of pregnancy on the results of initial investigations
The chest X-ray can show diaphragmatic elevation with increased lung markings and prominent pulmonary vasculature.

The ECG may appear unchanged during pregnancy, or the axis can be deviated to the left. Inferior T waves may appear flattened or inverted.

Plasma volume increases throughout pregnancy, with a smaller increase in red cell volume, thus there is a physiological anaemia. The white blood cell count can rise during pregnancy.

Fibrinogen levels are mildly elevated, but thrombin and activated partial thromboplastin times can be shortened. Antithrombin III levels are reduced while factors VII, VIII and IX are increased.

Levels of creatinine and urea are significantly reduced, because of an increase in glomerular filtration rate and renal blood flow. Glycosuria is common during pregnancy.

THE STRUCTURED APPROACH TO THE PREGNANT PATIENT

The initial assessment of the pregnant patient remains unchanged but particular attention has to be paid to prompt resuscitation, as the integrity of the fetus depends on optimum assessment and management of the mother. There are specific components that need special attention, especially after considering the changes described above. These are detailed below:
- Cricoid pressure during assisted ventilation and subsequent intubation reduces the risk of aspiration of gastric contents.
- Endotracheal intubation may be more difficult. The combination of neck obesity and breast enlargement may prevent the insertion of the laryngoscope. This problem can be overcome by detaching the blade, which is then placed in the patient's mouth and reattached to the handle. As always, early recognition of the likely need for urgent intubation allows time to alert an expert in advanced airway management, thus reducing the need for immediate intervention in a desperate situation that may have been avoidable.
- Be wary of using the physiological tachypnoea as a marker of shock, in particular in the third trimester.
- Be wary of hypotension in the second trimester. Supine hypertension (described above) can be rapidly relieved by placing a wedge under the patient's right hip manually displacing the uterus to the left, off the vena cava.

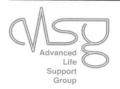

SPECIFIC MEDICAL EMERGENCIES IN PREGNANCY

Asthma

Asthma is the commonest chest disease in pregnancy. The acute management of this condition has already been described (Chapter 8) and no modification of this treatment is required in the acute phase. Both a pneumothorax and pneumomediastinum are rare complications of pregnancy, but are more common than in the non-pregnant state. They occur more commonly in labour, presumably due to raised intrathoracic pressure during straining, especially if there is an underlying lung condition.

The physical signs of a pneumothorax have already been described along with its subsequent management.

In contrast, a pneumomediastinum presents with chest pain and, if extensive, the patient may be shocked, due to tension pneumomediastinum. Most leaks are believed to follow rupture of an emphysematous bulla with air tracking into the mediastinum and subcutaneous tissues.

Chest X-ray features are diagnostic. Most leaks resolve spontaneously. Rarely, in the case of large airway leaks, thoracotomy may be required if the shocked patient does not respond to appropriate treatment.

Acute respiratory distress syndrome

This is a major cause of maternal mortality as it is the final common pathway for many obstetric complications. The overlap between the adult acute respiratory distress syndrome and the systemic inflammatory response syndrome has been described earlier in Chapter 10. The particular obstetric causes of this syndrome are listed in Table 23.1.

The management of these conditions has been described earlier, but often there is no treatment specific to the particular condition, e.g. amniotic fluid embolism.

Table 23.1 Obstetric causes of systemic inflammatory response syndrome

Aspiration of gastric content		Daily
Shock	Antepartum haemorrhage or postpartum haemorrhage	Weekly
Disseminated intravascular coagulation	Severe pre-eclampsia, amniotic fluid embolus, dead fetus syndrome, gram negative septicaemia,	Monthly
Infection	Acute pyelonephritis	Monthly
Hydatidiform mole		Annually

Pulmonary embolus

This is a major cause of maternal mortality. The diagnosis and management has been described in Chapter 8. However, particular points that are pertinent to the pregnant patient include the following:

• Pregnancy is a risk factor for venous thromboembolism.
• Stasis – the venous stasis in the lower limbs is caused by compression of the enlarging uterus. Increasing age and parity are important risk factors, as is caesarean section.
• Previous thromboembolism increases the risk of a similar problem during pregnancy.

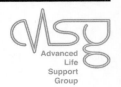

Other risk factors have been previously been described in Chapter 8.

The diagnosis of pulmonary embolus may be obvious clinically and be supported by appropriate clinical features, blood gas analysis and imaging.

However, massive pulmonary embolus has to be included in the differential diagnosis of shock. This has to be differentiated from an intra-abdominal cause of bleeding, especially if it occurs at the time of delivery. The latter will usually present with classic hypovolaemic shock, but remember that the relevant signs may be late in developing as the mother maintains her circulation at the expense of the fetus. The placenta is exquisitely sensitive to circulating catecholamines and rapid shut down of the uteroplacental unit will occur, jeopardising the fetus. Abdominal signs may also be present.

In contrast, the clinical features of pulmonary embolus may include signs of right-sided cardiac compromise, including a raised JVP, parasternal heave and a widely split second sound. According to the clinical picture, other less common conditions have to be considered in the shocked pregnant patient. These include dysrhythmia, myocardial infarction, pneumothorax/pneumomediastinum, aspiration of gastric contents and amniotic fluid embolism.

The management of pulmonary embolus in the pregnant patient does not differ from that described earlier. However, the clinical condition of the patient will dictate whether anticoagulation with heparin is appropriate. In the shocked patient, local facilities will dictate whether the management is thrombolysis or surgery. Subsequent treatment for the remainder of the pregnancy will be dictated by local protocol and discussion with the obstetrician and haematologist. Similarly, in patients who have known risk factors for thromboembolism, prophylaxis should be considered after discussion with a haematologist.

Heart disease in pregnancy

New onset of heart disease during pregnancy is rare. Patients with congenital heart disease will have been counselled carefully before pregnancy about potential problems and their solutions. Other cardiological conditions, including valvular disease, pre-existing cardiomyopathy and cardiac dysrhythmias are usually known before pregnancy and a careful management strategy is planned electively.

Occasionally, however, mitral stenosis may be detected for the first time during pregnancy. Management is unchanged from that described in Chapter 20. Digoxin and β blockers can be effective in controlling the ventricular rate. While diuretics can be used to reduce pulmonary oedema, it is important to avoid hypovolaemia.

Ischaemic heart disease is rare during pregnancy, but has a high mortality. Thrombolytic drugs are contraindicated in this situation.

Hypertension in pregnancy (and up to 2 weeks after delivery)

Hypertension in pregnancy can be caused by:
- pre-eclampsia syndrome due to the pregnancy
- pregnancy-induced hypertension which is transient, appears after midterm and resolves following delivery
- acute or chronic, pre-existing hypertension – classically towards the end of pregnancy
- due to an underlying medical condition not related to the pregnancy.

Thus all forms of hypertension in pregnancy, in particular those occurring after 20 weeks, should always be taken seriously. Diagnosis of the syndrome of

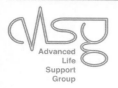

pre-eclampsia can be difficult. The risk factors for this condition are listed in the box below.

Risk factors for pre-eclampsia

Pregnancy
Multiple pregnancy
Age under 20 or over 35 years
Personal or family history of pre-eclampsia
Migraine
Pre-existing hypertension
Pre-existing renal disease

Clinical features of pre-eclampsia

- Hypertension
- Excessive weight gain
- Generalised oedema
- Ascites
- Epigastric pain
- Vomiting
- Hypertensive encephalopathy
- Cortical blindness

A patient with pre-eclampsia is usually asymptomatic. Epigastric pain suggests liver involvement. HELLP syndrome is a useful acronym to remember the components of haemolysis, elevated liver enzymes and low platelet count. However, none of the symptoms or signs are specific. Thus, the combination of hypertension, proteinuria and excessive weight gain should raise the suspicion of the pre-eclampsia syndrome. Not all of the clinical features listed above have to be present. Paradoxically, even hypertension and proteinuria do not appear to be essential components.

Clinical suspicion of pre-eclampsia syndrome can be supported by the results of the laboratory investigations, as listed in the box below.

Laboratory features of the pre-eclampsia syndrome

Proteinuria
Hyperuricemia
Hypocalcaemia
Thombocytopenia
Raised von Willebrand factor concentration
Reduced antithrombin III concentration
Haemolysis
Elevated liver enzymes – often with normal bilirubin

There are several important sequelae to the pre-eclampsia syndrome, most notably, tonic-clonic seizures or eclampsia(hence the use of the term pre-eclampsia). Other conditions are listed in the next box.

Sequelae to Pre-eclampsia

Tonic-clonic seizures
Cerebral haemorrhage
Cerebral oedema
Cortical blindness
Pulmonary oedema
Peripheral oedema
Acute respiratory distress syndrome
Disseminated intravascular coagulation
HELLP syndrome
Hepatic rupture or infarction
Renal cortical necrosis
Renal tubular necrosis
Fetal hypoxaemia/death

Key point

The sequelae to pre-eclampsia can arise before or after delivery

---

The management of pre-eclampsia syndrome is:

- Delivery – The placenta is the cause of the problem and therefore its removal is necessary.
- Control hypertension – this alone does not prevent the development of the pre-eclampsia syndrome. A variety of drugs are used according to local protocol. These may include hydralazine, labetalol and nifedipine. The complex nature of this syndrome often requires the involvement of multiple specialist colleagues.

Renal disease

This is uncommon in pregnancy. Acute renal injury is rare. It should be managed according to conventional guidelines, as described in Chapter 20. In late pregnancy in particular, this is usually associated with an underlying condition such as severe pre-eclampsia, eclampsia, prolonged intrauterine fetal death, amniotic fluid embolism or acute fatty liver.

Neurological problems

There is an increased incidence of ischaemic stroke during pregnancy and the puerperium. This is attributed to the mild hypercoagulable state that develops during the few weeks before and after delivery. This hypercoagulable state is attributed to the increased clotting factors, reduced level of antithrombin III and decreased fibrinolysis. However, it is important to exclude underlying procoagulant conditions, such as antithrombin III, protein C and protein S deficiencies, antiphospholipid antibodies, haemoglobinopathies and an underlying vasculitis. In young patients, an underlying cardiac cause, including embolic disease, has to be excluded.

In contrast, cerebral venous thrombosis occurs classically after delivery. The patient experiences a headache with progressive neurological deficit, fits and papilloedema. MRI is the investigation of choice.

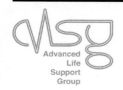

SUMMARY

Normal pregnancy results in changes in airway, breathing (manifest as tachypnoea) and circulation/cardiovascular (manifest as transient hypotension and tachycardia).

Haematological (physiological anaemia and a prothrombotic state) values also change.

Pregnancy is also a risk factor for conditions such as pre-eclampsia, eclampsia and amniotic fluid embolism. The gravid uterus and changes in the mother's body mass can cause mechanical complications, such as vena caval compression and airway management problems, which must be anticipated.

The potential effects of certain drugs on the fetus may need to be borne in mind when considering the risk-benefit ratio of some treatments.

However, in general, the principles of treatment remain the same as for the non-pregnant patient. Optimum treatment of the mother provides the optimum treatment for the fetus.

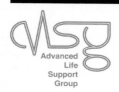

CHAPTER 24

The immunocompromised patient

OBJECTIVES

After reading this chapter you will be able to describe:
- why patients may have a compromised immune system and the infections they may incur
- a clinical approach to the immunocompromised patient.

SUSCEPTIBILITY TO INFECTION

Immunocompromised patients have alterations in phogocytic, humoral or cellular immunity that increase the risk of infection and reduce the ability to combat infection. Patient immunity may be impaired either temporarily or permanently due to:

- Immunodeficiency   congenital
                                    acquired (HIV)
- Immunosuppression   disease
                                    drugs
                                    radiation

The risk of infection is related to the:
- Cause (see box below)
- Duration
- Absolute neutrophil count (highest risk if neutrophils $<500/mm^3$).

High risk	**Haematological malignancies**
	AIDS patients with low CD4+ counts
	Bone marrow transplants
	Splenectomy/Splenic dysfunction
	Genetic disorders (e.g. severe compound immunodeficiency)
Intermediate risk	**Solid tumours/Chemotherapy**
	HIV/AIDS
	Solid organ transplant
Low risk	**Long-term corticosteroid use**
	Diabetes mellitus

CAUSE OF INFECTION

This will vary according to:
- Type of immunosuppression
- Degree of immunodeficiency
- Duration of immunodeficiency

Acute Medical Emergencies; The Practical Approach, 2nd edition.
Edited by Terence Wardle, Peter Driscoll, and Sue Wieteska.
© 2010 Blackwell Publishing Ltd.

Remember that as the immune system is impaired more than one organism/infection may be present. Hence a wide range of organisms can cause infection including:

- opportunistic organisms
- commensals
- *Candida albicans*
- *Cyclomegalovirus*
- nosocomial infections.

PRIMARY ASSESSMENT

This follows the structured ABC approach.

Particular importance must be placed on:

- universal precautions
- hypoxaemia due to pulmonary infections such as Pneumocystis Jiroveci
- shock due to volume depletion (e.g. increased insensible losses), poor diabetic control, fever, sepsis, haemorrhage
- confusion/focal neurological signs due to causes listed above
- sepsis, hypoglycaemia, intra-cranial infections
- fever. This is often the only symptom of infection and there is no pattern/periodicity.
- a thorough search of the skin and mucous membranes is essential for any clues/evidence of a rash.

Key point

A severely immunocompromised patient can have overwhelming infection without a fever

---

In addition to oxygen, fluids and other components of resuscitation, the following should be considered:

- manage in isolation
- intravenous broad-spectrum antibiotics – according to local policy
- antifungal agents to either treat or prevent secondary infection
- early liaison with specialists in microbiology, haematology, infectious diseases according to the clinical picture.

Investigations

The history and examination findings will govern the samples required including:

Blood	for bacterial cultures, atypical and viral serology, fungal cultures
Urine	gram stain culture, virology, antigens (e.g. legionella)
Stool	microscopy, cysts, ova, parasites
Nasal/throat swabs	culture
Sputum	culture, microscopy
Cerebrospinal fluid	culture, microscopy, cell count, PCR

SECONDARY ASSESSMENT

This should follow the usual format of:

1 'Phrased' history with particular reference to:
- underlying diseases

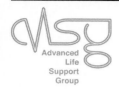

- previous surgery
- use of illicit drugs
- sexual history
- travel history
- alcohol use
- prescribed drugs
- nutrition
- immunisations
- chemoprophylaxis
- family history.

2 Thorough physical examination to identify:
- site of infection
- clues to the underlying cause.

Key point

The immunocompromised patient should be examined thoroughly every day

---

SUMMARY

The immunocompromised patient often presents as a medical emergency. Assessment should follow the structured approach. The common cause is immunosuppression (including chronic disease, malignancy and associated chemo/radiotherapy) and acquired immunodeficiency (including HIV). Severe neutropenia is the greatest risk factor. Early empirical treatment with antibiotics and antifungals is required as is early specialist consultation.

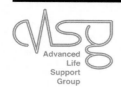

CHAPTER 25

The patient with acute spinal cord compression

OBJECTIVES

After reading this chapter you will be able to:
- understand why the diagnosis of acute spinal cord compression is delayed
- how to make this diagnosis earlier
- list the clinical features and underlying conditions associated with spinal cord compression
- describe the principles of management.

INTRODUCTION

This common condition often results in significant morbidity as the diagnosis is often delayed. A high index of suspicion is needed especially for patients with malignancy and back pain. The prognosis for recovery depends on the:
- severity of neurological deficit
- duration of deficit.

PATHOPHYSIOLOGY

The spinal cord is enclosed by a protective ring of bones, the vertebral column. Each bone comprises the vertebral body anteriorally and the lamina, pedicles and spinous process posteriorly. The spinal cord, covered by the thecal sac, extends from the base of the skull to the level of the first lumbar vertebra where it continues as the cauda equina, which is surrounded by cerebrospinal fluid. The thecal sac comprises the outermost layer is the dura and between the dura and the bone is the epidural space which normally contains fat and the venous plexus.

Causes of spinal cord compression
- Neoplastic   secondary = commonest
- Degenerative
- Trauma
- Inflammation   rheumatoid disease
- Infection   vertebral osteomyelitis (intraspinal)
- Haematoma   rare

Malignant spinal cord compression from secondary deposits is the commonest cause and is also a common complication of cancer affecting 5% of patients (bronchus, breast, renal, gastrointestinal, prostate, myeloma). The thoracic spine is most frequently involved (60%; lumbar-sacral 30%; cervical 10%) and arterial seeding of the bone probably accounts for most cases.

Acute Medical Emergencies; The Practical Approach, 2nd edition.
Edited by Terence Wardle, Peter Driscoll, and Sue Wieteska.
© 2010 Blackwell Publishing Ltd.

CLINICAL FEATURES

> **Key point**
>
> Early, prompt recognition is crucial to improve outcome

- Pain
- Weakness
- Numbness
- Loss of bladder and bowel function
- Ataxia

Pain is usually the first symptom in over 90% of patients and precedes neurological symptoms by 2 months. The pain is initially local, then radicular and is often worse on sitting.

Weakness is present in approximately 75% of patients. The pattern of weakness reflects the level of cord compression, e.g. above the conus will be pyramidal and symmetrical (affecting the corticospinal tract) involving preferentially, the flexors in the legs (and extensors in the arms if above the thoracic spine).

With cauda equina lesions the reflexes in the legs are reduced. Occasionally an isolated motor radiculopathy occurs with a lateral epidural deposit.

Numbness is ascending and nearly as common as weakness. When a sensory level is present it is often one to five levels below the level of the cord compression. Sensory loss in a 'saddle' distribution is common in cauda equina lesions. In contrast, lesions above the cauda equina result in sacral sparing (to pinprick). Sensory loss can also occur in a radicular distribution.

Loss of bladder and bowel function is usually a late finding due to an autonomic neuropathy.

Ataxia consider spinal cord compression in any patient with symptoms and signs of suspected or diagnosed malignancy who has back pain and an ataxic gait.

PRIMARY ASSESSMENT AND RESUSCITATION

Airway and cervical spine, are assessed and managed according to the details in Chapter 3, 'C' spine immobilisation is of paramount importance when pathology is suspected. If in doubt, always seek expert help from colleagues in emergency medicine and orthopaedics.

Breathing is rarely a problem unless the cord compression is marked and either above C6, potentially effecting the diaphragm (C3, 4, 5 – phrenic nerve), or proximal to the thoracic spine affecting intercostal muscles.

Circulation is assessed as described in Chapter 3. Particular potential 'C' problems include sepsis, autonomic dysfunction associated with malignancy and the numerous issues associated with 'trauma'. Although this topic is far too extensive to be considered in this manual, the management principles for shock are the same as those described in Chapters 3 and 9.

Disability is rarely a problem unless the following occur:
- Coexisting intracranial pathology (e.g. metastases)
- Metabolic sequelae to malignancy (e.g. hypercalcaemia, hyponatraemia, hypoglycaemia)
- Drug effects.

Exposure problems are rare, but pressure sores and associated sepsis should be actively sought.

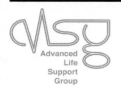

The other important management issue, although not resuscitation, is adequate analgesia. This not only is humane but will facilitate clinical examination and subsequent treatment.

The initial investigations have already been considered in detail (Chapters 3, 7, 9, 12 and 19). Magnetic resonance imaging is the modality of choice. CT with CT myelography is quicker but does not demonstrate clearly the spinal cord or epidural space. In contrast, MR produces excellent, accurate images of the cord and intramedullary pathology. It is also more sensitive than radioisotope bone scans at detecting bone metastases. However, MR is less likely to be well tolerated due to the duration of the scan. These tests are complimentary and the choice will depend on clinical need, patient preference, expert advice and the presence of 'metal implants'.

DIFFERENTIAL DIAGNOSIS

- Musculoskeletal pain
- Disc disease
- Spinal stenosis
- Spinal epidural abscess
- Vertebrae metastases without epidural extension
- Intramedullary metastases
- Malignant meningitis
- Malignant polyneuropathy

Management

Early referral to neurosurgery is essential. The precise management plan will vary according to the underlying cause, duration of symptoms/signs and the results of imaging.

There are some general principles:
- Pain management – usually opiates. Steroids may be beneficial in patients with malignancy
- Bed rest
- Anticoagulation – especially for patients with reduced mobility and cancer.
- Prevention of constipation – constipation can be due to limited mobility, analgesia, hypercalcaemia and autonomic dysfunction.

SUMMARY

Acute spinal cord compression is a relatively common condition. The diagnosis is often delayed. A high index of suspicion is needed in susceptible patients – especially those with malignant disease. Back pain is the cardinal feature, along with weakness, numbness, loss of bowel and bladder function. Early referral to a neurosurgeon is crucial to improve outcome.

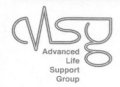
Advanced
Life
Support
Group

PART VI

Interpretation of Emergency Investigations

PART VI.

Interpretation of Emergency Investigations

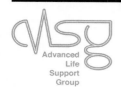

CHAPTER 26

Acid–base balance and blood gas analysis

OBJECTIVES

After reading this chapter you will be able to:
- describe the meanings of the common terms used in acid–base balance
- describe how the body removes carbon dioxide and acid
- explain the causes of an increased anion gap
- understand the system for interpreting a blood gas result.

TERMINOLOGY

It is important to understand the meaning of the terms commonly used when discussing acid–base balance.

Acids and bases

Key point

An acid is any substance which is capable of providing hydrogen ions (H^+)

Originally the word **'acid'** was used to describe the sour taste of unripe fruit. Subsequently many different meanings have led to considerable confusion and misunderstanding. This was not resolved until 1923 when the following definition was proposed.

A strong acid is a substance that will readily provide many hydrogen ions and conversely, a weak acid provides only a few. In the body we are mainly dealing with weak acids such as carbonic acid and lactic acid.

The opposite of an acid is a **base** and this is defined as any substance that 'accepts' hydrogen ions. One of the commonest bases found in the body is bicarbonate (HCO^{3-}).

The pH scale, acidosis, acidaemia, alkalosis and alkalaemia

The concentration of hydrogen ions in solution is usually very small, even with strong acids. This is particularly true when dealing with acids found in the body where the hydrogen ion concentrations are in the order of 40 nmol/l.

Key point

A nanomole = 1 billionth of a mole

Acute Medical Emergencies; The Practical Approach, 2nd edition.
Edited by Terence Wardle, Peter Driscoll, and Sue Wieteska.
© 2010 Blackwell Publishing Ltd.

To place this low concentration in perspective compare it with the concentration of other commonly measured electrolytes. For example, the plasma sodium is around **135 mmol/l**, i.e. 3 million times greater!

Dealing with such very small numbers is obviously difficult and so in 1909 the pH scale was developed. This scale has the advantage of being able to express any hydrogen ion concentration as a number between 1 and 14 inclusively. The pH of a normal arterial blood sample lies between 7.36 and 7.44 and is equivalent to a hydrogen ion concentration of 44–36 nmol/l respectively.

It is important to realise that when using the pH scale, the numerical value **increases** as the concentration of hydrogen ions **decreases** (Fig. 26.1). This is a consequence of the mathematical process that was used to develop the scale. Therefore an arterial blood pH below 7.36 indicates that the concentration of hydrogen ions has increased from normal. This is referred to as an **acidaemia**. Conversely, a pH above 7.44 would result from a reduction in the concentration of hydrogen ions. This condition is referred to as an **alkalaemia**.

In contrast, acidosis and alkalosis are terms used to denote the initial acid base disturbance at cellular level that if uncorrected would result in acidaemia and alkalaemia respectively.

Another important consequence of the derivation of the pH scale is that **small changes in pH mean relatively large changes in hydrogen ion concentration**; e.g. a fall in the pH from 7.40 to 7.10 means the hydrogen ion concentration has risen from 40 to 80 nmol/l; i.e. it has doubled.

Key point

Small changes in the pH scale represent large changes in the concentration of hydrogen ions

---

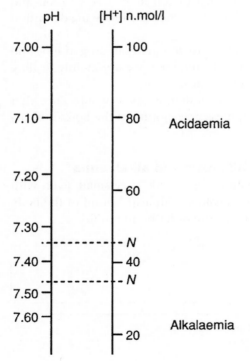

Fig. 26.1 The hydrogen ion scale.

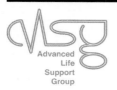

Summary

- Hydrogen ions are only present in the body in very low concentrations.
- As the hydrogen ion concentration increases the pH falls.
- As the hydrogen ion concentration falls the pH rises.
- An acidaemia occurs when the pH falls below 7.36 and an alkalaemia occurs when it rises above 7.44.

Buffers

Many of the complex chemical reactions occurring at a cellular level are controlled by special proteins called enzymes. These substances can only function effectively at very narrow ranges of pH (7.36–7.44). However, during normal activity the body produces massive amounts of hydrogen ions, which if left unchecked would lead to significant falls in pH. Clearly a system is required to prevent these hydrogen ions causing large changes in pH before they are eliminated from the body. This is achieved by 'buffers'. They 'take up' the free hydrogen ions in the cells and blood stream, thereby preventing a change in pH.

There are a variety of buffers in the body. The main intracellular ones are proteins, phosphate and haemoglobin. Extracellularly there are also plasma proteins and bicarbonate. Proteins 'soak up' the hydrogen ions like a sponge and transport them to their place of elimination from the body, mainly the kidneys. In contrast, bicarbonate reacts with hydrogen ions to produce water and carbon dioxide.

$$H^+ + HCO_3^- \Leftrightarrow H_2O + CO_2$$

The carbon dioxide is subsequently removed by the lungs.

With these common terms defined, let's consider why people can become acidaemic and how this can be corrected by the body.

ACID PRODUCTION AND REMOVAL

All of us, whether we are healthy or ill, produce large amounts of water, acid and carbon dioxide each day. A healthy adult will normally produce 1,5000,000 nmol of hydrogen ions each day as waste products generated when food is metabolised to release energy. This process occurs at a cellular level where these products initially accumulate. If this were left unchecked irreparable cellular damage would result.

The first acute compensatory mechanism is the intracellular buffering system. As described previously, this provides the cell with a temporary way of minimising the fluctuations in acidity. Subsequently, these waste products (i.e. carbon dioxide and hydrogen ions) are excreted into the blood stream where they are taken up by the extracellular buffers (Fig. 26.2).

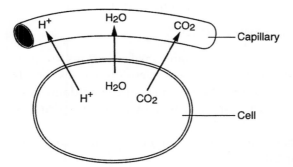

Fig. 26.2 Removal of waste products from cells.

However, this is only a temporary solution because there is only a limited amount of buffer. If this was the sum total of the body's defence to carbon dioxide and acids then the buffers would soon be saturated. Hence, a system is needed to remove these harmful substances from the body so that they do not reach toxic levels and, at the same time, regenerate the buffers. Fortunately, the body can eliminate these waste products removed mainly by the lungs and the kidneys.

Carbon dioxide removal (the respiratory component)

Carbon dioxide (CO_2) released from cells is transported in the blood to the lungs after diffusing into the alveoli is removed from the body during expiration (Fig. 26.3).

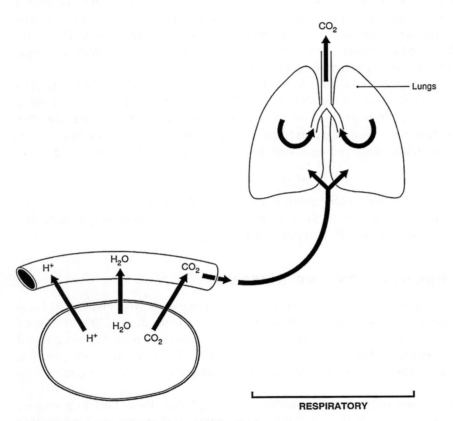

Fig. 26.3 Removal of carbon dioxide by the lungs.

If carbon dioxide production is faster than elimination or there is a blockage to its removal, then it will accumulate in the blood stream. In the plasma CO_2 reacts with water to produce hydrogen ions (H^+) and bicarbonate (HCO_3^-):

$$CO_2 + H_2O \Leftrightarrow H^+ + HCO_3^-$$

The greater the amount of carbon dioxide, the more hydrogen ions are produced. If this increase in plasma concentration of hydrogen ions causes the pH to fall below 7.36 then an acidaemia occurs. As the cause of the **acidaemia** in this case is a problem in the respiratory system, it is known as a **respiratory acidaemia**.

If a sample of arterial blood was taken immediately this occurred then the result given in Table 26.1 would be obtained.

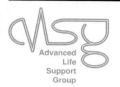

Table 26.1 Effect of a respiratory acidosis on blood gas analysis

	Normal	Respiratory acidaemia
pH	7.36–7.44	↓
PaCO$_2$	4.7–6.0 kPa	↑
	35–45 mm Hg	
Actual HCO$_3$$^-$	21–28 mmol/l	↑

Immediately after a rise in carbon dioxide the pH falls as H$^+$ ion concentration rises. There is a small rise in the concentration of actual bicarbonate.

As a by-product of the reaction between carbon dioxide and water, the actual bicarbonate concentration also increases by the same amount as the hydrogen ions. However, this increase is usually in the order of several nanomoles. As the normal concentration is 21–27 mmol (i.e. 21,000–27,000 nmol) the net increase in actual bicarbonate is very small. Consequently these changes in concentration are enough to change the pH scale but are not large enough to alter significantly the plasma bicarbonate concentration.

In a normal person at rest, the respiratory component will excrete at least 1,2000,000 nmol of hydrogen ions per day. It is therefore easy to see that there can be a rapid onset of acidosis during episodes of hypoventilation.

Acid removal (the metabolic component)

Acids are continuously produced as a result of cellular metabolism. The amount produced from normal metabolism is approximately 3,000,000 nmol/day. This acid load is soaked up by buffers in the blood stream so that they can be transported safely for elimination (Fig. 26.4).

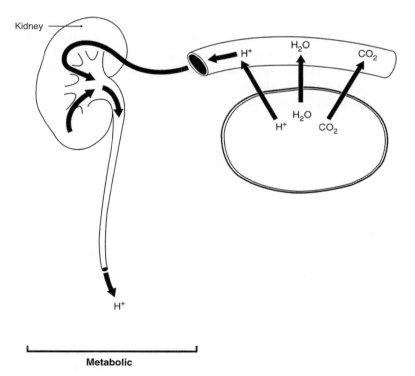

Fig. 26.4 Removal of hydrogen ions by the kidney.

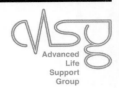

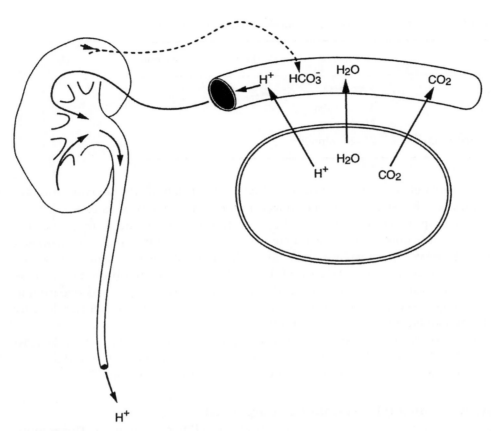

Fig. 26.5 Release of bicarbonate into the blood.

One of the buffers is bicarbonate. This is generated by the kidneys and released into the blood stream where it reacts with free hydrogen (Figure 26.5).

In certain circumstances, so much acid is produced by the cells that it exceeds the capacity of the protein buffers and bicarbonate. If this results in an accumulation of free hydrogen ions in the plasma so that the pH falls below 7.36 then an **acidaemia** has been produced. As this is a result of a defect in the metabolic system, it is termed a **metabolic acidaemia**.

If a sample of arterial blood was taken when this occurred then the result given in Table 26.2 would be obtained.

Table 26.2 Effect of a metabolic acidaemia (1)

	Normal	Metabolic acidaemia
pH	7.36–7.44	↓
$PaCO_2$	4.7–6.0 kPa	
	35–45 mm Hg	
Actual HCO_3^-	21–28 mmol/l	↓

An increase in carbon dioxide is too small to be observed because it is of the same order of magnitude as the increase in free hydrogen ion concentration, i.e. in nmol/l.

The actual bicarbonate level has fallen as a consequence of reacting with the free hydrogen ions to produce carbon dioxide and water. However, as noted

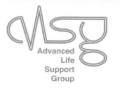

previously, this concentration is also affected by respiration. It follows that this concentration represents the effects of both the metabolic and respiratory systems. What is required therefore is a measure of the bicarbonate concentration resulting from only the metabolic system. This is why the blood analyser will also give a standard bicarbonate concentration as well (see results in Table 26.3).

Table 26.3 Effect of metabolic acidaemia (2)

	Normal	Metabolic acidaemia
pH	7.36–7.44	↓
$PaCO_2$	4.7–6.0 kPa	4.7–6.0 kPa
	35–45 mm Hg	35–45 mm Hg
Actual HCO_3^-	21–28 mmol/l	↓
Standard HCO_3^-	21–27 mmol/l	↓

The standard bicarbonate is an estimate of what the bicarbonate concentration would be, if the $PaCO_2$ were in the middle of the normal range. In other words, the contribution of any respiratory abnormality to HCO_3^- ion concentration is removed.

Base excess and base deficit

Both base excess and deficit are equivalent to the standard bicarbonate as another estimate of the contribution of the non-respiratory component to acid–base regulation; i.e. how much excess base (alkali) would be in the body if the $PaCO_2$ were in the middle of the normal range.

However, the difference from standard bicarbonate is that base excess and deficit take into account all the buffers in the blood sample and are considered a more accurate assessment of the metabolic component of acid–base status.

It follows that a **base excess** of 3 mmol/l means that 3 mmol of a strong acid had to be added to each litre of the original sample to get the pH to 7.4, with temperature kept at 37°C, and $PaCO_2$ kept at 5.3 kPa (40 mm Hg). Conversely a **base deficit** of 3 mmol/l means that 3 mmol of a strong base had to be added to each litre of the original sample to get the pH to 7.4 under the same conditions mentioned above.

For simplicity, many laboratories only use the term 'base excess'. A **negative** base excess is equivalent to base deficit. With the above examples, a base deficit of 3 mmol/l would be reported as a base excess of −3 mmol/l, and a true base excess of 3 mmol/l would be reported as a base excess of +3 mmol/l. The normal range of values for a base excess described in this way is −2 to +2 mmol/l.

> A base excess below −2.0 mmol/l indicates that there is a metabolic acidosis in the metabolic component to the acid–base balance.
> A base excess above +2.0 mmol/l indicates that there is a metabolic alkalosis in the metabolic component to the acid–base balance.

Considering these points it is possible to understand the results from the blood gas analysis of the respiratory and metabolic acidaemia cases discussed previously:

Respiratory acidaemia: see Table 26.4

Table 26.4 Effect of respiratory acidaemia

	Normal	Respiratory acidaemia
pH	7.36–7.44	↓
$PaCO_2$	4.7–6.0 kPa	↑
	35–45 mm Hg	
Actual HCO_3^-	21–28 mmol/l	↑
Standard HCO_3^-	21–27 mmol/l	–
Base Excess	−2 to +2 mmol/l	–

Metabolic acidaemia: see Table 26.5

Table 26.5 Effect of metabolic acidaemia

	Normal	Metabolic acidaemia
pH	7.36–7.44	↓
$PaCO_2$	4.7–6.0 kPa	4.7–6.0 kPa
	35–45 mm Hg	35–45 mm Hg
Actual HCO_3^-	21–28 mmol/l	↓
Standard HCO_3^-	21–27 mmol/l	↓
Base Excess	−2 to +2 mmol/l	↓

Summary

- CO_2 and metabolic acids are continuously produced by cell metabolism.
- The body has two methods of removing these waste products of metabolism and thereby maintain acid–base balance.
- Removal of CO_2 by the lungs regulates the respiratory component of the body's acid–base status.
- Excretion of H^+ ions and generation of HCO_3^- ions by the kidney are the main regulators of the metabolic component of acid–base balance.
- The actual bicarbonate concentration depends on both the respiratory and metabolic systems. In contrast, the standard bicarbonate and base excess are dependent only on the metabolic system.

The respiratory–metabolic link

The body therefore has two distinct methods of preventing the accumulation of hydrogen ions and the subsequent development of an acidaemia. As a further protection these two components are in balance (or equilibrium) so that each can **compensate** for a derangement in the other.

This link between the respiratory and metabolic systems is due to the presence of **carbonic acid** (H_2CO_3) (Fig. 26.6). The ability for each system to compensate for the other becomes more marked when the initial disturbance in one system is prolonged.

The production of carbonic acid depends on an enzyme called carbonic anhydrase that is present in abundance in the red cells and the kidneys. It is therefore ideally placed to facilitate the link between the respiratory and the metabolic systems.

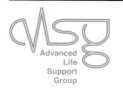

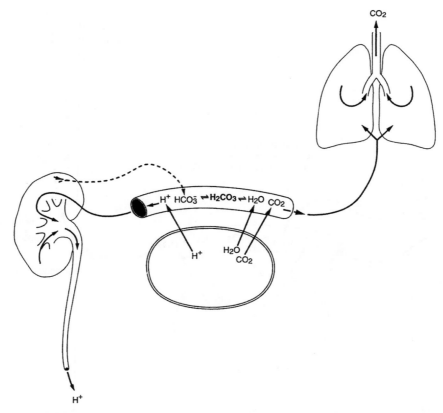

Fig. 26.6 Carbonic acid–bicarbonate buffers: acid production and its removal.

Let us consider how this link can help the body respond to an excess of either carbon dioxide or acid.

Example 1

In a patient with inadequate alveolar ventilation, e.g. chronic bronchitis, carbon dioxide accumulates. This will tend to cause a respiratory acidosis. Rather than the body existing in a chronic state of acidosis, the metabolic system can help compensate by increasing bicarbonate production by the kidneys. Using the carbonic acid link enables the removal of some of the excess carbon dioxide (Fig. 26.7 – see page 396). However, this takes several days to become effective as it depends on the increased production of enzymes in the kidney.

It is important to realise that in the acute situation **the body does not fully compensate**. Consequently, if an arterial blood sample is taken at this time, it will demonstrate that there is still a persistent but slight underlying acidaemia (Table 26.6).

Table 26.6 Underlying acidaemia

	Normal values	Effect of a respiratory acidaemia	Effect of metabolic compensation
pH	7.36–7.44	↓↓	↓
$PaCO_2$	4.8–5.3 kPa	↑	↑
	36–40 mm Hg		
Standard HCO_3^-	21–27 mmol/l	N	↑↑
Base excess	± 2 mmol/l	N	↑↑

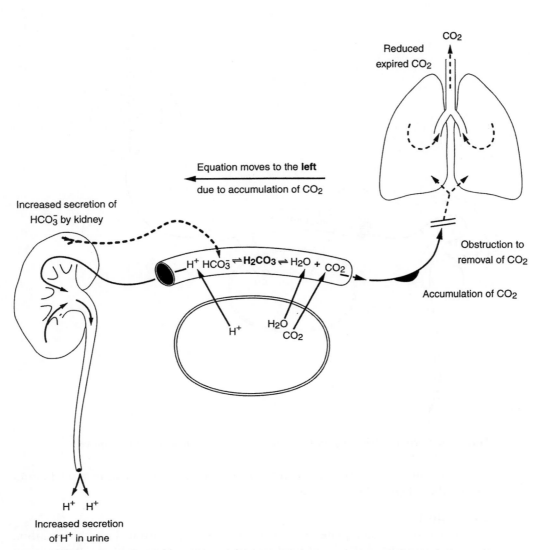

Fig. 26.7 Metabolic compensation for a respiratory acidosis (i.e. the metabolic system is compensating for the respiratory system).

Example 2

Diabetic patients sometimes develop a state of excess acid production known as **diabetic ketoacidosis**. The excess cellular acid is released into the plasma to be transported to the kidney for excretion. However, the kidneys are only able to excrete the additional acid load slowly and a metabolic acidosis develops. The kidneys are slowly stimulated to increase bicarbonate production. This will counteract the acidaemia but it takes several days. In the meantime, because of the carbonic acid link, some of the excess acid can be converted to carbon dioxide and eliminated by the respiratory system (Fig. 26.8).

This compensation occurs quickly because excess hydrogen ions are detected by special receptors in the brain which, in turn, increase the respiratory rate and depth within minutes (compare this with the slow response of the kidneys). This process enables the body to eliminate the extra carbon dioxide, providing that there is no obstruction to ventilation. The lowering of carbon dioxide levels in the blood encourages further free acid to be converted into carbonic acid and eventually carbon dioxide.

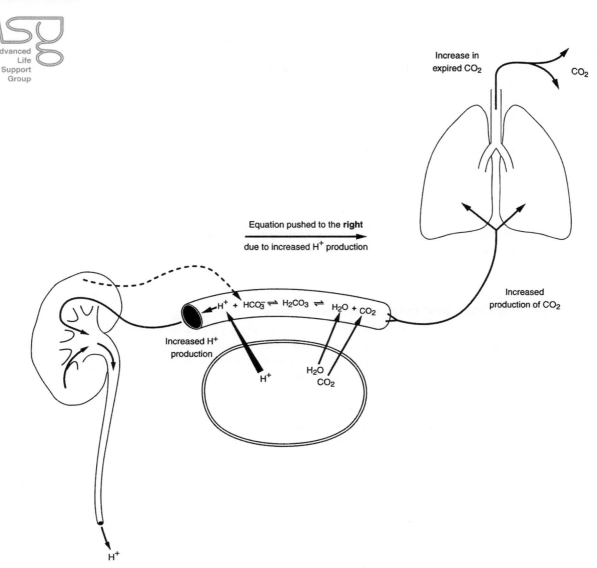

Fig. 26.8 Respiratory compensation for a metabolic acidaemia (i.e. the respiratory system is compensating for the metabolic system).

However, the body does not fully compensate in the acute situation. Therefore even after several hours, respiratory compensation will only be partial and the patient will still be slightly acidaemic (Table 26.7).

It must also be remembered that the degree to which the respiratory system can compensate depends on the work involved in breathing and the systemic effects of a low arterial concentration of carbon dioxide.

Table 26.7 Slight acidaemia

	Normal values	Effect of a metabolic acidosis	Effect of respiratory compensation
pH	7.36–7.44	↓↓	↓
$PaCO_2$	4.8–5.3 kPa	4.8–5.3 kPa	↓↓
	36–40 mm Hg	36–40 mm Hg	
Standard HCO_3^-	21–27 mmol/l	↓↓	↓
Base excess	± 2 mmol/l	↓↓	↓

Summary

- The metabolic component of the body's acid elimination mechanism can compensate for a respiratory acidosis by increasing the production of bicarbonate by the kidneys.
- Compensation by the metabolic component usually takes days to achieve.
- The respiratory component of the body's acid elimination mechanism can compensate for a metabolic acidosis by increasing ventilation of the lungs and hence eliminating carbon dioxide.
- Compensation by the respiratory component usually takes place within minutes.
- In the acute situation the body never fully compensates; therefore, the underlying acidaemia will remain.

Combined metabolic and respiratory acidaemia

Should both the metabolic and respiratory systems be defective or inadequate for the body's needs, then the accumulation of acid and carbon dioxide will be unchecked. An example of this particularly dire situation is seen in patients following a cardiorespiratory arrest. This results in the cells of the body producing lactic acid because they are being starved of oxygen. In addition, carbon dioxide accumulates in the cells and blood because it can no longer be excreted by the lungs due to the failure of ventilation (Fig. 26.9 – see page 399).

An arterial blood sample taken at this time would therefore demonstrate a combined respiratory and metabolic acidaemia (Table 26.8).

Table 26.8 Combined respiratory and metabolic acidaemia

	Normal values	Effect of respiratory and metabolic acidaemia
pH	7.36–7.44	↓ ↓ ↓ ↓
PaCO$_2$	4.8–5.3 kPa	↑ ↑
	36–40 mm Hg	
HCO$_3^-$	21–27 mmol/l	↓ ↓

CENTRAL VENOUS AND ARTERIAL BLOOD SAMPLES

So far we have concentrated on arterial blood analysis. This is blood that has had the benefit of passing through the lungs, where carbon dioxide can be eliminated and oxygen taken up. In contrast, central venous blood (i.e. blood in the right atrium) represents a mixture of all the blood returning to the heart from the body's tissues. It therefore has a high concentration of the body's waste products and low levels of oxygen (Table 26.9).

Compare these results with those following a cardiorespiratory arrest. In the absence of cardiopulmonary resuscitation blood will not flow through unventilated lungs. Therefore, the arterial sample and central venous sample will be **approximately the same**.

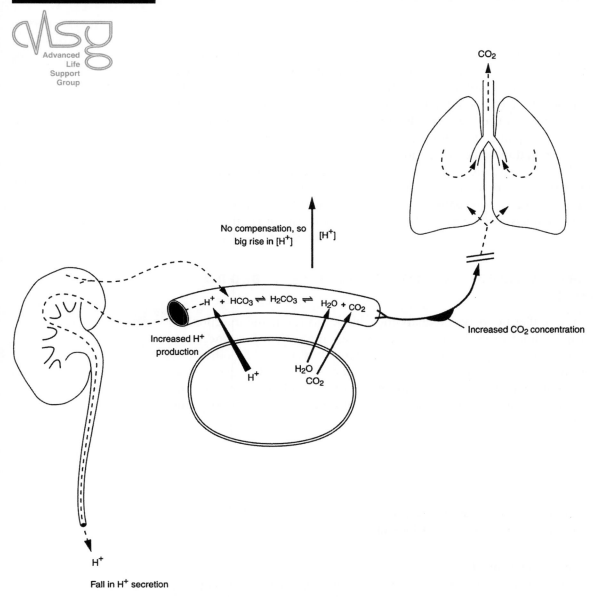

Fig. 26.9 Combined metabolic and respiratory acidosis.

In contrast, following endotracheal intubation, artificial ventilation and external chest compression, the carbon dioxide delivery to the alveoli is resumed. This is easily cleared by mechanical ventilation and some oxygen is taken up. The removal of carbon dioxide can be so effective that there is a marked reduction in

Table 26.9 Comparison of the composition of arterial and central venous blood

	Arterial blood	Central venous blood
pH	7.36–7.44	7.31–7.40
PaCO$_2$	4.8–5.3 kPa	5.5–6.8 kPa
	36–40 mm Hg	41–51 mm Hg
HCO$_3^-$	21–27 mmol/l	25–29 mmol/l
PaO$_2$ on air	Over 10.6 kPa	5.1–5.6 kPa
	Over 80 mm Hg	38–42 mm Hg

arterial carbon dioxide and the development of a paradoxical respiratory alkalosis (i.e. low arterial carbon dioxide despite high venous carbon dioxide and acidosis). Consequently, the arterial pH can be neutral, mildly acidotic or even alkalotic depending on how much carbon dioxide is being removed. In contrast, severe arterial acidosis in a patient receiving cardiopulmonary resuscitation indicates that resuscitation is inadequate, i.e. there is either inadequate blood flow to the lungs or inadequate ventilation or a combination of both.

The arterial sample taken during the resuscitation of a patient with a cardiorespiratory arrest is simply demonstrating the clinician's ability to remove carbon dioxide and add oxygen. The patient's true 'acid' state (i.e. pH, carbon dioxide and bicarbonate) is more accurately assessed by analysis of central venous blood.

A SYSTEMATIC APPROACH FOR ANALYSING A BLOOD GAS SAMPLE

There are many similarities between analysing a blood gas result and interpreting a rhythm strip. In both cases it is important to assess the patient first and to be aware of the clinical history and current medications. A review of the other laboratory investigations is also helpful. In the emergency situation, however, these data may not be immediately available. Consequently, you will have to interpret the initial results with caution and follow trends whilst the rest of the information is being obtained.

The system

> **History**
> Any symptoms due to the cause of an acid–base disturbance?
> Any symptoms as a result of an acid–base disturbance?
>
> **Results**
> Is there an acidaemia or alkalaemia?
> Is there evidence of a disturbance in the respiratory component of the body's acid–base balance?
> Is there evidence of a disturbance in the metabolic component of the body's acid–base balance?
> Is there a single or multiple acid–base disturbance?
> Is there any defect in oxygen uptake?
>
> **Integration**
> Do the suspicions from the history agree with the analysis of the results?

Is there an acidaemia or alkalaemia?

In most patients there will be an acute single acid–base disturbance. In these circumstances the body rarely has the opportunity to completely compensate for the alteration in hydrogen ion concentration. Consequently the pH will remain outside the normal range and thereby indicate the underlying acid–base disturbance.

> pH less than 7.36 = underlying acidaemia
> pH greater than 7.44 = underlying alkalaemia

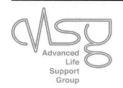

> In acute, single acid–base disturbances the body usually does not have time to fully compensate. The pH will therefore indicate the primary acid–base problem.

Nevertheless a normal pH does not necessarily mean the patient does not have an acid–base disturbance. In fact there are three reasons for a patient having a pH within the normal range:

- There is no underlying acid–base disturbance.
- The body has fully compensated for a single acid–base disturbance.
- There is more than one acid–base disturbance with equal but opposite effects on the pH.

Using your knowledge of the patient's history and examination you will have a good idea which of these options is the true answer. However, to confirm or refute your suspicions you will need to see if there are alterations in the respiratory and metabolic components of the body's acid–base balance. This entails reviewing the $PaCO_2$ and standard bicarbonate (or base excess) respectively.

Is the abnormality due to a defect in the respiratory component?

The $PaCO_2$ gives a good indication of ventilatory adequacy because it is inversely proportional to alveolar ventilation. When combined with pH it can be used to determine either if there is a problem with the respiratory system or if the respiratory component is simply compensating for a problem in the metabolic component.

For example: an arterial sample with a pH of 7.2 and a $PaCO_2$ concentration of 8.0 kPa (60 mm Hg). A pH of 7.2 indicates that there is an acidaemia. As the $PaCO_2$ is raised, this indicates that there is a **respiratory acidosis**. Consider now a patient with a similar pH but a $PaCO_2$ of 3.3 kPa (25 mm Hg). There is still an acidaemia but as the $PaCO_2$ is lowered, it would imply there is **respiratory compensation to a metabolic acidosis**. To confirm this, the metabolic component would need to be assessed.

Is the abnormality due to a defect in the metabolic component?

To determine the metabolic component, the concentration of bicarbonate is measured. In a similar situation to that described earlier, when the bicarbonate concentration is combined with pH one can determine if there is either a primary metabolic or compensatory metabolic problem.

Using the second example above, the standard bicarbonate was found to be 9.5 mmol/l and the base excess –10 mmol/l. Consequently, a pH of 7.2 and a $PaCO_2$ concentration of 3.3 kPa (25 mm Hg) is in keeping with the idea that this patient has a **respiratory compensation to a metabolic acidosis**.

Is there a single or multiple acid–base disturbance?

To narrow down the diagnosis even further we need to consider how much the $PaCO_2$ and bicarbonate (base excess) concentration has changed. If these changes fall within certain limits then there is usually only a single acid–base disturbance. Alternatively if they are outside this range then it is likely that the patient has more than one acid–base disturbance.

Take a moment to familiarise yourself with the layout of Flenley's graph (Fig. 26.10). In particular note the following:

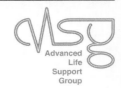

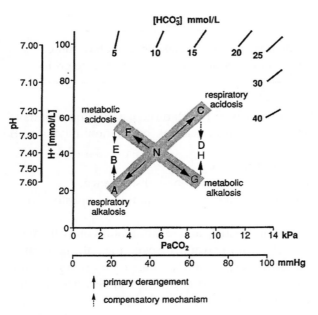

Fig. 26.10 Flenley's graph.

- The graph is showing how the pH alters with changes in $PaCO_2$.
- Cutting diagonally across the graph are lines which indicate the concentration of bicarbonate. These are known as isopleths.
- As the concentration of standard bicarbonate increases the gradient of the isopleths falls.
- The square box indicates the normal range for pH, $PaCO_2$ and actual bicarbonate concentration (N).
- Fanning out from this box are the possible ranges of normal responses you could expect with single acid–base disturbances.
- The bands representing the acute respiratory disturbances run approximately parallel to the isopleths. Respiratory acidaemia (C) and alkalaemia (A) will alter the pH and $PaCO_2$ but have little effect on the bicarbonate concentration. These bands do not include patients who have had long enough to develop metabolic compensation and so alter their bicarbonate concentrations. Such patients are represented in the chronic respiratory acidosis group (B and D).
- The band representing the metabolic disturbances runs across the isopleths. Therefore metabolic acidaemia (F) and alkalaemia (G) will alter the bicarbonate concentration as well as the pH and $PaCO_2$. These bands include the patients who are using respiratory compensation to counteract the pH changes. However, it does not include those patients who have had long enough to develop metabolic compensation (i.e. those who have a chronic metabolic disturbance (E and H)).

Using this graph you can plot the results from the blood gas analysis. If it lies within one of these bands then there is likely to be only one acid–base disturbance. However, if the results lie outside these normal ranges then there is likely to be more than one acid–base disturbance.

You have now finished the interpretation of the parameters in the blood gas analysis which provide information on the patient's acid–base balance. There is, however, one more important value which needs to be assessed in an arterial sample and that is the partial pressure of oxygen.

This is important because a failure to take up oxygen can lead to many adverse conditions including hypoxaemia. With regard to the acid–base balance,

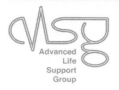

hypoxaemia can give rise to metabolic acidosis because it causes the cells to change to anaerobic metabolism and so produce excessive quantities of lactic acid.

Defect in oxygen uptake

By knowing the FiO_2 it is possible to predict what the PaO_2 would be if the patient was ventilating normally.

Since atmospheric pressure is 100 kPa (approximately 760 mm Hg), 1% is 1 kPa or 7.6 mm Hg. This would mean that inspiring 30% oxygen from a facemask would produce an inspired partial pressure of oxygen of 30 kPa (268 mm Hg). This should lead to an arterial concentration of around 20–25 kPa (152–257.6 mm Hg) because there is a normal drop of about 7.5 kPa (57 mm Hg) between the partial pressure of oxygen inspired at the mouth and that in the alveoli. A drop of significantly greater than 10 kPa (76 mm Hg) would imply that there is a mismatch in the lungs between ventilation of the alveoli and their perfusion with blood.

For example, an arterial PaO_2 of 32.9 kPa (250 mm Hg) in a patient breathing 40% oxygen is within normal limits. In contrast, an arterial PaO_2 of 23.7 kPa (180 mm Hg) in a patient breathing 50% oxygen indicates that there is a defect in the take-up of oxygen. An inspired oxygen of 50% will have a partial pressure of approximately 50 kPa. This would mean the expected PaO_2 would be at least $50 - 10 = 40$ kPa.

Example

Using this system for interpreting blood gases let us now consider the following case.

History

A 17-year-old girl who is normally in good health is found at home by her parents in a restless and confused state. She is pale, sweaty and hyperventilating.

Results

Whilst she was breathing room air, an arterial sample was taken for blood gas analysis. The results are given in Table 26.10.

Table 26.10 Example arterial blood sample

	Normal values	Patient's values
pH	7.36–7.44	7.10
$PaCO_2$	4.8–5.3 kPa	2.4 kPa
	36–40 mm Hg	18 mm Hg
Standard HCO_3	21–27 mmol/l	5.5 mmol/l
Base excess	±2 mmol/l	−14 mmol/l
PaO_2	Over 12.0 kPa	14 kPa
	Over 90 mm Hg*	105 mm Hg*

*On room air.

Analysis

History

Hyperventilation may be a primary problem (e.g. anxiety) or compensation for an underlying metabolic acidaemia. You would therefore suspect from the history

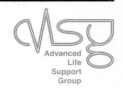

that there could be either a respiratory alkalaemia or a metabolic acidaemia with respiratory compensation. With regard to acid–base balance you can also deduce from the history that this is an acute event. It is therefore unlikely that there would be sufficient time for any metabolic compensation in either of the possible acid–base disturbances suspected.

Systematic analysis of the blood gas results
Is there an acidaemia or alkalaemia?

- As the pH is below 7.36 there is an acidaemia.

Is there evidence of a disturbance in the respiratory component of the body's acid–base balance?

- Yes, the $PaCO_2$ is low. In the light of the pH, this indicates there is either respiratory compensation to a metabolic acidosis or a combination of a big metabolic acidosis and smaller primary respiratory alkalosis.

Is there evidence of a disturbance in the metabolic component of the body's acid–base balance?

- Yes, the bicarbonate concentration is low and the base excess is very negative. In the light of the pH and $PaCO_2$ this supports the two possibilities suggested in the previous question.

Is there a single or multiple acid–base disturbance?

- Using Fig. 26.10 (see page 402) you can see that the results lie within the metabolic acidaemia band. This would imply that the patient has a metabolic acidaemia with respiratory compensation and has not had time to develop metabolic compensation.

Is the PaO_2 uptake abnormal?

- The expected PaO_2 when breathing room air is over 12.0 kPa (over 90 mm Hg). There is, therefore, no evidence of any problem in oxygen uptake in this patient.

Integrate the clinical findings with the data interpretation

The clinical and data analyses tally. This girl has a metabolic acidaemia with respiratory compensation. Your next move would be to determine what is the cause of the acidaemia. This involves further tests which are selected in the light of the patient's history and physical examination. A useful initial screen is to determine the anion gap.

ANION GAP

Derivation

The body needs to ensure that electroneutrality is maintained because an imbalance would impair cellular function. This means the total number of negatively charged particles (anions) and positively charged particles (cations) must be equal.

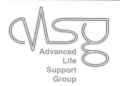

We can therefore write that in the circulation:

Total concentration of anions = total number of cations

You will be aware that only some of the anions and cations are routinely measured. We can therefore adjust the above equation to:

> **Total concentration of measured anions + Total concentration of unmeasured anions**
> **=**
> **Total concentration of measured cations + Total concentration of unmeasured cations**

If we use the symbol [ ] to indicate concentration, and insert the anions and cations which are routinely measured, the equation becomes:

$$[\text{Actual HCO}_3{}^-] + [\text{Cl}^-] + [\text{Total unmeasured anions}]$$
$$= [\text{Na}^+] + [\text{H}^+] + [\text{K}^+] + [\text{Total unmeasured cations}]$$

This equation can be rearranged to read:

$$[\text{Total unmeasured anions}] - [\text{Total unmeasured cations}]$$
$$= ([\text{Na}^+] + [\text{H}^+] + [\text{K}^+]) - ([\text{Actual HCO}_3^-] + [\text{Cl}^-])$$

The equation is rearranged this way because the total number of unmeasured anions is usually bigger than its cation counterpart. This difference is known as the anion **gap**. Consequently the equation becomes:

$$\text{Anion gap} = ([\text{Na}^+] + [\text{H}^+] + [\text{K}^+]) - ([\text{Actual HCO}_3^-] + [\text{Cl}^-])$$

Thinking back you will remember that the actual concentration of hydrogen ions is tiny compared to the other electrolytes. In addition, the concentration of potassium in plasma is small because it is mainly located inside the cells of the body. We can therefore remove these two concentrations from the equation without producing any significant errors. As a result the equation becomes:

$$\text{Anion gap} = [\text{Na}^+] - ([\text{Actual HCO}_3^-] + [\text{Cl}^-])$$

> **Key point**
>
> **The anion gap is the difference in concentration between the unmeasured anions and cations**

The normal range for the anion gap is 6–18 mmol/l

This value is obviously very dependent on the method used to measure the electrolytes. Chloride assessment in particular is being changed. As a result some departments will work on the newer normal range of anion gap which is 7 ± 4 mmol/l. It is therefore important that you find out from your laboratory what they consider the normal range to be.

Types of anion gap

Considering how the anion gap is derived it is easy to understand how it can be altered by changes in the concentration of unmeasured anions, unmeasured cations or a combination of the two.

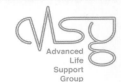

Increase in the unmeasured anions	Decrease in the unmeasured cations
Metabolic acidosis	Hypokalaemia
Hyperalbuminaemia	Hypomagnesaemia
Marked alkalosis	Hypocalcaemia
Therapy with substances which produce unmeasured anions (e.g. sodium citrate, lactate or acetate. It also applies to excessive doses of penicillins particularly carbenicillin and ticarcillin)	

Key point

The most common cause of an increase in the anion gap is metabolic acidosis

---

Anion gap and metabolic acidosis

Metabolic acidoses can be divided into those with a wide anion gap or a normal anion gap. Widening of the anion gap results from an increase in the acid load on the body. In contrast, metabolic acidoses with a normal anion gap are produced by conditions leading to either the loss of bicarbonate or where the kidneys are unable to excrete the normal daily acid load.

Key points

Conditions with a widened anion gap include metabolic acidoses due to increases in the acid load on the body.

Conditions with a normal anion gap include metabolic acidoses due to either a loss of bicarbonate or impaired elimination of a normal acid load

---

METABOLIC ACIDOSIS WITH A WIDE ANION GAP

The most likely metabolic acidosis you will come across is one giving rise to an increase in the anion gap. In these conditions a metabolic acidosis is produced because the actual bicarbonate concentration falls:

$$\text{Anion gap} \uparrow = [Na^+] - ([HCO_3^-] \downarrow + [Cl^-])$$

Nevertheless, it is important to remember that metabolic acidosis represents only one of several causes of an increase in anion gap. In most cases though, these non-acidotic causes produce only a small increase in the anion gap.

Key point

An increased anion gap needs to be put into clinical context because this will enable the most appropriate investigations to be selected to confirm the diagnosis

---

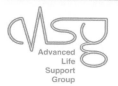

Table 26.11 Causes of metabolic acidosis with an increased or normal anion gap

Increased anion gap		Normal anion gap	
M	Methanol	D	Diuretic – potassium sparing
E	Ethylene glycol	I	Intestinal fistula
D	Diabetic ketoacidosis	A	Acetozolamide
I	Isoniazid	R	Renal tubular acidosis (I and II)
C	Cachexia	R	Renal failure
A	Alcohol	H	Hypo-aldosteronism
L	Lactic acidosis	O	Oral resin (cholestryamine)
T	Toluene	E	Entero-ureterostomy
R	Renal failure/rhabdomyolysis	A	Alimentary feeding
I	Iron		
P	Paraldehyde		
S	Salicylate		

Causes

A metabolic acidosis with a widened anion gap is common because it is produced by several common clinical conditions. These can be remembered by the mnemonic 'medical trips' (Table 26.11). In contrast, a metabolic acidosis with a normal anion gap is uncommon. The causes can be remembered with the mnemonic 'diarrhoea'.

The young girl's blood sample was analysed further by measuring the appropriate electrolyte concentrations. In this case these were found to be:

- Na^+ 135 mmol/l
- K^+ 5.0 mmol/l
- HCO_3 10 mmol/l
- Cl^- 95 mmol/l

Using this information it is possible to determine the anion gap:

$$\text{Anion gap} = [\text{Sodium}] - [\text{Bicarbonate} + \text{Chloride}]$$
$$= [135] - [10 + 95]$$
$$= 30 \text{ mmol/l}$$

Therefore the 17-year-old patient has a metabolic acidaemia with a wide anion gap.

The most likely cause of a metabolic acidosis with an increased anion gap in a previously healthy adolescent is an overdose or diabetic ketoacidosis. Consequently the salicylate and blood sugar levels must be checked in this patient.

SUMMARY

The body's system for removing the carbon dioxide and acid produced by metabolism has both a respiratory and metabolic component. These are linked by the effects of carbonic acid that enables one component to compensate for a defect in the other.

In acute medical emergencies one or both of these systems are often defective. Using a systemic approach to blood gas analysis you can determine where the problem lies. In the common structure of a metabolic acidosis, the use of the anion gap can also be helpful in identifying a specific cause.

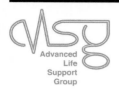
Advanced
Life
Support
Group

CHAPTER 27

Dysrhythmia recognition

OBJECTIVES

After reading this chapter you will be able to:
- understand the origin and pathways of electrical activity in the heart
- recognise which patients require this activity to be monitored and how it should be done
- understand the system for analysing electrical activity recorded on a rhythm strip.

CARDIAC ELECTRICAL ACTIVITY: ITS ORIGIN AND ORGANISATION

The sinoatrial node (SAN) is a specialised area of cardiac muscle that generates spontaneously a continuous sequence of regularly timed waves of electrical activity known as depolarisations. These radiate through both atria, inducing contraction. The ability of the SAN to spontaneously depolarise is termed pacemaker activity, and may also be seen in other areas of the heart, usually at slower rates. As the wave of depolarisation spreads through the atria it gives rise to the 'P' wave on the electrocardiogram (ECG). Normally the P wave has a duration of 0.08–0.12 s, (80–120 ms).

Atrial depolarisation normally finishes by converging on a specialised collection of cells called the atrioventricular node located at the base of the right atrium. This delays the transmission of the depolarising wave to the ventricles and gives rise to a significant proportion of the PR interval. The latter is measured on the ECG tracing from the start of the P wave to the first deflection of QRS complex (0.12–0.20 s, 120–200 ms).

After the atrioventricular node, the wave of depolarisation is conducted through the fibrous atrio-ventricular barrier via the bundle of His. At the proximal part of the muscular intraventricular septum this splits into the right and left bundle branches, with the latter subsequently separating into anterior and posterior divisions (fascicles). These, in turn, terminate in small (Purkinje) fibres which transmit the electrical impulse to the non-specialised ventricular myocardium. The passage of the impulse through the ventricular conduction system is rapid compared with the atrioventricular node and is represented by the QRS complex (<0.12 s, <120 ms) on the ECG.

Following stimulation, the myocardial cells recover their normal resting electrical potential in an active biochemical process called repolarisation. The atrial repolarisation wave is usually obscured by the QRS, but the ventricular repolarisation gives rise to the T wave. For most of the period of repolarisation the ventricles remain unresponsive (or 'refractory') to further electrical stimulation. A diagram of the conducting system and its relationship to the ECG is shown in Fig. 27.1.

Acute Medical Emergencies; The Practical Approach, 2nd edition.
Edited by Terence Wardle, Peter Driscoll, and Sue Wieteska.
© 2010 Blackwell Publishing Ltd.

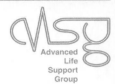

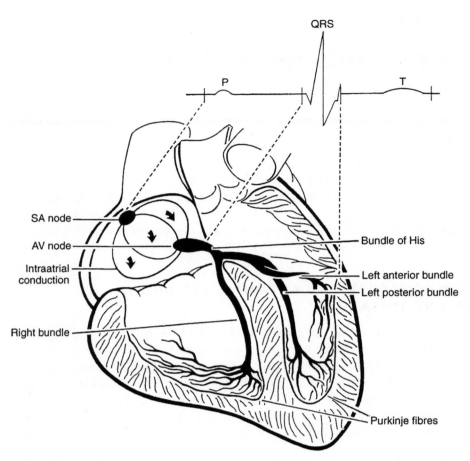

Fig. 27.1 The conduction system of the heart and its relationship to the electrocardiogram.

The T wave is sometimes followed by a U wave, which is a rounded deflection in the same direction as the T wave. Its exact genesis is unclear but it becomes more prominent in hypokalaemia, hypercalcaemia and may be inverted in ischaemic heart disease.

The QT interval is measured from the beginning of the QRS complex to the end of the T wave. Consequently it represents the total time for ventricular depolarisation and repolarisation. Nevertheless, prolongation of this interval is mainly associated with clinical conditions that delay ventricular repolarisation. This increases the period of time where the ventricles are susceptible to lethal dysrhythmias (see later).

It is important to realise that the duration of the QT interval is directly dependent on age and sex and inversely related to the heart rate. The latter is calculated by most ECG machines and expressed as the corrected QT interval so the heart rate has been considered (normal range 0.35–0.42 s, 350–420 ms).

PATHOLOGY OF THE CONDUCTING SYSTEM

The origin and spread of depolarisation through the heart can be affected by ischaemia, drugs, trauma and abnormal metabolic conditions. This can lead to spontaneous depolarisation originating from abnormal areas of the heart and spreading by an abnormal route. The ECG can be used in these situations to help locate the affected sites.

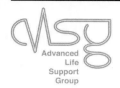

Many parts of the specialised conducting system have the ability to initiate a wave of depolarisation, and thus have potential pacemaker activity, but do so at varying rates. The eventual heart rate is determined by the part of the conducting system that has the fastest intrinsic rate of depolarisation, normally the sinoatrial node. After the sinoatrial node, the next fastest part is usually the junctional tissue near the atrioventricular node, which will then take over as the cardiac pacemaker, followed in turn by the bundle of His and ultimately the terminal fibres of the His-Purkinje system in the ventricular myocardium.

Occasionally a pathological focus develops in the heart which has a faster intrinsic rate of depolarisation when compared with the sinoatrial node. As a consequence, this focus will replace the sinoatrial node as the cardiac pacemaker.

CAUSES OF DYSRHYTHMIA

Increasing the heart rate

An increase in heart rate occurs normally as a result of emotion, exercise and fear. The effect is mediated by the sympathetic nervous system which acts on the sinoatrial node to increase its rate of depolarisation. However, an increase in the heart rate can also result from the following pathological reasons:

- automaticity
- re-entry
- both.

Automaticity

Automaticity is the ability to depolarise spontaneously. This is a common feature of cells in the conducting system and certain areas of myocardium. As mentioned previously, the sinoatrial node usually has the fastest rate of spontaneous depolarisation and therefore acts as the dominant pacemaker.

Re-entry

Re-entry occurs when there is a dual conducting system between the atria and the ventricles. This can be either within the atrioventricular node or bypassing it (e.g. Wolff–Parkinson–White and Lown–Ganong–Levine syndromes). One pathway (A) only allows conduction in a single direction (unidirectional block or a longer refractory period) and the other (B) has a slow conduction rate (Fig. 27.2). In response to a premature beat, the impulse has to go down the slow pathway (B). This is because the fast pathway (A) has not repolarised from the previous beat and is therefore unable to conduct the electrical impulse. This increase in transit time allows A to repolarise so that the impulse can be conducted opposite to the normal direction of flow. This gives B sufficient time to repolarise and so be able to be stimulated by the retrograde impulse which has travelled along A. Consequently a self-sustaining cycle of electrical impulses is created.

Both

Automaticity and re-entry can act together.

Slowing of the heart

A reduction in the heart rate is a normal physiological response during sleep, at rest, and in the athletic individual. The heart rate can also fall in certain pathological conditions when the rate of depolarisation of the intrinsic cardiac pacemaker and/or the conducting system has been reduced. Degenerative fibrosis is the most

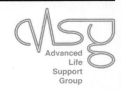

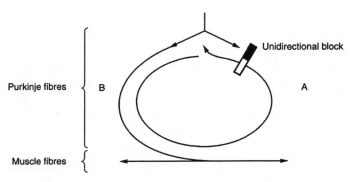

Fig. 27.2 The origin of a circus movement.

common cause but ischaemic heart disease, drugs and other diseases (e.g. hypothyroidism, jaundice) can also be responsible.

MONITORING CARDIAC ELECTRICAL ACTIVITY

In the acute situation cardiac electrical activity is usually assessed continuously by an ECG monitor connected to the patient by a standard system of electrical leads (Fig. 27.3).

Cardiac ECG monitors

Although there are many different types of cardiac monitor, the majority have common features including a screen for displaying the cardiac rhythm and a way to print a copy of it. This is commonly known as the 'rhythm strip'. Most models also incorporate a heart rate meter which is triggered by the QRS complexes and a device to automatically store a record of the ECG should the heart rate fall

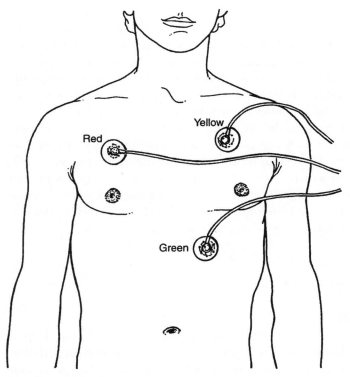

Fig. 27.3 Monitoring by the electrocardiogram.

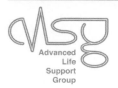

outside certain preset limits. Lights and audible signals may also provide additional indications of the heart rate.

Modern monitoring systems are usually digital. This enables the machine to perform complex functions such as computer aided rhythm analysis, automatic and semiautomatic defibrillation, and electronic storage of the signal for review and analysis.

Leads

Lead I measures the voltage between the right and left shoulder. It gives a good view of the left lateral aspect of the heart and the QRS complex but does not necessarily give a good picture of the P wave (Fig. 27.4).

Lead II measures the voltage between the right shoulder and left leg. It is the most commonly used lead for monitoring the cardiac rhythm. As it is in line with the mean frontal cardiac axis, it gives a good view of both QRS complexes and P waves. (Fig. 27.4).

Lead III measures the voltage between the left shoulder and left lower chest (or leg). It is rarely an advantage in dysrhythmia recognition but it does give a good view of the inferior aspect of the heart (Fig. 27.4).

The remaining leads are not used during routine monitoring or the initial management of a cardiac arrest. They are, however, required for definitive dysrhythmia analysis and determining the position of the cardiac axis. The MCL1 lead measures the voltage between the right pectoral area (VI position) and the left shoulder. This gives a good view of the QRS complex and the P wave, but it is not commonly used.

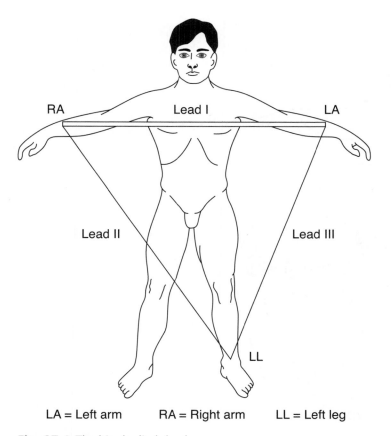

LA = Left arm   RA = Right arm   LL = Left leg

Fig. 27.4 The bipolar limb leads.

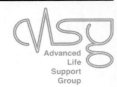

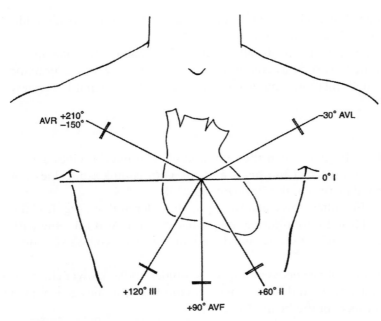

Fig. 27.5 The standard lead view of the heart.

Leads I, II, III and AVR, AVL, and AVF look at the heart in the vertical plane (Fig. 27.5).

Leads V1–6 view the heart in the horizontal plane such that V1 and V2 look at the right ventricle, V3 and V4 the interventricular septum and V5 and V6 mainly the left ventricle (Fig. 27.6).

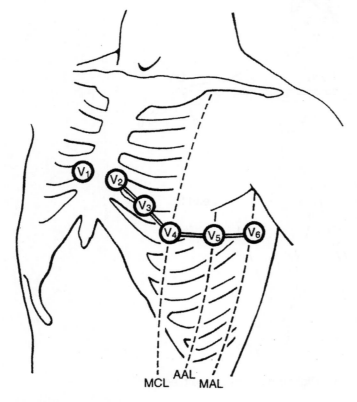

Fig. 27.6 The chest leads.

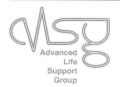

Practical points

ECG monitoring should be used on all patients presenting with chest pain, syncope, dizziness, collapse, hypotension, palpitations and cardiac arrest.

ECG machines record at a standard speed of 25 mm/s. Calibrated recording paper is used so that each large square (5 mm) is equivalent to 0.2 s (200 ms) and each small square (1 mm) is equivalent to 0.04 s (40 ms). The amplitude of the trace is standardised at 1 mV/cm and most machines have the capability of testing this (Fig. 27.7).

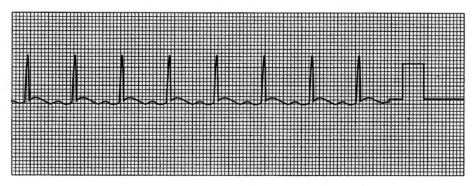

Fig. 27.7 Voltage calibration of the electrocardiogram.

To minimise electrical interference the electrodes should be all of the same type, applied over bone rather than muscle and positioned such that they are equidistant from one another. Hair should be removed from the areas where the electrodes are to be attached and the skin cleaned with alcohol to dissolve surface oil. The electrodes should be positioned on the patient's chest so that they will not interfere with any other activities, such as external cardiac massage.

Adhesive silver/silver chloride electrodes give the best signal and, if readily available, are preferable to defibrillation paddles even for the first 'quick look' in cardiac arrest. Another advantage is that paddles will only give a reading when they are in position and, therefore, are not practical for continuously assessing the rhythm. They also may fail to transmit the ECG signal following defibrillation and this may give a false impression of asystole. Nevertheless, if paddles are used, it is essential that they be placed over gel pads to ensure good electrical contact.

Ensure that the QRS height is sufficient to stimulate the rate meter by adjusting the gain control. However, this should not be so excessive as to cause artefacts on the monitor. The user needs to be aware how much the monitor trace is larger or smaller than normal.

Any activity, such as drug use or carotid sinus massage, should be recorded on the rhythm strip as it happens. This helps greatly in the later analysis of the dysrhythmia.

A common problem is artefact produced by the patient's movements, strenuous respiratory effort or if subjected to external cardiac compression. As the latter is usually sufficient to completely mask the patient's own cardiac rhythm, it must be stopped for 3–5 s so that the cardiac arrest rhythm can be analysed (see later).

It is important to realise that the leads used to monitor dysrhythmias are not the optimum ones for recording changes in the ST segment and the T wave. A 'diagnostic' setting may be required to reproduce ST displacement accurately but this produces more baseline wandering.

Ideally, old notes should be obtained and previous ECGs studied. The recording of a full 12-lead ECG should be done with any arrhythmia which does not cause loss of consciousness as this recording may provide vital evidence for future management.

A SYSTEMATIC APPROACH TO INTERPRETING A RHYTHM STRIP

Avoid the temptation to simply 'eye ball' the rhythm strip produced by the ECG monitor. Instead, develop a system so that clues and multiple problems are not missed.

Systematic approach to interpreting a rhythm strip

How is the patient?

Is there any electrical activity?

| No | Asystole |
| Yes | Not asystole |

Are there recognisable complexes?

| No | Ventricular fibrillation |
| Yes | Not ventricular fibrillation |

What is the ventricular rate?

What is the rhythm?

   Regular

   Regular irregularity

   Irregular irregularity

Are the P waves uniform?

   Shape

   Timing – Early or later than normal

Is there atrial flutter? (flutter waves, ventricular rate 150/min with 2:1 block)

Are there the same number of P waves as QRS complexes?

Yes	What is the PR interval?
No	Is the PR interval constant?
	Is the RR interval constant?

Is the QRS duration normal (less than 3 small squares, 0.12 s, 120 ms)?

Yes	Normal ventricular conduction
No	Abnormal ventricular conduction
	Shape
	Timing – Early or later than normal
	Frequency
	Ventricular tachycardia:
	Supraventricular tachycardia with aberrant ventricular conduction
	Torsade de pointes
	Idioventricular rhythm:
	Agonal rhythm

Basic principles

It is helpful to remember the following basic principles when you are interpreting the rhythm strip.

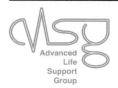

If the depolarisation wave is moving towards the electrode then an upward (positive) deflection is seen on the monitor.

If the depolarisation wave is moving away from the electrode then a downward (negative) deflection is seen on the monitor.

The next box contains one of the many systems that have been developed to enable health care workers to interpret a rhythm strip from lead II in the acute situation. It is an effective system based on a series of questions which pick out the most life-threatening dysrhythmias first.

1. How is the patient?

> **Key point**
>
> **Always remember: Treat the patient, not the rhythm**

It is extremely important to assess the patient before making a diagnosis and suggesting a treatment from a single rhythm strip. For example, a patient who is not breathing and has no palpable pulse is suffering from a cardiorespiratory arrest irrespective of what the monitor shows. For example, if the arrest occurs despite normal (or near normal) electrical activity then pulseless electrical activity (PEA; previously called electro-mechanical dissociation) exists.

2. Is there any electrical activity?

If there is no electrical activity, check:

- connections   to monitor
                           to patient
- QRS gain
- leads I and III.

If there is still no electrical activity diagnose asystole (Fig. 27.8). However, beware that a completely flat tracing, without any baseline wandering, is usually caused by not connecting the patient's leads.

Occasionally P waves can be detected, indicating that atrial activity is still present (ventricular standstill, P wave asystole). This may occurs, transiently, shortly after the onset of ventricular asystole, or during Stokes–Adams syncope, and is associated with a better prognosis than when P waves are absent.

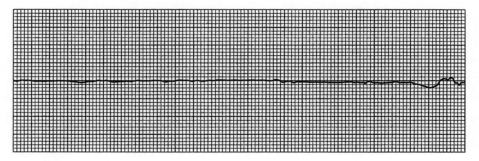

Fig. 27.8 Asystole.

3. Are there any recognisable complexes?

If there are no recognisable complexes, diagnose ventricular fibrillation (Fig. 27.9).

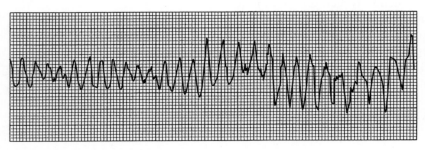

Fig. 27.9 Ventricular fibrillation.

Ventricular fibrillation is a totally chaotic rhythm because small areas of the myocardium depolarise in a random fashion. Initially, the amplitude of the waveform is large and the dysrhythmia is known as 'coarse ventricular fibrillation'. Over time 'fine ventricular fibrillation' develops because the amplitude diminishes and the tracing becomes flatter. Eventually asystole results.

It may be difficult to determine when the patient has made the transition from fine ventricular fibrillation to asystole. This is made more difficult by the presence of any baseline wandering and electrical interference. In such cases the rhythm should be reassessed taking the precautions listed for asystole. In addition, all contact with the patient should cease briefly (less than 5 s) so that a reliable tracing can be gained without interference.

> **Key point**
>
> The presence or absence of the commonest cardiac arrest rhythms will have been determined by answering these first three questions. As these require immediate treatment further interpretation of the ECG assumes that these rhythms have been excluded

4. What is the ventricular rate?

This can be calculated as follows:

Ventricular rate = 300/number of large squares between consecutive R waves

Fig. 27.10 demonstrates a ventricular rate of 75/min.

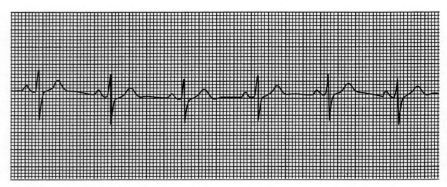

Fig. 27.10 Sinus rhythm.

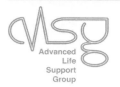

Any rhythm that has a ventricular rate greater than 100 is called a 'tachycardia'. The most common tachycardia is sinus tachycardia which has, by definition, one P wave before each QRS and usually has a rate of 100–130 beats/min (Fig. 27.11) and is due to physiological causes. In contrast, a ventricular rate less than 60/min is called a bradycardia. Sinus bradycardia is a common type of bradycardia that has a P wave before each QRS.

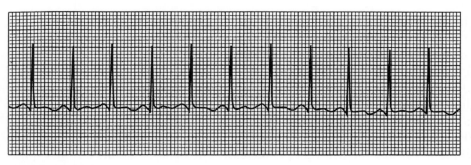

Fig. 27.11 Sinus tachycardia.

Supraventricular tachycardias (SVT) (Fig. 27.12) can be divided into two groups depending on whether it results from re-entry or enhanced automaticity. However, in the absence of finding an atrial premature beat (see later) before the tachycardia starts, it is not possible on routine ECG monitoring to distinguish between these two mechanisms.

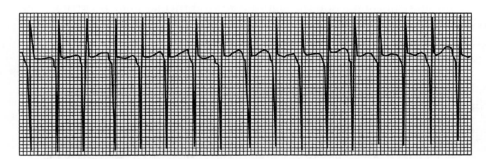

Fig. 27.12 Supraventricular tachycardia.

In a supraventricular tachycardia, the QRS complexes are narrow unless there is an aberrant conduction through the ventricles producing widening of the QRS complex (see later).

5. What is the rhythm?

To answer this question correctly it is important to inspect carefully an adequate length of the rhythm strip tracing. In this way it will be possible to detect subtle variations in rhythm.

Assessment of the regularity of the rhythm is made by comparing the RR intervals of adjacent beats at different places in the tracing. Callipers or dividers are very useful for this but it is also possible to obtain an accurate result by marking the peaks of four adjacent R waves on a piece of paper. This must be done precisely because rhythm irregularity becomes less marked as the heart rate increases. The paper is then moved along the strip to see if the RR gaps correspond. If they do then the rhythm is regular. As interpretation of a fast heart rate can be difficult, a further rhythm strip recorded during carotid sinus massage may help by temporarily slowing the heart rate.

Sinus rhythm is diagnosed when:
- the P waves have a normal duration (2–3 small squares, 0.08–0.12 s or 80–120 ms)
- the PR interval has a normal and consistent duration (3–5 small squares, 0.12–0.20 s or 120–200 ms)
- the heart rate is between 60 and 100/min
- a P wave precedes each QRS complex.

Usually successive RR intervals are constant but occasionally, in healthy young individuals, the RR interval varies with respiration. Nevertheless the P wave shape and PR interval remain the same. This variation in the RR interval is called sinus arrhythmia and results from the inhibition of the cardioinhibitory centre during inspiration causing the heart rate to increase. The opposite occurs during expiration.

If the RR interval is irregular, it is important to decide whether there is either an 'irregular irregularity' with no recognisable pattern or RR intervals of 'regular irregularity', when the variation in the RR intervals repeats in a regular fashion. In the latter case the relationship between the P waves and the QRS waves assumes special importance and will be discussed in greater detail later.

When an irregular irregularity in the RR interval is associated with a constant QRS shape, the likely diagnosis is atrial fibrillation (AF) (Fig. 27.13). Atrial fibrillation is due to atrial depolarisation in a disorganised fashion at a rate of 350–600/min with conduction through the atrioventricular node occurring at an irregular rate. There are no P waves with AF, but the baseline may vary between fine and course fluctuations in different parts of the strip.

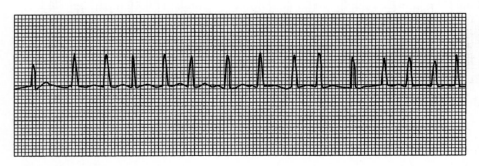

Fig. 27.13 Atrial fibrillation.

6. Are the P waves uniform?

Normal P waves have a duration of 2–3 small squares (0.08–0.12 s or 80–120 ms.) and a vertical deflection of less than 2.5 mm. They can be distinguished from the larger T waves.

It is important to check the whole strip for P waves because they may be hidden in the QRS complex or T wave, producing inconsistent and abnormal 'lumps and bumps' (Fig. 27.14). Repeating the tracing using a different lead (V1, MCL1 or III) can also help identify apparently missing P waves.

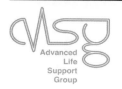

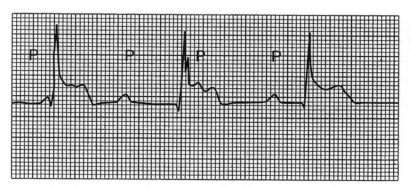

Fig. 27.14 P waves hidden in the QRS complex.

Occasionally, hidden P waves can be revealed in patients with a regular tachycardia by slowing the ventricular rate by either vagal stimulation (e.g. carotid sinus massage) or drugs (see atrial flutter)

Abnormal shaped P (i.e. 'ectopic') waves indicate that the direction of depolarisation through the atria is abnormal and consequently has not been initiated by the sinoatrial node. They have two possible sources.

Premature beats: As these usually originate in the atria and, rarely, from the atrioventricular junction they are known as atrial and junctional premature beats, respectively.

A distinguishing feature of a premature beat is the coupling interval, i.e. the time period between the normal P wave and the abnormal one (P'). This is shorter than that between two normal P waves (PP) because the myocardial focus giving rise to the premature atrial beat, depolarises before the sinoatrial node (Fig. 27.15). The coupling interval is constant if the premature beat is always produced from the same focus.

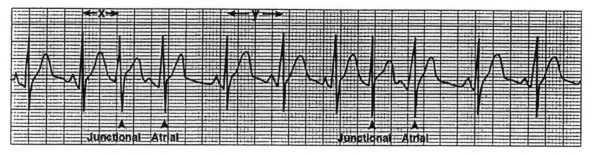

Fig. 27.15 Ectopic P waves.

The premature P wave (P') (Fig. 27.15) blocks the SAN from discharging and so disturbs the subsequent rhythm of P wave production. This can be demonstrated on the rhythm strip by noting the interval between the normal P waves on either side of the ectopic beat. This distance (X) is less than twice the normal PP interval (Y).

The abnormal focus may produce single or multiple premature beats. A tachycardia is defined as having three or more such beats occurring in rapid succession. If they occur in discrete self-terminating runs, they are described as being paroxysmal. When they occur in longer runs, the abnormal focus may take over completely and not allow any normal (SAN-generated) P waves to occur for a prolonged period of time. In these cases it is important to study the whole rhythm strip to determine if a normal PP interval can be found.

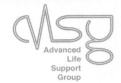

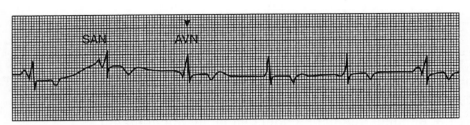

Fig. 27.16 Escape P waves.

Escape beats: If the sinoatrial node fails to generate electrical impulse then another part of the conduction system will discharge instead. This gives rise to an escape beat (Fig. 27.16). As it occurs later than expected, the coupling interval between the normal and escape P wave is longer than the normal (SAN-generated) PP interval.

Key points

Premature beat	Reduced coupling interval
Escape beat	Increased coupling interval

---

7. Is there atrial flutter?

In this condition the atria are depolarising at 250–350 beats/min but in most cases the rate is very close to 300 beats/min (i.e. one per large square). This atrial activity gives rise to regular 'F' (flutter) waves which gives the baseline a characteristic 'saw-tooth' appearance (Fig. 27.17).

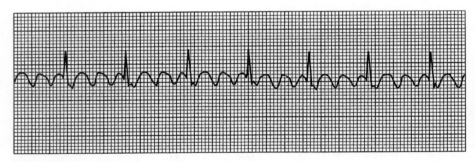

Fig. 27.17 Atrial flutter.

Only rarely does the atrio-ventricular node conduct all the atrial impulses to the ventricles, and atrial flutter is often associated with 2:1 atrio-ventricular block, giving a typical ventricular rate of 150/min, with flutter waves largely hidden in the QRS and T waves making the diagnosis difficult. Any regular tachycardia of 150/min should raise the suspicion of atrial flutter. When there are higher degrees of atrio-ventricular block flutter waves are more evident facilitating the diagnosis. Nevertheless the QRS complexes, which result, have a normal shape if the remaining part of the conduction system has not been altered. In cases where the diagnosis is in doubt, vagal stimulation can be used to increase temporarily the degree of atrioventricular node block so that flutter waves can be seen.

8. Are the number of P and QRS waves the same?

If the number of P and QRS waves are the same, measure the PR interval.

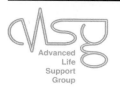

First-degree heart block

There are the same number of P waves as QRS complexes but the PR interval is constant and longer than 1 large square, 0.2 s (200 ms) (Fig. 27.18). This condition is an ECG diagnosis and generally does not progress to more serious forms of heart block. It can, however, result from digoxin and β blockers.

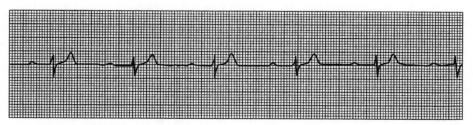

Fig. 27.18 First-degree block.

If the number of P waves is greater than the number of QRS complexes then the patient has either second- or third-degree heart block. To distinguish between them the PR interval must be examined.

Second-degree heart block – Mobitz type I (Wenckebach)

The PR interval progressively lengthens, until a P wave is not followed by a QRS complex. The atrioventricular node then recovers and the next PR interval reverts to the previous shortest conduction time. This rhythm is therefore distinguished by having both varying PR and RR intervals (Fig. 27.19). In some cases this phenomenon is physiological; in others, however, it can be the result of inferior myocardial infarction, digoxin or myocarditis.

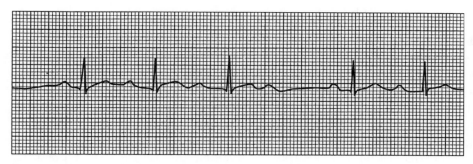

Fig. 27.19 Second-degree block – Mobitz type I.

Second-degree heart block – Mobitz type II

There is an intermittent non-conduction of some P waves but the PR interval remains constant (Fig. 27.20). However, it may be of a normal or prolonged duration. Mobitz type II is much more likely to progress to third-degree heart block

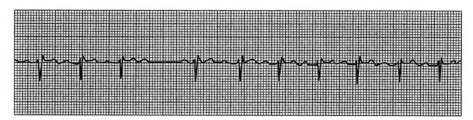

Fig. 27.20 Second-degree block – Mobitz type II.

than type I and there is a higher chance of developing asystole or ventricular dysrhythmias (see later). It is usually associated with a broad QRS complex due to bundle branch block.

Third-degree (complete heart block)

This results in total dissociation between the depolarisation of the atria and the ventricles with each beating independently (Fig. 27.21). As a consequence, there is no consistent relationship between the P waves and the QRS complexes on the ECG trace. The PR interval is, therefore, completely erratic but the PP and RR intervals are constant. Where complete heart block is associated with broad QRS complexes there is a greater risk of ventricular standstill.

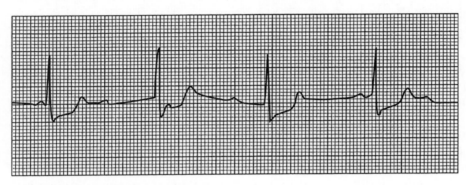

Fig. 27.21 Third-degree (complete) block.

Summary

The different types of heart block are summarised in Table 27.1.

Table 27.1 The different types of heart block

Block	P:QRS	PR interval	RR interval
First degree	Equal	Constant and prolonged	Constant
Second degree – type I	P > QRS	Variable	Variable
Second degree – type II	P > QRS	Constant	Variable
Third degree (complete)	P > QRS	Variable	Constant

9. Is the QRS duration normal?

The normal duration for the QRS is less than 3 small squares, 0.12 s (120 ms) or less. This can only occur if the ventricular depolarisation originates from above the bifurcation of the bundle of His. Broader complexes occur as a result of:
- ventricular premature beats
- ventricular escape beats
- bundle branch blocks
- left ventricular hypertrophy
- aberrant conduction.

Ventricular premature beats or ectopics

Ventricular premature beats present as bizarre, wide complexes with abnormal ST and T waves (Fig. 27.22). Unlike the normal situation, ventricular depolarisation

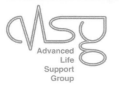

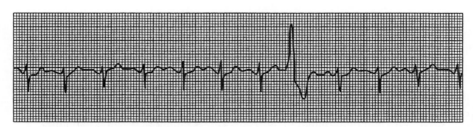

Fig. 27.22 Ventricular ectopic.

is premature thereby reducing the interval between the normal and abnormal beats (RR interval).

In contrast to atrial premature beats, ventricular premature beats neither alter nor reset the sinoatrial node. Consequently, the frequency of the P waves will continue undisturbed by the abnormal ventricular activity. There is, therefore, usually a compensatory pause after the ventricular premature beat. As a result the next P wave occurs at the normal time.

A ventricular premature beat discharging during the repolarisation phase of the ventricle runs the risk of precipitating ventricular fibrillation. The chances of this are thought to be higher if the beat occurs close to the T wave. This is known as the R-on-T phenomenon (Fig. 27.23).

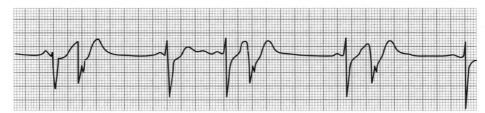

Fig. 27.23 R-on-T ectopic.

When there is more than one ventricular premature beat, specific terms are used if other features exist.

Multifocal ventricular ectopics are seen when the ventricular premature beats vary in shape from beat to beat (Fig. 27.24). This may or may not represent a

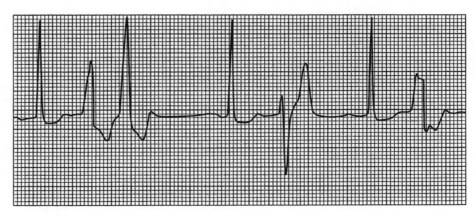

Fig. 27.24 Multifocal ventricular ectopics.

number of separate foci but it does indicate a significant increase in ventricular excitability and a higher chance of deteriorating into ventricular fibrillation.

Bigeminy is seen when a normal QRS complex is followed by a ventricular premature beat (Fig. 27.25).

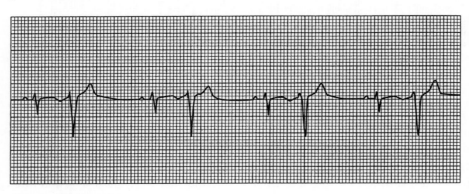

Fig. 27.25 Bigeminy.

Trigeminy occurs when two normal consecutive QRS complexes are followed by a ventricular premature beat (Fig. 27.26).

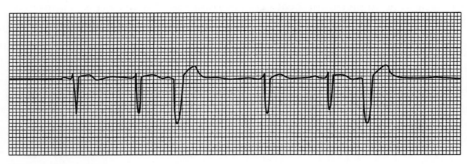

Fig. 27.26 Trigeminy.

A couplet is seen when there are two ventricular ectopic beats in a row (Fig. 27.27).

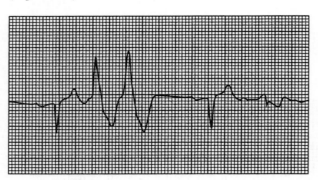

Fig. 27.27 Couplets.

Ventricular escape beats

These occur when the sinoatrial node and atrioventricular node can no longer generate an electrical impulse or stimulate the ventricles. In such circumstances the ventricles have to rely on their own intrinsic pacemaker (see earlier in the chapter). Consequently the heart rate is slow and the RR interval is longer than

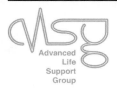

normal. If P waves exist they do not have any connection to the QRS (see 'Third-degree heart block').

The QRS complex can be narrow or wide depending on where the source of the ventricular pacemaker is located. An escape focus near the atrioventricular node will result in a rate of around 50/min with narrow complexes as they are conducted via the bundle of His. This can result from congenital abnormalities but is also associated with inferior myocardial infarction.

A ventricular focus from a more distal site in the atrioventricular node will produce an intrinsic rate of around 30/min (see later in this chapter). However, the QRS complexes will be wide (3 small squares, 0.12 s, 120 ms or more) because conduction through the ventricles is not by the normal pathway. This can result from congenital abnormalities as well as from anterior and inferior myocardial infarction. These patients have a worse prognosis than those with a narrow QRS as they have a greater risk of ventricular standstill.

Aberrant conduction with supraventricular premature stimulation

The QRS is abnormal because the premature atrial impulse gets to either the atrioventricular node or the ventricles before they have had a chance to repolarise. Consequently, the conduction through the ventricles is abnormal and the resulting QRS complex is broad and abnormal in shape. Occasionally the shape of the QRS varies from beat to beat because the conduction pathway through the ventricles is not consistent. The PR interval is normal or slightly prolonged in this condition.

10. Is there ventricular tachycardia?

This occurs when there are three or more consecutive ventricular premature beats, with a rate greater than 100/min. It is said to be sustained if it lasts more than 30 s (Fig. 27.28). Ventricular tachycardia produces a regular, or almost regular, rhythm with a constantly abnormally wide QRS complex. The rate is usually between 140 and 280 beats/min. This may be slower when the patient is treated with an anti-arrhythmic drug, particularly amiodarone, which may slow the rate rather than correct the abnormal rhythm.

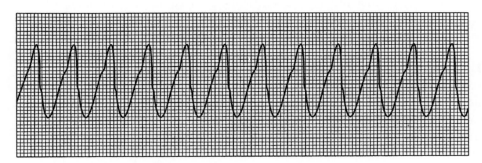

Fig. 27.28 Ventricular tachycardia.

A regular, broad QRS complex tachycardia can also be due to a supraventricular rhythm with an aberrant conduction, but this is rare. A broad complex tachycardia is ventricular tachycardia until proven otherwise. Occasionally the abnormal QRS complexes exist before the supraventricular tachycardia starts and the increase in rate simply reflects the increase in rate of stimulation from the atria. Alternatively, the complexes may only become abnormal once the supraventricular tachycardia starts. In these circumstances the normal conducting system cannot repolarise quickly enough for the new wave of depolarisation from the atria. As a

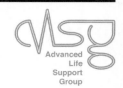

consequence the ventricles depolarise abnormally, manifested as a bundle branch block pattern and this is reflected in the abnormal QRS shape.

Distinguishing between ventricular tachycardia and supraventricular tachycardia with aberrant conduction can be difficult. A search must therefore be made for specific features.

The following favour VT:

- Evidence of independent P wave activity, including capture beats and fusion beats
- Concordant QRS polarity in chest leads (all QRS deflections in the chest leads in the same direction —- up or down)
- Wide QRS complex: greater than $3^{1}/_{2}$ small squares, 0.14 s (140 ms)

The following favour SVT with aberrant conduction:

- QRS morphology shows clear bundle branch block pattern.
- QRS morphology shows no change in pattern from that in sinus rhythm.

The most sensitive discriminator however is the patients past history, particularly of a previous myocardial infarction. It is perverse to assume that a patient who has previously suffered a myocardial infarct and who now presents with a broad complex tachycardia has developed, late in life, an unusual variant of supraventricular tachycardia rather than a typical ventricular dysrhythmia which might be expected given the previous cardiac history.

Fusion beats are produced when the atrial electrical impulse partially depolarises the ventricular muscle, which is also partially depolarised by the ventricular premature beat. The result is a normal P wave followed by an abnormal QRS complex. Capture beats occur in the context of atrioventricular dissociation, when the atrial electrical impulse completely depolarises the ventricle before it is depolarised by the ventricular premature beat. The effect is a normal QRS complex in the midst of the sequence of broad QRS complexes. Both fusion and capture beats are seen most frequently when the rate of the tachycardia is relatively slow.

Further clues as to the origin of the broad complex tachycardia come from studying the patient's 12-lead ECG, previous ECG tracings and medical notes. It is, therefore, essential that attempts be made to obtain these records. However, even after careful ECG evaluation it may still be impossible to distinguish between ventricular tachycardia and a supraventricular tachycardia with an aberrant conduction. In these cases, and especially after myocardial infarction, it is always safer to assume a ventricular origin for a broad complex tachycardia.

11. Is there *torsade de pointes* (polymorphic ventricular tachycardia)?

This is a type of ventricular tachycardia where the cardiac axis is constantly changing in a regular fashion (Fig. 27.29 – see page 429).

Torsade de pointes can occur spontaneously, but it can also result from ischaemic heart disease, hypokalaemia and certain drugs which prolong the QT interval including tricyclic antidepressants and class Ia and III anti-arrhythmic agents. This condition can end spontaneously or degenerate into ventricular fibrillation. Interestingly, ventricular fibrillation may have a similar pattern, particularly soon after its onset, but this is usually short lived.

Furthermore, ventricular fibrillation has a far more random appearance and greater variability in QRS morphology.

Atrial fibrillation in the presence of a Wolff–Parkinson–White type of accessory pathway that bypasses the atrioventricular node, may permit rapid transmission of atrial impulses to the ventricles. The resulting broad complex tachycardia may have a ventricular rate so fast that cardiac output falls dramatically, and the

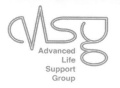

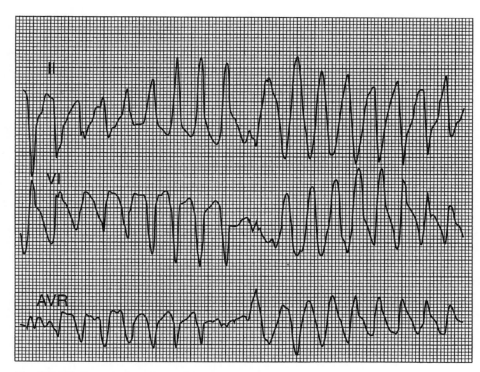

Fig. 27.29 *Torsade de pointes*, showing axis change.

rhythm can decay into ventricular fibrillation. It is one of the causes of sudden cardiac death in young people. The ECG appearances of this pre-excited atrial fibrillation are of a very rapid but irregular, broad complex tachycardia that may show marked variability in the QRS complexes. However, the QRS complexes do not show the twisting axis characteristic of *torsade de pointes*. Furthermore, it is often possible to recognise occasional normally conducted beats.

12. Is there an idioventricular rhythm?
This occurs when the ventricles have taken over as the cardiac pacemaker due to failure of the sinoatrial node, atria or atrioventricular node. In view of the ventricles' slow intrinsic rate of depolarisation the heart rate is usually slow (<40 beats/min). However, it can be accelerated and produce rates up to 100 beats/min.

Acute idioventricular rhythm commonly occurs after a myocardial infarction.

An agonal rhythm is characterised by the presence of slow, irregular, wide ventricular complexes of varying morphology. This rhythm is usually seen during the latter stages of unsuccessful resuscitation attempts. The complexes gradually slow and often become progressively broader before all recognisable electrical activity is lost.

SUMMARY

The electrical activity of the heart is highly organised and monitoring of this activity should be done in a particular way to minimise the chances of artefacts. By using a systematic approach it is possible to interpret ECG rhythm strips effectively. It is important to remember to treat the patient and not the monitor.

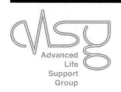

Advanced
Life
Support
Group

CHAPTER 28

Chest X-ray interpretation

OBJECTIVES

After reading this chapter you will be able to:
- describe an effective system for non-radiologists to interpret chest X-rays.

INTRODUCTION

To aid understanding, the chapter will begin by reviewing important anatomical features and considering how each particular area can be affected.

It is important that a systematic method is followed when studying any X-ray, so that subtle and multiple pathologies are not missed. Once the patient's details have been checked use the system recommended for chest X-ray interpretation shown in the box.

The 'AABCS' approach to radiographic interpretation

A – Adequacy
A – Alignment
B – Bones
C – Cartilage and joints
S – Soft tissue

Most patients require only one good quality film and the ideal is a posteroanterior view taken in the X-ray department. The clinical condition of acutely ill patients usually prohibits this. Thus an antero-posterior view is taken in the resuscitation room or on the ward. This enables monitoring and treatment to be continued because the film cartridge is placed behind the patient lying on the trolley or bed. However, the apparent dimensions of the heart shadow are altered as a result of this projection.

INTERPRETATION OF FRONTAL CHEST RADIOGRAPHS

Adequacy
Check the patient details are correct and the date and time of the study.

Having made sure it is the correct radiograph, check the side marker and look for any details written or stamped on the film. This will tell you if the film is posteroanterior or anteroposterior, erect, semi-erect or supine. Assess the exposure, by looking at the midthoracic intervertebral discs and noting if they are just visible through the mediastinal density. In overexposed films all the intervertebral discs are seen and the radiograph appears generally blacker. In contrast, underexposure gives rise to poor definition of structures and boundaries.

Acute Medical Emergencies; The Practical Approach, 2nd edition.
Edited by Terence Wardle, Peter Driscoll, and Sue Wieteska.
© 2010 Blackwell Publishing Ltd.

The film should show the lung apices and bases including the costophrenic recesses, the lateral borders of the ribs and peripheral soft tissues. The right hemidiaphragm should reach the anterior end of the right sixth/seventh rib or the ninth/tenth rib posteriorly on full inspiration. Poor inspiration (diaphragm higher than anterior fifth rib) affects the lower zone vessels such that they are compressed and appear more prominent. This in turn leads to vague lower zone shadowing. In addition, the heart appears enlarged because the diaphragms are high and the heart lies more horizontally.

Alignment

This is determined by looking at the relationship between the spinous processes of the upper thoracic vertebrae and the medial aspects of the clavicles. The ends of both clavicles should be equidistant from the central spinous process.

As with adequacy, alignment of the patient to the X-ray can significantly alter the size and shape of the chest contents on the radiograph. For example, if the patient is rotated there is distortion of the mediastinal contours as well as inequality in the transradiancy of the hemithoraces.

In addition to postural and rotational artefacts, remember the configuration of the patient's chest wall can give rise to abnormal appearances. For example, pectus excavatum can alter the size, shape and position of the mediastinum, as well as producing inequality in the transradiancy of the lungs.

Bones

The posterior, lateral and anterior aspects of each rib must be examined in detail. This can be done by tracing out the upper and lower borders of the ribs from the posterior costochondral joint to where they join the anterior costal cartilage at the midclavicular line. The internal trabecular pattern can then be assessed. Some people find this easier to do with the X-ray on its side.

Finish assessing the bones by inspecting the visible vertebrae, the clavicles, scapulae and proximal humeri. However, for full assessment specific views must be obtained.

Cartilage and joints

Calcification in the costal cartilage and larynx is common in the elderly. Occasionally the glenohumeral joints are seen on the chest X-ray. They may show either degenerative or inflammatory changes or calcification in the rotator cuff.

Soft tissue

The soft tissue can be considered in three parts:
- Mediastinum
- Lungs and diaphragm
- Extrathoracic soft tissues

Mediastinum

The mediastinum normally occupies the centre of the chest radiograph and has a well-defined margin. You should consider the upper, middle (hilar) and lower (heart) parts of the mediastinum.

Upper mediastinum

Check the position of the trachea. This should be central.

The upper left mediastinal shadow is formed by the left subclavian artery. This normally gives rise to a curved border which fades out where the vessels enter the neck. The left outer wall of the trachea is not visible in this area because

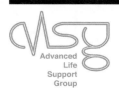

the subclavian vessels separate the trachea from the aerated lung. Inferiorly, the left paratracheal region is interrupted by both the aortic knuckle and the main pulmonary artery with the space between the two being known as the 'aortopulmonary window'. The aortic knuckle should be well defined. Note the presence of any calcification.

Middle mediastinum

The hilar shadows are produced mainly by the pulmonary arteries and veins. The major bronchi can be identified as air-containing structures but the bronchial walls are commonly only visible when seen end on. Though a contribution is made to these shadows by the hilar lymph nodes, they cannot be identified separately from the vascular shadows. The left hilum is usually higher than the right.

Any lobulation of the hilar shadow, local expansion or increase in density compared with the opposite side indicates a central mass lesion. Central enlargement of the pulmonary arteries may mimic mass lesions but the vascular enlargement is usually bilateral, accompanied by cardiomegaly and forms a branching shadow.

Lower mediastinum

The overall position, size and shape of the heart should be noted. Normally the cardiac shadow can have a transverse diameter which is up to 50% of the transverse diameter of the chest on a posteroanterior film. Cardiomyopathy or pericardial effusion can both give rise to a globular heart shadow but further diagnostic clues are usually available from the clinical history and examination.

The heart borders can then be assessed. The heart silhouette should be sharp and single with loss of a clear border indicating neighbouring lung pathology. If the borders are ill-defined then there is likely to be pathology in the adjacent lung. If the right heart border is lost then there may be right middle lobe consolidation. If the left heart border is not clear then there may be left upper lobe consolidation. A double outline suggests pneumomediastinum/pneumopericardium. With a pneumomediastinum, a translucent line can usually be seen to extend up into the neck and be accompanied by subcutaneous emphysema.

Inspection of the heart is completed by checking for calcification (valves and pericardium), prosthetic values, intravascular stents and retrocardiac abnormalities, e.g. hiatus hernia, increased density or the presence of foreign bodies and oesophageal metal stents.

Lungs and diaphragm
Lungs

These are best assessed initially by standing back from the radiograph so that you can compare the overall size and translucency of both hemithoraces. A number of changes may be seen.

Reduced volume: The commonest cause of lung volume loss is lobar collapse. When complete, these give rise to dense white shadows in specific locations and are usually accompanied by hilar displacement, increased radiolucency in the remaining lobes and reduction in the vascular pattern due to compensatory emphysema. When the collapse is incomplete, consolidation in the remaining part of the lobe is evident.

Reduced density: The transradiancy of both lungs should be equal and their outer edges should extend out to the ribs laterally and the diaphragm below. Any separation indicates that there is a pneumothorax. Within the normal lungs the only identifiable structures are blood vessels, end on bronchi and the interlobar fissures. Air trapping gives rise to increased translucency and flattening of the dome of the diaphragm. In extreme cases the mediastinum may be displaced to the contralateral side.

Increased density: There are several causes for an increase in pulmonary density. In consolidation the density is restricted to either part or all of a pulmonary lobe as a result of the air being replaced with fluid. With segmental consolidation the density is rounded and the edges blurred. When the whole of the lobe is involved the interface with neighbouring soft tissues is lost. This can lead to alteration in the outline of the heart and diaphragm depending on the location of the lobe (silhouette sign) (see earlier).

Pleural fluid is seen initially as blunting of the costophrenic angle. As more accumulates, the fluid level is easier to make out. However, if the patient is supine the fluid collects posteriorly and gives rise to a general ground-glass appearance on the affected side. Consequently, an effusion may be missed until it is large or the frontal and erect chest radiograph is carried out.

Pulmonary oedema presents as generalised fluffy air space shadowing which can be accompanied by Kerley B lines due to interstitial lymphatic congestion.

The position, configuration and thickness of the fissures should also be checked – anything more than a hairline thickness should be considered abnormal. To visualise a fissure the X-ray beam needs to be tangential; therefore, only the horizontal fissure is evident on the frontal film, and then only in 50% of the population. It runs from the right hilium to the sixth rib in the axilla. The azygos fissure is seen in approximately 1% of the population. The oblique fissures are only identified on the lateral view.

Diaphragm

The diaphragm must be checked for position, shape and clarity of the cardio-phrenic and costophrenic angles. The outline of the diaphragm is normally a smooth curve with the highest point medial to the midline of the hemithorax. Lateral peaking, particularly on the right, suggests a subpulmonary effusion or a haemothorax in the appropriate clinical setting.

In the vast majority of patients the right diaphragm is higher than the left. However, elevation of either side can result from pathology in the chest (anything reducing lung volume), abdomen or damage to the phrenic nerve. In this situation the patient's history will be very helpful in distinguishing between these possible causes.

The upper surface of the diaphragm is normally clearly outlined by air in the lung except where it is in contact with the heart and pericardial fat. Loss of clarity may indicate collapse or consolidation of the lower lobe. It could also indicate diaphragmatic rupture.

Extrathoracic soft tissue

Start at the top with the neck and supraclavicular area, and continue down the lateral wall of the chest on each side. Note any foreign bodies and subcutaneous emphysema. The latter is often seen in the cervical region and appears as linear transradiancies along tissue planes. When gross it may interfere with the assessment of the underlying lung. Finally, check under the diaphragm for abnormal structures or free gas.

Presence and position of any medical equipment

The position and presence of any invasive medical equipment must be assessed while the radiograph is examined so that potential complications can be identified. It is important to check specifically that the following are correctly placed: endo-tracheal tube, CVP line, chest drain, pacing wire and naso-gastric tube. A further chest X-ray should be done after any of these devices have been placed to confirm position and exclude complications relating to insertion.

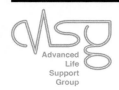

Reassess commonly missed areas

Once the system described above has been completed, it is important to re-evaluate those areas where pathology is often overlooked. These include:

- the lung apices
- behind the heart shadow
- under the diaphragm
- peripheral soft tissues.

This is particularly important if your eye has been drawn to an obvious abnormality in another area.

SUMMARY

Summary of the system for assessing frontal chest radiographs

Assess the adequacy of the film
  Patient's personal details
  Date and time of study
  Projection of the X-ray beam
  Exposure of the film (Penetration)
  Area of the chest on the film
  Degree of inspiration
Assess the alignment of the film

Assess the bones	Spine	
	Scapulae, clavicles	
	Humeri	
	Ribs	

Assess the cartilage and joints
Assess the soft tissue

Mediastinum	Upper	
	Middle (hilar)	
	Lower (heart)	
	Foreign bodies	
Lungs and diaphragm	Lungs	Size
		Density
		Fissures
		Nodules
		Opacifications
		Foreign bodies
	Diaphragm	Position
		Shape
		Clarity of the angles
		Foreign bodies
		Air – under the diaphragm
Medical Equipment	Position	

Reassess commonly missed areas of the film
  Apices
  Behind the heart
  Under the diaphragm
  Peripheral soft tissues

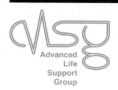

CHAPTER 29

Haematological investigations

OBJECTIVES

After reading this chapter you will be able to:
- identify which haematological tests are useful in the acute medical patient
- describe the rational use of such tests
- use test results to aid further clinical management.

INTRODUCTION

A full blood count is probably the commonest laboratory investigation that is requested because it is a 'routine test'. There is, however, no such commodity as a routine test and you should be able to justify requesting any investigation. A similar situation, though much less common, exists when requesting assessment of the components of the clotting cascade. It is, therefore, important that you critically appraise your requests and also interpret all the available information provided by a full blood count and not just the haemoglobin as often occurs.

RULES

When interpreting haematological results, always request investigations and interpret results in light of clinical findings.
- Beware of: the isolated abnormality
            bizarre results
            results that do not fit with the clinical picture.
- If in doubt:
  - Repeat the test.
  - Always seek corroborative evidence from: clinical findings
                                            other test results.
  - Always observe serial results for trends.

REVISION

Many haematological disorders are identified by, or suggested by, an abnormality in the full blood count. The result usually relates to three major cell lines in peripheral blood:
- Erythrocytes
- Leucocytes
- Platelets

In addition, there is a wealth of numerical information describing these cell lines that is often ignored – at the clinician's peril. This information, generated by automatic haematology counters, should be used to the clinician's advantage, hence the need for revision of some of the key cell count components.

Acute Medical Emergencies; The Practical Approach, 2nd edition.
Edited by Terence Wardle, Peter Driscoll, and Sue Wieteska.
© 2010 Blackwell Publishing Ltd.

HAEMOGLOBIN LEVEL

The normal levels of haemoglobin are 15 ± 2 g/dl (150 ± 20 g/l) for men and 14 ± 2 g/dl (140 ± 20 g/l) for women. In the acute medical patient a raised haemoglobin often indicates dehydration or polycythaemia. The latter is commonly associated with chronic respiratory disease rather than the rare polycythaemia rubra vera. In contrast, the haemoglobin level may be low, indicating anaemia. However, remember that in patients with acute blood loss the haemoglobin level may be normal initially, until either compensatory measures fail or haemodilution occurs.

> **Key point**
>
> Anaemia is not a diagnosis, but a 'symptom' of an underlying disease

The red cell count is quoted by some laboratories, but this has little diagnostic value in the acute medical patient. However, the combination of haemoglobin and red cell count can be used to derive the mean cell haemoglobin (MCH). This gives a reliable indication of the amount of haemoglobin per red cell and is measured in picograms (normal range 29.5 ± 2.5 pg). The mean cell haemoglobin concentration (MCHC) represents the concentration of haemoglobin in grams per decilitre (100 ml) of erythrocytes (normal range 33 ± 1.5 g/dl). This is obtained by dividing the haemoglobin concentration by the packed cell volume. A low mean cell haemoglobin concentration is due to a low haemoglobin content in the red cell mass and indicates deficient haemoglobin synthesis. Thus the red cells will appear pale (hypochromic).

Remember that high mean cell haemoglobin concentrations do not occur in red cell disorders because the haemoglobin concentration is already near saturation point in normal red cells. The mean cell haemoglobin concentration, unlike the mean cell haemoglobin, assesses the degree of haemoglobinisation of the red cells irrespective of their size and is useful in assessing the extent of under-haemoglobinisation. The packed cell volume (PCV or haematocrit) represents a proportion (by volume) of whole blood occupied by the red cells and is expressed as a percentage (normal range for men $47 \pm 7\%$, women $42 \pm 5\%$). The packed cell volume or haematocrit is always elevated in polycythaemia irrespective of the cause. However, this may only be relative when haemoconcentration occurs as a result of fluid loss producing a decrease in plasma volume. The packed cell volume is therefore reduced in the presence of excess extracellular fluid and raised in fluid depletion. The mean cell volume (MCV) measured in femtolitres (normal range 85 ± 10 fl) indicates erythrocyte size. Thus, it is increased in patients with macrocytic disorders (e.g. vitamin B_{12}/folate deficiency) and reduced in the presence of microcytes (e.g. iron deficiency anaemia).

It is important to realise that red cell indices indicate the average size and degree of haemoglobinisation of red cells. They are, therefore, only of value if combined with a blood film examination that will augment the information about the relative uniformity of changes in either cell size or haemoglobin concentration.

THE BLOOD FILM

The benefits of the blood film have already been described. Some of the common terms used to describe cell morphology are listed in the next box.

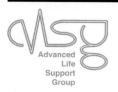

Morphological terms on blood cell reports

Red cells

Pale cells	Hypochromia indicating defective haemoglobinisation or haemoglobin synthesis
Macrocytes	Large cells, abnormal red cell production, premature release, megaloblastic erythropoiesis, haemolysis
Anisocytes	Variation in cell size
Poikilocytes	Variation in cell shape
Schistocytes/Burr cells	Fragmented forms, usually indicate red cell trauma
Sickle cells	Sickling disorders

White cells

Hypersegmented neutrophils	Vitamin B_{12} or folate deficiency
Left shift neutrophils	Neutrophils are being prematurely released
Toxic granulation	Increased neutrophil cytoplasmic granularity usually associated with underlying infection
Atypical lymphocytes	Likely viral infection
Blast cells	Usually indicate leukaemia

Platelets

Clumping	Often causing an artificially low platelet count

RED CELL ABNORMALITIES

Red cell abnormalities can be classified as alterations in either number or morphology.

Alteration in number

An increase in red cells is described as polycythaemia (see earlier). In contrast, anaemia is described as diminished oxygen carrying capacity of the blood due to a reduction either in the number of red cells or in the content of haemoglobin or both. This may be due to deficient red cell production and/or excessive loss. Although there is some overlap between these conditions, this classification does provide a convenient way of considering this condition (see the next box).

Another useful way of classifying anaemias is on the basis of the MCV/MCH:

Classifying anaemia

Low MCV/MCH	Normal MCV/MCH	Raised MCV
Iron deficiency	Chronic disease	Vitamin B_{12} deficiency
Chronic disease	Acute haemorrhage	Folate deficiency
Thalassaemia	Mixed picture, e.g. iron and folate deficiency	Alcohol use
	Aplastic anaemia	Haemolysis
		Hypothyroidism

An anaemia with a coexistent reduction in both white cells and platelets is referred to as pancytopenia. Causes of pancytopenia include aplastic anaemia, bone marrow infiltration (e.g. lymphoma, leukaemia, myelofibrosis, myeloma) and hypersplenism.

Alteration in morphology

An anaemia with reduced mean cell volume, mean cell haemoglobin and mean cell haemoglobin concentration, i.e. microcytic hypochromic anaemia, is highly suggestive of iron deficiency. Therefore a serum ferritin should be requested before treatment with iron is started.

However, if there is coexistent thrombocytosis then this type of anaemia could indicate ongoing blood loss or inflammation. If none of these conditions are evident then it is possible that the microcytic hypochromic picture is a manifestation of thalassaemia, which is rare in the UK. In contrast, an anaemia with raised mean cell volume and mean cell haemoglobin is suggestive of a variety of conditions including a deficiency in vitamin B_{12} and/or folic acid, hypothyroidism and alcohol use. An anaemia with normal mean cell volume, mean cell haemoglobin and mean cell haemoglobin concentration, i.e. a normochromic normocytic anaemia, can reflect chronic disease (e.g. inflammation, myeloma), acute blood loss or haemolysis.

Haemolysis is usually associated with a normochromic normocytic anaemia although some of the red cells can be large due to the release of a large number of immature red cells, i.e. reticulocytes. The latter can also occur following haemorrhage or in response to treatment with iron, folic acid and vitamin B_{12}. The comment polychromasia (grey/blue tint to cells) is often recorded on the full blood count indicating a reticulocyte response. A formal count of these cells can also be done.

Haemolytic anaemia is a term that describes a group of anaemias of differing cause, which are all characterised by abnormal destruction of red cells. The questions asked to identify the cause of haemolysis are shown in the box.

These questions can be used to produce a 'user-friendly' classification of haemolytic anaemia as shown in the next box.

Three key questions in the diagnosis of haemolytic anaemia

- Is it an inherited or acquired disorder?
- Is the location of the abnormality within the red cells (intrinsic) or outside (extrinsic)?
- Are the red cells prematurely destroyed in the blood stream (intravascular) or outside in the spleen and liver (extravascular)?

LABORATORY DIAGNOSIS OF HAEMOLYTIC ANAEMIA

The most likely clue is a normochromic normocytic anaemia with prominent reticulocytes. Other laboratory results include:
- unconjugated hyperbilirubinaemia (thus a lack of bilirubin in the urine)
- low haptoglobin (a glycoprotein that binds to free haemoglobin and is thus usually full saturated in haemolysis)

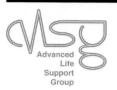

- haemoglobin and haemosiderin can be detected in the urine with intravascular haemolysis, because the haptoglobin which usually 'mops up' free haemoglobin is saturated.

Congenital disorders

More specific tests will be requested after taking a comprehensive history as this is likely to provide clues to underlying inherited disorders. The presence of hereditary spherocytosis or elliptocytosis will be seen on the blood film.

The thalassaemias are a heterogeneous group of disorders affecting haemoglobin synthesis; they will be diagnosed from the medical history, clinical examination, blood film and haemoglobin electrophoresis to identify structural haemoglobin variants. In addition, the presence of sickle cell syndromes will be diagnosed from the clinical history, in particular that of the family, and the presentation with haemolysis, vascular occlusive crises and sequestration crises. Under these circumstances the blood film is likely to show the presence of sickle shaped cells. Haemoglobin electrophoresis may reveal an abnormal haemoglobin such as in sickle cell anaemia with no detectable haemoglobin A.

The two common abnormalities of red cell metabolism resulting in haemolysis are glucose-6-phosphate dehydrogenase deficiency and pyruvate kinase deficiency. As well as the features of intravascular haemolysis described earlier, specific enzyme levels can also be measured to produce a definitive diagnosis.

Acquired disorders

Autoimmune haemolytic anaemia

Autoimmune haemolytic anaemia is a form of acquired haemolysis with a defect outside the red cell. The bone marrow produces structurally normal red cells. These are prematurely destroyed by the production of an aberrant antibody (IgM or IgG) targeted against the red cell membrane. Once the autoantibody has bound with the antigen on the red cell the exact type of haemolysis is determined by the class of antibody as well as the surface antigen. It usually involves sequestration by the spleen leading to extravascular haemolysis or activation of complement leading to intravascular haemolysis. A simple classification of these conditions is either warm or cold depending on whether the antibody reacts better with red cells at 37°C or 4°C respectively.

Warm autoimmune haemolytic anaemia

This is the commonest form of haemolytic anaemia. The erythrocytes are coated with either IgG alone or IgG and complement or complement alone. Premature destruction of red cells usually occurs in the liver and spleen. Half of all warm autoimmune haemolytic anaemias are associated with other autoimmune conditions or lymphoma. The most characteristic laboratory abnormality is a positive direct antiglobulin test (DAT or Coombs test). As a reminder the DAT is where red cells are already sensitised and have immunoglobulin bound to their surface antigens. Addition of extrinsic antihuman globulin results in haemolysis, i.e. a positive direct Coombs test. In contrast, the indirect test is where normal red cells have to be sensitised in vitro by the addition of the test serum containing red cell antibodies. Finally antihuman globulin is added. Agglutination indicates the presence of red cell antibodies, as used in red cell typing.

Cold autoimmune haemolytic anaemia

This is generally associated with an IgM antibody. Isoimmune haemolytic anaemia may occur with rhesus or ABO incompatibility, and in the context of

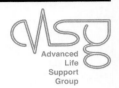

adult medicine this may follow a blood transfusion reaction. It can also follow infection with mycoplasma or Epstein–Barr virus.

Drug-induced haemolytic anaemia
There are three mechanisms of haemolysis:
- Drug-antibody complex (e.g. quinine) induces complement, leading to erythrocyte destruction.
- Drug-red cell complex (e.g. penicillin) acts as an antigen to which antibodies are formed, leading to erythrocyte destruction.
- A drug (e.g. methyldopa) induces production of an erythrocyte autoantibody, leading to erythrocyte destruction.

Non immune/traumatic haemolytic anaemia
Non-immune and traumatic haemolytic anaemia is most frequently manifested by a microangiopathic picture. This is one of the most frequent causes of haemolysis and describes intravascular destruction of red cells in the presence of an abnormal microcirculation. Causes of microangiopathic haemolytic anaemia are listed in the next box.

Causes of microangiopathic haemolytic anaemia

Disseminated intravascular coagulation
Valve prosthesis
Malignancy
Severe infections
Glomerulonephritis
Vasculitis
Accelerated (malignant) hypertension

WHITE CELLS

Total and differential leucocyte count
The total white count varies markedly as there is a diurnal rhythm with minimal counts occurring in the morning. This may rise during the rest of the day or following stress, eating or during the menstrual cycle.

The total leucocyte count is $(7 \pm 3) \times 10^9/l$. This comprises:
- neutrophils $(2–7) \times 10^9/l$ (40–80% of total count)
- lymphocytes $(1–3) \times 10^9/l$ (20–40% of total count)
- monocytes $(0.2–1) \times 10^9/l$ (2–10% of total count)
- eosinophils $(0.04–0.4) \times 10^9/l$ (1–6% of total count)
- basophils $(0.02–0.1) \times 10^9/l$ (<2% of total count)

Disorders of leucocytes
There are many conditions that will affect both the total and differential white cell count. Common disorders are listed in Tables 29.1–29.4.

Basophils rarely have any significance in the acute medical setting.

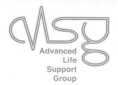

Table 29.1 Disorders of neutrophils

Raised number	Bacterial infection
	Myeloproliferative disease
	Tissue damage
	Malignancy
	Drugs, e.g. prednisolone
Reduced numbers	Chemicals
(production failure)	Severe infection
	Drugs, e.g. carbimazole
	Marrow infiltration by malignant tumour or marrow fibrosis
	Specific deficiencies of vitamin B_{12} and folic acid
	Peripheral sequestration/hypersplenism
	Shock

Table 29.2 Disorders of lymphocytes

Raised numbers (lymphocytosis)	Viral infection, especially glandular fever*
	Chronic lymphatic leukaemia
	Typhoid fever
	Brucellosis
Reduced numbers (lymphopenia)	Corticosteriods
	Viral infections*
	Cytotoxic drugs
	Ionising radiation

*In suspected viral infections a blood film may show changes in lymphocyte numbers and morphology.

Table 29.3 Disorders of monocytes

Raised numbers	Infective endocarditis
	Typhus fever
	Malaria
	Kala-azar
	Systemic lupus erythematosus
	Certain clinical poisonings, e.g. trichloroethylene

Table 29.4 Disorders of eosinophils

Raised numbers	Parasitic infections
	Atopy including asthma and drug sensitivity
	Chronic eczema
	Malignant tumours, e.g. Hodgkin's disease

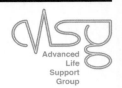

Haematological malignancies
Chronic myelocytic leukaemia

This is a myeloproliferative disease characterised by increased numbers of neutrophils and their precursors. The clinical features include weight loss, night sweats, pruritus and splenomegaly. It can occur in all age groups but the peak incidence is in middle age and it affects both sexes equally. The disease is associated with Philadelphia chromosomal translocation. Blood results show a leukocytosis, mainly neutrophils; platelet count is variable and anaemia may be a feature. There may also be a low leucocyte alkaline phosphatase score and raised urate.

Treatment consists of hydroxyurea, interferon and allopurinol to prevent gout. Allogeneic stem cell transplantation is an option for patients under 50 years of age.

Chronic lymphocytic leukaemia

This is a B-cell lymphoproliferative disease. Clinical features include lymphadenopathy, night sweats, weight loss and moderate splenomegaly. It is a disease of the elderly and is more common in men. Blood results show a lymhocytosis; anaemia and thrombocytosis may also be a feature.

Treatment consists of chemotherapy with chlorambucil and steroids.

Acute leukaemia

These leukaemias can be classified as lymhpoblastic or myeloblastic. They can occur as primary leukaemias or may follow previous chronic leukaemias that have transformed into an acute (more aggressive) type. Acute lymphoblastic leukaemia (ALL) is common in childhood.

Acute myeloblastic leukaemia is more common in the elderly. Clinical features are those of bone marrow failure and occur over a relatively short period of time. They include bruising, bleeding and infection. Lymphadenopathy and hepatosplenomegaly are common in ALL.

Treatment comprises chemotherapy and stem cell transplantation.

Lymphoma

There are two types: Hodgkin's (HL) and non-Hodgkin's (NHL).

HL is characterised by malignant cells called Reed–Sternberg cells which appear to be derived from B cells. There is an association with Epstein–Barr infection. There is a bimodal distribution of cases in young adulthood and in later life. Features include lymphadenopathy which is usually cervical and weight loss, night sweats and pruritus. Some patients complain of lymph node pain in association with alcohol consumption.

NHL is the term used to describe tumours of lymphoid tissue **without** the characteristic Reed–Sternberg cells. This disease is the most common haematological malignancy. Features include lymphadenopathy, abdominal pain, anaemia, sweating and weight loss.

Blood results usually show an anaemia (normochromic, normocytic), leucocytosis, raised ESR, raised LDH and abnormal LFTs. NHL specifically may cause a pancytopenia and a peripheral blood lymphocytosis.

Treatment for both types of lymphoma involves chemotherapy, radiotherapy and stem cell support/transplantation. There is a very complicated staging system for lymphomas which is beyond the scope of this book and treatment depends on the stage of the disease.

Multiple myeloma

Multiple myeloma is a malignant disease of plasma cells characterised by a monoclonal paraprotein in the urine/serum, boney involvement and an excess of

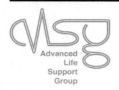

plasma cells in the bone marrow. It is a disease of the elderly and is slightly more common in men. Features include bone pain, hypercalcaemia, bone marrow failure, immune failure, renal failure and amyloidosis.

Blood results show anaemia and a paraprotein in the serum and/or Bence–Jones proteins in the urine; a blood film shows rouleaux and the bone marrow shows an excess of plasma cells.

Treatment may be conservative or with chemotherapy.

PLATELETS

There is a marked variation in the normal platelet count ranging from 150 to 400×10^9/l. Common platelet disorders are listed in the next box.

Disorders of platelets

Raised number (thrombocytosis)	Inflammation, e.g. Crohn's disease
	Haemorrhage
	Essential thrombocytosis (rare)
	Polycythaemia rubra vera (rare)
Reduced number (thrombocytopenia)	Deficient production, e.g. hypoplasia
	Replacement with leukaemic cells or fibrosis
	Dyshaemopoiesis secondary to vitamin B_{12} deficiency
	Increased destruction of platelets, e.g. drugs or autoimmune
	Sequestered in the spleen
	Increased consumption (disseminated intravascular coagulation)

Thrombocytopenia is a common finding. The risk of spontaneous haemorrhage is unusual unless the platelet count falls below 20×10^9/l.

COAGULATION

The physiological pathway of blood coagulation is an interlinked cascade of factors which most doctors learn for examinations. The basic principles are three activation pathways (intrinsic, extrinsic and alternative) which have a final common pathway. These pathways are summarised in Fig. 29.1 (see over).

Blood clotting is a vital defence mechanism that is regulated to ensure adequate and appropriate activation.

The major inhibitors of coagulation circulating in the plasma are:

- antithrombin III. This is the most potent inhibitor of the terminal proteins of the cascade, particularly factor X and thrombin. Its activity is greatly increased by interaction with heparin
- protein C is a vitamin K-dependent plasma protein which inactivates cofactors Va and VIIIa as well as stimulating fibrinolysis. Protein C is converted to an active enzyme from interaction with thrombin. Protein S is a cofactor for protein C
- fibrinolytic systems. This system for fibrin digestion is shown in Fig. 29.2. Fibrin clots are broken down by plasmin that is produced from plasminogen by 'activator enzymes'. Plasmin also inhibits thrombin generation, thus acting as an anticoagulant. In addition, fibrin degradation products have a similar effect.

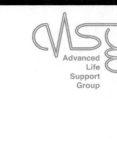

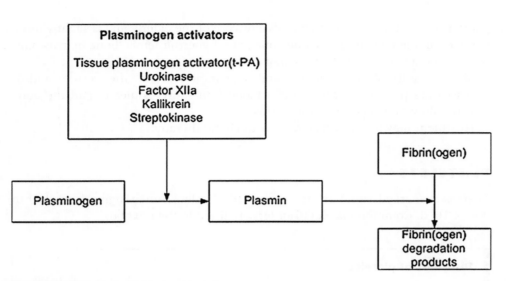

Fig. 29.1 Pathways of blood coagulation.
Streptokinase is an exogenous activator usually from B haemolytic streptococci

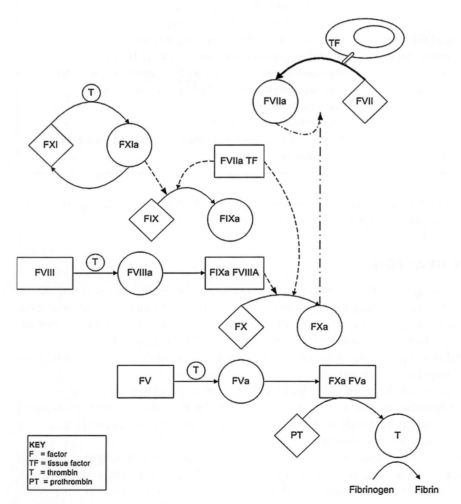

Fig. 29.2 The fibrinolytic system.
Dotted lines = enzyme action on substrates; Solid lines = conversion of protein from one
active state to another

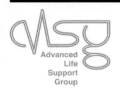

Fibrinolysis is also under strict control. Circulating plasmin is inactivated by the protease inhibitor δ2-antiplasmin.

Tests for the assessment of coagulation

In most acute medical situations, an assessment of the coagulation cascade only requires:

- prothrombin time: – a measure of the function of the extrinsic pathway
- activated partial thromboplastin time – assesses the intrinsic pathway
- assessments of fibrinolysis, e.g. fibrinogen level, fibrin degradation product level or D-dimer quantitation – are often used as markers of thromboembolism disseminated intravascular coagulation.

The common causes of prolonged prothrombin and activated partial thromboplastin times are listed in the box.

Common causes of prolonged prothrombin (PTT) and activated partial thromboplastin (APTT) times

PTT	APTT
Warfarin	Heparin
Liver disease	Haemophilia
Vitamin K deficiency	von Willebrand's disease
Disseminated intravascular coagulation	Liver disease
	Lupus anticoagulant syndrome

D-dimer

A D-dimer fragment is generated when cross linked fibrin in thrombi is broken down by plasmin. There are assays available which can detect the precence of D-dimers using monoclonal antibodies. This test is fairly non-specific and can be raised in the presence of a blood clot but also in infection/inflammation. Therefore it tends to be a more useful test if the result is negative. There is good evidence to show that a negative D-dimer test can help rule out a PE/DVT in low risk cases.

SUMMARY

A limited number of haematological investigations are required in the acutely ill medical patient. Much of the information available is often underused; therefore, a thorough understanding of the morphology and normal values of, in particular, red cells is extremely useful. A blood film is an underused investigation that can yield significant relevant information in the acute medical setting. These initial investigations, combined with a 'phrased' history, will influence the selection of subsequent haematological tests.

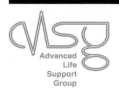
Advanced
Life
Support
Group

CHAPTER 30

Biochemical investigations

OBJECTIVES

After reading this chapter you will be able to:
- understand the importance of interpreting urea, electrolyte and creatinine results in light of clinical findings
- systematically assess urea, electrolyte and creatinine results
- use these results to aid your clinical management.

INTRODUCTION

Urea, electrolytes and creatinine are commonly requested laboratory investigations. All too often there is little thought about why these investigations have been requested and what the abnormalities, in particular of the electrolytes, may indicate. This chapter will provide a systematic approach to the assessment of such investigations, but before this is described there are certain rules which have to be obeyed.

RULES FOR THE INTERPRETATION OF UREA, ELECTROLYTES AND CREATININE

- Always interpret the results in the light of clinical findings.
- Beware: the isolated abnormality
              bizarre results
              results that do not fit the clinical picture.
- If in doubt, repeat the test.
- Always seek corroborative evidence from: clinical findings
                                               other test results.
- Always observe serial results for trends.

GUIDELINES FOR INTERPRETATION OF UREA, ELECTROLYTES AND CREATININE

A review of essential facts.

Urea

Blood urea provides an assessment of glomerular function. However, it can be influenced by many exogenous factors including food intake, fluid balance, gastrointestinal haemorrhage, drugs and liver function. Normal plasma urea is 4.6–6.0 mmol/l.

Acute Medical Emergencies; The Practical Approach, 2nd edition.
Edited by Terence Wardle, Peter Driscoll, and Sue Wieteska.
© 2010 Blackwell Publishing Ltd.

Creatinine

This provides a better indication of renal function. Plasma creatinine levels are proportional to muscle mass. Creatinine gives a reasonable indication of changes in glomerular filtration, provided the body weight remains stable. Normal plasma creatinine is 60–125 μmol/l.

Potassium

This is the most important intracellular cation and only approximately 2% of the total body potassium is found in the extracellular fluid. Normal plasma potassium is 3.5–5.0 mmol/l.

Bicarbonate

Bicarbonate is an important anion. Normal plasma bicarbonate is 24–28 mmol/l. In a venous blood sample the bicarbonate provides a useful, but crude, indication of the acid–base status.

Sodium

Sodium is the major extracellular cation and is intimately related to water balance. The normal plasma sodium is 135–145 mmol/l.

A SYSTEMATIC EXAMINATION OF UREA, ELECTROLYTES AND CREATININE

It is impossible to provide an accurate diagnosis purely by assessing a patient's urea, creatinine and electrolytes. However, this system, especially when viewed with a patient's clinical picture, will help to discriminate between many of the common conditions.

A systematic approach comprises:

- assessment of the patient's urea and creatinine
- the relationship between the urea and creatinine
- assessment of potassium, bicarbonate and sodium.

Examine the urea and creatinine; five common patterns can be seen, as described below.

All results will fall into one of these five broad categories and each will be examined.

Pattern		Diagnoses
↑↑ Urea	↑↑ Creatinine	Renal failure
↓ Urea	↓ Creatinine	Fluid overload
Urea < creatinine		Low protein diet
		Liver failure
		Dialysis
Urea > creatinine		Fluid depletion, e.g. dehydration, fever, trauma
		Drugs, e.g. diuretics
		Elevated protein, e.g. diet, gastrointestinal bleed, catabolism
Urea normal	Creatinine normal	Check for any electrolyte abnormality

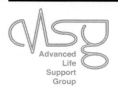

Urea raised and creatinine raised

The most common diagnosis would be renal failure. Therefore confirmatory evidence should be sought.

- Check plasma potassium: This will remain normal until the glomerular rate has fallen below 10 ml/min. Hyperkalaemia is common, but can be secondary to a metabolic acidosis, catabolism or haemolysis.
- Check bicarbonate: This is often reduced reflecting the acidosis associated with uraemia or a failure of bicarbonate secretion.
- Check serum sodium: This may be normal but is often low due to overhydration and dilution. To provide further information, plasma osmolality along with urine, sodium, osmolality and urea should be measured to distinguish between acute and established renal failure.

Urea low and creatinine low

This commonly results from fluid overload.

- Check potassium, bicarbonate and sodium. Low values would be expected. The basic problem is that sodium is retained but to a significantly lesser extent than the degree of water retention. This is often referred to as hyponatraemia with clinically normal extracellular fluid volume. This commonly results from two mechanisms.
- Increased water intake, e.g. excess intravenous fluids, excess drinking (both pathological and psychological polydipsia) and water absorption during bladder irrigation.
- Inability to excrete water, e.g. SIADH, adrenocortical insufficiency, hypothyroidism and drugs that reduce renal diluting capacity, e.g. diuretics. Under these circumstances there is water retention but body sodium is normal with possibly only small increase in extracellular fluid volume which will be undetected clinically. In contrast, if both extracellular fluid sodium and water are increased, but more water is retained than sodium, hyponatraemia will result with expansion of the extracellular fluid volume producing oedema. Note that the discriminating factor between these conditions is based on the clinical presence of oedema.

   Hyponatraemia with expansion of the extracellular volume occurs with cardiac, renal and liver failure. The urine sodium can provide further clues, in particular, in the patient who is hyponatraemic with an increased extracellular volume where the urine sodium is usually less than 10 mmol/l (except in renal failure).

   An interesting variant is beer drinker's hyponatraemia. Beer has a low sodium content. If in excess of 5 litres is consumed daily then hyponatraemia may result, usually with a clinically normal extracellular volume.

Urea less than creatinine

Low urea in relation to the creatinine usually indicates low protein diet or rarely liver failure or post dialysis. Low urea in liver disease is usually attributed to reduced synthesis.

- Check potassium
  - normal with low protein diet and post dialysis
  - normal in liver disease unless diuretics are used
  - low in liver disease with diuretic use.

Urea greater than creatinine

These results suggest fluid depletion, e.g. associated with dehydration, fever, infection or trauma. Drugs, in particular diuretics, can induce a similar problem. An alternative explanation is increased protein which may be from a dietary source, following a gastrointestinal haemorrhage, or secondary to catabolism.

- Check potassium
  low values would suggest gastrointestinal fluid loss
  high values are likely to indicate incipient renal failure or potassium sparing diuretic
- Check sodium
  low values indicate hyponatraemia with reduced extracellular fluid volume reflecting reduced intake (rare), usually attributed to inappropriate replacement of gastrointestinal fluid loss with 5% dextrose only.
  The major cause is excessive sodium loss which is usually:
- from the gastrointestinal tract secondary to vomiting, diarrhoea, fistulae or intestinal obstruction
- from the kidney, e.g. during the diuretic phase of acute tubular necrosis
- due to excess diuretic therapy (including mannitol or the osmotic effect of hyperglycaemia)
- due to postobstructive diuresis
- due to adrenocortical insufficiency or severe alkalosis where increased urinary loss of bicarbonate necessitates an accompanying cation, usually sodium.
  In addition, salt may be lost:
- from the skin in severe sweating, burns or erythroderma
- in association with inflammation of the peritoneum or pancreas
- following the removal of serous effusions, e.g. ascites.

The key feature to remember is that salt loss is always associated with loss of water and other ions, in particular, potassium. However, it is often easy to underestimate the loss of salt if another solute such as glucose is present in excess, i.e. hyperglycaemia. This will tend to retain fluid within the extracellular fluid and the severity of the situation will be only unmasked when the hyperglycaemia is treated. The urine sodium again will provide a good indicator in that it will be less than 10 mmol/l in all conditions, unless there is an intrinsic salt losing problem with the kidneys.

Urea normal and creatinine normal

Therefore exclude any electrolyte abnormality.

- Check potassium – high; secondary to haemolysis, increased intake (usually iatrogenic) or redistribution, e.g. with acidosis or muscle injury
  Under these situations the serum sodium is normal.

Hyperkalaemia may also be present because of reduced excretion, e.g. with acute renal failure or the use of potassium sparing diuretics. Again the sodium is usually normal although it can be reduced in the former because of dilution.

- An elevated potassium in the presence of reduced sodium is suggestive of adrenal insufficiency.

The commonest cause of a low potassium is a metabolic alkalosis; therefore check the bicarbonate level.

Potassium may be lost from the gastrointestinal tract, e.g. with diarrhoea or malabsorption. Under these circumstances the serum sodium is usually normal. In contrast, renal loss, associated with either diuretic therapy or cardiac or liver failure, is accompanied by hyponatraemia. A normal urea and creatinine with low potassium and high sodium combined means that excess of glucocorticoid and mineral corticoid hormones has to be excluded.

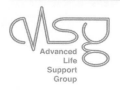

- Check bicarbonate – high, when associated with metabolic alkalosis and hypokalaemia.
- Check sodium – hyponatraemia in the context of normal urea, creatinine and potassium is related to the extracellular fluid volume (see earlier).

Pseudohyponatraemia is a trap for the unwary. Sodium is present only in the aqueous phase of plasma. If there is an associated abnormal amount of lipid the water volume will be reduced and the measured sodium will be low. This result will be spurious because of the high proportion of lipid. In nephrotic syndrome or diabetes mellitus; e.g. 1 litre of plasma may comprise 600 ml of water and 400 ml of lipid with a measured sodium of 120 mmol/l. The true calculated value of sodium, however, when expressed according to the volume of water, is 120 mmol/l of sodium in 600 ml of water; and this equates to 200 mmol/l. Although this is an extreme example, it indicates that if such problems are not identified, inappropriate treatment may occur. A way to clarify this situation is to measure urine sodium and chloride which are low in true hyponatraemia.

SUMMARY

Abnormalities in urea, electrolytes and creatinine are common in acutely ill patients. These guidelines must be interpreted in the light of clinical findings. They will, however, facilitate the diagnosis of common conditions.

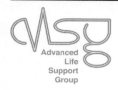

Advanced
Life
Support
Group

PART VII
Practical Procedures

PART VII

Practical Procedures

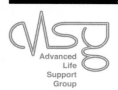
Advanced
Life
Support
Group

CHAPTER 31

Practical procedures: airway and breathing

PROCEDURES

- Oropharyngeal airway insertion
- Nasopharyngeal airway insertion
- Ventilation via a Laerdal pocket mask
- Orotracheal intubation
- Insertion of a laryngeal mask airway
- Needle cricothyroidotomy
- Needle thoracocentesis
- Aspiration of pneumothorax
- Aspiration of pleural fluid
- Chest drain insertion

OROPHARYNGEAL AIRWAY

Equipment
- A series of oropharyngeal (Guedel) airways (sizes 1, 2, 3, 4)
- Tongue depressor
- Laryngoscope

Procedure
The correct size of airway is selected by comparing it with the vertical distance from the angle of the mandible to the centre of the incisors. The airway is inserted in adults and older children as follows:

1 Open the patient's mouth and check for debris. This may be inadvertently pushed into the larynx as the airway is inserted
2 Insert the airway into the mouth either (a) 'upside down' (concave uppermost) as far as the junction between the hard and soft palates and rotate through 180° or (b) use a tongue depressor or the tip of a laryngoscope blade to aid insertion of the airway 'the right way up' under direct vision.
3 Insert so that the flange lies in front of the upper and lower incisors or gums in the edentulous patient (Fig. 31.1).
4 Check the patency of the airway and ventilation by 'looking, listening and feeling'.

Complications
- Trauma resulting in bleeding
- Vomiting or laryngospasm: if the patient is not deeply unconscious and has not lost gag reflex.

Acute Medical Emergencies; The Practical Approach, 2nd edition.
Edited by Terence Wardle, Peter Driscoll, and Sue Wieteska.
© 2010 Blackwell Publishing Ltd.

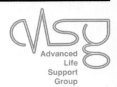

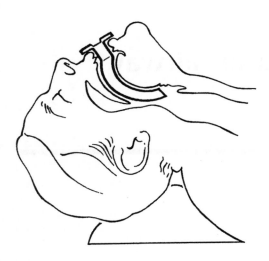

Fig. 31.1 Oropharyngeal airway *in situ*.

NASOPHARYNGEAL AIRWAY

Equipment
- A series of nasopharyngeal airways (sizes 6, 7, 8)
- Lubricant
- Safety pin

Procedure
Choose an airway approximately the same size as the patient's little finger or similar in diameter to the nares. Nasopharyngeal airways are designed to be inserted with the bevel facing medially. Consequently, the right nostril is usually tried first, using the following technique:
1 Lubricate the airway thoroughly.
2 Check the patency of right nostril.
3 Insert the airway bevel end first, along the floor of the nose (i.e. vertically in a supine patient) with a gentle twisting action.
4 When fully inserted, the flange should lie at the nares (Fig. 31.2).
5 Once in place insert a safety pin through the flange to prevent the airway being inhaled.
6 If the right nostril is occluded or insertion is difficult, use the left nostril.
7 Check the patency of the airway and ventilation by 'looking, listening and feeling'.

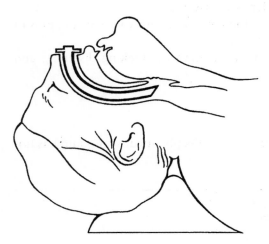

Fig. 31.2 Nasopharyngeal airway *in situ*.

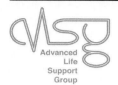

Complications

- Trauma resulting in bleeding
- Vomiting

Key point

Use the nasopharyngeal airway with caution in patients with a suspected base of skull fracture

---

LAERDAL POCKET MASK

Equipment

- Laerdal pocket mask
- Airway manikin

Procedure

The technique for using the mask is as follows.

1 With the patient supine, apply the mask to the patient's face using the thumbs and index fingers of both hands.

2 The remaining fingers are used to exert pressure behind the angles of the jaw (as for the jaw thrust) at the same time as the mask is pressed on to the face to make a tight seal (Fig. 31.3).

3 Blow through the inspiratory valve for 1–2 s, at the same time looking to ensure that the chest rises and then falls.

4 If oxygen is available, add via the nipple at 12–15 l/min.

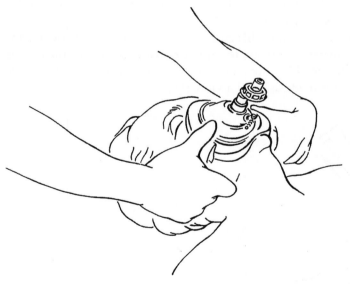

Fig. 31.3 Laerdal pocket mask.

OROTRACHEAL INTUBATION

Equipment

- Laryngoscope: most commonly with a curved (Macintosh) blade
- Tracheal tubes: females 7.5–8.0 mm internal diameter, 21 cm long
  males 8.0–9.0 mm internal diameter, 23 cm long

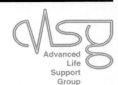

- Syringe, to inflate the cuff
- Catheter mount, to attach to ventilating device
- Lubricant for tube, water soluble, preferably sterile
- Magill forceps
- Introducers, malleable and gum elastic, for difficult cases
- Adhesive tapes or bandages for securing tube
- Ventilator
- Suction
- Stethoscope

Procedure

1 Whenever possible, ventilate the patient with 100% oxygen, using a bag–valve–mask device before intubation. During this time, check the equipment and ensure that all components are complete and functioning, particularly the laryngoscope, suction and ventilating device.

2 Choose a tracheal tube of the appropriate length and diameter, and check the integrity of the cuff.

3 Position the patient's head to facilitate intubation; flex the neck and extend the head at the atlantooccipital joint ('sniffing the morning air' position), provided there are no contraindications. This is often made easier by having a small pillow under the patient's head.

4 Hold the laryngoscope in your left hand, open the patient's mouth and introduce the blade into the right-hand side of the mouth, displacing the tongue to the left.

5 Pass the blade along the edge of the tongue. The tip of the epiglottis should be seen emerging at the base of the tongue.

6 Advance the tip of the blade between the base of the tongue and the anterior surface of the epiglottis (vallecula).

7 The tongue and epiglottis are then **lifted** to reveal the vocal cords; **note that the laryngoscope must be lifted in the direction that the handle is pointing and not levered** by movement of the wrist, as this might damage the teeth and will not provide as good a view (Fig. 31.4).

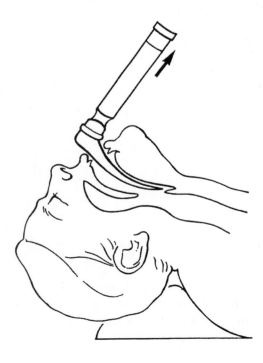

Fig. 31.4 Laryngoscopy.

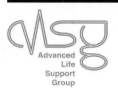

8 Introduce the tracheal tube from the right-hand side of the mouth and insert it between the vocal cords into the larynx under direct vision, until the cuff just passes the cords.

9 Once the tube is in place, inflate the cuff sufficiently to provide an airtight seal between the tube and the trachea. (As an initial approximation, the same number of millilitres of air can be used as the diameter of the tube in millimetres, and adjusted later.)

10 Attach a catheter mount to the tube and ventilate. Ensure that the tube is in the correct position and confirm ventilation of both lungs, by:
- looking for bilateral chest movement with ventilation
- listening for breath sounds bilaterally in the midaxillary line
- listening for gurgling sounds over the epigastrium, which may indicate inadvertent oesophageal intubation
- measuring the carbon dioxide in the expired gas. This will be greater than 0.2% in gas leaving the lungs providing there is a spontaneous circulation or good quality cardiopulmonary resuscitation in progress. Less than 0.2% indicates oesophageal placement of the tube.

Manoeuvres to assist with intubation

Occasionally, when the larynx is very anterior, direct pressure on the thyroid cartilage by an assistant may aid visualisation of the cords (not to be confused with cricoid pressure). However, despite this manoeuvre, in a small percentage of patients only the very posterior part of the cords (or none) can be seen and passage of the tracheal tube becomes difficult. In these cases, a gum elastic introducer can often be inserted into the larynx initially and then the tracheal tube slid over the introducer into the larynx. However, remember that the patient must be oxygenated between attempts at intubation.

Complications

- All the structures encountered from the lips to the trachea may be traumatised.
- When the degree of unconsciousness has been misjudged, vomiting may be stimulated.
- A tube that is too long may pass into a main bronchus (usually the right), causing the opposite lung to collapse, thereby severely impairing the efficiency of ventilation. This is usually identified by the absence of breath sounds and reduced movement on the unventilated side.
- The most dangerous complication associated with tracheal intubation is unrecognised oesophageal intubation. Ventilation may appear adequate, but in fact the patient is not receiving oxygen and is rapidly becoming hypoxaemic. If in doubt, take it out and ventilate the patient using a bag–valve–mask.

INSERTION OF THE LARYNGEAL MASK AIRWAY (LMA)

Equipment

- Laryngeal mask airway:

Size	Cuff volume
• 5 – large adult	40 ml
• 4 – adult male	30 ml
• 3 – adult female	20 ml

- Lubricant
- Syringe to inflate cuff
- Adhesive tape to secure laryngeal mask airway
- Suction
- Ventilating device

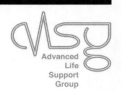

Procedure

- Whenever possible, ventilate the patient with 100% oxygen using a bag–valve–mask device before inserting the laryngeal mask airway. During this time, check that all the equipment is present and working, particularly the integrity of the cuff.
- Deflate the cuff and lightly lubricate the back and sides of the mask.
- Tilt the patient's head (if safe to do so), open the mouth fully, and insert the tip of the mask along the hard palate with the open side facing, but not touching the tongue (Fig. 31.5a).
- Insert the mask further, along the posterior pharyngeal wall, with your index finger initially providing support for the tube (Fig. 31.5b). Eventually resistance is felt as the tip of the laryngeal mask airway lies at the upper end of the oesophagus (Fig. 31.5c).
- Fully inflate the cuff using the air-filled syringe attached to the valve at the end of the pilot tube using the volume of air shown in the earlier box (Fig. 31.5d).

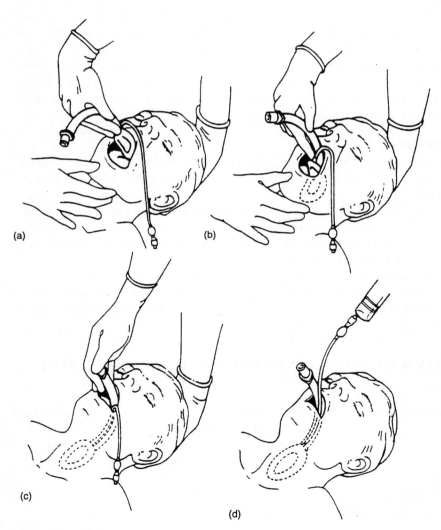

Fig. 31.5 Insertion of the laryngeal mask airway.

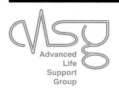

- Secure the laryngeal mask airway with adhesive tape and check its position during ventilation as for a tracheal tube.
- If insertion is not accomplished in less than 30 s, reestablish ventilation using a bag–valve–mask.

Complications
- Incorrect placement is usually due to the tip of the cuff folding over during insertion. The laryngeal mask airway should be withdrawn and reinserted.
- Inability to ventilate the patient, because the epiglottis has been displaced over the larynx. Withdraw the laryngeal mask airway and reinsert ensuring that it closely follows the hard palate. This may be facilitated by the operator or an assistant lifting the jaw upwards. Occasionally, rotation of the laryngeal mask airway may prevent its insertion. Check that the line along the tube is aligned with the patient's nasal septum; if not, reinsert.
- Coughing or laryngeal spasm is usually due to attempts to insert the laryngeal mask airway into a patient whose laryngeal reflexes are still present.

Intubation via the laryngeal mask airway
Insert an introducer through the laryngeal mask airway into the trachea, remove the laryngeal mask airway and then pass the tracheal tube over the introducer into the trachea. Alternatively, a small diameter cuffed tracheal tube (6.0 mm) may be passed directly through a size 4 laryngeal mask airway into the trachea. An intubating LMA (ILMA) is now available and this can accommodate a size 7 or 8 tracheal tube.

NEEDLE CRICOTHYROIDOTOMY

It is important to realise that this technique is a temporising measure, while preparing for a definitive airway.

Equipment
- Venflons 12–14 gauge
- Jet insufflation equipment
- Oxygen tubing with either a three-way tap or a hole cut in the side
- 20-ml syringe
- Gloves (sterile)

Procedure
1 Place the patient supine with the head slightly extended.
2 Identify the cricothyroid membrane as the recess between the thyroid cartilage (Adam's apple) and cricoid cartilage (approximately 2 cm below the 'V'-shaped notch of the thyroid cartilage) (Fig. 31.6).
3 Puncture this membrane vertically using a large bore (12–14 gauge) intravenous cannula attached to a syringe.
4 Aspiration of air confirms that the tip of the cannula lies within the tracheal lumen.
5 Angle the cannula at 45° caudally and advance over the needle into the trachea (Fig. 31.7).

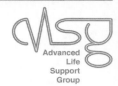

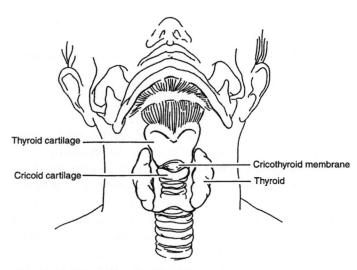

Fig. 31.6 Cricothyroidotomy: relevant anatomy.

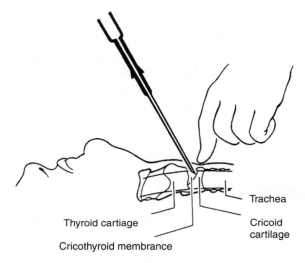

Fig. 31.7 Needle cricothyroidotomy.

6 Attach the cannula to an oxygen supply at 12–15 l/min either via a 'Y' connector or a hole cut in the side of the oxygen tubing. Oxygen is delivered to the patient by occluding the open limb of the connector or side hole for 1 s and then releasing for 4 s.

7 Expiration occurs passively through the larynx. Watch the chest for movement and auscultate for breath sounds, although the latter are difficult to hear.

8 If satisfactory, secure the cannula in place to prevent it being dislodged.

An alternative method of delivering oxygen is to use jet ventilation. This involves connecting the cannula to a high pressure oxygen source (4 bar, 400 kPa, 60 psi) via luerlock connectors or by using a Sanders injector. The same ventilatory cycle is used.

Complications

- Asphyxia
- Pulmonary barotrauma
- Bleeding
- Oesophageal perforation

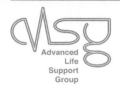

- Kinking of the cannula
- Subcutaneous and mediastinal emphysema
- Aspiration

Occasionally, this method of oxygenation will disimpact a foreign body from the larynx, allowing more acceptable methods of ventilation to be used.

There are two important facts to remember about transtracheal insufflation of oxygen:

- Firstly, it is not possible to deliver oxygen via a needle cricothyroidotomy using a self-inflating bag and valve. This is because these devices do not generate sufficient pressure to drive adequate volumes of gas through a narrow cannula. In comparison, the wall oxygen supply will provide a pressure of 400 kPa (4000 cm H_2O), which overcomes the resistance of the cannula.
- Secondly, expiration cannot occur through the cannula or through a separate cannula inserted through the cricothyroid membrane. The pressure generated during expiration is generally less than 3 kPa (30 cm H_2O), which is clearly much less than the pressure required to drive gas in initially. Expiration must occur through the upper airway, even when partially obstructed. If the obstruction is complete, then the oxygen flow must be reduced to 2–4 l/min to avoid the risk of barotrauma, in particular the creation of a tension pneumothorax

NEEDLE THORACOCENTESIS

Equipment
- Alcohol swab
- Intravenous cannula (minimum 16 gauge)
- 20-ml syringe
- Gloves (sterile)

Procedure
1 Identify the second intercostal space in the midclavicular line on the side of the pneumothorax (the opposite side to the direction of tracheal deviation).
2 Swab the chest wall with surgical preparation or an alcohol swab.
3 Attach the syringe to the cannula.
4 Insert the cannula into the chest wall, just over the rib, aspirating all the time.
5 If air is aspirated, remove the needle, leaving the plastic cannula in place.
6 Tape the cannula in place and proceed to chest drain insertion (see later) as soon as possible.

> **Key point**
>
> If needle thoracocentesis is attempted, and the patient does not have a tension pneumothorax, the chance of causing a pneumothorax is 10–20%. Patients must have a chest X-ray, and will require chest drainage if ventilated

Complications
- Local haematoma
- Lung laceration

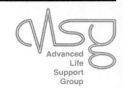

ASPIRATION OF PNEUMOTHORAX

Equipment
- Alcohol swab
- Intravenous cannula (minimum 16 gauge)
- 20-ml syringe
- Three-way tap
- Gloves (sterile)

Procedure
The equipment is the same as for needle thoracocentesis, plus a three-way tap.
1 Explain to the patient the nature of the procedure.
2 Use appropriate aseptic techniques.
3 Identify the second intercostal space in the midclavicular line.
4 After appropriate skin preparation, infiltrate the area with 1% lignocaine.
5 Insert a large (14 or 16 gauge) cannula, remove the central trochar and attach a three-way tap and 50-ml syringe.
6 Continue to aspirate until resistance is encountered or the patient experiences discomfort or coughing.

Key point

Aspiration of 2 litres of air may suggest a persistent air leak; the procedure should be abandoned and a formal chest drain insertion considered

---

Complications
- As for needle thoracocentesis

ASPIRATION OF PLEURAL FLUID

Equipment
- Skin preparation
- Local anaesthetic
- 5-ml syringe with orange, blue and green hubbed needles
- 50-ml syringe with three-way tap
- 16-gauge cannula

Procedure
It is recommended by the National Patient Safety Agency (NPSA) that pleural fluid aspiration should be done under ultrasound control.
1 Explain to the patient the nature of the procedure and obtain written consent.
2 Identify the appropriate side for aspiration of pleural fluid using the ultrasound probe.
3 Clean the skin.
4 After raising the skin bleb, the local anaesthetic is injected via the orange hubbed needle. Introduce the larger blue hubbed needle over the superior aspect of the rib through the intercostal tissues down to the pleura.
5 Always aspirate before injecting to ensure that a blood vessel has not been traumatised.

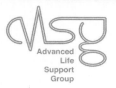

6 For a diagnostic aspiration a green hubbed 21-gauge needle can be inserted through this anaesthetised area into the pleural space, and fluid aspirated into a 30-ml syringe.

7 In contrast, fluid can be aspirated after insertion of a large cannula through this area and attaching the syringe to the cannula via a three-way tap.

Failure of aspiration

Attempted aspiration either too high or too low
Thickened pleura
Pleural tumour
Viscid empyema fibrinous exudate
Dry tap for reasons described above
Haematoma
Bleeding
Pneumothorax

Complications
- As for needle thoracocentesis

Chest drain insertion

(a) Seldinger technique

Equipment
- Skin preparation and surgical drapes
- Local anaesthetic
- Scalpel
- Scissors
- Seldinger chest drain kit comprising guide wire, dilator, over the wire drain
- Suture
- Underwater seal
- 10-ml syringe with orange, blue and green needles

Procedure
1 Confirm correct side for insertion.
2 Identify relevant landmarks (usually the fifth intercostal space anterior to the midaxillary line) on the side of the pneumothorax.
3 Identify relevant landmarks.
4 Swab the chest with skin preparation.
5 Use local anaesthetic – as described above.
6 Make a 'stab' incision (approximately 0.5 cm).
7 Insert the introducer cannula with an attached syringe; aspirate gently as you advance the cannula.
8 Remove syringe.
9 Insert wire through the cannula.
10 Remove cannula, maintaining wire position.
11 Advance dilator over wire, ensuring you hold the free end of the wire before advancing the dilator into the chest. Ensure the dilator moves freely (if not the drain will be difficult to insert).

12 Remove the dilator.

13 Insert the drain over the wire as per Step 9.

14 Remove the wire.

15 Connect the drain to an underwater seal.

16 Ensure either the tube is fogging (in patient with pneumothorax) or fluid is draining (pleural effusion).

17 Secure the drain.

18 X-ray the patient's chest.

(b) Dissection technique

Equipment
- Skin preparation and surgical drapes
- Local anaesthetic
- Scalpel
- Scissors
- Large clamps ×2
- Chest drain tube without trochar
- Suture
- Underwater seal
- 10-ml syringe with orange, blue and green needles

Procedure
1 Confirm correct side for insertion.

2 Identify relevant landmarks (usually the fifth intercostal space anterior to the midaxillary line) on the side with the pneumothorax.

3 Swab the chest wall with surgical preparation or an alcohol swab.

4 Use local anaesthetic if necessary – as described earlier.

5 Make a 2–3 cm transverse skin incision along the line of the intercostal space, towards the superior edge of the sixth rib (thereby avoiding the neurovascular bundle).

6 Bluntly dissect through the subcutaneous tissues just over the top of the rib, and puncture the parietal pleura with the tip of the clamp.

7 Put a gloved finger into the incision and clear the path into the pleura.

8 Advance the chest drain tube into the pleural space **without** the trochar.

9 Ensure that the tube is in the pleural space by listening for air movement, and by looking for fogging of the tube during expiration.

10 Connect the chest drain tube to an underwater seal.

11 Suture the drain in place, and secure with tape.

12 Obtain a chest X-ray.

Complications
- Damage to intercostal nerve, artery or vein
- Introduction of infection
- Tube kinking, dislodging or blocking
- Subcutaneous emphysema
- Persistent pneumothorax due to faulty tube insertion, leaking around chest drain, leaking underwater seal, bronchopleural fistula
- Failure of lung to expand due to blocked bronchus
- Anaphylactic or allergic reaction to skin preparation

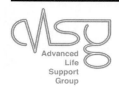

Advanced
Life
Support
Group

CHAPTER 32

Practical procedures: circulation

PROCEDURES

- Peripheral venous cannulation
- Central venous cannulation:
  - ○ Internal jugular vein
  - ○ Subclavian vein
  - ○ Femoral vein
  - ○ Seldinger technique

VENOUS ACCESS

Venous access is an essential part of managing any acutely ill patient. It is an invasive procedure that must not be treated with complacency.

Vascular access can be achieved via several routes:
- percutaneous cannulation of a peripheral vein
- following surgical exposure of a vein in the 'cutdown' technique
- percutaneous cannulation of a central vein
- intraosseous route.

Success is optimised and complications minimised when the operator understands the:
- local anatomy
- equipment
- technique
- complications.

PERIPHERAL VENOUS CANNULATION

The antecubital fossa is the commonest site for peripheral venous cannulation.

The cephalic vein passes through the antecubital fossa on the lateral side and the basilic vein enters very medially just in front of the medial epicondyle of the elbow. These two large veins are joined by the **median cubital or antecubital vein**. The median vein of the forearm also drains into the basilic vein (Fig. 32.1).

Although the veins in this area are prominent and easily cannulated, there are many other adjacent vital structures which can be easily damaged.

Acute Medical Emergencies; The Practical Approach, 2nd edition.
Edited by Terence Wardle, Peter Driscoll, and Sue Wieteska.
© 2010 Blackwell Publishing Ltd.

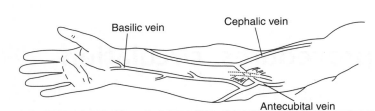

Fig. 32.1 Veins of the forearm and antecubital fossa.

The most popular device for peripheral intravenous access is the cannula over needle, available in a wide variety of sizes, 12–27 gauge. It consists of a plastic (PTFE or similar material) cannula which is mounted on a smaller diameter metal needle, the bevel of which protrudes from the cannula. The other end of the needle is attached to a transparent 'flashback chamber', which fills with blood, indicating that the **needle** bevel lies in the vein. Some devices have flanges or 'wings' to facilitate attachment to the skin. All cannulae have a standard Luer-Lock fitting to attach a giving set and some have a valved injection port attached through which drugs can be given.

Equipment
- Alcohol swab
- Intravenous cannulae
- Tourniquet
- Tape
- Commercial fixing system
- Gloves (need not be sterile)

Procedure
1 Choose a vein capable of accommodating a large cannula, preferably one that is both visible and palpable. The junction of two veins (see Figure 32.2) is often a good site as the 'target' is relatively larger and more stable.
2 Encourage the vein to dilate as this increases the success rate of cannulation. In the limb veins use a tourniquet that stops venous return but permits arterial flow. Further dilatation can be encouraged by gently tapping the skin over the vein. If the patient is cold and vasoconstricted, if time permits, topical application of heat from a towel soaked in warm water can cause vasodilatation.
3 If time permits, the skin over the vein should be cleaned. Ensure there is no risk of allergy if iodine-based agents are used. If alcohol-based agents are used, they must be given time to work (2–3 min), ensuring that the skin is dry before proceeding further.
4 In the conscious patient, consider infiltrating a small amount of local anaesthetic into the skin at the point chosen using a 22–25-gauge needle,

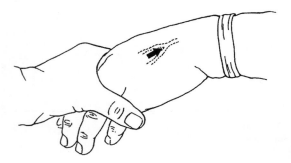

Fig. 32.2 Vein immobilised.

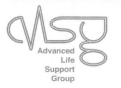

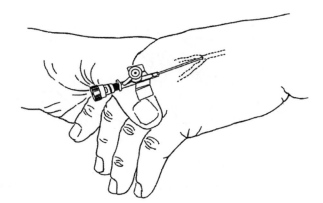

Fig. 32.3 Cannula inserted (note the flashback of blood).

particularly if a large (>1.2-mm, 18-gauge) cannula is to be used. This reduces the pain of cannulation, therefore making the patient less likely to move and less resistant to further attempts if the first is unsuccessful!

5 If a large cannula is used, insertion through the skin may be facilitated by first making a small incision with either a 19-gauge needle or a scalpel blade, taking care not to puncture the vein.

6 Immobilise the vein to prevent displacement by the advancing cannula. Pull the skin over the vein tight, with your spare hand (Fig. 32.2).

7 Hold the cannula firmly, at an angle of 10–15° to the skin and advance through the skin and then into the vein. Often a slight loss of resistance is felt as the vein is entered. This should be accompanied by the appearance of blood in the flashback chamber of the cannula (Fig. 32.3). However, the appearance of blood only indicates that the tip of the needle is within the vein, not necessarily any of the cannula.

8 Whilst keeping the skin taut, the next step is to reduce the angle of the cannula slightly and advance it a further 2–3 mm into the vein. This is to ensure that the first part of the plastic cannula lies within the vein. Care must be taken at this point not to push the needle out of the back of the vein.

9 Withdraw the needle 5–10 mm into the cannula so that the point no longer protrudes from the end. Often as this is done, blood will flow between the needle body and the cannula, confirming that the tip of the cannula is within the vein (Fig. 32.4).

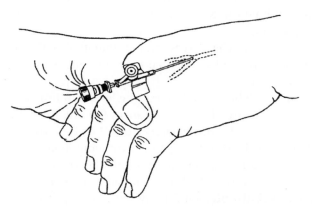

Fig. 32.4 Cannula with needle slightly withdrawn.

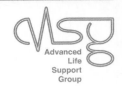

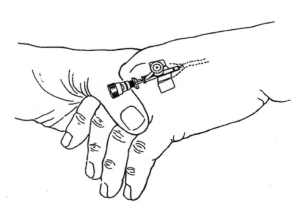

Fig. 32.5 Cannula fully inserted.

10 Advance the combined cannula and needle along the vein. The needle is retained within the cannula to provide support and prevent kinking at the point of skin puncture (Fig. 32.5).

11 Insert the cannula as far as the hub, release the tourniquet and remove the needle and place in a sharps bin.

12 Confirm that the cannula lies within the vein either by attaching an intravenous infusion, ensuring that it runs freely, or by injecting saline. Watch the tissues around the site for any signs of swelling that may indicate that the cannula is incorrectly positioned. Finally, secure the cannula in an appropriate manner.

Complications

- Failed cannulation is the most common, usually as a result of pushing the needle completely through the vein. It is inversely related to experience.
- Haematomata are usually secondary to the above with inadequate pressure applied to prevent blood leaking from the vein after the cannula is removed. They are made worse by forgetting to remove the tourniquet!
- Extravasation of fluid or drugs is commonly a result of failing to recognise that the cannula is not in the vein before use. Placing a cannula over a joint or prolonged use to infuse fluids under pressure also predisposes to leakage. The faulty cannula must be removed. Damage to the surrounding tissues will depend primarily on the nature of the extravasated fluid.
- Damage to other local structures is secondary to poor technique and lack of knowledge of the local anatomy.
- The plastic cannula can shear, allowing fragments to enter the circulation. This is usually a result of trying to reintroduce the needle after it has been withdrawn. The safest action is to withdraw the whole cannula and attempt cannulation at another site with a new cannula.
- The needle may fracture as a result of careless excessive manipulation with the finer cannulae. The fragment will have to be removed by either an interventional vascular radiologist or a surgeon.
- Inflammation of the vein (thrombophlebitis) is related to the length of time the vein is cannulated and the irritation caused by the substances flowing through it. High concentrations of drugs and fluids with extremes of pH or high osmolality are the main causes. Once a vein shows signs of thrombophlebitis, i.e. tender, red and the flow rate is deteriorating, the cannula must be removed to prevent subsequent infection or thrombosis which may spread proximally.
- To reduce the risk of thromobophlebitis/infection, many hospitals have a policy for peripheral venous access which states that cannulae should be changed

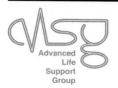

every 3 days and that the date of insertion should be written on the securing tape and in the patient's records.

CENTRAL VENOUS CANNULATION

Catheterisation of a central vein is relatively easy. As with all procedures, it is best learned under supervision (NICE guidelines advise ultrasound guidance). However, in an acutely ill patient, it may be necessary for someone to catheterise a central vein safely and quickly. Therefore an easy technique is required that has a high success rate with few complications.

Central venous cannulation is a common technique in acutely ill patients for:
- drug delivery
- central pressure monitoring
- pacing
- inserting a pulmonary artery flotation catheter
- parenteral nutrition.

Equipment
- Skin preparation
- Local anaesthetic
- 10-ml syringe with blue and green needles
- Appropriate catheter for central venous cannulation (see 'Seldinger technique')
- Suture
- Tape
- No 11 blade
- Ultrasound probe
- Gloves (sterile)

Procedure
Many approaches and different types of equipment have been described to secure central venous access. This chapter describes three approaches – internal jugular, subclavian and femoral – using a single standard technique. Whenever possible for neck vein access, place the patient in a head-down position to dilate the vein and reduce the risk of air embolus. This has been found to be successful in both experienced and inexperienced hands. No further justification of the choice is offered. For those already skilled at central venous cannulation using a different technique (**with an acceptable rate of complications**), carry on!

The internal jugular vein – paracarotid approach
At the level of the thyroid cartilage, the internal jugular vein (Fig. 32.6 – see over) runs parallel to the carotid artery in the carotid sheath and therefore rotation of the head, obesity and individual variations in anatomy have less effect on the location of the vein.

1 Place the patient in the supine position, arms at their side and the head in a neutral position.
2 Standing at the head of the patient identify the thyroid cartilage and use the fingers of the left hand to palpate the carotid pulse. The right internal jugular vein is the one most commonly used initially.
3 Identify the apex of a triangle formed by the two heads of sternoclavicular muscle (the base is the clavicle).
4 Under aseptic conditions, infiltrate with 1% lignocaine.

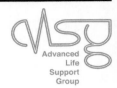

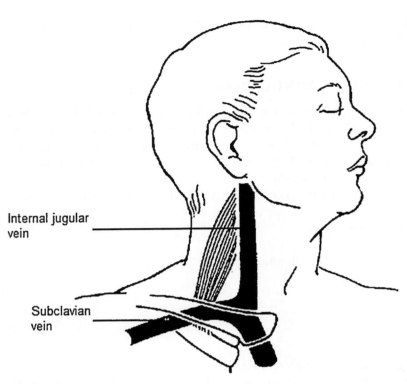

Internal jugular vein

Subclavian vein

Fig. 32.6 The course of the central veins of the neck.

5 With the fingers of the left hand 'guarding' the carotid artery, insert a needle 0.5 cm lateral to the artery. Inject 0.5–1 ml of air to expel any skin plug in the needle tip.

6 Advance the needle slowly caudally, parallel to the sagittal plane at an angle of 45° to the skin, aspirating at all times.

7 Confirm entry into the vein by blood entering the syringe. Introduce the catheter via a guide wire as described later.

8 If the vein is not entered at the first attempt, then subsequent punctures should be directed slightly more laterally (never medially towards the artery).

Although a chest X-ray should be taken it is less urgent than when using the subclavian vein, as the catheter is more likely to be correctly positioned and the incidence of pneumothorax is much lower with this approach.

The subclavian vein – infraclavicular approach

1 Place the patient in supine position, with arms at their side and head turned away from the side of the puncture. Occasionally it may be advantageous to place a small support (a 500 ml bag of fluid!) under the scapula of the side of approach, to raise the clavicle above the shoulder.

2 Standing on the same side as that to be punctured (usually the right), identify the midclavicular point and the suprasternal notch.

3 Under aseptic conditions infiltrate with 1% lignocaine.

4 Insert the needle 1 cm below the midclavicular point and inject 0.5–1 ml of air to expel any skin plug in the needle tip. Advance the needle posterior to the clavicle towards a finger in the suprasternal notch. Keep the syringe and needle horizontal during advancement. Aspirate at all times.

5 Blood entering the syringe will confirm entry into the vein. Introduce the catheter via a guide wire as already described.

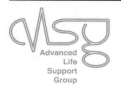

6 A chest X-ray should be taken as soon as possible to exclude a pneumothorax and confirm the correct position of the catheter.

The femoral vein

1 Place the patient in a supine position.

2 Under aseptic conditions, palpate the femoral artery (midinguinal point). The femoral vein lies directly medial to the femoral artery (remember lateral to medial structures are femoral nerve, artery, vein, space).

3 Infiltrate the puncture site with local anaesthetic.

4 While palpating the femoral artery insert the needle over the femoral vein parallel to the sagittal plane at an angle of 45° to the skin, aspirating at all times. A free flow of blood entering the syringe will confirm entry into the vein.

5 Advance the guide wire through the needle as described below.

Complications

- Venous thrombosis
- Injury to artery or nerve
- Infection
- Arteriovenous fistula
- Air embolism

In addition, attempts at internal jugular or subclavian vein access may cause pneumothorax, haemothorax and chylothorax.

SELDINGER TECHNIQUE

Equipment

- Skin cleaning swabs
- Lignocaine 1% for local anaesthetic with 2-ml syringe and 23-gauge needle
- Syringe and heparinised 0.9% saline
- Seldinger cannulation set: syringe
  needles
  Seldinger guide wire
  cannula

- Suture material
- Prepared infusion set
- Tape
- No 11 blade
- Gloves (sterile)

Procedure

Although initially described for use with arterial cannulation, this technique is very suitable for central venous cannulation and is associated with an increased success rate. It relies on the insertion of a guide wire into the vein over which a suitable catheter is passed. As a relatively small needle is used to introduce the wire, damage to adjacent structures is reduced.

Having decided which approach to use (see earlier), the skin must be prepared and towelled. Full aseptic precautions are necessary as a 'no-touch' technique is impossible.

1 Check and prepare your equipment; in particular, identify the floppy end of the guide wire and ensure free passage of the guide wire through the needle.

2 Attach the needle to a syringe and puncture the vein.

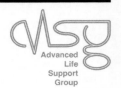

3 After aspirating blood, remove the syringe taking care to avoid the entry of air (usually by placing a thumb over the end of the needle).

4 Insert the floppy end of the guide wire into the needle and advance 4–5 cm into the vein.

5 Remove the needle over the wire, taking care not to remove the wire with the needle.

6 Load the catheter on to the wire, ensuring that the proximal end of the wire protrudes from the catheter. Holding the proximal end of the wire, insert the catheter and wire together into the vein. It is important never to let go of the wire!

7 Remove the wire holding the catheter in position.

8 Reattach the syringe and aspirate blood to confirm placement of the catheter in the vein.

If it is difficult to insert the wire, the needle and wire must be removed together. Failure to do this may damage the tip of the wire as it is withdrawn past the needle point. After 3 min gentle pressure to reduce bleeding, the needle can be reintroduced.

It is a good idea to make a small incision in the skin to facilitate the passage of the catheter.

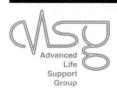

Advanced
Life
Support
Group

CHAPTER 33

Practical procedures: medical

> ## PROCEDURES
>
> - Joint aspiration
> - Balloon tamponade of oesophageal varices
> - Lumbar puncture
> - Blood cultures
> - Insertion of pulmonary arterial flotation (Swan–Ganz) catheter
> - Pulmonary capillary wedge pressure

JOINT ASPIRATION

Diagnostic indications
- Suspected septic arthritis
- Crystal induced synovitis
- Haemarthrosis

Therapeutic indications
- Tense effusions
- Septic effusions
  - Recurrent aspiration
  - Lavage (rare)
- Haemarthrosis
- Steroid injection

Contraindications
- Overlying skin infection/cellulitis

Equipment
- Antiseptic solution, e.g. ethanol, povidone iodine
- Swabs
- Sterile gloves
- Syringes: 5, 10, 20 ml
- Needles: large joint (21 gauge) green
- Small joint (23 gauge) blue

Procedure
1 Explain to the patient what you are going to do, and obtain written consent.
2 Identify the bony margins of the joint space.
3 Ensure you have all the appropriate materials required.
4 Using a sterile technique prepare the skin.

Acute Medical Emergencies; The Practical Approach, 2nd edition.
Edited by Terence Wardle, Peter Driscoll, and Sue Wieteska.
© 2010 Blackwell Publishing Ltd.

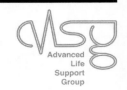

5 Inject a small amount of local anaesthetic (1% lignocaine) into the skin over the joint to be aspirated.

6 Gently insert the needle into the joint space. Normally a green needle (21 gauge) will suffice for most joints, but for finger and toe joints a blue (23-gauge) needle is advised.

7 Aspirate fluid and send for microbiological assessment, crystals, cytology, protein, lactate dehydrogenase (LDH), and glucose estimation.

Specific procedures
Knee joint aspiration
1 Ensure the patient is as comfortable as possible.
2 Slightly flex the knee to ensure relaxation of the quadriceps muscles.
3 Palpate the posterior edge of the patella medially or laterally. Using the general technique, described earlier, insert the needle horizontally or slightly downwards into the joint between the patella and femur (often a slight resistance is felt when the needle penetrates the synovial membrane).

Shoulder joint aspiration
This joint is easier to access through an anterior approach although a lateral and posterior approach's are also possible. The anterior approach will be described.
1 Ensure that the patient is seated with their arm relaxed against the side of the chest.
2 Palpate the space between the head of the humerus and the glenoid cap, about 1 cm below the coracoid process.
3 Using the procedure described earlier, insert the needle into the space with a slight medial angle (it should enter the joint easily and to almost the length of the green needle).

Complications
- Reaction to topical skin preparation.
- Inappropriate puncture of blood vessels or nerves.
- Introduction of infection into joint space.

BALLOON TAMPONADE OF OESOPHAGEAL VARICES
Equipment
- Sengstaken–Blakemore tube
- Two spigots
- 60-ml bladder syringe
- Saline/Contrast media
- Tongue depressors
- Tape
- Pressure gauge
- Suction
- Drainage bags

Procedure
Variceal bleeding can be controlled by balloon compression either at the cardia or within the oesophageal lumen. A large number of devices are available for this purpose. The commonest is a Sengstaken–Blakemore tube that has been modified to allow aspiration of gastric and oesophageal contents as well as inflation of gastric and oesophageal balloons.

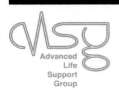

Insertion of the tube usually occurs in conscious patients and, therefore, the nasal route is advocated. Unfortunately this can make insertion difficult but is subsequently better tolerated by the patient. If the airway is in jeopardy, ensure that it is cleared and secured before attempting to insert the tamponade tube. If the patient has an endotracheal tube *in situ*, the oral route is advocated. Although you may be faced with torrential bleeding from oesophageal varices, ensure that you have all the equipment available before you attempt insertion of this tube and, more importantly, that the associated oesophageal and gastric balloons will inflate and remain inflated.

It is important to realise that tamponade tubes are difficult to introduce and they require meticulous supervision whilst inflated.

1 Lubricate the tube with water-soluble jelly.

2 Providing that there are no contraindications, insert the tube into the right nostril using a technique similar to that described for nasopharyngeal airway insertion in Chapter 30. Ensure you direct the tube backwards (not superior or inferior).

3 Advance the tube gently. It will follow the contour of the oropharynx into the oesophagus.

4 Advance the tube until you reach the 50-cm mark (note that the tube has 5-cm graduations). Advancing the tube to at least 50 cm will, in most patients, ensure that it is in the stomach. Aspiration of blood does not, however, verify this.

5 Inflate the gastric balloon with 200 ml of air or alternatively 200 ml of water-soluble contrast material. Gentle traction of the nasal end of the tube will ensure that the inflated gastric balloon is adjacent to the cardia and gastro-oesophageal junction.

6 Tape the balloon to the side of the patient's face. Often inflation of the gastric balloon, with gentle traction, is all that is required to stem variceal bleeding as the feeding vessel to the varices, the left gastric vein, is tamponaded by this manoeuvre. If this fails to control the bleeding then inflate the oesophageal balloon with air to 4.5–5.4 kPa (30–40 mm Hg) using a pressure gauge. If a specific pressure gauge is not available then it is possible to adapt a sphygmomanometer for this purpose.

7 Ensure that both gastric and oesophageal aspiration ports are draining freely. Both the gastric and oesophageal balloons seal automatically once inflated by one-way valves. Continuous oesophageal suction reduces the risk of aspiration.

8 Deflate the balloon after 24 h. This will reduce the risk of oesophageal mucosal ulceration and perforation.

It is important to realise that balloon tamponade is only a temporising procedure and once the bleeding has stopped the patient should have a repeat endoscopy to assess and treat varices.

Complications

- Aspiration, especially without continuous aspiration of the oesophageal port
- Hypoxaemia, if the balloon is inadvertently inserted into the trachea
- Tracheal rupture, as above
- Oesophageal rupture. The procedure is performed blindly and with the presence of a hiatus hernia or an oesophageal stricture it is possible for the Sengstaken–Blakemore tube to coil in the oesophagus. Inflation produces catastrophic results
- Mucosal ulceration in the oesophagus and stomach
- Failure to stop variceal haemorrhage

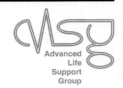

LUMBAR PUNCTURE

Indications
- Suspected meningitis
- Subarachnoid haemorrhage
- Encephalitis
- Benign intracranial hypertension

Contraindications
A lumbar puncture should not be done in the unconscious patient until a CT scan has excluded a mass lesion. Failure to do this may precipitate central/uncal herniation as cerebrospinal fluid is drained via the lumbar puncture needle. Furthermore, a diagnosis of subarachnoid haemorrhage on CT will negate the need for lumbar puncture. However, CT scans can miss a small subarachnoid bleed and as this often heralds subsequent catastrophic haemorrhage, a lumbar puncture must be done in any patient who has a clinical history suggestive of subarachnoid haemorrhage and a negative CT scan.

Equipment
- Antiseptic solution
- Gauze swabs
- Sterile drapes and gloves
- 1% lignocaine (max 5 ml)
- 5 ml syringe
- Needles: 25 gauge (orange)
                    21 gauge (green)
- Lumbar puncture needles
- Manometer
- Collection bottles
- Tape

Procedure
1 Explain to the patient what you are going to do, and obtain written consent.
2 Place the patient in the left lateral position, ensuring that their back, in particular the lumbar spine, is parallel to the edge of the bed. The hips and knees should be flexed to greater than 90° and the knees separated by one pillow. Ensure that the head is supported on one pillow and that the patient's cervical and thoracic spine are gently flexed.
3 Check that you have all the necessary equipment.
4 Identify the fourth lumbar vertebra, i.e. a line drawn between the top of the iliac crests.
5 Thoroughly cleanse the skin using an aseptic technique.
6 Identify the interspace between the second and third or third and fourth lumbar vertebrae (hence the spinal cord will not be damaged). In the midline, inject a small amount of 1% lignocaine to raise a skin bleb.
7 Through the skin bleb, advance a green needle and ensuring that the blood vessel has not been punctured. Inject 1 ml local anaesthetic into the interspinous ligament in the respective interspace. Too much local anaesthetic will cause damage to these tissues and produce profound discomfort.
8 Using a sterile spinal needle advance through the anaesthetised tissues, directing the needle slightly cephalad and maintaining a midline position.

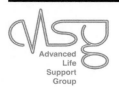

9 As you enter the subarachnoid space, a sudden change in resistance on advancing the needle is felt. Then gently remove the inner trochar and watch for a drop of cerebrospinal fluid appearing at the end of the needle. If this does not occur, replace the central trochar and advance the needle again, until a change in resistance is felt. Repeat the procedure until cerebrospinal fluid is seen.

10 Attach the manometer and measure the pressure of the cerebrospinal fluid.

11 Place five drops of cerebrospinal fluid sequentially in three tubes for red cell count, then five drops in a further two for microscopy culture and sensitivity. Similar samples should be taken for protein estimation, spectroscopy, virology, and glucose (the latter should be placed in a fluoride tube).

12 Note the colour of the cerebrospinal fluid, i.e. whether it is clear, opalescent or yellow (Remember xanthochromia is a spectroscopic diagnosis).

13 Remove the needle. Occasionally, postlumbar puncture headache may result which necessitates simple analgesia with paracetamol.

Complications

- Failure to obtain cerebrospinal fluid may be due to incorrect anatomical positioning, 'a dry tap', degenerative or inflammatory changes in the lumbar spine
- Nerve root pain when inserting the needle – usually transient
- Introduction of sepsis
- Bleeding
- Headache
- Coning

BLOOD CULTURES

Indications

- Pyrexia of unknown origin
- Sepsis
- Suspected infective endocarditis

Procedure

- Thoroughly cleanse the skin, ideally with an alcohol-based solution.
- Whilst this is evaporating to dryness wash your hands thoroughly; under aseptic conditions don surgical gloves.
- At the previously prepared site perform a venepuncture and aspirate 40 ml of blood.
- Thoroughly cleanse the top of the blood culture bottle.
- Insert 10 ml of blood into each blood culture bottle.

INSERTION OF PULMONARY ARTERIAL FLOATATION (SWAN-GANZ) CATHETER

Indications

1 Measurement of pulmonary capillary wedge pressure (PCWP)

2 Pulmonary artery end diastolic pressure (PAEDP)

3 Cardiac output

Equipment

See Central venous cannulation

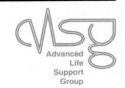

The Catheter

This is a balloon tipped device which has a single distal hole. It can be inserted at the bedside without X-ray control or under fluoroscopy.

The balloon serves two purposes. Firstly as soon as the catheter is inserted into a central vein, inflation of the balloon with air will ensure that it acts as a sail navigating the catheter through the tricuspid and pulmonary valves. Changes in the pressure tracing, as described later, will enable these structures to be identified. Secondly, once the catheter is inserted into a small pulmonary artery, the balloon may then be inflated, occluding the artery proximally. This will leave the catheter tip exposed to the PCWP.

Catheter Insertion

Using central venous access as described earlier advance the catheter into a large vein. If an insertion sheath is used, ensure it is one size larger than the catheter, to ensure passage of the deflated balloon through the insertion sheath.

1 Advance the catheter into the vein and connect to transducer.
2 Inflate the balloon.
3 Slowly advance the catheter tip, guided by the blood flow.
4 Advance the catheter through into the pulmonary artery bed, trying to find a position which gives a good pulmonary artery tracing with the balloon deflated and a good wedge pressure with the balloon inflated.
5 X-ray the chest.

Alternatively, the catheter can be inserted under fluoroscopic control. It is, however, still important to ensure that a good pulmonary artery tracing is obtained with the balloon deflated, and a good wedge pressure is obtained with the balloon inflated.

Measurement

Specific details of pulmonary capillary wedge pressure measurement will vary according to the equipment available. There are, however, certain common features, in particular:

1 Most equipment is designed for continuous monitoring, as such it is precalibrated. Therefore the only major adjustment is to zero the transducer to atmospheric pressure before recording. To do this, ensure that the catheter is connected via a three-way tap to the manometer line, the other portholes of the three-way tap should be connected to a flushing system and to the air. Ensure that in setting up the equipment all air bubbles are removed from the system.
2 Move the three-way tap to ensure that blood cannot flow back from the catheter to the transducer but that the final port of the three-way tap is open to the air.
3 Adjust the tracing on the monitor to zero.
4 Close the transducer sidearm and open the transducer to the catheter. Ideally allow approximately 30 min for the transducer to warm up.

Measurements are made with the patient flat and the transducer at the angle of Louis. You will note that during measurements the pressure swings related to respiration will induce a biphasic nature to the pulmonary wedge pressure. It is therefore important the mean wedge pressure is utilised.

It is always important to:

• check the transducer level
• check the system is set at zero
• check that wedging does not occur.

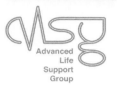

Problems

1 Failure to wedge – reposition the catheter
2 Flat/damp trace – unblock catheter. Ensure that there is no air in the system and that the transducer is not open to both the patient and air. Flush the system – usually a hand flush of 1 ml of saline is required, but ensure that no air is introduced
3 Over wedging – occasionally the catheter is lodged in a pulmonary artery, unfortunately the diameter of this vessel is less than that of the balloon and does not allow accurate pressure recording. This usually manifests by a fluctuating, steadily increasing pressure trace. Ideally deflate the balloon and reposition the catheter.

Pulmonary capillary wedge pressure

This can be recorded as described above, along with pressures in the pulmonary artery, right ventricle and right atrium (Table 33.1).

The PCWP is an indirect reflection of left arterial pressure (LAP). This in turn is similar to left ventricular end diastolic pressure (LVEDP).

In certain acute medical conditions the PCWP does not accurately reflect LVEDP. With pulmonary venous obstruction, e.g. pulmonary emboli or raised intrathoracic pressure (for instance intermittent positive pressure ventilation) the PCWP is less than the LVEDP – thus PCWP is a particularly useful measurement in patients with poor left ventricular function and it may be used to optimise fluid therapy.

Table 33.1 Normal pressure ranges

Site	Pressure (mm Hg)
Right atrium (mean)	−1 to +6
Right ventricle	0 to 25
Pulmonary artery (mean)	10 to 20
Pulmonary capillary wedge pressure (mean)	8 to 15

CARDIAC OUTPUT

Cardiac output may be assessed using the Fick equation which relates cardiac output (CO) to oxygen uptake (VO_2). In this manner cardiac output equals oxygen uptake divided by the difference in arteriovenous oxygen content.

$$\text{Cardiac output} = \frac{\text{Oxygen uptake}}{\text{Arteriovenous oxygen content difference}}$$

$$\text{Therefore CO (1/min)} = \frac{VO_2 \text{ (ml/min)}}{CaO_2 - CvO_2 \text{ (ml/l)}}$$

To obtain these values a true mixed venous sample of blood must be taken from the tip of the pulmonary artery. This will allow the difference in the arteriovenous oxygen content to be assessed.

Complications

As with central venous access
Pulmonary parenchymal damage

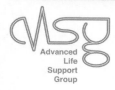

Advanced
Life
Support
Group

PART VIII

Appendix

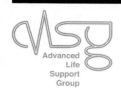
Advanced Life Support Group

Appendix: drugs commonly used in the management of medical emergencies

Drug	Indications	Dose and route	Notes
N-Acetyl cysteine	Paracetamol poisoning	IV infusion 150 mg/kg over 15 min then 50 mg/kg over 4 h, then 100 mg/kg over 16 h	Most effective if given less than 8 h post overdose. Requirement for treatment based on blood paracetamol levels at least 4 h post ingestion. Nomogram available on data sheet or British National Formulary. Treat at lower levels for at risk patients – alcoholics, anorexics and patients on liver enzyme inducing drugs
	Renal dysfunction in a patient with decompensated liver disease		Same dose for hepatorenal failure – continue 100 mg/kg every 16 h until improvement
Aciclovir	Herpes simplex encephalitis, varicella zoster virus in immunocompromised	100 mg/kg IV 8 hourly	Most effective if started at onset of infection. Can be used orally, topically or intravenously at lower dose for immunocompetent adults with herpes infections or prophylaxis in immunocompromised patients
Adenosine	Cardioversion of paroxysmal supraventricular arrhythmias	3–12 mg by rapid IV injection (see notes)	Do not use in Wolff–Parkinson–White syndrome with atrial fibrillation as increased conduction via accessory pathways may result in circulatory collapse or ventricular fibrillation. Use lower initial dose (0.5–1 mg) if heart transplant patient or patient taking dipyridamole (avoid use unless essential). Antagonised by theophyllines

Acute Medical Emergencies; The Practical Approach, 2nd edition.
Edited by Terence Wardle, Peter Driscoll, and Sue Wieteska.
© 2010 Blackwell Publishing Ltd.

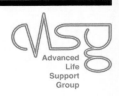

Drug	Indications	Dose and route	Notes
Adrenaline	Cardiac arrest	1 mg IV	Improves circulation achieved by chest compressions. Central line is the preferred route
		2 mg ETT	
	Anaphylaxis	0.5 ml 1 in 1000 IM	ECG monitoring necessary. Will frequently require adrenaline infusion after (see inotropic support next)
	Inotropic support	0.1–0.5 μg/kg/min IV	Give by continuous infusion (through dedicated line to avoid boluses). Predominantly increases cardiac output at lower doses. Also causes vasoconstriction at higher doses
Aminophylline	Acute severe asthma	5 mg/kg IV over 20 min	Do not give this initial loading dose to patients on oral theophyllines
		0.5 mg/kg/h IV	Vary infusion rate according to plasma theophylline levels (aim for 10–20 mg/l)
Amiodarone	Ventricular tachycardia, atrial fibrillation and flutter, supraventricular tachycardia	300 mg IV over 20–60 min, followed by 1200 mg/24 h IV	Effective antiarrhythmic with many complications. When given intravenously must be via a central venous catheter. Hypotension or cardiovascular collapse possible with rapid administration
Atenolol	Myocardial infarction	5–10 mg IV, followed by 50 mg orally at 15 min and 12 h, then 100 mg each day	Early use of atenolol post myocardial infarction reduces mortality. Should not be given to patients with a high degree of heart block, hypotension or overt left ventricular failure
Atropine	Asystole	3 mg IV	Used once only in the management of asystole
		6 mg ETT	
	Bradycardia	0.5 mg IV	Use incremental doses of 0·5 mg up to a maximum of 3 mg
Benzylpenicillin	Meningococcal septicaemia	2.4 g IV 4 hourly	Give immediately if meningococcal septicaemia suspected. If possible do blood cultures first. Do not delay for lumbar puncture
	Community acquired pneumonia	1–2 g qds	

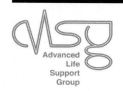

Drug	Indications	Dose and route	Notes
Clarithromycin	Atypical pneumonia, other infections in penicillin allergic patients	500 mg IV 12 hourly	Similar spectrum of activity to erythromycin but slightly greater activity and higher tissue levels
			Fewer gastrointestinal side effects than erythromycin
	Community acquired pneumonia		Can be given orally
Diazepam	Fitting	5–10 mg IV, repeated if necessary 10–20 mg rectally	May cause respiratory depression and hypotension. Use of flumazenil to reverse this may precipitate further seizures. Use rectal route if IV access not easily attainable
Digoxin	Atrial fibrillation	500 μg IV over 30 min	Loading dose. Do not give if patient taking digoxin
		62.5–500 μg/day orally or IV	Used to control ventricular response rate. Does not cause chemical cardioversion. Maintenance dose. Be wary that arrhythmias may be caused by digoxin toxicity
Dobutamine	Cardiogenic shock	2.5–20 μg/kg/min	Inodilator. Give by continuous infusion. May cause paradoxical hypotension with increasing doses as a result of tachycardia and vasodilatation
Dopamine	Shock with inadequate urine output	1–3 μg/kg/min	Used as an adjunct to inotropic support. Increases renal blood flow and urine output
Frusemide	Pulmonary oedema secondary to left ventricular dysfunction	50–100 mg IV	Works initially by vasodilator effect, and later as diuretic. Use with extreme caution in hypotensive patients as severe hypotension may develop. Consider use in conjunction with inotropic support
			In the acutely anuric patient, bumetanide may be a better alternative as excretion of the drug into the tubule is not required. Higher doses required in patients on large oral doses of a loop diuretic or with known renal impairment

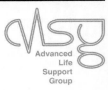

Drug	Indications	Dose and route	Notes
Glucagon	Hypoglycaemia	1 mg SC/IV/IM	Mobilises glycogen from the liver. If not recovered within 10 min give IV glucose
	β-Blocker overdose	50–150 μg/kg IV	Useful in shock refractory to atropine therapy in patients with β-blocker overdose. Is only available as 1 mg vials. Total dose required is up to approximately 10 mg
Glyceryl trinitrate	Pulmonary oedema secondary to left ventricular dysfunction	1–10 mg/h IV	In hypotensive patients, use only in conjunction with inotropic support
	Ischaemic chest pain	500 μg sublingual	If chest pain not rapidly relieved by nitrates, myocardial infarction should be excluded and alternative diagnoses considered
		1–5 mg buccal	
		1–10 mg/h IV	
Hydrocortisone	Anaphylaxis and angiooedema Bronchospasm	100–300 mg IV	Of secondary benefit as onset of action delayed for several hours. Use in more severely affected patients
	Acute adrenocortical insufficiency	100 mg IV 6–8 hourly	
Ipratropium bromide	Acute asthma	500 μg nebulised 4 hourly	Indicate in life-threatening asthma in conjunction with a β2-agonist. In severe acute asthma use as a second line treatment. Beneficial in a small group of patients with chronic obstructive pulmonary disease
Lignocaine	Ventricular tachycardia	100 mg IV 1–4 mg/min	Commonly used to treat ventricular tachycardia
			Myocardial depressant. Use cautiously if impaired left ventricular function. Treat underlying cause of arrhythmia – usually myocardial ischaemia
	Local anaesthetic	3 mg/kg maximum	Infiltrate locally or perineurally. Facilitates procedures – large IV line, intercostal tube insertion, lumbar puncture. Increased dose (7 mg/kg) may be used if infiltrated with adrenaline (not fingers, toes, nose, ears or penis)

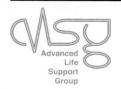

Drug	Indications	Dose and route	Notes
Lorazepam	Status epilepticus	4 mg IV	May cause respiratory depression or apnoea. Longer duration of action compared to diazepam
Metronidazole	Anaerobic infections including clostridium difficile	IV 500 mg 3 times daily	Avoid alcohol
Morphine	Myocardial infarction	2.5–20 mg IV (titrate against response)	Anxiolysis and analgesia reduce catecholamine levels, decreasing heart rate, afterload and hence myocardial oxygen consumption
	Pulmonary oedema	2.5–10 mg IV	Acts as above. Also effects on pulmonary vasculature reduce left ventricular preload
	Pain	2.5–20 mg IV (titrate against response)	Diamorphine is an alternative as may cause less hypotension and nausea. Powerful analgesic
			May cause respiratory depression
Naloxone	Opiate poisoning	0.4–2 mg IV 4 μg/min IV (increase dose as required to maintain required response)	Deliberate self-harm, iatrogenic or recreational use of opiates may result in respiratory arrest. Beware opiates with long half lives, especially methadone. IV infusion should be used if long acting opiate involved or recurrent coma or respiratory depression
Phenytoin	Status epilepticus	15 mg/kg loading dose IV at <50 mg/min	Second line drug in status epilepticus.
		Maintenance 100 mg IV 6–8 hourly	Phenytoin offers theoretical advantages as it can be infused rapidly. May cause central nervous system or cardiovascular depression, more marked with rapid infusion rates
Salbutamol	Acute asthma	2.5–5 mg nebulised as required	β_2-agonist. Nebulise with high concentrations of inspired oxygen
		250 μg IV	In severe or life-threatening acute asthma not responding to nebulised β_2-agonist, IV therapy is indicated. Consider need for anaesthetic help. Infusions of salbutamol are used following IV bolus
		3–20 μg/min IV	

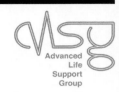

Drug	Indications	Dose and route	Notes
Streptokinase	Myocardial infarction	1.5 million units IV over 1 h	Reduces mortality post myocardial infarction
			Indicated when potential benefits outweigh risks
			Risks mainly relate to haemorrhage (see Chapter 10)
Tazocin	Community acquired pneumonia, chest infection or urinary sepsis in the acutely ill	4.5 g Tazocin EF every 8 h	
tPA	Myocardial infarction	15 mg bolus followed by 50 mg over 30 min, then 35 mg over 60 min IV	See streptokinase. May have mortality benefits in some subgroups compared to streptokinase. Use dictated by local protocols, commonly including patients with anterior myocardial infarction or hypotension related to myocardial infarction
	Pulmonary embolism	10 mg bolus followed by 90 mg over 2 h	Use in haemodynamically significant pulmonary embolus or pulmonary embolus causing severe hypoxaemia despite high FiO_2

IM, intramuscular; IV, intravenous; ETT, endotracheal tube; SC, subcutaneous; tPa, tissue plasminogen activator.

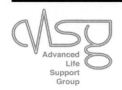

Answers to time out questions

CHAPTER 2: RECOGNITION OF THE MEDICAL EMERGENCY

Time Out 2.1 (see page 7)
This time out has allowed to reflect on your own practice and prioritise the importance of the components of your assessment.

Time Out 2.2 (see page 11)
Ensure that your list of clinical features is in a logical order.

CHAPTER 3: A STRUCTURED APPROACH TO MEDICAL EMERGENCIES

Time Out 3.1 (see page 24)
The primary assessment would comprise:

- Airway – assess patency. As the patient is talking no intervention at this stage is required except for high concentration of inspired oxygen (FiO_2 0.85).
- Breathing – assess rate, effort and symmetry of respiration. Look for an elevated JVP whilst palpating the trachea for tug or deviation. Percuss the anterior chest wall in upper, middle and lower zones, and in the axillae. Listen to establish whether breath sounds are absent, present or masked by added sounds. As no abnormality has been detected arterial oxygen saturation can be measured using the pulse oximeter.
- Circulation – assess pulse – rate, rhythm and character; blood pressure and capillary refill time. If there is no evidence of shock, a single cannula is inserted and blood taken for baseline haematological and biochemical values including a serum glucose. A bedside measurement of glucose is also important. Continuous monitoring of pulse, blood pressure and ECG will provide valuable baseline information as will a 12-lead ECG. The BM stix shows the glucose to be 1.2 mmol/l. The patient is therefore immediately treated with 250 ml 10% dextrose while the assessment continues.
- Disability – assessment of pupils – mildly dilated, symmetrical and slowly reacting to light. GCS 13/15: E4, V4, M5, no obvious lateralising signs.
- Exposure – no evidence of acute skin rash. Core temperature 36.8°C.

This assessment would be repeated and the patient would be monitored until the blood glucose had returned to normal. If the patient's conscious level did not change, however, treatment would continue to prevent secondary brain injury while reassessment and further investigations were requested. In contrast, if the patient's condition did improve then it would be appropriate to start the secondary assessment.

Acute Medical Emergencies; The Practical Approach, 2nd edition.
Edited by Terence Wardle, Peter Driscoll, and Sue Wieteska.
© 2010 Blackwell Publishing Ltd.

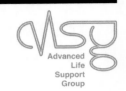

Time Out 3.2 (see page 28)

Primary assessment:

a Reassess the patient

b Shock – likely hypovolaemic

c Continue with high concentrations of inspired oxygen and give a fluid challenge, then reassess the patient. Correction of hypovolaemia restores sinus rhythm.

CHAPTER 4: AIRWAY ASSESSMENT

Time Out 4.1 (see page 40)

- Look – paradoxical (see-saw movement of the chest and abdomen in complete obstruction due to increased respiratory effort), accessory muscle use.
- Listen – stridor indicates upper airway obstruction, wheezes usually signify obstruction of the lower airways. Crowing accompanies laryngeal spasm while snoring indicates that the pharynx is partially occluded by the tongue. Gurgling usually signifies presence of semi-solid material.
- Feel – for expired air against the side of your cheek, chest movement, the position of trachea, any tracheal tug and the presence of subcutaneous emphysema.

CHAPTER 5: BREATHING ASSESSMENT

Time Out 5.1 (see page 53)

a

　i This is the amount of air inspired per breath and is equivalent to 7–8 ml/kg bodyweight or 500 ml for the 70-kg patient.

　ii This is the amount of air inspired each minute and is calculated by multiplying the respiratory rate by the tidal volume.

$$15 \text{ breaths/min} \times 500 \text{ ml} = 7.5 \text{ l/min}$$

b Alveolar ventilation can be calculated from the respiratory rate × (tidal volume – anatomical dead space). The anatomical dead space is constant. However as the respiratory rate increases, the amount of inspired air per breath or tidal volume is reduced. Therefore, as the respiratory rate increases in particular over 20 breaths/min, the tidal volume is reduced dramatically as is the alveolar ventilation. For further details the reader is referred to Chapter 5.

c This is shown in Chapter 5. The important feature however is that the relationship between the PaO_2 and O_2 saturation of haemoglobin is not linear. This means that haemoglobin O_2 saturation is initially well maintained over a very wide arterial oxygen concentration from 50 to 100 mm Hg.

d

　○ Airway obstruction

　○ Breathing

　　– bronchospasm, pulmonary oedema, tension pneumothorax

　　– critical oxygen desaturation.

CHAPTER 6: CIRCULATION ASSESSMENT

Time Out 6.1 (see page 63)

Please see Fig. 6.2.

Time Out 6.2 (see page 64)

- History of asystole

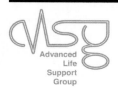
Advanced
Life
Support
Group

- When there is any pause ≥3 s in the presence of Mobitz Type II or complete heart block with wide QRS complexes. Clinical features that indicate treatment with atropine include cardiac failure, systolic blood pressure ≤90 mm Hg, heart rate <40 beats/min, presence of ventricular arrhythmias compromising blood pressure.

Time Out 6.3 (see page 65)

There are many ways to remember the causes of shock and one system in use is the preload, pump, afterload, (peripheral classification often referred to as the three Ps). Preload causes of shock are due to hypovolaemia that may be real, e.g. following haemorrhage, profuse diarrhoea or vomiting; and apparent, due to venodilation following treatment with intravenous nitrates. In addition, venous return can be obstructed by a gravid uterus, severe asthma or tension pneumothorax. Pump problems include severe left or right ventricular failure, cardiac tamponade. Peripheral or afterload causes are associated with widespread vasodilation (reduced systemic vascular resistance) seen with anaphylaxis, systemic inflammatory response syndrome including septicaemia and toxaemia and neurogenic shock.

CHAPTER 7: DISABILITY ASSESSMENT

Time Out 7.1 (see page 84)

See Fig. 7.5 showing dermatomes.

CHAPTER 8: THE PATIENT WITH BREATHING DIFFICULTIES

Time Out 8.1 (see page 89)

Key components of the assessment so far:
  Airway:
- Look
- Listen
- Feel
  Breathing:
- Look – colour, sweating, posture, respiratory effort, rate and symmetry
- Feel – tracheal position, tracheal tug, chest expansion
- Percuss
- Listen.

Time Out 8.2 (see page 90)

a Rapid primary assessment and treatment with:

  A High concentrations of inspired oxygen
  B Assessment indicates pulmonary oedema
  C Supports the diagnosis of left ventricular failure with hypotension therefore cardiogenic shock, so the patient requires intravenous access and, after appropriate bloods have been taken including markers of myocardial damage, inotropes should be started.

b Investigations should include a full blood count to ensure that there is no anaemia, baseline renal function and blood glucose, chest X-ray and 12-lead ECG. The patient will also require appropriate monitoring including pulse oximetry and continuous ECG.

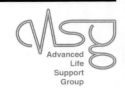

Time Out 8.3 (see page 96)

a This is a chronic inflammatory condition resulting in reversible narrowing of the airways.

b A susceptible airway in which bronchospasm may occur precipitated by IgE mast cell degranulation or exposure to environmental factors which will induce chronic inflammation. Bronchial contraction, mucosal oedema, increased mucous production and epithelial cell damage will drive the inflammatory response and exacerbate the airway narrowing. Persisting inflammation will induce collagen deposition under the basement membrane.

c Airway narrowing.

d It reduces the forced expiratory volume and peak expiratory flow rate. There is also increased functional residual capacity due to air trapping but no change in total lung capacity. Thus because of increased airways resistance, the work of breathing is increased and hence the patient feels breathless. In addition, in an acute attack some of the airways may be blocked by mucous plugs resulting in hypoxemia due to ventilation perfusion mismatch. This will also increase the work of breathing.

e By giving high concentrations of inspired oxygen.

Nebulised – (a) salbutamol 5 mg or terbutaline 10 mg; (b) ipratroprium bromide 0.5 mg or given via an oxygen driven nebuliser.

Intravenous – (a) hydrocortisone 200 mg; (b) salbutamol 250 µg over 10 min. Alternatively terbutaline or aminophylline can be used.

Chest X-ray to exclude a pneumothorax.

f The conditions are:
  i Hypoxaemia (PaO_2 <8 kPa despite FiO_2 >0.6)
  ii Hypercapnia ($PaCO_2$ >6 kPa)
  iii Exhaustion
  iv Altered conscious level
  v Respiratory arrest

Time Out 8.4 (see page 101)

a *Streptococcus pneumoniae*

b The patient may experience prodromal features of malaise, anorexia, myalgia, arthralgia and headache; there may also be a history of pyrexia and sweating. In addition, the patient will have had a cough productive of sputum and experience breathlessness, possible pleuritic pain and even haemoptysis. One third of patients may develop herpes simplex labialis. It is important to remember however that elderly patients may remain afebrile.

c High concentration of inspired oxygen, titrated to the arterial blood gas results, intravenous fluids and antibiotics according to local policy such as benzylpenicillin 1.2 g qds and clarithromycin 1 g daily.

d High risk factors in patients with pneumonia are summarised as the CURB 65 score (see table on page 105).

Time Out 8.5 (see page 106)

a This is pneumonia developing more than 48 h after admission to hospital.

b Those patients who are ill, bed-bound and who have impaired consciousness. This may be exacerbated by an inability to clear bronchial secretions, e.g. after a general anaesthetic or thoracic and abdominal surgery where coughing is impaired. The risk of a post operative pneumonia is also exacerbated in the

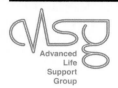

elderly and those patients who have a history of smoking, obesity and underlying chronic illness.

c Make sure that they are on supplemental oxygen and intravenous fluids along with an appropriate antibiotic regime. As there is a wide range of potential organisms, an early liaison with a microbiologist is advocated. Appropriate antibiotic regimes include tazocin, metronidazole plus gentamicin. If pseudomonas is suspected then either ceftazidime or ticarcillin may be required.

Time Out 8.6 (see page 107)
See Fig. 8.6 on page 103.

Time Out 8.7 (see page 108)
Larger emboli that block larger branches of the pulmonary artery provoke a rise in pulmonary artery pressure and rapid shallow respiration. Tachypnoea is also a reflex response to activation of vagal innovated luminal stretch receptors and interstitial J-receptors within the alveolar and capillary network.

CHAPTER 9: THE PATIENT WITH SHOCK

Time Out 9.1 (see page 125)
a The five factors are:
  i Concentration of oxygen reaching the alveoli
  ii Pulmonary perfusion
  iii Adequacy of pulmonary gas exchange
  iv Capacity of blood to carry oxygen
  v Blood flow to the tissues
b The sympathetic nervous system can help in several ways – increasing venous return by reducing the diameter of the veins and hence the capacity of the venous system; positively inotropic and the positively chronotropic effect.

Time Out 9.2 (see page 145)
a Clear, and if necessary, secure airway
  Give high concentrations of inspired oxygen
b Measure SpO_2
  Check for signs of aspiration
  Monitor respiratory rate
  Book chest X-ray
c Intravenous access × 2, start fluid replacement in one and take bloods from the other for FBC, U&E, glucose, clotting profile, cross match 4 units.
  Monitor pulse, blood pressure, 12-lead ECG and urine output
  Liaise with gastroenterologist/upper GI surgeon
  Subsequent management will depend on the response to fluid resuscitation, ongoing haemorrhage, change in physical/monitored signs.

CHAPTER 11: THE PATIENT WITH ALTERED CONSCIOUS LEVEL

Time Out 11.1 (see page 168)
a Consciousness is a function of the integrated action of the brain. The two interlinked key areas are the reticular formation and the cerebral cortex.

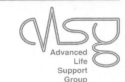

b This assessment comprises:
- Pupillary response
- Eye movement
- Corneal response
- Respiratory pattern.

Time Out 11.2 (see page 185)

a These develop on medium sized arteries at the base of the brain and the commonest sites are the distal internal carotid/posterior communicating artery and the anterior communicating artery complex.

b Intracranial saccular aneurysm and arterio venous malformation

c Greater than 12 h

d 25%

e *Streptococcus pneumoniae* and *Neisseria meningitidis*

f The immunocompromised patients including those with the human immuno deficiency virus; immigrants from Pakistan, India, Africa and the West Indies; alcoholics and intravenous drug users; patients with previous pulmonary tuberculosis.

g Gustatory and olfactory hallucinations, amnesia, expressive dysphasia, temporal lobe seizures, anosmia and behavioural abnormalities. This specific symptom complex occurs because herpes simplex encephalitis involves primarily the temporal and frontal cortex.

h Cerebral malaria should be considered a differential diagnosis of any acute febrile illness until it can be excluded by – definite lack of exposure, repeat examination of blood smears, following a therapeutic trial of antimalarial chemotherapy.

i Non-neurological features of *Plasmodium falciparum* infection include anaemia, spontaneous bleeding from the GI tract, jaundice, hypoglycaemia, shock, oliguria, acute renal failure and pulmonary oedema.

j Although intracranial abscesses can be caused by infection from sinuses or penetrating trauma, intracerebral abscesses can also follow septicaemia due to infective endocarditis, pulmonary abscess and bronchiectasis. Extradural abscesses are difficult to diagnose and may present with a localised headache in association with mastoiditis and sinusitis. In contrast, subdural and intracerebral abscesses present with headache, vomiting, impaired consciousness and neurological signs.

k An extradural haematoma follows a tear to the middle meningeal artery. It is a classic sequence of events after the head injury when the patient becomes unconscious, develops a lucid interval and then becomes comatosed. In contrast, subdural haematoma usually occurs in patients who are over anticoagulated or following falls in the elderly or alcoholic patients. Intracerebral haematoma occurs spontaneously and the clinical features and signs will be dictated by the area of the brain that has been affected.

CHAPTER 12: THE 'COLLAPSED' PATIENT

Time Out 12.1 (see page 201)

a Stroke is a syndrome characterised by an acute onset of focal, but occasionally global, loss of function lasting more than 24 h. This can be brought about by a number of causes including reduction in cerebral blood flow along a known vascular pathway affecting neurological tissue, generalised cerebral hypoperfusion from whatever cause and localised vascular disease.

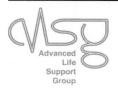

b The patient should have a rapid primary assessment with reference to a serum glucose estimation.

CHAPTER 14: THE PATIENT WITH A HEADACHE

Time Out 14.1 (see page 221)

a These can be classified as intracranial – e.g. meningitis, encephalitis and sub-arachnoid haemorrhage, or extracranial – e.g. acute sinusitis, acute viral illness, malaria or typhoid.

b Weakness usually affects the proximal and distal limb muscles equally, wasting occurs but is not prominent, reflexes are diminished or absent. Sensation may be unaffected although there may be variable loss.

Time Out 14.2 (see page 226)

a Initial diagnosis includes acute sinusitis, cervical spondylosis, giant cell arteritis and acute glaucoma.

b Acute sinusitis – orbital cellulitis/abscess, meningitis, cerebral abscess, osteomyelitis and cavernous sinus thrombosis.

Cervical spondylosis – spinal cord compression.

Giant cell arteritis – visual problems including blindness ischaemia/infarction of the heart, intestine and brain; acute glaucoma. Ischaemia of the optic nerve and retina.

Time Out 14.3 (see page 231)

a Tension headache – diffuse, commonly at the vertex frequently bilateral and described as a pressure tight band or squeezing. Usually starts in the morning and increases throughout the day. There is no vomiting and no visual disturbance.

Migrainous headaches can be paroxysmal, unilateral, bilateral and are often described as throbbing. In the minority of patients 20% will develop visual aura or some sensory disturbance.

Cluster headaches – unilateral with ipsilateral corneal injection, nasal congestion, and possibly a transient Horner's syndrome. The headache is usually centred around the orbit and lasts for between 30 min and 2 h each day for between 4 and 16 weeks.

b A lumbar puncture must be considered in any patient who has an acute onset of a headache that is new, progressive and awakes them from a sleep, especially those people who have a history suggestive of coital migraine.

CHAPTER 15: THE PATIENT WITH ABDOMINAL PAIN

Time Out 15.1 (see page 238)

a The differential diagnosis is:

  i Consider:
  - Leaking abdominal aortic aneurysm
  - Gastrointestinal bleeding (e.g. bleeding peptic ulcer)
  - Acute pancreatitis
  - Severe gastroenteritis
  - Cardiogenic shock (acute myocardial infarction)
  - Small bowel infarction (mesenteric artery occlusion)
  - Sepsis (e.g. colonic perforation, pneumonia)

ii Consider:
- Ectopic pregnancy
- Gastrointestinal bleeding (e.g. bleeding peptic ulcer)
- Acute pancreatitis
- Severe gastroenteritis/ulcerative colitis
- Diabetic ketoacidosis
- Ruptured spleen (spontaneous rupture occurs rarely in infectious mononucleosis)
- Sepsis (e.g. lower lobe pneumonia, meningococcal septicaemia)
- Acute adrenal insufficiency.

b The management priorities are:
- Is the airway unprotected and is there a risk of aspiration (particularly in the patient with vomiting and/or a depressed level of consciousness)? If so, secure the airway. Start high concentrations of inspired oxygen by facemask with a non-rebreathing reservoir bag.
- Examine the chest. Is ventilation and gas exchange adequate? If not, consider the need for intubation and ventilation (e.g. in patients with severe acute pancreatitis or septic shock).
- Assess degree of circulatory failure. Obtain vascular access with two large bore (peripheral) cannulae; take samples for blood cross match, baseline haematology and biochemistry (including amylase and glucose stick test), blood gas analysis, and – when appropriate – coagulation screen, β-hCG pregnancy test and sickle cell screen. For hypovolaemia initiate fluid resuscitation with 0.9% saline, followed by blood for haemorrhagic shock.
- 12-lead ECG if myocardial infarction/arrhythmia/pulmonary embolism suspected; urgent chest X-ray for pneumonia or other chest pathology; establish monitoring of SaO_2, ECG and BP.
- Perform abdominal, rectal and – if indicated – vaginal examination.
- Urgent surgical or gynaecological referral and/or other emergency treatment (analgesia, antibiotics), as appropriate.
- Consider the need for nasogastric tube and/or urinary catheter.
- Perform/arrange a portable ultrasound scan where this may confirm the diagnosis (e.g. suspected abdominal aortic aneurysm).

Reassess and go on to complete the secondary assessment.

Time Out 15.2 (see page 254)
Adverse prognostic factors in acute pancreatitis (within 48 h):
- Age >55 years
- White blood cell count >15 × 10^9/l
- Blood glucose >10 mmol/l (no diabetic history)
- Serum urea >16 mmol/l (no response to IV fluids)
- PaO_2 <8 kPa
- Serum calcium <2.0 mmol/l
- Serum albumin <32 g/l
- Lactate dehydrogenase >600 U/l.

CHAPTER 16: THE PATIENT WITH HOT RED LEGS OR COLD WHITE LEGS

Time Out 16.1 (see page 263)
Post-operative, immobile, pregnant patients, women on the oral contraceptive pill, family history of coagulopathy.

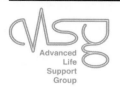

Time Out 16.2 (see page 268)

- Arterial emboli tend to occur at the bifurcation of arteries. These will depend on the extent of the occlusion of the circulation and the degree of colateral circulation.
- Medical features include pain, pallor, pulselessness, parathesia, paralysis and perishing cold.
- In contrast, a closed compartment syndrome is caused by a swollen or a contused muscle or bleeding into the muscle from inside a rigid fascial envelope. Pain and parasthesia are early symptoms but the affected limb may also be pale and cool with slow capillary refill. However the presence of a distal pulse does not help diagnosis.

CHAPTER 17: THE PATIENT WITH HOT AND/OR SWOLLEN JOINTS

Time Out 17.1 (see page 280)

There are many algorithms but the important step is the first step which is to exclude a septic arthritis.

CHAPTER 18: THE PATIENT WITH A RASH

Time Out 18.1 (see page 292)

a The four categories are:
- **i** Urticaria
- **ii** Erythema
- **iii** Purpura and vasculitis
- **iv** Blistering disorders

b The reader is referred to Chapter 18 for the algorithms for each of these conditions.

CHAPTER 20: ORGAN FAILURE

Time Out 20.1 (see page 318)

The immediate management comprises a rapid primary assessment to ensure airway patency. Her FiO_2 should be increased to 0.85. Breathing must be reassessed to exclude life-threatening bronchospasm, tension pneumothorax and pulmonary oedema. She should be treated with nebulised bronchodilators including salbutamol and ipratropium, along with intravenous hydrocortisone and a bronchodilator. An urgent chest X-ray is required. The result is a right-sided pneumothorax. Whilst there are no clinical features to indicate underlying tension, even a small pneumothorax in a person with pre-existing chest disease can cause rapid decompensation. Therefore a chest drain is also required.

Time Out 20.2 (see page 341)

a The causes are:
- **i** Acute asthma; pulmonary embolus; cardiac, e.g. dysrhythmia; neurological, e.g. status epilepticus; neuromuscular, e.g. myasthenia gravis.
- **ii** The commonest cause is ischaemic heart disease. Others include valvular pathology, acute hypertension, cardiomyopathy.
- **iii** Any chronic neurological disorder can have the final common pathway of brain failure. Dementia is another cause. These are not acute medical emergencies, however, the important point is to be able to differentiate these

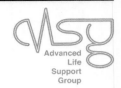

conditions from potentially treatable problems such as a patient with an acute confusional state or underlying depression.

iv These may be classified as prerenal, intrinsic renal or post renal conditions. The commonest group is the prerenal, which usually arises as secondary to hypovolaemia. The second most common cause is post-renal or obstructive uropathy, e.g. in association with prostatic pathology. Intrinsic renal disease in comparison is rare.

v Acute liver failure is usually caused by drugs such as an overdose of paracetamol and with increasing frequency of Ecstacy. It can also occur in pregnancy. Acute on chronic liver failure is commonly caused by alcoholic liver disease.

vi The causes of endocrine failure will depend on the particular gland that is affected and also the hormone or hormones that are not being produced. Irrespective of these conditions considered, there are common features that influence all aspects of the primary assessment.

CHAPTER 21: THE ELDERLY PATIENT

Time Out 21.1 (see page 354)

10%

CHAPTER 22: TRANSPORTATION OF THE SERIOUSLY ILL PATIENT

Time Out 22.1 (see page 366)

A 27-year-old mechanic with a subarachnoid haemorrhage is stable with a respiration rate of 14/min, sinus tachycardia 110/min, BP 120/70, blood glucose by BM stick test 7 mmol/l, GCS 15/15 PERLA. The decision has been made to transfer this patient to the local neurological centre for assessment before surgery.

Assessment

Male, 27, clinical details as described above.
- What is the problem?
  Diagnosis – subarachnoid haemorrhage.
- What has been done?
  Prevention of secondary brain injury, CT scan and lumbar puncture.
- What was the effect?
  Maintaining the status quo and preventing secondary brain injury.
- What is needed now?
  Transfer for further assessment.
  There are potential problems that may arise during transfer:

Airway – obstruction, hypoxaemia

Breathing – hypocarbia respiratory arrest

Circulation – cardiac arrest, dysrhythmia, hypoglycaemia, hyponatremia

Disability – deterioration in Glasgow Coma Score, fit, extension of subarachnoid haemorrhage, development of raised intracranial pressure.

Control

A comprehensive assessment by the clinician in charge and the decision has been made to transfer the patient to hospital for further investigation.

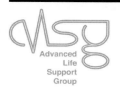

Communication

With:

The consultant

Intensive care consultant

Patient's relatives

Accepting consultant

Ambulance control

Communication also includes determining the lines of responsibility and using the assessment questions to provide a structure to tell the receiving team the salient points before transfer. In addition, the reason for transfer and what is needed for the receiving centre should be explained.

Evaluation

The need for specialist care has already been determined as part of the initial assessment.

Package and preparation

The patient has been stabilised before transfer and all baseline blood tests including arterial gases have been requested, reviewed and appropriate action taken. All relevant equipment monitoring and treatment has been pre-packed and checked. Furthermore, this also includes contingency equipment that should be required in case the patient deteriorates and incurs one of the problems that were listed earlier. The neurosurgical centre is 30 miles away by motorway with no predicted problems and a stable patient, so the decision has been made to transport by ambulance.

Personnel

The ambulance crew

One doctor

One nurse

Part of the regular transfer team has been briefed and have the appropriate personnel. Ensure all personal equipment is available and working. The ambulance should have appropriate monitoring equipment and back up systems including oxygen should any problems arise. Shortly before transfer, all the patient's documentations have been photocopied and appropriate forms are available to record the patient's condition during transfer.

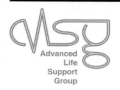

Index

Note: Page numbers in **bold** type refer to figures; those in *italic* refer to tables or boxed material.

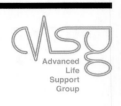
Advanced Life Support Group

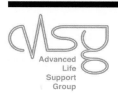

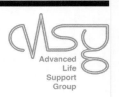

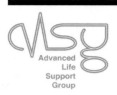

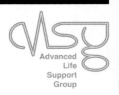

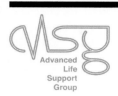

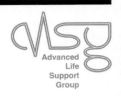

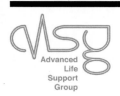

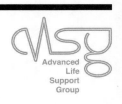

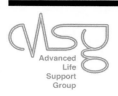

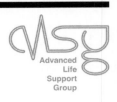

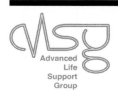

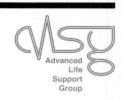

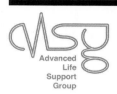

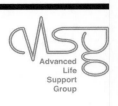

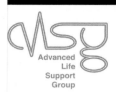

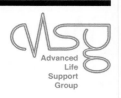

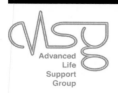

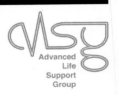

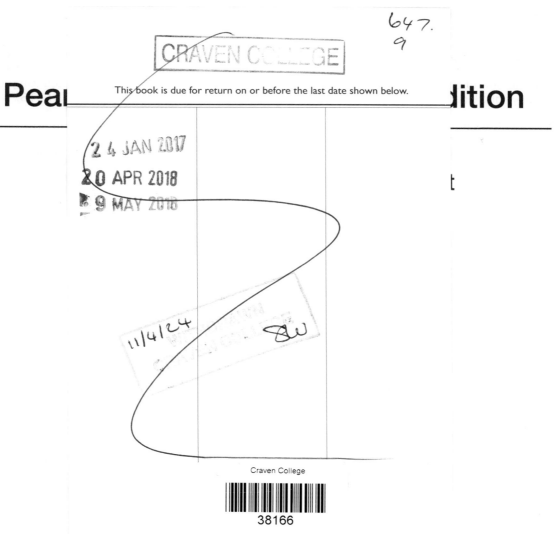

Pea... ...dition

t

PEARSON®

Pearson Education Limited
Edinburgh Gate
Harlow
Essex CM20 2JE
England and Associated Companies throughout the world

Visit us on the World Wide Web at: www.pearsoned.co.uk

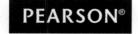 ISBN 10: 1-292-02101-2
ISBN 13: 978-1-292-02101-0

British Library Cataloguing-in-Publication Data
A catalogue record for this book is available from the British Library

Printed in Great Britain by Ashford Colour Press Ltd

Table of Contents

Introducing Hospitality

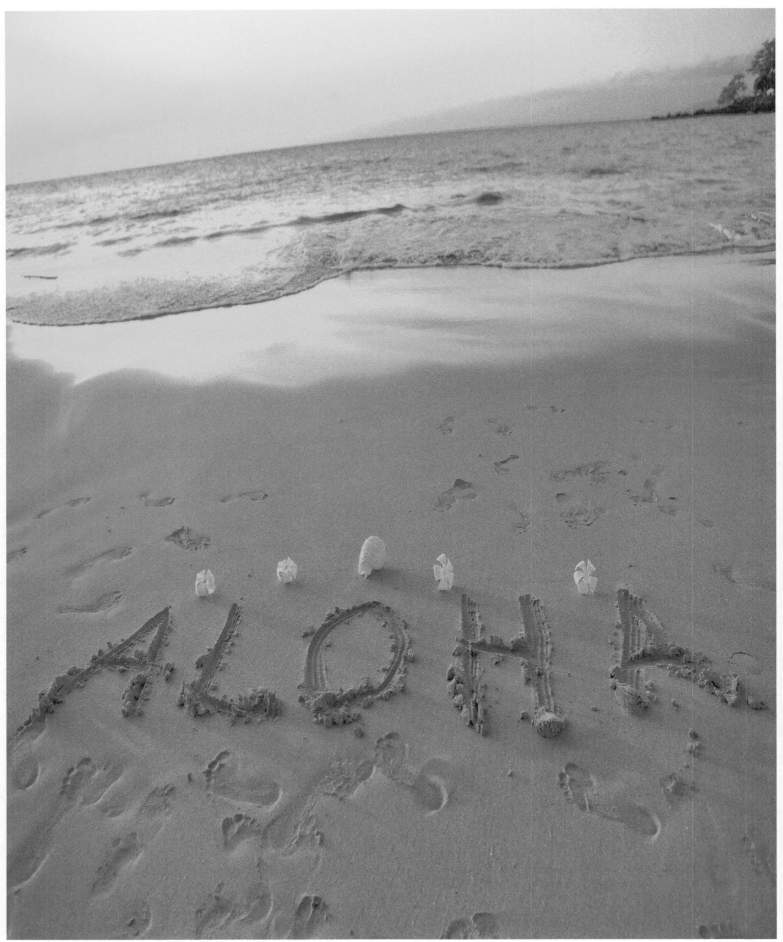

Introducing Hospitality

OBJECTIVES

After reading and studying this chapter, you should be able to:

- Describe the characteristics of the hospitality industry.

- Explain corporate philosophy.

- Discuss why service has become such an important facet of the hospitality industry.

- Suggest ways to improve service.

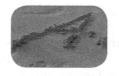 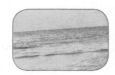  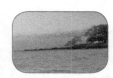

Prelude

Hospitality through the Ages[1]

The concept of hospitality is as old as civilization itself. Its development from the ancient custom of breaking bread with a passing stranger to the operations of today's multifaceted hospitality conglomerates makes fascinating reading, and interesting comparisons can be made with today's hospitality management.

The word *hospitality* comes from *hospice,* an old French word meaning "to provide care/shelter for travelers." The most famous hospice is the Hospice de Beaune in the Burgundy region of France, also called the Hotel Dieu or the House of God. It was founded as a charity hospital in 1443 by Nicolas Rolin, the Chancellor of Burgundy, as a refuge for the poor.

The hospital is still functioning, partly because of its role in the wine world. Throughout the centuries, several Burgundian landowners have donated vineyards to the Hospice to help pay for maintaining its costs. Every Fall, the wines from these vineyards—about a hundred acres of vines—are sold at a colorful wine auction on the third Thursday in November, which determines the prices for the next year's Burgundy wines.

Ancient Times

The Sumerians (who lived in what is now Iraq) were the first to record elements of hospitality in about 4,500 years B.C.E. They moved from being hunter-gatherers to growing crops, which, due to surpluses, they were able to trade. More time became available for other activities such as writing, inventing money, creating pottery, making tools, and producing beer, which was probably safer to drink than water! Taverns served several beers, and as with today, provided a place for locals to relax and enjoy each other's company.

Between 4,000 and 2,000 B.C.E., early civilizations in Europe, China, Egypt, and India all had some elements of hospitality offerings, such as taverns and inns along the roadside.

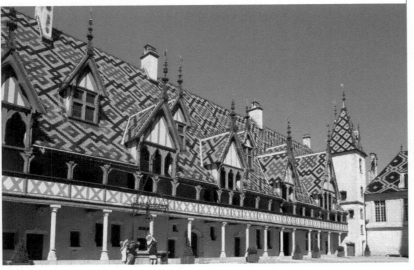

The Hospice de Beaune.

Greece and Rome

Mention of hospitality—in the form of taverns—is found in writings dating back to ancient Greece and Rome, beginning with the Code of Hammurabi (circa 1700 B.C.E.). The Code required owners to report guests who planned crimes in their taverns. The penalty for not doing so was death, making tavern-keeping a hazardous occupation. The death penalty could also be imposed for watering the beer!

Increased travel and trade made some form of overnight accommodations an absolute necessity. Because travel was slow and journeys long and arduous, many travelers depended solely on the hospitality of private citizens.[2] In the Greek and Roman empires, inns and taverns sprang up everywhere. The Romans constructed elaborate and well-appointed inns on all the main roads. They were located about twenty-five miles apart. To ensure that fresh horses were available for officials and couriers of the Roman government, these inns could only be used with special government documents granting permission. By the time Marco Polo traveled to the Far East, there were 10,000 inns, the best of which were in China.[3]

Some wealthy landowners built their own inns on the edges of their estates. These inns were run by household slaves. Nearer the cities, inns and taverns were run by freemen or by retired gladiators who would invest their savings in the "restaurant business" in the same way that so many of today's retired athletes open restaurants. The first "business lunch" is reputed to have been the idea of Seqius Locates, a Roman innkeeper; in 40 B.C.E. Locates devised the idea for ships' brokers, who were often too busy to go home for their midday meals.

Medieval Times

On the European continent, Charlemagne established rest houses for pilgrims in the eighth century; the sole purpose of several orders of knighthood was to protect pilgrims and to provide hospitality for pilgrims on their routes. One such rest house, an abbey at Roncesvalles, advertised services such as a warm welcome at the door, free bread, a barber and a cobbler, cellars full of fruit and almonds, two hospices with beds for the sick, and even a consecrated burial ground.

In 1282, the innkeepers of Florence, Italy, incorporated a guild, or an association for the purpose of business. The inns belonged to the city, which sold three-year leases at auction. They must have been profitable, because by 1290, there were eighty-six innkeepers as members of the guild.

In England, the stagecoach became the favored method of transportation. A journey from London to the city of Bath took three days, with several stopovers at inns or taverns that were also called post houses. Today, the journey from London to Bath takes about one and a half hours by car or train. As travel and travelers increased during the Middle Ages, so did the number of wayside inns in Europe; yet, they were primitive affairs by today's standards. Guests often slept on mattresses in what today would be the inn's lobby. As the quality of the inns improved, more people began to travel. Many of the travelers were wealthy people, accustomed to the good life; their expectations demanded that inns be upgraded.

In the late sixteenth century, a type of eating place for commoners called an *ordinary* began to appear in England. These places were taverns serving a fixed-price, fixed-menu meal at a long common table. Ordinary diners could not be choosy, nor did they often question what they were eating. Frequently, the main dish served was a long-cooked, highly seasoned meat-and-vegetable stew. Culinary expertise was limited by the availability and cost of certain ingredients. Few diners had sound teeth—many had no teeth at all—so the meal had to be able to be gummed as well as being edible. Fresh meat was not always available; spoiled meat was often the rule rather than the exception. Spices helped not only to preserve meat but also to disguise the flavor of gamey or "high" meat.

Coffee Houses

During the sixteenth century, two "exotic" imports began to influence the culinary habits of Western Europe: coffee and tea. These beverages, so integrated into the twenty-first century way of life, were once mere curiosities. Travelers to Constantinople (now Istanbul, Turkey) enjoyed coffee there and brought it back to Europe.

During the seventeenth century, coffeehouses sprang up all over Europe. By 1675, the city-state of Venice had dozens of coffee houses, including the famous Café Florian on the piazza San Marco, still filled to capacity today. The first English coffee house was opened in 1652. Coffee houses, the social and literary centers of their day and the predecessor of today's cafés and coffee shops, served another, even more useful (though less obvious), purpose: They helped to sober up an entire continent.

In a day when water was vile, milk dangerous, and carbonated beverages centuries in the future, alcoholic drinks were the rule, rather than the exception. Adults drank amounts measured in gallons. Queen Elizabeth I's ladies-in-waiting, for instance, were allowed a breakfast allowance of two gallons of ale. Drunkenness was rampant.

The New World

There is some evidence that a tavern was built in Jamestown, Virginia, during the early days of the settlement. It was in Boston where the first ordinary was recorded—Cole's Ordinary—in 1663. After Cole's, the next recorded ordinary was Hudson's House, in 1640.[4] The Dutch built the first known tavern in New York—the Stadt Huys—in 1642. Early colonial American inns and taverns are steeped as much in history as they are in hospitality. The next year, Kreiger's Tavern opened on Bowling Green in New York City. During the American Revolution, this tavern, then called the King's Arms, became the Revolutionary headquarters of British General Gage.

The even more famous Frauncis Tavern was the Revolutionary headquarters of General George Washington and was the place where he made his famous Farewell Address. It is still operating today. As the colonies grew from scattered settlements to towns and cities, more and more travelers appeared, along with more accommodations to serve them. The inn, tavern, or ordinary in the colonies soon became a gathering place for residents, a place where they could catch up

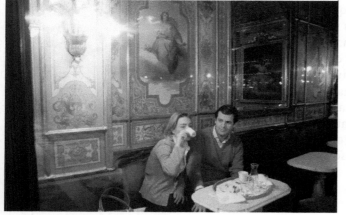

Café Florian, St. Marks Square, Venice, Italy.

on the latest gossip, keep up with current events, hold meetings, and conduct business. The innkeeper was often the most respected member of the community and was always one of its more substantial citizens. The innkeeper usually held some local elected office and sometimes rose much higher than that. John Adams, the second president of the United States, owned and managed his own tavern between 1783 and 1789.

The Revolutionary War did little to change the character of these public places. They maintained their position as social centers, political gathering places, newsrooms, watering holes, and travelers' rests; now, however, these places were going by different names—hotels—that reflected a growing French influence in the new nation.

The French Revolution

The French Revolution took place at approximately the same time as the American colonies were fighting for their independence. Among many other effects, the French Revolution helped to change the course of culinary history. M. Boulanger, "the father of the modern restaurant," sold soups at his all-night tavern on the Rue Bailleul. He called these soups *restorantes* (restoratives), which is the origin of the word *restaurant*. One dish was made of sheep's feet in a white sauce, another was *boulangere* potatoes—a dish in use today—made of sliced potatoes cooked in stock, which was baked in the bread baker's oven after the bread was done.[5]

The French Revolution, 1789–1799, changed the course of culinary history. Because nearly all the best chefs worked for the nobility, who were deposed or literally "lost their heads," the chefs lost their employment. Many chefs immigrated to America, especially to New Orleans, a French enclave in America. Others scattered throughout Europe or immigrated to Quebec, a French-speaking province of Canada. The chefs brought their culinary traditions with them. Soon the plain, hearty fare of the British and the primitive cooking of the Americans were laced with *sauces piquantes* (sauces having a pleasantly sharp taste or appetizing flavor) and *pots au feu* (French beef stew). In 1784, during a five-year period as an envoy to France, Thomas Jefferson acquired a taste for French cuisine. He later persuaded a French chef to come to the White House to lend his expertise. This act stimulated interest in French cuisine and enticed U.S. tavern owners to offer better quality and more interesting food.

Over time, New Orleans was occupied by Britain, Spain, France, and America, and one interesting restaurant there, the Court of the Two Sisters, has the names of prisoners of various wars inscribed on the walls of its entrance.

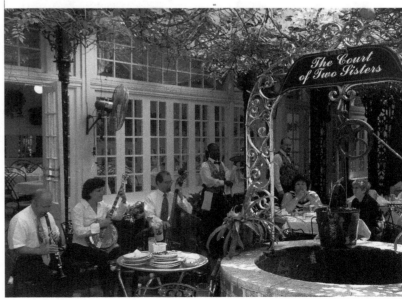

The Court of the Two Sisters.

The Nineteenth Century

Restaurants continued to flourish in Europe. In 1856, Antoine Carême published *La Cuisine Classique* and other volumes detailing numerous dishes and their sauces. The grande cuisine offered a carte (or list) of suggestions available from the kitchen. This was the beginning of the à la carte menu. In 1898 the Savoy Hotel opened in London. The general manager was the renowned César Ritz (today, the Ritz-Carlton hotels bear his name) and the chef de cuisine was August Escoffier. Between them, they revolutionized hotel restaurants. Escoffier was one of the greatest chefs of all time. He is best known for his classic book *Le Guide Culinaire,* which simplified the extraordinary works of Carême. He also installed the brigade de cuisine system in the kitchen.

Americans used their special brand of ingenuity to create something for everyone. By 1848, a hierarchy of eating places existed in New York City. At the bottom was Sweeney's "sixpenny eating house" on Ann Street, whose proprietor, Daniel Sweeney, achieved questionable fame as the father of the "greasy spoon." Sweeney's less than appetizing fare ("small plate sixpence, large plate shilling") was literally slid down a well-greased counter to his hungry guests, who cared little for the social amenities of dining.

The famous Delmonico's was at the top of the list of American restaurants for a long time. The Delmonico family owned and operated the restaurant from 1827 until 1923, when it closed due to Prohibition, The name *Delmonico's* was synonymous with fine food, exquisitely prepared and impeccably served—the criteria by which all like establishments were judged. Delmonico's served Swiss-French cuisine and became the focal point of American gastronomy (the art of good eating). Delmonico's is also credited with the invention of the bilingual menu, Baked Alaska, Chicken à la King, and Lobster Newberg. The Delmonico steak is named after the restaurant. More and more, eating places in the United States and abroad catered to residents of a town or city and less to travelers; the custom of eating out for its own sake had arrived.

Thirty-five restaurants in New York City have now celebrated their one-hundredth birthdays. One of them, PJ Clarke's established in 1884, is a "real" restaurant-bar that has changed little in its hundred years of operation. On entering, one sees a large mahogany bar, its mirror tarnished by time, the original tin ceiling, and the tile mosaic floor. Memorabilia ranges from celebrity pictures to Jessie, the house fox terrier that customers had stuffed when she died and who now

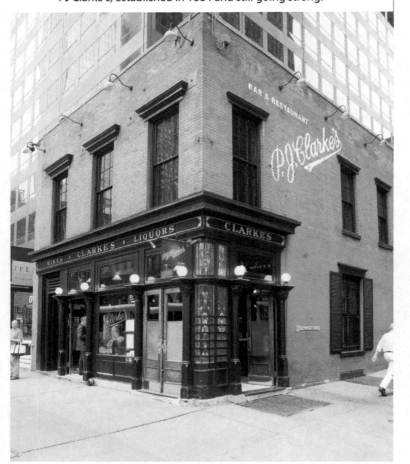

PJ Clarke's, established in 1884 and still going strong.

stands guard over the ladies' room door. Guests still write down their own checks at lunchtime, on pads with their table numbers on them (this goes back to the days when one of the servers could not read or write and struggled to remember orders).[6]

Many American cities had hotel palaces: Chicago had the Palmer House, New Orleans had the St. Charles, St. Louis had the Planter's Hotel, Boston had The Lenox, and San Antonio had The Menger. As the railroads were able to transport passengers to exotic locations like South Florida, hotels such as The Breakers in Palm Beach were built to accommodate the guests.

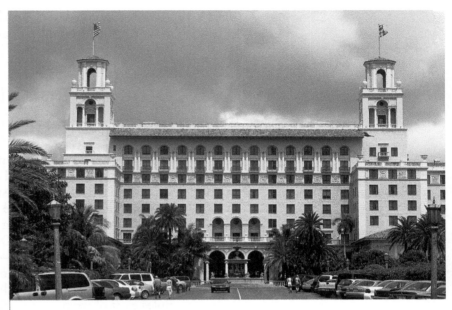
The Breakers, Palm Beach, Florida.

The Twentieth Century

In 1921, Walter Anderson and Billy Ingraham began the White Castle hamburger chain. The name White Castle was selected because white stood for purity and castle for strength. The eye-catching restaurants were nothing more than stucco building shells, a griddle, and a few chairs. People came in droves, and within ten years, White Castle had expanded to 115 units.[7]

The Four Seasons restaurant opened in 1959 as the first elegant American restaurant that was not French in style. The Four Seasons was the first restaurant to offer seasonal menus. With its modern architecture and art as a theme, Joe Baum, the developer of this and many other successful restaurants, understood why people go to restaurants—to be together and to connect to one another. It is very important that the restaurant reinforce why guests chose it in the first place. Restaurants exist to create pleasure, and how well a restaurant meets this expectation of pleasure is a measure of its success.[8]

Following World War II, North America took to the road. There was a rapid development of hotels, motels, fast food, and coffee shops. The 1950s and 1960s also saw an incredible growth in air transportation. Cross-continental flights were not only more frequent, but took much less time. Many of the new jets introduced in this period helped develop tourism worldwide. Hotels and restaurant chains sprang up to cater to the needs of the business and leisure traveler as well as city residents.

In the 1980s, hospitality, travel, and tourism continued to increase dramatically. The baby boomers began to exert influence through their buying power. Distant exotic destinations and resorts became even more accessible. The 1990s began with the recession that had started in 1989. The Gulf War continued the downturn that the industry had experienced. As hospitality and tourism companies strived for profitability, they downsized and consolidated. From 1993 until 9/11, the economic recovery proved very strong and hospitality businesses expanded in North America and abroad, particularly in Europe and China.

Welcome to You, the Future Hospitality Industry Leaders!

The hospitality industry is a fascinating, fun, and stimulating one in which to enjoy a career, plus you get compensated quite well and have excellent advancement opportunities. We often hear from industry professionals that it (the industry) gets in your blood—meaning we become one with the hospitality industry. On countless class industry visits, the persons speaking to the class said that they wouldn't change their job—even if they had a chance. Only one speaker said, "You must be nuts if you want to work in this industry"—of course, he was joking! But there are some realities you need to be aware of, and they are discussed in the section titled, "Characteristics of the Hospitality Industry," found later in this chapter. Many examples exist of people graduating and being offered positions that enable them to gain a good foundation of knowledge and experience in the industry. Possible career paths are illustrated in Figure 1. In most cases, it does not take long for advancement opportunities to come along. Let's begin our journey with a look at *service spirit*, which plays a crucial role in the success of our industry, no matter what your position or title is.

Ever think about why Marriott International is so successful? Well, one of the reasons is given by Jim Collins writing in the foreword to Bill Marriott's book, *The Spirit to Serve: Marriott's Way*. Collins says Marriott has *timeless core values and enduring purpose*, including the belief that its people are number one: "Take care of Marriott people and they will take care of the guests." Also, Marriott's commitment to continuous improvement and good old-fashioned dedication to hard work and having fun while doing it provide a foundation of stability and enduring character. Collins adds that Marriott's core purpose— making people away from home feel that they are among friends and are really wanted—serves as a fixed point of guidance and inspiration.

So, where does *hospitality spirit* fit into all this? It's simple—it begins with each and every time we have a guest encounter. People with a *service spirit* are happy to do something extra to make a guest's experience memorable. The hospitality spirit means that it is our passion to give pleasure to others, or as one human resources director, Charlotte Jordan, calls it, "creating memorable experiences for others and being an ambassador of the world, adding warmth and caring."[9] Every day we encounter guests who rely on us for service, which can make or break their experience. We want to "wow" guests and have them return often with their friends. Yes, we are in the people business, and it's "we the people" who succeed in the hospitality industry when we take pride in the words of the Ritz-Carlton hotel company: We are ladies and gentlemen taking care of ladies and gentlemen.

The **National Restaurant Association (NRA)** forecasts a need for thousands of supervisors and managers for the hospitality and tourism industries. Are you wondering if there's room in this dynamic industry for you? You bet! There's room for everyone. The best advice is to consider what you love to do most and get some experience in that area—to see if you really like it—because our

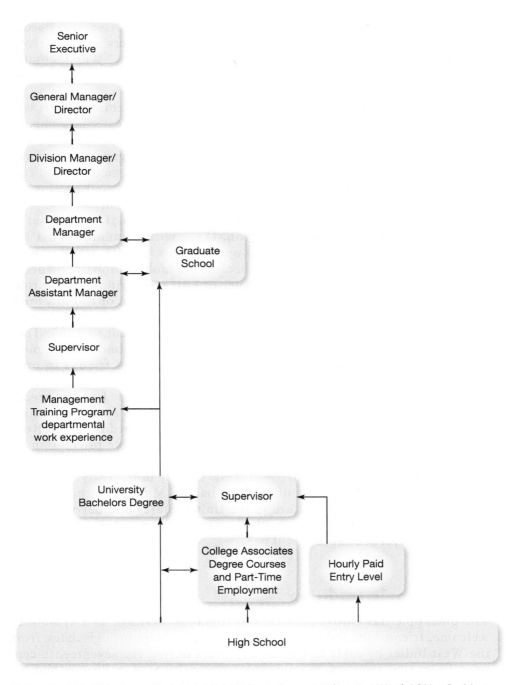

Figure 1 • A Possible Career Path in the Hospitality Industry. Is Education Worth It? You Bet! Just Think—Over a Career, the Difference in Salary between an Associate and a Bachelor's Degree Is $500,000. Yes, That's Half a Million Bucks!

(*Source:* U.S. Census Bureau Average Lifetime Earnings—Different Levels of Education.)

industry has some distinct characteristics. For starters, we are in the business of giving service. When Kurt Wachtveilt, thirty-year veteran general manager of the Oriental Hotel in Bangkok, Thailand—considered by many to be one of the best hotels in the world—was asked, "What is the secret of being the best?"

he replied, "Service, service, service!" But what is service? *Service* is defined in *Webster's New World Dictionary* as "the act or means of serving." To serve is to "provide goods and services for" and "be of assistance to." With thousands of guest encounters each day, it is critical to give our guests exceptional service at each encounter. And that's the challenge!

The hospitality industry can also be a good choice for entrepreneurs who prefer to do their own thing, whether it be running a bar, catering company, restaurant, or night club; being involved in event management; or being a tour guide or wedding planner or whatever. The prospects are good for starting a successful endeavor. Think about it: You could begin with one restaurant concept, open a second, and then begin to franchise. Whatever your dreams and goals, the hospitality industry likely has an opportunity for you.

Consider that a company like Marriott International started out as a small root beer place, in Washington, D.C., with a counter and a few stools. And that an immigrant, who opened up a hot dog stand outside Dodger Stadium in Los Angeles later became the multimillionaire owner of a chain restaurant (Karl Kartcher, owner of Carl's Jr.). And that a former dishwasher, Ralph Rubio, now owns the successful chain of Rubio's Fresh Mexican Grill quick-service restaurants, which have sold more than 50 million fish tacos since the opening of the first restaurant in 1983. Then there is Peter Morton, who, in the early 1970s, lived in London, and, missing American food, borrowed $60,000 from family and friends to open the Great American Disaster. It was an immediate success, with a line of customers around the block. Morton quickly realized that London needed a restaurant that not only served American food but also embodied the energy and excitement of music past and present. He opened the Hard Rock Cafe and offered a hearty American meal at a reasonable price in an atmosphere charged with energy, fun, and the excitement of rock and roll.[10] More recently, Howard Schultz, who while in Italy in the early 1980s was impressed with the popularity of espresso bars in Milan, saw the potential to develop the coffee bar culture in the United States and beyond. There are now well over 16,000 Starbucks locations.[11] Any ideas on what the next hot entrepreneurial idea will be?

The Pineapple Tradition

The pineapple has enjoyed a rich and romantic heritage as a symbol of welcome, friendship, and **hospitality**. Pineapples were brought back from the West Indies by early European explorers during the seventeenth century. From that time on, the pineapple was cultivated in Europe and became the favored fruit to serve to royalty and the elite. The pineapple was later introduced into North America and became a part of North American hospitality as well. Pineapples were displayed at doors or on gateposts, announcing to friends and acquaintances: "The ship is in! Come join us. Food and drink for all!"

Since its introduction, the pineapple has been internationally recognized as a symbol of hospitality and a sign of friendliness, warmth, cheer, graciousness, and conviviality.

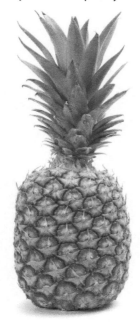

The pineapple is the symbol of hospitality.

The Interrelated Nature of Hospitality and Tourism

The hospitality and **tourism** industries are the largest and fastest-growing industry groupings in the world. One of the most exciting aspects of this industry is that it is made up of so many different professions. What picture comes to mind when you think about a career in hospitality and tourism? Do you picture a chef, a general manager, owners of their own businesses, a director of marketing, or an event manager? The possibilities are many and varied, ranging from positions in restaurants, resorts, air and cruise lines, theme parks, attractions, and casinos, to name a few of the several sectors of the hospitality and tourism industries (see Figures 2 and 3).

James Reid, a professor at New York City Technical College, contributed his thoughts to this section. As diverse as the hospitality industry is, there are some powerful and common dynamics, which include the delivery of services and products and the guests' impressions of them. Whether an employee is in direct contact with a guest (**front of the house**) or performing duties behind the scenes (**heart of the house**), the profound and most challenging reality of working in this industry is that hospitality employees have the ability to affect the human experience by creating powerful impressions—even brief moments of truth—that may last a lifetime. (A "moment of truth" is an industry expression used to describe a guest and an associate meeting, as when a guest walks into a restaurant.)

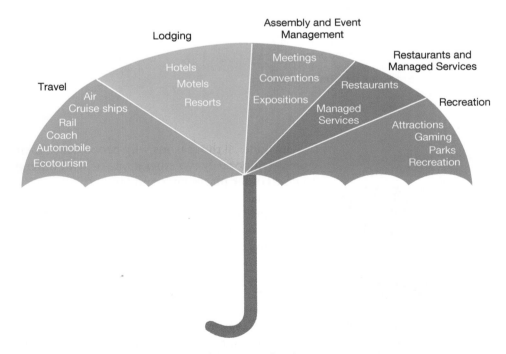

Figure 2 • Scope of the Hospitality and Tourism Industries.

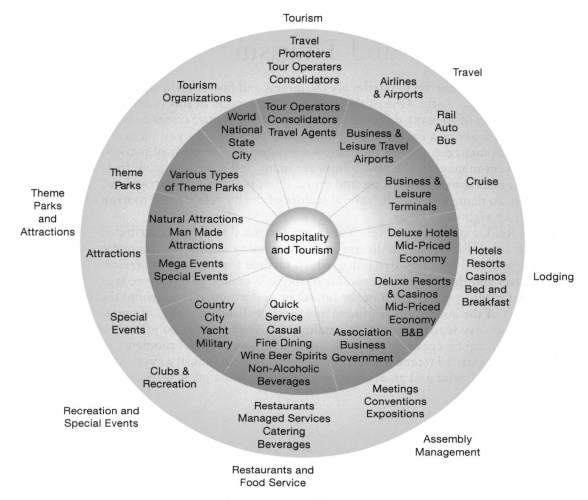

Figure 3 • The Interrelated Nature of Hospitality, Travel, and Tourism.

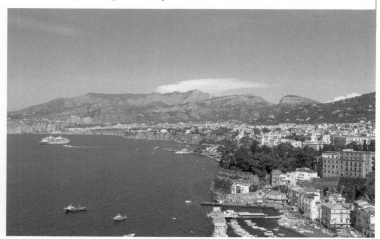

The interrelated nature of hospitality and tourism means that we would fly here, stay in a restaurant, and eat in a restaurant.

Imagine all the reasons why people leave their homes temporarily (whether alone or with others) to go to other places near and far.

People travel for many reasons. A trip away from home might be for vacation, for work, to attend a conference, or maybe even to visit a college campus, just to name a few. Regardless of the reason, under the umbrella of travel and tourism, many professions are necessary to meet the needs and wants of people away from home. Think of the many people who provide services to travelers and who have the responsibility of representing their communities and creating experiences that, when delivered successfully, are pleasurable and memorable for travelers. These people welcome, inform, comfort, and care for tourists and are collectively a part of a process that can positively affect human lives and well-being.

The hotel business provides career opportunities for many associates who help make reservations and greet, assist, and serve guests in hospitality operations of varied sizes and in locations all over the world. Examples include a husband and wife who operate their own bed and breakfast (B&B) in upstate Vermont. This couple provides the ideal weekend retreat for avid skiers during a frosty February, making their guests want to return year after year. Another ex-

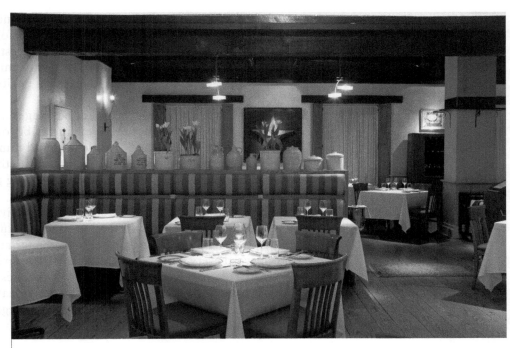

Gramercy Tavern, a Danny Meyer, Union Square Hospitality Group Restaurant.

ample is the hundreds of employees necessary to keep the 5,505-room MGM Grand in full swing 365 days a year! Room attendants, engineers, front-desk agents, food servers, and managers are just a few of the positions that are vital to creating experiences for visitors who come to Las Vegas from around the globe.

The restaurant business is also a vital component under the travel and tourism umbrella. People go to restaurants to fulfill diverse needs and wants. Eating is a biological need that restaurants accommodate, but restaurants and the people who work in them fulfill numerous other human desires, such as the need for socialization and to be entertained.

Gramercy Tavern restaurant in New York City may be the perfect location for a certain group of friends to celebrate a twenty-first birthday. The individual guest who turned twenty-one may remember this fête for a lifetime because the service and food quality were excellent and added value to the experiences for all the celebrants. For this kind of collective and powerful impression to be made, many key players are needed to operate and support the service-delivery system: several front-of-the-house staff members, such as the food servers, bartenders, greeters, managers, and bus attendants; plus the back-of-the-house employees, such as the chefs, dishwashers, food purchaser, and stewards (to name a few). All these people had to coordinate a variety of activities and responsibilities to create this dynamic, successful, and, for the restaurant ownership, profitable event.

In managed services, foodservices are provided for airlines, military facilities, schools, colleges and universities, health care operations, and business and industry. These foodservice operations have the dual challenge of meeting the needs and wants of both the guests and the client (i.e., the institution that hired the foodservices). The employees who are part of foodservices enterprises have responsibilities very much like those of other restaurant operations. The quality of food products delivered in an airline, for example, may be the key to winning passengers back in the future and creating positive word-of-mouth promotion that attracts new customers.

Since history has been recorded, beverages have provided a biological need that has expanded the beverage menu far beyond water alone! Whether it is the cool iced tea garnished with lemon and mint served poolside at a Riviera resort or the champagne toast offered at a fiftieth wedding anniversary party in Boston, beverages play a major role in satisfying people and adding to the many celebrations of life.

As with food products, the creation and delivery systems for beverage products are vital components of the hospitality industry. These operations involve many people who consumers rarely see: the farmer in Napa Valley who tends to the vineyard every day of the year, the coffee bean harvester in Colombia, the sake server in Tokyo, or the orchard owner who crates oranges in Florida. These individuals behind the scenes have diverse and crucial responsibilities so that guests, whether in a resort, an office, a hospital, a college, or a roadside snack bar, can have the quality of products they want.

TECHNOLOGY SPOTLIGHT

The Increasing Importance of Technology to the Hospitality Industry

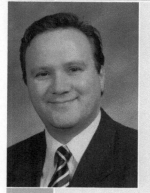

Cihan Cobanoglu, Ph.D., Dean, School of Hotel and Restaurant Management, University of South Florida, Sarasota-Manatee

Think about the last travel reservation that you made—did you book your travel online? Did you check consumer reviews on the hotel or restaurant? Studies show that as many as 55% of consumers now use the Internet to book their travel, a percentage that vastly changes the landscape of the hospitality industry. In fact, technology could be the thin line between a successful business and bankruptcy for many organizations. In 2011, only four out of every ten restaurants that open will still be operating in three years. One of the main reasons for the high failure rate is the lack of control in a slim profit-margin industry. With technology, hospitality and tourism businesses can attempt to control costs and generate success. Technology used to be accepted as a cost center by hospitality and tourism organizations. However, in today's world, technology is a strategic enabler. Technology has become such a vital tool that it is hard to imagine a hotel, resort, theme park, cruise ship, restaurant, or airline company running without it.

Consider this: In a typical full-service hotel, there are about 65 different technology applications. This number is around 35 for a limited-service hotel. Hotels are finding new ways to use technology for a strategic advantage. Consider this example: Mandarin Oriental is keeping track of the fruits eaten by the guest. These records are kept in the guest's profile. Next time the guest visits the hotel, when a fruit basket is sent, it is dominated by the fruits that guest likes. This creates a "wow" factor since it is not directly solicited, rather, quietly observed and recorded with the help of proper training and technology.

Similarly, restaurants use more than 30 different technology applications to provide faster, more cost efficient and productive business operations for guests and staff. Airline companies use complex central reservation and yield-management tools. Travel agencies depend on global reservation system networks to operate. Cruise ships employ different technology and navigation systems to operate in an efficient and fast way. Theme parks use different biometric technologies to keep track of their guests and staff members.

The Airline industry became a commodity a long time ago. In the contemporary age, travelers do not necessarily care about which carrier will take them from point A to point B. Price seems to be the most important factor in selecting an air carrier. The hotel industry is showing similar symptoms. In the age where hospitality and tourism products are becoming a commodity, technology is becoming a true differentiator. Hoteliers like in the example of Mandarin Oriental are turning to technology to differentiate themselves so that they do not become a commodity in the eyes of guests. Many studies already showed that high-speed Internet is one of the most important in-room amenities that enable guest satisfaction in a hotel. In this new age of technology, it is very important for hospitality and tourism students to understand all different technology applications out there to be able to compete in a tough market environment.

Characteristics of the Hospitality Industry

Hospitality businesses are open 365 days a year and 24 hours a day. No, we don't have to work all of these days, but we do tend to work longer hours than people in other industries. Those on their way to senior positions in the hospitality industry, and many others for that matter, often work ten hours a day. However, because of managerial burnout, there is a trend in the industry of reducing working hours of managers to fifty hours a week to attract and retain members of Generation X and the Millennial Generation. Evenings and weekends are included in the workweek—so we have to accept that we may be working when others are enjoying leisure time.

The hospitality industry depends heavily on shift work. Early in your career, depending on the department, you will likely work on a particular shift. Basically, there are four shifts, beginning with the morning shift, so you may be getting up as early as 6:00 A.M. to get to the shift that starts at 7:00 A.M. The midshift is usually from 10:00 A.M. to 7:00 P.M.; the evening shift starts at 3:00 P.M. and goes on until 11:00 P.M.; and finally there is the night shift that begins at 11:00 P.M. and lasts until 7:30 A.M. Supervisors and managers often begin at 8:00 A.M. and work until 6:00 or 8:00 P.M. Success does not come easily.

In the hospitality industry, we constantly strive for outstanding **guest satisfaction**, which leads to guest loyalty and, yes, profit. Our services are mostly

intangible, meaning the guest cannot "test drive" a night's stay or "taste the steak" before dining. Our product is for the guest's use only, not for possession. Even more unique, for us to produce our product—hospitality—we must get the guest's input. Imagine General Electric building a refrigerator with the customer in the factory, participating in the actual construction of the product! Seems preposterous, yet we do it every single day, numerous times per day, and in a uniquely different way each time. This is referred to as the **inseparability** of production and consumption of the service product, which presents a special challenge because each guest may have his or her own requests.

The other unique dimension of our industry is the **perishability** of our product. For example, we have 1,400 rooms in inventory—that is, available to sell—but we sell only 1,200 rooms. What do we do with the 200 unsold rooms? Nothing. We have permanently lost 200 room-nights and their revenue. This example illustrates that in the hospitality industries we are in business to make a **return on investment** for owners and/or shareholders and society. People invest money for us to run a business, and they expect a fair return on their investment. Now, the amount that constitutes a fair return can be debated and will depend on the individual business circumstances. The challenge increases when there is an economic downturn or, worse, a recession, such as we have recently experienced. Then, the struggle is to make more money than is spent, known as keeping one's head above water!

▶ Check Your Knowledge

1. List and describe the four shifts in the hospitality industry.
2. Identify and explain two differences between the hospitality business and other business sectors.

Each year, the National Restaurant Association (NRA) invites the best and brightest students from universities and colleges to participate in the annual restaurant show in Chicago. The highlight of the show is the "Salute to Excellence" day when students and faculty attend forums, workshops, and a gala award banquet with industry leaders. Coca-Cola and several other corporations involved in the industry sponsor the event.

During the day, students are invited to write their dreams on a large panel, which is later displayed for all to enjoy. Here are a few of one of the previous year's hopes and dreams:

- To help all people learn and grow (Jason P.)
- To be the best I can (NMC)
- To establish a chain of jazz cafés in six years and go public in ten years (Richard)
- To successfully please my customers (J. Calicendo)
- To be happy and to make others happy, too

- To put smiles on all faces
- To be one of the most creative chefs—I would like to be happy with everything I create
- To make a difference in the lives of people through food! (Mitz Dardony)
- To be successful professionally, socially, and financially (Marcy W.)
- To preserve our natural resources by operating a restaurant called Green (Kimberley Mauren)
- Anything I do I like to do it in such a way that I can always be meaningful to people (Christian Ellis-Schmidt)
- To reach the top because I know there is a lot of space up there (P. W., Lexington College)
- To use the knowledge that I've gained throughout my career and pass it on to others in hopes of touching their lives in a positive way! To smile and to make smiles. (Armey P. DaCalo)
- I want to be prosperous in my desire to achieve more than $. Happiness and peace are the keys to life. (D. McKinney)
- To teach and be as good as those who have taught me (Thomas)

So what are your dreams and goals? Take a moment to think about your personal dreams and goals. Keep them in mind and look back on them often. Be prepared to amend them as you develop your career.

Careers

There are hundreds of career options for you to consider, and it's fine if you are not yet sure which one is for you. In Figure 3 you can see the major hospitality industry segments: lodging, restaurants and foodservice, recreation and special events, assembly management, theme parks and attractions, travel, and tourism. For instance, lodging provides career opportunities for many associates who make reservations, greet, assist, and serve guests in hotels, resorts, and other lodging operations all over the world. Among the many examples are the operators of a B&B in upstate New York who cater to seasonal guests. Another example is the hundreds of employees necessary to keep the City Center in Las Vegas operational.

Figures 4, 5, and 6 show a career ladder for lodging management and food and beverage management and the rooms division in mid-sized and large hotels. Figure 7 shows a career ladder for restaurant management. Information relating to careers comes from the U.S. Census Bureau's statistic of lifetime salaries by education level,[12] which indicates that high school graduates earn $1.2 million, Associate degree holders earn $1.6 million, Bachelor's degree holders earn $2.1 million, and Master's degree holders earn $2.5 million. Now, these numbers are based on 1999 data, so the good news is that they are going to be much higher for you! Speaking of salaries, Figure 8 is a salary guide for hospitality positions.

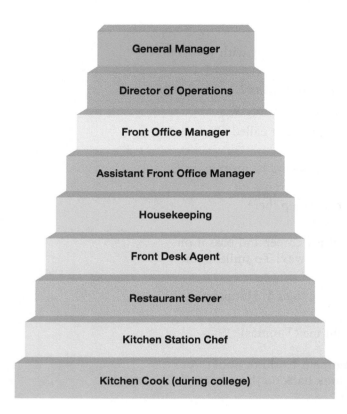

Figure 4 • Lodging Management Career Ladder.

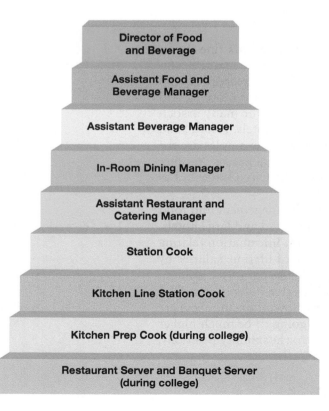

Figure 5 • Lodging Food and Beverage Career Ladder.

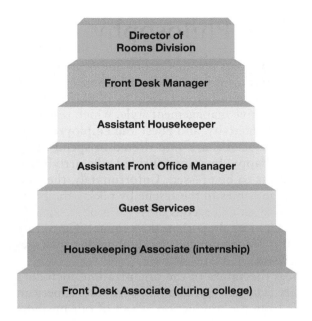

Figure 6 • Lodging Rooms Division Career Ladder.

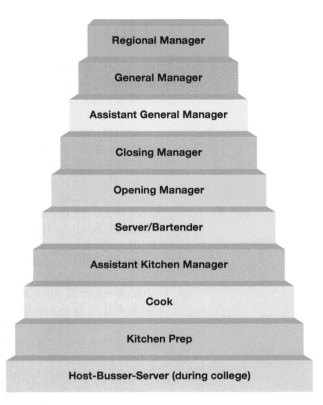

Figure 7 • Restaurant Management Career Ladder.

Hospitality Salaries

President of a Chain Lodging Company	$250,000–500,000
President of a Chain Restaurant Company	$175,000–450,000
Vice President of a Lodging Company	$150,000–250,000
Hotel/Resort General Manager	$75,000–175,000
Country Club General Manager	$100,000–350,000
Vice President of a Restaurant Company	$75,000–150,000
Restaurant General Manager	$40,000–80,000
Hotel or Resort Rooms Division Director	$50–80,000
Hotel/Resort Human Resources Director	$50,000–80,000
Hotel or Resort Food and Beverage Director	$55,000–100,000
Hotel/Resort Catering Manager	$50,000–90,000
Assistant Restaurant Manager	$25,000–40,000
Hotel Front Office Manager	$30,000–60,000
Hotel/Resort Executive Housekeeper	$30,000–75,000
Hotel/Resort Assistant Food and Beverage Manager	$35,000–60,000
Hotel/Resort Executive Chef	$40,000–90,000
Restaurant Chef	$30,000–80,000
Front Desk Agent	$16,000–25,000
Servers	$20,000–40,000
Cooks	$20,000–30,000

Figure 8 • A Guide to Hospitality Salaries.

Hospitality Industry Philosophy

Current **hospitality industry philosophy** has changed from one of managers' planning, organizing, implementing, and measuring to that of managers' counseling associates, giving them resources, and helping them to think for themselves. The outcome is a more participative management style, which results in associate **empowerment**, increased productivity, and guest and employee satisfaction. For example, Ritz-Carlton associates are empowered to spend up to $2,000 to make a guest completely happy. Imagine a bride-to-be arriving at a hotel and sending her wedding dress to be pressed. Unfortunately, the iron burns the dress. Luckily, the concierge comes to the rescue by taking the bride to a wedding dress store, where they select a gorgeous dress for around $1,800, and the bride is happy because it is a nicer dress than the original. Corporate philosophy has strong links to quality leadership and the **total quality management (TQM)** process. (TQM is discussed in a later section.)

Corporate philosophy embraces the values of the organization, including ethics, morals, fairness, and equality. The new paradigm in corporate American hospitality is the shift in emphasis from the production aspect of our business to the focus on guest-related services. The philosophy of "whatever it takes" is winning over "it's not my job." Innovation and creativity are winning over "that's the way we've always done it." Successful organizations are those that are able to impart corporate philosophies to employees and guests alike. Disney Corporation, as discussed later in the chapter, is a good example of a corporation that has a permeating corporate philosophy.

Service Philosophy Is a Way of Life

J. W. (Bill) Marriott Jr. is chairman of the board of directors of Marriott International. Marriott's web site defines the "Marriott Way" as "about serving the associates, the guest, and the community." These ideals serve as the cornerstone for all Marriott associates who strive to fulfill the "Spirit to Serve."[16] The values originate from deep inside the people themselves—authentic, bone deep, and passionately held. Marriott's **core values** include the belief that people are number one ("Take care of Marriott people and they'll take good care of Marriott guests"), a commitment to continuous improvement and overcoming adversity, and a good old-fashioned dedication to hard work and having fun while doing it.

Marriott's core values drive the culture. Similarly, regardless of which service organization we work for, our culture influences the way we treat associates, guests, and the community, and that affects the success of everyone. In the words of J. W. Marriott Jr., "Culture is the life-thread and glue that links our past, present, and future."[17]

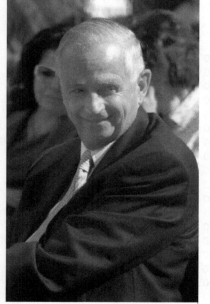

J.W. (Bill) Marriott Jr.

Sustainable Hospitality

Sustainable development is a holistic concept based on a simple principle. As outlined in the 1987 Brundtland Commission Report titled, "Our Common Future." The Bruntland Commission, formally the World Commission on Environment and Development, was convened by the United Nations to address the growing concern "about the accelerating deterioration of the human environment."[13] The concept of sustainability involves "development that meets the needs of the present without compromising the ability of future generations to meet their own needs."

Sustainability is the ability to achieve continuing economic prosperity while protecting the natural resources of the planet and providing a high quality of life for its people and future generations.[14] Operators of hospitality businesses have generally embraced the concept of sustainable hospitality and are increasingly operationalizing it. As an example in the lodging industry, the Willard InterContinental's Sustainable Development initiative is showing substantial results. The program's chief goals are based on profits, people, and planet. The first goal is to find ways to operate the hotel according to the idea of a "triple bottom line," which embodies profitable operation combined with attention to the people who use and work in the hotel and with a focus on careful stewardship of resources.[15]

▶ Check Your Knowledge

1. Describe Marriott's "Spirit to Serve."
2. What is corporate philosophy?

Success in Service

What must happen to achieve success in service? Given that approximately 70 percent of the U.S. and Canadian economies and an increasing percentage of other countries' are engaged in **service industries**, it is critical to offer guests exceptional service, but what is exceptional service? *Service* is defined in *Webster's New World Dictionary* as "the act or means of serving." To serve is to "provide goods and services for" and "be of assistance to."

This is the *age of service*, and the hospitality industry is getting revamped because guest expectations have increased and the realization is that "*we buy loyalty with service.*"[18] With thousands of guest encounters, or moments of truth, each day, it is critical to incorporate service excellence in each hospitality organization. Some corporations adopt the expression, "If you're not serving the guest, you had better be serving someone who is." This is the essence of teamwork: Someone in the **back of the house** also called the **heart of the house** is serving someone in the **front of the house**, who is serving the guest.

A guest is anyone who receives or benefits from the output of someone's work. The external guest is the guest most people think of in the traditional sense. The satisfaction of external guests ultimately measures a company's success, because they are the people who are willing to pay for its services. The internal guests are the people inside a company who receive or benefit from the output of work done by others in the company, for example, the server or busser preparing the restaurant to serve lunch has been "served" by the dishwasher, who has prepared clean plates, knives, forks, spoons, and glassware.

For success in service, we need to do the following:

1. Focus on the guest.
2. Understand the role of the guest-contact employee.
3. Weave a service culture into education and training systems.
4. Emphasize high-touch as well as high-tech.
5. Thrive on change—constantly improve the guest experience.

As hospitality professionals, we need to recognize a variety of guest-related situations and act to relieve them or avoid them. Imagine how an associate can win points by showing empathy—that is, putting him- or herself in someone else's shoes—in the following situation: A party of two ladies arrives for lunch one cool January day at an upscale Florida water-front hotel. They decide it would be nice to have lunch on the terrace. A server from the adjacent lounge notices the guests, and upon learning of their request to have lunch on the terrace, quickly lays up a table for them, brings them hot tea, takes their order, and then goes to the laundry to have two blankets put in the dryer for a couple of minutes to take out to the ladies to keep them warm. Little did the server realize who the guests were—travel writers for the *New York Times* who described their outstanding experience in an article that brought praise to the hotel and its service.

Another key objective in the service equation is to encourage guest loyalty. We not only need to keep guests happy during their stay but also to keep them

INTRODUCING J. W. (BILL) MARRIOTT JR.

Chairman and Chief Executive Officer, Marriott International

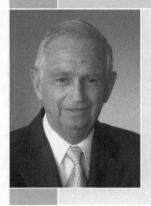

Bill Marriott is the son of J. W. Marriott, founder of Marriott International, a company that began as a nine-stool root beer stand in Washington, D.C., in 1927. Bill was an Eagle Scout and recipient of the Distinguished Eagle Scout Award who, during and after high school, worked various positions in his parents' Hot Shoppes restaurant chain. He graduated from the University of Utah with a Bachelor of Science degree in finance and served as an officer in the Navy before joining the Marriott Corporation in 1956.

Bill Marriott has had an enormous influence on the hospitality industry with years of dedicated service. He is an example of the Spirit to Serve, the title of his well-worth-reading book. Under Marriott's lead, Marriott International has grown from a family restaurant business to a global lodging company of over 3,000 managed and franchised properties of 18 brands, ranging from economy limited-service brands up to full-service luxury hotels and resorts, as well as executive apartments, conference centers, and golf courses in 67 countries and territories.[19]

Mr. Marriott continues his father's tradition of visiting two to three hundred hotels a year. He is passionate about quality and service and can quickly tell how good a general manager (GM) is by the reaction of associates to him or her when the GM is walking the halls of the property. If the associates smile and greet the GM with a cheerful good morning, he knows he has a great GM, but if the associates look down and don't say anything, he knows that there is a problem.

Bill Marriott also cares passionately about Marriott associates by giving them the best possible working conditions, competitive wages and salaries, and excellent benefits. Marriott also provides outstanding training programs to help associates do a great job and to retain the best associates. One of the often used quotes from Mr. Marriott is, "I want our associates to know that there really is a guy named Marriott who cares about them."[20] A central part of Marriott's core values is that attention to detail, quite simply, leads to high customer satisfaction, to repeat business—and to good profits and attractive returns for stockholders and property owners.[21]

returning—with their friends, we hope! It costs several times more to attract new guests than it does to retain existing ones. Imagine how much more profitable a hospitality business would be if it could retain just 10 percent of its guests as loyal guests. Losing a guest equates to losing much more than one sale; it has the potential to be a loss of a lifetime guest. Consider a $40 restaurant dinner for two people. If the guests return twice a month over several years—say, ten—the amount they have contributed to the restaurant quickly becomes huge ($9,600). If they bring their friends, this amount is even higher. Can you remember your worst service experience? Also, can you remember your best service experience?

We know that service is a complex yet critical component of the hospitality industry. In their book, *Service America!*, Albrecht and Zemke suggest two basic kinds of service: "Help me!" and "Fix it."[22] "Help me!" refers to guests' regular and special needs, such as, "Help me find the function room" or, "Help me to get a reservation at the best restaurant in town." "Fix it" refers to services such as, "Please fix my toilet; it won't flush" or, "Please fix the TV so that we can watch the World Series."

Moments of Truth

"Moments of truth" is a term coined by Jan Carlson. When Carlson became president of Scandinavian Airline System (SAS), it was ranked at the bottom of the European airline market. He quickly realized that he had to spend a lot of time on the front line coaching SAS associates in how to handle guest encounters, or as he called them, "moments of truth." As a result of his efforts, SAS was soon ranked at the top of the European airlines for service. Service commitment is a total organizational approach that makes the quality of service, as perceived by the customer, the number one driving force for the operation of the business.[23]

FOCUS ON SERVICE

Hospitality Is Offering a Cup of Kindness

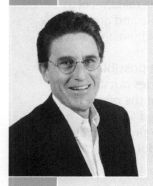

William B. Martin, Cal Tech–Monterey Bay

Customer service is a central focus of hospitality. It is what hospitality is all about—what we do. If you are interested in a hospitality career, it is important to understand and learn as much as possible about customer service and particularly how to be successful at it. Your success will come from a complete understanding of hospitality.

Let's begin by exploring why we provide hospitality. Why are hospitality businesses in business? What is the primary purpose of a foodservice operation? A lodging establishment? A travel- or tourism-related business? Is it just for the money? Many of you might answer an easy yes to this question. But as you will see, hospitality is much more than just about money. Money is important, but it is important as a means and as a necessary ingredient to help us get to where we want to go. Money is not the primary reason for hospitality. Then what is the primary purpose of hospitality?

Our job, first and foremost, is to enhance the lives of those people (guests, customers, passengers, etc.) to whom we are dedicated to serve. Yes, it is that simple (and complex at the same time). Our job is to make the lives of others better in a small way or big way; it makes no difference. Whatever it is, we are out to make people's lives on this planet a little bit better, or maybe even a lot better. This is our purpose. It is where we find meaning. We in the hospitality industry are about enhancing the lives of others—period. Ultimately, that is what makes it all worthwhile.

With that said, where does customer service fit in? Good question. If you are a sharp student, you've already got it. You can readily see that if the purpose of hospitality is to enhance the lives of others, the way we do that is through service. And what is service? It is how we go about treating our guests—how we make (or fail to make) their lives better by how we treat them. And we can go a long way toward treating them well by simply offering them a cup of kindness.

What does this mean? What does it take to be kind? What do we have to do? How do we enhance the lives of others through kindness? We begin by *understanding* what it is that they need. The problem is that all of our guests come to us with many needs. Some we can meet, some we can't. But of all the needs they come with, four of them are specifically hospitality related. If you can work toward helping them satisfy these needs, you can go a long way toward making their lives better through kindness. Quality customer service demands that service providers understand what it is that customers want. Kindness, after all, comes through understanding. Kindness is demonstrated by making everyone feel *welcome*.

Quality customer service requires that we make all guests feel *comfortable*—that we provide the assurance that they will be taken care of, and follow through. They don't need to worry; they are in good hands. In short, when we can do this we are filling their cups with more kindness. Whether they deserve it or not, they should be made to feel important. Why? Because, we all have a *need to feel important*. This is a part of our job. Moreover, it is another important way we can show kindness to our guests.

We need to stay focused on the primary purposes of hospitality. We need to understand the power of kindness and the importance of satisfying the four basic customer service needs of our guests. In the final analysis, hospitality and customer service success are found in our ability to enhance the lives of others through how we treat them—with a little cup of kindness.

Every hospitality organization has thousands of moments of truth every day. This leads to tremendous challenges in maintaining the expected levels of service. Let's look at just some of the moments of truth in a restaurant dining experience[24]:

1. Guest calls the restaurant for a table reservation.
2. Guest tries to find the restaurant.
3. Guest parks.
4. Guest is welcomed.
5. Guest is informed that the table is not ready.
6. Guest either waits or goes to the lounge for a cocktail.
7. Guest tries to attract the bartender's attention for a cocktail because there are no seats available.
8. Guest is called over a loudspeaker or paged.
9. Guest is seated at the table.
10. Server takes order.
11. Server brings beverages or food.
12. Server clears food or beverages.
13. Server brings check.
14. Guest pays for meal.
15. Guest departs restaurant.

From your own experiences, you can imagine just how many moments of truth there are in a restaurant dining experience.

▶ Check Your Knowledge

1. What is the purpose of a mission statement?
2. Why is service so important?
3. What is a moment of truth?

The Focus on Service

Giving great service is a very difficult task; few businesses give enough priority to training associates in how to provide service. We suffer from an overreliance on technology so that service providers are often not motivated to give great service. For example, when checking a guest into the hotel, the front-desk associate may greet the guest but then look down at the computer for the remainder of the service encounter, even when asking for the guest's name. Or consider the reservations associate who says nothing when asked for a specific type of guest room because he is waiting for the computer to indicate availability.

To help improve service in the hospitality industry, the Educational Foundation of the NRA, one of the hospitality industry's leading associations, developed a number of great programs that will enhance your professional development. Further information may be obtained from the NRA's web site (**www.restaurant.org**).

Among the various programs and courses is one titled Foodservice Leadership. Effective leaders are those who make things happen because they have developed the knowledge, skills, and attitude required to get the most out of the people in their operation. Leadership involves change; in fact, change is the one thing we can be sure of in the coming years. Our guests are constantly changing; so is technology, product availability, and, of course, our competition.

The American Hotel & Lodging Association (AH&LA) offers a great variety of information on service-related topics including **best practices**, which give details of the most effective techniques in lodging operations. One area of interest is the Green Resource, where innovative means of going green are shared to improve the carbon footprint and the "bottom line."[25]

One way in which leaders involve employees in the process of improving guest service is through TQM and empowerment.

Service and Total Quality Management

The increasingly open and fiercely competitive marketplace is exerting enormous pressure on service industries to deliver superior service. Inspired by rising guest expectations and competitive necessity, many hospitality companies have jumped on the service quality bandwagon. W. Edwards Deming is credited with launching the Total Quality movement. He was best known for his work in Japan, where in the 1950s and onward, the quality of Japanese products was not good. He taught top Japanese management how to improve design—through the use of statistical methods he reduced the number of defects—and thus service, product quality, testing, and sales. Dr. Deming made a significant contribution to the improvement of Japanese products.[26]

The Malcolm Baldrige National Quality Award is the highest level of national recognition for quality that a U.S. company can receive. Named after former commerce secretary Malcolm Baldrige, who was a champion of quality movement as a way of improving U.S. commerce, the award promotes an understanding of quality excellence, greater awareness of quality as a critical competitive element, and the sharing of quality information and strategies.

The Ritz-Carlton Hotel Company, the only hospitality company to win two Malcolm Baldrige National Quality Awards, in 1992 and 1999, was founded on principles of excellence in guest service. The essence of this philosophy was refined into a set of core values collectively called the Gold Standards. The credo is printed on a small laminated card that all employees must memorize or carry on their person at all times when on duty. The card lists the three steps of service:

1. A warm and sincere greeting; use the guest name, if and when possible.

2. Anticipation and compliance with guests' needs.

3. Fond farewell; give them a warm good-bye and use their names if and when possible.

The quality movement began at the turn of the century as a means of ensuring consistency among the parts produced in the different plants of a single company so that they could be used interchangeably. In the area of service, TQM is a participatory process that empowers all levels of employees to work in groups to establish guest service expectations and determine the best way to meet or exceed these expectations. Notice that the term *guest* is preferred over the term *customer*. The inference here is that if we treat customers like guests, we are more likely to exceed their expectations. One successful hotelier has insisted for a long time that all employees treat guests as they would like to be treated themselves.

TQM is a continuous process that works best when managers are also good leaders. A successful company will employ leader–managers who create a stimulating work environment in which guests and employees (sometimes called internal guests: One employee serves another employee, who in turn serves a guest) become integral parts of the mission by participating in **goal** and objective setting.

Implementing TQM is exciting because after everyone becomes involved, there is no stopping the creative ways employees will find to solve guest-related problems and improve service. Other benefits include cost reductions and increased guest and employee satisfaction, leading ultimately to increased profits.

The Employee Promise

At the Ritz-Carlton, our Ladies and Gentlemen are the most important resource in our service commitment to our guests.

By applying the principles of trust, honesty, respect, integrity, and commitment, we nurture and maximize talent to the benefit of each individual and the company.

The Ritz-Carlton fosters a work environment where diversity is valued, quality of life is enhanced, individual aspirations are fulfilled, and the Ritz-Carlton mystique is strengthened.

I am proud to be Ritz-Carlton

1. I build strong relationships and create Ritz-Carlton guests for life.
2. I am always responsive to the expressed and unexpressed wishes and need of our guests.
3. I am empowered to create unique, memorable, and personal experiences for our guests.
4. I understand my role in achieving the Key Success Factors, embracing Community Footprints, and creating The Ritz-Carlton Mystique.
5. I continuously seek opportunities to innovate and improve the Ritz-Carlton experience.
6. I own and immediately resolve any guest problems.
7. I create a work environment of teamwork and lateral service so that the needs of our guests and each other are met.
8. I have opportunity to continuously learn and grow.
9. I am involved in the planning of the work that affects me.
10. I am proud of my professional appearance, language, and behavior.
11. I protect the privacy and security of our guests, my fellow employees, and the company's confidential information and assets.
12. I am responsible for uncompromising levels of cleanliness and creating a safe and accident-free environment.

A DAY IN THE LIFE OF RYAN LASHWAY

Assistant Manager, Mar Vista Dockside Restaurant, Longboat Key, Florida

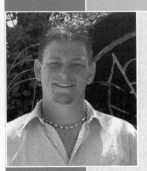

To describe a typical day of work for me at the Mar Vista, I must first tell you a little bit about the restaurant. Located on Sarasota Bay on the north end of Longboat Key in historic Longbeach Village, the Mar Vista has existed for over 60 years. Built in the early 1940s, "The Pub" was originally a bait and tackle shop until the 1950s, when the owners started selling hamburgers and beer to the local fishermen crowd. The Mar Vista operated like this until coming under the ownership of Ed Chiles of the Chiles Group Corporation in 1990. Chiles is the son of former governor of Florida Lawton Chiles and also owns the Beachhouse and Sandbar restaurants on Anna Maria Island. The Mar Vista is an authentic part of Old Florida, and our history and ambiance make it a fun and relaxing place. Our goal at the Mar Vista is to provide our guests with the finest in food and courteous,

(continued)

A DAY IN THE LIFE OF RYAN LASHWAY *(continued)*

prompt service. For further information about the Chiles Group Corporation, visit our web site at **www.groupersandwich.com**.

A typical day for a manager at the Mar Vista goes like this:

8:30 A.M. Arrive and check the premises for any unusual activity. Unlock the doors and turn on all lights and A/C units. Check to see that the overnight cleaning crew has done a thorough job, especially in the kitchen, restrooms, and behind the bars. Then, look at the schedules to see which employees are working on any given day and make ready for the kitchen staff's arrival at 9:00 A.M.

9:00 A.M. Upon arrival, the kitchen staff is entered into our in-house computer system so that their hours for the day will be recorded. Towels and cleaning materials must also be supplied for the entire staff. The restrooms must be checked and stocked with hand towels, liquid soap, and toilet paper. The premises are then walked again and the grounds checked for trash. All windows and mirrors must be cleaned.

10:30 A.M. The wait staff and bar staff arrive. The cash banks for the bar must be counted and paired up for daily use. The safe in the manager's office must then be opened and the money from the previous day made ready for pickup by our financial officer. The kitchen manager must then be met with to discuss the daily specials. Upon agreement of the best use for food items, the specials must then be printed and inserted into the menus.

11:30 A.M. Open for lunch business. Throughout the day, management focuses on customer relations and making sure the restaurant runs smoothly. Incoming paperwork from deliveries for the kitchen and bar must be fully documented, and all incoming orders must be checked in and signed for. Any problems with food orders or guest service must be handled in such a way that the customer is never scorned; return business is the primary focus. In general, the customers are always right, and in this business we must do whatever is necessary to keep them happy.

3:00 P.M. Toward the end of the lunch shift, servers are finishing their daily work and will require checkout forms to do their money drops. Managers must check each server out individually and make sure that all side work is completed and that the restaurant will be ready for the next shift crew arriving at 4:00 P.M. Managers must meet with the kitchen manager again and prepare the dinner specials. The P.M bartender will also be arriving and will require a night bank, while the A.M. bartender will need to be checked out and his or her bank checked for correct money transactions.

5:00 P.M. Dinner begins and the night manager arrives. Discuss the events and highlights of the day with the P.M. manager and notify him or her of any problems.

Then it's off to rest up and prepare to do it again tomorrow!

Top executives and line managers are responsible for the success of the TQM process; when they commit to ownership of the process, it will be successful. Focused commitment is the foundation of a quality service initiative, and leadership is the critical component in promoting commitment. Achieving TQM is a top-down, bottom-up process that must have the active commitment and participation of all employees, from the top executives down to those at the bottom of the corporate ladder. The expression "If you are not serving the guest, then you had better be serving someone who is" still holds true today.

The difference between TQM and quality control (QC) is that QC focuses on error detection, whereas TQM focuses on error prevention. QC is generally based on industrial systems and, because of this, tends to be product oriented rather than service oriented. To the guest, services are experiential; they are felt, lived through, and sensed. The moment of truth is the actual guest contact.

The nature of business has changed. Leaders empower employees who welcome change. Empowerment is a feeling of partnership in which employees feel responsible for their jobs and have a stake in the organization's success. Empowered employees tend to do the following:

- Speak out about their problems and concerns.
- Take responsibility for their actions.
- Consider themselves a network of professionals.
- Accept the authority to make their own decisions when serving guests.

To empower employees, managers must do the following:

1. Take risks.
2. Delegate.
3. Foster a learning environment.
4. Share information and encourage self-expression.
5. Involve employees in defining their own vision.
6. Be thorough and patient with employees.

CORPORATE PROFILE

Marriott International, Inc.[27]

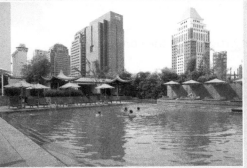

Marriott International is a leading worldwide hospitality company. Its heritage is traced back to a root beer stand opened in Washington, D.C., in 1927 by J. Willard and Alice S. Marriott. Today, Marriott International has more than 3,500 lodging properties in the United States and 67 other countries and territories. Marriott International operates and franchises hotels under the following tiers of brands:

Luxury Tier: Bulgari Hotels and Resorts, a collection of sophisticated, intimate luxury properties tucked away in exclusive destinations

The Ritz-Carlton Hotel Company, LLC: The worldwide symbol for the finest in hotel and resort accommodations, dining, and service. Two-time recipient of the Malcolm Baldrige National Quality Award, offering signature service amenities, fine dining, 24-hour room service, twice-daily housekeeping, fitness centers, business centers, and concierge services.

(continued)

CORPORATE PROFILE (continued)

JW Marriott Hotels and Resorts: The most elegant and luxurious Marriott brand, offering business and leisure travelers a deluxe level of comfort and personal service

Autograph Collection: A collection of high-personality, independent hotels, powered by the world-class platforms of Marriott International

Lifestyle/Boutique: EDITION was created in partnership with boutique hotel pioneer Ian Schrager to introduce a new brand with as many as one hundred hotels that have perfected a highly personal, intimate, and rarified experience for each guest.

Renaissance Hotels invite guests to "stay interesting" at distinctive hotels offering unique, locally relevant architecture and design, destination restaurants and bars, and off-the-radar travel experiences worldwide.

- **Signature Brand: Marriott Hotels and Resorts:** The flagship brand of quality-tier, full-service hotels and resorts with features such as fully equipped fitness centers, gift shops, swimming pools, concierge levels, business centers, meeting facilities, and high-speed Internet.

- **Select Service & Extended Stay Brands: Courtyard by Marriott:** A moderately priced lodging brand designed by business travelers for business travelers that has recently increased the number of downtown locations, often through conversions of historical buildings. Features include 80 to 150 guest rooms, high-speed Internet access, restaurants, lounges, meeting spaces, central courtyards, exercise rooms, swimming pools, and 24-hour access to food.

- **SpringHill Suites by Marriott:** A moderately priced, all-suite lodging brand that offers up to 25 percent larger-than-standard hotel rooms. Features include complimentary continental breakfast, self-serve business centers, indoor pools, whirlpool spas, high-speed Internet access, and exercise rooms.

- **Fairfield Inn by Marriott:** A consistent, quality lodging at an affordable price. Features include spacious guest rooms, daily complimentary breakfast, and swimming pools. Future plans call for exercise rooms.

- **Residence Inn by Marriott:** Designed as a home away from home for travelers staying five or more nights, it includes a residential atmosphere with spacious accommodations. Features include complimentary hot breakfasts, evening hospitality hours, swimming pools, sport courts, personalized grocery shopping, guest suites with separate living and sleeping areas, fully equipped kitchens, and work spaces with data ports and voice mail.

- **Towne Place Suites by Marriott:** A midpriced, extended-stay brand that provides all the comforts of home in a residential atmosphere.

- **Marriott Executive Apartments:** A corporate housing brand designed to meet the needs of business executives on an overseas assignment for thirty days or more by offering residential accommodations with hotel-like amenities.

In addition to these brands there are also several Vacation Clubs, which are offered on a fractional ownership basis.

Marriott has been ranked the number-one most admired company in the lodging industry by *Fortune* for the past five years and also one of the "100 Best Companies to Work For" for the past seven years.

▶ Check Your Knowledge

1. List five attributes, traits, and characteristics of a leader.
2. What is the Malcolm Baldrige National Quality Award?

The Disney Approach to Guest Service

The Disney mission statement is simple: "We create Happiness." Disney is regarded as one of the excellent corporations throughout the text. The following discussion, adapted from a presentation given by Susan Wilkie to the Pacific chapter of the Council on Hotel Restaurant and Institutional Education (CHRIE) conference outlines Disney's approach to guest service.

When conceiving the idea to build Disneyland, Walt Disney established a simple philosophical approach to his theme park business, based on the tenets of quality, service, and show. The design, layout, characters, and magic of Disneyland grew out of Walt's successful experience in the film industry. With Disneyland, he saw an opportunity to create a whole new form of entertainment: a three-dimensional live show. He wanted Disneyland to be a dynamic, ever-changing experience.

To reinforce the service concept, Disney has *guests*, not *customers*, and *cast members*, not *employees*. These terms set the expectations for how guests will be served and cared for while at the park or resort. This commitment to service means the following:

- Disney clearly understands its product and the meaning of its brand.
- It looks at the business from the guests' perspective.
- It considers creating an exceptional experience for every individual who enters its gates to be its responsibility.

Disney executives say that "our inventory goes home at night." Disney's ability to create a special brand of magic requires the talents of thousands of people fulfilling many different roles. But the heart of it is the frontline cast members. So, what is it that makes the service at Disney so great? The key elements of Disneyland guest services include the following:

- Hiring, developing, and retaining the right people
- Understanding its product and the meaning of the brand
- Communicating the traditions and standards of service to all cast members
- Training leaders to be service coaches
- Measuring guest satisfaction
- Recognizing and rewarding performance

  Disney has used profile modeling but says it all comes down to a few simple things:

- Interpersonal relationship–building skills
- Communication
- Friendliness

Disney uses a forty-five-minute team approach to interviewing called *peer interviews*. In one interview, there may be four candidates and one interviewer. The candidates may include a homemaker returning to the workforce, a teacher looking for summer work, a retiree looking for a little extra income, and a teenager looking for a first job. All four candidates are interviewed in the same session. The interviewer is looking for how they individually answer questions but also how well they interact with each other—a good indicator of their future onstage treatment of guests.

The most successful technique used during the forty-five-minutes is to *smile*. The interviewer smiles at the people being interviewed to see if they *return the smiles*. If they don't, it doesn't matter how well they interview—they won't get the job.

On the first day at work, every new Disney cast member participates in a one-day orientation program at the Disney University, "Welcome to Show Business." The main goal of this experience is to learn the Disney approach to helpful, caring, and friendly guest service.

How does this translate into action? When a guest stops a street sweeper to ask where to pick up a parade schedule and the sweeper not only answers the question but recites the parade times from memory, suggests the best viewing spots on the parade route, offers advice on where to get a quick meal before parade time, *and* ends the interaction with a pleasant smile and warm send-off, people can't help but be impressed. It also makes the sweepers feel their jobs are interesting and important—which they are!

I AM YOUR GUEST

We can all find inspiration from these anonymous words about people who make our business possible:

- ✓ *I am your guest.* Satisfy my needs, add personal attention and a friendly touch, and I will become a "walking advertisement" for your products and services. Ignore my needs, show carelessness, inattention, and poor manners, and I will cease to exist as far as you are concerned.
- ✓ *I am sophisticated.* Much more so than I was a few years ago. My needs are more complex. It is more important to me that you appreciate my business; when I buy your products and services, I'm saying you are the best.
- ✓ *I am a perfectionist.* When I am dissatisfied, take heed. The source of my discontent lies in something you or your products have failed to do. Find that source and eliminate it or you will lose my business and that of my friends as well. For when I criticize your products or services, I will talk to anyone who will listen.
- ✓ *I have other choices.* Other businesses continually offer "more for my money." You must prove to me again and again that I have made a wise choice in selecting you and your company above all others.

The Show is why people go to Disneyland. Each land tells a unique story through its theme and attention to detail, and the cast members each play a role in the Show. The most integral component of the training is the traditions and standards of guest service. The first of these is called the *Personal Touch*. The cast members are encouraged to use their own unique style and personality to provide a personal interaction with each guest. One of the primary ways Disney accomplishes this is through name tags. Everyone, regardless of position, goes by his or her first name. This tradition was started by Walt and continues today. It allows cast members to interact on a more personal level with guests. It also assists internally, by creating an informal environment that facilitates the flow of open communication and breaks down some of the traditional barriers.

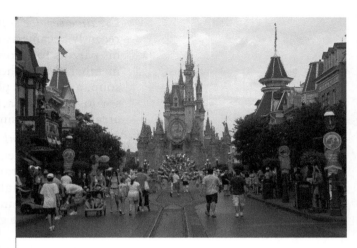

Cinderella's castle soaring above tourists at Walt Disney World, Orlando, Florida.

Opening Disneyland

Imagine what Walt Disney had to overcome to open Disneyland. Disneyland opened on July 17, 1955, to the predictions that it would be a failure. And, in truth, everything that could go wrong did. Just to give an example, here is what happened on opening day:

- Plumbers went on strike.
- Tickets were duplicated.
- Attractions broke down.
- There was a gas leak in Fantasyland.
- The asphalt on Main Street didn't harden in time, so in the heat of July, horses' hooves and women's high heels stuck in the street.

As Walt once said, "You may not realize it when it happens, but a kick in the teeth might be good for you." Walt had his fair share of challenges, one of which was obtaining financing to develop Disneyland—he had to deal with more than 300 banks.

So what is the Disney service model?

It begins with a smile. This is the universal language of hospitality and service. Guests recognize and appreciate the cast members' warmth and sincerity.

Make eye contact and use body language. This means stance, approach, and gestures. For instance, cast members are trained to use *open* gestures for directions, not pointed fingers, because open palms are friendlier and less directive.

Respect and welcome all guests. This means being friendly, helpful, and going out of the way to *exceed* guests' expectations.

Value the magic. This means that when they're on stage, cast members are totally focused on creating the magic of Disneyland. They don't talk about personal problems or world affairs, and they don't mention that you can find Mickey in more than one place.

Initiate guest contact. Cast members are reminded to initiate guest contact actively. Disney calls this being aggressively friendly. It's not enough to be responsive when approached. Cast members are encouraged to take the first step with guests. They have lots of little tricks for doing this, such as noticing a guest's name on a hat and then using the name in conversation or kneeling to ask a child a question.

Creative service solutions. For example, one Disneyland Hotel cast member recently became aware of a little boy who had come from the Midwest with his parents to enjoy the park and then left early because he was ill. The cast member approached the supervisor with an idea to send the child chicken soup, a character plush toy, and a get-well card from Mickey. The supervisor loved the idea, and all cast members are now allowed to set up these arrangements in similar situations without a supervisor's approval.

End with a "thank you." The phrases cast members use are important in creating a service environment. They do not have a book of accepted phrases; rather, through training and coaching, cast members are encouraged to use their own personality and style to welcome and approach guests, answer questions, anticipate their needs, thank them, and express with sincerity their desire to make the guest's experience exceptional.

Taken individually, these might sound pretty basic. But taken together, they help define and reinforce the Disney culture. After initial cast member training is completed, these concepts must be applied and continually reinforced by leaders who possess strong coaching skills. Disney uses a model called the *Five Steps of Leadership* to lead the cast member performance.

Each step in the leadership model is equally important in meeting service and business goals. Each leader must do the following:

1. Provide clear expectations and standards.
2. Communicate these expectations through demonstration, information, and examples.
3. Hold cast members accountable for their feedback.
4. Coach through honest and direct feedback.
5. Recognize, reward, and celebrate success.

To supplement and reward the leadership team, Disney provides technical training to every new manager and assistant manager. In addition, the management team also participates in classes at the Disney University to learn the culture, values, and the leadership philosophy necessary to be successful in the Disney environment.

Disney measures the systems and reward process by distributing 1,000 surveys to guests as they leave Disneyland and 100 surveys to guests who stayed at each of the Disney hotels. The guests are asked to take the surveys home and mail them back to Disney. In return, their names are entered for a drawing for a family weekend package at the park and hotel.

Feedback from the surveys has been helpful in improving the guest experience. For example, as a result of the surveys, the entertainment division realized that the opportunity to interact with a character was a key driver to guest satisfaction. So, the entertainment team designed a brochure, "The Characters Today," which is distributed at the main entrance daily. This brochure allows guests to maximize their opportunity to see the characters. This initiative has already raised guest satisfaction by ten percentage points.

Cast members are also empowered to make changes to improve service. These measures are supplemented by financial controls and "mystery shoppers" (when people use the services like any other guest, but they are really employed to sample the service and report their findings) that allow Disney to focus resources on increasing guest satisfaction. The reward system does not consist of just the hard reward system we commonly think of, such as bonuses and incentive plans, important though they are. Recognition is not a one-size-fits-all system. Disney has found that noncash recognition is as powerful as, if not more powerful than, a recognition tool in many situations. Some examples follow:

- Disney recognizes milestones of years of service. They use pins and statues and have a formal dinner for cast members and guests to reinforce and celebrate the value of their experience and expertise at serving Disney's guests.

- Throughout the year, Disney hosts special social and recreational events that involve the cast members and their families in the product.

- Disney invites cast members and their families to family film festivals featuring new Disney releases to ensure that they are knowledgeable about the latest Disney products.

- The Disneyland management team hosts the Family Christmas Party in the park after hours. This allows cast members to enjoy shopping, dining, and riding the attractions. Management dresses in costumes and runs the facilities.

Career Paths

Now that we know that the hospitality industries are the largest and arguably the fastest growing in the world, let's explore some of the many **career paths** available to graduates. The concept of career paths describes the career progression available in each segment of the hospitality industry. A career path does not always go in a straight line, as sometimes described in a career ladder. You could liken it to jumping into a swimming pool: You get wet whichever end you jump in and then you might swim over to the other side—but not always in a straight line. It's like that in the hospitality industry, also. We may begin in one area and later find another that is more attractive. Opportunities come our way and we need to be prepared to take advantage of them. To illustrate, take Barbra. A few years ago, she was a hospitality management graduate who was not very outgoing, so she decided to take a position in the hotel accounting office. A few years later, we visited the hotel where she was working, and to our pleasant surprise, we found a smiling Barbra welcoming us as the front office manager. After a few more years, she moved into the food and beverage department and then the marketing department, and is now a general manager.

Progression means that we can advance from one position to another. In the hospitality industry we don't always use straight-line career ladders because we need experience in several areas before becoming, say, a general manager, director of human resources, catering manager, meeting planner, or director of marketing. The path to general manager in a hotel may go through food and beverage, rooms division, marketing, human resources, or finance and accounting, or, more likely, a combination of these, because it is better to have experience in several areas (cross-training). The same is true for restaurants. A graduate with service experience will need to spend some time in the kitchen learning each station and then bartending before becoming an opening or closing assistant or manager, general manager, area manager, regional director, vice president, and president.

Sometimes we want to run before we can walk. We want to progress quickly. But remember to enjoy the journey as much as the destination. If you advance too quickly, you may not be ready for the additional responsibility, and you may not have the skills necessary for the promotion. For instance, you cannot expect to become a director of food and beverage until you really know "food and beverage": this means spending a few years in the kitchen. Otherwise, how can you relate to an executive chef? You have to know how the food should be prepared and served. You have to set the standards—not have them set for you. Be prepared because you never know when an opportunity will present itself.

Career Goals

You may already know that you want to be a director of accounting, an event manager, a director of marketing, or of food and beverage, or a restaurant owner. If you are not sure of which career path to pursue, that's OK. Now is the time to explore the industry to gain the information you need to decide which career path to follow. A great way to do this is through internships and work experience. Some suggest trying a variety of jobs rather than sticking to the same one.

If we follow the interrelated nature of hospitality, travel, and tourism in Figure 2 or 3, we can see some of the numerous career options in various industry segments.

Is the Hospitality Industry for You?

In this chapter, we described some characteristics of the hospitality industry. Due to the size and scope of the hospitality industry, career prospects are gradually improving. We also know that it is an exciting and dynamic industry with growth potential, especially when the economy is strong. In the hospitality industry we are often working when others are at leisure—think of the evening or weekend shift; however, in some positions and careers, many evenings and weekends can be yours to enjoy as you wish. (Accounting, marketing and sales, human resources, and housekeeper are some examples).

The hospitality industry is a service industry; this means that we take pride in caring about others as well as ourselves. Ensuring that guests receive outstanding service is a goal of hospitality corporations. This is a business that gets into your blood! It is mostly fun, exciting, and seldom dull, and an industry in which almost everyone can succeed. So, what does it take to be successful in the hospitality industry? The personal characteristics, qualities, skills, and abilities you'll need are honesty, hard work, being a team player, being prepared to work long hours spread over various shifts, the ability to cope with stress, good decision-making skills, good communication skills, being dedicated to exceptional service, and having a passion and desire to exceed guest expectations. Leadership, ambition, and the will to succeed are also important and necessary for career success.

Recruiters look for *service-oriented* people, who "walk their talk," meaning they do what they say they're going to do. Good work experience, involvement in on-campus and professional organizations, a positive attitude, a good grade point average—all show a commitment to an individual's studies. Career-minded individuals who have initiative and are prepared to work hard and make a contribution to the company, which has to make a profit, are what companies are looking for.

Self-Assessment and Personal Philosophy

The purpose of completing a self-assessment is to measure our current strengths and weaknesses and to determine what we need to improve on if we are going to reach our goals. Self-assessment helps establish where we are now and shows us the links to where we want to go, our goals. In a self-assessment, we make a list of our positive attributes. For example, we may have experience in a guest-service position; this will be helpful in preparing for supervisory and managerial positions. Other positive attributes include our character and all the other things that recruiters look for, as listed previously.

We also make a list of areas where we might want to make improvements. For example, we may have reached a certain level of culinary expertise, but need more experience and a course in this specialty. Or you may want to improve your Spanish-language skills because you will be working with Spanish-speaking colleagues. Your *philosophy* is your beliefs and the way you treat others and your work. It will determine who you are and what you stand for. You may state that you enjoy giving excellent service by treating others as you would like to be treated and that you believe in honesty and respect.

A great web resource for self-assessment is www.queendom.com; this site provides self-assessment quizzes.

Now Is the Time to Get Involved

For your own enjoyment and personal growth and development, it is very important to get involved with on-campus and professional hospitality and tourism organizations and participate in the organization of events. Recruiters notice the difference between students who have become involved with various organizations and students who have not, and they take that into consideration when assessing candidates for positions with companies. Becoming involved will show your commitment to your chosen career and will lead you to meet interesting peers and industry professionals who can potentially help you along your chosen career path. You will develop leadership and organizational skills that will help you in your career.

Professional Organizations

Professional organizations include becoming a student member of CHRIE (www. chrie.org). You can also access the excellent Webzine *Hosteur*, which is published especially for students; CHRIE offers its members free access. The NRA (www. restaurant.org) is another organization to join. You will likely find several NRA magazines and publications to be very helpful. The NRA and your state restaurant association are affiliated, and both have trade shows; the NRA hosts the Salute to Excellence, a day of activities that culminates with a gala dinner. Only two students from each school are invited to this special event; make sure you're one of them, as it is well worth it. The AH&LA (www.ahla.com) is a good organization to belong to if you are interested in a career in the lodging segment of the industry. Benefits of AH&LA memberships include access to the organization's career center, which is powered by Hcareers.com, the largest online database of career opportunities in the lodging industry; a subscription to *Lodging* magazine, a leading industry publication with news, product information, and current articles on industry-related topics; subscriptions to *Lodging News*, *Lodging Law*, *Lodging H/R* e-newsletters; and use of the AH&LA's information center—helpful for those pesky term papers! And you receive scholarship information, too!

The International Special Events Society (ISES; www.ises.com) includes over 3,000 professionals representing special event producers, from festivals to trade shows. Membership brings together professionals from a variety of special events disciplines. The mission of ISES is to educate, advance, and promote the special events industry and its network of professionals, along with related issues.

The Professional Convention Management Association (PCMA; www.pcma.org) is a great resource for convention management educational offerings and networking opportunities. The National Society of Minorities in Hospitality (NSMH; www.nsmh.org) has a membership of several hundred minority hospitality majors who address diversity and multiculturalism as well as career development via events and programs.

Trends in Hospitality and Tourism

There is a healthy increase in hospitality and tourism not only in North America but around the world. We can identify a number of trends that are having and will continue to have an impact on the hospitality industry. Some, like diversity, have already been realized and are sure to increase in the future. Here, in no particular order, are some of the major trends that hospitality professionals indicate as having an influence on the industry.

- *Globalization.* We have become the global village that was described a few years ago. We may have the opportunity to work or vacation in other countries, and more people than ever travel freely around the world.

- *Safety and security.* Since September 11, 2001, we have all become more conscious of our personal safety and have experienced increased scrutiny at airports and federal and other buildings. But it goes beyond that; terrorists kidnap tourists from their resorts and hold them for ransom, thugs mug them, and others assault them. Security of all types of hospitality and tourism operations is critical, and disaster plans should be made for each kind of threat. Personal safety of guests must be the first priority.

- *Diversity.* The hospitality industry is one of the most diverse of all industries; not only do we have a diverse employee population, but we also have a diverse group of guests. Diversity is increasing as more people with more diverse cultures join the hospitality workforce.

- *Service.* It is no secret that service is at the top of guests' expectations, yet few companies offer exceptional service. World-class service does not just happen; training is important in delivering the service that guests have come to expect.

- *Technology.* Technology is a driving force of change that presents opportunities for greater efficiencies and integration for improved guest service. However, the industry faces great challenges in training employees to use the new technology and in standardization of software and hardware design. Some hotels have several systems that do not talk to each other, and some reservation systems bounce between 7 and 10 percent of sales nationally.

- *Legal issues.* Lawsuits are not only more frequent, but they cost more if you lose and more to defend. One company spent several million dollars just to defend one case. Government regulations and the complexities of employee relations create increased challenges for hospitality operators.
- *Changing demographics.* The U.S. population is gradually increasing, and the baby boomers are retiring. Many retirees have the time and money to travel and utilize hospitality services.
- *Price–value.* Price and value are important to today's more discerning guests.
- *Social media.* This phenomenon has grown rapidly, allowing people to connect for social and business communications.
- *Sanitation.* Sanitation is critical to the success of any restaurant and foodservice operation. Guests expect to eat healthy foods that have been prepared in a sanitary environment.

CASE STUDY

Being Promoted from Within

One month ago, Tom was promoted from line cook to kitchen manager. It was a significant step up in his life. He felt that his promotion was well deserved, as he had always been a hard worker. Tom never had a second thought about going the extra mile for his employer. He felt that since he had seniority in the kitchen and was friendly with everyone in the back of the house, he would be sure to get the respect he deserved from everyone for whom he had responsibility. About three weeks into his new position, Tom found that this was not the case. Several back-of-the house employees had become careless about their responsibilities after Tom were promoted. They were coming to work late, wearing unlaundered uniforms, and becoming more and more sloppy with their plate presentations. Every day at work, Tom was becoming more frustrated and upset. He knew that the employees were never careless about these matters with their previous supervisor.

Discussion Questions

1. What are some possible reasons for the back-of-the house employees' carelessness?
2. How should Tom assess the current situation?
3. If you were Tom's supervisor, what advice would you have given him before he started his new position?

Career Information

Do you know exactly where you want to be in five or ten years? The best advice is to follow your interests. Do what you love to do and success will soon come. Often, we assess our own character and personality to determine a suitable path. Some opt for the accounting and control side of the tourism business; others, perhaps with more outgoing personalities, vie for sales and marketing; others prefer operations, which could be either in back or in front of the house. Creating your own career path can be an exciting and a challenging task. However, the travel and tourism industry is generally characterized as dynamic, fun, and full of challenges and opportunities. And remember, someone has to run Walt Disney World, Holland American Cruise Lines, Marriot Hotels and Resorts, B&Bs, restaurants, and be the airport manager.

The anticipated growth of tourism over the next few years offers today's students numerous career opportunities in each section of the industry, as well as increasing job stability. There are many general things that can be said about a career in the hospitality industry. For example, a regular 8:30 A.M. to 4:30 P.M. job is not the norm; nearly all sectors operate up to 24 hours a day, 365 days a year—including evenings, weekends, and holidays. The good news is that nearly all sectors are experiencing growth and should continue to do so over the next few years.

CASE EXAMPLE

How to Treat Prospective Associates

One of the many jobs I have had through my career was working for the Stamford Marriott, where I experienced firsthand how a world-class human resources (HR) department executed a well-devised HR plan. I should first start by describing this hotel: It is a 500-room hotel that is full service and always busy. We had about twenty-five to thirty employees in the kitchen alone; the banquet and service staff represented another forty people, and there were probably another one hundred people employed as housekeepers, room service, front desk, bellman, maintenance, HR, and management. The Marriott Corporation has very high standards for the employees they hire, and getting a job with Marriott is not as easy as it might appear to be. My first experience with the Marriott was its HR department. I applied to the job from a listing at the school I was attending in Hyde Park, New York. The listing stated they needed a cook to work long weekend hours and they would accept applications Monday through Friday between 2:00 and 4:00 P.M. I chose to go on Tuesday at 2:00 P.M. and leave my application. When I arrived, I was greeted by one of the HR employees, who gave me the application and offered me a soda while I filled out the application. After filling out the paperwork, I handed it to the employee and thought that they would probably contact me if they were interested, but as I turned to leave, the HR employee asked me to stay. Amanda, the HR director, asked me to come into the office for a prescreening, where I was asked questions about prior experience, my education, and my plans for the future. Amanda kept using terms like *team members* and *family*. After a short time, Amanda had the sous chef come down to talk to me, and he asked me questions about my passions and hobbies. I began to feel as if they might hire me, but the sous chef said he needed to send the chef down to talk to me. By now, I had been in the HR office for over an hour. The chef came down and asked me to take a trip up to the restaurant on the top floor. It was empty and it was just the two of us. He began by telling his story about how he made it to where he is today. I began to feel that this was a big decision for the hotel; the entire staff was sizing me up to see if they wanted me to work with them. The chef said he would like to have me on his staff, but there was one more person I would need to talk to. A few minutes later, I was in the office of the hotel manager, feeling very nervous. The hotel manager stood up, introduced himself, and asked me why I chose the Marriott, as if I had this plan all along to work for this corporation. I answered that it was because of the company's excellent reputation. The hotel manager said he thought I would fit in well with his team. After finishing all my interviews, I was escorted back down to Amanda, who finished my paperwork, took me on a tour of the hotel, and introduced me to the entire staff. As I walked through the hotel, there was not one person I passed who did not say hi and introduce themselves.

So why did I walk you through the interview process at the Marriott? I realized after my experience with human resources (HR) that it was their mission to make sure they had the right person for the job. The planning to make sure that every applicant was interviewed by at least three managers and the interest in my future goals and future with the company was very impressive. Amanda was able to free up three very important people and it was with pleasure that those managers interviewed me. I was trained in my job for two weeks before I went solo, and Amanda checked on me three times in my first two weeks. The employees at this Marriott loved their jobs and did not have to be prodded to do what they were supposed to do. We all felt grateful to be working with a company that cared so much about their employees. The quality of work that these employees produced was incredible, and everyone watched everyone else to make sure that the standards stayed high and that guest satisfaction was our main focus.

In the planning stages of this HR department, the long-term or strategic plan was to hire only the right person for each position; they also took extra care in the hiring process to make sure that the person fit the Marriott team. The personnel for that Marriott were chosen by the managers of HR and were handpicked; when they found a person to fit the mold. they took extra time with the applicant to make sure everything lined up. The Marriott used the exemption form of management and were able to use this style because of the quality of the employees they would hire. The job descriptions were clearly defined so that employees knew what their job entailed, and all employees were thoroughly trained.

Having a plan in place allows companies like the Marriott to choose the best people, they become proactive instead of reactive, they are ready to hire a good person because the system is in place to allow the interviews, and the training is in place so the employee does not become frustrated. The HR manager knows that checking on the employee in the first week helps build confidence in the employee that if he or she has problems he or she has somewhere to go. My experience with the Marriott was an experience that I will never forget.

Courtesy of Joseph Moreta.

Summary

1. The hospitality and tourism industries are the largest and fastest-growing industries in the world.
2. Now is a great time to be considering a career in the hospitality and tourism field because thousands of supervising managers are needed for this dynamic industry.
3. Common dynamics include delivery of services and guest impressions of them.
4. Hospitality businesses are open 365 days a year and 24 hours a day and are likely to require shift work.
5. One essential difference between the hospitality business and other businesses is that in hospitality we are selling an intangible and perishable product.
6. Corporate philosophy is changing from managers' planning, organizing, implementing, and so on, to that of managers' counseling associates, giving them resources, and helping them to think for themselves.
7. Corporate philosophy embraces the values of the organization, including ethics, morals, fairness, and equality. The philosophy of "do whatever it takes" is critical for success.
8. Corporate culture refers to the overall style or feel of the company, or how people relate to one another and their jobs.
9. A mission statement is a statement of central purposes, strategies, and values of the company. It should answer the question, "What business are we in?"
10. A goal is a specific target to be met; objectives or tactics are the actions needed to accomplish the goal.
11. Total quality management has helped improve service to guests by empowering employees to give service that exceeds guest expectations.

Key Words and Concepts

corporate philosophy
empowerment
front of the house
goal
guest satisfaction
heart of the house

hospitality
inseparability
intangible
National Restaurant
 Association (NRA)
perishability

total quality management
 (TQM)
tourism
sustainability
return on investment

Review Questions

1. Why is service so critical in the hospitality and tourism industries?
2. Describe and give an example of the following:
   Mission statement
   Moment of truth

3. What is the Disney service model?
4. Explain why Ritz-Carlton won the Malcolm Baldrige award.

Internet Exercises

1. Organization: **World Travel and Tourism Council**
   Web site: **www.wttc.org**
   Summary: The World Travel and Tourism Council (WTTC) is the global business leaders' forum for travel and tourism. It includes all sectors of industry, including accommodation, catering, entertainment, recreation, transportation, and other travel-related services. Its central goal is to work with governments so that they can realize the full potential economic impact of the world's largest generator of wealth and jobs: travel and tourism.
   (a) Find the latest statistics or figures for the global hospitality and tourism economy.

2. Organization: **Ritz-Carlton Hotels**
   Web site: **www.ritzcarlton.com**
   Summary: The Ritz-Carlton is renowned for its elegance, sumptuous surroundings, and legendary service. With seventy-four hotels in twenty-three countries worldwide, a majority of them award winning, the Ritz-Carlton reflects one hundred years of tradition.
   (a) What is it about Ritz-Carlton that makes it such a great hotel chain?

3. Organization: **Disneyland and Walt Disney World**
   Web site: **disneyland.disney.com** and **disneyworld.disney.com**
   (a) Compare and contrast Disneyland's and Walt Disney World's web sites.

Apply Your Knowledge

1. Write your personal mission statement.

2. Suggest ways to improve service in a hospitality business.

Suggested Activities

1. Where are you going? Take a moment to think about your future career prospects. Where do you want to be in five, ten, or twenty years?
2. Prepare some general hospitality- and career-related questions, and interview two supervisors or managers in the hospitality industry. Share and compare the answers with your class next session.

Endnotes

1. This section draws on: *Hospitality through the Ages.* (Corning, NY: Corning Foodservice Products: Corning Foodservice Products, February 1972), 2–34.
2. William S. Gray and Salvatore C. Liquori, *Hotel and Motel Management and Operation* (Englewood Cliffs, NJ: Prentice Hall, 1980), 4–5, quoted in John R. Walker, *Introduction to Hospitality,* 2nd ed. (Upper Saddle River, NJ: Prentice Hall, 1999), P5.
3. John R. Walker, *Introduction to Hospitality,* 2nd ed. (Upper Saddle River, NJ: Prentice Hall, 1999), P5.
4. Garvin R. Nathan, *Historic Taverns of Boston: 370 Years of Tavern History in One Definitive Guide* (Lincoln, NE: iUniverse, 2006), 3.
5. Linda Glick Conway, ed., *The Professional Chef,* 5th ed. (Hyde Park, NY: The Culinary Institute of America, 1991), 5.
6. Ibid.
7. John Mariani, *America Eats Out* (New York: William Morrow, 1991), 122–124.
8. Martin E. Dorf, *Restaurants That Work* (New York: Whitney Library of Design, 1992), 9.
9. Personal conversation with Charlotte Jordan, May 6, 2007.
10. Nathan Cobb, *Boston Globe Magazine*, June 4, 1989, quoted in John R. Walker, *The Restaurant from Concept to Operation*, 6th ed. (New York: John Wiley and Sons, 2012), 59.
11. Starbucks Coffee Company, *Our Heritage*, www.starbucks.com/about-us/our-heritage (accessed January 14, 2011); and Starbucks Coffee Company, *Company Profile,* http://assets.starbucks.com/assets/company-profile-feb10.pdf (accessed January 18, 2011).
12. Robert Longley, *Lifetime Earnings Soar with Education: Masters Degree Worth $2.5 Million Income Over a Lifetime,* http://usgovinfo.about.com/od/moneymatters/a/edandearnings.htm (accessed February 3, 2011).
13. NGO Committee on Education, United Nations, *Our Common Future, Chairman's Foreword*, http://www.un-documents.net/ocf-cf.htm (accessed February 15, 2011).
14. Sustainable Hospitality Group, *What Is Sustainability?* http://www.sustainablehg.com/sustainable-hospitality-group/sustainability.htm#whatis (accessed February 14, 2011).
15. Hervé Houdré, Center for Hospitality Research, *Sustainable Hospitality: Sustainable Development in the Hotel Industry*, www.hotelschool.cornell.edu/research/chr/pubs/perspective/perspective-14924.html (accessed February 14, 2011).
16. Marriott International, Inc., *Core Values*, www.marriott.com/corporateinfo/culture/coreValues.mi (accessed January 18, 2011).
17. Marriott, *Marriott Culture*, www.marriott.com/corporateinfo/culture/coreCulture.mi (accessed January 18, 2011).
18. Mohamed Gravy, General Manager Holiday Inn Sarasota, address to University of South Florida students, Tampa, Florida, February 8, 2010.
19. Marriott International, Inc., *J.W. Marriott, Jr.*, www.marriott.com/corporateinfo/culture/heritage JWMarriottJR.mi (accessed May 27, 2011).
20. Ibid.
21. JW Marriott Jr and Kathi Ann Brown, *The Spirit to Serve: Marriott's Way* (New York: Harper Collins, 1997), 34.
22. Karl Albrecht and Ron Zemke, *Service America!* (Homewood, IL: Dow Jones-Irwin, 1985), 2.
23. Karl Albrecht, *At America's Service* (New York: Warner Books, 1992), 13.
24. Albrecht, *At America's Service*, 27.
25. American Hotel & Lodging Association, *AH&LA Green Resource Center*, http://www.ahla.com/green.aspx (accessed February 3, 2011).
26. Phil Cohen, "Deming's 14 Points," *HCi*, http://www.hci.com.au/hcisite2/articles/deming.htm (accessed January 14, 2011).
27. Marriott International, Inc., *Brands*, http://www.marriott.com/hotel-development/marriott-brands.mi (accessed August 10, 2011).

Glossary

Corporate philosophy The core beliefs that drive a company's basic organizational structure.

Empowerment The act of giving employees the authority, tools, and information they need to do their jobs with greater autonomy.

Front-of-the-house Comprises all areas with which guests come in contact, including the lobby, corridors, elevators, guest rooms, restaurants and bars, meeting rooms, and restrooms. Also refers to employees who staff these areas.

Goal A specific result to be achieved; the end result of a plan.

Guest satisfaction The desired outcome of hospitality services.

Heart of the house The back of the house.

Hospitality 1. The cordial and generous reception of guests. 2. A wide range of businesses, each of which is dedicated to the service of people away from home.

Inseparability The interdependence of hospitality services offered.

Intangible Something that cannot be touched.

National Restaurant Association (NRA) The association representing restaurant owners and the restaurant industry.

Perishability The limited lifetime of hospitality products; for example, last night's vacant hotel room cannot be sold today.

Return on Investment (ROI) An important financial measure that determines how well management uses business assets to produce profit. It measures the efficiency with which financial resources available to a company are employed by management. ROI 5 Annual Profit divided by Average Amount Invested. *See also* ROA.

Total quality management (TQM) A managerial approach that integrates all of the functions and related processes of a business such that they are all aimed at maximizing guest satisfaction through ongoing improvement.

Tourism Travel for recreation or the promotion and arrangement of such travel.

Photo Credits

Credits are listed in the order of appearance.

The Hotel Business

From Chapter 2 of *Introduction to Hospitality Management,* Fourth Edition. John R. Walker. Copyright © 2013 by Pearson Education, Inc. Published by Pearson. All rights reserved.

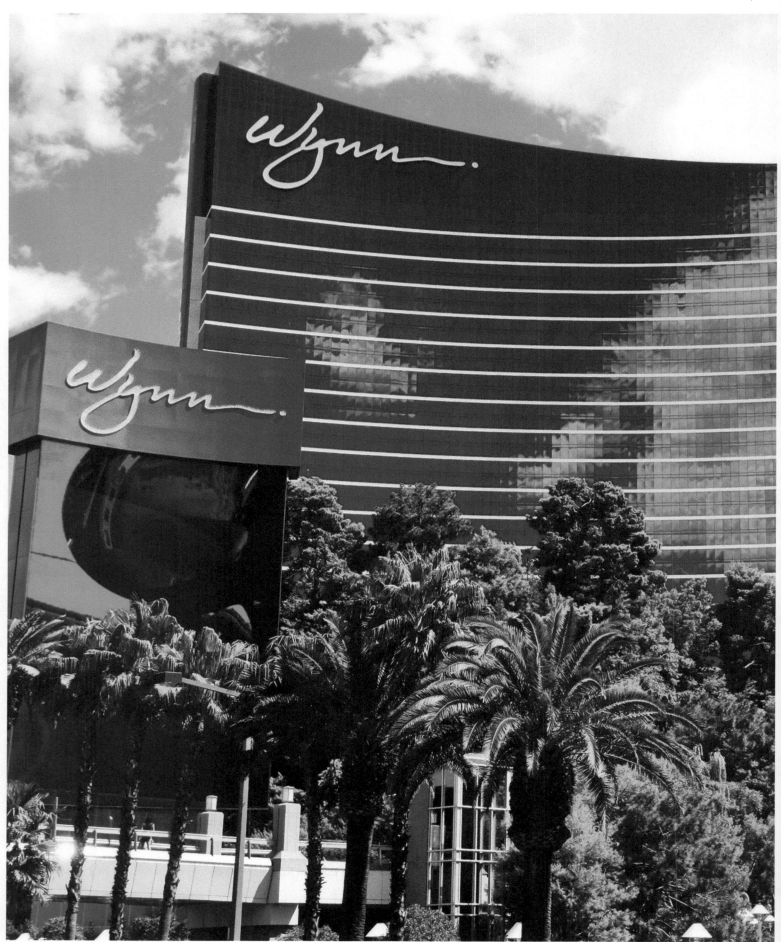

The Hotel Business

OBJECTIVES

After reading and studying this chapter, you should be able to:

- Describe hotel ownership and development via hotel franchising and management contracts.

- Classify hotels by type, location, and price.

- Discuss the concept and growth of vacation ownership.

- Name some prestigious and unusual hotels.

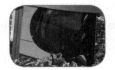
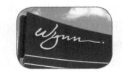
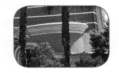
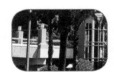

A Brief History of Innkeeping in the United States[1]

1634—Samuel Coles Inn opens on Washington Street and is the first tavern in Boston; it is later named the Ships Tavern.

1642—The City Tavern in New York City is built by the the West India Company.

1775—The Green Dragon in Boston becomes the meeting place of American Revolutionaries. Patrick Henry calls the taverns of colonial America the "cradles of liberty."

1790—The first use of the word *hotel* in America is at Carre's Hotel, 24 Broadway, New York City.

1801—The Francis Union Hotel in Philadelphia opens in a former presidential mansion.

1801–1820—Taverns are rechristened as *hotels* following a surge in popularity of all things French.

1824—The Mountain House, the first of the large resort hotels in the Catskills, eventually has 300 rooms and accommodates 500 persons.

1829—The Tremont House in Boston appears. Designed from cellar to eaves to be a hotel, it has three stories and 170 rooms. This hotel is known for several firsts: the first bellboys, the first inside water closets (toilets), the first hotel clerk, the French cuisine on a Yankee menu, the first menu card in this country, the first annunciators in guest rooms, the first room keys given to the guests, and the first guests checked in at a dedicated reception area—previously they checked in at the bar.

1834—The Astor House, New York City's first palatial hotel, has rooms furnished in black walnut and Brussels carpeting.

1846—The first centrally heated hotel, the Eastern Exchange Hotel, opens in Boston.

1848—Safety deposit boxes are provided for guests by the New England Hotel in Boston.

1852—Electric lights dazzle guests for the first time in New York City's Hotel Everett and at Chicago's Palmer House in 1894.

1859—The first passenger elevator goes into operation in the Old Fifth Avenue Hotel; upper rooms are sometimes more expensive than those on lower floors.

1875—The Palace Hotel in San Francisco is billed as the "world's largest hotel"; floor clerks are installed along with four elevators.

1880–1890s—There is a resort boom in Florida, New England, Virginia, Pennsylvania, and Atlantic City.

1887—The Ponce de León Hotel, in St. Augustine, is built; it is the first luxury hotel in Florida.

1888—The Del Coronado Hotel is built; it is the first luxury resort in California.

1892—The Brown Palace Hotel in Denver is built with "gold money" to be as fine as any hotel back east. The Brown Palace focuses on catering to business people and is regarded as one of the first convention hotels.

1908—The Statler Hotel in Buffalo, New York, is established by Elsworth Milton Statler, and is considered by many to be the premier hotelier of all time (his story makes interesting reading—try Googling him). The Statler hotel is the first to introduce keyholes for safety, electric light switches, private baths, ice water, and the delivery of a morning newspaper. The hotel is also constructed so as to have bathrooms backing onto each other; this enables the plumbing to go up or down one shaft along with protected electrical wiring. The Statler Inn at Cornell University is built with money from the Statler foundation.

1919—Conrad Hilton opens the Mobley Hotel in Cisco, Texas.

1920—There are 12 million cars in America, and auto camping becomes a national pastime as cities open up camps for people to stay at.

1922—Cornell University begins a hotel and restaurant program.

1929 to 1945—During the Great Depression and World War II, hotel occupancy drops and several hotels are lost by owners—others just manage to survive.

1946—The Golden Nugget and the Flamingo open in Las Vegas, prompting a boom in hotel construction that continues to this day.

1950s and 1960s—More interstate highways are constructed and more motels and hotels are established for the ordinary person, not just the rich.

1954—Kemmons Wilson opens the first Holiday Inn.

1966—The ice and vending machines make their debuts in InterContinental hotels.

1967—The Atlanta Hyatt Regency Hotel, designed by John Portman with an atrium and an indoor garden, opens.

1960s—Westin introduces 24-hour room service.

1960s and 1970s—Hotels begin to develop internationally.

1970s—Hotels are hit hard by the energy crisis—there is little development. Cable TV arrives; it later evolves into Internet access.

1975—Hyatt introduces concierge lounges for its VIP guests.

1980s—The electric key card is introduced, and hotels begin to accept major credit cards as payment.

1980s and 1990s—Hotel chains develop more rapidly internationally.

1980s and 1990s—Hotel chains develop hotels in several tiers/price points to appeal to different market segments.

1990s—Voice mail and in-room Internet connections are introduced.

2000s—Boutique hotels come of age, and LEED (Leadership in Energy and Environmental Design) hotels are constructed. Sustainability becomes increasingly more important.

THE AMERICAN HOTEL & LODGING ASSOCIATION

Dedicated to Serving the Interests of Hoteliers

For over one hundred years, the American Hotel & Lodging Association (AH&LA) has been an advocate for all matters relating to lodging. The AH&LA represents 50,800 properties with 4,762,095 guestrooms, $127.2 billion in sales, $53.50 revenue per available room (Rev Par), and an average occupancy rate of 54.7 percent. As a nonprofit trade association, the AH&LA exists to help the lodging industry prosper, with national advocacy on Capitol Hill, public relations and image management, education, research, and information. The AH&LA also has several programs that benefit members, among which are a comprehensive Green Resource Center; diversity programs and advice for helping members improve their diversity initiatives; technology resources and initiatives to help members improve their technology efforts; social media advice, including resources for Facebook, blogs, Twitter, Yelp (the number-one travel application for the iPhone) and Four Square (another way for consumers to write reviews, leave suggestions, and talk about hotels), and LivingSocial, Groupon, Buy With Me, and so on, online resources for leveraging the collective buying power to which more than 20 million people subscribe, with electronic promotions sent daily.

The AH&LA has conventions, the main one being in New York City in November. Additionally, there are state chapters and conventions that are recommended for you to attend as they offer several interesting presentations and discussions on lodging topics.

FOCUS ON DEVELOPMENT

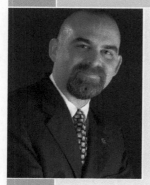

Dr. Chad M. Gruhl, Associate Chair and Associate Professor at Denver State University

Dr. Chad Gruhl is a hotel expert working for such places as the Waldorf Astoria in New York City, Trump Plaza Hotel and Casino in Atlantic City, New Jersey, Hotel InterContinental in Chicago, and Residence Inn by Marriott in three states.

There has been a tremendous amount of development in the hotel industry that has taken place in the past thirty years. The large hotel corporations discovered that if they targeted specific markets, they would be able to increase market share for particular segments. For example, in the early 1980s Marriott International focused primarily on its major hotel chain, full-service Marriott Hotels. Later in the 1980s, Marriott began expanding and developing other concepts in order to capture a larger market share:

1983—Created and opened Courtyard by Marriott (mid-economy segment)

1984—Entered into the timeshare segment of hospitality (now the largest in the world)

1987—Acquired Residence Inn by Marriott (extended-stay segment)

1987—Created the concept of Fairfield by Marriott (economy segment)

1995—Purchased Ritz-Carlton Hotels (high-end segment)

1997—Opened TownePlace Suites (select extended-stay segment), Fairfield Suites (economy segment), and Marriott Executive Residence Brand (residence segment)

1999—Acquires ExecuStay (corporate housing segment)

Today Marriott International flies 18 flags with over $10 billion in sales, 192,000 employees, over 5,000 eating places, and over 3,000 lodging properties in 67 countries and territories in the world.

Do these large companies do it all themselves? Meaning, Do they operate, own, and expand the corporate name all by themselves? The answer is, absolutely not. The largest hotel companies have expanded their companies at very fast rates through franchising. This is one of the primary sources of income for most large hotel and restaurant companies.

For example, to apply for an InterContinental Hotel and Resorts flag (the right to use their name), it costs $500 per room with a $75,000 minimum for the initial cost and application fee. After the hotel opens, it costs 5 percent of revenue for royalty fees and another 3 percent for marketing fees. In other words, it is very expensive to fly a major hotel flag. So why would anyone develop a hotel where they fly another company's flag? The answer is simple: The major hotel companies have very large reservation systems and brand recognition that brings people to that hotel once the hotel opens its doors.

There are eight large corporate hotel companies that fly approximately 75 percent of all U.S. hotels. Behind each large corporation are only a few of the larger flags that they own:

1. **Wyndham Hotels:** Days Inn, Howard Johnson, Ramada, Super 8
2. **Choice Hotels:** Comfort Inns, Quality Inns, Clarion, Econo Lodge
3. **Accor:** Sofitel, Novotel, Mercure, Ibis, Motel 6, Formule 1
4. **InterContinental Hotel Group:** Crowne Plaza, Holiday Inn, Staybridge Suites
5. **Marriott International:** Ritz-Carlton, Renaissance, Courtyard, Fairfield Inns, Residence Inns
6. **Blackstone:** Hilton Hotels, Waldorf Astoria, DoubleTree, Embassy Suites, Hampton Inns
7. **Carlson Hospitality:** Radisson Hotels, Country Inns, Park Inn, TGI Fridays
8. **Starwood:** Sheraton Hotels, Four Points, St. Regis, Le Meridien Hotels, W Hotels, Westin Hotels

There are many development and franchising opportunities in the hotel and restaurant world. You, too, can make your mark on the industry.

Hotel Development and Ownership

Franchising and management contracts are the two main driving forces in the development and operation of the hotel business. After the potential of franchising caught on, there was no stopping American ingenuity. In about a half century, the hotel business was changed forever, and here is how it happened.

Franchising

Franchising in the hospitality industry is a concept that allows a company to expand more rapidly by using other people's money than if it had to acquire its own financing. The company, or franchisor, grants certain rights to the franchise—for example, the rights to use its trademark, signs, proven operating systems, operating procedures and possibly reservations system, marketing know-how, purchasing discounts, and so on—for a fee. In return, the franchisee agrees by signing the franchise contract to operate the restaurant, hotel, or franchised outlet in accordance with the guidelines set by the franchisor. Franchising is a way of doing business that benefits both the franchisor—who wants to expand the business rapidly—and the franchisee—who has financial backing but lacks specific expertise and recognition. Some corporations franchise by individual outlets and others by territory. North America is host to more than 180 hotel brand extensions and franchised hotel brands.

Franchising hotels in the United States began in 1907, when the Ritz Development Company franchised the Ritz-Carlton name in New York City.[2] Howard Johnson began franchising his hotels in 1954—he had since 1927 successfully franchised the "red roof" restaurants. Holiday Inn (now a part of InterContinental Hotels Group [IHG], one of the largest lodging enterprises in the world) also grew by the strategy of franchising: In 1952, Kemmons Wilson, a developer, had a disappointing experience while on a family vacation when he had to pay for an extra room for his children. Therefore, Wilson decided to build a moderately priced family-style hotel.

Each room was comfortably sized and had two double beds; this enabled children to stay for free in their parents' rooms. In the 1950s and early 1960s, as the economy grew, Holiday Inn grew in size and popularity. Holiday Inns eventually added restaurants, meeting rooms, and recreational facilities. They upgraded the furnishings and fixtures in the bedrooms and almost completely abandoned the original concept of being a moderately priced lodging operation.

One of the key factors in the successful development of Holiday Corporation was that it was one of the first companies to enter the midprice range of the market. These inns, or motor hotels, were often located away from the expensive downtown sites, near important freeway intersections and the more reasonably priced suburbs. Another reason for their success was the value they offered: comfort at a reasonable price, avoiding the expensive trimmings of luxury hotels.

At about this time, a new group of budget motels emerged. Motel 6 (so named because the original cost of a room was $6 a night) in California slowly spread across the country, as did Days Inn and others. Cecil B. Day was in the construction business and found Holiday Inns too expensive when traveling on vacation with his family. He bought cheap land and constructed buildings of no more than two stories to keep the costs down. These hotels and motels, primarily for commercial travelers and vacationing families, were located close to major highways and were built to provide low-cost lodging without frills. Some of these buildings were modular constructions. Entire rooms were built elsewhere, transported to the site, and placed side by side.

It was not until the 1960s that Hilton and Sheraton began to franchise their names. Franchising was the primary growth and development strategy of hotels and motels during the 1960s, 1970s, and 1980s. However, franchising presents two major challenges for the franchisor: maintenance of quality standards and avoidance of financial failure on the part of the franchisee.

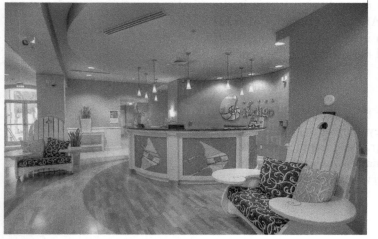

The colorful lobby of a Hotel Indigo, a franchised InterContinental Hotels Group concept.

It is difficult for the franchise company to state in writing all the contingencies that will ensure that quality standards are met. Recent franchise agreements are more specific in terms of the exterior maintenance and guest service levels. Franchise fees vary according to the agreements worked out between the franchisor and the franchisee; however, an average agreement is based on 3 or 4 percent of room revenue.

The world's leading franchisors of hotels are Wyndham Worldwide with 597,674 rooms in 7,160 hotels; Choice Hotels International, ranked second with 487,410 rooms in 6,000 hotels; and InterContinental Hotels and Resorts with 646,679 rooms in 4,400 hotels.[3]

Franchising provides both benefits and drawbacks to the franchisee and franchisor. The benefits to the franchisee are as follows:

- A set of plans and specifications from which to build
- National advertising
- A centralized reservation system (CRS)
- Participation in volume discounts for purchasing furnishings, fixtures, and equipment
- Listing in the franchisor's directory
- Low fee percentage charged by credit card companies

The drawbacks to the franchisee are as follows:

- Franchisees must pay high fees, both to join and ongoing.
- Central reservations generally produce between 17 and 26 percent of reservations.
- Franchisees must conform to the franchisor's agreement.
- Franchisees must maintain all standards set by the franchisor.

The benefits to the franchise company are as follows:

- Increased market share and recognition
- Up-front fees

The drawbacks to the franchise company are as follows:

- The need to be very careful in the selection of franchisees
- Difficulty in maintaining control of standards

Franchising continues to be a popular form of expansion both in North America and the rest of the world. However, there are always a few properties that lose their right to franchise by not maintaining standards.

Factors propelling franchise growth include the following:

- Fresh looks (curb appeal)
- Location near highways, airports, and suburbs

- Expansion in smaller cities throughout the United States
- New markets located in proximity to golf courses and other attractions
- Foreign expansion and a move to increase brand awareness

Is There a Franchise in Your Future?[4]

Many of you may not realize the pervasiveness of franchised operations in the United States. Predictions are that more than 50 percent of all retail sales in the United States (including restaurants) will soon be transacted through franchised units. Furthermore, franchises are available not only in the hotel, restaurant, travel, and recreation industries, but also in a large variety of other businesses that might interest you. These businesses include automotive tires and parts, retailing of all kinds, mail and copy services, janitorial and decorating services, personnel agencies, and so on. Today, many franchises can be operated from home by those interested in lifestyle changes.

If you end up working for a hospitality-related organization after graduation, chances are that your career will be influenced by franchising. You may work directly for a franchisor (the company that sells a franchised concept to an entrepreneur), whether on the corporate staff (for example, training, franchise consulting) or in an operations position in a franchisor-owned unit. Many franchisors own their own units that they use to test new operational or marketing ideas and to demonstrate the viability of the business to potential franchisees (the entrepreneurs who buy the franchised unit).

Alternatively, you may work for a franchisee. Some franchisees are small businesses, owning only one or a few units. Other franchisees are large corporations, owning hundreds of units and doing hundreds of millions of dollars in sales every year. For instance, RTM, Inc., owns and operates more than 600 Arby's restaurants. Additionally, it owns and franchises two midsized chicken restaurants, Lee's Famous Recipe Chicken and Mrs. Winner's Chicken and Biscuits. Working for a company as large as RTM would be similar to working for a large franchisor.

A third way that franchising may involve you is through ownership. Rather than starting your own independent business after college, you may want to consider buying a franchise. Several advantages can result. First, by working with a larger company you get the benefits of its experience in running the business that you have chosen to enter. Many of the mistakes that a new entrepreneur may make have already been overcome by your franchisor. The company might provide cash flow. The company might also provide other support services at little or no cost, such as marketing and advertising, site selection, construction plans, assistance with financing, and so on. All this assistance leads to a second key reason for buying a franchise—reducing your risk of failure. Franchising is probably less risky than starting your own business from scratch.

Consider the following factors that many franchisors seek. Are you strongly motivated to succeed and do you have a past history of business success, even if it is in a different business? Do you have a significant sum of money as well as access to credit? Are you willing to accept the franchisor's values, philosophy, and ways of doing business, as well as its technical assistance? Do you have the full support of your immediate family as you develop your business? Are you willing to devote substantially all of your working time to the business?

CORPORATE PROFILE

Wyndham Worldwide—A Collection of Hotel Brands

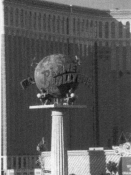

Wyndham Hotels and Resorts, Days Inn, Howard Johnson, Ramada, Knights Inn, Super 8, Travelodge, Baymont Inns & Suites, Microtel Inns and Suites, Hawthorn Suites, and Wingate by Wyndham, totaling 7,160 hotels in 66 countries.[5]

As a franchisor, the company licenses the owners and operators of independent businesses to use Wyndham brand names, without taking on big business risks and expenses. Wyndham does not operate hotels, but instead provides coordination and services that allow franchisees to retain local control of their activities. At the same time, franchisees benefit from the economies of scale of widely promoted brand names and well-established standards of service, national and regional direct marketing, co-marketing programs, and volume purchasing discounts.

All brands share extensive market research, use proprietary reservation systems and a room inventory tracking system, which is extremely technology intensive and eliminates waste. By monitoring quality control and extensively promoting the brand names, Wyndham offers its independent franchise owners franchise fees that are relatively low compared to the increased profitability they gain.

Through franchising, the company limits its own risks and is able to keep overhead costs low. Wyndham also limits the volatility in the business as best as they can because fees come from revenue, not the franchisee's profitability. A further advantage of being a franchiser of such dimension is that the company is even more protected from the cyclical nature of the economy than are other franchise ventures.

Wyndham Vacation Ownership is the largest vacation ownership business when measured by the number of vacation ownership interests. Wyndham Vacation Ownership develops, markets, and sells vacation ownership interests and provides consumer financing to owners through its three primary consumer brands: Wyndham Vacation Resorts, WorldMark by Wyndham, and Wyndham Vacation Resorts Asia Pacific.[6]

Wyndham Vacation Ownership has developed or acquired approximately 150 vacation ownership resorts throughout the United States, Canada, Mexico, the Caribbean, and the South Pacific that represent approximately 20,000 individual vacation ownership units and more than 830,000 owners of vacation ownership interests.[7]

Wyndham Exchange and Rentals helps to deliver vacations to more than 3.8 million members in approximately 100 countries. Wyndham provides exclusive access for specified periods to more than 87,000 vacation properties, including vacation ownership condominiums, traditional hotel rooms, villas, cottages, bungalows, campgrounds, city apartments, second homes, fractional resorts, private residence clubs, condominium hotels, and yachts. With a portfolio of more than thirty brands, Wyndham delivers unique vacation experiences to over 4 million leisure-bound families each year.[8]

Wyndham has been named to the Diversity Inc. twenty-five noteworthy companies that are raising diversity management leaders. Wyndham has also been ranked among the best one hundred greatest companies in America by *Newsweek* magazine, who also ranked Wyndham among the top one hundred greenest companies in America.

Franchising does have some disadvantages, as noted by many former franchisees. Your expectations of success may not be met. Perhaps the business did not have the potential that you expected, or perhaps you were not willing to invest the time needed. In a few cases, an overzealous or dishonest franchisor representative has misled franchisees.

As a franchisee, your freedom is somewhat restricted. You must operate within the constraints set out by your franchise agreement and the operational standards manual. Although there may be some room for you to express your creativity and innovation, it is generally limited. This may mean that, over time, the work might become monotonous and unchallenging, yet you have a long-term commitment to the company because of the franchise agreement that you signed. Your failure to consistently follow the franchisor's methods for running the business could result in the termination of your contract and your forced removal from the business.

Finally, the franchisor may not be performing well, thereby hurting your local business. Also, they may allow other franchisees to open units so near to your operation that your business is adversely affected.

Buying a franchise can be a very rewarding business experience in many ways. But like any other business venture, it requires research and a full discussion with family, friends, and business advisors, such as your accountant and attorney. You should carefully weigh whether you are psychologically suited to be a franchisee. Perhaps you perform more effectively in a corporate structure as an employee. Perhaps you are better suited to starting your own business from scratch. A careful analysis can help you make an informed decision. Buying a franchise such as Subway, Cold Stone Creamery, or Sea Master cruises is a lot cheaper—as in a few thousand dollars—compared to $1 million–plus for a hotel or even a McDonald's. A key question to be answered before you buy a franchise is whether you are better suited to being a franchisee or an independent entrepreneur.

Referral Associations

Referral associations offer similar benefits to properties as franchises, albeit at a lower cost. Hotels and motels with a referral association share a CRS and a common image, logo, or advertising slogan. In addition, referrals may offer group-buying discounts to members, as well as management training and continuing education programs. Each independent hotel refers guests to each

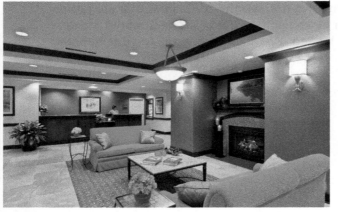

A hotel lobby.

of the other member hotels. Hotels and motels pay an initial fee to join a referral association. Size and appearance standards are less stringent than those in a franchise agreement; hence, guests may find more variation between the facilities than between franchise members.

Preferred Hotels and Resorts Worldwide is a consortium of 185 independent, luxury hotels and resorts united to compete with the marketing power of chain operations. It promotes the individuality, high standards, hospitality, and luxury of member hotels. It also provides marketing support services and a reservation center.

With the decrease in airline commissions, referral organizations—especially those at the luxury end of the market—are well placed to offer incentives to agents to book clients with the referral group's hotels. An example is awarding trips to the property for every ten rooms booked. Another is when the referral hotels offer, for instance, a 20 percent commission to travel agents during slow periods.

Three luxury Boston-area preferred properties—the Boston Harbor Hotel, the Bostonian Hotel, and the Charles Hotel in Cambridge, Massachusetts—joined together in promoting a St. Patrick's Day weekend package. Preferred Hotels in Texas—the Mansion on Turtle Creek and Hotel Crescent Court in Dallas, La Mansion Del Rio South in San Antonio, and the Washington Hotel in Fort Worth—launched a major, year-long promotion that includes a tie-in with major retail, credit card, and airline partners.

In addition to regional marketing programs, the referral associations that handle reservations for members have joined Galileo International's Inside Availability Service. This gives agents access to actual rates and room availability that are not always available information on the standard central reservation system (CRS) databases.

Leading Hotels of the World (LHW) was set up in 1928 as Luxury Hotels of Europe and Egypt by 38 hotels, including the London Savoy; the Hotel Royal in Evian, France; and the Hotel Negresco in Nice, France—each was interested in improving its marketing. The organization operated by having hotels advise their guests to use the establishments of fellow members. It then opened a New York office to make direct contact with wealthy American and Canadian travelers wishing to visit Europe and Egypt.

LHW, which is controlled by its European members, acts as an important marketing machine for its members, especially now, with offices around the world providing reservations, sales, and promotional services. All the hotels and offices are connected by a central computer reservation system called ResStar. The number of reservations members receive from Leading Hotel members varies from place to place, but with 420 member hotels, it must be beneficial.

Like LHW, Small Luxury Hotels of the World (SLH) is another marketing consortium in which seventy-nine independently owned and managed hotels and resorts are members. For more than thirty-five years, it has sought to market and sell its membership to the travel industry and to provide an inter-hotel networking system for all members. Each hotel is assessed and regularly checked to ensure that it maintains the very highest standards. Figure 1 shows the largest hotel chains in terms of number of rooms, number of countries represented, and total hotels.

Management Contracts

Management contracts have been responsible for the hotel industry's rapid boom since the 1970s. They became popular among hotel corporations because little or no up-front financing or equity is involved. Hotel management companies often form a partnership of convenience with developers and owners who generally do not have the desire or ability to operate the hotel. The management company provides operational expertise, marketing, and sales clout, often in the form of a CRS.

Company	Number of Guest Rooms	Number of Countries	Total Hotels
InterContinental Hotels Group (InterContinental Hotels & Resorts, Crowne Plaza Hotels & Resorts, Hotel Indigo, Holiday Inn Hotels & Resorts, Holiday Inn Express, Staybridge Suites, Candlewood Suites)	646,679	100	4,400
Wyndham Worldwide (Super 8, Days Inn, Ramada, Wyndham Hotels & Resorts, Baymont Inn & Suites, Wingate Inn, Travelodge, Howard Johnson, AmeriHost Inn, Knights Inn, Villager Lodge, Hawthorn Suites, Microtel Inns and Suites)	597,674	66	7,160
Marriott International (Marriott Hotels & Resorts, JW Marriott Hotels & Resorts, Renaissance Hotels & Resorts, Courtyard, Residence Inn, Fairfield Inn, Marriott Conference Centers, TownePlace Suites, SpringHill Suites, Ritz-Carlton	595,461	70	3,500
Hilton Hotels Corporation (Conrad, DoubleTree, Embassy Suites, Hampton Hotels, Hilton, Hilton Garden Inn, Homewood Suites, Scandic, Waldorf Astoria Collection)	585,060	81	3,600
Choice Hotels International (Comfort Inn, Comfort Suites, Quality, Sleep Inn, Clarion, Cambria Suites, MainStay Suites, Econo Lodge, Rodeway Inn, Suburban Extended Stay Hotel, Ascend)	487,410	35	6,000
Accor (Sofitel, Red Roof Inn, Motel 6, Studio 6, Novotel, Suitehotel, Ibis, Etap, Formule 1, Ibis, Orbis, Sofitel, Pullman, M Gallery, All Seasons Hotels)	475,433	90	4,000
Best Western International	308,447	80	4,000
Starwood Hotels & Resorts Worldwide (St. Regis, The Luxury Collection, Sheraton, Westin, Four Points by Sheraton, element, Le Meridien, W Hotels, aloft)	308,447	80	4,000
Carlson Hospitality Worldwide (Regent Hotels & Resorts, Radisson Hotels & Resorts, Park Plaza Hotels & Resorts, Country Inns & Suites by Carlson, Park Inn Hotels)	159,129	77	938
Global Hyatt Corporation (Hyatt Hotels & Resorts, Hyatt Place, Hyatt Summerfield Suites, Park Hyatt, Grand Hyatt, Hyatt Regency)	134,296	45	434

2010 Hotels.

Figure 1 • The Largest Hotel Chains in Terms of Number of Rooms, Number of Countries, and Total Hotels.

Some companies manage a portfolio of properties on a cluster, regional, or national basis. Even if the hotel corporation is involved in the construction of the hotel, ownership generally reverts to a large insurance company or other large corporation. This was the case with the La Jolla, California, Marriott Hotel. Marriott Corporation built the hotel for about $34 million, and then sold it to Paine Webber, a major investment banking firm, for about $52 million on completion. Not a bad return on investment!

The management contract usually allows for the hotel company to manage the property for a period of five, ten, or twenty years. For this, the company receives as a management fee, often a percentage of gross and/or net operating profit, usually about 2 to 4.5 percent of gross revenues. Lower fees in the 2-percent range are more prevalent today, with an increase in the incentive fee based on profitability. Some contracts begin at 2 percent for the first year, increase to 2.5 the second, and to 3.5 the third and for the remainder of the contract.[9]

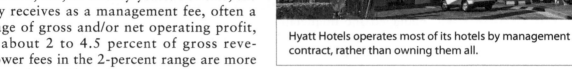
Hyatt Hotels operates most of its hotels by management contract, rather than owning them all.

Today, many contracts are for a percentage of sales and a percentage of operating profit. This is normally 2 + 2 percent. Increased competition among management companies has decreased the management contract fees in the past few years. In recent years, hotel companies increasingly have opted for management contracts because considerably less capital is tied up in managing as compared with owning properties. This has allowed for a more rapid expansion of both the U.S. and international markets.

Recent management contracts have called for an increase in the equity commitment on the part of the management company. In addition, owners have increased their operational decision-making options to allow them more control over the property. General managers have increased responsibility to owners who also want their share of profit.

Today, hotel management companies exist in an extremely competitive environment. They have discovered that the hotel business, like most others, has changed and they are adapting accordingly. Today's hotel owners are demanding better bottom-line results and reduced fees. Management companies are seeking sustainability and a bigger share of the business. With international expansion, a hotel company entering the market might actively seek a local partner or owner to work within a form of joint venture.

▶ Check Your Knowledge

1. What main factor changed the nature of the hotel industry? What impact does it have today?

2. In your own words, define *franchising* and *management contracts*.

Real Estate Investment Trust

Real estate investment trusts (REITs) have existed since the 1960s. In those early days, they were mostly mortgage holders. But in the 1980s, they began to own property outright, often focusing on specific sectors such as hotels, office buildings, apartments, malls, and nursing homes. A REIT must have at least 75 percent of its assets in real estate. Today, about 300 REITs, with a combined market value of $70 billion, are publicly traded. Investors like them because they do not pay corporate income tax and instead are required to distribute at least 95 percent of net income to shareholders. In addition, because they trade as stocks, they are much easier to get into or out of than are limited partnerships or the direct ownership of properties. In the hotel industry, REITs are clearly where the action is. As with any investment, the investor is looking for a reasonable return on the investment. Anyone can buy stocks of REITs or other publically traded companies; first, it is wise to ensure that the company is well managed and financially sound before putting any money down. The leading REIT corporations are Patriot American Hospitality, Wyndham Hotels, and Starwood Lodging Trust.

INTRODUCING CONRAD HILTON AND HILTON HOTELS CORPORATION

"King of Innkeepers" and Master of Hotel Finance

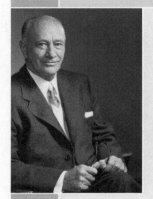

Before he was 18, Conrad Hilton had worked as a trader, a clerk, a bellboy, and a pianist. By age 25, he had worked in politics and banking.

In 1919, while visiting Cisco, Texas, Conrad Hilton had intended to take advantage of the oil boom by buying a small bank. Instead, he found bank prices prohibitive and hotels so overbooked he could not find a place to sleep. When one owner in Cisco complained he would like to sell his property in order to take advantage of the oil boom, Hilton struck a deal. He bought the Mobley Hotel with an investment of $5,000. Hilton rented rooms to oil industry prospectors and construction workers. Because of high demand for accommodations and very little supply, Hilton rented rooms in eight-hour shifts, for 300-percent occupancy. On some occasions, he even rented out his own room and slept in a lobby chair.

Because Hilton knew the banking business well and had maintained contacts who would lend him money for down payments on properties, he quickly expanded to seven Texas hotels. Hilton's strategy was to borrow as much money as possible to expand as rapidly as possible. This worked well until the Great Depression of the early 1930s. Hilton was unable to meet the payments on his properties and lost several of them but did not declare bankruptcy.[1]

Hilton, like many great leaders, even during the Depression years had the determination to bounce back. To reduce costs, he borrowed money against his life insurance and even formed an alliance with the National Hotels Corporation.

Hilton's success was attributed to two main strategies: (1) hiring the best managers and letting them have total autonomy and (2) being a careful bargainer who, in later years, was careful not to overextend his finances. Conrad Hilton had begun a successful career in the banking business before he embarked on what was to become one of the most successful hotel careers ever.

Hilton's business and financial acumen is legendary. The *New York Times* described Conrad Hilton as "a master of finance and a cautious bargainer who was careful not to overfinance" and as someone who had "a flawless sense of timing."[2] In 1954, Conrad acquired the Statler Hotel Company for $111 million, which at the time was the world's most expensive real estate transaction.

Hilton was the first person to notice vast lobbies with people sitting in comfortable chairs but not spending any money. So he added the lobby bar as a convenient meeting place and leased out space for gift shops and newsstands. Most of the additional revenue from these operations went directly to the bottom line. Today, Hilton Hotels Corporation includes Conrad Hotels, DoubleTree, Embassy Suites Hotels, Hampton Inn and Hampton Inns & Suites, Hilton Hotels, Hilton Garden Inn, Hilton Grand Vacation, Homewood Suites by Hilton, and the Waldorf Astoria Collection. These brands total thousands of hotels in cities all over the world, and "Be my guest" is still the gracious and warm way guests are received. There are 3,600 Hilton brand hotels today, and they are owned by the Blackstone Group.[3]

[1] Paul R. Dittmer and Gerald G. Griffen, *The Dimensions of the Hospitality Industry: An Introduction* (New York: Van Nostrand Reinhold, 1993), 91–92; and Conrad Hilton, *Be My Guest* (New York: Prentice Hall Press, 1957), 184–199.

[2] Joan Cook, "Conrad Hilton, Founder of Hotel Chain, Dies at 92," *New York Times,* January 5, 1979, sec. 11.

[3] Hilton worldwide, *Home Page,* www.hiltonworldwide.com (accessed February 17, 2011).

Hotel Development

Hotel ownership and development is very **capital intensive**. It takes millions of dollars to develop a property. New hotels are built as a business venture by a developer, and because the developer expects to make a **fair return on the** (substantial) **investment**, a **feasibility study** is done to assess the viability of the project—this is required by lenders. The feasibility study examines the market area's demand and supply, including any potential or real competition in the pipeline. The feasibility study determines the degree to which the proposed hotel project would be financially successful. Revenue projections based on anticipated occupancy, average daily rate, and revenue per available room are presented. The feasibility study also helps determine the type of hotel that would best suit the market and is used by the developer to obtain financing for the project. One of the most important documents is a **Summary Operating Statement**, which details revenues and expenses for a period; an example of a Summary Operating Statement is given in Figure 2. Also of interest is the source and disposition of the industry dollar. An example is given in Figure 3.

In Figure 2, note that close to 70 percent of a hotel's revenue and most of the profit comes from the sale of rooms. About 26 percent of revenue comes from food and beverage sales. In Figure 3 we can see that the average hotel room revenue is slightly different, at 66.6 percent. Each hotel will have a slight variation on these figures according to its own individual circumstances. Note in Figure 3 how high the percentage of wages, salaries, and benefits are at 46.7 percent.

Obviously, there needs to be a gap in the market in which a segment is currently not being served (for example, the hip, lifestyle boutique hotels such as Hotel Indigo), plus, a new hotel is expected to take some business away from existing properties if the room rates are close in price. There are two views on new hotels versus remodeled hotels as far as room rates and profits are concerned. It is often difficult for a

CONSOLIDATED INCOME WITH VARIANCES
For the Twelve Months Ending December 31, 2010

YEAR TO DATE

	ACTUAL	%	BUDGET	%	VARIANCE	PRIOR YEAR	%	VARIANCE
TOTAL ROOMS OCCUPIED	52,985	74.1%	50,784	71.0%	2,201	52,168	72.9%	817
TOTAL ROOMS AVAILABLE	71,540		71,540		0	71,540		0
TOTAL A.D.R	$219.68		$204.21		$15.47	$206.50		$13.18
REVPAR	$162.70		$144.96		$17.74	$150.58		$12.12
DEPARTMENTAL REVENUE								
ROOMS	11,639,641	61.5%	10,370,540	61.3%	1,269,101	10,772,724	61.5%	866,917
FOOD	4,532,944	23.9%	4,226,134	25.0%	306,810	4,253,435	24.3%	279,509
BEVERAGE	1,788,711	9.4%	1,563,904	9.2%	224,807	1,510,419	8.6%	278,292
TELEPHONE	42,877	0.2%	44,148	0.3%	(1,271)	46,914	0.3%	(4,037)
OTHER INCOME	316,945	1.7%	112,760	0.7%	204,185	332,427	1.9%	(15,483)
MINI BAR	75,281	0.4%	76,684	0.5%	(1,403)	76,963	0.4%	(1,683)
PARKING	536,839	2.8%	518,751	3.1%	18,088	531,325	3.0%	5,515
TOTAL REVENUE	18,933,238	100.0%	16,912,921	100.0%	2,020,317	17,524,208	100.0%	1,409,030
DEPARTMENTAL INCOME								
ROOMS	8,865,555	76.2%	7,744,979	74.7%	1,120,576	8,019,679	74.4%	845,876
FOOD	863,133	19.0%	863,366	20.4%	(233)	789,310	18.6%	73,823
BEVERAGE	1,243,380	69.5%	1,077,443	68.9%	165,937	1,027,144	68.0%	216,235
TELEPHONE	(89,252)	−208.2%	(97,428)	−220.7%	8,176	(119,963)	−255.7%	30,712
OTHER INCOME	217,118	68.5%	11,076	9.8%	206,042	227,147	68.3%	(10,028)
MINI BAR	25,401	33.7%	19,063	24.9%	6,338	19,034	24.7%	6,367
PARKING	312,343	58.2%	310,943	59.9%	1,400	401,540	75.6%	(89,197)
TOTAL DEPARTMENTAL INCOME	11,437,678	60.4%	9,929,442	58.7%	1,508,236	10,363,890	59.1%	1,073,788
UNDISTRIBUTED OPERATING EXPENSES								
ADMINISTRATIVE & GENERAL	1,506,103	8.0%	1,364,085	8.1%	142,018	1,466,980	8.4%	39,123
SALES AND MARKETING	1,154,957	6.1%	1,090,337	6.4%	64,620	1,028,346	5.9%	126,612
FRANCHISE FEE	1,011,621	5.3%	919,238	5.4%	92,383	951,431	5.4%	60,191
PROPERTY MAINTENANCE	597,253	3.2%	523,475	3.1%	73,778	552,043	3.2%	45,210
UTILITIES	404,098	2.1%	386,663	2.3%	17,435	391,568	2.2%	12,530
TOTAL UNDISTRIBUTED OPER EXPS	4,674,032	24.7%	4,283,798	25.3%	390,234	4,390,367	25.1%	283,665
GROSS OPERATING PROFIT	6,763,646	35.7%	5,645,644	33.4%	1,118,002	5,973,524	34.1%	790,122
MANAGEMENT FEES	378,665	2.0%	338,336	2.0%	40,329	350,485	2.0%	28,180
INCOME BEFORE FIXED CHARGES	6,384,981	33.7%	5,307,308	31.4%	1,077,673	5,623,039	32.1%	761,942
FIXED CHARGES								
PROPERTY TAXES - PERSONAL	135,223	0.7%	160,848	1.0%	(25,625)	153,082	0.9%	(17,858)
INSURANCE	29,714	0.2%	67,400	0.4%	(37,686)	66,375	0.4%	(36,661)
INTEREST	11,056	0.1%	43,921	0.3%	(32,865)	7,644	0.0%	3,412
BASE RENT	4,829,181	25.5%	4,829,184	28.6%	(3)	4,720,939	26.9%	108,242
PERCENTAGE RENT	810,036	4.3%	153,790	0.9%	656,246	426,217	2.4%	383,819
OWNERS EXPENSES	29,704	0.2%	0	0.0%	29,704	(152,875)	−0.9%	182,580
EXTRAORDINARY EXPENSES	89,431	0.5%	0	0.0%	89,431	0	0.0%	89,431
OUTSIDE ACCOUNTING FEES	17,485	0.1%	18,000	0.1%	(515)	35,803	0.2%	(18,318)

Figure 2 • A Full-Service Hotel Summary Operating Statement.

(PFK Hospitality Research, Sage Hospitality.)

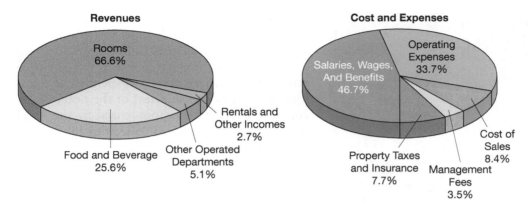

Figure 3 • Source and Disposition of the Industry Dollar.
(Courtesy of PKF Hospitality Consulting.)

new property to make a profit for a few years because of the higher cost of construction and the need to become known and to gain a good market share. On the other hand, a remodeled hotel has the cost of remodeling to pay for plus higher operating costs for energy and maintenance, so the two options tend to cancel each other out.

Today, many larger hotels are developed as part of a mixed-use project. The hotel could be near or next to a convention center, business, or attraction. The hotel may also have a residential component (as in residencies if it's a Ritz Carlton or a condotel) and may include a spa.

Older hotels are generally renovated about every seven years. This is bacause they become dated and would otherwise lose market share, which equals profit. Older hotels have an advantage over new ones—or should have an advantage as a result of positive recognition in the market. Additionally, much or all of their mortgage may be paid off, so their debt service is likely easier on the cash flow than it is for a new hotel. Older hotels may have more charm, but they are more expensive to maintain. Older hotels should also have built up repeat business through guest loyalty, something a new hotel needs to do.

Kimpton hotels have an amazing collection of boutique properties. In 1981, Bill Kimpton pioneered the boutique hotel concept in the United States. His dream was to provide weary travelers with a haven of comfort, service, security, and style. According to Market Metrix Hospitality Index,™ Kimpton has the highest customer satisfaction scores (higher than 93 percent) and emotional attachment scores (89 percent) of any hotel company operating in the United States.[10]

Hotel chains are introducing new brands to their portfolio as they identify market segment needs. Marriott has the Autograph collection of diverse independent hotels—boutique Arts, Iconic historic, Boutique Chic, Luxury Redefined, and Retreat properties.[11] Starwood has almost one hundred Aloft hotels. and Hyatt has introduced Andaz, also a boutique style-hotel which is vibrant yet relaxed, with each hotel reflecting the unique cultural scene and spirit of the surrounding neighborhood.[12]

The Economic Impact of Hotels

Hotels provide substantial **direct** and **indirect economic impact** to the communities in which they are located. For direct impact, consider a hotel that has an average of 240 guests a night who spend $250 at the hotel and in restaurants

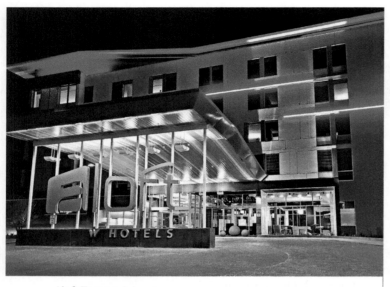

Aloft Tempe, Arizona.

and stores in the community. That would mean $240 × $250 × 365 days = $21.9 million a year infused into the local economy.

The indirect impact comes from the ripple effect, this is where money is spent by the employees (wages and salaries) of the hotel in the community. It is also money used by the hotel to purchase all the items to service the guests. Communities also benefit from the Transient Occupancy Tax (TOT), otherwise known as the bed tax. Interestingly, the TOT tax averages 12.62 percent in the United States, or $12.39 a night nationwide.[13] In addition, the hotel and its guests and employees also pay local taxes on the purchases they make. This all adds up to a considerable economic impact. Every dollar collected by a hotel eventually recycles, or multiplies itself, creating many levels of economic activity in communities. This multilevel economic activity generated by a hotel's business is estimated by using economic multipliers for revenues, wages and salaries, and employment. If we take just the revenue impact, we can see that if a hotel's annual sales are $4,250,000 and the revenue multiplier for that area is 1.979, then the total revenue impact for the year would be $8,410,750. If we consider the employment impact, we note that if the example hotel has 160 employees and the employment multiplier for the area is 1.62, then the hotel will generate 259 jobs in the area.[14] Figure 4 illustrates the multiplier effect of hotels.

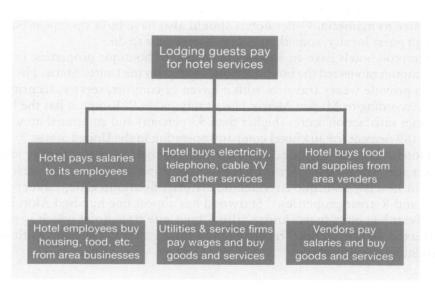

Figure 4 • The Multiplier Effect of Hotel Dollars on a Community.

(Courtesy of the American Hotel and Lodging Association.)

Classification of Hotels

According to the AH&LA, in 2010 the U.S. lodging industry consisted of 50,800 hotels and motels, with a total of 4,762,095 rooms. The average revenue per available room was $53.50 and the average occupancy was 54.7 percent.[15] Unlike many other countries, the United States has no formal government classification of hotels. However, the American Automobile Association (AAA) classifies hotels by diamond award, and the Mobil Travel Guide offers a five-star award.

The AAA has been inspecting and rating the nation's hotels since 1977. About 3 percent of the 59,000 properties inspected annually throughout the United States, Canada, and Mexico earn the five-diamond award, which is the association's highest award for excellence. In 2011, the five-diamond award was bestowed on 179 lodgings in the United States, Canada, the Caribbean and Mexico—an increase of 100 in the last ten years.[16] AAA uses descriptive criteria to evaluate the hotels that it rates (see Figure 5).

- One-diamond properties have simple roadside appeal and the basic lodging needs.
- Two-diamond properties have average roadside appeal, with some landscaping and a noticeable enhancement in interior decor.
- Three diamonds carry a degree of sophistication through higher service and comfort.
- Four diamonds have excellent roadside appeal and service levels that give guests what they need before they even ask for it.
- Five-diamond properties have the highest service levels, sophistication, and offerings.

Hotels may be classified according to location, price, and type of services offered. This allows guests to make a selection on these categories as well as personal criteria. Following is a list of hotel classifications:

City center. Luxury, first-class, midscale, economy, suites

Resort. Luxury, midscale, economy suites, condominium, timeshare, convention

Airport. Luxury, midscale, economy, suites

Freeway. Midscale, economy suites

Casino. Luxury, midscale, economy

Full service.

Convention.

Economy.

Extended stay.

Bed and breakfast.

General	◇	◇◇	◇◇◇	◇◇◇◇	◇◇◇◇◇
	Simple roadside appeal	Average roadside appeal	Very good roadside appeal	Excellent roadside appeal	Outstanding roadside appeal
	Limited landscaping	Some landscaping	Attractive landscaping	Professionally planned landscaping	Professional landscaping with a variety of foliage and stunning architecture
Lobby	Adequate size with registration, front desk, limited seating, and budget art, if any	Medium size with registration, front desk, limited seating, carpeted floors, budget art, and some plants	Spacious with front desk, carpeted seating area arranged in conversation groupings, good-quality framed art, live plants, luggage carts, and bellstation	Spacious or consistent with historical attributes; registration and front desk above average with solid wood or marble; ample seating area with conversation groupings and upscale appointments including tile, carpet, or wood floors; impressive lighting fixtures; upscale framed art and art objects; abundant live plants; background music; separate check-in/-out; bellstation	Comfortably spacious or consistent with historical attributes; registration and front desk above average; ample seating with conversation groupings and upscale appointments; impressive lighting fixtures; variety of fine art; abundant plants and fresh floral arrangements; background music; separate check-in/-out; bellstation that may be part of concierge area; concierge desk
Guestrooms	May not reflect current industry standards	Generally reflect current industry standards	Reflect current industry standards	Reflect current industry standards and provide upscale appearance	Reflect current standards and provide luxury appearance
Service	Basic attentive service	More attentive service	Upgraded service levels	High service levels and hospitality	Guests are pampered by flawless service executed by professional staff

Figure 5 • Summary of AAA Diamond Rating Guidelines.

(Reprinted from http://www.aaasouth.com/travel/diamond_ratings.aspx?Link_Source=diamond&From_Page=AAA.com&zip=32836, by permission of AAA.)

Alternatively, the hotel industry may be segmented according to price. Figure 6 gives an example of a national or major regional brand-name hotel chain in each segment.

City Center Hotels

City center hotels, by virtue of their location, meet the needs of the traveling public for business or leisure reasons. These hotels could be luxury, midscale, business, suites, economy, or residential. They offer a range of accommodations and services. Luxury hotels offer the ultimate in decor, butler service, concierge and special concierge floors, secretarial services, the latest Wi-Fi or in-room technology, computers, fax machines, beauty salons, health spas, 24-hour room

Economy $49–$69	Midprice $69–$125	Upscale $125–$225	Luxury $150–$450	All-Suites $109–$225
Holiday Inn Express	Holiday Inn Fairfield Inn		Crowne Plaza Hotel InterContinental	
Fairfield Inn	Courtyard Inn Residence Inn	Courtyard Inn Marriott Residence Inn	Marriott Marquis Ritz-Carlton	Marriott Suites
Days Inn		Omni	Renaissance	
EconoLodge	Radisson Inn	Radisson		Radisson Suites
Ramada Limited	Ramada Inn	Ramada		Ramada Suites
	Sheraton Inn Four Points	Sheraton	Sheraton Grande	Sheraton Suites
Sleep Inn	American Inn	Hyatt	Grand Hyatt Hyatt Regency Hyatt Park	Hyatt Suites
Comfort Inn	Quality Inn Wingate	Clarion Hotels		Quality Suites Comfort Suites
Extended Stay America	Hilton Inn	Hilton	Hilton Towers	Hilton Suites
Thrift Lodge	DoubleTree Club	DoubleTree		DoubleTree Suites
Travelodge Hotels	Travelodge Hotels	Forte Hotels	Forte Hotels	
Motel 6	Country Inn & Suites	Westin	Westin	Spring Hill Suites
Super 8	La Quinta			
	Red Roof Inn			Homewood Suites by Hilton
	Best Western			Hampton Suites
	Hampton Inn			Embassy Suites

Note: Some brands' price ranges may overlap because of location and seasonal pricing.

Figure 6 • Hotels by Price Segment.

service, swimming pools, tennis courts, valet service, ticket office, airline office, car rental, and doctor/nurse on duty or on call.

Generally, they offer a signature restaurant, coffee shop, or an equivalent recognized name restaurant; a lounge; a named bar; meeting and convention rooms; a ballroom; and possibly a fancy night spot. The Drake Hotel in Chicago is an example of a city center luxury hotel. An example of a midpriced hotel in New York City is the Ramada Hotel; an economy hotel is the Day's Inn; a suites property is the Embassy Suites.

Resort Hotels

Resort hotels came of age with the advent of rail travel. Increasingly, city dwellers and others had the urge to vacation in locations they found appealing. Traveling to these often more exotic locations became a part of the pleasure experience. In the late 1800s, luxury resort hotels were developed to accommodate the clientele that the railways brought. Such hotels include the famous Greenbrier at White Sulphur Springs, West Virginia; the Hotel del Coronado near San Diego, California; the Breakers in Florida; and the Homestead at Hot Springs, Virginia.

The leisure and pleasure travelers of those days were drawn by resorts, beaches, or spectacular mountain scenery. At first, many of these grand resorts were seasonal. However, as automobile and air travel made even the remote resorts more accessible and an increasing number of people could afford to visit, many resorts became year-round properties.

Resort communities sprang up in the sunshine belt from Palm Springs to Palm Beach. Some resorts focus on major sporting activities such as skiing, golf, or fishing; others offer family vacations. Further improvements in both air and automobile travel brought exotic locations within the reach of the population.

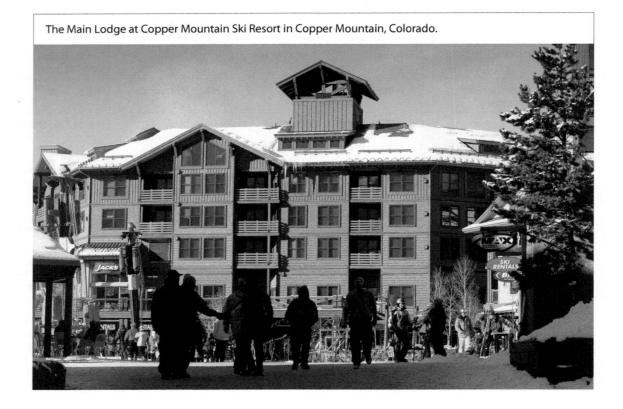

The Main Lodge at Copper Mountain Ski Resort in Copper Mountain, Colorado.

Europe, the Caribbean, and Mexico became more accessible. As the years passed, some of the resorts suffered because the public's vacation plans changed.

The traditional family month-long resort vacation gave way to shorter, more frequent getaways of four to seven days. The regular resort visitors became older; in general, the younger guests preferred the mobility of the automobile and the more informal atmosphere provided by the newer and more informal resorts.

Hyatt hotels have organized a program consisting of a variety of activities for children, thereby giving parents an opportunity either to enjoy some free time on their own or join their children in fun activities. Many resort hotels began to attract conventions, conferences, and meetings so that they could maintain or increase occupancy, particularly during the low and shoulder seasons.

Guests go to resorts for leisure and recreation. They want a good climate—summer or winter—in which they can relax or engage in recreational activities. Because of the remoteness of many resorts, guests are a kind of "captured clientele," who may be on the property for days at a time. This presents resort managers with some unique operating challenges. Another operating challenge concerns seasonality: Some resorts either do not operate year-round or have periods of very low occupancy. Both present challenges in attracting, training, and retaining competent staff.

Many guests travel considerable distances to resorts. Consequently, they tend to stay longer than they do at transient hotels. This presents a challenge to the food and beverage manager to provide quality menus that are varied and are presented and served in an attractive, attentive manner. To achieve this, resorts often use a cyclical menu that repeats itself every fourteen to twenty-one days. Also, they provide a wide variety and number of dishes to stimulate interest. Menus are now more health conscious—lighter and low in saturated fats, cholesterol, salt, and calories.

The food needs to be presented in a variety of ways. Buffets are popular because they give guests the opportunity to make choices from a display of foods. Barbecues, display cooking, poolside dining, specialty restaurants, and reciprocal dining arrangements with nearby hotels give guests even more options.

With increased global competition, not only from other resorts but also from cruise lines, resort managers are challenged to both attract guests and to turn those guests into repeat business, which traditionally has been the foundation of resort viability.

To increase occupancies, resorts have diversified their marketing mix to include conventions, business meetings, sales meetings, incentive groups, sporting events, additional sporting and recreational facilities, spas, adventure tourism, ecotourism, and more.

Because guests are cocooned in the resort, they expect to be pampered. This requires an attentive, well-trained staff; hiring, training, and retaining a competent staff present a challenge in some remote areas and in developing countries.

There are a number of benefits to operating resorts. The guests are much more relaxed in comparison to those at transient hotels, and the resorts are located in scenically beautiful areas. This frequently enables staff to enjoy a better quality of life than do their transient hotel counterparts. Returning guests tend to treat associates like friends. This adds to the overall party-like atmosphere, which is prevalent at many of the established resorts.

INTRODUCING VALERIE FERGUSON

Regional Vice President of Loews Hotels, Past Chair of the American Hotel & Lodging Association and Regional Vice President of Loews Hotels

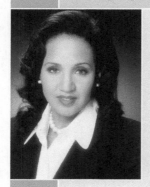

To most, "making it big" seems like a regular statement and a task easily achieved. To Valerie Ferguson, well, it comes with a lot of work, dedication, and heart. She speaks often about seizing opportunities and adding self-interest to what you do for your career.

For this African American woman, life wasn't always easy. As the managing director of Loews Philadelphia Hotel and regional vice president of Loews Hotels, she has a lot to say about what got her where she is now.

One of her most important role models was her father, Sam Ferguson. She says, "My father and I had a great relationship in which he supported me, but in which he never put any images in front of me about what I should shoot for."

After high school, Valerie applied to and was accepted at the University of San Francisco, where she earned a degree in government. Eventually realizing that law wasn't where her heart was, she decided to move out to Atlanta where she got a job as a nighttime desk clerk at the Hyatt Regency. She fell in love with the hotel industry and saw it as a challenge. Soon enough, though, she realized that the challenges she was really facing were issues of race and gender. She explains, "I was raw in my approach to the business world, but I soon came to realize that it takes more than working hard. To succeed, a person must be able to proclaim his or her goals."

Her success comes from being out there and connecting with people and society. Valerie is past chair of the American Hotel & Lodging Association (AH&LA) board and still serves on the Diversity Committee. She is also past associate director of the National Restaurant Association. She is a director on the boards of the Pennsylvania Travel Council, Philadelphia Workforce Investment, Communities in Schools, and the Educational Institute.

Valerie was nominated general manager of the year for the Hyatt Hotels Corporation. Through the years, she has managed several hotels for Hyatt and Ritz-Carlton. Her outstanding work and devotion to the hospitality and lodging industry have not gone unrewarded. She was named one of the Top 100 Black Women in Corporate America by *Ebony* magazine. She was named one of the Top 100 Black Women of Influence by the Atlanta Business League Pioneers. She was also named one of the 100 Most Influential Women in Travel by *Travel Agent* magazine. Other honorary awards for her work in the lodging industry were the 1998 National Association for the Advancement of Colored People (NAACP) Southeast Region Trailblazer Award for Business, the Martin Luther King Jr. Drum Major for Justice Award from Coretta Scott King and the Women of the Southern Christian Leadership Conference (SCLC). Ed Rabin, executive vice president of Hyatt and an early Ferguson mentor, says, "From the get-go, she demonstrated an ability and willingness to understand and learn the business and win over guests, colleagues, and peers in the process."

When Loews was being opened, Valerie was thrilled with the adventure of being with a still-growing company. President and CEO of Loews Jonathan Tisch became a close friend as they served together on the board of the American Hotel and Lodging Association (AH&LA). In 1994, Valerie ran for a seat on the AH&LA's executive committee and eventually succeeded Tisch as chair. She was the first African American and second woman to serve as AH&LA chair.

She comments on the hospitality industry: "The hospitality industry is one of the last vestiges of the American dream, where you can enter from very humble beginnings and end up a success." The great relationship she has with people has been a great contribution to her well-deserved success.

Ferguson has come a long way in her career. She is proud of what she is doing and doesn't believe that she has stopped climbing the ladder of success. She is fighting to make other women and minority members realize that there is a whole world of opportunities out there and they should set their goals high. She believes that equality of opportunity "should not come as the result of a mandate of the federal government or as the result of pressure from groups outside this industry. The impetus for change must come from within the hearts and souls of each of us."

Sources: Lodging 23, no. 5 (January 1998); Loews Hotels and Resorts, *Welcome to Loews Hotels*, www.loewshotels.com accessed (October 26, 2011); American Hotel & Lodging Association, *Officers: valerie ferguson*, ww.ahma.com/about/officers/ferguson.htm (accessed May 14, 2005; site now discontinued); www.findarticles.com/cf_0_/mv0VOU/1998_July_30/50216477/pl/article.jhtml; Robert A. Nozar, "Newsmaker Interview: Valerie Ferguson," *Hotel & Motel Management*, November 1998, www.hotel-online.com/Neo/SpecialReports1998/Nov98_Ferguson.html (accessed October 26, 2011).

Airport Hotels

Many airport hotels enjoy high occupancy because of the large number of travelers arriving and departing from major airports. The guest mix in airport hotels consists of business, group, and leisure travelers. Passengers with early or late flights may stay over at the airport hotel, whereas others rest while waiting for connecting flights.

Airport hotels are generally in the 200- to 600-room size and are full service. To care for the needs of guests who may still feel as if they are in different time zones, room service and restaurant hours may be extended or even offered around the clock. More moderately priced hotels have vending machines.

As competition at airport hotels intensified, some added meeting space to cater to businesspeople who want to fly in, meet, and fly out. Here, the airport hotel has the advantage of saving the guests from having to go downtown. Almost all airport hotels provide courtesy van transportation to and from the airport.

Convenient locations, economical prices, and easy and less costly transportation costs to and from the airport are some reasons why airport hotels are becoming intelligent choices for business travelers. Airport hotels can mean a bargain for groups, especially considering that the transportation to the hotel and back from the airport is usually free or is very inexpensive, says Brian Booth, director of sales and marketing at the Dallas Hyatt Regency Airport Hotel. One of the most conveniently located hotels in the country is the Miami International Airport Hotel, which is located within the airport itself.

Freeway Hotels and Motels

Freeway hotels and motels came into prominence, with the help of the Interstate Highway Act, in the 1950s and 1960s. They are smaller than most hotels—usually fewer than fifty rooms—and are frequently mom-and-pop establishments or franchised (such as Motel 6). As Americans took to the open road, they needed a convenient place to stay that was reasonably priced with few frills. Guests could simply drive up, park outside the office, register, rent a room, and park outside the room. Over the years, more facilities were added: lounges, restaurants, pools, vending machines, game rooms, and satellite TV.

Motels are often clustered near freeway off ramps on the outskirts of towns and cities. Today, some are made of modular construction and have as few as eleven employees per hundred rooms. These savings in land, construction, and operating costs are passed on to the guest in the form of lower rates.

Casino Hotels

The casino hotel industry is now coming into the financial mainstream, to the point that, as a significant segment of the entertainment industry, it is reshaping the U.S. economy. The entertainment and recreation sector has become a very important engine for U.S. economic growth, providing a boost to consumer spending, and thus creating tremendous prosperity for the industry. One of the fastest-growing sectors of the entertainment field is gaming.

The gaming business is strictly for adults; in addition to gaming, a multinational fine cuisine for dining, health spas for relaxation, dance clubs, and dazzling shows are available. Casino hotels are now marketing themselves as business hotels. They include in their rooms work space, Wi-Fi, a fax, a copier, and computer data ports. Other amenities include a full-service business center, travel bureau, and room service. Larger casino hotels also attract conventions, which represent a lucrative business. There are now more than 150 hotels in Native American tribal land. They cater to an increasing number of guests who want to stay and be entertained as well as gamble.

Convention Hotels

Convention hotels provide facilities and meet the needs of groups attending and holding conventions. Apart from this segment of the market, convention hotels also attract seasonal leisure travelers. Typically, these hotels exceed 500 guest rooms and include larger public areas to accommodate hundreds of people at any given time. Convention hotels have many banquet areas within and around the hotel complex. These hotels have a high percentage of double occupancies, and rooms have double queen-sized beds. Convention hotels may also offer a concierge floor to cater to individual guest needs. Round-the-clock room service, an in-house laundry, a business center, a travel desk, and an airport shuttle service are other amenities found in convention hotels.

Full-Service Hotels

Another way to classify hotels is by the degree of service offered: full-service, economy, extended-stay, and all-suite hotels. Full-service

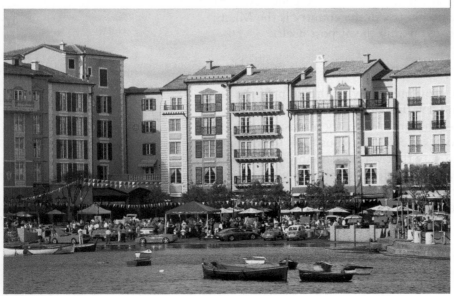
The Universal Portofino Bay Hotel in Orlando, Florida, is a popular convention hotel modeled after Portofino, Italy.

hotels offer a wide range of facilities, services, and amenities, including many that were mentioned under the luxury hotel category: multiple food and beverage outlets including bars, lounges, and restaurants; both formal and casual dining; and meeting, convention, and catering services. Business features might include a business center, secretarial services, fax, in-room computer hookups, and so on.

Most of the major North American cities have hotel chain representation, such as Four Seasons, Hilton, InterContinental, Choice, Hyatt, Marriott, Omni, Wyndham, Radisson, Loews, and Starwood. Each of these chains has a portfolio of brands in different market segment: deluxe, such as Marriott's Ritz-Carlton and the JW Marriott; luxury, such as Renaissance; luxury boutique, such as Edition and Autograph, a collection of high-personality independent hotels.

Economy/Budget Hotels

After enjoying a wave of growth for most of the last twenty years, the economy hotel segment may be close to the saturation point. There are about 25,000 properties in this segment with many market categories. The economic law of supply and demand rules: If an area has too many similar properties, then price wars usually break out as they try to attract guests. Some will attempt to differentiate themselves and stress value rather than discounting. This adds to the fascination of the business.

An economy or budget hotel offers clean, reasonably sized and furnished rooms without the frills of full-service hotels. Popular brands in this market sector are Hampton Inn, Fairfield Inn, Holiday Inn Express, Best Western, Travelodge, Motel 6, Microtel, Days Inn, Choice's Sleep Inn, Roadway Inn and Econo Lodge, Wingate, Super 8, Baymont Inn, and Country Inn. These properties do not have restaurants or offer substantial food and beverages, but they do offer guests a continental breakfast in the lounge or lobby.

These chains became popular by focusing on selling beds, not meals or meetings. This enabled them to offer rates about 30 percent lower than the midpriced hotels can. Economy properties, which represent about 15 percent of total hotel rooms, have experienced tremendous growth.

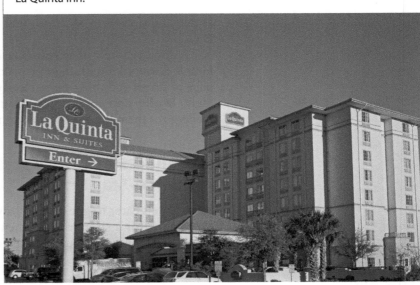

La Quinta Inn.

Boutique Hotels

Boutique hotels offer a different lodging experience compared to mid- to large chain hotels. Boutique hotels have a unique architecture, style, decor, and size. They are smaller than their chain competitors, with about 25 to 125 rooms and a high level of personal service. Some examples of boutique hotels are the trendy South Beach retro types, Kimpton Hotels, Joie de Vivre

A DAY IN THE LIFE OF SEAN BAKEWELL

Guest Services Supervisor, Palmer House Hilton, Chicago

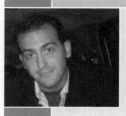

The Palmer House has 1,639 rooms and is considered North America's longest continuously run hotel. It was built in 1871 and two weeks later burned to the ground in the Great Chicago Fire. It was rebuilt and was considered the world's only fireproof hotel in 1875. The hotel has many unique features, such as prohibition-era tunnels in the basement leading to the Chicago river, many original Tiffany decorative pieces, and a score of celebrities past and present who have entertained in our famed Empire room. The hotel has an art deco–style design and is truly unique.

As a Guest Services Supervisor, I primarily oversee the bell desk. I supervise around thirty employees–both the doormen and bellmen. Our bellmen must follow Hilton Hotel's standards; these include welcoming each guest to the hotel, offering luggage assistance, using the guest's name if possible, escorting guests to their rooms, pointing out key amenities in the room, offering to fill the ice bucket, asking the guests to please call the bell desk if they require anything during their stay, and inviting the guests back to stay with us again.

Besides maintaining and upholding the Hilton standards for bellmen and doormen, there are other responsibilities of the position. I do the payroll for the department. This involves monitoring time-clock punches and ensuring each employee has taken a lunch break. Many groups that stay in the hotel desire that we deliver items to guests staying in their group block. These items can include gift bags, gift baskets, newsletters, newspapers, and wedding gift bags. There are charges for these services, and each bellmen gets paid per item they deliver. It's my responsibility that the bellmen receive the materials, the correct rooming lists for such groups, and the correct amount of money for delivering these items. We call these distributions. Some bellmen can earn an extra thousand dollars a month doing these distributions.

The bellmen and doormen are both union positions. It is my responsibility to make sure that the hotel is living up to their side of the union contract. This affects disciplinary actions, payroll, and scheduling. Another aspect of my job is to handle guest concerns. This involves talking to upset guests and finding ways to satisfy their concerns. Examples include broken luggage, wrong luggage being delivered to the room, and poor attitude from the staff.

I have worked for Hilton for over three years. I started as a Guest Service Agent, which is essentially a front desk agent. After two years of being a Guest Service Agent, I was promoted to the supervisory position. I majored in hospitality business at Michigan State University. My best advice to any hospitality student is simply to start working and gain experience.

Hotels, Edition from Marriott, and the avant-garde hotel George in Washington, D.C.

A good example of a chain boutique hotel is Hotel Indigo, an InterContinental Hotels Group. Hotel Indigo provides an oasis where guests can escape the hectic pace of travel and think more clearly, work more productively, rest more refreshingly. It offers an environment that doesn't just shelter guests, but inspires and reenergizes them. That's the idea behind Hotel Indigo.[17]

Extended-Stay Hotels and All-Suites
Extended-Stay Hotels

Some hotels cater to guests who stay for an extended period. They do, of course, take guests for a shorter time when space is available; however, the majority of guests are long term. Guests take advantage of a reduction in room rates based on the length of their stay. The mix of guests is mainly business and professional/technical guests, or relocating families.

Candlewood Suites, Extended Stay America, Homestead Studio Suites, Hawthorn Suites, Baymont Inns and Suites, Residence Inns, and Homewood Suites are popular brands in this segment of the lodging industry. These properties offer full kitchen facilities and shopping services or a convenience store on the premises. Complimentary continental breakfast and evening cocktails are served in the lobby. Some properties offer a business center and recreational facilities.

All-suites extended-stay hotels typically offer approximately 25 percent more space for the same amount of money as the regular hotel in the same price range. The additional space is usually in the form of a lounge and possibly a kitchenette area.

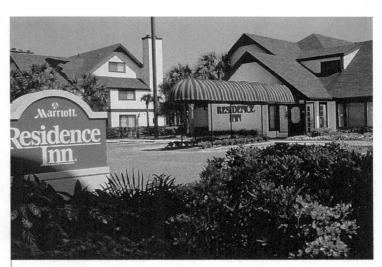

Residence Inn is a market leader in the extended-stay segment of the lodging industry.

Embassy Suites, owned and operated by Hilton Hotels Corporation; Residence Inns, Fairfield Suites, and Town-Place Suites, all by Marriott; Extended Stay America; Homewood Suites; and Guest Quarters are among the popular brands in the all-suites, extended-stay segment of the lodging industry. Several of the major hotel chains have all-suites extended-stay subsidiaries, including Radisson, Choice Hotels (which dominate the economy all-suites segment with Comfort and Quality Suites), Sheraton Suites, Hilton Suites, Homegate Studios, and Suites by Wyndham Hotels. These properties provide a closer-to-home feeling for guests who may be relocating or attending seminars or who are on work-related projects that necessitate a stay of greater than about five days.

There are now almost 2,500 all-suites extended-stay properties. Many of these properties have business centers and offer services such as grocery shopping and laundry/dry cleaning. The designers of extended-stay properties realize that guests prefer a homelike atmosphere. Accordingly, many properties are built to encourage a community feeling, which allows guests to interact informally.

Condotels and Mixed-Use Hotels

As the word suggests, a condotel is a combination of a hotel and condominium. Developers build a hotel and sell it as condo units, which the owners can pool for use as hotel rooms and suites. The hotel operating company gets a cut of the money from renting the units and so does the owner. The owner of the condo unit may have exclusive right to the use of the unit for a fixed period of time (usually one month); other than that, the hotel operating company knows that it can rent out the condos.

Some new hotels are developed as mixed-use properties, meaning that a hotel may also have "residences"—real condos that people use, so they are not for renting like condotel—along with amenities such as a spa and sports facilities. Mixed-use hotels can also be a part of a major urban or resort development, which may include office buildings, convention centers, sporting facilities, or shopping malls.

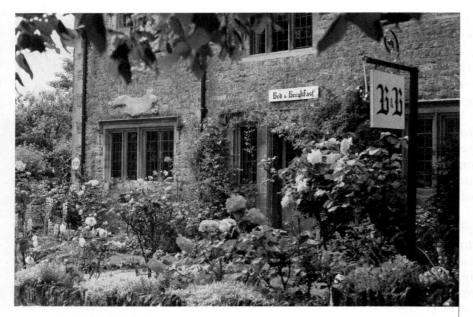

A Bed and Breakfast in Yorkshire, England.

Bed and Breakfast Inns

Bed and breakfast inns, or B&Bs as they are familiarly known, offer an alternative lodging experience to the normal hotel or motel. According to *TravelASSIST* magazine, B&B is a concept that began in Europe and started as overnight lodging in a private home. A true B&B is an accommodation with the owner, who lives on the premises or nearby, providing a clean, attractive accommodation and breakfast, usually a memorable one. The host also offers to help the guest with directions, restaurants, and suggestions for local entertainment or sightseeing.

There are many different styles of B&Bs with prices ranging from about $30 to $300 or more per night. B&Bs may be quaint cottages with white picket fences leading to gingerbread houses, tiny and homey, with two or three rooms available. On the other hand, some are sprawling, ranch-style homes in the Rockies; multistoried town homes in large cities; farms; adobe villas; log cabins; lighthouses; and many stately mansions. The variety is part of the thrill, romance, and charm of the B&B experience.[18]

There are an estimated 25,000 bed and breakfast places in the United States alone. B&Bs have flourished for many reasons. Business travelers are growing weary of the complexities of the check-in/checkout processes at some commercial hotels. With the escalation of transient rates at hotels, an opportunity has been created to serve a more price-sensitive segment of travelers. Also, many leisure travelers are looking for accommodation somewhere between a large, formal hotel and staying with friends. The B&Bs offer a homelike atmosphere. They are aptly called "a home away from home." Community breakfasts with other lodgers and hosts enhance this feeling. Each B&B is as unique as its owner. Décor varies according to the region of location and the unique taste of its owner. The owner of the bed and breakfast often provides all the necessary labor, but some employ full- or part-time help.

▶ Check Your Knowledge

1. What characteristics do the following hotel segments encompass?
    a. City center hotels
    b. Resort hotels
    c. Airport hotels
    d. Freeway hotels and motels

e. Full-service hotels

f. Economy/budget hotels

g. Extended-stay hotels

h. Bed and breakfast inns

Best, Biggest, and Most Unusual Hotels and Chains

So, which is the best hotel in the world? The answer may depend on whether you watch the Travel Channel or read polls taken by a business investment or travel magazine. Magazines like *Travel + Leisure* and web sites like Trip Advisor invite readers to vote for their favorite hotels and then they publish the list, so it's more of a popularity poll. However, the results are interesting and are not split into several categories: best in Asia, best in the Caribbean, best romantic, best city, and so on. One recent list had the Golden Well, Prague, Czech Republic, as number one, whereas another had Oberoi Vanyavilas, Rajasthan, India. High on the list was the Fairmont Mara Safari Club, Masai Mara, Kenya, and the Earth Lodge at Sabi Sabi Private Game Reserve, Kruger National Park, Southern Africa. The Oriental Hotel in Bangkok, Thailand, has been rated number one in the world; so, too, has the Regent of Hong Kong, the Mandarin Oriental of Hong Kong, and the Connaught of London. Each "list" picks other hotels. The largest hotel in the world is the Izmailovo Hotel in Moscow with 7,500 rooms, followed by the 7,372-room MGM Grand in Las Vegas and the Venetian Hotel, also in Las Vegas, which has 7,117 rooms.

The Best Hotel Chains

The Ritz-Carlton and the Four Seasons are generally rated the highest-quality large chain hotels. The Ritz-Carlton Hotel Company has received all the major awards the hospitality industry and leading consumer organizations can bestow. It has received the Malcolm Baldrige National Quality Award from the United States Department of Commerce—the first and only hotel company to win the award and the first and only service company to win the award two times, in 1999 and 1992. Ritz-Carlton has long been recognized as the best luxury hotel chain in the industry. Amanresorts has been awarded the Zagat best hotel group in the world, and Rosewood Hotels and Resorts have several outstanding properties.

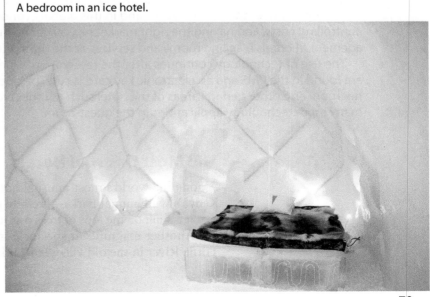

A bedroom in an ice hotel.

TECHNOLOGY SPOTLIGHT

The Use of Technology in Property Management

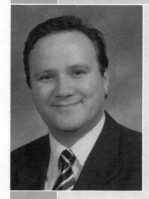

Cihan Cobanoglu, Ph.D., Dean, School of Hotel and Restaurant Management, University of South Florida, Sarasota-Manatee

Technology has become an inseparable part of the hotel business. In a typical full-service hotel, there are about sixty-five different technology applications. This number is around thirty-five for a limited-service hotel. The use of technology starts even before a guest checks in to a hotel. More than half of the hotel guests book their hotel rooms electronically. This means that guests use either direct or indirect reservation/distribution channels. Direct reservation/distribution channels include walk-in, phone call to the hotel, hotel's web site, and hotel chain's web site (central reservation system). Indirect reservation/distribution channels include online travel agencies such as Expedia.com, Travelocity.com, Orbitz.com, and opaque travel agencies where the consumer does not know the brand of the hotel until after the purchase is completed. These opaque online travel agencies include priceline.com and Hotwire.com. A distribution/reservation system typically performs the following basic functions: (1) selling individual reservations, (2) selling group reservations, (3) displaying room availability and guest lists, (4) tracking advance deposits, (5) tracking travel agent bookings and commissions, and (6) generating confirmation letters and e-mails and various reports.

Each hotel has a property management system (PMS). The functions of the PMS are enabling guest reservations, enabling guest check-in/out, enabling staff to maintain guest facilities, keeping accounting for a guest's financial transactions, and tracking guest activities. The PMS is often interfaced to central reservation systems and global reservation systems. This way, when a guest makes a reservation from a hotel chain's web site such as Hilton.com or Marriott.com, the reservation is automatically transferred to the hotel's property reservation system. This interface allows the hotel to control the room inventory on a real-time basis and to manage the revenue management process efficiently. The revenue management module of the PMS also uses advanced technology systems. Hotels use the revenue management system to calculate the rates, rooms, and restrictions on sales in order to best maximize the return. These systems measure constrained and unconstrained demand along with pace to gauge which restrictions—for example, length of stay, nonrefundable rate, or close to arrival. Revenue management teams in the hotel industry have evolved tremendously over the last ten years, and in this global economy, targeting the right distribution channels, controlling costs, and having the right market mix plays an important role in yield management. Yield management in hotels is selling rooms and services at the right price, at the right time, to the right people.

The use of technology continues after the reservation. When the guest checks in, the reservation details are found in the PMS and an electronic key card is cut. The guest can use this electronic card to access his or her room and other general areas of the hotel such as fitness room, pool area, and concierge club. There are many more technology applications in the guest-room.

The Most Unusual Hotels

Among the world's most unusual hotels are ones like the Treetops Hotel in one of Kenya's wild animal parks—literally in the treetops. The uniqueness of the hotel is that it is built on the tops of trees overlooking a wild animal watering hole in the park.

Another magnificent spectacle is the Ice Hotel, situated on the shores of the Torne River in the old village of Jukkasjäsvi in Swedish Lapland. The Ice Hotel is built from scratch on an annual basis with a completely new design, new suites, new departments, even the "Absolut Ice Bar," a bar carved in ice with ice glasses and ice plates. The Ice Hotel can accommodate more than one hundred guests, with each room having its own distinct style. The hotel also has an ice chapel, an ice art exhibition hall, and, believe it or not, a cinema.

Australia boasts an underwater hotel at the Great Barrier Reef, where guests have wonderful underwater views from their rooms.

Japan has several unusual hotels. One is a cocoon-like hotel, called Capsule Hotel, in which guests do not have a room as such. Instead, they have a space of about 4 feet by 7 feet. In this space is a bed and a television—which guests almost have to operate with their toes! Such hotels are popular with people who get caught up in the obligatory late-night drinking with the boss and with visiting professors, and who find them the only affordable place to stay in expensive Tokyo.

The highest hotel in the world, in terms of altitude, is nestled in the Himalayan mountain range at an altitude of 13,000 feet. Weather permitting, there is a marvelous view of Mount Everest. As many as 80 percent of the guests suffer from nausea, headaches, or sleeplessness caused by the altitude. No wonder the hottest-selling item on the room-service menu is oxygen—at $1 a minute.

Vacation Ownership

From its beginnings in the French Alps in the late 1960s, **vacation ownership** has become the fastest-growing segment of the U.S. travel and tourism industry, increasing in popularity at the rate of about 15 percent each year.

Vacation ownership offers consumers the opportunity to purchase fully furnished vacation accommodations in a variety of forms, such as weekly intervals or in points-based systems, for a percentage of the cost of ownership. For a one-time purchase price and payment of a yearly maintenance fee, purchasers own their vacation either in perpetuity (forever) or for a predetermined number of years. Owners share both the use and cost of upkeep of their unit and the common grounds of the resort property. Vacation ownership purchases are typically financed through consumer loans of five to ten years duration, with terms dependent on the purchase price and the amount of the buyer's down payment. The average cost of a vacation ownership is $14,800–$18,500.[19]

Vacation clubs, or point-based programs, provide the flexible use of accommodations in multiple resort locations. With these products, club members purchase points that represent either a travel-and-use membership or a deed real estate product. These points are then used like money to purchase accommodations during a season, for a set number of

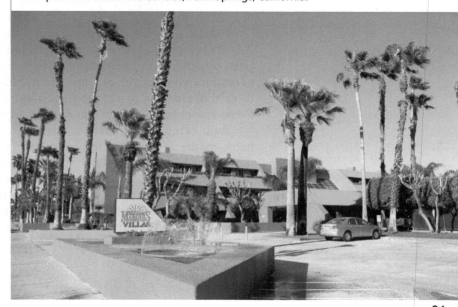

Marquis Villas timeshare condos, Palm Springs, California.

days at a participating resort. The number of points needed to access the resort accommodation varies by the members' demand for unit size, season, resort location, and amenities.

Henry Silverman, formerly of Avis Budget–which owns the Indianapolis, Indiana–based Resort Condominiums International (RCI)–said that a timeshare is really a two-bedroom suite that is owned, rather than a hotel room that is rented for a transient night. A vacation club, on the other hand, is a "travel-and-use" product. Consumers do not buy a fixed week, unit size, season, resort, or number of days to vacation each year. Instead, they purchase points that represent currency, which is used to access the club's vacation benefits. An important advantage to this is the product's flexibility, especially when tied to a point system. Disney Vacation Club is one major company that uses a point system. General manager Mark Pacala states, "The flexibility of choosing among several different vacation experiences is what sets the Disney Vacation Club apart from many similar plans. The vacation points system allows members to select the type of vacation best suited to their needs, particularly as those needs change from year to year." Each year, members choose how to use their vacation points, either for one long vacation or for a series of short getaways.[20]

The World Tourism Organization has called timeshares one of the fastest-growing sectors of the travel and tourism industry. Hospitality companies are adding brand power to the concept with corporations such as Marriott Vacation Club International, the Walt Disney Company, Hilton Hotels, Hyatt Hotels, Choice Hotels, InterContinental, and even the Ritz-Carlton and Four Seasons participating in an industry that has grown rapidly in recent years. Still, only about 4 percent of all U.S. households hold vacation ownership. RCI estimates that the figure could rise to 10 percent within the next decade for households with incomes of more than $75,000. It is not surprising that hotel companies have found this to be a lucrative business.

RCI, the largest vacation ownership exchange (that allows members to exchange vacations with other locations), has more than 2.8 million member families living in 200 countries. There are 3,700 participating resorts, and members can exchange vacation intervals for vacations at any participating resort, and to date, RCI has arranged exchange vacations for more than 54 million people.[21] Vacation ownership is popular at U.S. resorts from Key West in Florida to Kona in Hawaii and from New York City and Las Vegas to Colorado ski resorts.

Interval World is a vacation exchange network made up of more than 2,000 resorts and more than 1.6 million member families worldwide. Interval does not own or manage any of the resorts, but rather provides members— vacation owners from around the world—with a variety of exchange services to enhance their vacation experiences. Members can exchange a stay at their home resort for a stay at one of the timeshares supported by Interval World.

By locking in the purchase price of accommodations, vacation ownership helps ensure future vacations at today's prices at luxurious resorts with amenities, service, and ambience that rival any of the world's top-rated vacation destinations. Through vacation exchange programs, timeshare owners can travel to other popular destinations around the world. With unparalleled flexibility and fully equipped condominiums that offer the best in holiday luxury, vacation ownership puts consumers in the driver's seat, allowing them to plan and enjoy vacations that suit their lifestyle.

Timeshare resort developers today include many of the world's leading hoteliers, publicly held corporations, and independent companies. Properties that combine vacation ownership resorts with hotels, adventure resorts, and gaming resorts are among the emerging timeshare trends. The reasons for purchasing most frequently cited by current timeshare owners are the high standards of quality accommodations and service at the resorts where they own and exchange, the flexibility offered through the vacation exchange opportunities, and the cost effectiveness of vacation ownership. Nearly one-third of vacation owners purchase additional intervals after experiencing ownership. This trend is even stronger among long-time owners: More than 40 percent of those who have owned for eight years or longer have purchased additional intervals within the timeshare.

Travel the World through Exchange Vacations

Vacation ownership offers unparalleled flexibility and the opportunity for affordable worldwide travel through vacation ownership exchange. Through the international vacation exchange networks, owners can trade their timeshare intervals for vacation time at comparable resorts around the world. Most resorts are affiliated with an exchange company that administers the exchange service for its members. Typically, the exchange company directly solicits annual membership. Owners individually elect to become members of the affiliated exchange company. To exchange, the owner places his or her interval into the exchange company's pool of resorts and weeks available for exchange and, in turn, chooses an available resort and week from that pool. The exchange company charges an exchange fee, in addition to an annual membership fee, to complete an exchange. Exchange companies and resorts frequently offer their members the additional benefit of saving or banking vacation time in a reserve program for use in a different year.

International Perspective

We are all part of a huge global economy that is splintered into massive trading blocks, such as the European Union (EU) and the North American Free Trade Agreement (NAFTA) among Canada, the United States, and Mexico, with a total population of 441 million consumers.[22]

The EU, with a population of more than 501 million people in twenty-seven nations, is an economic union that has removed national boundaries and restrictions not only on trade but also on the movement of capital and labor.[23] The synergy developed between these twenty-seven member nations is beneficial to all and is a form of self-perpetuating development. As travel, tourism, commerce, and industry have increased within the European Economic Community (EEC), which could soon expand by another five nations, and more in the future, so has the need for hotel accommodations.

In the Middle East, in countries like Dubai and Abu Dhabi, United Arab Emirates, several very impressive hotels

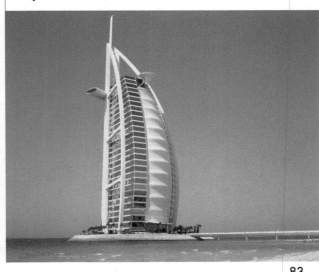

Burj Al Arab hotel, Dubai, United Arab Emirates.

and resorts have been added as part of a strategy to encourage more tourism to and within the region and the world. Once the airport is capable of handling several international flights daily, then soon hotels are built to cater to the traveler's needs. Now, these cities are gateways to the region and host international conferences.

NAFTA will likely be a similar catalyst for hotel development in response to increased trade and tourism among the three countries involved. But Argentina, Brazil, Chile, and Venezuela may also join an expanded NAFTA, which would become known as the Americas Trading Bloc.

It is easy to understand the international development of hotels given the increase in international tourism trade and commerce. The growth in tourism in Pacific Rim countries is expected to continue at the same rate as in recent years. Several resorts have been developed in Indonesia, Malaysia, Thailand, and Vietnam, and China and India have both seen hotel growth. Further international hotel development opportunities exist in Eastern Europe, Russia, and the other republics of the former Soviet Union, where some companies have changed their growth strategy from building new hotels to acquiring and renovating existing properties.

In Asia, Hong Kong's growth has been encouraged by booming economies throughout Southeast Asia and the kind of tax system for which supply-siders hunger. The Hong Kong government levies a flat 16.5 percent corporate tax, a 15 percent individual income tax, and no tax on capital gains or dividends. Several hotel corporations have their headquarters in Hong Kong. Among them are Mandarin Oriental, Peninsula, and Shangri-La, all world-renowned for their five-star status. They are based in Hong Kong because of low corporate taxation and the ability to bring in senior expatriate executives with minimal bureaucratic difficulty.[24]

In developing countries, once political stability has been sustained, hotel development quickly follows as part of an overall economic and social progression. An example of this is the former Eastern European countries and former Soviet republics that for the past few years have offered development opportunities for hotel corporations.

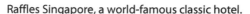

Raffles Singapore, a world-famous classic hotel.

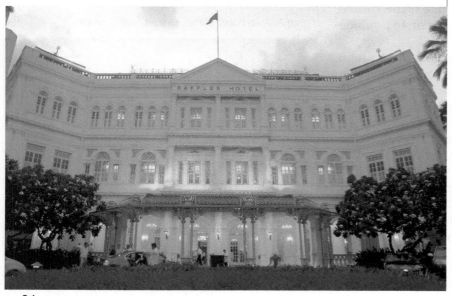

Sustainable or Green Lodging

Today, of necessity, developers are more environmentally conscious because it can cost far more not only to build a lodging facility but also to run it if it is not sustainable. By using local materials, a new hotel or resort can save money on the cost of materials plus the cost of transporting those materials from a distance, or even importing them. Given the weak U.S. dollar, it increases costs if materials must be imported.

The cost of energy has increased so much in recent years that lodging construction now incorporates ways of using natural lighting and building energy-efficient buildings. Energy-efficient buildings require far less air-conditioning than do conventional buildings because they use materials such as darkened glass and lower-wattage lighting that produces lower temperatures.

How can hotels, motels, lodges, and resorts become more sustainable? Reducing and eliminating waste can produce the biggest positive environmental impact. This can be accomplished through a number of practices, including sustainable lighting and water conservation. A property with 300 guest rooms can spend $300,000 per year on electricity and $50,000 on natural gas, and another $60,000 annually on water and sewer.[25]

Lighting can account for 30 to 40 percent of commercial electricity consumption. This can be reduced by the following strategies:

- Use lighting only when necessary—employ motion detectors.
- Use energy-efficient fixtures and lamps.
- Use low-wattage lighting for signs and décor.
- Avoid over-lighting wherever possible.

Water conservation is another method that can greatly reduce waste. Today, many hotels are replacing showerheads, toilets, and faucets with low-flow water devices. Low-flow showerheads can save 10 gallons of water every five minutes of showering. That means a savings of over $3,000 annually if one hundred people shower each day, and water and sewer costs are one cent per gallon.[26] Other water conservation methods include only washing full loads of dishes and laundry, serving drinking water by request only, asking guests to consider reusing towels, and restricting lawn watering.

Fairmont Hotels and Resorts[27] are among the leading sustainable lodging companies whose projects fall into three key areas: (1) minimizing the company's impact on the environment by making ongoing operational improvements, mainly in waste management and energy and water conservation; (2) working at a corporate level to foster high-profile partnerships and accreditations that help promote environmental issues and to share its stewardship message; and (3) to follow best practices, which include working at individual properties to develop innovative ways to reduce the carbon footprint of hotels.

Career Information

A variety of career options are directly and indirectly related to hotel development and classification. Some examples include working in the corporate office to develop hotels or searching out locations, negotiating the deals, and/or organizing the construction or alterations. This involves knowledge of operations plus expertise in marketing, feasibility studies, finance, and planning.

Similarly, consulting firms like PKF have interesting positions for consultants who provide specialized services in feasibility studies, marketing, human resources, and accounting and finance due diligence (a check to ensure that the cost of purchasing a property is reasonable and that all systems are in working order). Working for a consulting firm usually requires a master's degree plus operational experience in an area of specialty. AAA and Mobil both have inspectors who check hotel standards. Inspectors are required to travel and write detailed reports on the properties at which they stay.

Good advice comes from Jim McManemon, general manager of the Ritz-Carlton, Sarasota, Florida: "It is important to have a love of people, as there is so much interaction with them. I also suggest working in the industry to gain experience. Actually, it is a good idea to work in various departments while going to school so you can either join a management-training program or take a supervisory or assistant management position upon graduation. Work hard, be a leader, and set an example for the people working with you."[28]

Go to the university relations web site for Wyndham Hotels and scroll down to see what advice is given: www.wyndhamworldwide.com/careers/university.html.

Trends in Hotel Development

- *Capacity control.* Refers to who will control the sale of inventories of hotel rooms, airline seats, auto rentals, and tickets to attractions. Presently, owners of these assets are in control of their sale and distribution, but increasingly control is falling into the hands of those who own and manage global reservation systems and/or negotiate for large buying groups. Factors involved in the outcome will be telecommunications, software, available satellite capacity, governmental regulations, limited capital, and the travel distribution network.

- *Safety and security.* Important aspects of safety and security are terrorism, the growing disparity between the haves and have-nots in the world, diminishing financial resources, infrastructure problems, health issues, the stability of governments, and personal security.

- *Assets and capital.* The issues concerning assets and capital are rationing of private capital and rationing of funds deployed by governments.

- *Technology.* An example of the growing use of *expert systems* (a basic form of artificial intelligence) would be making standard operating procedures available online, twenty-four hours a day, and establishing yield management systems designed to make pricing decisions. Other examples include increasing numbers of smart hotel room and communications ports to make virtual office environments for business travelers and the impact of technology on the structure of corporate offices and individual hotels.

- *New management.* The complex forces of capacity control, safety and security, capital movement, and technology issues will require a future management cadre that is able to adapt to rapid-paced change across all the traditional functions of management.

- *Globalization.* A number of U.S. and Canadian chains have developed and are continuing to develop hotels around the world. International companies are also investing in the North American hotel industry.

- *Consolidation.* As the industry matures, corporations are either acquiring or merging with each other.

- *Diversification within segments of the lodging industry.* The economy segment now has low-, medium-, and high-end properties. The extended-stay market has a similar spread of properties, as do all the other hotel classifications.

CASE STUDY

In recent years, several new lodging brands have been introduced by leading hotel chains to the market. Among the names of these brands are DoubleTree, Candlewood Suites, Homewood Suites, Mainstay, Spring Hill Suites, and so on. In addition, there is Hyatt, which recently purchased AmeriSuites, which it has renovated and now calls Hyatt Place.

A hot trend in lodging development is condo hotels, called condotels. With condotels, a developer can more quickly raise the funds necessary from investors than from other traditional sources such as banks and finance houses. As a result, it makes sense for developers to encourage investors by offering an arrangement for owners to have exclusive use of the unit for a fixed number of days a year (typically 30–60 days) and for the hotel company to rent out the units/rooms for the remainder of the year. The cost of development is high and ranges from an average of $800 to $900 per square foot up to a high of $1,400. Projects such as the Residences at MGM Grand Las Vegas, which sold more than $1 billion, or the Hard Rock Hotel and Casino, also in Las Vegas, which launched 1,300 units in less than ten weeks, are amazing. Other areas of the United States are good existing or potential markets for condotel development.

Despite the rave reviews on Wall Street for condotels, there are some unresolved issues. With time, who will develop and pay for the replacement of furniture fixtures and equipment (FF&E)? What are the association dues and what form will the relationship take between owners, the developer, and the hotel company? There are the additional complexities for the hotel operator—such as space for meetings, restaurants, and recreation—and how many rooms will be available on any given night. Yet, the payoffs for both individual investors–owners and hotel operating companies—are good to great. With 78 million baby boomers ready to retire, the prospects look very good to all concerned.

Discussion Questions

1. So what is in a name? Is Hyatt right to use the name Hyatt Place?
2. Is InterContinental or Hilton wrong not to include their name, as in Hilton Hampton Inn or Hampton Inn by Hilton? What is your opinion?
3. Which other areas of the United States are good potential locations for condotels and why?
4. Will condotels split into various segments like other lodging properties have?

- *Rapid growth in vacation ownership.* Vacation ownership is the fastest-growing segment of the lodging industry and is likely to continue growing as the baby boomers enter their fifties and sixties.
- *An increase in the number of spas and the treatments offered.* Wellness and the road to nirvana are in increasing demand as guests seek release from the stresses of a fast-paced lifestyle.
- *Gaming.* An increasing number of hotels are coming online that are related to the gaming industry.
- *Mixed-use properties.* An increasing number of hotels are being developed as multiuse properties, meaning hotels with residences (condominiums), spas, and recreational facilities.
- *Sustainable lodging development.* There is increasing development of lodging facilities with environmentally designs, construction, and operating procedures.

Summary

1. Improved transportation has changed the nature of the hotel industry from small, independently owned inns to big hotel and lodging chains that are operated using concepts such as franchising and management contracts.
2. Hotels can be classified according to location (city center, resort, airport, freeway), types of services offered (casino, convention), and price (luxury, midscale, budget, and economy). Hotels are rated by Mobil and AAA (five-star or five-diamond rankings).
3. Vacation ownership offers consumers the opportunity to purchase fully furnished vacation accommodations, similar to condominiums, sold in a variety of forms, such as weekly intervals or point-based systems, for only a percentage of the cost of full ownership. According to the World Tourism Organization, timeshares are one of the fastest-growing sectors of the travel and tourism industry.
4. Every part of the world offers leisure and business travelers a choice of unusual or conservative accommodations that cater to personal ideas of vacation or business trips.
5. The future of tourism involves international expansion and foreign investment, often in combination with airlines, and with the goal of improving economic conditions in developing countries. It is further influenced by increased globalization, as evidenced by such agreements as NAFTA.

Key Words and Concepts

capital intensive
fair return on investment
feasibility study
direct economic impact

indirect economic impact
franchising
management contracts
real estate investment trusts (REITs)

referral associations
vacation ownership

Review Questions

1. What are the advantages of (a) management contracts and (b) franchising? Discuss their impacts on the development of the hotel industry.
2. Explain how hotels cater to the needs of business and leisure travelers in reference to the following concepts: (a) resorts, (b) airport hotels, and (c) vertical integration.
3. Explain what vacation ownership is. What are the different types of timeshare programs available for purchase?

Internet Exercises

1. Organization: **Hilton Hotels**
   Web site: **www.hiltonworldwide.com**
   Summary: Hilton Hotels Corporation and Hilton International have a worldwide alliance to market Hilton. Hilton is recognized as one of the world's best-known hotel brands. Collectively, Hilton offers more than 3,600 hotels in more than 66 countries, truly a major player in the hospitality industry.
   (a) What are the different hotel brands that can be franchised through Hilton Hotels Corporation?
   (b) What are your views on Hilton's portfolio and franchising options? click on "Hilton Worldwide Brands."

2. Organization: *Hotels* **Magazine**
   Web site: **www.hotelsmag.com**
   Summary: *Hotels* magazine is a publication that offers vast amounts of information on the hospitality industry with up-to-date industry news, corporate trends, and nationwide developments.
   (a) What are some of the top headlines currently being reported in the industry?
   (b) Click on "Print Magazine Archives," click on the icon for the October 2010 edition, and then go to page 22 of the online magazine. Browse through the corporate rankings and industry leaders. List the top five hotel corporations and note how many rooms each one has.

Apply Your Knowledge

1. From a career perspective, what are the advantages and disadvantages of each type of hotel?
2. If you were going into the lodging sector, which type of property would you prefer to work at and why?

Suggested Activities

1. Identify which kind of hotel you would like to work at and give reasons why.

Endnotes

1. http://www.bostonhistorycollaborative.org/BostonFamilyHistory/ancestors/english/eng_1650.html (accessed February 16, 2011); Donald E. Lundberg, *The Hotel and Restaurant Business*, 6th ed. (New York: Van Nostrand Reinhold, 1994), 28–29; John Caprarella, et al.: *The History of Lodging: The Hotel in America*, 2002.

2. New York Architecture, *The Plaza Hotel*, www.nyc-architecture.com/MID/MID056.htm (accessed October 26, 2011).

3. Source company web sites and "HOTELS' 325," *Hotels*, October 2010, www.marketingandtechnology.com/repository/webFeatures/HOTELS/2010giants.pdf (accessed February 23, 2011).

4. This section is courtesy of Robert Kok, Professor, Johnson and Wales University.

5. Wyndham Worldwide, *Wyndham Hotel Group*, www.wyndhamworldwide.com/about/wyndham_hotel_group.cfm (accessed February 22, 2011).

6. WorldMark by Wyndham, *About Wyndham*, www.worldmarkbywyndham.com/about/ (accessed February 22, 2011).

7. Ibid.

8. Wyndham Worldwide, *Wyndham Exchange & Rentals*, www.wyndhamworldwide.com/about/wyndham_exchange_and_rentals.cfm (accessed February 22, 2011).

9. Personal conversation with Bruce Goodwin, President of Goodwin and Associates hotel consultants, May 4, 2011.

10. Kimpton Hotels & Restaurants, *About Us*, www.kimptonhotels.com/about-us/about-us.aspx (accessed February 22, 2011).

11. Marriott International, Inc., *Our Brands: Autograph Collection*, www.marriott.com/corporateinfo/glance.mi#brand4 (accessed February 18, 2011).

12. Hyatt Corporation, *Our Brands: Andaz*, www.hyatt.com/hyatt/about/our-brands/andaz.jsp (accessed February 18, 2011).

13. American Hotel & Lodging Association, *Press Release: 2008 Study on Hotel Room Taxes Quantifies Economic Impact*, www.ahla.com/pressrelease.aspx?id=22524 (accessed on February 24, 2011).

14. Adapted from the American Hotel & Lodging Association's Economic Impact of Hotels and Motels.

15. American Hotel & Lodging Association, *AH&LA Lodging Industry Profile (LIP) Archive: 2010*, www.ahla.com/content.aspx?id=30505 (accessed February 18, 2011).

16. Barbara De Lollis, "AAA Announces Five Diamond Hotels for 2011," *USA Today Travel*, http://travel.usatoday.com/hotels/post/2011/01/aaa-five-diamond-awards-hotels-restaurants/138554/1 (accessed February 18, 2011).

17. InterContinental Hotels Group, *Hotel Indigo: Our Story*, www.ichotelsgroup.com/h/d/in/1/en/c/2/content/dec/teaser/in/1/en/lp/read_our_story.html (accessed October 26, 2011).

18. "What Is a Bed and Breakfast Inn?" *TravelASSIST*, January 1996, www.travelassist.com/mag/a88.html (accessed October 26, 2011).

19. Great Escapes, *Home Page*, www.greatescapesonline.com/Visitor/Ownership.aspx (accessed February 19, 2011); Resort Condominiums International, *About Us*, www.rci.com/RCI/prelogin/aboutUs.do (accessed February 19, 2011).

20. Lynn Sheldon, "Timeshare Concept Adopted by Hotel Industry," *Rhode Island Roads*, www.riroads.com/archive/timesharehotels.htm (accessed October 26, 2011).

21. Resort Condominiums International, *RCI Milestones*, www.rci.com/RCI/RCIW/RCIW_index?body=RCIW_Milestone&action=aboutrci (accessed October 26, 2011).

22. NAFTANOW.org, *Fast Facts: North American Free Trade Agreement*, www.naftanow.org/facts/default_en.asp (accessed February 24, 2011).

23. Matej Hruska, "EU Population Tops 500 Million," *Bloomberg Businessweek*, July 29, 2010, www.businessweek.com/globalbiz/content/jul2010/gb20100729_623637.htm (accessed on February 24, 2011).

24. Personal conversation with Leonard Gordon, March 15, 2006.

25. N.C. Division of Pollution Prevention and Environmental Assistance (DPPEA), *Hotel/Motel Waste Reduction: Facilities Management*, www.p2pays.org/ref/14/13910.pdf (retrieved February 24, 2011).

26. Ibid.

27. Fairmont Hotels & Resorts, Green Partnership Program, www.fairmont.com/EN_FA/AboutFairmont/environment/GreenPartnershipProgram/ (accessed February 25, 2011).

28. Personal interview with Jim McManemon, General Manager, Ritz-Carlton, Sarasota, Florida, and Chris Bryant, Guest Services Manager, Grand Hyatt, Tampa Bay, Florida, February 26, 2011.

Glossary

Capital intensive   Something requiring a lot of capital.

Fair return on investment   A reasonable return for the amount invested.

Franchising   A concept that allows a company to expand quickly by allowing qualified people to use the systems, marketing, and purchasing power of the franchiser.

Indirect economic impact   An economic impact that is not direct.

Management contract   A written agreement between an owner and an operator of a hotel or motor inn by which the owner employs the operator as an agent (employee) to assume full responsibility for operating and managing the property.

Real Estate Investment Trust (REIT)   A method that enables small investors to combine their funds and protects them from the double taxation levied against an ordinary corporation or trust; designed to facilitate investment in real estate in much the same way a mutual fund facilitates investment in securities.

Referral associations   Associations that refer guests to other participating members.

Vacation ownership   Offers consumers the opportunity to purchase fully furnished vacation accommodations in a variety of forms, such as weekly intervals or points in point-based systems, for a percentage of the cost of full ownership.

Photo Credits

Credits are listed in the order of appearance.

Rooms Division Operations

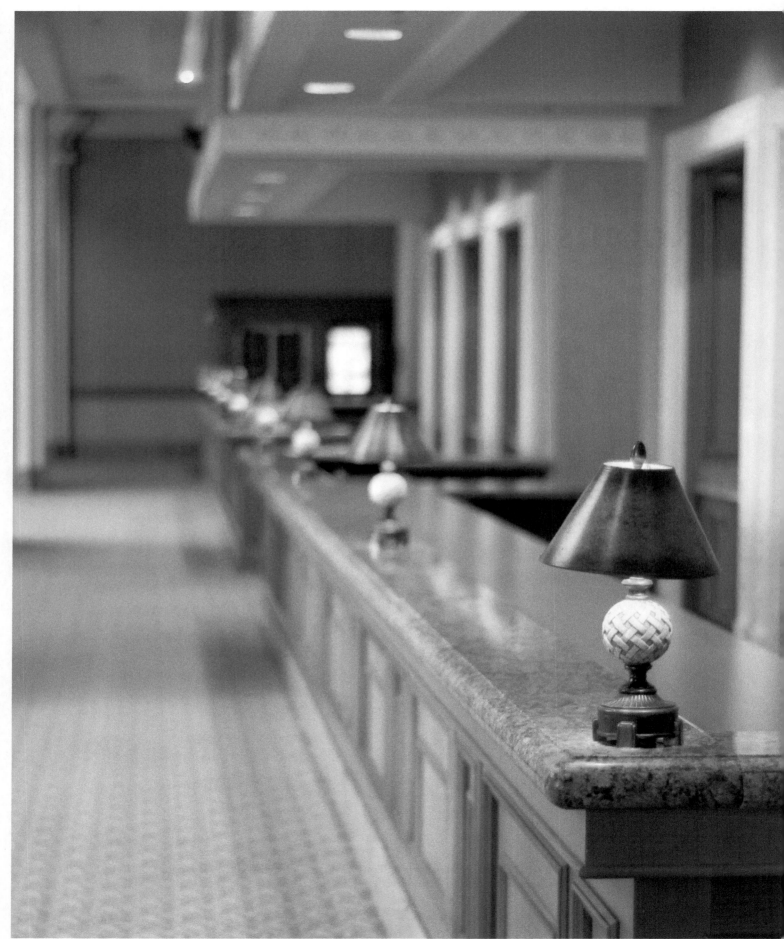

Rooms Division Operations

OBJECTIVES

After reading and studying this chapter, you should be able to:

- Outline the duties and responsibilities of key executives and department heads.

- Draw an organizational chart of the rooms division of a hotel and identify the executive committee members.

- Describe the main functions of the rooms division departments.

- Describe property management systems and discuss yield management.

- Calculate occupancy percentages, average daily rates, and actual percentage of potential rooms revenue.

- Outline the importance of the reservations and guest services functions.

- List the complexities and challenges of the concierge, housekeeping, and security/loss prevention departments.

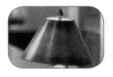 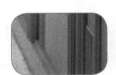 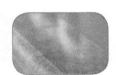 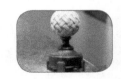

This chapter examines the function of a hotel and the many departments that constitute a hotel. It also helps to explain why and how the departments are interdependent in successfully running a hotel.

The Functions and Departments of a Hotel

The primary function of a hotel is to provide lodging accommodation. A large hotel is run by a general manager and an executive committee that consists of the key executives who head the major departments: rooms division director, food and beverage director, marketing and sales director, human resources director, chief accountant or controller, and chief engineer or facility manager. These executives generally have a regional or corporate counterpart with whom they have a reporting relationship, although the general manager is their immediate superior.

A hotel is made up of several businesses or **revenue centers** and **cost centers**. A few thousand products and services are sold every day. Each area of specialty requires dedication and a quality commitment for each department to get little things right all the time. Furthermore, hotels need the cooperation of a large and diverse group of people to perform well. James McManemon, the general manager (GM) of the elegant Ritz-Carlton Sarasota hotel, calls it "a business of details."[1]

Hotels are places of glamour that may be awe inspiring. Even the experienced hotel person is impressed by the refined dignity of a beautiful hotel like a Ritz-Carlton or the artistic splendor of a Hyatt. The atmosphere of a hotel is stimulating to a hospitality student. Let us step into an imaginary hotel to feel the excitement and become a part of the rush that is similar to show business, for a hotel is live theater and the GM is the director of the cast of players.

Hotels, whether they are chain affiliated or independent properties, exist to serve and enrich society and at the same time make a profit for the owners. Frequently, hotels are just like pieces of property on a Monopoly board. They often make or lose more money with equity appreciation or depreciation than through operations. Hotels have been described as "people palaces." Some are certainly palatial, and others are more functional. Hotels are meant to provide all the comforts of home to those away from home.

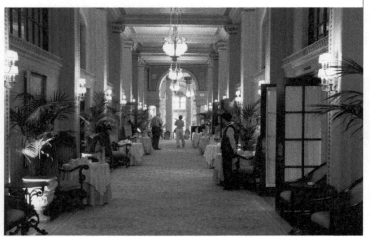

The Grand Hall in the Willard InterContinental, Washington, D.C. It was at this hotel that the term *lobbyist* was coined when then-President Grant would retire after dinner to an armchair in the lobby. People would approach him and try to gain his support for their causes.

Management Structure

Management structure differs among larger, midscale, and smaller properties. The midscale and smaller properties are less complex in their management structures than are the larger ones. However, someone must be responsible for each of the key result areas that make the operation successful. For example, a small property may not have a director of human resources, but each department head will have general day-to-day operating responsibilities for the human resources function. The manager has the ultimate responsibility for all human resources decisions. The same scenario is possible with each of the following areas: engineering and maintenance, accounting and finance, marketing and sales, food and beverage management, and so on.

Role of the Hotel General Manager

Hotel general managers have a lot of responsibilities. They must provide owners with a reasonable return on investment, keep guests satisfied and returning, and keep employees happy. This may seem easy, but because there are so many interpersonal transactions and because hotels are open every day, all day, the complexities of operating become challenges that the general manager must face and overcome. The GM not only focuses on leading and operating the hotel departments but also on aspects of the infrastructure, from room atmosphere to security.

Larger hotels can be more impersonal. Here, the general manager may only meet and greet a few VIPs. In the smaller property, it is easier—though no less important—for the GM to become acquainted with guests to ensure that their stay is memorable and to secure their return. One way that experienced GMs can meet guests, even in large hotels, is to be visible in the lobby and food and beverage (F&B) outlets at peak times (checkout, lunch, check-in, and dinner time). Guests like to feel that the GM takes a personal interest in their well-being. Max Blouet, who was general manager of the famous George V Hotel in Paris for more than thirty years, was a master of this art. He was always present at the right moment to meet and greet guests during the lunch hour and at the evening check-in. Great hoteliers always remember they are hosts.

The GM is ultimately responsible for the performance of the hotel and the employees. The GM is the leader of the hotel. As such, she or he is held accountable for the hotel's level of profitability by the corporation or owners.

To be successful, GMs need to have a broad range of personal qualities. Among those most often quoted by GMs are the following:

- Leadership
- Attention to detail
- Follow-through—getting the job done
- People skills
- Patience
- Ability to delegate effectively

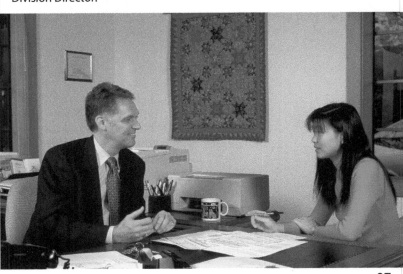

A General Manager discussing the "forecast" with a Rooms Division Director.

INTRODUCING CESAR RITZ

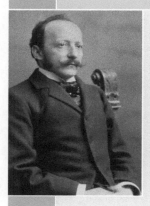

Cesar Ritz was a legend in his own time; like so many of the early industry leaders, he began at the bottom and worked his way up through the ranks. In his case, it did not take long to reach the top because he quickly learned the secrets of success in the hotel business. His career began as an apprenticed hotel keeper at the age of fifteen. At nineteen, he was managing a Parisian restaurant. Suddenly, he quit that position to become an assistant waiter at the famous Voisin restaurant. There he learned how to pander to the rich and famous. In fact, he became so adept at taking care of the guests—remembering their likes and dislikes, even their idiosyncrasies—that a guest would ask for him and would only be served by him.

At twenty-two, he became manager of the Grand National Hotel in Lucerne, Switzerland, one of the most luxurious hotels in the world. The hotel was not very successful at the time Ritz became manager, but with his ingenuity and panache, he was able to attract the "in" crowd to complete a turnaround. After eleven seasons, he accepted a bigger challenge, the Savoy Hotel in London, which had only been open a few months and which was not doing well. Cesar Ritz became manager of one of the most famous and luxurious hotels in the world at the age of thirty-eight.

Once again, his flair and ability to influence society quickly made a positive impression on the hotel. To begin with, he made the hotel a cultural center for high society. Together with Escoffier as executive chef, he created a team that produced the finest cuisine in Europe in the most elegant of surroundings. He made evening dress compulsory and introduced orchestras to the restaurants. Cesar Ritz would spare no expense to create the lavish effect he sought. On one occasion, he converted a riverside restaurant into a Venetian waterway, complete with small gondolas and gondoliers singing Italian love songs.[2]

Both Ritz and Escoffier were dismissed from the Savoy in 1897. Ritz was implicated in the disappearance of over 3,400 pounds of wine and spirits.[3] In 1898, Ritz opened the celebrated Hotel Ritz in the Place Vendome, Paris, France. The Hotel Ritz Madrid in Madrid, Spain, opened in 1910, inspired by King Alfonso XIII's desire to build a luxury hotel to rival the Ritz in Paris. Ritz enjoyed a long partnership with Escoffier, the famous French chef and father of modern French cooking.[4]

Ritz considered the handling of people as the most important of all qualities for a hotelier. His imagination and sensitivity to people and their wants contributed to a new standard of hotel keeping. The Ritz name remains synonymous with refined, elegant hotels and service.[5] However, Ritz drove himself to the point of exhaustion, and at age fifty-two, he suffered a nervous breakdown. So, this is a lesson for us not to drive ourselves too much to the point of exhaustion.

A successful GM selects and trains the best people. A former GM of Chicago's Four Seasons Hotel deliberately hired division heads who knew more about what they were hired for than he did. The GM sets the tone—a structure of excellence—and others try to match it. Once the structure is in place, each employee works to define the hotel's commitment to excellence. General managers need to understand, empathize, and allow for the cultures of both guests and employees. Progressive general managers empower associates to do anything legal to delight the guest.

The Executive Committee

The general manager, using input from the **executive committee** (Figure 1), makes all the major decisions affecting the hotel. These executives, who include the directors of human resources, food and beverage, rooms division, marketing and sales, engineering, and accounting, compile the hotel's occupancy forecast together with all revenues and expenses to make up the budget. They generally meet once a week for one or two hours—although the Ritz-Carlton has a daily lineup at 9 A.M.—and might typically cover some of the following topics:

Guest satisfaction

Employee satisfaction

Total quality management

Occupancy forecasts

Sales and marketing plans

Training

Major items of expenditure

Renovations

Ownership relations

Energy conservation

Recycling

New legislation

Profitability

Some GMs rely on input from the executive committee more than others do, depending on their leadership and management style. These senior executives determine the character of the property and decide on the missions, goals,

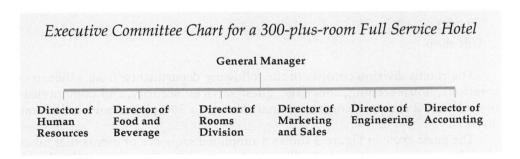

Executive Committee Chart for a 300-plus-room Full Service Hotel

General Manager

| Director of Human Resources | Director of Food and Beverage | Director of Rooms Division | Director of Marketing and Sales | Director of Engineering | Director of Accounting |

Figure 1 • Executive Committee Chart.

and objectives of the hotel. For a chain hotel, this will be in harmony with the corporate mission.

In most hotels, the executive committee is involved with the decisions, but the ultimate responsibility and authority rests with the GM. One major role of the committee is communicator, both up and down the line of authority. This helps build interdepartmental cooperation. Not all lodging operations will have an executive committee—obviously, there is no need for one at a small motel, lodge, or a B&B.

▶ Check Your Knowledge

1. What is the role of the general manager?
2. Who is a member of the executive committee and what topics does this person deal with?

The Departments

In larger hotels, the rooms division has several departments that all work together to please guests. In midsize and smaller properties, those departments may be reduced in size and number, but they still need to serve guests.

Rooms Division

The rooms division director is held responsible by the GM for the efficient and effective leadership and operation of all the rooms division departments. They include concerns such as the following:

Financial responsibility for rooms division

Employee satisfaction goals

Guest satisfaction goals

Guest services

Guest relations

Security

Gift shop

The **rooms division** consists of the following departments: front office, reservations, housekeeping, concierge, guest services, security, and communications. Figure 2 shows the organizational chart for a 300-plus-room hotel rooms division.

The guest cycle in Figure 3 shows a simplified sequence of events that takes place from the moment a guest calls to make a reservation until he or she checks out.

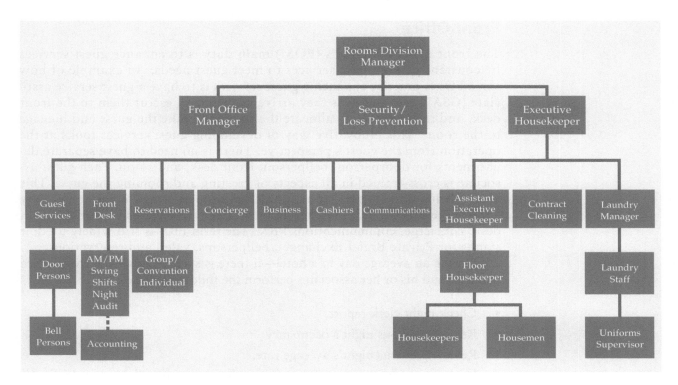

Figure 2 • Rooms Division Organizational Chart.

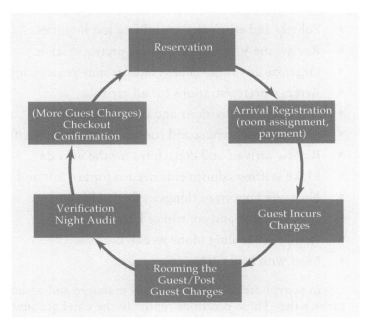

Figure 3 • The Guest Cycle.

Front Office

The front office manager's (FOM) main duty is to enhance guest services by constantly developing services to meet guest needs. An example of how some FOMs practice enhancing guest services is to have a guest service associate (GSA) greet guests as they arrive at the hotel, escort them to the front desk, and then personally allocate the room and take the guest and luggage to the room. This innovative way of developing guest services looks at the operation from the guest's perspective. There is no need to have separate departments for doorperson, bellperson, front desk, and so on. Each guest associate is cross-trained in all aspects of greeting and rooming the guest. This is now being done in smaller and midsized properties as well as at specialty and deluxe properties. Guest service associates are responsible for the front desk, concierge, communications/PBX (The term PBX is still widely used; it stands for Private Brand Exchange), bellpersons, valet, and reservations.

During an average day in a hotel—if there is such a thing—the front office manager and his or her associates perform the following duties:

- Check night clerk report.
- Review previous night's occupancy.
- Review previous night's average rate.
- Look over market mix and determine what rooms to sell at what price.
- Handle checkouts and check-ins.
- Check complimentary rooms.
- Verify group rooms to be picked up for the next thirty days.
- Review arrivals and departures for the day.
- Politely and efficiently attend to guest inquiries.
- Review the VIP list and prepare preregistration.
- Organize any room changes guests may request and follow up.
- Arrange preregistrations for all arrivals.
- Attend rooms divisions and operations meeting.
- Advise housekeeping and room service of flowers/fruit for VIPs.
- Review arrivals and departures for the next day.
- Make staffing adjustments needed for arrivals and departures.
- Note any important things in the log book.
- Check issuing and control of keys.
- Review scheduling (done weekly).
- Meet with lead GSAs (done daily).

In some hotels, the reservations manager and associates report to the director of sales. These positions report to the chief accountant: night auditor, night audit associates, and cashiers.

The front office has been described as the hub or nerve center of the hotel. It is the department that makes a first impression on the guest and one that the guest relies on throughout his or her stay for information and service. Positive first impressions are critical to the successful guest experience. Many guests arrive at the hotel after long, tiring trips. They want to be met by someone with a warm smile and a genuine greeting. If a guest should have a negative experience when checking into a hotel, he or she will be on guard in encounters with each of the other departments. The position description for a guest service agent details the work performed. Position descriptions for the three main functions of the front office are as follows:

1. *To sell rooms.* The hotel departments work like a team in a relay race. Sales or reservations staff make up room sales until the evening before the guest's arrival. At 6:00 P.M., when the reservations office closes, all the expected arrivals and available rooms are then handed over to the front desk P.M. shift. Reservations calls after 6:00 P.M. may either be taken by the front desk staff or the 1–800 number. The front desk team will try to sell out (achieve 100 percent occupancy) by selling the remaining rooms to call-in or walk-in guests—and of course the frantic calls from preferred guests who need a favor!

   Upselling occurs when the guest service agent/front desk clerk suggestively sells the features of a larger room, a higher floor, or perhaps a better view. **Yield management** originated in the airline industry where demand also fluctuates. Basically, a percentage of guests who book and send in a deposit in advance will be able to secure a room at a more reasonable price than can someone booking a room with just three days' notice. The price will be even higher for the booking at three days' notice if demand is good.

   Many other factors influence the hotel's ability to sell out. Chief among these are *demand*—the number of people needing rooms—and *supply*—the number of available rooms. A good example is the New York Hotel Convention. This event takes place in a city that has a high demand for hotel rooms in proportion to its inventory (number of available rooms). Because there is a fairly constant demand for rooms in New York, special events tend to increase demand to a point that forces up **room rates**. (See Figure 4.) Another example comes from the airline industry, which always seems to raise prices at the peak travel times (Thanksgiving, Christmas, Easter, and the summer vacation times). They only offer special fares when school is in session. Revenue management is explained in more detail later in this chapter.

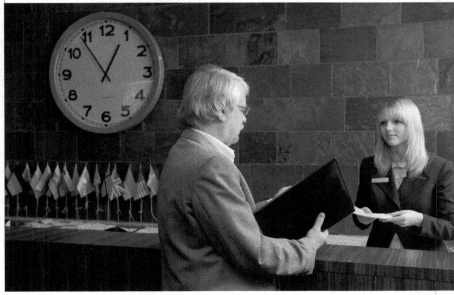

A front office manager taking care of a guest request.

FOCUS ON ROOMS DIVISION

Rooms Division with Charlie Adams

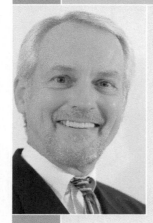

From the early days of primitive inns to our modern super hotels, like the Izmailovo Hotel with 7,500 rooms in Moscow, employees are the crucial ingredient to a hotel or motel's success. Even with extraordinary advances in technology and the globalization of lodging in the 21st century; lodging remains fundamentally a people business and it is the employees who are responsible for the appearance, image and reputation of a lodging facility.

The rooms division is considered the "center" of hotel activity because it is accountable for revenue, customer service, and departmental forecasting. Room sales are the primary source of income for most hotels and almost 100% of the revenue for many select service or budget hotels. The rooms division has the most guest contacts because it is comprised of reservations, front office, housekeeping and uniformed services. The reservations department provides the needed accurate information for other departments to use to forecast for upcoming events and guest needs; along with scheduling the proper staffing levels in the hotel.

Starting your career in the rooms division of a hotel is an exciting, demanding and rewarding experience. You will be part of a team whose overall responsibility is the well-being of guests and ensuring their expectations are met and they have a memorable experience. As a room division employee you will be part of several interconnected functions which include: front desk, housekeeping, reservations, concierge, guest services, security and communications. The following are some important tips for success in fulfilling the company's promise to each guest:

Front Desk Here is where the first and last impressions are always made! At the front desk it is important to be personable, confident, and patient because your guests will vary in temperament, needs and expectations. Always remember a friendly, calm and positive attitude are your best tools even in trying situations. Multi-tasking becomes an art form at front desk calling on all of your communication, typing and computer skills.

Housekeeping Perception is reality and cleanliness is always at the top of a guest's expectations. In housekeeping it is the attention to details, the eye for the out of place, the worn or frayed that keeps it real for guests. It is a demanding work area with much physical labor that is essential to guest satisfaction. Your work is done mostly behind the curtain, out of guest view, but noticed and appreciated when they enter to fresh towels, a made bed and a flawlessly clean room. This is where you should start your lodging management career because it is the most demanding and least popular department among new hospitality graduates and yet it is the best training ground for early lodging management success!

Reservations How do you convey a smile over the phone? You must as you begin the process of the guest cycle. Reservations calls for total command of the keyboard, awareness of hotel revenue goals , upcoming events, room availability but above all listen, truly **listen**, to the guest so you can match their requests with the hotels services. The promise begins with you and you must never write a check that the front desk can cash at check-in.

Concierge A job that calls for diplomacy, ability to wheel-n-deal and just a touch of magic. Your role is to accommodate the guest needs during their stay. It calls for an encyclopedic memory of restaurants, theater offerings, key points of interest and current city events. The ability to develop a vast network of connections throughout the hospitality community in your area is essential to serve your guests and see to their every wish. Your reward as a successful concierge is that no two days are ever the same and there are always new and different challenges, opportunities and rewards.

Guest Services more commonly referred to as uniformed services; consist of valet, doorperson and bellperson positions. All jobs essential to first and last impressions that set the tone for the quality of service. A congenial disposition that projects a true spirit of helpfulness will disarm any initial guest trepidation. It also calls for thorough comprehension of the hotel, its layout, rooms and amenities. It is work that demands immaculate grooming (especially the uniform), standing for long hours and physical activity. In uniform, you are the hotel to the guest.

Major hotel chains offer a number of different room rates, including the following:

rack rate
corporate
association rate
government
encore
cititravel
entertainment cards
AAA
AARP (American Association of Retired Persons)
wholesale
group rates
promotional special

The rack rate is the rate that is used as a benchmark quotation of a hotel's room rate. Let us assume that the Hotel California had a rack rate of $135. Any discounted rate may be offered at a percentage deduction from the rack rate. An example would be a corporate rate of $110, an association rate of $105, and AARP rate of $95—certain restrictions may apply. Group rates may range from $95 to $125 according to how much the hotel needs the business.

Throughout the world there are three main plans on which room rates are based:

AP/American Plan—room and three meals a day
MAP/Modified American Plan—room plus two meals
EP/European Plan—room only, meals extra

Figure 4 • The Types of Room Rates Offered by Hotels.

---

2. *To maintain balanced guest accounts.* This begins with advance deposits, opening the guest folio (account), and posting all charges from the various departments. Most hotels have **property management systems (PMSs)** (property management systems are explained in more detail later in this chapter) and point-of-sale terminals (POS), which are online to the front office.

   This means that guest charges from the various outlets are directly debited to the guest's folio. Payment is either received on guest checkout or transferred to the **city ledger** (a special account for a company that has established credit with the hotel). This means that the account will be sent and paid within a specified time period.

3. *To offer services such as handling mail, faxes, messages, and local and hotel information.* People constantly approach the front desk with questions.

Front desk employees need to be knowledgeable about the various activities in the hotel. The size, layout, and staffing of the front desk will vary with the size of the hotel. The front desk staff size of a busy 800-room city center property will naturally differ from that of a country inn. The front desk is staffed throughout the twenty-four hours by three shifts.

The evening shift duties are the following:

1. Check the log book for special items. (The log book is kept by guest contact; associates at the front office note specific and important guest requests and occurrences such as requests for room switches or baby cribs.)
2. Check on the room status, number of expected checkouts still to leave, and arrivals by double-checking registration cards and the computer so that they can update the forecast of the night's occupancy. This will determine the number of rooms left to sell. Nowadays, this is all part of the capability of the PMS.
3. Handle guest check-ins. This means notifying the appropriate staff of any special requests guests may have made (e.g., nonsmoking room or a long bed for an extra-tall guest).
4. Take reservations for that evening and future reservations after the reservations staff have left for the day.

Night Auditor

A hotel is one of the few businesses that balances its accounts at the end of each business day. Because a hotel is open twenty-four hours every day, it is difficult to stop transactions at any given moment. The **night auditor** waits until the hotel quiets down at about 1:00 A.M., and then begins the task of balancing the guests' accounts receivable. The process of night auditing is as follows:

1. The night audit team runs a preliminary reconciliation report that shows the total revenue generated from room and tax, banquets and catering, food and beverage outlets, and other incidentals (phone, gift shop, etc.).
2. All errors on the report are investigated.
3. All changes are posted and balanced with the preliminary charges.
4. A comparison of charges is carried out, matching preliminary with actual charges.
5. Totals for credit card charges, rooms operations, food and beverages, and incidentals are verified.
6. The team "rolls the date"—they go forward to the next day.

Other duties of the night audit staff include the following:

1. Post any charges that the evening shift was not able to post.
2. Pass discrepancies to shift managers in the morning. The room and tax charges are then posted to each folio and a new balance shown.

3. Run backup reports so that if the computer system fails, the hotel will have up-to-date information to operate a manual system.

4. Reconcile point-of-sale and PMS to guest accounts. If this does not balance, the auditor must balance it by investigating errors or omissions. This is done by checking that every departmental charge shows up on guest folios.

5. Complete and distribute the daily report. This report details the previous day's activities and includes vital information about the performance of the hotel.

6. Determine areas of the hotel where theft could potentially occur.

Larger hotels may have more than one night auditor, but in smaller properties these duties may be combined with night manager, desk, or night watchperson duties.

CORPORATE PROFILE

Hyatt Hotels

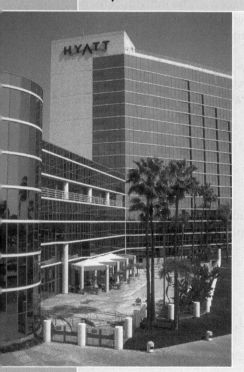

When Nicholas Pritzker emigrated with his family from the Ukraine to the United States, he began his career by opening a small law firm. His outstanding management skills led to the expansion of the law firm, turning it into a management company. Pritzker purchased the Hyatt House motel next to the Los Angeles International Airport in 1957.

Today, Hyatt is an international brand of hotels within the Global Hyatt Corporation, a multibillion-dollar hotel management and development company. It is among the leading chains in the hotel industry, with close to 8 percent of the market share.[6] Hyatt has earned worldwide fame as the leader in providing luxury accommodations and high-quality service, targeting especially the business traveler, but strategically differentiating its properties and services to identify and market to a very diverse clientele. This differentiation has resulted in the following types of hotels:

1. *Grand Hyatt* features distinctive luxury hotels in major gateway cities.

2. The *Hyatt Regency Hotels* represent the company's core product. They are usually located in business city centers and are regarded as five-star hotels.

3. *Hyatt Resorts* are vacation retreats. They are located in the world's most desirable leisure destinations, offering the "ultimate escape from everyday stresses."

4. The *Park Hyatt Hotels* are smaller, European-style, luxury hotels. They target the individual traveler who prefers the privacy, personalized service, and discreet elegance of a small European hotel.

(continued)

5. *Hyatt Place* is a lifestyle 125- to 200-room property located in urban, airport, and suburban areas. Signature features include The Gallery, which offers a coffee and wine bar and a 24/7 kitchen where travelers can find freshly prepared food.

6. *Hyatt Vacation Club* offers vacation ownership, vacation rentals, and mini vacations.

7. *Summerfield Suites* is an extended-stay brand of 125- to 200-room all-suite properties that provide the feel of a condominium but with complementary full breakfast and evening social. Locations are urban, airport, and suburban.

8. *Andaz* is a casual, stylish, boutique-style hotel; each hotel reflects the unique cultural scene and spirit of the surrounding neighborhood.

The Hyatt Hotels Corporation is characterized by a decentralized management approach, which gives the individual general manager a great deal of decision-making power, as well as the opportunity to use personal creativity and, therefore, stimulate differentiation and innovation. The development of novel concepts and products is perhaps the key to Hyatt's outstanding success. For example, the opening of the Hyatt Regency Atlanta, Georgia, with its atrium lobby gave the company instant recognition throughout the world. The property's innovative architecture, designed by John Portman, revolutionized the common standards of design and spacing, thus changing the course of the lodging industry.

A further positive aspect of the decentralized management structure is the fact that the individual manager is able to be extremely guest responsive by developing a thorough knowledge of the guests' needs and thereby providing personalized service—fundamental to achieving customer satisfaction. This is, in fact, the ultimate innkeeping purpose, which Hyatt attains at high levels.

The other side of Hyatt's success is the emphasis on human resources management. Employee satisfaction, in fact, is considered to be a prerequisite to external satisfaction. Hyatt devotes enormous attention to employee training and selection. What is most significant, however, is the interaction among top managers and operating employees.

The company operates 453 hotels and resorts in forty-three countries worldwide.

The **daily report** contains key operating ratios such as **room occupancy percentage (ROP)**, which is the number of rooms occupied divided by the number of rooms available:

$$\frac{\text{Rooms Occupied}}{\text{Rooms Available}}$$

Thus, if a hotel has 850 rooms and 622 are occupied, the occupancy percentage is $622 \div 850 = 73$ percent.

The **average daily rate** is calculated by dividing the rooms revenue by the number of rooms sold:

$$\frac{\text{Rooms Revenue}}{\text{Rooms Sold}}$$

If the rooms revenue is $75,884 and the number of rooms sold is 662, then the ADR is $114.63. The ADR is, together with the occupancy percentage, one of the key operating ratios that indicates the hotel's performance. See Figure 5 for an example of a daily report.

Room occupancy percentage (ROP):

If total available rooms are	850
And total rooms occupied are	622

Then:

Occupancy percentage = (622 / 850) × 100 = 73%

Average daily rate:

If rooms revenue is	$75,884
And total number of rooms sold is	622

Then:

$$\text{Average daily rate} = \frac{75,884}{662} = \$114.63$$

A more recently popular ratio to gauge a hotel rooms division's performance is the percentage of potential room's revenue, which is calculated by determining potential rooms revenue and dividing the actual revenue by the potential revenue.

While these figures are of great importance to running a successful hotel, the most important of the lodging ratios is **revenue per available room** (REV PAR), which is discussed in the next section.

Revenue Management

Revenue management is used to maximize room revenue at the hotel. It is based on the economics of supply and demand, which means that prices rise when demand is strong and drop when demand is weak. Naturally, management would like to sell every room at the highest rack rate. However, this is not a reality, and rooms are sold at discounts from the rack rate. An example is the corporate or group rate. In most hotels, only a small percentage of rooms are sold at rack rate. This is because of conventions and group rates and other promotional discounts that are necessary to stimulate demand.

What revenue management does is allocate the right type of room to the right guest at the right price so as to maximize revenue per available room.[7] Thus, the purpose of revenue management is to increase profitability. Generally, the demand for room reservations follows the pattern of group bookings, which are made months or even years in advance of arrival, and individual bookings, which mostly are made a few days before arrival. Figures 6 and 7 show the pattern of individual and group room reservations. Revenue management examines the demand for rooms over a period of a few years and determines the extent of demand for a particular room each night. This includes busy period, slow periods, and holidays. The computer program figures out a model of that

Clarion Hotel Bayview

Daily Management Report Supplement
January 2007

Daily Report
January 2007

Occupancy%	Today	Avg or %	M–T–D Avg or %		Y–T–D Avg or %	
Rack Rooms	9	2.9%	189	3.37	189	3.37
Corporate Rooms	0	0.0%	103	1.83	103	1.83
Group Rooms	274	87.8%	2,379	42.36	2,379	42.36
Leisure Rooms	3	1.0%	395	7.03	395	7.03
Base Rooms	23	7.4%	348	6.14	345	6.14
Government Rooms	2	0.6%	32	.57	32	.57
Wholesale Rooms	1	0.3%	121	2.15	121	2.15
No-Show Rooms		0.0%	0	.00	0	.00
Comp Rooms	0	0.0%	37	.66	37	.66
Total Occ Rooms & Occ %	312	100%	3,601	64.12	3,601	64.12
Rack	$1,011	$112.33	17,207	91.04	17,207	91.04
Corporate	$0	ERR	8,478	82.31	8,478	82.31
Group	$22,510	$82.15	178,066	74.85	178,066	74.85
Leisure	$207	$69.00	24,985	63.25	24,985	63.25
Base	$805	$35.00	12,063	34.97	12,063	34.97
Govt	$141	$70.59	2,379	74.34	2,379	74.34
Wholesale	$43	$43.00	5,201	42.98	5,201	42.98
No-Show/Comp/Allowance	$0		−914	−24.69	−914	−24.69
Total Rev & Avg Rate	$24,717	$79.22	247,466	68.72	247,466	68.72

Hotel Revenue

	Today		M–T–D Avg or %		Y–T–D Avg or %	
Rooms	$24,717		247,466	77.46	247,466	77.46
Food	$1,400		37,983	11.89	37,983	11.89
Beverage	$539		9,679	3.03	9,679	3.03
Telephone	$547		5,849	1.83	5,849	1.83
Parking	$854		11,103	3.48	11,103	3.48
Room Svc II	$70		1,441	.45	1,441	.45
Other Revenue	$1,437		963	1.87	963	1.87
Total Revenue	$29,563		319,484	100.00	319,484	100.00

Figure 5 • A Hotel Daily Report.

Clarion Hotel Bayview

Daily Management Report Supplement	Daily Report
January 2007	January 2007

Cafe 6th & K	Today	Avg or %	M–T–D Avg or %		Y–T–D Avg or %	
Cafe Breakfast Covers	88	57.1%	1,180	47.12	1,180	47.12
Cafe Lunch Covers	43	27.9%	674	26.92	674	26.92
Cafe Dinner Covers	23	14.9%	650	25.96	650	25.96
Total Cafe Covers	154	100.0%	2,504	100.00	2,504	100.00
Cafe Breakfast	$608	$6.91	7,854	6.66	7,854	6.66
Cafe Lunch	$246	$5.72	5,847	8.67	5,847	8.67
Cafe Dinner	$227	$9.86	4,309	6.63	4,309	6.63
Gaslamp Lounge Food			2,431	3.74	2,431	3.74
Total Rev/Avg Check	$1,081	$7.02	20,440	8.16	20,440	8.16
Banquets						
Banquet Breakfast Covers	0	ERR	154	13.24	154	13.24
Banquet Lunch Covers	0	ERR	134	11.52	134	11.52
Banquet Dinner Covers	0	ERR	254	21.84	254	21.84
Banquet Coffee Break Covers	0	ERR	621	53.40	621	53.40
Total Banquet Covers	0	ERR	1,163	100.00	1,163	100.00
Banquet Breakfast	$0	ERR	980	6.36	980	6.36
Banquet Lunch	$0	ERR	2,997	22.36	2,997	22.36
Banquet Dinner	$0	ERR	4,530	17.84	4,530	17.84
Banquet Coffee Break	$0	ERR	1,093	1.76	1,093	1.76
Total Rev/Avg Check	$0	ERR	9,600	8.25	9,600	8.25
Room Service						
Room Service Breakfast Covers	13	40.6%	324	48.00	324	48.00
Room Service Lunch Covers	3	9.4%	53	7.85	53	7.85
Room Service Dinner Covers	16	50.0%	298	44.15	298	44.15
Total Covers	32	100.0%	675	100.00	675	100.00
Room Service Breakfast	$119	$9.13	2,665	8.22	2,665	8.22
Room Service Lunch	$29	$9.77	418	7.89	418	7.89
Room Service Dinner	$171	$10.67	2,907	9.75	2,907	9.75
Total Rev/Avg Check	$319	$9.96	5,990	8.87	5,990	8.87

Figure 5 • A Hotel Daily Report. *(continued)*

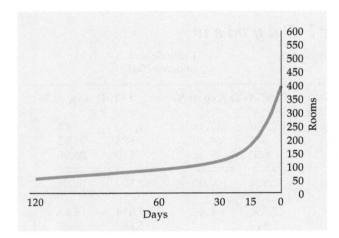

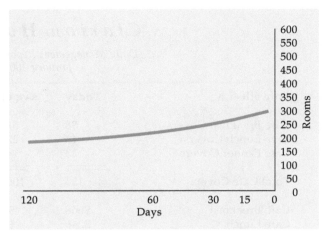

Figure 6 • Individual Room Booking Reservations Curve.
(*Source:* Personal correspondence with Jay R. Schrock, May 18, 2007.)

Figure 7 • Group Booking Curve.

demand, which is then used to guestimate future demand so that management can determine pricing levels to set.

Because group reservations are booked months, even years, in advance, revenue management systems can monitor reservations and, based on previous trends and current demand, determine the number and type of rooms to sell at what price to obtain the maximum revenue.

The curve in Figure 6 indicates the pattern of few reservations being made 120 days prior to arrival. Most of the individual room bookings are made in the last few days before arrival at the hotel. The revenue management program monitors the demand and supply and recommends the number and type of rooms to sell for any given day, and the price for which to sell each room.

With revenue management, not only will the time before arrival be an important consideration in the pricing of guest rooms, but also the type of room to be occupied.

The application of revenue management in hotels is still being refined to take into consideration factors such as multiple nights' reservations and incremental food and beverage revenue. If the guest wants to arrive on a high-demand night and stay through several low-demand nights, what should the charge be?

Revenue management has some disadvantages. For instance, if a businessperson attempts to make a reservation at a hotel three days before arrival and the rate quoted to maximize revenue is considered too high, this person may decide to select another hotel and not even consider the first hotel when making future reservations.

Revenue per available room, or **REV PAR**, was developed by Smith Travel Research. It is calculated by dividing room revenue by the number of rooms available.

For example, if room sales are $50,000 in one day for a hotel with 400 available rooms, then the REV PAR formula is $50,000 divided by 400, or a REV PAR of $125.

Hotels use REV PAR to see how they are doing compared to their competitive set of hotels. Hotel operators use REV PAR as an indicator of a hotel's revenue management program. One of the ways that REV PAR is used is for comparison to other properties in a competitive set on the Smith Travel Star Report.

Smith Travel Report (STR Global) is the publisher of the STAR reports, a benchmarking suite that tracks one hotel's occupancy, average daily rate, and REV PAR against a competitive set of hotels for comparison purposes. The information provided helps identify if a particular property is gaining or losing market share and helps the organization make necessary corrections to its management, marketing, and sales strategies. The STR STAR reports are used extensively in the lodging industry as the best tool for revenue management.[8]

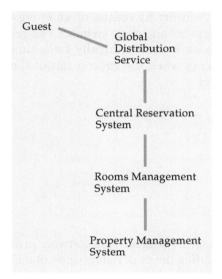

Figure 8 • The Sequence and Relationships of a Hotel Guest Reservation.

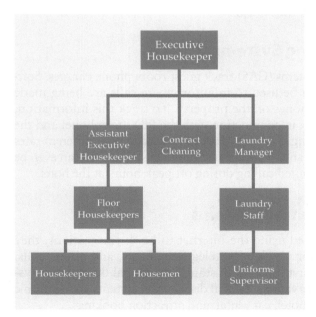

Figure 9 • Housekeeping Department Organization Chart.

▶ Check Your Knowledge

1. What is the rooms division director responsible for?
2. Describe the duties performed by the front office manager (FOM).
3. What is the Rack Rate and what other types of room rates are there?
4. How do you calculate the room occupancy percentage and the average daily rate?

Energy Management Systems

Technology is used to extend guest in-room comfort by means of an energy management system. Passive infrared motion sensors and door switches can reduce energy consumption by 30 percent or more by automatically switching off lights and air-conditioning, thus saving energy when the guest is out of the room. Additional features include the following:

- Room occupancy status reporting
- Automatic lighting control
- Minibar access reporting
- Smoke detector alarm reporting
- Central electronic lock control
- Guest control amenities

Because of increasing energy costs, some operators are installing software programs that will turn off nonessential equipment during the peak billing times of day (utility companies' charges are based on peak usage). Hospitality operators can save money by utilizing this type of energy-saving software to reduce their energy costs.

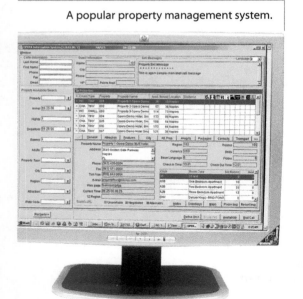

A popular property management system.

Call Accounting Systems

Call accounting systems (CAS) track guest room phone charges. Software packages can be used to monitor where calls are being made and from which phones on the property. To track this information, the CAS must work in conjunction with the PBX (telephone) and the PMS. Call accounting systems today can be used to offer different rates for local guest calls and long-distance guest calls. The CAS can even be used to offer discounted calling during off-peak hours at the hotel.

Guest Reservation Systems

Before hotels started using the Internet to book reservations, they received reservations by letters, telegrams, faxes, and phone calls. Airlines were the first industry to start using **global distribution systems (GDS)** for reservations. Global distribution systems are electronic markets for travel, hotel, car rental, and attraction bookings.

A **central reservation system (CRS)** houses the electronic database in the **central reservation office (CRO)**. Hotels provide rates and availability information to the CRO usually by data communication lines. This automatically updates the CRS so that guests get the best available rate when they book through the central reservation office. Guests instantly receive confirmation of their reservation or cancellation. The hotel benefits from using a central reservation system. With such a system, hotels can avoid overselling rooms by too large a margin. The CRS database can also be used as a chain or individual property marketing tool because guest information can easily be stored. A CRS can also provide yield management information for a hotel. The more flexible a central reservation system is, the more it will help with yield management. For example, when demand is weak for a hotel, rates will need to drop to increase reservations and profitability. When demand is higher, the hotel can sell room rates that are closer to the rack rate (*rack rate* is the highest rate quoted for a guestroom, from which all discounts are offered).

A CRS can be used in several areas of a hotel. If a hotel has a reservations department, the terminals or personal computers in that department can be connected to the central reservation system. It is also important for front desk employees to have access to the CRS so that they know what the hotel has available because they may need to book rooms for walk-ins who don't have reservations. Constant communication back and forth is needed between the central reservation system and the front office and reservations department. Managers who are the decision makers in the hotel will also use the system to forecast and set pricing for rooms and different amenities.

Hotels can use other forms of technology to facilitate reservation systems. Several companies offer an **application service provider (ASP)** environment that can deliver a complete booking system tied to the hotel's inventory in real time via the Web. One operator, Paul Wood of the El Dorado Hotel in Santa Fe, New Mexico, says that he simply went to the ASP web site and put in a promotional corporate rate for the summer, and the same day he started seeing reservations coming in with that code. After a few months, bookings were up 3 percent over the previous year.

Billing Guests

Hospitality businesses today seek to obtain the most high-speed and reliable computer systems they can afford that they can use to bill their guests without delay. Fast access to guests' accounts is required by large hotels because of their high priority of guest satisfaction (no lineups at checkout).

Billing guests has become much easier with the aid of computers. Billing guests can be a long process if information technologies are not used to complete transactions. PMSs aid large hotels to make faster transactions and provide a more efficient service to their guests. These systems help the hospitality associates bill their guests within seconds.

Some hotels utilize software that enables guests to check and approve their bills by using the TV and remote control, thus avoiding the need to line up at the cashier's desk to check out. A copy of the final bill is then mailed to the guest's home address.

Security

Each business in the hospitality industry offers some sort of security for their guests and employees. Peace of mind that the hotel or restaurant is secure is a key factor in increasing guest satisfaction. Security is one of the highest concerns of guests who visit hospitality businesses. Hospitality information technology systems include surveillance systems in which cameras are installed in many different areas of the property to monitor the grounds and help ensure guest safety. These cameras are linked directly to computers, televisions, and digital recorders, which helps security teams keep an eye on the whole property.

Recent technological advances have produced electronic door locking systems, some of which even offer custom configurations of security and safety. Guest room locks are now capable of managing information from both magstripe and smart cards simultaneously. From the hotel's point of view, a main advantage of this kind of key is that the hotel knows who has entered the room and at what time because the system can trace anyone entering the room.

In-room safes can now be operated by key cards. Both systems are an improvement on the old metal keys. Even smarter safes use biometric technology such as the use of thumbprints or retina scans to verify a user's identity.

Guest Comfort and Convenience

Hotels provide guest comfort and convenience to maintain a home-away-from-home feeling for their guests. Hotels receive recognition when they provide many additional in-room services and amenities for their guests, such as dining, television, telephones, Internet connections, minibars, and hygiene products. These amenities help provide a cozy experience for the guest. Many other services can be provided outside of the rooms, such as swimming pools, massages, fine dining, postal services, and meeting space. Other services are provided to suit the demands of all types of guests; a concierge and business center, for example.

Hotels communicate with many entities to provide services for their guests. Some companies offer creative solutions to hotels for enhanced in-room services for guests. Sprint InSite with KoolConnect Interactive Media has created a product that provides many services to the guest from just one supplier. Services include Internet access and e-mail; movies, music, and games on demand; hotel and concierge services; special promotions; advertising; travel planning; feedback from guests; and customer support. All these services aid hotels in fulfilling guest demands. Sprint states, "Build loyalty and promote business retention by enhancing the overall quality-of-visit for your guest."[9] Play Stations and video games are also a part of the technology-based guest amenities.

▶ Check Your Knowledge

1. What functions does the PMS perform?

2. What is revenue management? How is revenue management applied in the hotel industry?

TECHNOLOGY SPOTLIGHT

Hotel Information Technology

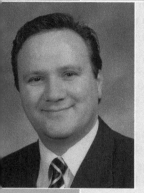

Cihan Cobanoglu, Ph.D., Dean, School of Hotel and Restaurant Management, University of South Florida, Sarasota-Manatee

"Home away from home!" This is how we would like to express what hotels means to our guests. For this to happen, we must provide technologies that guests use at home. Of course, the main purpose of the guestroom has never changed: to provide a clean, safe place to spend the night. In 1970, for the first time, hoteliers put ice-cube makers and small refrigerators inside the guestroom. In the beginning, not all rooms had these amenities. Usually, those rooms that had these special amenities were charged more than the other rooms. In 1972, the first models of telephone systems were introduced to the guestroom. In those days, there was only one telephone line for the entire hotel; therefore, guests sometimes waited long hours before they could place a call. In 1975, after color TV was well established in homes, hotels started to offer it. In the beginning, some hotels advertised that they had color TV to differentiate themselves from the competition and charged extra for rooms with TV. In 1980, the Hotel Billing Information System (HOBIC) was introduced. In 1981, it became legal for hotels to profit from phone calls. This is when call-accounting systems exploded in the hotel industry. In 1986, electronic door-keys were introduced, increasing the security and the convenience of guests. Interface between TV systems and property management systems was established in 1990 so that the guests can see their bills through the TV. With that, in 1993, guests were able to check out from their room by using the TV. In 1995, high-speed Internet access was available in hotel rooms. After 2000, hotels started to use voice-over Internet Protocol (IP) phoning systems, high-definition TV, wireless Internet access, interactive entertainment systems, smart-energy management systems, and many other systems.

In today's modern hotel rooms, it is possible to see the following technologies that make the guest stay a more comfortable one: (1) electronic locking system, 2) energy management and climate control systems, 3) fire alarm and security systems, 4) in-room minibars, 5) in-room safe boxes, 6) guestroom phone systems, 7) voice-mail/wake-up systems, 8) in-room entertainment systems, 9) guestroom control panels, and 10) self check-in/check-out systems.

Let's look into the future to see what the guestroom might look like then:

You just booked a hotel room from your smart phone with a voice command. When you go to check in to the hotel, you see that check-in desk is replaced with a "hospitality desk." As soon as you arrive to the hotel, your phone is showing you a map of the hotel rooms, asking you to make a choice. Once you make your choice, your phone becomes your electronic key card. When you wave your phone, the door opens and the 100-percent sustainable room welcomes you with your preferred wall color (thanks to nano-paint) and your favorite song. When you turn on the TV with your voice command, you see your favorite and local TV channels (thanks to Internet TV) and your video library from your home phone. The picture frame shows the pictures from your Facebook page. Your sheets and towels will be changed based on the "green" preferences such as to change the bed sheet and towels every three days and bring the temperature of the room 10 degrees down or up based on the season when you are not in the room. When you need help, you connect to a virtual concierge to get any kind of information about the hotel and the area. The wardrobe door generates power when you open and close the door for lighting. When you use the restroom, the smart toilet checks your health and sends you a digital report to your e-mail. Does this sound like a nice dream? Actually, this is a description of next-generation hotel.

Reservations

The reservations department is headed by the reservations manager who, in many hotels today, is on the same level as the front office manager and reports directly to the director of rooms division or the director of sales. This emphasizes the importance of the sales aspects of reservations and encompasses yield management. Reservations is the first contact for the guest or person making the reservation for the guest. Although the contact may be by telephone, a distinct impression of the hotel is registered with the guest. Because of this, exceptional telephone manners and telemarketing skills are necessary. Because some guests may be shopping for the best value, it is essential to sell the hotel by emphasizing its advantages over the competition.

The reservation department generally works from 8:00 A.M. to 6:00 P.M. Depending on the size of the hotel, several people may be employed in this important department. The desired outcome of the reservations department is to exceed guest expectations when they make reservations. This is achieved by selling all of the hotel rooms for the maximum possible dollars and avoiding possible guest resentment of being overcharged. Reservations originate from a variety of sources:

1. The Internet
2. Corporate/1-800 numbers
3. Travel agents
4. Telephone to the same property
   a. Fax
   b. Letter
   c. Cable
5. Meeting planners
6. Tour operators
7. Referral from another company property
8. Airport telephone
9. Walk-in

Clearly, reservations are of tremendous importance to the hotel because of the potential and actual revenue realized. Many hotel chains have a 1-800 number that a prospective guest may call without charge to make a reservation at any of the company properties in the United States and internationally. The corporate central reservations system allows operators to access the inventory of room availability of each hotel in the chain. Once a reservation has been made, it is immediately deducted from the inventory of rooms for the duration of the guest stay. The central reservations system interfaces with the hotel's inventory and simultaneously allows reservations to be made by the individual hotel reservations personnel. A number of important details need to be recorded when taking reservations.

Confirmed reservations are reservations made with sufficient time for a confirmation slip to be returned to the client by mail or fax. Confirmation is generated by the computer printer and indicates confirmation number, dates of arrival and departure, type of room booked, number of guests, number of beds,

118

type of bed, and any special requests. The guest may bring the confirmation slip to the hotel to verify the booking.

Guaranteed reservations are given when the person making the reservation wishes to ensure that the reservation will be held. This is arranged at the time the reservation is made and generally applies in situations when the guest is expected to arrive late. The hotel takes the credit card number, which guarantees payment of the room, of the person being billed. The hotel agrees to hold the room for late arrival. The importance of guaranteed reservations is that the guest will more likely cancel beforehand if unable to show up, which gives more accurate inventory room count and minimizes no-shows.

Another form of guaranteed reservations is advance deposit/advance payment. In certain situations, for example, during a holiday, to protect itself against having empty rooms (no-shows), the hotel requires that a deposit of either one night or the whole stay be paid in advance of the guest's arrival. This is done by obtaining the guest's credit card number, which may be charged automatically for the first night's accommodation. This discourages no-shows. Corporations that use the hotel frequently may guarantee all of their bookings so as to avoid any problems in the event a guest arrives late, remembering that in cities where the demand is heavy, hotels release any nonguaranteed or nonpaid reservations at 4:00 P.M. or 6:00 P.M. on the evening of the guest's expected arrival.

Communications CBX or PBX

The communications CBX or PBX includes in-house communications; guest communications, such as pagers and radios; voice mail; faxes; messages; and emergency center. Guests often have their first contact with the hotel by telephone. This underlines the importance of prompt and courteous attention to all calls because first impressions last.

The communications department is a vital part of the smooth running of the hotel. It is also a profit center because hotels generally add a 50-percent charge to all long-distance calls placed from guest rooms. Local calls cost about $0.75 to $1.25, plus tax, but many hotels offer local calls for free.

Communications operates twenty-four hours a day; in much the same way as the front office does, having three shifts. It is essential that this department be staffed with people who are trained to be calm under pressure and who follow emergency procedures.

Guest Services/Uniformed Services

Because first impressions are very important to the guest, the guest service or uniformed staff has a special responsibility. The guest service department or **uniformed staff** is headed by a guest services manager who may also happen to be the bell captain. The staff consists of door attendants and bellpersons and the concierge, although in some hotels the concierge reports directly to the front office manager.

Door attendants are the hotel's unofficial greeters. Dressed in impressive uniforms, they greet guests at the hotel front door, assist in opening/closing automobile doors, removing luggage from the trunk, hailing taxis, keeping the hotel entrance clear of vehicles, and giving guests information about the hotel and the local area in a courteous and friendly way. People in this position generally receive many gratuities (tips); in fact, years ago, the position was handed down from father to son or sold for several thousand dollars. Rumor has it that this is one of the most lucrative positions in the hotel, even more lucrative than the general manager's.

A DAY IN THE LIFE OF DENNY BHAKTA

Revenue Manager Hilton Hotels San Diego

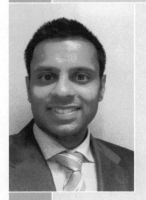

Revenue Management is a strategic function in maximizing room revenue (REV PAR) along with growing market share. REV PAR and market share are the two primary barometers used in the industry to grade a Revenue Manager's competency. It is essential for Revenue Managers to have a system in place for daily business reviews to formulate winning strategies. Daily duties include:

1. Analyzing Data: A Revenue Manager must develop a reporting system for daily monitoring. In recent years, the larger hotel brands have developed proprietary Revenue Management systems that provide on-demand reporting of historical data, future position and the ability to apply real time pricing changes to future nights. Understanding past performance can uncover various business trends over high and low demand periods. It is critical to understand the effectiveness of previous pricing strategies to better position the hotel on future nights. The general public can view rates and book rooms up to 365 days into the future. Therefore the Revenue Manager must monitor daily pickup in reservations and regrets for future nights and make necessary adjustments to enhance speed to market. Each hotel will have different booking windows (or lead times) for their Transient & Group business. For example, the San Diego market has a majority of Transient bookings that occur within 120 days to arrival, whereas the Group business is booked many months out, and in some cases several years in advance. The primary booking window must be analyzed on a daily basis and adjusted accordingly. The longer booking windows can be analyzed periodically with the Director of Sales to equip the Sales team with rates to book group business based on the hotel's revenue goals.

2. Mix of Business Assessment: Finding the right balance of Occupancy and ADR could yield the greatest REV PAR and greatly influenced by the mix of business. It is composed of two primary customer segments: Transient (individual travelers for business or leisure) and Groups which are bookings with 10 more rooms per night (i.e. conventions, company meetings, etc). Hotels can differ with mixes of business based on location, number of rooms, and event space. Convention hotels may have a desired mix of 80 percent Group and 20 percent Transient to achieve their optimum point of profit. Whereas small to midsize hotels may have a need for greater Transient business, all of which are key factors in formulating effective pricing strategies. Although the majority of Group business will be booked further in advance, those rates are also determined by the Revenue Manager and Director of Sales based on historical trends and future business needs.

3. Competitor Analysis: It is always valuable to know what the competition is doing. Revenue Management is part science and part craft. With the advancement in technology, companies such as Smith Travel Research and The Rubicon Group have created essential tools that allow hoteliers and Revenue Managers to determine their position in the marketplace. Smith Travel Research produced the STAR report that is routed on a weekly and monthly basis. This report allows a hotel to choose a competitive set, which then compares the hotel's actualized results by segment versus the competitive set, resulting in market share indexes for Occupancy, ADR and REV PAR. Although it is every hotel's goal to capture fair market share (dollar for dollar), it is a greater priority to gain share by outperforming the competition. The Rubicon Group created a "Market Vision" tool that provides the competitors rates and Occupancy levels up to 365 days into the future which can determine peaks and valleys in market demand.

4. Distribution Channels: It is crucial to know where the business is coming from, and how to increase production from the right channels. Most hotel brands have a central reservations systems, which is powered by their website and land based call centers. In addition, there are thousands of travel agencies that book rooms into hotel, which includes: online agencies (i.e. Expedia & Travelocity) and land based agencies (i.e. AAA Travel & American Express Travel). The major agencies will have Regional Market Managers that will supply market share data along with insight on any future developments that could be very beneficial to a hotel's strategy. A great Revenue Manager will establish daily communications with the large agencies to gain knowledge and to leverage hotel placement on their websites. Customers will not book you if they can't find you. The same applies to land based travel agents which are generally serviced by the hotel's Sales & Marketing team, who can be great resources in looking into the future. Greater market intelligence can equate to sound decision making.

5. Pricing Strategies: There is no right and wrong to the number of times rates should be adjusted on any given night. However, a greater understanding of market dynamics will come from a balance of historical knowledge and future market intelligence.

Lastly, the questions will always be asked: could we have done something different to maximize REV PAR? It is the Revenue Manager's responsibility to answer the question with integrity. Successful General Managers will appreciate the honesty and will have greater confidence level in a Revenue Manager that can determine both strengths and weaknesses in their own strategies.

The bellperson's main function is to escort guests and transport luggage to their rooms. Bellpersons also need to be knowledgeable about the local area and all facets of the hotel and its services. Because they have so much guest contact, they need a pleasant, outgoing personality. The bellperson explains the services of the hotel and points out the features of the room (lighting, TV, air-conditioning, telephone, wake-up calls, laundry and valet service, room service and restaurants, and the pool and health spa).

Concierge

The **concierge** is a uniformed employee of the hotel who has her or his own separate desk in the lobby or on special concierge floors. The concierge is a separate department from the front office room clerks and cashiers.

Luxury hotels in most cities have concierges. New York's Plaza Hotel has 800 rooms and a battery of ten concierges who serve under the direction of Thomas P. Wolfe. The concierge assists guests with a broad range of services such as the following:

- Tickets to the hottest shows in town, even for the very evening on the day they are requested. Naturally, the guest pays up to about $150 per ticket.
- A table at a restaurant that has no reservations available.
- Advice on local restaurants, activities, attractions, amenities, and facilities.
- Airline tickets and reconfirmation of flights.
- VIP's messages and special requests, such as shopping.

Less frequent requests are:

- Organize a wedding on two days' notice
- Arrange for a member of the concierge department to go to a consulate or embassy for visas to be stamped in guests' passports
- Handle business affairs

What will a concierge do for a guest? Almost anything, *Condé Nast Traveler* learned from concierges at hotels around the world. Among the more unusual requests were the following:

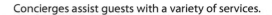
Concierges assist guests with a variety of services.

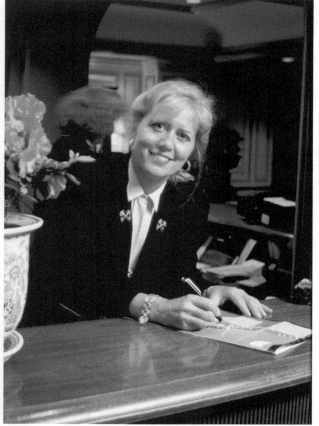

1. Some Japanese tourists staying at the Palace Hotel in Madrid decided to bring bullfighting home. Their concierge found bulls for sale, negotiated the bulls' purchase, and had them shipped to Tokyo.

2. After watching a guest pace the lobby, the concierge of a London hotel, now operating the desk at the Dorchester, asked the pacer if he could help. The guest was to be married within the hour, but his best man had been detained. Because he was dressed up anyway, the concierge volunteered to substitute.

3. A guest at the Hotel Plaza Athenee in Paris wanted to prevent her pet from mingling with dogs from the "wrong side" of the boulevard while walking. Madame requested that the concierge buy a house in a decent neighborhood so that her pampered pooch might stroll in its garden unsullied. Although the dog continued to reside at the hotel, Madame's chauffeur shuttled him to the empty house for his daily constitutional.

Concierges serve to elevate a property's marketable value and its image. They provide the special touch services that distinguish a "top property." To make sure they can cater to a guest's precise needs, concierges should make sure that they know precisely what the guest is looking for budget-wise, as well as any other parameters. Concierges must be very attentive and must anticipate guest needs when possible. In this age of highly competitive top-tier properties and well-informed guests, only knowledgeable concierge staff can provide the services to make a guest's stay memorable. As more properties try to demonstrate enhanced value, a concierge amenity takes on added significance.

The concierge needs not only a detailed knowledge of the hotel and its services, but also of the city and even international details. Many concierges speak several languages; most important of all, they must want to help people and have a pleasant, outgoing personality. The concierges' organization, which promotes high professional and ethical standards, is the Union Professionelle des Portiers des Grand Hotels (UPPGH), more commonly called the *Clefs d' Or* (pronounced clays-dor) because of the crossed gold-key insignia concierges usually wear on the lapels of their uniforms.

Housekeeping

The largest department in terms of the number of people employed is housekeeping. Up to 50 percent of the hotel employees may work in this department. Because of the hard work and comparatively low pay, employee turnover is very high in this essential department. The person in charge is the executive housekeeper or director of services. Her or his duties and responsibilities call for exceptional leadership, organization, motivation, and commitment to maintaining high standards. The logistics of servicing large numbers of rooms on a daily basis can be challenging. The importance of the housekeeping department is underlined by guest surveys that consistently rank cleanliness of rooms number one.

The four major areas of responsibilities for the executive housekeeper are as follows:

1. Leadership of people, equipment, and supplies
2. Cleanliness and servicing the guest rooms and public areas
3. Operating the department according to financial guidelines prescribed by the general manager
4. Keeping records

An example of an executive housekeeper's day might be as follows:

7:45 A.M. **Walk the lobby and property with the night cleaners and supervisors**

Check the housekeeping logbook

Check the forecast house count for number of checkouts

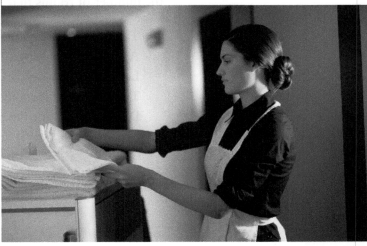

A housekeeper checks the linens on her cart. Attention to detail is important in maintaining standards.

Check daily activity reports, stayovers, check-ins, and VIPs to ensure appropriate standards

Attend housekeepers' meeting

Meet challenges

Train new employees in the procedures

Meet with senior housekeepers/department managers

Conduct productivity checks

Check budget

Approve purchase orders

Check inventories

Conduct room inspections

Review maintenance checks

Interview potential employees

6:00 P.M. Attend to human resource activities, counseling, and employee development

Perhaps the biggest challenge of an executive housekeeper is the leadership of all the employees in the department. Further, these employees are often of different nationalities. Depending on the size of the hotel, the executive housekeeper is assisted by an assistant executive housekeeper and one or more housekeeping supervisors, who in turn supervise a number of room attendants or housekeeping associates (see Figure 9). The assistant executive housekeeper manages the housekeeping office. The first important daily task of this position is to break out the hotel into sections for allocation to the room attendants' schedules.

The rooms of the hotel are listed on the floor master. If the room is vacant, nothing is written next to the room number. If the guest is expected to check out, then SC will be written next to the room number. A stayover will have SS, on hold is AH, out of order is OO, and VIPs are highlighted in colors according to the amenities required.

If 258 rooms are occupied and 10 of these are suites (which count as two rooms), then the total number of rooms to be allocated to room attendants is 268 (minus any no-shows). The remaining total is then divided by 17, which is the number of rooms that each attendant is expected to make up.

Total number of rooms occupied	258
Add 10 for the suites	+10
Less any no-shows	−3
Total number of rooms and suites occupied	= 265
Divided by 17 for the number of rooms that each attendant is expected to make up	17
	$265 \div 17 = 16$

Therefore, sixteen attendants are required for that day.

Figure 10 shows a daily attendant's schedule. To reduce payroll costs and encourage room attendants to become "stars," a number of hotel corporations have empowered the best attendants to check their own rooms. This has reduced the need for supervisors. Notice in Figure 10 how the points are weighted for various items. This is the result of focus groups of hotel guests who explained the things about a room that are important to them. The items with the highest points were the ones that most concerned the guests.

The housekeeping associates clean and service between fifteen and twenty rooms per day, depending on the individual hotel characteristics. Servicing a room takes longer in some older hotels than it does in some of the newer properties. Also, service time depends on the number of checkout rooms versus stay-overs because servicing checkouts takes longer. Housekeeping associates begin their day at 8:00 A.M., reporting to the executive or assistant executive housekeeper. They are assigned a block of rooms and given room keys, for which they must sign and then return before going off duty.

The role of the executive housekeeper may vary slightly between the corporate chain and the independent hotel. An example is the purchasing of furnishings and equipment. A large independent hotel relies on the knowledge and experience of the executive housekeeper to make appropriate selections, whereas the chain hotel company has a corporate purchase agent (assisted by a designer) to make many of these decisions.

The executive housekeeper is responsible for a substantial amount of record keeping. In addition to the scheduling and evaluation of employees, an inventory of all guest rooms and public area furnishings must be accurately maintained with the record of refurbishment. Most of the hotel's maintenance work orders are initiated by the housekeepers who report the maintenance work. Many hotels now have a computer linkup between housekeeping and engineering and maintenance to speed the process. Guests expect their rooms to be fully functional, especially at today's prices. Housekeeping maintains a perpetual inventory of guest room amenities, cleaning supplies, and linens.

Amazingly, it took about 2,000 years, but hotels have figured out that guests spend most of their stay on a bed, so they are introducing wonder beds and heavenly beds to allow guests to enjoy sweet dreams—but hopefully not miss that pesky wake-up call. Around the country, guest rooms are getting a makeover that includes new mattresses with devices that allow one side to be set firmer than the other side or on an incline. Other room amenities include new high-definition or plasma TVs, WiFi services, and room cards that activate elevators.

Productivity in the housekeeping department is measured by the person-hours per occupied room. The labor costs per person-hour for a full-service hotel ranges from $2.66 to $5.33, or twenty minutes of labor for every occupied room in the hotel. Another key ratio is the labor cost, which is expected to be 5.1 percent of room sales. Controllable expenses are measured per occupied rooms. These expenses include guest supplies such as soap, shampoo, hand and body lotion, sewing kits, and stationery. Although this will vary according to the type of hotel, the cost should be about $2.00 per room. Cleaning supplies should be approximately $0.50 and linen costs $0.95, including the purchase and laundering of all linen. These budgeted costs are sometimes hard to achieve. The executive housekeeper may be doing a great job controlling costs, but if the sales department discounts rooms, the room sales figures may come in below

Housekeepers Guest Room Self–Inspection Rating

Inspection Codes:

P – POLISH	R – REPLACE	E – WORK ORDER	S – SOAP SCUM	SM – SMEAR
SA – STAIN	H – HAIR	D – DIRT	DU – DUST	M – MISSING

PART I – GUEST ROOM		S			U	COMMENTS
Entry, door, frame, threshold, latch				1		
Unusual odor OR smoke smell				3		
CLOSET, doors, louvers–containing				1		
Hangers, 8 suits, 4 skirts, 2 bags w/ invoices				2		
Two (2) robes, with info card				2		
Extra TP & FACIAL				1		
One (1) luggage rack				1		
Current rate card				1		
VALET	Shoe Horn & Mitt			2		
DRESSER	LAMP/ SHADE/ BULB			2		
	ICE BUCKET, LID, TRAY			2		
	TWO (2) WINE GLASSES			2		
	Room Service MENU			2		
MINIBAR	TOP, FRONT, 2 Wine glasses/ price list			1		
SAFE	KEY IN SAFE, SIGN			5		
CHECK BEHIND DRESSER				2		
DRAWERS	BIBLE AND BUDDHIST BOOK			1		
	PHONE BOOKS, ATT DIRECTORY			1		
TELEVISION	ON & OFF, CH 19 BEHIND			1		
COFFEE TABLE	REMOTE CONTROL/TEST 1			2		
	T.V. LISTINGS/BOOK MARK			1		
	GLASS TOP/LA JOLLA BOOK			1		
CARPET	VACUUM, SPOTS?			2		
SOFA	UNDER CUSHION/ BEHIND			2		
3 W LAMP	BULB, SHADE, & CORD			1		
WINDOWS	GLASS, DOOR, LATCH—C BAR?			2		
CURTAINS	Pull — check seams			1		
PATIO	2 CHAIRS, TABLE & DECK			3		
DESK	2 CHAIRS, TOP, BASE, & LAMP/SHADE			5		
	GREEN COMPENDIUM			3		
	Waste paper can			1		
BED	Tight, Pillows, bedspread			5		
	Check Under/SHEETS, PILLOWS			3		
HVAC	Control, setting, vent			1		
SIDE TABLES	Lamps & shade			2		
	Telephone, MESSAGE LIGHT			1		
	Clock Radio CORRECT TIME?			1		
MIRRORS	LARGE MIRROR OVER DRESSER			1		
PICTURES	ROOM ART WORK			1		
WALLS	Marks, stains, etc.			3		

Numbers in rating column range from 1 (least important) to 5 (most important).

Figure 10 • Housekeepers Guest Room Self-Inspection Form.

Housekeepers Guest Room Self–Inspection Rating

Inspection Codes:

P – POLISH	R – REPLACE	E – WORK ORDER		S – SOAP SCUM	SM – SMEAR
SA – STAIN	H – HAIR	D – DIRT		DU – DUST	M – MISSING

PART II – BATHROOM		S			U	COMMENTS
BATH TUB/SHOWER						
	GROUT/TILE & EDGE			2		
	ANTISLIP GRIDS			2		
	SIDE WALLS			1		
	SHOWER HEAD			1		
	WALL SOAP DISH			1		
	CONTROL LEVER			1		
	FAUCET			1		
	CLOTHESLINE			1		
	SHOWER ROD, HOOKS			1		
	SHOWER CURTAIN/ LINER			2		
VANITY	TOP, SIDE, & EDGE			1		
	SINK, TWO FAUCETS			3		
	3 GLASSES, COASTERS			2		
	WHITE SOAP DISH			1		
	FACIAL TISSUE & BOX			1		
AMENITY BASKET						
	1 SHAMPOO			1		
	1 CONDITIONER			1		
	1 MOISTURIZER			1		
	2 BOXED SOAP			1		
	1 SHOWER CAP			1		
MIRROR	LARGE & COSMETIC			2		
WALLS, CEILING, & VENT				2		
TOILET	TOP, SEAT, BASE, & LIP			2		
OTHER	TOILET PAPER, fold			1		
	SCALE AND TRASH CAN			2		
	FLOOR, SWEPT AND MOPPED			3		
	TELEPHONE			1		
BATH LINENS, racks						
	THREE (3) WASH CLOTHS			1		
	THREE (3) HAND TOWELS			1		
	THREE (3) BATH TOWELS			1		
	ONE (1) BATH MAT			1		
	ONE (1) BATH RUG			1		
LIGHT SWITCH				1		
DOOR	FULL LENGTH MIRROR			1		
	HANDLE/LOCK			1		
	THRESHOLD			1		
	PAINTED SURFACE			1		

Figure 10 • Housekeepers Guest Room Self-Inspection Form. (*continued*)

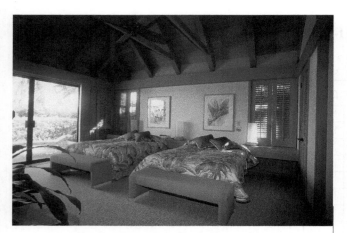

A Room at the Mauna Lani Resort on the Kohala Coast ready for guests.

budget. This would have the effect of increasing the costs per occupied room.

Another concern for the executive housekeeper is accident prevention. Insurance costs have skyrocketed in recent years, and employers are struggling to increase both employee and guest safety. It is necessary for accidents to be carefully investigated. Some employees have been known to have an accident at home but go to work and report it as a work-related injury to be covered by workers' compensation. To safeguard themselves to some extent, hotels keep sweep logs of the public areas; in the event that a guest slips and falls, the hotel can show that it does genuinely take preventative measures to protect its guests.

The **Occupational Safety and Health Administration (OSHA)**, whose purpose it is to ensure safe and healthful working conditions, sets mandatory job safety and health standards, conducts compliance inspections, and issues citations when there is noncompliance. Additionally, the U.S. Senate Bill 198, known as the **Employee Right to Know**, has heightened awareness of the storage, handling, and use of dangerous chemicals. Information about the chemicals must be made available to all employees. Great care and extensive training is required to avoid dangerous accidents.

The executive housekeeper must also minimize loss prevention. Strict policies and procedures are necessary to prevent losses from guest rooms. Some hotels require housekeeping associates to sign a form stating that they understand they may not let any guest into any room. Such action would result in immediate termination of employment. Although this may seem drastic, it is the only way to avoid some hotel thefts.

Laundry

Increasingly, hotels are operating their own laundries. This subdepartment generally reports to the executive housekeeper. The modern laundry operates computerized washing/drying machines and large presses. Dry cleaning for both guests and employees is a service that may also come under the laundry department. Hotels are starting to get away from in-house dry cleaning because of environmental concerns.

Sustainable Lodging

Green Hotel Initiatives

The environmentally conscious companies are not only helping to avoid further environmental degradation but are also saving themselves money while being good corporate citizens. Operationally, hotels have been recycling for years and saving water and chemicals by leaving cards in guest rooms saying that sheets will be changed every third day unless otherwise requested. Some hotels move the top sheet down to the bottom on the second or third day. Likewise, a card in the bathroom explains to guests that if they want a towel changed to leave it on the floor. Hotels have been quick to realize that the life of sheets and towels has been greatly extended, thus increasing savings.

The wattage of lighting has been reduced and long-life and florescent bulbs are saving thousands of dollars a year per property. Air-conditioning units can now control the temperature of a room through body-motion sensing devices that even pick up people's breathing. These devices can automatically shut off the air-conditioning unit when guests are out of their rooms. Savings are also being made with low-flow toilets and showerheads that have high-pressure low-volume flows of water.

Ecoefficiency, also generally termed *green*, is based on the concept of creating more goods and services while using fewer resources and creating less waste and pollution. In other words, it means doing more with less. So what does this have to do with your bottom line? Ecoefficiency helps hotels provide better service with fewer resources; reducing the materials and energy-intensity of goods and services lowers the hotel's ecological impact and improves the bottom line. It's a key driver for overall business performance.[10] Figure 11 shows a model for the implementation of sustainable lodging practices.

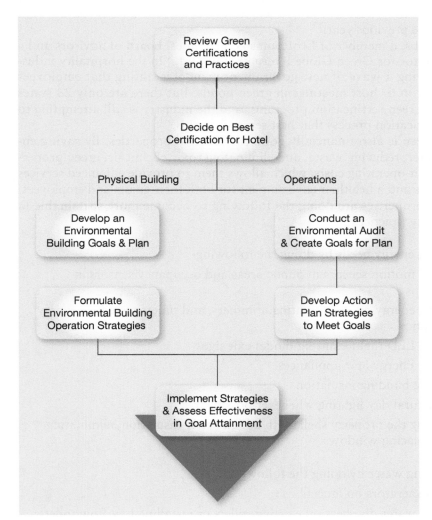

Figure 11 • A Model for the Implementation of Sustainable Lodging Practices.

Triple bottom line, sometimes called the TBL or 3P approach (people, planet, and profits), requires thinking in three dimensions, not one. It takes into account ecological and societal performance in addition to financial. Today, quantifiable environmental impacts include consumption of finite resources, energy usage, water quality and availability, and pollution emitted. Social impacts include community health, employee and guest safety, education quality, and diversity.[11]

Sustainable lodging, also known as green hotels, has become a powerful movement. The American Hotel and Lodging Association (AH&LA) and various state associations are leading the way with operational suggestions for best practices that lead to a green certification. Both corporations and independent properties are increasingly becoming greener in their operating practices. Sustainable Lodging & Restaurant–certified facilities develop goals and identify people in their organizations to find new opportunities to improve their operations through education, employee ideas, and guest feedback.

J.D. Power and Associates' 2009 North America Hotel Guest Satisfaction Index Study, which surveyed over 66,000 guests who stayed in North American hotels between May 2008 and June 2009, found that guests' awareness of their hotel's green programs increased significantly in 2009. Sixty-six percent of guests said they were aware of their hotel's conservation efforts, up from 57 percent the previous year.[12]

Ray Hobbs, a member of EcoRooms & EcoSuites' board of advisors and a certified auditor for Green Globe International, said, "In the hospitality industry, we're seeing a wave of new government mandates stating that employees can only stay in or host meetings in green hotels. But there are only 23 states with official green certification programs, and the industry is still attempting to find the certification process that best serves its needs."[13]

Being green is also financially good for certified properties. By saving energy and water, reducing waste, and eliminating toxic chemicals, green properties lower their operating costs, which allows them to provide enhanced services to their guests and a healthier environment for both their guests and employees. Sustainable properties are doing the following to become more sustainable in their operating practices[14]:

- Reducing energy needs by doing the following:

  Installing motion sensors in public areas and occupancy sensors in guestrooms

  Installing energy-efficient lighting, dimmers, and timers to reduce energy consumption

  Installing LED (light emitting diode) exit signs

  Installing Energy Star appliances

  Increasing building insulation

  Using natural day lighting whenever possible

  Tightening the property shell, with added/better insulation, eliminating leaks, replacing windows

- Conserving water by doing the following:

  Installing aerators on faucets

  Installing water diverters on existing toilets or installing low-flow toilets

Installing low-flow showerheads

Implementing towel and linen reuse programs

Landscaping with native plants

Using timers/moisture sensors in landscape watering

Changing lawn watering to encourage deeper root growth

- Reducing waste by doing the following:

  Providing recycling areas for guests and staff

  Purchasing postconsumer recycled paper and buying in bulk

  Serving meals with cloth napkins and reusable china and dinnerware

  Using refillable soap/shampoo dispensers in bathrooms

  Recycling usable furniture, etc., at "dump stores" or through charity

  Reusing old towels and linens as cleaning rags

  Asking vendors to minimize packaging

  Recycling cooking grease

  Composting food and lawn waste

- Reducing hazardous waste by doing the following:

  Properly disposing of fluorescent lighting, computers, and other electronic equipment

  Participating in local hazardous waste collection days

  Using low VOC (volatile organic compound) paints, carpets, and glues

  Using rechargeable batteries

  Using energy-efficient shuttle vans

  Using environmentally friendly cleaning products

  Another hotel company has a plan for its sustainability[15]:
  HTI Explore Green Options for Business at the Hutchinson Hotel

Guest Shuttle

Free shuttle service to area attractions is provided; the vehicle is either a hybrid car or a 15-passenger van for bigger groups.

Guest Bicycles

Bicycles are available for guest use in warm weather. Excellent bicycle-route maps are provided for those who want to explore the city on two wheels.

Greening the Guestroom

Guest rooms offer an opportunity for greening. Sustainable hotels do the following[16]:

- Give guests an option to have the towels and linens changed every other day, or less frequently, rather than every day. Surveys have shown that more than 90 percent of guests like the option.

- Encourage staff to close drapes and turn off lights and air conditioning when rooms are unoccupied.
- Install water-efficient fixtures, such as showerheads, aerators, and low-flow toilets in each room.
- Use refillable soap and shampoo dispensers.
- Encourage guests to recycle by providing clearly marked recycling bins for cans, bottles, and newspapers.
- Install energy-efficient lighting fixtures in each room. Compact fluorescent fixtures can be screwed into many existing lamps and ceiling fixtures. To prevent theft, many hotels are installing new fixtures with compact fluorescent lamps hardwired into the fixture.
- Consider purchasing Energy Star–labeled TVs and other energy-efficient appliances.
- Clean rooms with environmental cleaners to improve indoor air quality and reduce emissions of VOCs.
- Use placards in the room to inform your guests about your green efforts. Why not tell them a hotel can save 13.5 gallons of freshwater by choosing not to replace bath towels and linen daily?
- Use an opt-out approach to linen and towel reuse (this can save a 250-room hotel more than $15,000 per year).
- If a hotel adopts these and other measures every year, it would amount to savings of thousands of dollars. Consider also the gains for hotels that adopt and practice sustainable operations. In the case of Washington, D.C., it has been estimated that the hotel gained $800,000 of incremental group business as a result of having sustainable meeting and event management at the property.

▶ Check Your Knowledge

1. Describe the different types of reservations that guests make at hotels.
2. What is the role played by uniformed services?
3. Explain the responsibilities of an executive housekeeper.

Security/Loss Prevention

Providing guest protection and loss prevention is essential for any lodging establishment regardless of size. Violent crime is a growing problem, and protecting guests from bodily harm has been defined by the courts as a reasonable expectation from hotels. The security/loss division is responsible for maintaining security alarm systems and implementing procedures aimed at protecting the personal property of guests and employees and the hotel itself.

A comprehensive security plan must include the following elements:

Security Officers

- These officers make regular rounds of the hotel premises, including guest floors, corridors, public and private function rooms, parking areas, and offices.
- Duties involve observing suspicious behavior and taking appropriate action, investigating incidents, and cooperating with local law enforcement agencies.

Equipment

- Two-way radios between security staff are common.
- Closed-circuit television cameras are used in out-of-the-way corridors and doorways, as well as in food, liquor, and storage areas.
- Smoke detectors and fire alarms, which increase the safety of the guests, are a requirement in every part of the hotel by law.
- Electronic key cards offer superior room security. Key cards typically do not list the name of the hotel or the room number. So, if lost or stolen, the key is not easily traceable. In addition, most key card systems record every entry in and out of the room on the computer for further reference.

Safety Procedures

- Front desk agents help maintain security by not allowing guests to reenter their rooms once they have checked out. This prevents any loss of hotel property by guests.
- Security officers should be able to gain access to guest rooms, store rooms, and offices at all times.
- Security staff develop **catastrophe plans** to ensure staff and guest safety and to minimize direct and indirect costs from disaster. The catastrophe plan reviews insurance policies, analyzes physical facilities, and evaluates possible disaster scenarios, including whether they have a high or low probability of occurring. Possible disaster scenarios may include fires, bomb threats, earthquakes, floods, hurricanes, and blizzards. The well-prepared hotel develops formal policies to deal with any possible scenario and trains employees to implement chosen procedures should they become necessary.

Identification Procedures

- Identification cards with photographs should be issued to all employees.
- Name tags for employees who are likely to have contact with guests not only project a friendly image for the property, but are also useful for security reasons.

Trends in Hotel and Rooms Division Operations

- *Diversity of work force.* All the pundits are projecting a substantial increase in the number of women and minorities who will not only be taking hourly paid positions, but also supervising and management positions as well.

- *Increase in use of technology.* Reservations are being made by individuals over the Internet. Travel agents are able to make reservations at more properties. There is increasing simplification of the various PMSs and their interface with POS systems. In the guest room, increasing demand for high-speed Internet access, category 5 cables, and in some cases equipment itself is anticipated.

- *Continued quest for increases in productivity.* As pressure mounts from owners and management companies, hotel managers are looking for innovative ways to increase productivity and to measure productivity by sales per employee.

- *Increasing use of revenue management.* The techniques of revenue management will increasingly be used to increase profit by effective pricing of room inventory.

- *Greening of hotels and guest rooms.* Recycling and the use of environmentally friendly products, amenities, and biodegradable detergents will increase.

- *Security.* Guests continue to be concerned about personal security. Hotels are constantly working to improve guest security. For example, one hotel has instituted a women-only floor with concierge and security. Implementation of security measures will increase.

- *Diversity of the guest.* More women travelers are occupying hotel rooms. This is particularly a result of an increase in business travel.

- *Compliance with the ADA.* As a result of the Americans with Disabilities Act (ADA), all hotels must modify existing facilities and incorporate design features into new constructions that make areas accessible to persons with disabilities. All hotels are expected to have at least 4 percent of their parking space designated as "handicapped." These spaces must be wide enough for wheelchairs to be unloaded from a van. Guest rooms must be fitted with equipment that can be manipulated by persons with disabilities. Restrooms must be wide enough to accommodate wheelchairs. Ramps should be equipped with handrails, and meeting rooms must be equipped with special listening systems for those with hearing impairments.

- *Use of hotels' web sites.* Hotel companies will continue to try to persuade guests to book rooms using the hotel company web site rather than via an

Internet site such as Hotels.com because the hotel must pay about $20 for each room booking from such sites.

- *In-room technology.* Hotels are upgrading in-room technology.

Career Information

Hotel management is probably the most popular career choice among seniors who are graduating from hospitality educational programs. The reason for this popularity is tied to the elegant image of hotels and the prestige associated with being a general manager or vice president of a major lodging chain. Managing a hotel is a complex balancing act that involves keeping employees, guests, and owners satisfied while overseeing a myriad of departments, including reservations, front desk, housekeeping, maintenance, accounting, food and beverage, security, concierge, and sales. To be a GM, a person must understand all of the various functions of a hotel and how their interrelationship makes up the lodging environment. The first step down this career path is to get a job in a hotel while you are in college.

Once you become proficient in one area, volunteer to work in another. A solid foundation of broad-based experience in the hotel will be priceless when you start your lodging career. Some excellent areas to consider are the front desk, night audit, food and beverage, and maintenance. Another challenging but very important place to gain experience is in housekeeping. It has been said that if you can manage the housekeeping department, the rest of lodging management is easy. An internship with a large hotel chain property can also be a powerful learning experience. There is simply no substitute for being part of a team that operates a lodging property with several hundred rooms. You may hear about graduates being offered "direct placement" or "manager in training" (MIT) positions. (There are several name variations for these programs.) Direct placement means that when you graduate, you are offered a specific position at a property. An MIT program exposes you to several areas of the hotel over a period of time. Then you are given an assignment based on your performance during training. Neither one is better from a career standpoint.

Another important consideration of a lodging career is your wardrobe. In a hotel environment, people are judged based on their appearance. A conservative, professional image is a key to success. Clothes are the tools of the lodging professional's trade, and they are not inexpensive. Begin investing in clothes while you are in school. Buy what you can afford, but buy items of quality. Stay away from trendy or flashy clothes that will quickly be out of fashion. When you take a position, you can expect to work around fifty hours per week. The times you work may vary. You can expect to have a starting salary of between $30,000 and $34,000. Some hotel chains will assist with moving expenses and may even offer a one-time signing bonus. However, try not to focus too much on the money; instead, try to find a company that you feel comfortable with and that will allow you opportunities for advancement. Figure 12 shows a career path in lodging management.

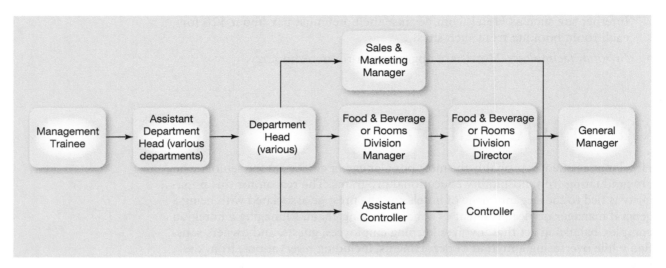

Figure 12 • A Career Path in Lodging Management.

Courtesy of Dr. Charlie Adams, Texas Tech University.

CASE STUDY

Checking Out a Guest

A guest walked up to the front desk agent in an upscale hotel, ready to check out. As she would usually do when checking out a guest, the agent asked the guest what his room number was. The guest was in a hurry and showed his anxiety by responding, "I stay in a hundred hotel rooms and you expect me to remember my room number?"

The agent then asked for the guest's name, to which he responded, "My name is Mr. Johnstein." After thanking him, the agent began to look for the guest's last name, but the name was not listed in the computer. Because the man had a heavy accent and the agent assumed that she had misunderstood him, she politely asked the guest to spell his last name. He answered, "What? Are you an idiot? The person who checked me in last night had no problem checking me in." Again, the agent looked on the computer to find the guest.

The guest, becoming even more frustrated, said, "I have a plane to catch and it is ridiculous that it has to take this long to check me out. I also need to fax these papers off, but I need to have them photocopied first." The agent responded, "There is a business center at the end of the counter that will fax and photocopy what you need." The guest replied, "If I wanted your opinion, I would have asked you for it. Haven't you ever heard of customer service? Isn't this a five-star hotel? With your bad attitude, you should be working in a three-star hotel. I can't believe they let you work here at the front desk. Haven't you found my name yet?"

The agent, who was beginning to get upset, asked the guest again to spell out his full name. The guest only replied, "Here are my papers I want faxed if you are capable of faxing them." The agent reached to take the papers, and the guest shouted, "Don't grab them from my hand! You have a bad attitude, and if I had more time, I would talk to someone about getting you removed from your position to a hotel where they don't require such a level of customer service." The agent was very upset, but kept herself calm to prevent the guest from getting angrier.

The agent continued to provide service to the guest, sending the faxes and making the photocopies he had requested. Upon her return, the agent again asked the guest to repeat his last name because he had failed to spell it out. The guest replied by spelling out his name, "J-o-h-n-s-t-o-n-e." The agent was finally able to find his name on the computer and checked him out while he continued to verbally attack her. The agent finished by telling the guest to have a nice flight.

Discussion Questions

1. Is it appropriate to have the manager finish the checkout? Or should the front desk agent just take the heat?
2. Would you have handled the situation in the same manner?
3. What would you have done differently?

CASE STUDY

Overbooked: The Front-Office Perspective

Overbooking is an accepted hotel and airline practice. Many question the practice from various standpoints, including ethical and moral. Industry executives argue that there is nothing more perishable than a vacant room. If it is not used, there is no chance to regain lost revenue. Hotels need to protect themselves because potential guests frequently make reservations at more than one hotel or are delayed and, therefore, do not show up.

The percentage of no-shows varies by hotel and location but is often around 5 percent. In a 400-room hotel, that is 20 rooms, or an average loss of approximately $2,600 per night. Considering these figures, it is not surprising that hotels try to protect themselves by overbooking.

Hotels look carefully at bookings: Whom they are for, what rates they are paying, when they were made, whether they are for regular guests or from a major account (a corporation that uses the hotel frequently), and so on.

Jill Reynolds, the front-office manager at the Regency La Jolla, had known for some time that the 400-room hotel would be overbooked for this one night in October. She prepared to talk with the front-desk associates as they came on duty at 7:30 in the morning, knowing it would be a challenge to sell out without "walking" guests. Seldom does a hotel sell out before having to walk a few guests.

The hotel's policy and procedure on walking guests enables the front desk associates to call nearby hotels of a similar category to find out if they have rooms available to sell. If it is necessary to walk a guest, the associate explains to the guest that, regrettably, no rooms are available because of fewer departures than expected. The associate must explain that suitable accommodations have been reserved at a nearby hotel and that the hotel will pay for the room and transportation to and from the hotel. Usually, guests are understanding, especially when they realize that they are receiving a free room and free transportation.

On this particular day, the house count indicates that the hotel is overbooked by thirty rooms. Three or four nearby, comparable hotels had rooms available to sell in the morning. Besides walking guests, Jill considers other options—in particular "splitting" the fifteen suites with connecting parlors. If the guests in the suites do not need the parlor, it is then possible to gain a few more "rooms" to sell separately; however, rollaway beds must be placed in the rooms. Fortunately, eight parlors were available to sell.

Discussion Question

1. If you were in the same situation, what would you do?

CASE STUDY

Overbooked: The Housekeeping Perspective

It is no secret that in all hotels the director of housekeeping must be able to react quickly and efficiently to any unexpected circumstances that arise. Stephen Rodondi, executive housekeeper at the Regency in La Jolla, California, usually starts his workday at 8:00 A.M. with a department meeting. These morning meetings help him and the employees to visualize their goals for the day. On this particularly busy day, Rodondi arrives at work and is told that three housekeepers have called in sick. This is a serious challenge for the hotel because it is overbooked and has all its 400 rooms to service.

Discussion Question

1. What should Stephen do to maintain standards and ensure that all the guest rooms are serviced?

Source: Courtesy of Stephen Rodondi, Executive Housekeeper, Hyatt Regency, La Jolla, Ca.

Bob Weil, director of food and beverage at the Longboat Key Club and Resort, Sarasota, Florida, offers the following advice: "Be passionate about what you do and be in touch with the people you work with. I tour the property every day to get a feeling for the challenges our team may have—it's important to be in tune with what's going on." Another piece of advice is to never stop cooking and to maintain your fitness so that you can be a high-energy person. Students can expect many rewards in the hospitality business, but remember, it's a long journey, a process. You need to experience all levels in order to become a complete leader.

Summary

1. A big hotel is run by a general manager and an executive committee, which is represented by the key executives of all the major departments, such as rooms division, food and beverage, marketing, sales, and human resources.

2. The general manager represents the hotel and is responsible for its profitability and performance. Because of increased job consolidation, he or she also is expected to attract business and to empathize with the cultures of both guests and employees.

3. The rooms division department consists of front office, reservations, housekeeping, concierge, guest services, and communications.

4. The front desk, as the center of the hotel, sells rooms and maintains balanced guest accounts, which are completed daily by the night auditor. The front desk constantly must meet guests' needs by offering services such as mailing, faxing, and messages.

5. PMSs, centralized reservations, and yield management have enabled hotels to work more efficiently and to increase profitability and guest satisfaction.

6. The communications department, room service, and guest services (such as door attendants, bellpersons, and the concierge) are vital parts of the personality of a hotel.
7. Housekeeping is the largest department of the hotel. The executive housekeeper is in charge of inventory, cleaning, employees, and accident and loss prevention. The laundry may be cleaned directly in the hotel or by a hired laundry service.
8. The electronic room key and closed-circuit television cameras are basic measures provided to protect the guests and their property.

Key Words and Concepts

application service provider (ASP)
average daily rate (ADR)
call accounting systems (CAS)
catastrophe plans
central reservation office (CRO)
central reservation system (CRS)
city ledger
concierge
confirmed reservations
cost centers
daily report
Employee Right to Know
executive committee
global distribution systems (GDS)

guaranteed reservations
night auditor
Occupational Safety and Health Administration (OSHA)
productivity
property management systems (PMS)
revenue management
revenue centers
revenue per available room (REV PAR)
room occupancy percentage (ROP)
room rates
rooms division
uniformed staff
yield management

Review Questions

1. Briefly define the purpose of a hotel. Why is it important to empathize with the culture of guests?
2. List the main responsibilities of the front office manager.
3. How did Michelle Riesdorf become general manager of a Spring Hill Suites property?
4. What are the advantages and disadvantages of yield management?
5. Why is the concierge an essential part of the personality of a hotel?
6. Explain the importance of accident and loss prevention. What security measures are taken to protect guests and their property?

Internet Exercises

1. Organization: **Global Hyatt Corporation**
   Web site: **www.hyatt.com**
   Summary: Global Hyatt Corporation is a multibillion-dollar hotel management company. Together with Hyatt International, the company has about 8 percent of the hotel industry market share. Hyatt is recognized for its decentralized management approach, in which general managers are given a great deal of the management decision-making process. Click the "About Hyatt" tab, and click "Careers" under the "For Job Seekers" section. Then click on "mgmt training program" and take a look at the Management Training Program that Hyatt has to offer.

   (a) What is Hyatt's management training program?
   (b) What requisites must applicants meet to qualify for Hyatt's management training program?

2. Organization: **Hotel Jobs**
   Web site: **www.hoteljobs.com**
   Summary: Hoteljobs.com is a web site that offers information to recruiters, employers, and job seekers in the hospitality industry.
   (a) What different jobs are being offered under "Job Search" and which one, if any, interests you?
   (b) Post your résumé online.

Apply Your Knowledge

1. If you were on the executive committee of a hotel, what kinds of things would you be doing to ensure the success of the hotel?

2. Your hotel has 275 rooms. Last night 198 were occupied. What was the occupancy percentage?

Suggested Activities

1. Go to a hotel's web site and find the price of booking a room for a date of your choice. Then, go to one of the web sites (Hotels.com, Expedia, Travelocity, etc.) that "sell" hotel rooms and see how the price there compares with the price on the hotel's web site.

Endnotes

1. James E. McManemon, address to University of South Florida students, March 26, 2010.
2. Richard A. Wentzel, "Leaders of the Hospitality Industry or Hospitality Management," *An Introduction to the Industry*, 6th ed. (Dubuque, IA: Kendall/Hunt, 1991), 29.
3. Allen Brigid, "Ritz, César Jean (1850–1918)," in *Oxford Dictionary of National Biography*

(Oxford: Oxford University Press, May 2006), **www.oxforddnb.com** [site requires password], (accessed March 4, 2011).

4. F. Ashburner, "Escoffier, Georges Auguste (1846–1935)," *Oxford Dictionary of National Biography* (Oxford: Oxford University Press May 2006), **www.oxforddnb.com** [site requires password], (accessed March 4, 2011).

5. Donald E. Lundberg, *The Hotel and Restaurant Business*, 4th ed. (New York: Van Nostrand Reinhold, 1984), 33–34.

6. Personal conversation with Rollie Teves, July 20, 2007.

7. Personal correspondence with Jay R. Schrock, Ph.D., Dean, School of Hotel and Restaurant Management, University of South Florida, Sarasota-Manatee, January 18, 2011.

8. STR Global, *Products*, http://www.strglobal.com/Products/Product_Overview.aspx (accessed March 3, 2011).

9. Personal conversation with Bruce Lockwood, March 16, 2006.

10. Susan Patel, *Triple Bottom Line and Eco-Efficiency: Where to Start?*, EcoGreenHotel, **www.ecogreenhotel.com/green_hotel_news_Triple-Bottom-Line-and-Eco-Efficiency.php** (accessed February 26, 2011).

11. Ibid.

12. "Green Hotel Certification Programs Snowball, Sparks Confusion," *Sustainable Travel*, **http://blog.sustainabletravel.com/green_hotel_certification_prog_1.html** (accessed February 26, 2011).

13. Ibid.

14. New Hampshire Sustainable Lodging & Restaurant Program, Home Page, **www.nhslrp.org/** (accessed February 26, 2011).

15. Q Hotel and Spa, *Green Is Good*, **www.theqhotel.com/content.php?content_id=1**, (accessed February 26, 2011).

16. Pennsylvania Green Hotels & Motels, *Tourism and the Environment: Greening Your Hotel Operations*, **www.dep.state.pa.us/dep/deputate/pollprev/industry/hotels/operations.htm**, (accessed February 26, 2011).

Glossary

Application service provider (ASP)   Delivers a complete booking system tied to the hotel's inventory in real time via the Internet.

Average daily rate (ADR)   One of the key operating ratios that indicates the level of a hotel's performance. The ADR is calculated by dividing the dollar sales by the number of rooms rented.

Call accounting system (CAS)   A system that tracks guest room phone charges.

Catastrophe plan   A plan to maximize guest and property safety in the event of a disaster.

Central reservations office (CRO)   The central office of a lodging company, where reservations are processed.

Central reservations system (CRS)   A reservation system that is commonly used in large franchises to connect their reservation systems with one another; enables guests to call one phone number to reserve a room at any of the chain properties.

City ledger   A client whose company has established credit with a particular hotel. Charges are posted to the city ledger and accounts are sent once or twice monthly.

Concierge   A uniformed employee of a hotel who works at a desk in the lobby or on special concierge floors and answers questions, solves problems, and performs the services of a private secretary for the hotel's guests.

Confirmed reservation   A reservation made by a guest that is confirmed by the hotel for the dates they plan to stay.

Cost centers   Centers that cost money to operate and do not bring in revenue.

Daily report   A report prepared each day to provide essential performance information for a particular property to its management.

Employee right to know   Per U.S. Senate Bill 198, information about chemicals must be made available to all employees.

Executive committee   A committee of hotel executives from each of the major departments within the hotel; generally made up of the general manager, director of rooms division, food and beverage director, marketing and sales director, human resources director, accounting and/or finance director, and engineering director.

Global Distribution Systems (GDS)   A system that can distribute the product or service globally.

Guaranteed reservations   If rooms are available on guest demand, the hotel guarantees the guests rooms on those days.

Night auditor   The individual who verifies and balances guests' accounts.

Productivity   The amount of product, goods or services produced by employees.

Property management system (PMS)   A computerized system that integrates all systems used by a lodging property, such as reservations, front desk, housekeeping, food and beverage control, and accounting.

Revenue centers   Centers that produce revenue.

Revenue management   The management of revenue.

Revenue per available room (Rev par)   Total Rooms Revenue for Period divided by Total Rooms Available During a Period.

Room division   The departments that make up the rooms division.

Room occupancy percentage (ROP)   The number of rooms occupied divided by rooms available; a key operating ratio for hotels.

Room rates   The various rates charged for hotel rooms.

Uniformed staff   Front of the house staff.

Yield management   The practice of analyzing past reservation patterns, room rates, cancellations, and no-shows in an attempt to maximize profits and occupancy rates and to set the most competitive room rates.

Photo Credits

Credits are listed in the order of appearance.

Tara Flake/Shutterstock
Angus Osborn/DK Images
Bonnie Kamin/PhotoEdit
akg-images/Newscom
Roberts Ratuts/Fotolia LLC
Dr. Charlie Adams Texas Tech University

Myrleen Ferguson-Cate/PhotoEdit, Inc.
MICROS
Denny Bhakta
Klehr & Churchill /Riser/Getty Images
stefanolunardi/Shutterstock
Rob Reichenfeld/DK Images

Food and Beverage Operations

From Chapter 4 of *Introduction to Hospitality Management,* Fourth Edition. John R. Walker. Copyright © 2013 by Pearson Education, Inc. Published by Pearson. All rights reserved.

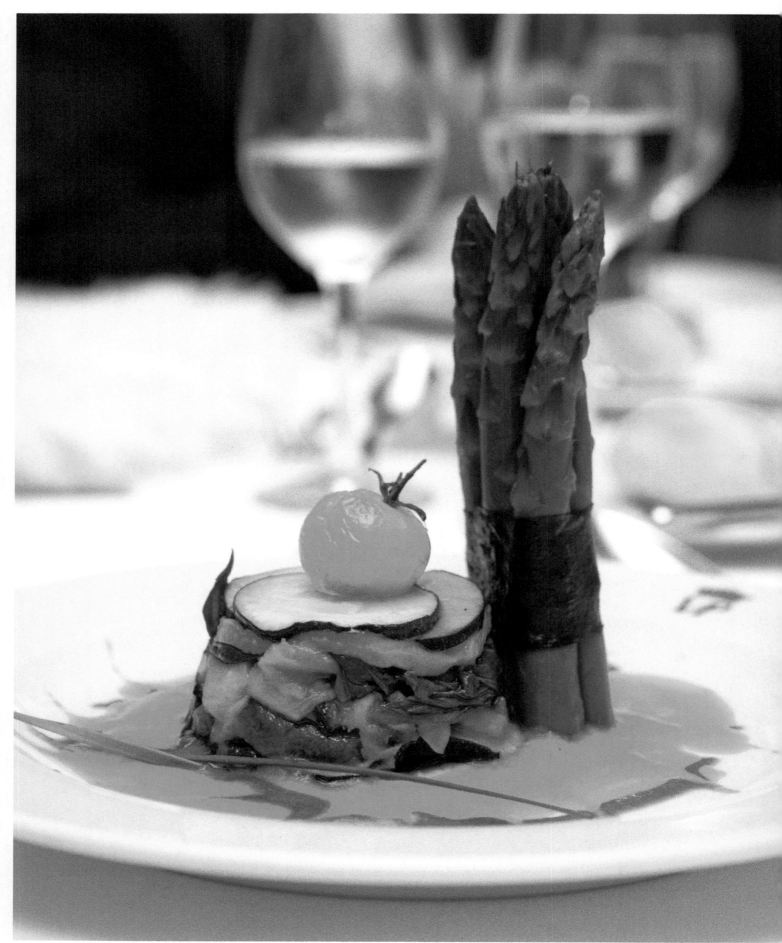

Food and Beverage Operations

OBJECTIVES

After reading and studying this chapter, you should be able to:

- Describe the duties and responsibilities of a food and beverage director and other key department heads.

- Describe a typical food and beverage director's day.

- State the functions and responsibilities of the food and beverage departments.

- Perform computations using key food and beverage operating ratios.

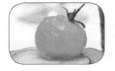
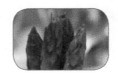
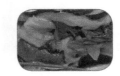
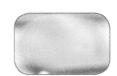

Food and Beverage Management

In the hospitality industry, the food and beverage division is led by the **director of food and beverage.** He or she reports to the general manager and is responsible for the efficient and effective operation of the following departments:

- Kitchen/Catering/Banquet
- Restaurants/Room Service/Minibars
- Lounges/Bars/Stewarding

Figure 1 illustrates a food and beverage organization chart.

The position description for a director of food and beverage is both a job description and a specification of the requirements an individual needs to do the job. In recent years, the skills needed by a food and beverage director have grown enormously, as shown by the following list of responsibilities:

- Exceeding guests' expectations in food and beverage offerings and service
- Leadership
- Identifying trends
- Finding and keeping outstanding employees
- Training
- Motivation
- Budgeting
- Cost control

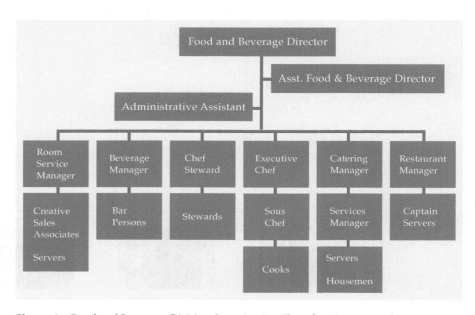

Figure 1 • Food and Beverage Division Organization Chart for a Large Hotel.

- Finding profit from all outlets
- Having a detailed working knowledge of the front-of-the-house operations

These challenges are set against a background of stagnant or declining occupancies and the consequent drop in room sales. Therefore, greater emphasis has been placed on making food and beverage sales profitable. Traditionally, only about 20 percent of the hotel's operating profit comes from the food and beverage divisions. In contrast, an acceptable profit margin from a hotel's food and beverage division is generally considered to be 25 to 30 percent. This figure can vary according to the type of hotel. For example, according to Pannell Kerr Forster, an industry consulting firm, all-suite properties achieve a 7 percent food and beverage profit (probably because of the complimentary meals and drinks offered to guests).

A typical food and beverage director's day might look like the following:

8:30 A.M.	Check messages and read logs from outlets and security. Tour outlets, especially the family restaurant (a quick inspection).
	Check the breakfast buffet, reservations, and the shift manager.
	Check daily specials.
	Check room service.
	Check breakfast service and staffing.
	Meet the executive chef and purchasing director.
	Meet executive steward's office to ensure that all equipment is ready.
	Meet banquet service office to check on daily events and coffee break sequence.
10:00 A.M.	Work on current projects: new summer menu, pool outlet opening, conversion of a current restaurant with a new concept, remodeling of ballroom foyer, installation of new walk-in freezer, and analysis of current profit-and-loss (P&L) statements. Plan weekly food and beverage department meetings.
11:45 A.M.	Visit kitchen to observe lunch service and check the "12:00 line," including banquets.
	Confer with executive chef.
	Check restaurants and banquet luncheon service.
1:00 P.M.	Have working lunch in employee cafeteria with executive chef, director of purchasing, or director of catering.
1:30 P.M.	Meet with human resources to discuss current incidents.
2:30 P.M.	Check messages and return calls. Telemarket to attract catering and convention business.
	Conduct hotel daily menu meeting.
3:00 P.M.	Go to special projects/meetings.
5:30 P.M.	Tour cocktail lounges.

	Check for staffing.
	Review any current promotions.
	Check entertainment lineup.
6:00 P.M.	Check special food and beverage requests/requirements of any VIPs staying at the hotel.
	Tour kitchen.
	Review and taste.
8:00 P.M.	Review dinner specials.
	Check the restaurant and lounges.

A food and beverage director's typical day starts at 8:00 A.M. and ends at 8:00 P.M., unless early or very late events are scheduled, in which case the working day is even longer. Usually, the food and beverage director works Monday through Saturday. If there are special events on Sunday, then he or she works on Sunday and takes Monday off. In a typical week, Saturdays are used to catch up on reading or specific projects.

The director of food and beverage eats in his or her restaurants at least twice a week for dinner and at least once a week for breakfast and lunch. Bars are generally visited with clients, at least twice per week. The director sees salespersons regularly because they are good sources of information about what is going on in the industry and they can introduce leads for business. The director attends staff meetings, food and beverage meetings, executive committee meetings, interdepartmental meetings, credit meetings, and P&L statement meetings.

To become a food and beverage director takes several years of experience and dedication. One of the best routes is to gain work experience or to participate in an internship in several food and beverage departments while attending college. This experience should include full-time, practical kitchen work for at least one to two years to master the core concepts, followed by varying periods of a few months in purchasing, stores, cost control, stewarding, and room service. Stewarding is responsible for back-of-the-house areas such as dishwashing and issuing and inventorying china, glassware, and cutlery. Stewarding duties include maintaining cleanliness in all areas. Additionally, a year spent in each of the following work situations is helpful: restaurants, catering, and bars. After these departmental experiences, and once you master the core competencies, you can likely serve as a department manager, preferably in a different hotel from the one in which the departmental experience was gained. This prevents the awkwardness of being manager of a department in which the person was once an employee and also offers the employee the opportunity to learn different things at different properties.

▶ Check Your Knowledge

1. What are the skills and responsibilities of a food and beverage director?
2. Describe a food and beverage director's day.

INTRODUCING GEORGE GOLDHOFF

Vice President of Food and Beverage, Beau Rivage Resort and Casino, Biloxi, Mississippi

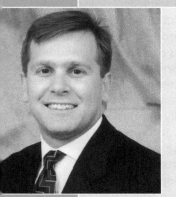

Being hired as the pot washer for the Old Homestead Country Kitchen at the early age of fifteen hardly seemed to herald the beginnings of an auspicious career in the hospitality industry. But to George Goldhoff, with his high energy and natural leadership skills, he had found the perfect environment in which to excel. The sense of family and camaraderie between the staff members and the interaction with guests, mixed with the intensity of performance and deadlines, have never lost their appeal. Excellence in service would become his lifelong pursuit.

Fast-forward twenty years. As director of food and beverage at Bellagio of MGM/Mirage, Inc., in Las Vegas, George was responsible for the quality assurance, personnel development, and financial performance of seventeen restaurants and ten bars, with 3,000 employees and more than $200 million in revenues. His responsibilities may have increased since his pot washer days, but the core message in his service training remains intact: sincerity toward the guest and anticipation of guest needs. His approach to service is simple: Greet all guests with a smile, make sure they are comfortable, offer them something to eat and drink. These service basics, simple instructions given to him as a five-year-old by his parents, have stayed with him. Playing host at one of his parents' dinner parties, he learned early the power of a sincere smile and the rewarding experience of pleasing others. Little did he or his parents intuit that one day his child's play would evolve into a rewarding career in hospitality.

As one of the original members of the opening team for the Bellagio, George drew from his extensive and varied food and beverage background to make the Bellagio's opening a success. In 1983 George graduated from Schenectady County Community College as a dean's list student and recipient of an athletic scholarship award. He continued on to the University of Massachusetts where he earned his B.S. degree in hotel, restaurant, and travel administration. His acceptance to these two institutions, after having dropped out of high school, instilled in George the self-confidence in his abilities and the technical skills necessary to achieve his goals. For a young man without a high school diploma who was often characterized as wild and rebellious, it was a revelation, an awakening to his potentials and the realization that he could accomplish great things. His introduction to corporate culture was as an assistant front office manager and Hyatt corporate trainee in Savannah, Georgia.

Upon completion of his training, he moved to beautiful Tahoe in 1988, where he was able to combine his love for restaurants and sports. An all-around athlete, adhering to the work hard, play hard principle, he pursued speed skiing competitions at the highest levels. He stayed on as general manager of Rosie's Café for two and a half years. However, growing tired of the small town confines of Tahoe City and with the singular challenges of Rosie's Café becoming undemanding, George acted on a friend's advice, contacted a mutual friend, and took a job on a 750-foot merchant ship. For the next six months George sailed around the world cooking breakfast, lunch, and dinner for a crew of twelve, while visiting ports in Gibraltar, Malta, Egypt, the United Arab Emirates, Kuwait, and Saudi Arabia. In 1990, aspiring to be a major player not just in skiing, but in the restaurant arena as well, he sought grander, more sophisticated restaurants to manage.

George's ambitions led him to the Plaza Hotel in New York, where he started as an assistant beverage director. George immersed himself in his new position with his usual high-voltage energy and infectious enthusiasm, earning him nicknames such as the Golden Boy and Mr. Hollywood. It did not take long for George to be recognized for his positive attitude and management abilities. Within six months, he was promoted to manager of the stately Oak Room, the youngest manager in the restaurant's ninety-year history. Within a two-year period, he was promoted to managing four of the Plaza Hotel's five à la carte restaurants.

Holding to his personal belief that "you are the company you keep," he has always endeavored to associate with the highest quality restaurateurs and organizations. In 1993, he realized one of his dreams—the

(continued)

INTRODUCING GEORGE GOLDHOFF *(continued)*

opportunity to work with the legendary Joe Baum—managing the famous Rainbow Room in Rockefeller Center. His commitment to service, the evident pride he takes in his work, and his high standard of ethics earned George praise from Joe Baum as being his best maître d' ever. Such a high compliment could have gone to his head. However, George is not one to sit back and take it easy. Instead, he set even higher standards and focused his energies on new goals. He quotes his old boss and industry idol Joe Baum as saying, "Values and standards are those you make for yourself. You don't have to be as good as the other guy. You have to be better—a lot better."

Against the advice of well-meaning family and peers, he left the Rainbow Room in 1997 to enroll in the MBA program at Columbia University. This was no easy decision, considering George was happily married at this point, with one child and another on the way. However, he has never been afraid to take risks, and is not one to fear taking on new challenges. In fact, his adventurous and go-getter nature revels in change. With the same self-confidence, resourcefulness, and ability to focus on multiple tasks he, not surprisingly, took first place in Columbia's Business Plan competition and was the recipient of the prestigious Eugene Lang Entrepreneurial Initiative Fund. Armed with his MBA degree and newly acquired business skills, he was ready for his next adventure.

Even before he had graduated, he was tapped by Stephen Rushmore, founder and president of Hospitality Valuation Services, to work with him as a consultant and valuation analyst. Here he was afforded the opportunity to incorporate his academic learning, fresh ideas, and extensive hotel background into his work. He created the 1996 Hotel Valuation Index (HVS), which was later published in the *Cornell Quarterly*. Ever the entrepreneur, he left HVS in 1997 to establish his own venture, The Irish Coast, Inc., creating and implementing the Guinness Irish pub concept. He jumped into the task of perfecting the Irish pub ambience of warmth, comfort, and congeniality, the heart of hospitality. Hence, it was only a matter of time before he would find himself in Las Vegas, the "Hospitality Capital of the World." In 1998, he signed on with Mirage Resorts to open the ultimate luxury resort and casino, Bellagio.

For George, it's all about service. Excellence in customer satisfaction and a genuine concern for his staff and coworkers have been his guiding principles. Characterized by colleagues as a dreamer, he has the rare ability to communicate his vision and to motivate and inspire others into executing that vision, making it a reality. The ability to instill in those around him the desire to strive beyond and stretch past their comfort zones is just one of his leadership characteristics. His motivational secret is to "constantly remind the staff that their job is precious, even if they've been doing it year after year." He maintains that the key to service is to "know one's job and to remember that a little kindness goes a long way to making people happy. A guest always knows if someone doesn't care."

In addition to starting up and overseeing the entire food and beverage operations for the hotel, he was chosen to represent Mirage Resorts in Focus Las Vegas, a leadership development program of the Las Vegas Chamber of Commerce. Making a difference in others' lives has always been one of the appealing factors of being in the hospitality field. He has always felt personally rewarded when he can give back to others, such as promoting a new busperson, building up someone else's self-esteem, watching people gain confidence in themselves and take pride in their work. He concedes he did not reach his position on his own, but with the assistance of many caring mentors. Always mindful and appreciative of those who have helped him throughout his career, he enjoys helping others discover their own potential. He considers human relations to be one of his strengths and regards staff development to be one of his greatest priorities as a leader. Empowering frontline employees is essential to maintaining a restaurant's competitive edge: "Give them the tools and let them do the job."

George has great expectations for himself and those around him and is not afraid of hard work. In fact, he works with a passion. The long hours and the intensity do not faze him. His adaptability to different situations, his ability to relate to a variety of personalities and temperaments, and his keen sense of humor serve him well both in front and back of the house. With his winning smile and straightforward demeanor, he sets his sights on a promising future and the many adventures ahead.

Kitchen

A hotel kitchen is under the charge of the **executive chef** or chef in smaller and medium-sized properties. This person, in turn, is responsible to the director of food and beverage for the efficient and effective operation of kitchen food production. The desired outcome is to exceed guests' expectations in the quality and quantity of food, its presentation, taste, and portion size, and to ensure that hot food is served hot and cold food is served cold. The executive chef operates the kitchen in accordance with company policy and strives to achieve desired financial results.

Some executive chefs are now called **kitchen managers**; they even serve as food and beverage directors in midsized and smaller hotels. This trend toward "right-sizing," observed in other industries, euphemistically refers to restructuring organizations to retain the most essential employees. Usually, this means cutting labor costs by consolidating job functions. For example, Michael Hammer is executive chef and food and beverage director at the 440-room Hilton La Jolla in Torrey Pines, California. Mike is typical of the new breed of executive chefs: His philosophy is to train his sous chefs, *sous* being a French word meaning "under," to make many of the operating decisions. He delegates ordering, hiring, and firing decisions; sous chefs are the ones most in control of the production and the people who work on their teams. By delegating more of the operating decisions, he is developing the chefs de partie (or stations chefs) and empowering them to make their own decisions. As he puts it, "No decision is wrong—but in case it is unwise, we will talk about it later."

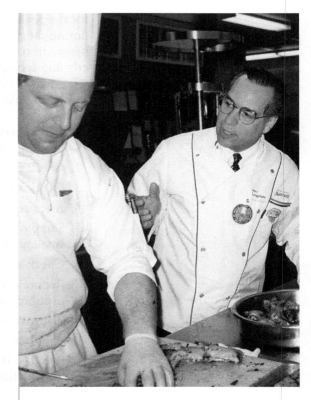

The executive chef of a very large hotel manages the kitchen and may not do much cooking.

Mike spends time maintaining morale, a vital part of a manager's responsibilities. The kitchen staff is under a great deal of pressure and frequently works against the clock. Careful cooperation and coordination are the keys to success. He explains that he does not want his associates to "play the tuba"—he wants them to conduct the orchestra. He does not hold food and beverage department meetings; instead he meets with groups of employees frequently, and problems are handled as they occur. Controls are maintained with the help of software that costs their standard recipes, establishes **perpetual inventories**, and calculates potential food cost per outlet. Today, executive chefs and food and beverage directors look past food cost to the actual profit contribution of an item. For example, if a pasta dish costs $3.25 and sells for $12.95, the contribution margin is $9.70. Today, there are software programs such as ChefTec that offer software solutions for purchasing, ordering, inventory control, and recipe and menu costing; ChefTec Plus offers perpetual inventory, sales analysis, theoretical inventory reports, and multiple profit centers.

Controlling costs is an essential part of food and beverage operations and, because labor costs represent the most significant variable costs, staffing becomes an important factor in the day-to-day running of the food and beverage locations. Labor cost benchmarks are measured by covers-per-person-hour. For example, in stewarding, it should take no more than one person per hour to clean 37.1 covers. Mike and his team of outlet managers face interesting challenges, such as staffing for the peaks and valleys of guest needs at breakfast. Many guests want breakfast during the peak time of 7:00 to 8:30 A.M., requiring organization to get the right people in the right place at the right time to ensure that meals are prepared properly and served in a timely manner.

At the Hilton La Jolla–Torrey Pines, Executive Chef Hammer's day goes something like the following:

1. Arrive between 6:00 and 7:00 A.M. and walk through the food and beverage department with the night cleaners.
2. Check to make sure the compactor is working and the area is clean.
3. Check that all employees are on duty.
4. Ask people what kind of challenges they will face today.
5. Sample as many dishes as possible, checking for taste, consistency, feel, smell, and overall quality.
6. Check walk-ins.
7. Recheck once or twice a day to see where the department stands production-wise—this helps reduce or eliminate overtime.
8. Approve schedules for food and beverage outlet.
9. Keep a daily update of food and beverage revenues and costs.
10. Forecast the next day's, week's, and month's business based on updated information.
11. Check on final numbers for catering functions.

Financial results are generally expressed in ratios, such as **food cost percentage**—the cost of food divided by the amount of food sales. A simple example is the sale of a hamburger for $1.00. If the cost of the food is $0.30, then the food cost percentage is 30 percent, which is about average for many hotels. The average might be reduced to 27 percent in hotels that do a lot of catering. As discussed later in this section, in determining the food and beverage department's profit and loss, executive chefs and food and beverage directors must consider not only the food cost percentage, but also the **contribution margin** of menu items. The contribution margin is the amount contributed by a menu item toward overhead expenses and is the difference between the cost of preparing the item and its selling price.

Another important cost ratio for the kitchen is labor cost. The **labor cost percentage** may vary depending on the amount of convenience foods purchased versus those made from scratch (raw ingredients). In a kitchen, the labor cost percentage may be expressed as a **food sales percentage**. For example, if food sales total $1,000 and labor costs total $250, then labor costs may be expressed as a percentage of food sales by the following formula:

$$\frac{\text{Labor Cost}}{\text{Food Sales}}, \quad \text{therefore} \quad \frac{\$250}{\$1,000} = 25\% \text{ labor cost}$$

Labor management is controlled with the aid of programs such as TimePro from Commeg Systems. TimePro is a time, attendance, and scheduling package that provides an analytical tool for managers and saves time on forecasting and scheduling.

CORPORATE PROFILE

Marilyn Carlson, CEO of Carlson Companies

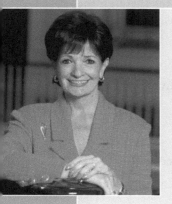

Based in Minneapolis, Carlson's brands and services employ about 170,000 people in nearly 150 countries and territories. Led by Chairperson and Chief Executive Officer Marilyn Carlson Nelson, Carlson Companies continues to build on a cornerstone set by her father, Curt Carlson, nearly 70 years ago: developing long-lasting relationships with clients.

The history of Carlson Companies is one of the classic business success stories in the American free-enterprise system. Starting in 1938 with merely an idea and $55 of borrowed capital, entrepreneur Curtis L. Carlson founded the Gold Bond Stamp Company in his home city of Minneapolis, Minnesota. His trading stamp concept, designed to stimulate sales and loyalty for food stores and other merchants, proved to be right for the times and swept the nation in a wave of dramatic growth.

Through the years, Carlson diversified into hotels, travel, and other related businesses. In the 1960s, Carlson and several other partners collectively bought an interest in the original Radisson Hotel in downtown Minneapolis. Eventually, Carlson became sole owner of the hotel brand and expanded it around the globe.

Among the names in the Carlson family of brands and services are Radisson Hotels & Resorts, Park Plaza Hotels & Resorts, Country Inn & Suites by Carlson, Park Inn hotels, T.G.I. Friday's, and Carlson Wagonlit Travel.

Carlson Hospitality Worldwide encompasses 1,085 hotels in 77 countries, 900 restaurants in 60 countries, and is the world's leading travel management company. Under the banner of Ambition 2015, Carlson has established the following ambitions for its brands:

By 2015 we want our brands to be the leading brand in their segment.

We want to become the number-one hospitality company to work for.

We want to become the number-one hospitality company to invest with.

For Carlson hotels, the Ambition 2015 strategy entails growing the hotel portfolio by at least 50 percent to reach 1,500 hotels in operation by 2015. The hotel strategy is centered around five major themes[1]:

Establish a clear, compelling position for each brand.

Operationalize the brand promises.

Accelerate development.

Win the revenue battle.

Build a global team and organization.

For the restaurant brand T.G.I. Friday's, the Ambition 2015 is focused on driving the growth of this iconic brand. It has three major priorities[2]:

Boost same store sales at existing domestic stores.

Pressure domestic development in a targeted fashion.

Accelerate international growth.

In addition to global business success, Carlson Companies is also recognized as a top employer. Both *Fortune* and *Working Mother* magazines have rated the company as one of their "100 Best Places to Work in America."

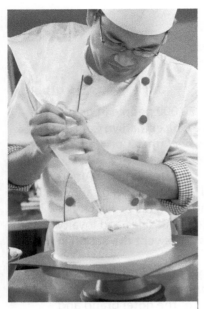

A Pastry Chef.

An executive chef has one or more **sous chefs**. Because so much of the executive chef's time is spent on administration, sous chefs are often responsible for the day-to-day running of each shift. Depending on size, a kitchen may have several sous chefs: one or more for days, one for evenings, and another for banquets.

Under the sous chefs is the **chef tournant**. This person rotates through the various stations to relieve the **station chef** heads. These stations are organized according to production tasks, based on the classic "brigade" introduced by Escoffier. The **brigade** includes the following:

Sauce chef, who prepares sauces, stews, sautés, hot hors d'oeuvres
Roast chef, who roasts, broils, grills, and braises meats
Fish chef, who cooks fish dishes
Soup chef, who prepares all soups
Cold larder/pantry chef, who prepares all cold foods: salads, cold hors d'oeuvres, buffet food, and dressings
Banquet chef, who is responsible for all banquet food
Pastry chef, who prepares all hot and cold dessert items
Vegetable chef, who prepares vegetables (this person may be the fry cook and soup cook in some smaller kitchens)

Soup, cold larder, banquets, pastry, and vegetable chefs' positions may be combined in smaller kitchens.

▶ Check Your Knowledge

1. What is a food cost percentage and how is it calculated?
2. What is a contribution margin?
3. How is labor cost percentage calculated?

A DAY IN THE LIFE OF JIM GEMIGNANI

Executive Chef, Marriott Hotel

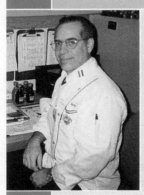

Jim Gemignani is executive chef at the 1,500-room Marriott Hotel in San Francisco. Chef Jim, as his associates call him, is responsible for the quality of food, guest, and associate satisfaction and for financial satisfaction in terms of results. With more than 200 associates in eight departments, Chef Jim has an interesting challenge. He makes time to be innovative by researching food trends and comparative shopping. Currently, American cuisine is in, as are freestanding restaurants in hotels. An ongoing part of American cuisine is the healthy food that Chef Jim says has not yet found a niche.

Hotels are building identity into their restaurants by branding or creating their own brand name. Marriott, for example, has Pizza Hut pizzas on the room service menu. Marriott hotels have created their own tiers of restaurants. JW's is the formal restaurant, Tuscany's is a northern Italian–themed restaurant, the American Grill has replaced the old coffee shop, and Kimoko is a Japanese restaurant. As a company, Marriott decided to go nationwide with the first three of these concepts. This has simplified menus and improved food quality and presentation, and yet regional specials allow for individual creativity on the part of the chef.

When asked about his personal philosophy, Chef Jim says that in this day and age, one needs to embrace change and build teams; the guest is an important part of the team. Chef Jim's biggest challenge is keeping guests and associates happy. He is also director of food service outlets, which now gives him a front-of-the-house perspective. Among his greatest accomplishments are seeing his associates develop—twenty are now executive chefs—retaining 96 percent of his opening team, and being voted Chef of the Year by the San Francisco Chef's Association.

Chef Jim's advice: "It's tough not to have a formal education, but remember that you need a combination of 'hands-on' and formal training. If you're going to be a leader, you must start at the bottom and work your way up; otherwise, you will become a superior and not know how to relate to your associates."

Food Operations

A hotel may have several restaurants or no restaurant at all; the number and type of restaurants varies as well. A major chain hotel generally has two restaurants: a signature or upscale formal restaurant and a casual coffee shop–type restaurant. These restaurants cater to both hotel guests and to the general public. In recent years, because of increased guest expectations, hotels have placed greater emphasis on food and beverage preparation and service. As a result, there is an increasing need for professionalism on the part of hotel personnel.

Hotel restaurants are run by **restaurant managers** in much the same way as other restaurants. **Restaurant managers** are generally responsible for the following:

- Exceeding guest service expectations
- Hiring, training, and developing employees
- Setting and maintaining quality standards
- Marketing
- Banquets
- Coffee service
- In-room dining, minibars, or the cocktail lounge
- Presenting annual, monthly, and weekly forecasts and budgets to the food and beverage director

Some restaurant managers work on an incentive plan with quarterly performance bonuses. Hotel restaurants present the manager with some interesting challenges because hotel guests are not always predictable. Sometimes they will use the hotel restaurants, and other times they will dine out. If they dine in or out to an extent beyond the forecasted number of guests, problems can arise. Too many guests for the restaurants results in delays and poor service. Too few

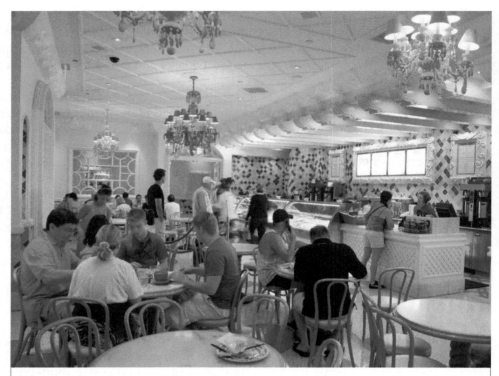

The Gelato Cafe, an Italian style cafe in the Bellagio Hotel.

guests means that employees are underutilized, which can increase labor costs unless employees are sent home early. A restaurant manager keeps a diary of the number of guests served by the restaurant on the same night the previous week, month, and year.

The number (house count) and type of hotel guest (e.g., the number of conference attendees who may have separate dining arrangements) should also be considered in estimating the number of expected restaurant guests for any meal. This figure is known as the **capture rate**, which, when coupled with historic and banquet activity and hotel occupancy, will be the restaurant's basis for forecasting the number of expected guests.

Most hotels find it difficult to coax hotel guests into the restaurants. However, many continuously try to convert foodservice from a necessary amenity to a profit center. The Royal Sonesta in New Orleans offers restaurant coupons worth $5 to its guests and guests of nearby hotels. Another successful strategy, adopted by the Plaza Athénée in New York, is to show guests the restaurants and explain the cuisine before they go to their rooms. This has prompted more guests to dine in the restaurant during their stay. At some hotels, the restaurants self-promote by having cooking demonstrations in the lobby: The "on-site" chefs offer free samples to hotel guests. Progressive hotels, such as the Kimco Hotel in San Francisco, ensure that the hotel restaurants look like freestanding restaurants with separate entrances.

FOCUS ON LODGING

Gracious Hospitality

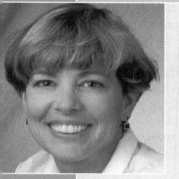

Catherine Rabb, Johnson and Wales University

I find great pleasure in seeing a well-managed hotel handling full occupancy, special events, and busy dining rooms with seemingly effortless grace. How welcoming it is for the traveler or for the guest at a special event to be served by professionals who embody the true spirit of gracious hospitality.

What the guest doesn't see is the complex network of interlocking relationships and intensive training necessary behind the scenes to make each day successful at any hotel. It has been said that hotels need to be like ducks—appearing to glide effortlessly along the surface, while paddling like the devil underneath! Every person in our operation is a critical component of our business. We sell food and beverages in a variety of ways, but in hospitality operations, the interaction with the guest becomes part of the product, with no room for returns if service is defective. We are only as good as our last meal, our last event, or our last contact with a guest. Service itself *is* the product.

As you will learn in this chapter, many different departments and people with diverse skills must work together efficiently. Hotels of different sizes and styles exist, so some operations need more people, and some need less; but for all hotels a dedication to providing the best available services and products is critical. This diverse group of people must work together to create a service product whose appearance is seamless. The coordination of people, talents, schedules, and needs is a complex ballet of intricate steps choreographed to create a seamless whole. A successful operation needs the talents of every member of the staff and welcomes the varied skills, energies, and ideas that their team brings to the table. Everyone, from the newest part-time employee to the manager, needs to be at the top of his or her game to reach the goal of service excellence.

The term *multitasking* has perhaps been overused in recent years; however, nowhere is the term better suited than to describe the routine tasks done by so many industry professionals. Whether we are chefs, bartenders, stewards, catering managers, or food and beverage directors, we all need a wide variety of skills and abilities to be successful in this challenging industry. We need the technical skills necessary to do the job: correct service techniques, food preparation skills, the ability to mix a perfect drink, or to set a room properly for a special event. We must also possess the ability to interact with our team members, each of whom is responsible for a different set of tasks performed under pressure. It is critical that we understand and master the fact that our business must make a profit, and we work hard to blend effective budgets and cost controls with our service goals. We continuously provide extensive, thorough, effective, and ongoing training for ourselves and our staff so that our team is knowledgeable, trained, and empowered to act in the best interest of the guest and, ultimately, our operation. Our knowledge of the legalities of operating a business must be extensive so that our operations and our staff are protected. We are competitive because our market is changing and challenging, and we continually strive to position our businesses to be competitive. We must be strong because the physical demands of the business can be demanding, and we must be self-aware, for doing a challenging job well means that we are able to take care of ourselves and our lives outside the hotel. We lead by example to inspire our teammates to do the very best job they can, whatever the circumstances. Terrific service requires terrific people who possess the ability to integrate these characteristics into every workday.

What type of people are drawn to this business? People who love a challenge. People who enjoy other people. People who love their work and take pride in their ability to create a beautiful banquet, a perfect soup, or a well-designed training program. People with a work ethic, honesty, and integrity that make them an example to others. People who love to learn. People who enjoy the fact that every day is different and brings different challenges. Perhaps someone like you!

Bars

Hotel bars allow guests to relax while sipping a cocktail after a hectic day. This opportunity to socialize for business or pleasure is advantageous for both guests and the hotel. Because the profit percentage on all beverages is higher than it is on food items, bars are an important revenue source for the food and beverage departments. The cycle of beverages from ordering, receiving, storing, issuing, bar stocking, serving, and guest billing is complex, but, unlike restaurant meals, a beverage can be held over if not sold. An example of a world-famous hotel bar is the King Cole Bar in the St. Regis Hotel in New York City. This bar has been a favored New York "watering hole" of the rich and famous for many years. The talking point of the bar is a painted mural of Old King Cole, the nursery rhyme character.

Bars are run by bar managers. The responsibilities of a bar manager include the following:

- Supervising the ordering process and storage of wines
- Preparing a wine list
- Overseeing the staff
- Maintaining cost control
- Assisting guests with their wine selection
- Proper service of wine
- Knowledge of beers and liquors and their service

Bar efficiency is measured by the **pour/cost percentage**. Pour cost is obtained by dividing the cost of depleted inventory by sales over a period of time. Food and beverage directors expect a pour cost of between 16 and 24 percent. Generally, operations with lower pour costs have more sophisticated control systems and a higher-volume catering operation. An example of this is an automatic system that dispenses the exact amount of beverage requested via a pouring gun, which is fed by a tube from a beverage store. These systems are expensive, but they save money for volume operations by being less prone to pilferage, overpouring, or other tricks of the trade. Their greatest savings comes in the form of reduced labor costs; fewer bartenders are needed to make the same amount of drinks. However, the barperson may still hand pour premium brands for show.

Hotel bars are susceptible to the same problems as other bars. The director of food and beverage must set strict policy and procedure guidelines and see to it that they are followed. In today's litigious society, the onus is on the operator to install and ensure **responsible alcoholic beverage service**, and all beverage service staff should receive training in this important area because it might limit the bar's liability. (The NRA offers Serve Safe alcohol.) If a guest becomes intoxicated and is still served alcohol or a minor is served alcohol and is involved in an accident involving someone else, then the server of the beverage, the barperson, and the manager may be liable for the injuries sustained by the person who was harmed, the third party.

Another risk bars encounter is **pilferage**. Employees have been known to steal or tamper with liquor. They could, for example, dilute drinks with water or colored liquids, sell the additional liquor, and pocket the money. There are several other ways to defraud a bar. One of the better known ways is to overcharge guests for beverages. Another is to underpour, which gives guests less for their money. Some bartenders overpour measures to receive larger tips. The best way to prevent these occurrences is to have a good control system, which should include **shoppers**—people who are paid to use the bar like regular guests, except they are closely watching the operation.

In a large hotel there are several kinds of bars:

Lobby bar. This convenient meeting place was popularized when Conrad Hilton wanted to generate revenue out of his vast hotel lobby. Lobby bars, when well managed, are a good source of income.

Restaurant bar. Traditionally, this bar is away from the hubbub of the lobby and offers a holding area for the hotel's signature restaurant.

A server carries Singapore Slings in the Long Bar at Raffles Hotel Singapore.

Service bar. In some of the very large hotels, restaurants and room service have a separate backstage bar. Otherwise, both the restaurant and room service are serviced by one of the regular beverage outlets, such as the restaurant bar.

Catering and banquet bar. This bar is used specifically to service all the catering and banquet needs of the hotel. These bars can stretch any operator to the limit. Frequently, several cash bars must be set up at a variety of locations; if cash wines are involved with dinner, it becomes a race to get the wine to the guest before the meal, preferably before the appetizer. Because of the difficulties involved in servicing a large number of guests, most hotels encourage inclusive wine and beverage functions, in which the guests pay a little more for tickets that include a predetermined amount of beverage service. Banquet bars require careful inventory control. The bottles should be checked immediately after the function, and, if the bar is very busy, the bar manager should pull the money just before the bar closes. The breakdown of function bars should be done on the spot if possible to help prevent pilferage.

The banquet bar needs to stock not only large quantities of the popular wines, spirits, and beers, but also a selection of premium spirits and after-dinner liqueurs. These are used in the ballroom and private dining rooms, in particular.

Pool bars. Pool bars are popular at resort hotels where guests can enjoy a variety of exotic cocktails poolside. Resort hotels that cater to conventions often put on theme parties one night of the convention to allow delegates to kick back. Popular themes that are catered around the pool might be a Hawaiian luau, a Caribbean reggae night, a Mexican fiesta, or Country and Western events. Left to the imagination, one could conceive of a number of theme events.

Minibars. Minibars or honor bars are small, refrigerated bars in guest rooms. They offer the convenience of having beverages available at all times. For security, they have a separate key, which may be either included in the room key envelope at check-in or withheld, according to the guest's preference. Minibars are typically checked and replenished on a daily basis. Charges for items used are automatically added to the guest folio.

Night clubs. Some hotels offer guests evening entertainment and dancing. Whether formal or informal, these food and beverage outlets offer a full beverage service. Live entertainment is very expensive. Many hotels are switching to operations with a DJ or where the bar itself is the entertainment (e.g., sports bar). Directors of food and beverage are now negotiating more with live bands, offering them a base pay (below union scale) and a percentage of a cover charge.

Sports bars. Sports bars have become popular in hotels. Almost everyone identifies with a sporting theme, which makes for a relaxed atmosphere that complements contemporary lifestyles. Many sports bars have a variety of games such as pool, football, bar basketball, and so on, which, together with satellite-televised sporting events, contribute to the atmosphere.

Casino bars. Casino bars and beverage service are there to keep people gambling by offering low-cost or free drinks. Some have lavish entertainment and light food offerings, which entice guests to enjoy the gaming experience, even when sustaining heavy losses.

Different types of bars produce revenue according to their location in the hotel and the kind of hotel in which they are located. Nightclubs, sports bars, and the banqueting department see bulk consumption of alcoholic beverages, and restaurant bars usually see more alcohol consumption than minibars and lounge bars.

▶ Check Your Knowledge

1. What departments does the food and beverage director oversee?
2. What are the responsibilities of a food and beverage director on a day-to-day basis?
3. Explain how the pour/cost percentage is used in a bar to measure efficiency.

Stewarding Department

The **chief steward** is responsible to the director of food and beverage for the following functions:

- Cleanliness of the back of the house (all the areas of the backstage that hotel guests do not see)
- Maintaining clean glassware, china, and cutlery for the food and beverage outlets
- Maintaining strict inventory control and monthly stock check
- Maintenance of dishwashing machines

- Inventory of chemical stock
- Sanitation of kitchen, banquet aisles, storerooms, walk-ins/freezers, and all equipment
- Pest control and coordination with exterminating company
- Forecasting labor and cleaning supplies

In some hotels, the steward's department is responsible for keeping the kitchen(s) clean. This is generally done at night to prevent disruption of the food production operation. A more limited cleaning is done in the afternoon between the lunch and dinner services. The chief steward's job can be an enormous and thankless task. In hotels, this involves cleaning up after several hundred people three times a day. Just trying to keep track of everything can be a headache. Some hotels

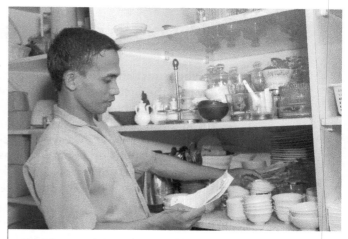

A chief steward checking the inventory.

have different patterns of glasses, china, and cutlery for each outlet. The casual dining room frequently has an informal theme, catering and banqueting a more formal one, and the signature restaurant, very formal place settings. It is difficult to ensure that all the pieces are returned to the correct places. It is also difficult to prevent both guests and employees from taking souvenirs. Strict inventory control and constant vigilance help keep pilferage to a minimum.

TECHNOLOGY SPOTLIGHT

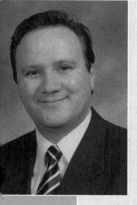

Cihan Cobanoglu, Ph.D., Dean, School of Hotel and Restaurant Management, University of South Florida, Sarasota-Manatee

Full-service hotels have several food and beverage operations. These may include breakfast, lunch, and dinner restaurants; lobby, pool, fitness club, spa, and snack bars; a night club and discothèque; and banquet/event rooms. In addition, hotels may have outlets such as gift shop. All of these transactions are managed by point-of-sale (POS) systems. A POS system can enhance decision-making, operational control, guest services, and revenues. A POS system is a network of cashier and server terminals that typically handles food and beverage orders, transmission of orders to the kitchen and bar, guest-check settlement, timekeeping, and interactive charge posting to guest folios. POS information can also be imported to accounting and food-cost/inventory software packages. A variety of reports can be generated, including open check (list of outstanding checks), cashier, voids/comps, sales analysis, menu mix, server sales summary, tip, labor cost, and so forth. Sophisticated POS systems can generate as many as 200 management reports. The advantages of using a POS system in a food and beverage operations include the following:

1. **Elimination of arithmetic errors:** A POS system may eliminate manual arithmetic calculations, therefore increasing guest satisfaction and tips. A study concluded that restaurants using handwritten checks have lower tipping and a substantial loss of potential revenue.

(continued)

2. **Improved guest check control:** In an industry where the failure rate among restaurants is about 60% within the first three years, controlling costs and revenue is critical. A POS system allows for all transactions to be recorded, allowing less room for fraud. Failure to audit missing checks and to reconcile guest check sales with cash register readings often results in a lower sales volume and higher cost ratios. With a POS system, a server must place the order through a server terminal for it to be printed in the kitchen or bar. This ensures the recording of all sales and provides line cooks with legible orders. It also electronically tracks open checks, settled checks, voids, comps, discounts, and sales for each server, as well as employee meals.

3. **Increased average guest check:** Since orders are transmitted to the kitchen printer, travel time to the kitchen is reduced. This allows more time for suggestive selling and servicing guests. Also, a POS system provides a detailed summary for each server, listing average guest check, items sold, and total sales. This information can be used for job evaluations, motivational programs (for example, wine contest), and assessing merchandising skills (for example, average guest check and item sales) and server efficiency (for example, sales per hour).

4. **Faster reaction to trends:** A POS system can provide a wealth of information on a real-time basis. Most POS systems can easily track sales and cost information by time period (for example, hourly, daily, weekly), employee, meal period, register, outlet, table, and menu item. This allows a restaurant operator to quickly spot and react to problematic areas affecting profitability, such as a declining average guest check during lunch, excessive labor hours in the kitchen, a changing menu mix, or sluggish liquor sales.

5. **Reduced labor costs and greater operational efficiency**: An efficient POS system should be able to increase operational efficiency, therefore allowing staff members to have higher levels of productivity. In the long term, this may result in reduced labor costs.

In addition to the POS system, some of the applications for a restaurant include table management systems, home delivery, frequent-dining and gift card programs, inventory control systems, and menu management systems.

Catering Department

Throughout the world's cultural and social evolution, numerous references have been made to the breaking of bread together. Feasts or banquets are one way to show one's hospitality. Frequently, hosts attempted to outdo one another with the extravagance of their feasts. Today, occasions for celebrations, banquets, and catering include the following:

- State banquets, when countries' leaders honor visiting royalty and heads of state
- National days
- Embassy receptions and banquets
- Business and association conventions and banquets
- Gala charity balls
- Company dinner dances
- Weddings

The term *catering* has a broader scope than does *banquet*. **Banquet** refers to groups of people who eat together at one time and in one place. **Catering** includes a variety of occasions when people may eat at varying times. However, the terms are often used interchangeably.

For example, catering departments in large, city-center hotels may service the following events in just one day:

- A Fortune 500 company's annual shareholders' meeting
- An international loan-signing ceremony
- A fashion show
- A convention
- Several sales and board meetings
- Private luncheons and dinner parties
- A wedding or two

Naturally each of these requires different and special treatment. Hotels in smaller cities may cater the local chamber of commerce meeting, a high school prom, a local company party, a regional sales meeting, a professional workshop, and a small exhibition.

Catering may be subdivided into on-premise and off-premise. In off-premise catering, the event is catered away from the hotel. The food may be prepared either in the hotel or at the event. The organization chart in Figure 2 shows how the catering department is organized. The dotted lines show cooperative reporting relationships, and continuous lines show a direct reporting relationship. For example, the banquet chef reports directly to the executive chef, but must cooperate with the director of catering and the catering service manager.

The **director of catering** (**DOC**) is responsible to the food and beverage director for selling and servicing, catering, banquets, meetings, and exhibitions in a way that exceeds guests' expectations and produces reasonable profit. The director of catering has a close working relationship with the rooms division manager because the catering department often brings conventions, which require rooms, to the hotel. There is also a close working relationship with the executive chef. The chef plans the banqueting menus, but the catering manager must ensure that they are suitable for the clientele and practical from a service point of view. Sometimes they work together in developing a selection of menus that will meet all the requirements, including cost and price.

The director of catering must be able to do the following:

1. Sell conventions, banquets, and functions.
2. Lead a team of employees.
3. Together with input from team members, make up departmental goals and objectives.
4. Set individual and department sales and cost budgets.

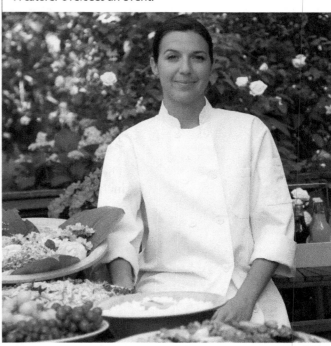

A caterer oversees an event.

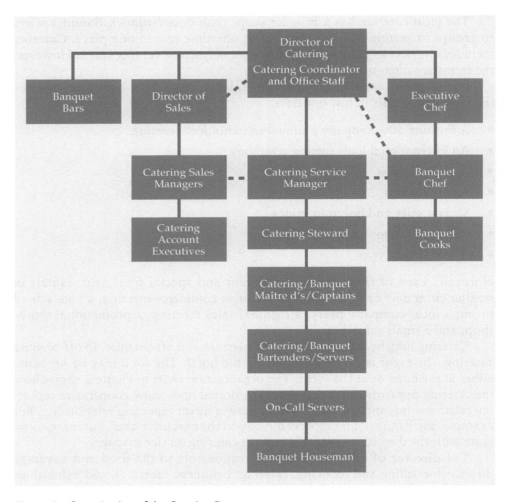

Figure 2 • Organization of the Catering Department.

5. Set service standards.
6. Ensure that the catering department is properly maintained.
7. Be extremely creative and knowledgeable about food, wine, and service.
8. Be very well versed in the likes, dislikes, and dietary restrictions of various ethnic groups, especially Jewish, Middle Eastern, and European.

Position Profile

The director of catering is required to have a variety of skills and abilities, including the following:

• A thorough knowledge of food and beverage management, including food preparation and service
• Ability to sell conventions, functions, and banquets
• Ability to produce a profit
• Ability to develop individual and department sales and cost budgets

Leadership

- Lead a team of employees.
- Set departmental mission, goals, and objectives.
- Train the department members in all facets of operations.
- Set service standards.
- Ensure that the catering department is properly maintained.

The catering department is extremely complex and demanding; the tempo is fast and the challenge to be innovative is always present. The director of catering in a large city hotel should, over the years, build up a client list and an intimate knowledge of the trade shows, exhibitions, various companies, groups, associations, and social, military, education, religious, and fraternal market (SMERF) organizations. This knowledge and these contacts are essential to the director of catering's success, as is the selection of the team members.

The main sales function of the department is conducted by the director of catering (DOC) and catering sales managers (CSMs). Their jobs are to optimize guest satisfaction and revenue by selling the most lucrative functions and exceeding guests' food and beverage and service expectations.

The DOC and catering sales managers obtain business leads from a variety of sources, including the following:

Hotel's director of sales. He or she is a good source of event bookings because he or she is selling rooms, and catering is often required by meetings and conventions.

General managers. These are good sources of leads because they are very involved in the community.

Corporate office sales department. If, for example, a convention were held on the East Coast one year at a Marriott hotel, and by tradition the association goes to the West Coast the following year, the Marriott hotel in the chosen city can contact the client or meeting planner. Some organizations have a selection of cities and hotels bid for major conventions. This ensures a competitive rate quote for accommodations and services.

Convention and visitors bureau. Here is another good source of leads because its main purpose is to seek out potential groups and organizations to visit that city. To be fair to all the hotels, they publish a list of clients and brief details of their requirements, which the hotel catering sales department may follow up on.

Reading the event board of competitive hotels. The event board is generally located in the lobby of the hotel and is frequently read by the competition. The CSM then calls the organizer of the event to solicit the business the next time.

Rollovers. Some organizations, especially local ones, prefer to stay in the same location. If this represents good business for the hotel, then the DOC and GM try to persuade the decision makers to use the same hotel again.

Cold calls. During periods of relative quiet, CSMs call potential clients to inquire if they are planning any events in the next few months. The point is to entice the client to view the hotel and the catering facilities. It is amazing how much information is freely given over the telephone.

The most frequent catering events in hotels are the following:

- Meetings
- Conventions
- Dinners
- Luncheons
- Weddings

For meetings, a variety of room setups are available, depending on a client's needs. The most frequently selected meeting room setups are as follows:

Theater style. Rows of chairs are placed with a center group of chairs and two aisles. Figure 3 shows a **theater-style room seating** setup with equipment centered on an audiovisual platform. Sometimes multimedia presentations, requiring more space for reverse-image projections, reduce the room's seating capacity.

Classroom style. As the name suggests, tables, usually slim 18-inch ones, are used because meeting participants need space to take notes. **Classroom-style seating** usually takes about three times as much space as theater style and takes more time and labor to set up and break down. Figure 4 shows a classroom-style setup.

Horseshoe style. **Horseshoe-style room seating** (Figure 5) is frequently used when interaction is sought among the delegates, such as training sessions and workshops. The presenter or trainer stands at the open end of the horseshoe with a black or white board, flip chart, overhead projector, and video monitor and projector.

Dinner style. Dinners are generally catered at round tables of eight or ten persons for large parties and on boardroom-style tables for smaller numbers. Of course, there are variations of the **dinner-style room seating** setup (see Figure 6).

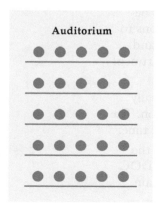

Figure 3 • Theater-Style Seating.

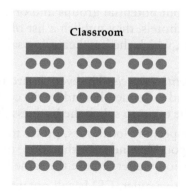

Figure 4 • Classroom-Style Seating.

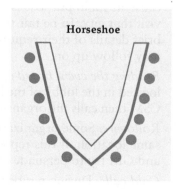

Figure 5 • Horseshoe-Style Seating.

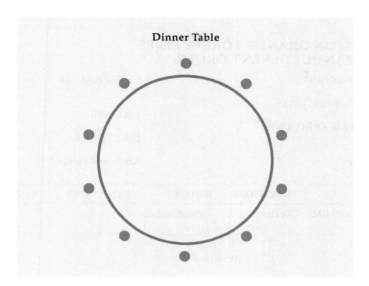

Dinner Table

Figure 6 • Dinner-Style Seating.

Catering Event Order

A **catering event order (CEO)**, which may also be called a **banquet event order (BEO)**, is prepared/completed for each function to inform not only the client but also the hotel personnel about essential information (what needs to happen and when) to ensure a successful event.

The CEO is prepared based on correspondence with the client and notes taken during the property visits. Figure 7 shows a CEO and lists the room's layout and decor, times of arrival, if there are any VIPs and what special attention is required for them, bar times, types of beverages and service, cash or credit bar, time of meal service, the menu, wines, and service details. The catering manager or director confirms the details with the client. Usually, two copies are sent, one for the client to sign and return and one for the client to keep.

An accompanying letter thanks the client for selecting the hotel and explains the importance of the function to the hotel. The letter also mentions the guaranteed-number policy. This is the number of guests the hotel will prepare to serve and will charge accordingly. The guaranteed number is given about seven days prior to the event. This safeguards the hotel from preparing for 350 people and having only 200 show up. The client, naturally, does not want to pay for an extra 150 people—hence, the importance of a close working relationship with the client. Contracts for larger functions call for the client to notify the hotel of any changes to the anticipated number of guests in increments of ten or twenty.

Experienced catering directors ensure that there will be no surprises for either the function organizer or the hotel. This is done by calling to check on how the function planning is going. One mistake catering directors sometimes make is accepting a final guest count without inquiring as to how that figure was determined. This emphasizes the fact that the catering director should

SHERATON GRANDE TORREY PINES
BANQUET EVENT ORDER

POST AS:	WELCOME BREAKFAST	CHERI WALTER
EVENT NAME:	MEETING	
GROUP:	CROCKER AND ASSOCIATES	
ADDRESS:	41 MAIN ST	BILLING:
	BOWLING GREEN, OHIO 43218	
PHONE:	(619) 635-4627	DIRECT BILL
FAX:	(619) 635-4528	
GROUP CONTACT:	Dr. Ken Crocker	Amount Received:
ON-SITE-CONTACT:	same	

DAY	DATE	TIME	FUNCTION	ROOM	EXP	GTE	SET	RENT
Fri	January 25, 2013	7:30 AM – 12:00 PM	Meeting	Palm Garden	50			250.00

BAR SET UP:

N/A

WINE:

FLORAL:

MENU:

MUSIC:

7:30 AM CONTINENTAL BREAKFAST

Freshly Squeezed Orange Juice, Grapefruit Juice, and
   Tomato Juice
Assortment of Bagels, Muffins, and Mini Brioche
Cream Cheese, Butter, and Preserves
Display of Sliced Seasonal Fruits
Individual Fruit Yogurt
Coffee, Tea, and Decaffeinated Coffee

PRICE:_____

AUDIO VISUAL:
–OVERHEAD PROJECTOR/SCREEN
–FLIPCHART/MARKERS
–VCR/MONITORS

PARKING:

HOSTING PARKING, PLEASE PROVIDE VOUCHERS

11:00 AM BREAK

Refresh Beverages as needed

LINEN:
HOUSE

SETUP:
–CLASSROOM-STYLE SEATING
–HEAD TABLE FOR 2 PEOPLE
–APPROPRIATE COFFEE BREAK SETUP
–(1) 6' TABLE FOR REGISTRATION AT ENTRANCE
     WITH 2 CHAIRS, 1 WASTEBASKET

All food and beverage prices are subject to an 18% service charge and 7% state tax. Guarantee figures, cancellations, changes must be given 72 hours prior or the number of guests expected will be considered the guarantee. To confirm the above arrangements, this contract must be signed and returned.

ENGAGOR SIGNATURE _____   DATE _____

BEO # 003069

Figure 7 • Catering Event Order.

(Courtesy of Sheraton Grande Torrey Pines.)

be a consultant to the client. Depending on the function, the conversion from invitations to guests is about 50 percent. Some hotels have a policy of preparing for about 3 to 5 percent more than the anticipated or guaranteed number. Fortunately, most events have a prior history. The organization may have been at a similar hotel in the same city or across the country. In either case, the catering director or manager will be able to receive helpful information from the catering director of the hotel where the organization's function was held previously.

The director of catering holds a daily or weekly meeting with key individuals who will be responsible for upcoming events. Those in attendance should be the following:

Director of catering

Executive chef and/or banquet chef

Beverage manager or catering bar manager

Catering managers

Catering coordinator

Director of purchasing

Chief steward

Audiovisual representative

The purpose of this meeting is to avoid any problems and to be sure that all key staff know and understand the details of the event and any special needs of the client.

Catering Coordinator

The **catering coordinator** has an exacting job in managing the office and controlling the "bible," or function diary, now on computer. He or she must see that the contracts are correctly prepared and must check on numerous last-minute details, such as whether flowers and menu cards have arrived.

Web-enabled technology tools such as Newmarket International's Delphi System (which is used at more than 4,000 properties) is a leader in delivering group, sales, catering, and banquet software for global travel and entertainment groups. One of the latest hotels to adopt the Delphi System is the Wynn Las Vegas, which installed the sales and catering systems Delphi Diagrams, MeetingBroker, and e-Proposal. The Delphi System can keep inventory current in real time because of its ability to interface with the property management system. The suite of Delphi products allows function space to be clearly and concisely managed, which increases guest satisfaction and profitability.

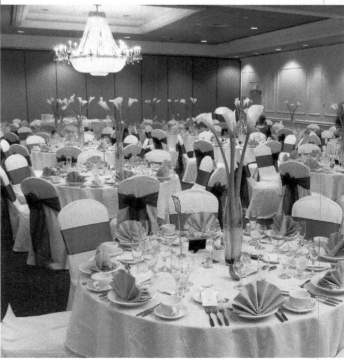

An elegant banquet room at a hotel.

A DAY IN THE LIFE OF JAMES McMANEMON

Food and Beverage Manager, Hyatt Regency

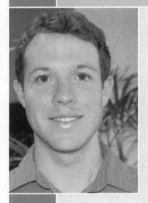

Friday—Start of a Busy Weekend

6:30 A.M.–8:00 A.M. (opening manager) When I arrive to work in the morning, the first thing I do is walk through the restaurant to ensure prompt opening. I make sure tables are properly set, the carpet is clean, lighting is set correctly, and that nothing is missing or broken. I check for all the little things that may seem trivial to the untrained eye but that don't go overlooked by our more observant guests. I call this "aesthetic detailing."

Next, I walk through the breakfast buffet to make sure it's fully stocked and meets corporate standards. We offer an array of breakfast items, including scrambled eggs, bacon and sausage, herbed potatoes, pancakes, homemade granola, steel cut oatmeal, fresh sliced fruit, an assortment of delicious cheeses, freshly baked pastries, and smoked salmon with all the fixings to load up your favorite bagel. The buffet comes with juice, coffee, or tea to drink. On average, approximately 60% of our breakfast guests choose the buffet every morning, many of whom have opted to include the buffet package in their daily room rate. This is a popular option for families on vacation, large groups with an appetite, and the typical business traveler who needs something quick in the morning.

Afterwards, I make my way over to the coffee bar to check that the barista is set up and ready to go for the coffee rush. We proudly brew Starbucks coffee, and offer all of their specialty coffees. Espresso, latte, Americano, macchiato—you name it and we'll make it. I will spend the next fifteen minutes talking to guests and conducting quality checks at each table to ensure that all of our guests' needs are being fulfilled and that they are enjoying their dining experience.

8:00 A.M.–8:30 A.M. Morning meeting for Operations Managers. At this time, the managers of each operation in the hotel meet in the General Manager's office to recap the previous day's business, as well as to discuss activity in each department for the current day. This meeting will include the Food and Beverage Manager, Banquets Manager, Housekeeping Manager, Front Office Manager, Sales and Catering Manager, Executive Chef, and General Manager.

I will routinely discuss amenities that need to be sent up to guests' rooms that day, groups in-house that we will see in one of the food and beverage outlets, reservations and parties we are expecting in the restaurant, and anything else that is relevant to the day's business. It just so happens that today the restaurant will be hosting a four-course dinner for thirty people, carefully crafted and paired with unique wines by our executive chef. I will receive the list of each course and will be in charge of creating a menu template and printing special menus for the event.

8:30 A.M.–11:00 A.M. Balance managing the breakfast shift with preparation paperwork. Besides creating the menu for the four-course dinner this evening, I must update each employee's clocks in and out from the previous day for payroll at the end of the week, purchase inventory that we will need for one of the outlets, and check and respond to any e-mails from fellow employees, potential clients, and so on.

11:00 A.M.–12:00 P.M. Once breakfast ends at 11 A.M., I will conduct a post-shift with my employees (servers, room service attendants, barista), in which I discuss how I felt the breakfast shift went that morning, along with anything else they would need to know for the upcoming lunch shift that day. I will make sure that side-work is completed in a timely manner and that room service has walked all of the floors in the hotel and picked up trays from breakfast. I will also meet with the incoming bartenders who are about to start their shift for the day. I am in charge of managing a lobby bar, a poolside bar, and a boathouse bar.

12:00 P.M.–2:00 P.M. Manage the lunch shift. This will entail expediting food on the line, once again talking with guests and conducting quality checks, assisting bartenders when one of the bars gets busy, and checking in on each of the various outlets from time to time.

2:00 P.M.–4:00 P.M. Complete any unfinished paperwork, and put the finishing touches on the four-course menu we will host this evening. Here is an idea of what we will be serving tonight:

First course: Lemon verbena smoked scallops with a cantaloupe caviar, micro mint leaves, and black lava sea salt, paired with the Four Vines "Naked" Chardonnay from Santa Barbara, California. This wine is "naked" in the sense that it's aged in stainless steel barrels and has never seen a splinter of oak. This is a very crisp wine with flavors of fresh tree fruits and hints of citrus.

Second course: Watermelon steak crusted with a warm and smoky spice blend, wild arugula, Humboldt fog cheese, and aged balsamic, paired with the Montes "Cherub" Rose of Syrah from Colchagua Valley, Chile. This is a cool and refreshing dry blush wine with a peppery aftertaste.

Third course: Espresso braised short rib with forest mushroom polenta and burnt leek chocolate pesto, paired with the Cinnabar "Mercury Rising" Meritage from Paso Robles, California. This is a bold and rounded red wine that combines Cabernet Sauvignon, Cabernet Franc, Merlot, and Petit Verdot.

Fourth course: Cinnamon plum tea panna cotta with amarena cherries, paired with the Bonterra Muscat from Lake County, California. This wine serves as the perfect accompaniment to the thick panna cotta and rich, syrupy cherries.

After the menu has been created and printed, I will show the servers how the restaurant should be set for this event. There should be a different glass for each wine, forks and knives for each course, and a spoon for dessert. The table decorum should be elegant but simple. We don't want to overwhelm our guests with gaudy decorations; the food and wine will speak for itself. This is how we make an impression.

4:00 P.M.–10:00 P.M. (closing manager) Manage the dinner rush. You must be the director of your employees. In addition to the party of thirty, there will be plenty of other guests in the restaurant for dinner this evening who will expect to receive a wonderful dining experience. We are likely to see some heavy action in the lobby bar, boathouse bar, and room service departments as well. The manager must balance the activity in each of these outlets to ensure a smooth and successful operation. This is like playing a game of chess. You know who all your players are (bartenders, servers, bussers, greeter, room service attendants), and you must use them as necessary to maintain a steady flow of business in order to provide quality service. This is the challenge in managing multiple food and beverage outlets, but it is also where the excitement lies.

10:00 P.M.–12:00 A.M. Once the dinner rush is over and the bars have died down, it's time to walk through each of the outlets and make sure they are properly set for the following morning, then finish the closing paperwork and call it a day. Although one manager does not typically stick around from sunrise until midnight, it has been known to happen on occasion. This is an industry that requires sacrifice of your time, and sometimes your patience. Describing a day in the life of a food and beverage manager is somewhat challenging, because each day is so different . . . and that's what I love about it.

Catering Services Manager

The **catering services manager (CSM)** has the enormous responsibility of delivering higher-than-expected service levels to guests. The CSM is in charge of the function from the time the client is introduced to the CSM by the director of catering or catering manager. This job is very demanding because several functions always occur simultaneously. Timing and logistics are crucial to the success of the operation. Frequently, there are only a few minutes between the end of a day meeting and the beginning of the reception for a dinner dance.

The CSM must be liked and respected by guests and at the same time be a superb organizer and supervisor. This calls for a person of outstanding character and leadership—management skills that are essential for success. The CSM has several important duties and responsibilities, including the following:

- Directing the service of all functions
- Supervising the catering housepersons in setting up the room
- Scheduling the banquet captains and approving the staffing levels for all events
- Cooperating with the banquet chef to check menus and service arrangements
- Checking that the client is satisfied with the room setup, food, beverages, and service
- Checking last-minute details
- Making out client bills immediately after the function
- Adhering to all hotel policies and procedures that pertain to the catering department, including responsible alcoholic beverage service and adherence to fire code regulations
- Calculating and distributing the gratuity and service charges for the service personnel
- Coordinating the special requirements with the DOC and catering coordinator

▶ Check Your Knowledge

1. What is the difference between banquets and catering?
2. What does SMERF stand for?
3. Where do the director of catering and the catering sales manager obtain their information?
4. What are the various styles used when setting up a meeting room? Give examples of when each style might be used.

Room Service/In-Room Dining

The term **room service** has for some time referred to all service to hotel guest rooms. Recently, some hotels have changed the name of room service to *in-room dining* to present the service as more upscale. The intention is to bring the dining experience to the room with quality food and beverage service.

A survey of members of the American Hotel & Lodging Association showed that 56 percent of all properties offer room service and that 75 percent of airport properties provide room service. Generally, the larger the hotel and the higher the room rate, the more likely it is that a hotel will offer room service.

Economy and several midpriced hotels avoid the costs of operating room service by having vending machines on each floor and food items such as pizza or Chinese food delivered by local restaurants. Conversely, some hotels prepare menus and lower price structures that do not identify the hotel as the provider of the food. As a result, the guests may have the impression that they are ordering from an "outside" operation when they are in fact ordering from room service.

The level of service and menu prices will vary from hotel to hotel. The Hilton at Torrey Pines, California, has butler service for all guest rooms without additional charge.

A few years ago, room service was thought of as a necessary evil, something that guests expected, but which did not produce profit for the hotel. Financial pressures have forced food and beverage directors to have this department also contribute to the bottom line. The room service manager has a difficult challenge running this department, which is generally in operation between sixteen and twenty-four hours a day. Tremendous effectiveness is required to make this department profitable. Nevertheless, it can be done. Some of the challenges in operating room service are as follows:

Delivering orders on time—this is especially important for breakfast, which is by far the most popular room service meal

Making room service a profitable food and beverage department

Avoiding complaints of excessive charges for room service orders

There are many other challenges in room service operation. One is forecasting demand. Room service managers analyze the front-desk forecast, which gives details of the house count and guest mix—convention, group, and others for the next two weeks. The food and beverage forecast will indicate the number of covers expected for breakfast, lunch, and dinner. The convention résumés will show where the convention delegates

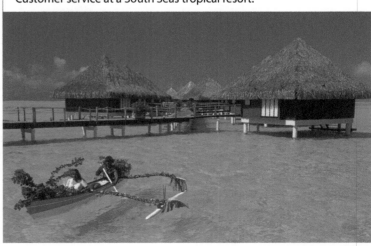

Customer service at a South Seas tropical resort.

are having their various meals. For example, the number of in-house delegates attending a convention breakfast can substantially reduce the number of room service breakfast orders.

Experience enables the manager to check if a large number of guests are from different time zones, such as the West or East Coasts or overseas. These guests have a tendency to get up either much earlier or much later than the average guest. This could throw room service demands off balance. Demand also fluctuates between weekdays and weekends; for example, city hotels may cater to business travelers, who tend to require service at about the same time. However, on weekends, city hotels may attract families, who will order room service at various times.

To avoid problems with late delivery of orders, a growing number of hotels have dedicated elevators to be used only by room service during peak periods. At the 565-room Stouffer Riviera Chicago, director of food and beverage Bill Webb has a solution: Rapid action teams (RAT) are designated food and beverage managers and assistants who can be called on when room service orders are heavy.

Westin Hotels recently introduced Service Express, an innovation that allows a customer to address all needs (room service, housekeeping, laundry, and other services) with a single call. In addition, new properties are designed with the room service kitchen adjacent to the main kitchen so that a greater variety of items can be offered.

Meeting the challenge of speedy and accurate communication is imperative to a successful room service operation. This begins with timely scheduling and ends with happy guests. In between is a constant flow of information that is communicated by the guest, the order taker, the cook, and the server.

Another challenge is to have well-trained and competent employees in the room service department. From the tone of voice of the order taker and the courteous manner with which the order is taken to the panache of the server for the VIP dinners, training makes the difference between ordinary service and outstanding service. With training, which includes menu tasting with wine and suggestive selling, an order taker becomes a room service salesperson. This person is now able to suggest cocktails or wine to complement the entree and can entice the guest with tempting desserts. The outcome of this is to increase the average guest check. Training also helps the setup and service personnel hone their skills to enable them to become productive employees who are proud of their work.

Sustainable Food and Beverage Operations

Practicing sustainable food and beverage operations can and does lead to a better bottom line. When operators save water and electricity, recycle, and purchase local produce, they help lessen the footprint of the operation. Guests are increasingly aware of the importance of sustainable operations of a food and beverage facility. They are pleased to see the greening of food and beverage operations and the use of local natural products, which helps reduce the cost of transportation and adds local flavor.

Michelle Leroux, director of sales and marketing at the Delta Chelsea Hotel in Toronto, has noticed a shift in the booking inquiries: "It isn't so much that having a 'green' or 'sustainable' meeting package sells additional pieces of business—it is more along the line that certain groups will not book at your hotel if you can't demonstrate knowledge and experience with sustainable meetings."[3]

According to Brita Moosmann, a consultant,[4] the best way to start the process of making food and beverage more sustainable and profitable is to conduct a comprehensive audit or evaluation of your food and beverage operation in order to provide a baseline in terms of energy efficiency and carbon footprint; they should be part of an overriding strategy that will provide an in-depth analysis of the organization's sustainable position. This evaluation also should measure the impact of the various elements on the organization's stakeholders and have a total quality approach regarding customer satisfaction. It is also advisable to obtain feedback to understand what is important to the local community.

Trends in Lodging Food and Beverage Operations

- Hotels are using branded restaurants instead of operating their own restaurants.
- Hotels are opting not to offer food and beverage outlets. These are usually smaller to midsized properties that may have restaurants on the same lot nearby.
- Restaurants and beverage outlets are being made more casual.
- Restaurants are being developed or remodeled with a theme. For example, one major hotel chain has adopted a northern Italian theme in all its restaurants.
- Menus are being standardized for all hotel restaurants in a chain.
- Many hotels are converting one of the beverage outlets into a sports-themed bar.
- Technology is being used to enhance guest services and control costs in all areas of a hotel, including guest ordering and payment, food production, refrigeration, marketing, management control, and communication.
- More low-fat and low-carb items are being added to menus.

CASE STUDY

Ensuring Guest Satisfaction

The Sunnyvale Hotel is operated by a major hotel management corporation. To ensure guest satisfaction, 300 survey forms each containing sixty-five questions are mailed to guests each month. Usually, about seventy of the forms are returned. The hotel company categorizes the guest satisfaction scores obtained into colored zones, with green being the best, then clear and yellow, and red being the worst. Scores can be compared with those of equivalent hotels.

The most recent survey indicated a significant decline for the Sea Grill Restaurant, with scores in the red zone. Guests' concerns were in the following areas: hostess attentiveness, spread of service, and quality of food.

On investigation, the director of food and beverage also realized that the name of the restaurant, Sea Grill, was not appropriate for the type of restaurant being operated. When asked, some guests commented that "it's a bit odd to eat breakfast in a fish place."

Discussion Question

1. What would you do, as director of food and beverage, to get the guest satisfaction scores back into the clear or green zones?

CASE STUDY

Friday Evening at the Grand Hotel's Casual Restaurant

Karla Gomez is the supervisor at the Grand Hotel's casual restaurant. Karla's responsibilities include overseeing five servers and two bussers, seating guests, and taking reservations. One Friday evening, the restaurant was very busy—all twenty tables were occupied, there was a substantial wait list, and there were people on standby. The service bar was almost full of guests, and most of the seated guests in the dining area had finished their entrées or were just beginning their desserts. They were not leaving, however, in part because of cold, rainy weather outside. The guests did not seem to be in a rush to leave the restaurant, but several of the guests waiting for tables were complaining about the long wait.

Discussion Question

1. What can Karla do to solve the problem?

Summary

1. The food and beverage department division is led by the director of food and beverage, who is responsible for the efficient operation of kitchen, catering, restaurants, bars, and room service; in addition, the director has to keep up with trends and preplan for special events.

2. A hotel kitchen is the responsibility of the executive chef, who is in charge of the quality and quantity of food, organization of the kitchen and his or her sous chefs, administrative duties, and careful calculation of financial results.

3. A hotel usually has a formal and a casual restaurant, which are either directly connected to the hotel or operated separately.

4. Bars are an important revenue source for a hotel, but they must adhere to strict guidelines to be profitable. Commensurate with its size, a hotel might have several kinds of bars, such as a lobby bar, a restaurant bar, a minibar, or even a night club.

5. The chief steward has the often unrewarded job of cleaning the kitchen, cutlery, plates, glasses, and backstage of the hotel and is in charge of pest control and inventory.

6. Catering is subdivided into on-premise and off-premise occasions, which may include meetings, conventions, dinners, luncheons, and weddings. According to the occasion, the type of service and room setup may vary. Catering involves careful planning and the interaction and cooperation of many people.

7. Room service offers the convenience of dining in the room, with quality food and beverage service, at a price acceptable to both the guest and the hotel.

Key Words and Concepts

banquet
banquet event order (BEO)
brigade
capture rate
catering
catering coordinator
catering event order (CEO)
catering services manager (CSM)
chef tournant
chief steward
classroom-style seating
contribution margin
dinner-style room seating
director of catering (DOC)
director of food and beverage
executive chef

food cost percentage
food sales percentage
horseshoe-style room seating
kitchen manager
labor cost percentage
perpetual inventory
pilferage
pour/cost percentage
responsible alcoholic beverage service
restaurant manager
room service
shopper
sous chef
station chef
theater-style room seating

Review Questions

1. Briefly describe the challenges a food and beverage director faces on a daily basis.
2. List the measures used to determine the food and beverage department's profit and loss.

3. Explain the problems a hotel faces in making the following departments profitable: restaurants, bars, and room service.
4. Explain the importance of the catering department for a hotel and list the responsibilities of a catering sales manager.

Internet Exercises

1. Organization: **Foodservice**
   Web site: **www.foodservice.com**
   Summary: Foodservice.com is a web site that focuses on the foodservice industry. It has links to employment, industry resources, foodservice, technology innovations, and much more.
   (a) Click the "Forums and Chat" icon. Go to the "Chef and Cooks Corner," and look at some of the latest posts. Bring your favorite one to the table (discuss in class).
   (b) Look at the most current articles on the food safety forum. What are the major concerns being addressed?

2. Organization: **National Restaurant Association**
   Web site: **www.restaurant.org**
   Summary: The National Restaurant Association is an organization devoted to representing, educating, and promoting the restaurant/hospitality industry.
   (a) Look under the "Education & Networking" tab. What does it mean to be "FMP Certified" and what are the eligibility requirements?
   (b) What are some of the upcoming events and what do they have to offer?

Apply Your Knowledge

1. If a casual dining restaurant in a four-star hotel forecasts 100 covers, how many servers, bussers, hosts, and assistant managers would you schedule on that particular day? Calculate the labor cost of these associates for that day if the manager(s) work from 1:00 P.M. to 11:00 P.M., the server(s) work from 4:00 P.M. to 11:00 P.M., the busser(s) work from 4:30 P.M. to 11:30 P.M., and the host(s) works from 4:00 P.M. to 11:00 P.M. Use minimum wage of

   $5.75 for calculations. Use the rate of $12 per hour for the assistant manager(s) and $6.50 for hosts.

2. Kitchen labor costs are an important ratio used to determine the efficiency of the food and beverage department. The labor cost for a banquet meal is $126.45 and the revenue for the banquet is $505.80. What is the labor cost percentage?

Suggested Activities

1. Contact a bar manager in your area. Discuss with him or her how to monitor pilferage and overpouring. Ask what the expected and actual pouring cost percentages are and how the manager deals with any variances.
2. Visit a hotel restaurant in your area. Make a note of how busy the establishment is. Does it seem to be staffed with the appropriate number of employees? Are guests being served in a timely manner? Think about why this specific restaurant may be overly crowded or overly vacant. What could or should be done differently? What seems to be working well?

Endnotes

1. Carlson, *Ambition 2015*, www.carlson.com/our-company/ambition-2015.php (accessed January 17, 2011).
2. Ibid.
3. Brita Moosmann, *Sustainable F&B Operations Can Create Valuable Profit Partner* http://www.hotelnewsnow.com/Articles.aspx/2235/ Sustainable-FB-operations-can-create-valuable-profit-partner (accessed March 9, 2011).
4. Ibid.

Glossary

Banquet   A formal dinner.

Brigade   A team of kitchen personnel organized into stations.

Capture rate   In hotel food and beverage practice, the number of hotel guests who use the food and beverage outlets.

Catering   The part of the food and beverage division of a hotel that is responsible for arranging and planning food and beverage functions for conventions and smaller hotel groups, and local banquets booked by the sales department.

Catering service manager (CSM)   Head of the catering services department.

Chef tournant   A chef who rotates the various stations in the kitchen to relieve the station chefs.

Chief steward   The individual in a hotel, club, or foodservice operation who is responsible for the cleanliness of the back of the house and dishwashing areas and for storage and control of china, glassware, and silverware.

Classroom-style meeting   A type of meeting setup generally used in instructional meetings, such as workshops.

Contribution margin   Key operating figure in menu engineering, determined by subtracting food cost from selling price as a measure of profitability.

DOC   Director of catering.

Executive chef   The head of the kitchen.

Food cost percentage   A ratio comparing the cost of food sold to food sales, which is calculated by dividing the cost of food sold during a given period by food sales during the same period.

Horseshoe-style room seating   A meeting room containing tables arranged in the shape of a U.

Kitchen manager   The individual who manages the kitchen department.

Labor cost percentage   Similar to food cost percentage, except that it relates to labor. The formula is: Labor costs divided by net sales multiplied by 100 equals the labor cost percentage.

Perpetual inventory   A running inventory that automatically updates itself.

Pilferage   Stealing.

Pour-cost percentage   Similar to food cost percentage, except used in beverage control.

Restaurant manager   The head of operations in a restaurant.

Room service   The cleaning of rooms and resupplying of materials (towels, soap, etc.) by the housekeeping staff.

Shoppers   People who are paid to use a bar as regular guests would, except that they observe the operation closely.

Sous chef (soo shef)   A cook who supervises food production and who reports to the executive chef; he or she is second in command of a kitchen.

Station chef   A chef in charge of a station.

Theater-style meeting seating   A meeting setup usually intended for a large audience that is not likely to need to take notes or refer to documents. It generally consists of a raised platform and a lectern from which the presenter addresses the audience.

Photo Credits

Credits are listed in the order of appearance.

Beverages

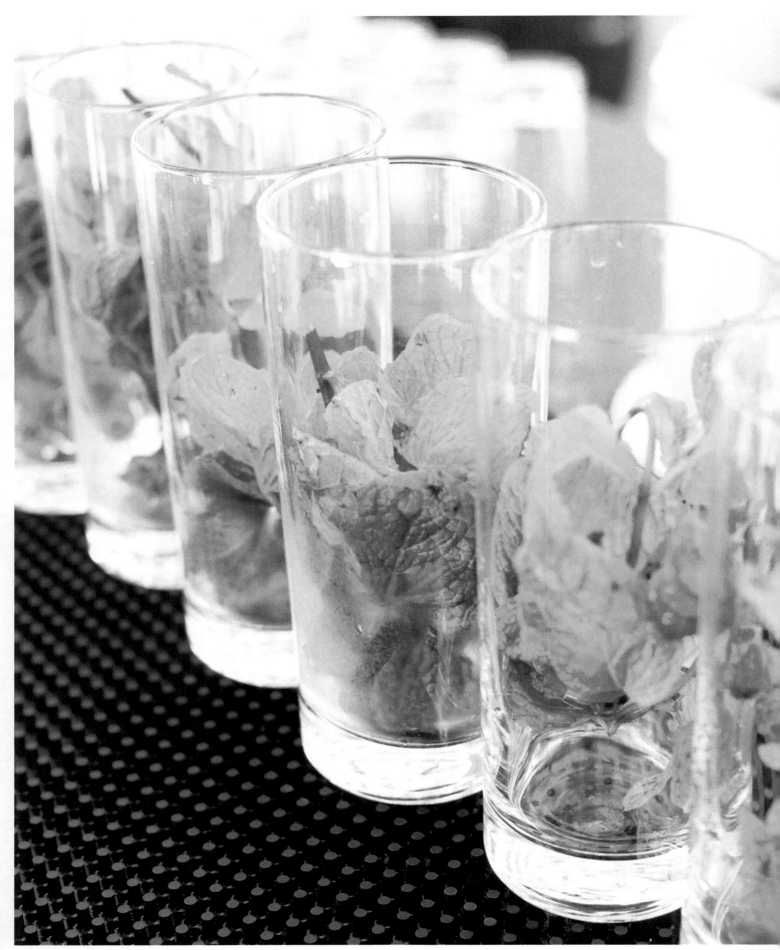

Beverages

OBJECTIVES

After reading and studying this chapter, you should be able to:

- List and describe the main grape varieties.

- Suggest appropriate pairings of wine with food.

- Identify the various types of beer.

- List the types of spirits and their main ingredients.

- Explain a restaurant's liability in terms of serving alcoholic beverages.

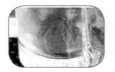
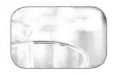
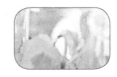
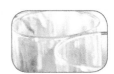

This chapter offers an overview of alcoholic and nonalcoholic beverages in the hospitality industry. Be sure that you realize the utmost importance of responsible beverage consumption and service. Arrange for a designated driver if you intend to have a drink. If you do drink alcoholic beverages, then stay with the same drink—don't mix them (two different types are grape and grain—that is, wine and spirits). That's when trouble really begins and hangovers are bad. Remember that moderation is the key to enjoying beverages, whether at a get-together with friends at a local restaurant or on a getaway for spring break. Examine the tragic alcohol-related auto and other accidents that too many people are involved in each year. Enjoy, but do not overindulge.

Serving beverages is traditional throughout the world. According to his or her culture, a person might welcome a visitor with coffee or tea—or bourbon. Beverages are generally categorized into two main groups: alcoholic and nonalcoholic. **Alcoholic beverages** *are further categorized as wines, beer, and spirits. Figure 1 shows these three categories.*

Wines

Wine is the fermented juice of freshly gathered ripe grapes. Wine may also be made from other sugar-containing fruits, such as blackberries, cherries, or elderberries. In this chapter, however, we will confine our discussion to grape wines. Wine may be classified first by color: red, white, or rose. Wines are further classified as light beverage wines, still wines, sparkling wines, fortified wines, and aromatic wines.

Light Beverage Wines

White, red, or rose table wines are "still" light beverage wines; such still table wines may come from a variety of growing regions around the world. In the United States, the premium wines are named after the grape variety, such

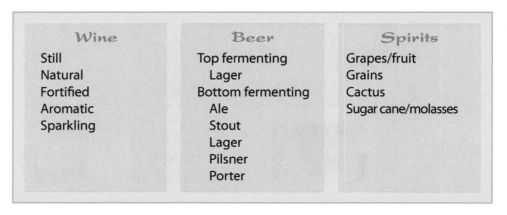

Wine	Beer	Spirits
Still	Top fermenting	Grapes/fruit
Natural	Lager	Grains
Fortified	Bottom fermenting	Cactus
Aromatic	Ale	Sugar cane/molasses
Sparkling	Stout	
	Lager	
	Pilsner	
	Porter	

Figure 1 • Alcoholic Beverages.

as chardonnay and cabernet sauvignon. This proved so successful that Europeans are now also naming their wines after the grape variety and their region of origin, such as Pouilly Fuisse and Chablis.

Sparkling Wines

Champagne, sparkling white wine, and sparkling rose wine are called the **sparkling wines**. Sparkling wines sparkle because they contain carbon dioxide. The carbon dioxide may be either naturally produced or mechanically infused into the wine. The best-known sparkling wine is champagne, which has become synonymous with celebrations and happiness.

Champagne became the drink of fashion in France and England in the seventeenth century. Originating in the Champagne region of France, the wine owed its unique sparkling quality to a second fermentation—originally unintentional—in the bottle itself. This process became known as *methode champenoise*.

The Benedictine monk Dom Perignon (1638–1715) was the cellar master for the Abbaye Hautvilliers and an exceptional wine connoisseur. He was the first to experiment with blending different wines to achieve the so-called *cuvee* (the basis of champagne production). He also revolutionized wine by retaining the resulting carbon dioxide in the bottles. Dom Perignon's methods were refined throughout the centuries and led to the modern method used in champagne production.

Champagne may, by law, only come from the Champagne region of France. Sparkling wines from other countries have *methode champenoise* written on their labels to designate that a similar method was used to make that particular sparkling wine.

Figure 2 explains how to handle and serve champagne.

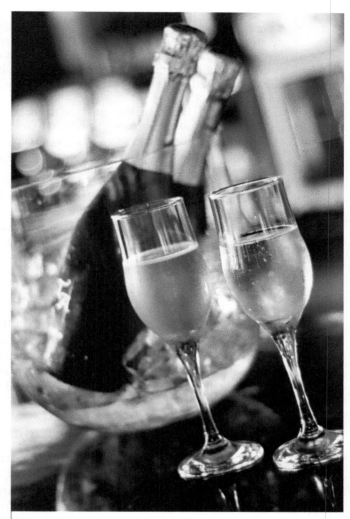

Bottles of champagne. Remember not to point the cork at anyone when opening the bottle; point it at the ceiling. In fact, a napkin should be placed over the cork, which is then held there while the bottle is gently twisted open. Champagne is served chilled in fluted glasses, which help the bouquet and effervescence last longer.

▶ Check Your Knowledge

1. Why is champagne served in fluted glasses?

2. How are alcoholic beverages categorized?

3. Why should you avoid mixing grape (wine) and grain (spirits) drinks?

4. Where should you point the cork of a champagne bottle when opening it?

Champagne should be stored horizontally at a temperature between fifty and fifty-five degrees Fahrenheit. However, it should be served at a temperature between forty-three and forty-seven degrees Fahrenheit. This is best achieved by placing the bottle in an ice bucket.

When serving champagne, there are some recommended steps to take to achieve the best results, as listed below.

1. If the bottle is presented in a champagne cooler, it should be placed upright in the cooler, with fine ice tightly packed around the bottle.
2. The bottle should be wrapped in a cloth napkin. Remove the foil or metal capsule to a point just below the wire, which holds the cork securely.
3. Hold the bottle firmly in one hand at a forty-five degree angle. Unwind and remove the wiring. With a clean napkin, wipe the neck of the bottle and around the cork.
4. With the other hand, grasp the cork so that it will not fly out. Twist the bottle and ease the cork out.
5. When the cork is out, retain the bottle at an angle for about five seconds. The gas will rush out and carry with it some of the champagne if the bottle is held upright.
6. Champagne should be served in two motions: pour until the froth almost reaches the brim of the glass. Stop and wait for the foam to subside. Then finish filling the glass to about three-quarters full.

Figure 2 • Handling and Serving Champagne.

Fortified Wines

Sherries, ports, Madeira, and Marsala are **fortified wines**, meaning that they have had brandy or wine alcohol added to them. The brandy or wine alcohol imparts a unique taste and increases the alcohol content to about 20 percent. Most fortified wines are sweeter than regular wines. Each of the groups of fortified wines has several subgroups with myriad tastes and aromas.

Aromatic Wines

Aromatized wines are fortified and flavored with herbs, roots, flowers, and barks. These wines may be sweet or dry. Aromatic wines are also known as aperitifs, which generally are consumed before meals as digestive stimulants. Among the better-known brands of aperitif wines are Dubonnet Red (sweet), Dubonnet White (dry), vermouth red (sweet), vermouth white (dry), Byrrh (sweet), Lillet (sweet), Punt e Mes (dry), St. Raphael Red (sweet), and St. Raphael White (dry).

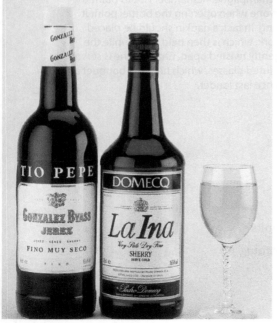

Sherry can be dry (fino), medium, or sweet. Pictured here are bottles of dry sherry with a glass. The lighter the color, the drier the sherry.

The History of Wine

Wine has been produced for centuries. The ancient Egyptians and Babylonians recorded using the fermentation process. The very first records about winemaking date back about 7,000 years. The Greeks received the vine from the Egyptians, and later the Romans contributed to the popularization of wine in Europe by planting vines in the territories they conquered.

The wine produced during these times was not the cabernet or chardonnay of today. The wines of yesteryear were drunk when they were young and likely to be highly acidic and crude. To help offset these deficiencies, people added different spices and honey, which made the wine at least palatable. To this day, some Greek and German wines have flavoring added.

The making of good wine is dependent on the quality of the grape variety, type of soil, climate, preparation of vineyards, and method of winemaking. Thousands of grape varieties exist, thriving in a variety of soil and climatic conditions. Different plants thrive on clay, chalky, gravelly, or sandy soil. The most important winemaking grape variety is the *Vitis vinifera*, which yields cabernet sauvignon, gamay, pinot noir, pinot chardonnay, and riesling.

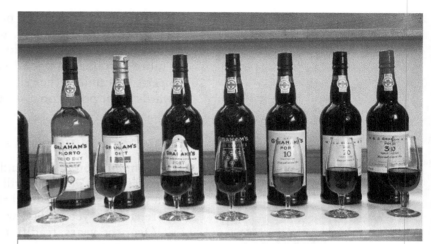

Port wines are generally red, fortified, and sweet. Vintage port is the most prized by port lovers. Port is typically served with cheese and biscuits at the end of a meal.

Making Wine

Wine is made in six steps: crushing, fermenting, racking, maturing, filtering, and bottling. Grapes are harvested in the autumn, after they have been scientifically tested for maturity, acidity, and sugar concentration. The freshly harvested grapes are taken to pressing houses, where the grapes are destemmed and crushed. The juice that is extracted from the grapes is called **must.**

The second step of the process is **fermentation** of the must, a natural phenomenon caused by yeasts on the skin of the grapes. Additional yeasts are added either environmentally or by formula. When exposed to air in the proper environment, the yeast multiplies. Yeast converts the sugar in the grapes to ethyl alcohol, until little or no sugar remains in the wine. The degree of sweetness or dryness in the wine can be controlled at the end of the fermentation process by adding alcohol, removing the yeast by filtration, or adding sulphur dioxide.

Red wine gains its color during the fermentation process from the coloring pigments of the red grape skins, which are put back into the must.

After fermentation has ceased, the wine is transferred to racking containers, where it settles before being poured into oak barrels or large stainless steel containers for the maturing process. Some of the better wines are aged in oak barrels, from which they acquire additional flavor and character during the barrel aging. Throughout the aging process, red wine extracts tannin from the wood, which gives longevity to the wine. Some white wine and most red wine are barrel-aged for periods ranging from months to more than two years. White wines that are kept in stainless steel containers are crisp, with a youthful flavor; they are bottled after a few months for immediate consumption.

After maturing, the wine is filtered to help stabilize it and remove any solid particles still in the wine. This process is called **fining.** The wine is then **clarified** by adding either egg white or bentonite, which sinks to the bottom of the vat. The wine then is bottled.

White grapes make white wines; the main white grapes are chardonnay, sauvignon blanc, riesling, pinot blanc, and gewürztraminer.

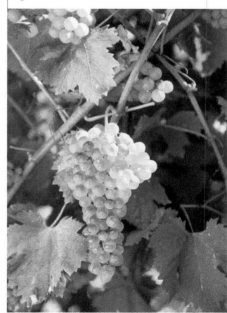

Fine **vintage** wines are best drunk at their peak, which may be a few years—or decades—away. Red wines generally take a few more years to reach their peak than do white wines. In Europe, where the climate is more variable, the good years are rated as vintage. The judgment of experts determines the relative merits of each wine-growing district and awards merit points on a scale of 1 to 10.

Matching Wine with Food

The combination of food and wine is one of life's great pleasures. We eat every day, so a gourmet will seek out not only exotic foods and vintage wines, but also simple food that is well prepared and accompanied by an unpretentious, yet quality, wine.

Over the years, traditions have developed a how-to approach to the marrying of wines and food. Generally, the following traditions apply:

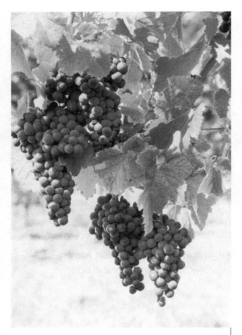

Red grapes make red wine; the main red grapes are cabernet sauvignon, merlot, merlot/cabernet sauvignon, pinot noir, and Shiraz.

- White wine is best served with white meat (chicken, pork, or veal), shellfish, and fish.
- Red wine is best served with red meat (beef, lamb, duck, or game).
- The heavier the food, the heavier and more robust the wine should be.
- Champagne can be served throughout the meal.
- Port and red wine go well with cheese.
- Dessert wines best complement desserts and fresh fruits that are not highly acidic.
- When a dish is cooked with wine, it is best served with that wine.
- Regional food is best complemented by wines of the region.
- Wines should never accompany salads with vinegar dressings, or curries; the tastes will clash or be overpowering.
- Sweet wines should be served with foods that are not too sweet.

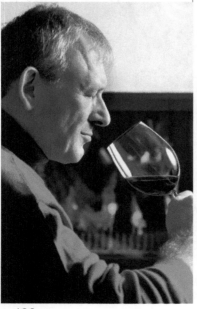

Sniffing the bouquet of the wine.

Figure 3 matches some of the better-known varietal wines with food.

Food and wine are described by texture and flavor. Textures are the qualities in food and wine that we feel in the mouth, such as softness, smoothness, roundness, richness, thickness, thinness, creaminess, chewiness, oiliness, harshness, silkiness, coarseness, and so on. Textures correspond to sensations of touch and temperature, which can be easy to identify—for example, hot, cold, rough, smooth, thick, or thin. Regarding the marrying of food and wine, light food with light wine is always a reliable combination. Rich food with rich wine can be wonderful as long as the match is not too rich. The two most important qualities to consider when choosing the appropriate wine are richness and lightness.

Flavors are food and wine elements perceived by the olfactory nerve as fruity, minty, herbal, nutty, cheesy, smoky, flowery, earthy, and so on. A person often determines flavors by using the nose as well as the tongue. The combination of texture and flavor is what makes food and wine a pleasure to enjoy; a good match between the food and wine can make occasions even more memorable. Figure 4 suggests the steps to be taken in **wine tasting**.

FOCUS ON WINES

Wine and Food Pairing

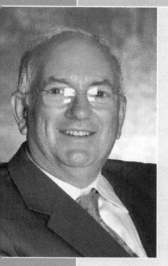

Jay R. Schrock, University of South Florida

The combination of food and wine is as old as the making of wine. It is truly one of the great pleasures in life. Food and wine are natural accompaniments and enhance the flavor and enjoyment of each other. The flavor of a wine consumed by itself will taste different than when it is imbibed with food. Much of the wine taste experience is actually perceived from the nose; hence, you will hear that "the wine has a good nose." In fact, wine experts, called *sommeliers*, say that 80 percent of the taste comes from the nose. The nose is where the flavors such as nuts, oak, fruits, herbs, spices, and all the other words used to describe wine come from. To improve the smell and taste of wine, we often decant it and serve it in stemware with large openings. The wine taster often swirls the wine to increase the aromas entering the nose.

Over the years, traditions have developed as to how to approach **wine and food pairing**. Remember, these are traditions and that food and wine pairing is a highly subjective and an inexact process. The traditional rules basically state that red wines are served with red meat and white wines are served with fish and poultry. These rules are still generally valid, but they don't take into consideration the complexity of today's multiethnic fusion cuisines, with their wide range of flavors and the corresponding wide range of wines from around the world that are now readily available to everyone. Today, you are more likely to hear of food and wine pairing suggestions, rather than the hard and fast traditional rules of the past.

The new tradition has begun:

1. When serving more than one wine at a meal, it's best to serve lighter wines before full-bodied ones. The drier wines should be served before sweeter wines. The exception is if a sweet-flavored food is served early in the meal. Serve wines with lower alcohol content before wines with higher alcohol content.

2. Pair light-bodied wines with lighter food and fuller-bodied wines with heaver, richer, or more flavorful foods. This is a restatement of the old red wine with red meat and white wine with fish and chicken suggestion.

3. Match flavors. A pinot noir goes well with duck, prosciutto, and mushrooms and a gewürztraminer is a well-suited accompaniment for ham, sausage, curry, and Thai and Indian food. Beware of pairing a wine with food that is sweeter than the wine. Most people agree that chocolate is the one exception. It seems to go with almost anything.

4. Delicately flavored foods that are poached or steamed should be paired with delicate wines.

5. Match regional wines with regional foods; they have been developed together and have a natural affinity for each other. The red sauces of Tuscany and the Chianti wines of the Tuscany region in Italy are an unbeatable combination.

6. Soft cheese such as Camembert and Brie pair well with a variety of red wine, including cabernet sauvignon, zinfandel, and red burgundy. Cabernet sauvignon also goes well with sharp, aged cheddar cheese. Pungent and intensely flavored cheeses, such as a blue cheese, are better with the sweeter eiswein (or icewine) or late-harvest dessert wines. Sheep and goat cheeses pair well with dry white wines, while red wine with fruit flavors goes best with milder cheeses.

Many of your restaurant guests may want to have wine with their dinner but are intimidated by the process or are afraid of the price. Set your guests' minds at ease when they are ordering wine. The know-it-all attitude will not work here; you are not trying to sell a used car or life insurance. You are trying to improve your guests' experience, the check average, and your tip. Make an honest suggestion, and try to explain the differences in wine choices. If guests are pondering two wines by the glass, do not just suggest the more expensive one; bring two glasses and let them taste. They will decide for themselves.

WINE	SMELL AND TASTE ASSOCIATED WITH WINE	FOOD PAIRING
Gewürztraminer (Alsace in France)	grapefruit, apple, nectarine, peach, nutmeg, clove, cinnamon	Thai, Indian, Tex-Mex, Szechwan, ham, sausage, curry, garlic
Chardonnay Chablis (Burgundy in France)	citrus fruit, apple, pear, pineapple, other tropical fruit	pork, salmon, chicken, pheasant, rabbit
Sauvignon Blanc Sancerre (Loire in France)	citrus fruit, gooseberry, bell pepper, black pepper, green olives, herbs	goat cheese, oysters, fish, chicken, pork, garlic
Pinot Blanc	citrus fruit, apple, pear, melon	shrimp, shellfish, fish, chicken
Pinot Noir Cote d' Or (Burgundy in France)	strawberry, cherry, raspberry, clove, mint, vanilla, cinnamon	duck, chicken, turkey, mushrooms, grilled meats, fish and vegetables, pork
Merlot Gamay (Beaujolais in France)	cherry, raspberry, plum, pepper, herbs, mint	beef, lamb, duck, barbecued meats, pork ribs
Cabernet Sauvignon Medoc (Bordeaux in France)	cherry, plum, pepper, bell pepper, herbs, mint, tea, chocolate	beef, lamb, braised, barbecued and grilled meats, aged cheddar, chocolate
Late harvest white wines	citrus fruit, apple, pear, apricot, peach, mango, honey	custard, vanilla, ginger, carrot cake, cheesecake, cream puffs, apricot cobbler

Figure 3 • Matching Wine with Food.

(Courtesy of Jay R. Schrock.)

Many restaurants have introduced wine tastings as special marketing events to promote the restaurant itself, or a particular type or label of wine. Wine tasting is more than just a process—it is an artful ritual. Wine offers a threefold sensory appeal: color, aroma, and taste. Wine tasting, thus, consists of three essential steps.

1. Hold the glass to the light. The color of the wine gives the first indication of the wine's body. The deeper the color, the fuller the wine will be. Generally, wines should be clear and brilliant.
2. Smell the wine. Hold the glass between the middle and the ring finger in a "cup-like" fashion and gently roll the glass. This will bring the aroma and the bouquet of the wine to the edge of the glass. The bouquet should be pleasant. This will tell much about what the taste will be.
3. Finally, taste the wine by rolling the wine around the mouth and by sucking in a little air—this helps release the complexities of the flavors.

Figure 4 • Wine Tasting.

► Check Your Knowledge

1. What are the names of the main white and red grape varieties used to make wine?

2. Cabernet sauvignon is best served with _____.

3. Chardonnay is best served with _____.

4. Why does a wine taster swirl the wine around the glass before tasting it?

5. What is the general guideline for serving wine with food?

Major Wine-Growing Regions

Europe

Germany, Italy, Spain, Portugal, and France are the main European wine-producing countries. Germany is noted for the outstanding Riesling wines from the Rhine and Moselle river valleys. Italy produces the world-famous Chianti. Spain makes good wine, but is best known for making sherry. Portugal also makes good wine, but is better known for its port.

France is the most notable of the European countries, producing not only the finest wines but also champagne and cognac. The two most famous wine-producing areas in France are the Bordeaux and Burgundy regions. The vineyards, villages, and towns are steeped in the history of centuries devoted to the production of the finest quality wines. They represent some of the most beautiful countryside in Europe and are well worth visiting.

In France, wine is named after the village in which the wine is produced. In recent years, the name of the grape variety has also been used. The name of the wine grower is also important; because the quality may vary, reputation understandably is very important. A vineyard might also include a chateau in which wine is made.

Within the Bordeaux region, wine growing is divided into five major districts: Medoc, Graves, St. Emilion, Pomerol, and Sauternes. The wine from each district has its own characteristics.

There are several other well-known wine-producing regions of France, such as the Loire Valley, Alsace, and Côtes du Rhône. French people regard wine as an important part of their culture and heritage.

United States and Canada

In California, viticulture began in 1769 when Junipero Serra, a Spanish friar, began to produce wine for the missions he started. At one time, the French considered California wines to be inferior. However, California is blessed with a near-perfect climate and excellent vine-growing soil. In the United States, the name of the grape variety is used to name the wine, not the village or chateau as used by the French. The better-known varietal white wines in the United States are chardonnay, sauvignon blanc, riesling, and chenin blanc; varietal red wines are cabernet sauvignon, pinot noir, merlot, Syrah, and zinfandel.

California viticulture areas are generally divided into three regions:

1. North and central coastal region
2. Great central valley region
3. Southern California region

The north and central coastal region produces the best wines in California. A high degree of use of mechanical methods allows for efficient, large-scale production of quality wines. The two best-known areas within this region are the

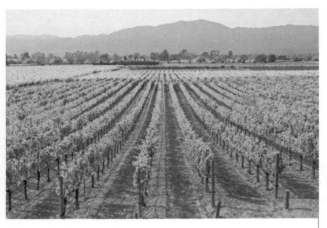

A Napa Valley vineyard.

Napa and Sonoma Valleys. The wines of the Napa and Sonoma Valleys resemble those of Bordeaux and Burgundy. In recent years, the wines from the Napa and Sonoma Valleys have rivaled and even exceeded the French and other European wines. The chardonnays and cabernets are particularly outstanding.

The Napa and Sonoma Valleys are the symbols as well as the centers of the top-quality wine industry in California.

Several other states and Canadian provinces provide quality wines. New York, Oregon, and Washington are the other major U.S. wine-producing states. In Canada, the best wineries are in British Columbia's Okanagan Valley and southern Ontario's Niagara peninsula. Both of these regions produce excellent wines.

Australia

Australia has been producing wines for about 150 years, but it is only in the last half-century that these wines have achieved the prominence and recognition they rightly deserve. Australian winemakers traveled to Europe and California to perfect the winemaking craft. Unlike France, with many rigid laws controlling wine growth and production, Australian winemakers use high technology

INTRODUCING ROBERT MONDAVI

Founder of Robert Mondavi Winery

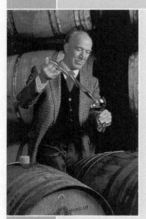

Since its founding in 1966, the Robert Mondavi Winery has established itself as one of the world's top wineries. Robert Mondavi, who recently passed away, was active as wine's foremost spokesperson, having greatly contributed to the wine industry throughout his successful life.

Robert Mondavi was born in 1913 to an Italian couple who had emigrated from the Marche region of Italy in 1910. His father, Cesare, became involved in shipping California wine grapes to fellow Italians. Extremely pleased with California, Cesare Mondavi decided to move to the Napa Valley and set up a firm that shipped fruit east. Robert Mondavi grew up among wines and vines and remained in his father's business.

Robert began by improving the family enterprise, adding to it the management, production, and marketing skills he learned at Stanford University, from which he graduated in 1936. Robert acknowledged the great business potential of the Napa Valley in the broader context of the California wine industry. What the firm needed was to be upgraded with innovations in technology to keep up with the changes in the overall business environment.

Mondavi had an ambitious dream that was realized when the Charles Krug Winery was offered for sale in 1943. The facility was purchased, and Robert knew that the strategy for success included well-planned marketing as well as the crucial winemaking expertise that the family already had.

Mondavi understood also the importance of the introduction of innovative processes that could place the winery in a competitive position. From the 1950s to the 1960s, he performed many experiments and introduced pivotal innovations. For example, Robert popularized new styles of wine, such as the chenin blanc, which was previously known as white pinot and was not doing well in the market. Mondavi changed the fermentation, turning it into a sweeter, more delicious wine. The name was also changed, and sales increased fourfold the following year.

Similarly, he noticed that the sauvignon blanc was a slow-selling wine. He began producing it in a drier style, called it fumé blanc, and turned it into an immediate success. Although the winery's operations were successful, Mondavi was still looking for a missing link in the chain. A trip to Europe, designed to study the finest wineries' techniques, convinced him to adopt a new, smaller type of barrel to age the wine, which he believed added a "wonderful dimension to the finished product."

In 1966, Robert Mondavi opened the Robert Mondavi Winery, which represented the fulfillment of the family's vision to build a facility that would allow them to produce truly world-class wines. In fact, since its establishment, the winery has led the industry, standing as an example of continuous research and innovation in winemaking, as well as a "monument to persistence in the pursuit of excellence."

Throughout the years of operation, the original vision remained constant: to produce the best wines that were the perfect accompaniments to food and to provide the public with proper education about the product. The Robert Mondavi Winery sponsors several educational programs, such as seminars on viticulture, a totally comprehensive tour program in the Napa Valley, and the great chefs program.

The Robert Mondavi Corporation was acquired by Constellation Brands in 2004, a leading international producer and marketer of beverages, selling nearly 90 million cases annually.

to produce excellent wines, many of which are blended to offer the best characteristics of each wine.

Australia has about sixty wine-growing regions, with diverse climates and soil types, mostly in the southeastern part of the continent, in New South Wales, Victoria, and South Australia, all within easy reach of the major cities of Sidney, Melbourne, and Adelaide. There are about 1,120 wineries in Australia. One of the larger and more popular wineries is Lindemans, which regularly receives accolades for its consistent quality and value. The leading red wines are cabernet sauvignon, cabernet-shiraz blends, cabernet-merlot blends, merlot, and shiraz. The leading white wines are chardonnay, semillon, sauvignon blanc, and semillon chardonnay. Among the better-known wine-growing areas is Hunter Valley in New South Wales, which produces semillon. When mature, this wine has a honey, nut, and butter flavor. The chardonnay is complex with a peaches-and-cream character. In recent years, Australian wines have shown exceptional quality and value, leading to increased sales in Europe, the United States, and Asia.

Wine also is produced in many other temperate parts of the world, most notably New Zealand, Chile, Argentina, and South Africa.

How to Read a Wine Label

Labeling requirements vary significantly from country to country. The local laws at the point of sale govern specific information that is required to be on the label where the wine is marketed, rather than where it is produced. This requirement often results in two different wine labels for the same wine. Then, if the wine is marketed where it was produced, it will have one wine label; if the wine is to be exported, it may have another version of the first wine label to meet the requirements of local laws. After the label is designed, it must be approved by the same government agency that controls wine production in that country, as well as the various government agencies that control the import and sale of the wine.[1]

In the United States, we label wines by their varietal grape and include the name of their region on the label. In Europe, wines tend to be labeled regionally rather than by varietal. The wine label on the front of the bottle generally has five headings:

1. The name of the vineyard
2. The grape variety
3. The growing area
4. The vintage
5. The producer

Wine labels are helpful in telling you a lot about what is in the bottle. Most wine bottles have two labels applied to each bottle. The front label is meant to attract your attention, while the back label may be used to provoke your senses. As an example, the label may state: "A wonderful aperitif, this smooth, elegant, wonderfully fruity wine . . . " The label may also include serving suggestions for pairing with food. These statements are not governed by law.[2]

Wine and Health

A glass of wine may be beneficial to health. This perspective was featured in the CBS news magazine program *60 Minutes*, which focused on a phenomenon called the French paradox. The French eat 30 percent more fat than Americans do, smoke more, and exercise less, yet they suffer fewer heart attacks—about one-third as many as Americans. Ironically, the French drink more wine than people of any other nationality—about 75 liters per person a year. Research indicates that wine attacks platelets, which are the smallest of the blood cells that cause the blood to clot, preventing excess bleeding. However, platelets also cling to the rough, fatty deposits on arterial walls, clogging and finally blocking arteries and causing heart attacks. Wine's flushing effect removes platelets from the artery wall. After the *60 Minutes* program was broadcast, sales of wine, particularly red wine, in the United States increased dramatically.

Sustainable Wine Production[3]

Environmentally and socially responsible grape growing and winemaking is not new, but what was once labeled a trend is now becoming an industry standard. Organic is a term given to environmentally friendly methods that use no chemicals or pesticides. Sustainability is defined as a holistic approach to growing and food production that respects the environment, the ecosystem, and even society.

The California Association of Wine Grape Growers has prepared a "Code of Sustainable Winegrowing Practices"; this is a 490-page voluntary self-assessment workbook covering everything from pest management to wine quality to water conservation to environmental stewardship. This tool allows growers and vintners to gauge how they are doing, and then to design and implement their own action plans.

A good example of sustainable winemaking is the Viansa Winery in California. It has long boasted a natural antipest team of bats, barn owls, and insectaries to keep its bug populations under control. The winery uses organic fungicide and has eliminated all herbicides.

Beer

Beer is a brewed and fermented beverage made from malted barley and other starchy cereals and flavored with hops. *Beer* is a generic term for a variety of mash-based, yeast-fermented brewed malt beverages that have an alcohol content mostly between 3.8 and 8 percent.[4] The term **beer** includes the following:

- Lager, the beverage that is normally referred to as beer, is a clear light-bodied, refreshing beer.
- Ale is fuller bodied and bitterer than lager.
- Stout is a dark ale with a sweet, strong, malt flavor.
- Pilsner is not really a beer. The term *pilsner* means that the beer is made in the style of the famous beer brewed in Pilsen, Czech Republic.

The Brewing Process

Beer is brewed from water, **malt, yeast,** and **hops.** The brewing process begins with water, an important ingredient in the making of beer. The mineral content and purity of the water largely determine the quality of the final product. Water accounts for 85 to 89 percent of the finished beer.

Next, grain is added in the form of malt, which is barley that has been ground to a coarse grit. The grain is germinated, producing an enzyme that converts starch into fermentable sugar.

The yeast is the fermenting agent. Breweries typically have their own cultured yeasts, which to a large extent determine the type and taste of the beer.

Mashing is the term for grinding the malt and screening out any bits of dirt. The malt then goes through a hopper into a mash tub, which is a large stainless steel or copper container. Here the water and grains are mixed and heated.

The liquid is now called **wort** and is filtered through a mash filter or lauter tub. This liquid then flows into a brewing kettle, where hops are added and the mixture is boiled for several hours. After the brewing operation, the hop wort is filtered through the hop separator or hop jack. The filtered liquid then is pumped through a wort cooler and into a fermenting vat where pure-culture yeast is added for fermentation.[5] The brew is aged for a few days prior to being barreled for draught beer or pasteurized for bottled or canned beer.

Today, marketing and distribution partnerships promote an even greater choice of beers for consumers. Among those available from Anheuser-Busch distributors are Löwenbräu and Beck's from Germany; Stella Artois and Hoegaarden from the Netherlands; Staropramen and Czechvar from the Czech Republic; Harbin from China;

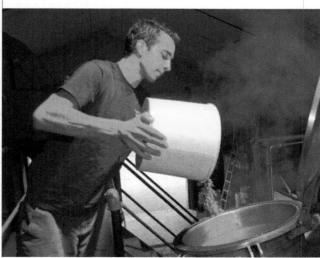

In the process of making beer, hops are added to the wort in the brew kettle.

and Landshark from Florida. Other interesting beverages include Michelob Ultra Dragon Fruit Peach, Michelob Ultra Fruit Pomegranate Raspberry, and Michelob Ultra Fruit Live Cactus.

Organic and Craft Beers, Microbreweries, and Brewpubs

The U.S. Department of Agriculture (USDA) established the National Organic Program in 1997, opening the door for organic beer. The guidelines for organic beer are the same as for all organic foods: The ingredients must be grown without toxic and persistent pesticides or synthetic fertilizers and in soil that has been free from such chemicals for at least three years. No genetically modified ingredients can be used in the brewing process. Studies show that organic farming reduces erosion and ground-water pollution and that it significantly reduces negative impacts on wildlife.[6]

The organic requirements lend themselves well to smaller breweries. An American craft brewery is a small, independent, and traditional brewery.[7] Craft beer showcases the different areas of the country and their seemingly distinct styles of beer and craft beer scenes. You can get an India Pale Ale (IPA) from anywhere, but there's a reason people will refer to a super hoppy, dry IPA as a "west coast IPA." Also, a lot of craft breweries only distribute in a small- to medium-sized area.[8] As craft brewers have come of age, little did the world know that their full-flavored craft beers would generate such passion and excitement.

Today is a great time to be a beer lover, and as a nation, we now have more beer styles and beer brands to choose from than any other market in the world.[9] Traditionally, a brewer has either an all-malt flagship (the beer that represents the greatest volume sold among that brewer's brands) or has at least 50% of its volume represented by either all-malt beers or by beers that use adjuncts to enhance rather than lighten flavor.[10]

The Brewers Association describes a microbrewery as a brewery that produces a limited amount (less than 15,000 barrels) of beer a year. A brewpub brews and sells beer on the premises and may also be known as a microbrewery if the production has a significant distribution beyond the premises.[11]

Sustainable Brewing

Breweries use a lot of resources yet have the potential to significantly reduce their environmental footprint. Here is how some brewers are reducing their footprint:[12]

- Efficient brewhouse: The brewery is as sustainable and efficient as possible, starting with the parts of the building that were reclaimed and recycled when the Full Sail brewery first opened in the old Diamond Fruit cannery in Oregon. Full Sail utilizes measures such as energy-efficient lighting and air compressors, and compresses the work week into four very productive days, which helps reduce water and energy consumption by 20 percent.

- Sustainable brew process: Pure water literally flows from the peaks that surround the brewery, so Full Sail takes care to conserve this precious resource. While average breweries consume six to eight gallons of water for every gallon of beer produced, Full Sail has reduced its consumption to a mere 3.45 gallons, and operates its own on-site wastewater treatment facility. Local farms supply the other essential ingredients for award-winning brews: 85 percent of hops and 95 percent of barley come straight from Northwest farms.

- Reduce-Reuse-Recycle: Full Sail uses 100 percent recycled paperboard on all its packaging (and was one of the first in the industry to commit to long-term purchasing of recycled paper products). Everything from office paper to glass to stretch wrap to wooden pallets is recycled. Even dairy cows are beneficiaries of brewery waste: 4,160 tons of spent grain and 1,248 tons of spent yeast are sent back to farmers every year to use as feed for cows.

- Community-wide practices: Full Sail purchases 140 blocks of Pacific Power Blue Sky renewable energy per month. This practice results in the reduction of 168 tons of carbon dioxide emissions, the equivalent of planting 33,000 trees. Full Sail also supports over 300 events and charities each year, with a focus on those in Oregon. Employees at the company have inspired environmental change among other businesses in the Hood River area as well. Full Sail was a founding member of the Hood River Chamber of Commerce's "Green Smart" program, an initiative that helps businesses and organizations within the Hood River watershed increase their productivity and profitability by improving resource efficiency and by reducing waste and pollution.

As the push for sustainability gains momentum, one only need to look down at the pint or mug he or she is holding to see how breweries are joining the growing green movement! Beer is the third most-consumed beverage in the world behind water and tea. Upon surveying a number of breweries, and sustainable brewing documents, BlueMap Inc. has determined 10 green steps every brewery should consider.[13]

Utilize Biochar Processing to Re-Use Spent Grains

Processing spent grains through pyrolisis (a process that burns grains to create Biochar, a valuable soil amendment), is a carbon-negative process: it creates heat and syngas while sequestering carbon. By doing so, pyrolisis decreases a brewery's carbon footprint.

Implement Water Use Reduction Measures

Water is one of the largest inputs in brewing. A brewery can conserve water by reducing lost steam, increasing the efficiency of wort production, increasing the life of water in boiler systems, and altogether preventing waste.

Implement Variable-Speed Fans or Motors

Many brewery processes have variable loads that are more efficiently served by variable-speed motors, fans, and drives. Where applicable, an upgrade in a brewery's fans and motors can offer substantial savings and have favorable pay back periods. Savings are only observed if loads vary.

Ensure a Regular Maintenance Regime

A regular maintenance regimen is a great way to cut down on energy inefficiencies. Regularly scheduled maintenance allows breweries to catch problems sooner and address them before excess energy is wasted. Also, keeping a system tuned up means that motors and pumps run at optimum speeds, controls are set properly, and control systems are turned on.

Capture Methane at On-Site Water Treatment Facilities

For breweries that process wastewater on-site, methane capture is a great way to regain value from a waste stream. Currently, closed systems and pond cover methane capture exist. These systems purify and burn methane onsite, which typically offsets the brewery's fuel costs while cutting costs.

Recapture CO_2 during Fermentation

Fermentation releases CO_2. Savvy breweries can capture this CO_2 and use it (instead of purchased CO_2) in the bottling process to carbonate their beer. This reduces both CO_2 released to the air and CO_2 purchasing costs.

Optimize Thermal Resources within the Brewing Process

Much of the brewing process consists of thermal processes: boiling and cooling liquids. Auditing the entire process can reveal ways to capture thermal resources and apply them to other brewing processes, thereby reducing energy and fuel costs of heating and cooling.

Implement Alternatives to Diatomaceous Earth (DE) Filtering

Though DE is a long-standing industry standard as a filter medium, health risks associated with DE (and potential problems regulating its use and disposal) are prompting some to seek alternatives. Where applicable, sheet filtering, cross flow filtration systems, and DE recycling systems can be used to avoid some of these flaws.

Optimize Refrigeration, Lighting, Construction, and Other Building Controls

Sustainable building is potentially one of the largest opportunities for a brewery to reduce energy consumption and curtail demand spikes (thereby minimizing fines). Management systems can be installed to green the lighting of spaces, maximize building functions, optimize chill systems, and stagger cooling loads.

Utilize Renewable Energy Technologies

Beer is made with hops, grain, water and yeast. What could be a more natural way to complement these natural ingredients than using sun or wind to power the beer brewing process? Renewable energy sources include geothermal, syngas, or biogas. When sized correctly, these technologies greatly reduce purchased electricity and fuel and can have very attractive payback periods.

By considering these 10 recommendations, the third-largest beverage industry in the world can reduce its overall ecological impact while in many cases save money.

Further examples of breweries around the country that are finding creative ways to reduce their carbon footprint are by installing wind and solar power. Colorado's New Belgium Brewery has an 870 panel solar array from which it gets 13 percent of its energy needs; Odell Brewing Company gets 39 percent of its energy needs.[14]

INTRODUCING ROB WESTFALL

Bar Manager, The Speakeasy, Siesta Key, Florida

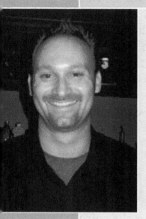

The Speakeasy has been a staple in Siesta Key's Village for over ten years. Known for its exceptional variety of live music, it is also a place where locals feel right at home. The Speakeasy features ice-cold air conditioning in a polished, clean environment. Located at the back of the room is our pool table with plenty of space to allow for professional play. Specialty drinks are another draw for patrons at The Speakeasy. Our menu is loaded with innovative cocktails that are tough to find in another establishment. Along with our extensive list of wines by the glass, we also offer many premium single-malt scotches, cognacs, and bourbons and a host of fine liqueurs. The Speakeasy is owned and operated by Café Gardens, which also owns the Daiquiri Deck located directly next door.

A typical day for a manager at The Speakeasy goes like this:

9:45 A.M. Arrive for manager meeting at the Daiquiri Deck. All Daiquiri Deck managers, the owners, and myself are present at this meeting. The meeting consists of a variety of issues. Typically, the first order of business is reviewing the numbers from the previous week. Numbers like net sales, cost of labor, cost of goods, and promotional costs are discussed. Additionally, budgets are a major concern every week. Budgets are set based on sales projections from the previous year and are very important to the success of the business. Next, we discuss any issues from the previous week. In the bar business, an "issue" could be just about anything from fights to vandalism. We find it extremely important to discuss all of these issues so that the management team is all on the same page.

11:00 A.M. Mondays are very important in the bar business. Inventory must be taken to ensure that costs are in line, and that you know what product you need. First, I take an inventory of all beverage products at The Speakeasy. Liquor, beer, wine, cigarettes, cigars, and mixers are all items that must be counted.

12:00 P.M. Upon completion of the inventory, it is time to put your orders together for the week. Knowing your usage is extremely important when placing an order. Buying in bulk is always superior to simply filling holes from week to week. Simply, it allows you more buying power and, essentially, more free goods.

1:00 P.M. Confirm band schedule. Booking bands and maintaining an entertainment schedule can sometimes be one of the most frustrating areas of the bar business. However, it can also be the most rewarding. The experience you gain from working with so many different types of entertainment is difficult to replace. The majority of bands show up on time and treat their job professionally, but there are a significant amount of them that do not. I call my bands to confirm their schedule on a weekly basis for this very reason.

2:00 P.M. Typically, there is always some bar maintenance that needs to be addressed. I always take a walk around and check everything out to make sure that everything is working property.

3:00 P.M. Work on any upcoming promotions and ensure their success. Spirit tastings, holidays, full-moon parties, and private parties are examples of these types of events.

4:00 P.M. Send memo to corporate office regarding what checks need to be written for entertainment that week. Ensure that each band has proper paperwork filled out for tax purposes.

5:00 P.M. Every day the staff needs to be reminded to step it up. Motivation comes from the top down. The bar business is a stage, and the bartenders are on a stage. The staff will typically need to be reminded of this on a consistent basis. Open lines of communication are very important and allow you to apply constructive criticism or accolades, as they are appropriate.

6:00 P.M. It's time to have a drink.

That's the management side of the bar. The nighttime is another animal entirely!

Spirits

A **spirit** or **liquor** is made from a liquid that has been fermented and distilled. Consequently, a spirit has a high percentage of alcohol, gauged in the United States by its proof content. **Proof** is equal to twice the percentage of alcohol in the beverage; therefore, a spirit that is 80 proof is 40 percent alcohol. Spirits traditionally are enjoyed before or after a meal, rather than with the meal. Many spirits can be consumed straight, or neat (without ice or other ingredients), or they may be enjoyed with water, soda water, juices, or cocktail mixes.

Fermentation of spirits takes place by the action of yeast on sugar-containing substances, such as grain or fruit. Distilled drinks are made from a fermented liquid that has been put through a distillation process.

Whiskies

Among the better-known spirits is whisky, which is a generic name for the spirit first distilled in Scotland and Ireland centuries ago. The word *whisky* comes from the Celtic word *visgebaugh*, meaning "water of life." Whisky is made from a fermented mash of grain to which malt, in the form of barley, is added. The barley contains an enzyme called diastase that converts starch to sugars. After fermentation, the liquid is distilled. Spirits naturally are white or pale in color, but raw whisky is stored in oak barrels that have been charred (burnt). This gives whisky its caramel color. The whisky is stored for a period of time, up to a maximum of twelve to fifteen years. However, several good whiskies reach the market after three to five years.

Most whiskies are blended to produce a flavor and quality that is characteristic of the brand. Not surprisingly, the blending process at each distillery is a closely guarded secret. There are four distinct whisky types that have gained worldwide acknowledgment throughout the centuries: Scotch whisky, Irish whisky, bourbon whisky, and Canadian whisky.

Scotch Whisky

Scotch whisky, or scotch, has been distilled in Scotland for centuries and has been a distinctive part of the Scots' way of life. From its origins in remote and romantic Highland glens, Scotch whisky has become a popular and international drink, its flavor appreciated throughout the world. Scotch became popular in the United States during the days of **Prohibition** (1919 to 1933) when it was smuggled into the country from Canada. It is produced like other whiskies, except that the malt is dried in special kilns that give it a smoky flavor. To be legally called Scotch whisky, the spirit must conform to the standards of the Scotch Whisky Act; only whisky made with this process can be called Scotch whisky. Some of the better-known quality-blended Scotch whiskies are Chivas Regal and Johnnie Walker Black, Gold, and Blue Labels.

A single malt Scotch whisky is the product of one specific distillery and has not been mixed with whisky from any other distilleries. Some whisky aficionados prefer a single malt Scotch, from which there are several brands to chose.

Irish Whiskey

Irish whiskey is spelled with an *e* and is produced from malted or unmalted barley, corn, rye, and other grains. The malt is not dried like it is in the production of Scotch whisky, which gives Irish whiskey a milder character, yet an excellent flavor. Two well-known Irish whiskies are Old Bushmill's Black Bush and Jameson's 12 Year Old Special Reserve.

Bourbon Whisky

Liquor was introduced in America by the first settlers, who used it as a medicine. Bourbon has a peculiar history. In colonial times in New England, rum was the most popular distilled spirit. After the break with Britain,

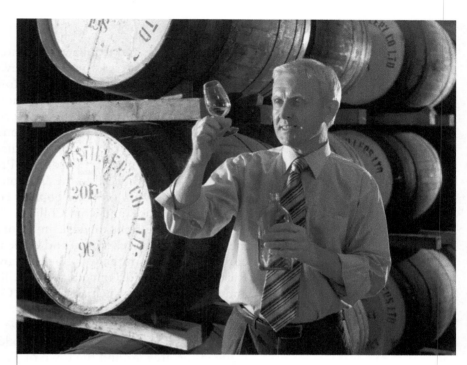

Checking the color of Johnnie Walker Scotch that is maturing in barrels.

settlers of Scottish and Irish background predominated. They were mostly grain farmers and distillers, producing whisky for barter. When George Washington levied a tax on this whisky, the farmers moved south and continued their whisky production. However, the rye crop failed, so they decided to mix corn, particularly abundant in Kentucky, with the remaining rye. The result was delightful. This experiment occurred in Bourbon County—hence the name of the new product.

Bourbon whisky is produced mainly from corn; other grains are also used, but they are of secondary importance. The distillation processes are similar to those of other types of whisky. Charred barrels provide bourbon with its distinctive taste. It is curious to note that barrels can only be used once in the United States to age liquor. Aging, therefore, occurs in new barrels after each distillation process. Bourbon may be aged up to six years to improve its mellowness. Among the better-known bourbon whiskies are Jack Daniels, Maker's Mark, and George Dickel.

Canadian Whisky

Like bourbon, Canadian whisky is produced mainly from corn. It is characterized by a delicate flavor that nonetheless pleases the palate. Canadian whisky must be at least four years old before it can be bottled and marketed. It is distilled at 70 to 90 percent alcohol by volume. Among the better-known Canadian whiskies are Seagram's and Canadian Club.

White Spirits

Gin, rum, vodka, and tequila are the most common of the spirits that are called **white spirits**. Gin, first known as Geneva, is a neutral spirit made from juniper berries. Although gin originated in Holland, it was in London that the word *Geneva* was shortened to gin, and almost anything was used to make it. Often gin was made in the bathtub in the morning and sold in hole-in-the-wall dram shops all over London at night. Obviously, the quality left a lot to be desired, but the poor drank it to the point of national disaster.[15] Gin also was widely produced in the United States during Prohibition. In fact, the habit of mixing something else with it led to the creation of the cocktail. Over the years, gin became the foundation of many popular cocktails (for example, martini, gin and tonic, gin and juice, and Tom Collins).

Rum can be light or dark in color. Light rum is distilled from the fermented juice of sugarcane, and dark rum is distilled from molasses. Rum comes mainly from the Caribbean islands of Barbados (Mount Gay), Puerto Rico (Bacardi), and Jamaica (Myers). Rums are mostly used in mixed frozen and specialty drinks such as rum and Coke, rum punches, daiquiris, and piña coladas.

Tequila is distilled from the *Agave tequilana* (a type of cactus), which is called *mezcal* in Mexico. Official Mexican regulations require that tequila be made in the area around the town of Tequila because the soil contains volcanic ash, which is especially suitable for growing the blue agave cactus. Tequila may be white, silver, or golden in color. The white is shipped unaged, silver is aged up to three years, and golden is aged in oak from two to four years. Tequila is mainly used in the popular margarita cocktail or in the tequila sunrise (made popular in a song by the Eagles rock group).

Vodka can be made from many sources, including barley, corn, wheat, rye, or potatoes. Because it lacks color, odor, and flavor, vodka generally is combined with juices or other mixers whose flavors predominate. To offer consumers more choices, vodka producers have popularized flavored vodkas with lemon, pepper, vanilla, raspberry, peach, pears, and mango, among others. Brand names of vodka producers are Absolut from Sweden, Stolichnaya (or Stoli for short) from Russia, Grey Goose from France, Tru Organic from the United Sates, and Van Gogh from the Netherlands.

Other Spirits

Brandy is distilled from wine in a fashion similar to that of other spirits. American brandy comes primarily from California, where it is made in column stills and aged in white-oak barrels for at least two years. The best-known American brandies are made by Christian Brothers and Ernest and Julio Gallo. Their brandies are smooth and fruity with a touch of sweetness. The best brandies are served as after-dinner drinks, and ordinary brandies are used in the well for mixed drinks.

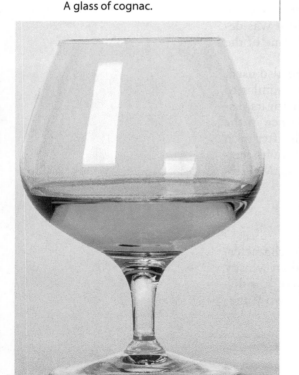
A glass of cognac.

Cognac is regarded by connoisseurs as the best brandy in the world. It is made only in the Cognac region of France, where the chalky soil and humid climate combine with special distillation techniques to produce the finest brandy. Only brandy from this region may be called cognac. Most cognac is aged in oak casks from two to four years or more. Because cognacs are blends of brandies of various ages, no age is allowed on the label; instead, letters signify the relative age and quality.

Brandies labeled as *VSOP* must be aged at least four years. All others must be aged in wood at least five years. Five years, then, is the age of the youngest cognac in a blend; usually, several others of older age are added to lend taste, bouquet, and finesse. About 75 percent of the cognac shipped to Canada and the United States is produced by four companies: Courvoisier, Hennessy, Martell, and Remy Martin.

Cocktails

The first cocktails originated in England during the Victorian era, but it wasn't until the 1920s and 1930s that cocktails became popular.

Cocktails are usually drinks made by mixing two or more ingredients (wines, liquors, fruit juices), resulting in a blend that is pleasant to the palate, with no single ingredient overpowering the others. Cocktails are mixed by stirring, shaking, or blending. The mixing technique is particularly important to achieve the perfect cocktail. Cocktails are commonly divided into two categories according to volume: short drinks (up to 3.5 ounces) and tall drinks (generally up to 8.5 ounces).

The secret of a good cocktail lies in several factors:

- The balance of the ingredients. No single ingredient should overpower the others.
- The quality of the ingredients. As a general rule, cocktails should be made from a maximum of three ingredients.
- The skill of the bartender. The bartender's experience, knowledge, and inspiration are key factors in making a perfect cocktail.

A good bartender should understand the effect and the "timing" of a cocktail. It is not a coincidence that many cocktails are categorized by when they are best served. There are aperitifs, digestifs, corpse-revivers, pick-me-ups, and so on. Cocktails can stimulate an appetite or provide the perfect conclusion to a fine meal.

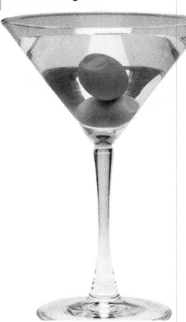

A martini cocktail served in a martini glass.

▶ Check Your Knowledge

1. Describe the different types of beer.
2. Describe the various spirits.

Nonalcoholic Beverages

Nonalcoholic beverages are increasing in popularity. In the 1990s and 2000s, a radical shift has occurred from the free-love 1960s and the singles bars of the 1970s and early 1980s. People are, in general, more cautious about the consumption of alcohol. Lifestyles have become healthier, and organizations such as Mothers Against Drunk Driving (MADD) have raised the social conscience about responsible alcohol consumption. Overall consumption of alcohol has decreased in recent years, with spirits declining the most.

In recent years, several new beverages have been added to the nonalcoholic beverage list. From Goji juice to passion fruit green tea, the nonalcoholic beverage world has been innovative in creating flavored teas and coffees and an ever-increasing variety of juices to satisfy all our tastes.

Nonalcoholic Beer

Guinness, Anheuser-Busch, and Miller, along with many other brewers, have developed beer products that have the same appearance as regular beer but that have a lower calorie content and approximately 95 to 99 percent of the alcohol removed, either after processing or after fermentation. The taste, therefore, is somewhat different from regular beer.

Coffee

Coffee is the drink of the present. People who used to frequent bars are now patronizing coffeehouses. Sales of specialty coffees exceed $4 billion a year. The Specialty Coffee Association of America estimates that there are more than 17,400 coffee cafés nationwide.[16]

Coffee first came from Ethiopia and Mocha, which is in the Yemen Republic. Legends say that Kaldi, a young Abyssinian goatherd, accustomed to his sleepy goats, noticed that after chewing certain berries, the goats began to prance about excitedly. He tried the berries himself, forgot his troubles, lost his heavy heart, and became the happiest person in "happy Arabia." A monk from a nearby monastery surprised Kaldi in this state, decided to try the berries too, and invited the brothers to join him. They all felt more alert that night during prayers![17]

In the Middle Ages, coffee found its way to Europe via Turkey but not without some objections. In Italy, priests appealed to Pope Clement VIII to have the use of coffee forbidden among Christians. Satan, they said, had forbidden his followers, the infidel Moslems, the use of wine because it was used in the Holy Communion and had given them instead his "hellish black brew." Apparently, the pope liked the drink, for he blessed it on the spot, after which coffee quickly became the social beverage of Europe's middle and upper classes.[18]

In 1637, the first European coffeehouse opened in England; within thirty years, coffeehouses had replaced taverns as the island's social, commercial, and political melting pots.[19] The coffeehouses were nicknamed *penny universities*, where any topic could be discussed and learned for the price of a pot of coffee.

The men of the period not only discussed business but actually conducted business. Banks, newspapers, and the Lloyd's of London Insurance Company began at Edward Lloyd's coffeehouse.

Coffeehouses were also popular in Europe. In Paris, Café Procope, which opened in 1689 and still operates today, has been the meeting place of many a famous artist and philosopher, including Rousseau and Voltaire (who are reputed to have drunk forty cups of coffee a day).

The Dutch introduced coffee to the United States during the colonial period. Coffeehouses soon became the haunts of the revolutionary activists plotting against King George of England and his tea tax. John Adams and Paul Revere planned the Boston Tea Party and the fight for freedom at a coffeehouse. This helped establish coffee as the traditional democratic drink of Americans.

Brazil produces more than 30 percent of the world's coffee, most of which goes into canned and instant coffee. Coffee connoisseurs recommend beans by name, such as arabica and robusta beans. In Indonesia, coffee is named for the island on which it grows; the best is from Java and is rich and spicy with a full-bodied flavor. Yemen, the country in which coffee was discovered, names its best coffee for the port of Mocha. Its fragrant, creamy brew has a rich, almost chocolaty aftertaste. Coffee beans are frequently blended by the merchants who roast them; one of the best blends, mocha java, is the result of blending these two fine coffees.

Coffee may be roasted from light to dark according to preference. Light roasts are generally used in canned and institutional roasts, and medium is the all-purpose roast most people prefer. Medium beans are medium brown in color, and their surface is dry. Although this brew may have snappy, acidic qualities, its flavor tends to be flat. Full, high, or Viennese roast is the roast preferred by specialty stores, where balance is achieved between sweetness and sharpness. Dark roasts have a fancy, rich flavor, with espresso the darkest of all roasts. Its almost-black beans have shiny, oily surfaces. All the acidic qualities and specific coffee flavor are gone from espresso, but its pungent flavor is a favorite of espresso lovers.

Decaffeinating coffee removes the caffeine with either a solvent or water process. In contrast, many specialty coffees have things added. Among the better-known specialty coffees are café au lait or caffè latte. In these cases, milk is steamed until it becomes frothy and is poured into the cup together with the coffee. A cappuccino is made with espresso, hot milk, and milk foam, which may then be sprinkled with powdered chocolate and cinnamon.[20]

Tea

Tea is a beverage made by steeping in boiling water the leaves of the tea plant, an evergreen shrub, or small tree, native to Asia. Tea is consumed as either a hot or cold beverage by approximately half of the world's population, yet it is second to coffee in commercial importance because most of the world's tea crop is consumed in the tea-growing regions. Tea leaves contain 1 to 3 percent caffeine. This means that weight for weight, tea leaves have more than twice as much caffeine as coffee beans. However, a cup of coffee generally has more caffeine than a cup of tea because one pound of tea leaves makes 250 to 300 cups of tea, whereas one pound of coffee beans makes only 40 cups of coffee.

CORPORATE PROFILE

Starbucks Coffee Company

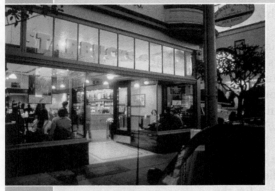

Operations

Starbucks Coffee Company (named after the first mate in Herman Melville's *Moby-Dick*) is the leading retailer, roaster, and brand of specialty coffee in North America. More than 7 million people visit Starbucks stores each week. In addition to its more than 17,000 retail locations, the company supplies fine dining, foodservice, travel, and hotel accounts with coffee and coffee-making equipment and operates a national mail-order division.

Locations and Alliances

Starbucks currently has 17,018 stores in fifty U.S. states and in fifty countries.[21] Starbucks has strategic alliances with United Airlines and is now the exclusive supplier of coffee on every United flight.

In addition, Specialty Sales and Marketing supplies Starbucks coffee to the health care, business and industry, college and university, and hotel and resort segments of the foodservice industry; to many fine restaurants throughout North America; and to companies such as Costco, Nordstrom, Starwood, Barnes and Noble, Hilton Hotels, Sodexho, ARAMARK, Compass, Wyndham, Borders, Radisson, Sysco, Safeway, Albertson's, Kraft Foods, Pepsico, and Marriott International.

Product Line

Starbucks roasts more than thirty varieties of the world's finest arabica coffee beans. The company's retail locations also feature a variety of espresso beverages and locally made fresh pastries. Starbucks specialty merchandise includes Starbucks private-label espresso makers, mugs, plunger pots, grinders, storage jars, water filters, thermal carafes, and coffee makers. An extensive selection of packaged goods, including unique confections, gift baskets, and coffee-related items, are available in stores and online.

Starbucks introduced Frappuccino blended beverages, a line of low-fat, creamy, iced coffee drinks. This product launch was the most successful in Starbucks history. The company also has a bottled version of Frappuccino, which is currently available in grocery stores and in many Starbucks retail locations.

A long-term joint venture between Starbucks Coffee and Breyer's Grand Ice Cream dishes up a premium line of coffee ice creams, with national distribution of several different flavors to leading grocery stores. Starbucks has become the number-one brand of coffee ice cream in the United States. Currently, ice cream lovers can choose from eight delectable flavors or two ice cream bars.

Community Involvement

Starbucks contributes to a variety of organizations that benefit AIDS research, child welfare, environmental awareness, literacy, and the arts. The company encourages its partners (employees) to take an active role in their own neighborhoods.

Starbucks fulfills its corporate social responsibility mission by reducing its environmental footprint on the planet. The company addresses three high-impact areas: sourcing of coffee, tea, and paper; transportation of people and products; and design and operations (energy, water, waste reduction, and recycling). Starbucks has developed relations with organizations that support the people and places that grow its coffee and tea, such as Conservation International, CARE, Save the Children, and the African Wildlife Foundation. Additionally, Starbucks has entered into a partnership with the U.S. Agency for International Development (USAID) and Conservation International to improve the livelihoods of small-scale coffee farmers through private sector approaches within the coffee industry that are environmentally sensitive, socially responsible, and economically viable. In 2005, Starbucks received the World Environment Center's Gold Medal for International Corporate Achievement in Sustainable Development.

Starbucks has received numerous awards for quality innovation, service, and giving.

The following list shows where the different types of tea originate:

China—oolong, orange pekoe

India—Darjeeling, Assams (also known as English breakfast tea), Dooars

Indonesia—Java, Sumatra

Carbonated Soft Drinks and Energy Drinks

Coca-Cola and Pepsi have long dominated the carbonated soft drink market. In the early 1970s, Diet Coke and Diet Pepsi were introduced and quickly gained popularity. The diet colas now command about a 10-percent market share. Caffeine-free colas offer an alternative, but they have not, as yet, become as popular as diet colas.

Energy drinks are beverages that are designed to give the consumer a burst of energy by using a combination of methylaxanthines (including caffeine), B vitamins, and exotic herbal ingredients. Energy drinks commonly include caffeine, guarana (extracts from the guarana plant), taurine, various forms of ginseng, maltodextrin, inositol, carnitine, creatine, glucuronolactone, and ginkgo biloba. Some contain high levels of sugar, while most brands also offer an artificially sweetened version. Red Bull is an example of a popular energy drink that originated in Thailand and that has a Japanese heritage. It was adapted to Australian tastes and in only a few years has become popular around the world. The claims are that Red Bull vitalizes the body and mind by supplying tired minds and exhausted bodies with vital substances that have been lost, while reducing harmful substances. It purports to provide immediate energy and vitamins to the consumer. Red Bull has a large market share in more than 100 countries.

Sales of energy drinks and shots are soaring, even as there are growing health concerns given the popularity of the high-caffeine drinks among young people. The dollar value of energy-drink sales rose 13.3 percent last year, thanks in part to a "significant boost" from energy-shot sales at convenience stores, according to a report from the market research firm SymphonyIRI Group.[22] American Beverage Association science chief Maureen Storey says energy drinks are no worse than coffee. A 16-ounce cup of Starbucks' Pike Place coffee, for instance, has 330 mg of caffeine. That size of latte has 160 mg—the same as a 16-ounce can of the energy drink Monster Energy, which bills

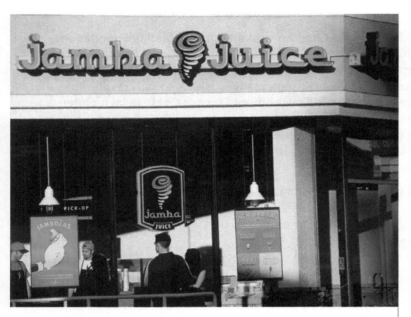

A juice bar.

itself as "a killer energy brew" that "you can really pound down." The federal Food and Drug Administration limits caffeine in soft drinks to 71 mg for 12 ounces but doesn't regulate the caffeine in energy drinks, coffee, or tea.[23]

Juices

Popular juice flavors include orange, cranberry, grapefruit, mango, papaya, and apple. Nonalcoholic versions of popular cocktails made with juices have been popular for years and are known as virgin cocktails.

Juice bars have established themselves as places for quick, healthy drinks. Lately, "smart drinks" that are supposed to boost energy and improve concentration have become popular. The smart drinks are made up of a blend of juices, herbs, amino acids, caffeine, and sugar and are sold under names such as Energy Plasma Blast and IQ Booster.

Other drinks have jumped on the healthy drink bandwagon, playing on the consumer's desire to drink something refreshing, light, and healthful. Often, these drinks are fruit flavored, giving the consumer the impression of drinking something healthier than sugar-filled sodas. Unfortunately, these drinks usually just add the flavor of the fruit and rarely have any nutritional value.

In addition, some drinks are created by mixing different fruit flavors to arrive at new, exotic flavors such as Passion-Kiwi-Strawberry and Mango-Banana Delight. Some examples of such drinks are Snapple and Tropicana Twister.

Sports enthusiasts also find drinks that professional athletes use and advertise available in stores. These specially formulated isotonic beverages are intended to help the body regain the vital fluids and minerals that are lost during heavy physical exertion. The National Football League sponsors Gatorade and encourages its use among its athletes. The appeal of being able to drink what the professionals drink is undoubtedly one of the major reasons for the success of Gatorade's sales and marketing. Other brands of isotonic beverages include Powerade and All Sport, which is sponsored by the National Collegiate Athletics Association.

Bottled Water

Bottled water was popular in Europe years ago when it was not safe to drink tap water. In North America, the increased popularity of bottled water has coincided with the trend toward healthier lifestyles.

In the 1980s, it was chic to be seen drinking Perrier (a sparkling water) or some other imported bottled water. Perrier, which comes from France, lost market share a few years ago when an employee tampered with the product.

Now the market leader is Evian (a spring water), which is also French. Domestic bottled water is as good as imported and is now available in various flavors that offer the consumer a greater selection.

Bottled waters are available as sparkling, mineral, and spring waters. Bottled water is a refreshing, clean-tasting, low-calorie beverage that will likely increase in popularity as a beverage on its own or to accompany another beverage such as wine or whisky.

Bars and Beverage Operations

From an operating perspective, bar and beverage management follows much the same sequence as does food management, as shown in the following list:

- Forecasting
- Determining what to order
- Selecting the supplier
- Placing the order
- Receiving the order
- Storing
- Issuing
- Serving
- Accounting
- Controlling

Bar Setup

Whether a bar is part of a larger operation (restaurant) or a business in its own right, the physical setup of the bar is critical to its overall effectiveness. There is a need to design the area in such a way that it not only is pleasing to the eye but it also is conducive to a smooth and efficient operation. This means that bar stations—where drinks are filled—are located in strategic spots, and that each station has everything it needs to respond to most, if not all, requests. All well liquors should be easily accessible, with popular call brands not too far out of reach. The brands that are less likely to be ordered (and more likely to be high priced) can be farther away from the stations. The most obvious place for the high-priced, premium brands is the back bar, a place of high visibility. Anyone sitting at the bar will be looking directly at the back bar, giving the customers a chance to view the bar's choices.

As for beer coolers, their location depends on the relative importance of beer to the establishment. In many places, beer is kept in coolers under the bar or below the back bar, and sample bottles or signs are displayed for customers. However, in many places, beer is the biggest seller, and bars may offer numerous brands from around the world. In such places, other setups may be used, such as standup coolers with glass doors so that customers can easily see all the varieties available. This is also true for draft beers.

Inventory Control

The beverage profitability of an organization is not a matter of luck. Profits result largely from the implementation and use of effective **inventory controls** by management and employees. Training is also important to ensure that employees treat inventory as cash and that they handle it as if it were their own money. Management's example will be followed by employees. If employees sense a lax management style, they may be tempted to steal. No control system can guarantee the prevention of theft completely. However, the better the control system, the less likely it is that there will be a loss.[24]

To operate profitably, a beverage operation manager needs to establish what the expected results will be. For example, if a bottle of gin contains twenty-five 1-ounce measures, it would be reasonable to expect twenty-five times the selling price in revenue. When this is multiplied for each bottle, the total revenue can be determined and compared to the actual revenue.

One of the critical areas of bar management is the design, installation, and implementation of a system to control possible theft of the bar's beverage inventory. Theft may occur in a number of ways, including the following:

- Giving away drinks
- Overpouring alcohol
- Mischarging for drinks
- Selling a call liquor at a well price
- Outright stealing of bar beverages by employees

As is the case with food operations, anticipated profit margin is based on the ratio of sales generated to related beverage costs. Bar management must be able to account for any discrepancies between expected and actual profit margins.

All inventory control systems require an actual physical count of the existing inventory, which may be done on a weekly or monthly basis, depending on the needs of management. This physical count is based on units. For liquor and wine, the unit is a bottle, either 0.750 or 1.0 liter; for bottled beer, the unit is a case of twenty-four bottles; for draft beer, the unit is one keg. The results of the most current physical count are then compared to the prior period's physical count to determine the actual amount of beverage inventory consumed during the period. This physical amount is translated into a cost or dollar figure by multiplying the amount consumed for each item by its respective cost per unit. The total cost for all beverages consumed is compared to the sales generated to result in a profit margin, which is then compared to the expected margin.

Management should design forms that can be used to account for all types of liquor, beer, and wine available at the bar. The listing of the items should follow their actual physical setup within the bar to facilitate easy accounting of the inventory. The forms should also have columns where amounts of each inventory item can be noted. A traditional way to account for the amount of liquor in a bottle is by using the "10" count, where the level of each bottle is marked by tenths; thus, a half-full bottle of well vodka would be marked as ".5" on the form. Similarly, for kegs of draft beer, a breakdown of 25, 50, 75, and 100 percent may be used to determine their physical count.

Beverage Management Technology

Technology for beverage management has improved with products from companies such as Scannabar (**www.scanbar.com**), which offer beverage operators a system that accounts for every ounce, with daily, weekly, or monthly results. The ongoing real-time inventory allows viewing results at any time and place, with tamperproof reliability interfaced with major point-of-sale (POS) systems.

The Scannabar liquor module has a bar-coded label on each bottle, making it easy to track bottles from purchase to recycle bin. Each bottle variety has the same scannbar, allowing for easy calibration. The bar-coded ribbon is used as a measuring tool to give accurate results. Inventory taking is done with a portable handheld radio-frequency bar code reader. Once the label is scanned, the level of alcohol in the bottle is recorded and the data are sent from the user's handheld reader to the computer in the office for real-time results.[25]

The wine module keeps control of all wines by region, variety, or vintage. After the wines have been configured within the directory, the procedure is that, when a wine is received, the variety is identified by scanning the bar code already on the bottle or is selected directly from the portable handheld radio-frequency bar code reader. A bar-coded tag is placed around the collar, which creates a unique identity for each bottle. Once the bottle is ready to be served, either at the table or at the bar, the bar-coded tag is removed from the bottle and scanned out of inventory. Scanning the tag around the neck of the bottle accomplishes inventory taking.[26]

The beverage system from AZ Bar America (**www.azbarusa.com**) offers a POS system that runs the operations behind the bar. It rings up the charge as the beverage is being poured while automatically removing the product from inventory.

Instead of holding up bottles and guessing what is left in them or even weighing each bottle at the end of shifts, the AZ2000 controller can at any time give a report of what was sold, who completed the transaction, how the system was used, and what the actual profits are by brand, transaction, or product group. The system can be remotely monitored from home or other location by dialing into the bar location; this is handy for making price changes and monitoring sales activity.

The AZ2000 is the heart of a dispensing system that interfaces with a variety of products: "spouts," a cocktail tower, beer, wine, juice, soft drink machines, and soda guns. The system even runs cocktail programming, so if the bartender does not know what goes into a certain drink, he or she can hit the cocktail button, and the system will tell the bartender what liquor bottle to pick up and will control the recipe pour amounts.[27]

TECHNOLOGY SPOTLIGHT

Using Technology to Control Beverage Costs

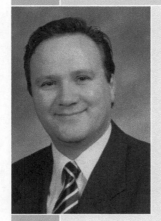

Cihan Cobanoglu, Ph.D., Dean, School of Hotel and Restaurant Management, University of South Florida, Sarasota-Manatee

Controlling costs in a food service operation is one of the key elements for being successful. Traditionally, the profit margins in the food service establishments are very slim (about 5 to 8 percent). This requires the restaurant owners and managers to be in control of the food and beverage costs at all times. There are several technology applications that will help food service operations to keep track and control costs. An important part of food service operations is beverage service and sales. Controlling beverage costs differs from controlling food costs. Food costs should be around 28 to 32 percent of the sales price, whereas beverage costs should be between 18 and 22 percent of the sales price. Every reduction in food and beverage cost percentage results in a higher gross profit. Beverage sales (alcoholic and non-alcoholic) are an easy way to increase profitability because the costs are lower and the gross margin is far greater for beverage than for food.

There are several technologies that will help operators to control beverage costs. One of them is AccuBar, which is a sophisticated beverage management program that uses personal digital assistants (PDAs) to scan the bar codes on the labels of liquor, beer, and wine bottles, as well as virtually any other items you may have in inventory. The PDA quickly collects counts to simplify tracking of (1) physical inventory, (2) receiving, (3) perpetual inventory, (4) supplier, (5) ordering, (6) transfers between locations, (7) banquet and event consumption, (8) large wine cellars, (9) requisitions, (10) empties, (11) variances, (12) slow-moving stock, (13) and cost of goods. Once the PDA has collected the data, it syncs with a PC (or wirelessly) to send the encrypted files to AccuBar's back-end software. From there, the user can log in through a secure web site to perform many of AccuBar's functions. Restaurant operators report 50- to 80-percent time savings when using the AccuBar system. That's a key benefit, because often it means the difference between a thorough, insightful inventory and one that has been rushed through after hours. And it can mean one manager efficiently completing the process with time to spare, instead of several burned-out managers having to work late or off hours.

Another way of tracking beverage costs is through a device that controls the dispensing of alcoholic beverages. In this system, each bottle is attached to a dispensing system with different measures of pours. As the bartender pours in to a glass, each pour is registered, therefore allowing full control of the beverage sales and keeping inventory. The disadvantage of this system is the low speed of service in a busy bar environment.

A new generation of beverage-dispensing control systems is the radio-frequency identification (RFID)–based systems. In this system, an RFID spout is assigned to each bottle in the bar, and every drink dispensed is automatically tracked in real time. Beverage Tracker by Capton (**www.beveragetracker.com**) uses RFID–enabled free-pour spouts, allowing bartenders to pour liquor without adjusting normal bar operations. Each spout contains an RFID microchip that wirelessly transmits pour data via radio frequency to a receiver. Every RFID microchip has a unique serial code, so each spout can be tracked individually. Beverage Tracker spouts are completely self-contained and hold the battery, electronics, transmitter, and microchip. They are water resistant and impact resistant so they can be cleaned like any other pour spout. They fit all major brands of liquor and are completely reprogrammable through a simple software update. Every event, including pours, placement on bottle, and placement off bottle, is date and time stamped and transmitted in real time. Beverage Tracker spouts transmit on a low-range AM spectrum (433 megahertz). With this system, the management can know the perpetual inventory (total inventory—all sales) at a given time.

Personnel Procedures

Another key component of internal control is having procedures in place for screening and hiring bar personnel. Employees must be experienced in bartending and cocktail serving and also must be honest because they have access to the bar's beverage inventory and its cash.

Bar managers may also implement several other procedures to control inventory and reduce the likelihood of employee theft. One popular method is the use of *spotters*, who are hired to act like typical bar customers, but who are actually observing the bartenders and/or cocktailers for inappropriate behavior, such as not taking money from customers or overpouring. Another method for checking bar personnel is to perform a bank switch in the middle of the shift. In some cases, employees steal from the company by taking money from customers without ringing it up on the register. They keep the extra money in the cash drawer until the end of the shift when they are cashing out, at which point they retrieve the stolen funds. To do a bank switch, the manager must "z-out" a bartender's cash register, take the cash drawer, and replace it with a new bank. The manager then counts the money in the drawer, subtracts the starting bank, and compares that figure to the one on the register's tape. If there is a significant surplus of funds, it is highly likely that the employee is stealing. If there is less than what is indicated on the tape, the employee may be honest but careless when giving change or hitting the buttons on the register. Either way, there is a potential for loss.

Restaurant and Hotel Bars

In restaurants, the bar is often used as a holding area to allow guests to enjoy a cocktail or aperitif before sitting down to dinner. This allows the restaurant to space out the guests' orders so that the kitchen can cope more effectively; it also increases beverage sales. The profit margin from beverages is higher than the food profit margin.

In some restaurants, the bar is the focal point or main feature. Guests feel drawn to having a beverage because the atmosphere and layout of the restaurant encourages them to have a drink. Beverages generally account for about 25 to 30 percent of total sales. Many restaurants used to have a higher percentage of beverage sales, but the trend toward responsible consumption of alcoholic beverages has influenced people to decrease their consumption.

Bars carry a range of each spirit, beginning with the *well* package. The well package is the least expensive pouring brand that the bar uses when guests simply ask for a "scotch and water." The *call* package is the group of spirits that the bar offers to guests who are likely to ask for a particular name brand. For example, guests may call for Johnnie Walker Red Label. An example of a premium scotch is Johnnie Walker Black Label, and a super premium scotch is Chivas Regal.

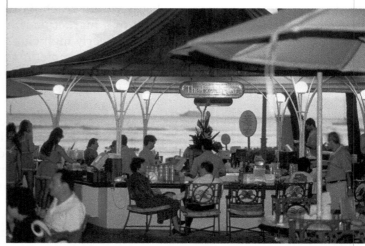

The Banyan Court bar at the Moana Hotel is a perfect venue for a "sundowner."

213

A popular method of costing each of the spirits poured is to calculate cost according to the following example:

A premium brand of vodka such as Grey Goose costs $32.00 per liter and yields twenty-five $1^1/_4$-oz shots that each sell for $5.50. Therefore, the bottle brings in $137.50. The profit margins produced by bars may be categorized as follows:

Liquor Pouring Cost % (approx.)	12
Beer	25
Wine	38

When combined, the sales mix may have an average pouring cost of 16 to 20 percent.

Most bars operate on some form of par stock level, which means that for every spirit bottle in use, there is a minimum par stock level of one, two, or more bottles available as a backup. As soon as the stock level falls to a level below the par level, more is automatically purchased.

Nightclubs

Nightclubs have long been a popular place to go to get away from the stresses of everyday life. From the small club in a suburban neighborhood to the world-famous clubs of New York, Las Vegas, and Miami's South Beach, all clubs have one thing in common: People frequent them to kick back, relax, and, more often than not, enjoy a wild night of dancing and partying with friends and strangers alike.

Like restaurant ownership, starting up a nightclub is a very risky business. But with the right education and proper planning, nightclub ownership can be a very profitable endeavor. As with most businesses in the hospitality industry, many believe that experience is more important than education and that you can learn as you go. However, when embarking on a journey as involved as owning a nightclub, a person with a degree and a high level of education is well ahead of the game.

The ability to read the market is key in developing a nightclub. When investing anywhere from $300,000 to $1 million in start-up costs, it is of utmost importance to be sure that the right spot is chosen and that a relevant market is within reach. Great nightclubs result from an accurate and calculated read of a marketplace, not by virtue of good luck. In fact, the number-one cause of early nightclub failure stems from an inaccurate read on the marketplace. For example, if an entrepreneur is interested in opening up a country line-dancing nightclub in an urban neighborhood, he or she may want to do extensive market research to be sure that members of the community even like country music.

When considering the prospect of a new nightclub, it is important to invest considerable time in the study of demographics, market attitude, and social dynamics of the proposed target. Many people tend to come up with a concept they are dead set on pursuing without really digging into the market. One should take all markets into account, even if the other markets may not seem relevant at the time. In the future, it may be these same markets that are being divided to come to the newer clubs that have just opened.

A new and exciting concept is a highly important factor in creating a nightclub. Some people feel that if one nightclub is doing well down the street, they will open the same type and be equally successful. This is not true. Variety is one of the keys to successful business. By offering patrons a fresh new opportunity, one can draw clientele away from the old clubs and into the new club.

Budgeting is another big factor in developing a nightclub. Although such an undertaking can be very costly, cutting corners in building and design will only hurt the business later. It is better to spend the money now and do it right than to have to spend more money for repairs later. Creating a budget should include all aspects of the operation, including, but not limited to, food and beverage, staffing and labor, licenses, building ramifications, décor, lighting, and entertainment.

Be sure to know all the legal issues that come with running a nightclub. For example, many laws exist on the sale and distribution of alcohol. In many instances, if a problem occurs involving a patron who was last drinking at the club, the problem can be considered the fault of the operation's management. Lawsuits can arise fairly easily, and it is highly important to be aware of such possibilities.

Nightclubs can be great experiences for both the patrons and the owner because revenues can be very high. However, it is important to remember the risks involved and work to minimize them.

Although this is only a brief discussion of the creation of a nightclub, the points given are quite important to successful operation. As with all business endeavors, the more one knows about the industry with which he or she is getting involved, the better off the business will be. For more information regarding the nightclub industry, go to **www.nightclub.com** or **www.nightclubbiz.com**.

Brewpubs and Microbreweries

Brewpubs are a combination brewery and pub or restaurant that brews its own fresh beer onsite to meet the taste of local customers. Microbreweries are craft breweries that produce up to 15,000 barrels (or 30,000 kegs) of beer a year. The North American microbrewery industry trend revived the concept of small breweries serving fresh, all-malt beer. Although regional breweries, microbreweries, and brewpubs account for only a small part of the North American brewing industry in terms of total beer production (less than 5 percent), they have a potentially large growth rate. One reason for the success of microbreweries and brewpubs is the wide variety of styles and flavors of beer they produce. On one hand, this educates the public about beer styles that have been out of production for decades and, on the other hand, helps brewpubs and restaurants meet the individual tastes and preferences of their local clientele.

Starting a brewpub is a fairly expensive venture. Although brewing systems come in a wide range of configurations, the cost of the equipment ranges from $200,000 to $800,000. Costs are affected by factors such as annual production capacity, beer types, and packaging. The investment in microbreweries and brewpubs is well justified by the enormous potential for returns. Microbreweries can produce a wide variety of ales, lagers, and other beers, the quality of which depends largely on the quality of the raw materials and the skill of the brewer. There are several regional brewpub restaurants of note, including Rock Bottom, which built its foundation on a tradition of fresh handcrafted beers and a diverse menu. It promotes itself as a place to gather with friends, drink the best beer around, enjoy a great meal, and share good times. John Harvard's has a famous selection of ales and lagers that are brewed on the premises according to the old English recipes brought to America in 1637 by John Harvard, after whom Harvard University is named. Gordon Biersch has several excellent brewery restaurants also offering handcrafted ales and beers along with a varied menu.

Sports Bars

Sports bars have always been popular but have become more so with the decline of disco and singles bars. They are places where people relax in the sporting atmosphere, so bar/restaurants such as Trophies in San Diego or Characters at Marriott hotels have become popular "watering holes." Satellite TV coverage of the top sporting events helps sports bars to draw crowds. Sports bars have evolved over the years into much more than corner bars featuring the game of the week. In the past, sports bars were frequented by die-hard sports fans and were rarely visited by other clientele. Today, the sports bar is more of an entertainment concept and is geared toward a more diverse base of patrons.

Sports bars were originally no more than a gathering spot for local sports fans when the home team played on TV. Now, such places have been transformed into mega-sports adventures, featuring musical entertainment, interactive games, and hundreds of TVs tuned in to just about every sport imaginable. "There are no more watering holes," says Zach Strauss, general manager of Sluggers World Class Sports Bar in Chicago. "Things have changed. People are more health conscious; nobody really drinks, drinks, drinks anymore. . . . You have to offer more than booze. People expect sports bars to have more personality, better food, and better service."[28]

Today's sports bars are attracting a much more diverse clientele. Now, more women and families are frequenting these venues, which provide a new prospect for revenue for bar owners. Scott Estes, founding partner of Lee Roy Selmon's restaurant in Tampa, Florida, has recognized that women are an increasing revenue force in the industry and has made adjustments to his restaurant to be sure to capitalize on this rapidly expanding market. Sports bars are also making changes in their establishments to become more family oriented. Lee Roy Selmon's main dining room, for example, is a TV-free environment. Many families go into sports bars and

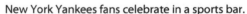
New York Yankees fans celebrate in a sports bar.

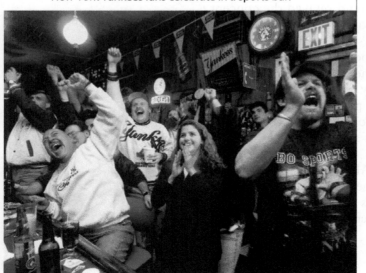

request a room with no TVs, so, recognizing that, an increasing number of owners have chosen to set aside a special place where families can eat uninterrupted by the noise of TV.

Another method of attracting bar patrons on slower nights is to offer games and family-friendly menus. Frankie's Food, Sports, and Spirits in Atlanta attracts families by hosting a sports-trivia game for teens. For the younger crowd, the restaurant provides a kids' menu every day and serves each pint-sized meal on upside-down Frisbees, which children can take home as souvenirs. Sports bars have also become the latest version of the traditional arcade. Many bars offer interactive video games where friends and families can compete against one another. Virtual reality games such as Indy 500 and other sports games are available at many establishments. Some venues have even gone a step farther and offer batting cages, bowling alleys, and basketball courts for their patrons to enjoy.

Another aspect of the sports bar that has changed drastically is the menu. Sports bars have a reputation for serving spicy chicken wings, hamburgers, and other typical bar fare. But just as sports bars have evolved in their entertainment offerings, so too have their menus. People's tastes have changed, causing sports bars to offer a more diverse menu. Today, guests can dine on a variety of foods, from filet mignon, to fresh fish, to gourmet sandwiches and pizza. Now people frequent sports bars as much for the great meal they will have as for the entertainment. In the past, sports bars usually had a few TVs that showcased games that would appeal to the area and big games such as the Super Bowl. The sudden increase in technology and TV programming available has made game viewing very different. The popularity of satellites and digital receivers has allowed bars to tune in to virtually dozens of events at any given time. Bars now have hundreds of TVs, and fans can watch games featuring every sport, team, and level of play around the world at any time of the day or night.

Burbank, California–based ESPN Zone has about 200 TVs in each of its locations so that fans can catch all the action. A handful of TVs are placed in the restaurant's bathrooms because The evolution of sports bars has turned the smoky corner bar into an exciting dining and sports experience. Customers who once rarely frequented the establishments, such as women and families, are now some of the biggest patrons, increasing both attendance and revenue at sports bars.

Coffee Shops

Another fairly recent trend in the beverage industry in the United States and Canada is the establishment of coffeehouses, or coffee shops. Coffeehouses originally were created based on the model of Italian bars, which reflected the deeply rooted espresso tradition in Italy. The winning concept of Italian bars lies in the ambiance they create, which is suitable for conversation of a personal, social, and business nature. A talk over a cup of coffee with soft background music and maybe a pastry is a typical scenario for Italians. Much of the same concept was re-created in the United States and Canada, where there was a niche in the beverage industry that was yet to be acknowledged and filled. The original concept was modified, however, to include a much wider variety of beverages and styles of coffee to meet the tastes of North American consumers. Consequently, the typical espresso/cappuccino offered by Italian bars has been expanded in North America to include items such as iced mocha, iced cappuccino, and so forth.

Students as well as businesspeople find coffeehouses a place to relax, discuss, socialize, and study. The success of coffeehouses is reflected in the establishment of chains such as Starbucks, as well as family-owned, independent shops.

Wireless cafés are a recent trend in the coffeehouse sector. Wireless cafés offer the use of computers, with Internet capability, for about $6 per hour. Guests can enjoy coffee, snacks, or even a meal while online. Reasonable rates allow regular guests to have e-mail addresses.

▶ Check Your Knowledge

1. Describe the bar setup.
2. How is inventory control conducted?
3. What is the average beverage pouring cost percentage?
4. What is a trend in sports bars?

Liquor Liability and the Law

Owners, managers, bartenders, and servers may be liable under the law if they serve alcohol to minors or to persons who are intoxicated. The extent of the liability can be very severe. The legislation that governs the sale of alcoholic beverages is called **dram shop legislation**. The dram shop laws, or civil damage acts, were enacted in the 1850s and dictated that owners and operators of drinking establishments are liable for injuries caused by intoxicated customers.

Some states have reverted back to the eighteenth-century common law, removing liability from vendors except in cases involving minors. Nonetheless, most people recognize that as a society we are faced with major problems of underage drinking and drunk driving.

To combat underage drinking in restaurants, bars, and lounges, a major brewery distributed a booklet showing the authentic design and layout of each state's driver's licenses. Trade associations such as the National Restaurant Association and the American Hotel & Lodging Association, together with major corporations, have produced a number of preventive measures and programs aimed at responsible alcohol beverage service. The major thrust of these initiatives is awareness programs and mandatory training programs, such as Serve Safe for Alcohol, that promote responsible alcohol service. Serve Safe for Alcohol is sponsored by the National Restaurant Association and is a certification program that teaches participants about alcohol and its effects on people, the common signs of intoxication, and how to help customers avoid drinking too much.

Other programs for responsible alcohol service and consumption include designated drivers, who only drink nonalcoholic beverages to ensure that they can drive friends home safely. Some operators give free nonalcoholic beverages to the designated driver as a courtesy.

One positive outcome of the responsible alcohol service programs for operators is a reduction in the insurance premiums and legal fees for beverage establishments, which had skyrocketed in previous years.

Trends in the Beverage Industry

- The comeback of cocktails
- Designer bottled water
- Microbreweries
- More wine consumption
- Increase in coffeehouses and coffee intake
- Increased awareness and action to avoid irresponsible alcoholic beverage consumption
- An increase in beverages to attract more female participation.
- An increase in the number and variety of "energy drinks"

CASE STUDY

Hiring Bar Personnel

As bar manager of a popular local night club, it is your responsibility to interview and hire all bar personnel. One of your friends asks you for a job as a bartender. Because he has experience, you decide to help him out and give him a regular shift. During the next few weeks, you notice that the overall sales for his shifts are down slightly from previous weeks when other bartenders worked that shift. You suspect he may be stealing from you.

Discussion Questions

1. What are your alternatives for determining whether your friend is, in fact, stealing?
2. If you determine that he has been stealing, how do you handle it?

CASE STUDY

Java Coffee House

Michelle Wong is manager of the Java Coffee House at a busy location on Union Street in San Francisco. Michelle says that there are several challenges in operating a busy coffeehouse, such as training staff to handle unusual circumstances. For example, one guest consumed a cup of coffee and ate two-thirds of a piece of cake and then said he didn't like the cake, so didn't want to pay for his order.

Another problem is suppliers who quote good prices to get her business and then, two weeks later, raise the price of some of the items.

Michelle says that the young employees she has at the Java Coffee House are her greatest challenge of all. According to Michelle, there are four kinds of employees—those who are lazy; those who are good but not responsible; those who steal; and those who are great and are no trouble.

Discussion Questions

1. What are some suggestions for training staff to handle unusual circumstances?
2. How do you ensure that suppliers are delivering the product at the price quoted?
3. What do you do with lazy employees?
4. What do you do with irresponsible employees?
5. How do you deal with employees who steal?

Summary

1. Beverages are categorized into alcoholic and nonalcoholic beverages. Alcoholic beverages are further categorized into spirits, wines, and beer.
2. Wine is the fermented juice of ripe grapes. It is classified as red, white, and rose, and we distinguish between light beverage wines, sparkling wines, and aromatic wines.
3. The six steps in making wine are crushing, fermenting, racking, maturing, filtering, and boiling. France, Germany, Italy, Spain, and Portugal are the main European wine-producing areas, and California is the main American wine-producing area.
4. Beer is a brewed and fermented beverage made from malt. Different types of beer include ale, stout, lager, and pilsner.
5. Spirits have a high percentage of alcohol and are served before or after a meal. Fermentation and distillation are parts of their processing. The most popular white spirits are rum, gin, vodka, and tequila.
6. Today people have become more health conscious about consumption of alcohol; nonalcoholic beverages such as coffee, tea, soft drinks, juices, and bottled water are increasing in popularity.
7. Beverages make up 20 to 30 percent of total sales in a restaurant, but managers are liable if they serve alcohol to minors. Programs such as designated driver and Serve Save for Alcohol and the serving of virgin cocktails have increased.

Key Words and Concepts

alcoholic beverage
beer
brandy
champagne
cognac
dram shop legislation
fermentation
fining
fortified wines
hops
inventory control
liquor
malt
mashing

must
nonalcoholic beverage
Prohibition
proof
sparkling wine
spirit
vintage
white spirits
wine
wine and food pairing
wine tasting
wort
yeast

Review Questions

1. What is the difference between fortified and aromatic wines? In what combination is it suggested to serve food and wine and why?
2. Describe the brewing process of beer. What is the difference between a stout and a pilsner?
3. Name and describe the main types of spirits.
4. Why have nonalcoholic drinks increased in popularity, and what difficulties do bar managers face when serving alcohol?
5. Describe the origin of coffee.
6. Describe the proper procedure for handling and serving champagne.
7. Describe the origin of cocktails. What constitutes a cocktail?
8. Describe a typical bar setup.

Internet Exercises

1. Organization: **Clos Du Bois**
   Web site: **www.closdubois.com**
   Summary: Clos Du Bois is one of America's well-known and loved wineries and is a premier producer of wines from Sonoma County in California. The winery was started in 1974 and since then has acquired many more vineyards and a name for itself. It now sells about a million cases of premium wine annually.

   (a) look at the suggested food and wine pairings. What can you serve with the Clos Du Bois North Coast sauvignon blanc? Compare it to what you already know about what to eat with sauvignon blanc.

   (b) The Clos Du Bois has been named Wine of the Year for nine years by *Wine & Spirits*. What is it about this wine that makes it so different from others?

2. Organization: **Siebel Institute of Technology**
   Web site: **www.siebelinstitute.com**
   Summary: Siebel Institute of Technology is recognized for its training and educational programs in brewing technology.

(a) What are some of the services that the Siebel Institute of Technology offers its students?
(b) List the career path options available through Siebel Institute of Technology.

Apply Your Knowledge

1. In groups, do a blindfold taste test with cans of Coke and Pepsi. See if your group can identify which is which and who likes Coke or Pepsi the most.
2. Complete a class survey of preference for Coke or Pepsi and share the results with your classmates.
3. Request a local wine representative to demonstrate the correct way of opening and serving a bottle of nonalcoholic wine. Then practice opening a bottle yourself.
4. What type of wine would be recommended with the following:
   (a) Pork
   (b) Cheese
   (c) Lamb
   (d) Chocolate cake
   (e) Chicken

Suggested Activities

1. Search the Internet for underage drinking statistics and related highway deaths in your state.
2. Mothers Against Drunk Driving (MADD) is a nonprofit organization working to stop drunk drivers and support victims of drunk drivers. Find out what impact MADD has had on society.
3. Create an outline for a sports bar concept.

Endnotes

1. Personal correspondence with Jay R. Schrock, Dean, School of Hotel and Restaurant Management, University of South Florida, March 26, 2011.
2. *Ibid.*
3. This section draws on Sarah Berkley, "Organic and Sustainable Wine Production Expanding Rapidly in California," Organic Consumers Association, http://www.organicconsumers.org/organic/wine012104.cfm, retrieved March 12, 2010.
4. Budweiser Brewing Company presentation, University of South Florida, Tampa, Florida, September 7, 2004.
5. *Ibid.*
6. Hottinger, Greg, "Organic Beer," O'Mama Report, Organic Trade Association, www.theorganicreport.com/pages/605_organic_beer.cfm.
7. Craft Beer, *Small, Independent Traditional* www.craftbeer.com/pages/beerology/small-independent-traditional (accessed March 21, 2011).
8. Drink Craft Beer, *Home Page*, www.drinkcraftbeer.com/ (accessed March 21, 2011).
9. Craft Beer, *Small, Independent Traditional* www.craftbeer.com/pages/beerology/small-independent-traditional (accessed March 21, 2011).

10. *Ibid.*
11. Brewers Association, *Home Page*, www.brewersassociation.org (accessed March 21, 2011).
12. Walker_ExpHosp_Chapter10cb[1].doc http://thefullpint.com/beer-news/oregon-honors-full-sail-brewing-for-sustainability, retrieved March 14, 2010.
13. Josh Amaris, "10 Steps toward Sustainability Every Brewery Should Consider," www.bluemapinc.com/articles/article_12_brewing.html and www.checkthemarkets.com/index.php?option=com_content& task=view&id=688&Itemid=98, retrieved March 15, 2010.
14. http://biggreenboulder.com/energy/sustainable- and http://biggreenboulder.com/energy/sustainable-brewing-in-colorado-not-done-impressing-you-yet/, retrieved March 15, 2010.
15. C. Katsigiris and M. Porter, *The Bar and Beverage Book*, 3rd ed. (New York: John Wiley and Sons, 2002), 139.
16. Personal correspondence with Susan Davis of the Specialty Coffee Association of America, August 26, 2005.
17. Ancora Coffee Roasters, "A Goat and a King: Coffee's Colorful History," *Coffee Class: History*, www.ancoracoffee.com/Class/History_Of_Coffee.aspx (accessed March 21, 2011).
18. Ancora Coffee Roasters, "Coffee's Trek across the World," *Coffee Class: History*,
19. www.ancoracoffee.com/Class/History_Of_Coffee.aspx (accessed March 21, 2011).
19. The Bean Shop, *History of Coffee*, www.thebeanshop.com/beanshop/default.asp?p=31. (accessed March 21, 2011).
21. Starbucks, *Starbucks Company Profile*, July 2011, http://assets.starbucks.com/assets/aboutuscompanyprofileq3201172811final.pdf (accessed November 3, 2001).
22. "Energy drink sales up despite health concerns," *Chicago Sun Times*, March 18, 2011, www.suntimes.com/lifestyles/health/4385825-423/energy-drink-sales-up-despite-health-concerns.html?print=true (accessed November 4, 2011).
23. *Ibid.*
24. Marnie Roberts, "Take me out to the sports bar," *Restaurants USA*, August 2011, www.restaurant.org/tools/magazines/rusa/magArchive/year/article/?ArticleID=515 (accessed March 19, 2011).
25. Scannabar, *Liquor Inventory Software*, (accessed March 19, 2011).
26. Scannabar, *Wine Inventory Software*, http://en.scannabar.com/products/wine-inventory/ (accessed March 19, 2011).
27. www.azbaramerica.com retrieved March 19, 2011.
28. Personal conversation with Zach Strauss, General Manager of Sluggers World Class Sports Bar in Chicago, May 4, 2007.

Glossary

Champagne   Sparkling wine made in the Champagne district of France.

Dram shop legislation   Laws and procedures that govern the legal operation of establishments that sell measured alcoholic beverages.

Fermentation   The chemical process in which yeast acts on sugar or sugar-containing substances, such as grain or fruit, to produce alcohol and carbon dioxide.

Fining   The process by which wine that has matured is filtered to help stabilize it and remove any solid particles still in the wine.

Fortified wine   Wine to which brandy or other spirits have been added to stop further fermentation or to raise its alcoholic content.

Hops   The dried, conical fruit of a special vine that imparts bitterness to beer.

Inventory control   A method for keeping track of all resources required to produce a product.

Malt   Germinated barley.

Mashing   In the making of beer, the process of grinding the malt and screening out bits of dirt.

Must   A mixture of grape pulp, skins, seeds, and stems.

Proof   A figure representing liquor's alcohol content.

Sparkling wine   Wine containing carbon dioxide, which provides effervescence when the wine is poured.

Spirits   Distilled drinks.

Vintage   The year in which a wine's grapes were harvested.

White spirits   Gin, rum, vodka, and tequila.

Wine   Fermented juice of grapes or other fruits.

Wort   In the making of beer, the liquid obtained after the mashing process.

Photo Credits

Credits are listed in the order of appearance.

Chris Howey/Shutterstock
bogdanhoda/Shutterstock
Linda Whitwam/Dorling Kindersley;
    Ian O'Leary/Dorling Kindersley
Ian O'Leary/Dorling Kindersley; Kzenon/Fotolia LLC
Jay R. Schrock
The Robert Mondavi Family of Wineries; Andy Z./Shutterstock
Chris Laurens/Alamy

Rob Westfall
Monty Rakusen Cultura/Newscom
Jules Selmes and Debi Treloar/DK Images
Stockbyte/Getty Images
Starbucks Coffee Company
Amy Etra/PhotoEdit
Rob Reichenfeld/DK Images

The Restaurant Business

From Chapter 6 of *Introduction to Hospitality Management,* Fourth Edition. John R. Walker. Copyright © 2013 by Pearson Education, Inc. Published by Pearson. All rights reserved.

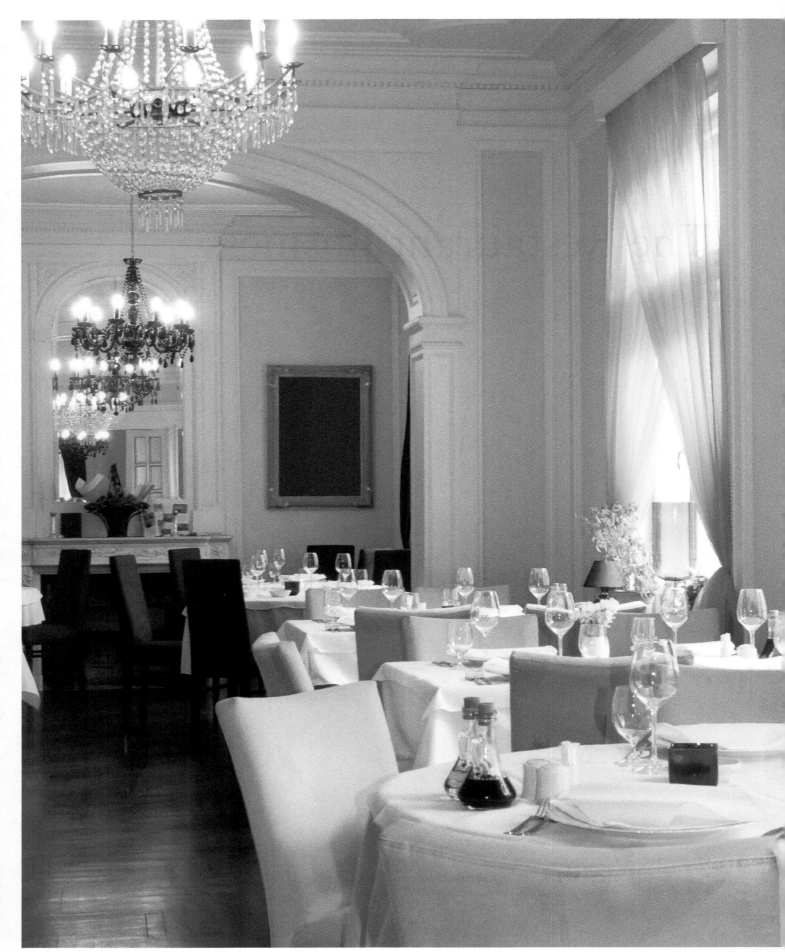

The Restaurant Business

OBJECTIVES

After reading and studying this chapter, you should be able to:

- Describe the different characteristics of chain and independent restaurants.

- Identify some of the top chain and independent restaurants.

- List the classifications of restaurants.

- Differentiate characteristics of chain and independent restaurants.

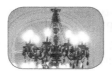
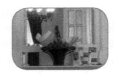
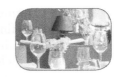
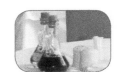

The Restaurant Business

Restaurants are a vital part of our everyday lifestyles; because we are a society on the go, we patronize them several times a week to socialize, as well as to eat and drink. Restaurants offer a place to relax and enjoy the company of family, friends, colleagues, and business associates and to restore our energy level before heading off to the next class or engagement. Actually, the word *restaurant* derives from the word *restore*. Today, there are more than 960,000 restaurants in the United States, with sales of $604 billion and 12.8 million employees (marking the restaurant business as the largest employer apart from the government!). The restaurant industry's share of the food dollar has risen to 47.5 percent. On a typical day, more than 130 million people in the United States are guests in restaurants and foodservice operations.[1]

As a society we spend an increasing amount, approaching 50 percent, of our food dollar away from home. Restaurants are a multibillion-dollar industry that provides employment and contributes to the nation's social and economic well-being. No discussion of restaurants can continue without talking about the main ingredient: food. So, let's take a brief look at our culinary heritage.

Classical Cuisine

North America gained most of its culinary legacy from France. Two main events were responsible for our culinary legacy coming from France. First was the French Revolution in 1793, which caused the best French chefs of the day to lose their employment because their bosses lost their heads! Many chefs came to North America as a result, bringing with them their culinary talents. The second event was when Thomas Jefferson, who in 1784 spent five years as envoy to France, brought a French chef to the White House when he became president. This act stimulated interest in French cuisine and enticed U.S. tavern owners to offer better quality and more interesting food.

No mention of classical cuisine can be made without talking about the two main initiators: Marie-Antoine Carême (1784–1833), who is credited as the founder of classical cuisine, and Auguste Escoffier, who is profiled later in this chapter. Carême was abandoned on the streets of Paris as a child, and then worked his way up from cook's helper to become the chef to the Prince de Talleyrand and the Prince Regent of England. He also served as head chef to the future King George IV of England, Tsar Alexander of Russia, and Baron de Rothschild. His goal was to achieve "lightness," "grace," "order," and "perspicuity" of food. Carême dedicated his career to refining and organizing culinary techniques. His many books contain the first really systematic account of cooking principles, recipes, and menu making.[2]

The other great contributor to classical cuisine, Auguste Escoffier (1846–1935), unlike Carême, never worked in an aristocratic household. Instead, he held forth in the finest hotels of the time: the Place Vendome in Paris and the Savoy and Carlton hotels in London. Escoffier is noted for his many contributions to cuisine, including simplifying the Grand Cuisine of Carême by reducing the number of flavors and garnishes and even simplifying the number of sauces to five "mother" or leading sauces. Escoffier brought simplicity and harmony to the Grand Cuisine. His many cookbooks are still in use today: *La Guide Culinaire* (1903) is a collection of more than 5,000 classic cuisine recipes;

in *Le Liver des Menus* (1912), he compares a great meal with a symphony; and *Ma Cuisine* (1934) contains more than 2,000 timeless recipes. All of his books emphasize the importance of mastering the techniques of cooking.[3]

This is an exciting time to be involved in the culinary arts and restaurant industry. Not only are new restaurant concepts and themes to fit a variety of tastes and budgets appearing on the scene, the culinary arts are being developed by several creative and talented chefs. It is important to realize that in this industry, we are never far from food. So, let's take a look at the recent development of **culinary arts**.

The main "ingredient" in a restaurant is cuisine, and one of the main foundations of classical French cooking, on which much of American cuisine is based, is the five **mother sauces**: bechamel, velouté, espagnole, tomato, and hollandaise. These elaborate sauces were essential accompaniments for the various dishes on the menu. Until about 1900, all menus were written in French—some still are—and regardless of whether a person was dining in a good hotel or restaurant in London or Lisbon, the intention was that the dish should be prepared in the same manner and taste similar to the French version. The travelers of the day either spoke French or had a knowledge of menu French.

Classical French cuisine was popular until the late 1960s and early 1970s, when **nouvelle cuisine** became popular. Nouvelle cuisine is a lighter cuisine than the classical French and is based on simpler preparations—with the aid of processors, blenders, and juicers—using more natural flavors and ingredients. Instead of thickening a sauce with a flour-based **roux**, a **purée** of vegetables could be used instead. Fresh is in, and this includes herbs for flavor. Nouvelle cuisine combines classical techniques and principles with modern technology and scientific research. "Simpler, quicker" quickly became more stylish, with plate presentation becoming a part of the chef's art. North American cooking had arrived. The bounties of Canada and the United States provided the basis for regional cuisine to flourish nationally. **Fusion**, the blending of flavors and techniques from two cuisines, became popular. For example, New England and Italian or Californian and Asian cuisines can be blended. For example, a Japanese recipe might be blended with a Mexican one to create a new hybrid recipe.

Many great chefs have influenced our recent culinary development. Among them are Julia Child, whose television shows did much to take the mystique out of French cooking and encourage a generation of homemakers to elevate their cooking techniques and skills. More recently, Anthony Bourdain on the Travel Channel with his excellent program titled *No Reservations* and Emeril "Bam" Lagasse and Bobby Flay via the Food Network have popularized cooking and the gourmand lifestyle.

Culinary schools have done an excellent job of producing a new generation of chefs who are making significant contributions to the evolving culinary arts. For example, Alice Waters at Chez Panisse, her restaurant in Berkeley, California, is credited with the birth of California cuisine. Waters uses only fresh produce bought from local farmers. Paul Prudhomme is another contemporary chef who has energized many aspiring chefs with his passion for basic cooking, especially cajun style.

Charlie Trotter, chef–owner of Charlie Trotter's in Chicago, who is considered by many to be America's finest chef–owner and king of fusion, said in one of his books:

After love there is only cuisine! It's all about excellence, or at least working towards excellence. Early on in your approach to cooking—or in running a restaurant—you have to determine whether or not you are willing to

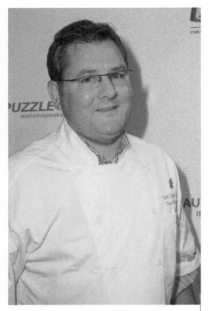

Charlie Trotter, one of America's finest restaurant chef–owners and king of fusion.

commit fully and completely to the idea of the pursuit of excellence. *I have always looked at it this way: if you strive for perfection—an all out assault on total perfection—at the very least you will hit a high level of excellence, and then you might be able to sleep at night. To accomplish something truly significant, excellence has to become a life plan.*[4]

Chef Trotter brings his knowledge and exposure together into a coherent view on what the modern fine-dining experience could be. He says, "I thought the blend of European refinement regarding the pleasures of the table, American ingenuity and energy in operating a small enterprise, Japanese minimalism and poetic elegance in effecting a sensibility, and a modern approach to incorporating health and dietary concerns would encompass a spectrum of elements through which I could express myself fully. Several years later, I find I am even more devoted than ever to this approach."[5]

Food Trends and Practices

As the level of professionalism rises for the chef of the twenty-first century, chefs will need a strong culinary foundation with a structure that includes multiculture cooking skills and strong employability traits, such as passion, dependability, cooperation, and initiative. Additional management skills include strong supervisory training, sense of urgency, accounting skills, sanitation/safety knowledge, nutritional awareness, and marketing/merchandising skills.

Not only are trans fats banned from many cities menus but, according to the National Restaurant Association's research, nearly three out of four Americans say they are trying to eat more healthfully in restaurants than they did two years ago. The **HealthyDiningFinder.com** web site is a great resource for those looking to make smart choices when dining out.[6] Among the early program members are Arby's, P. F. Chang's, Buca di Beppo, Cracker Barrel, Round Table Pizza, El Pollo Loco, and Famous Dave's.

The term *back-to-basic cooking* has been redefined to mean taking classical cooking methods and infusing modern technology and science to create healthy and flavorful dishes. Some examples of this include the following:

- Thickening soups and sauces by processing and using the food item's natural starches instead of traditional thickening methods

- Redefining the basic mother sauces to omit the béchamel and egg-based sauces and add or replace them with coulis, salsas, or chutneys

- Pursuing more cultural culinary infusion to develop bold and aggressive flavors

- Experimenting with sweet and hot flavors

- Taking advantage of the shrinking globe and disappearance of national borders to bring new ideas and flavors to restaurants

- Evaluating recipes and substituting ingredients for better flavor; that is, flavored liquid instead of water, infused oils and vinegars instead of nonflavored oils and vinegars

INTRODUCING AUGUSTE ESCOFFIER (1846–1935)

"Emperor of the World's Kitchens"

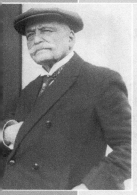

Auguste Escoffier is considered by many to be the patron saint of the professional cook. Called the "emperor of the world's kitchens," he is considered a reference point and a role model for all chefs. His exceptional culinary career began at the age of thirteen, when he apprenticed in his uncle's restaurant, and he worked until 1920, and retired to die quietly at home in Monaco in 1935. Uneducated, but a patient educator and diligent writer, he was an innovator who remained deeply loyal to the regional and bourgeois roots of French cookery. He exhibited his culinary skills in the dining rooms of the finest hotels in Europe, including the Place Vendome in Paris and the Savoy and Carlton hotels in London.

When the Prince of Wales requested something light but delicious for a late dinner after a night in a Monte Carlo casino, Auguste Escoffier responded with *poularde Derby*, a stuffed chicken served with truffles cooked in champagne, alternating with slices of butter-fried *foie gras*, its sauce basted with the juices from the chicken and truffles. Another interesting anecdote regarding the chef's originality in making sauces tells of a special dinner for the Prince of Wales and Kaiser Wilhelm. Escoffier was asked to create a special dish to honor such an occasion. Struggling with an apparent loss of creativity until the night before the event, the chef finally noticed a sack of overripe mangos, from which he created a sauce that he personally came out from the kitchen to serve. As he placed the plate on the table, he looked at the Kaiser and with a wicked smile said, "*zum Teufel*"—to the devil. Thus was born sauce diable, today a favorite classic sauce. Escoffier's insistence on sauces derived from the cooking of main ingredients was revolutionary at the time and in keeping with his famous instruction: *faités simple*—keep it simple.

In fact, in his search for simplicity, Escoffier reduced the complexity of the work of Carême, the "cook of kings and king of cooks," and aimed at the perfect balance of a few superb ingredients. In *Le Livre des Menus* (1912), Escoffier makes the analogy of a great dinner as a symphony with contrasting movements that should be appropriate to the occasion, the guests, and the season. He was meticulous in his kitchen, yet wildly imaginative in the creation of exquisite dishes. In 1903, Escoffier published *Le Guide Culinaire*, an astounding collection of more than 5,000 classic cuisine recipes and garnishes. Throughout the book, Escoffier emphasizes technique, the importance of a complete understanding of basic cookery principles, and ingredients he considers essential to the creation of great dishes.

Escoffier's refinement of Carême's *grand cuisine* was so remarkable it developed into a new cuisine referred to as *cuisine classique*. His principles have been used by successive generations, most emphatically by the *novelle cuisine* brigade. Francois Fusero, *chef de cuisine* at the Hotel Hermitage, Monte Carlo, and many others, regard Escoffier as their role model.

- Substituting herbs and spices for salt
- Returning to one-pot cooking to capture flavors
- Offering more healthy dining choices in restaurants

Today, being a chef is considered a profession that offers a variety of opportunities in every segment of the hospitality industry and anywhere in the world.

TECHNOLOGY SPOTLIGHT

Weighing Wi-Fi in Restaurants

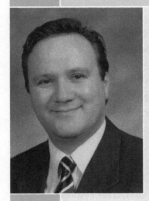

Cihan Cobanoglu, Ph.D., Dean, School of Hotel and Restaurant Management, University of South Florida, Sarasota-Manatee

Does Wi-Fi, or high-speed Internet access (HSIA), play a significant role in hotel guest satisfaction, and does it have a hand in hotel booking preferences? As per the 2009 Hotel Guest Technology Study, commissioned by the American Hotel & Lodging Association's technology and e-business committee and conducted by the University of Delaware, the answer to that question is a resounding yes. Yet if this question were to be applied to restaurants, would the results be the same? Is Wi-Fi service, whether it is free or comes with a fee, a determinant in customer retention? The University of Delaware conducted a follow-up study to understand the impact of Wi-Fi service in the restaurant environment.

Industry snapshot

Wi-Fi is increasingly becoming a must-have for public places, and consumers are demanding it. Over the past few years, IEEE 802.11 wireless networks have become increasingly deployed over a wide range of environments, with wireless local area networks (LANs) popping up in coffee shops, airports, hospitals, and restaurants. Most restaurants offer Wi-Fi service via the 802.11g standard (at 54 megabits per second) or the 802.11b standard (at 11 megabits per second). A small number of restaurants offer the newest Wi-Fi standard, 802.11n (at 100 megabits per second).

Restaurants that offer Wi-Fi services typically follow one of these three business models:

- For-a-Fee Model: The hot spot is offered by a location owner in partnership with a wireless Internet service provider to generate revenue through paid subscribers.

- Free-of-Charge Model: The hot spot is offered free to the customer with the cost being borne by the location provider.

- Hybrid Model: The hot spot is free to customers who purchase the service in the restaurant (for example, 30 minutes of free Internet for $10 spent in the restaurant). Even though more and more restaurants are offering Wi-Fi to their guests following one of the three business models, there is little research as to its impact on customer retention.

Study results

A survey was sent to roughly 1,000 American consumers, of which 257 people responded. The results showed that (1) Wi-Fi access has become an important amenity in restaurants and cafes in the United States; (2) tech-savvy customers prefer restaurants or cafés with Wi-Fi access; (3) customers prefer the free-of-charge Wi-Fi model over the paid models in restaurants; and (4) a stepwise regression model (a statistical technique used to identify the impact of a variable on other variables) showed that the following are predictors of the likelihood of a customer's return to a restaurant—Wi-Fi service availability, Wi-Fi service quality, the price of Wi-Fi service, the perceived risk of using Wi-Fi service, and the perceived value of Wi-Fi.

This study suggests that there is a positive correlation between Wi-Fi service and customer return visits. This finding makes more sense considering that 70 percent of respondents indicate utilizing a Wi-Fi–enabled device such as a laptop or PDA. Additionally, increasing numbers of consumers own dual-mode cell phones that allow phone conversations to be conducted over a Wi-Fi network for lower or no cost. Given these trends, it is likely that the demand for Wi-Fi access in public places such as restaurants will only increase.

This study also suggests that there is a negative correlation between the cost of Wi-Fi access in restaurants and customers' intentions to return. As the cost of restaurant Wi-Fi access increases, customers are less likely to return to that establishment. To offset this, Wi-Fi service should be offered to customers either free of charge or through a business model where customers are required to make a food or beverage purchase to access the free Wi-Fi service. This way, the cost of the service will be satisfied. The data also shows a positive correlation between perceived value of Wi-Fi and intention to return to a restaurant.

There also is a negative correlation between the perceived risk of using Wi-Fi at a restaurant and a guest's intention to return. There is little that restaurants can offer to address the perceived risk of using Wi-Fi in public networks. Users should be prepared to use their own tools to enable Wi-Fi security, such as secure socket layers and virtual private networks. However, restaurants can offer secure Wi-Fi access to their loyal customers through Wi-Fi protected access, which is an advanced encryption method for Wi-Fi access.

The study results indicate that restaurants could gain a positive return on their Wi-Fi investment. Restaurant owners and operators may do well to review the complete results and evaluate their high-speed Internet offering strategy.

Culinary Practices

In this new millennium, we are seeing culinary education setting the pace for dining exploration.[7] As you prepare for a career in the hospitality industry, you will find it imperative that you develop a strong culinary foundation. Within the structure of this you will need to develop cooking skills, strong employability traits, people skills, menu development skills, nutrition knowledge, sanitation/safety knowledge, accounting skills, and computer skills.

Before you can become a successful chef, you have to be a good cook. To be a good cook, you have to understand the basic techniques and principles of cooking. The art of cooking has not changed much in thousands of years. And, although the concept of cooking has not changed, science and technology have allowed us to improve the methods of food preparation. We still use fire for cooking: Grilling, broiling, and simmering are still popular methods of cooking.

To become a successful chef, you will need to learn all of the basic cooking methods in order to understand flavor profiles. As you look at recipes to cook, try to enhance the basic ingredient list to improve the flavor. As an example, always try to substitute a flavored liquid if water is called for in a recipe. It is also important to understand basic ingredient flavors so that you can improve flavor. The idea behind back-to-basic cooking means you evaluate your recipe and look for flavor improvement with each item.

Employability traits are those skills that focus on attitude, passion, initiative, dedication, sense of urgency, and dependability. These traits are not always traits that can be taught, but a good chef can demonstrate them by example. Most of the employers with job opportunities for students consider these skills to be more important than technical skills. The belief is that if you have strong employability traits, your technical skills will be strong.

One of the most important things to realize about the restaurant industry is that *you can't do it alone*. Each person in your operation has to work together for you to be successful. The most important ingredient in managing people is to *respect them*. Many words can be used to describe a manager (coach, supervisor, boss, mentor), but whatever term is used, you have to be in the game to be effective. Managing a kitchen is like coaching a football team—everyone

INTRODUCING RICHARD MELMAN

Chairman of the Board and Founder, Lettuce Entertain You Enterprises, Inc.

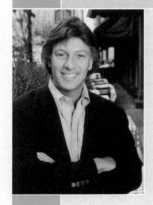

Richard Melman is founder and chairman of Lettuce Entertain You Enterprises, a Chicago-based corporation that owns and licenses seventy restaurants nationwide and in Japan.

The restaurant business has been Melman's life work, beginning with his early days in a family-owned restaurant and later as a teenager working in fast-food eateries and a soda fountain and selling restaurant supplies. After realizing that he wasn't cut out to be a college student and failing to convince his father that he should be made a partner in the family business, Melman met Jerry A. Orzoff, a man who immediately and unconditionally believed in Melman's ability to create and run restaurants. In 1971, the two opened R.J. Grunts, a hip burger joint that soon became one of the hottest restaurants in Chicago. Here, Melman and Orzoff presented food differently and with a sense of humor, creating the youthful and fun restaurant that was a forerunner in the trend toward dining out as entertainment that swept this country in the early 1970s.

Melman and Orzoff continued to develop restaurant concepts together until Orzoff's death in 1981. Through his relationship with Orzoff, Melman formulated a philosophy based on the importance of partners, of sharing responsibilities and profits with them, and of developing and growing together.[1]

To operate so many restaurants well, Lettuce has needed to hire, train, and develop people, and then to keep them happy and focused on excellence. Melman's guiding philosophy is that he is not interested in being the biggest or the best known—only in being the best he can be. He places enormous value on the people who work for Lettuce Entertain You Enterprises and feels tremendous responsibility for their continued success. Today, he has forty working partners, most of whom came up through the organization, and has 5,000 people working for him. Over the years, Melman has stayed close to the guests by using focus groups and frequent-diner programs. The group's training programs are rated among the best in the business, and Melman's management style is clearly influenced by team sports. He says, "There are many similarities between running a restaurant and a team sport. However, it's not a good idea to have ten all-stars; everybody can't bat first. You need people with similar goals—people who want to win and play hard."[2]

Melman's personal life revolves around his family. He and his wife Martha have been married for thirty years and have three children.[3]

[1]Marilyn Alva, "Does He Still Have It?" *Restaurant Business* 93, no. 4 (March 1, 1994), 104–111.
[2]Personal communication with Richard Melman, June 8, 2004.
[3]Lettuce Entertain You Restaurants, *Home Page*, www.leye.com, (accessed November 4, 2011).

must work together to be effective. The difference between a football team and a kitchen is that chefs/managers cannot supervise from the sidelines; they have to be in the game. One of my favorite examples of excellent people management skills is that of the general manager of a hotel who had the ware-washing team report directly to him. When asked why, he indicated that they are the people who know what is being thrown in the garbage, they are the people who know what the customers are not eating, and they are the people most responsible for the sanitation and safety of an operation. There are many components to managing people—training, evaluating, nurturing, delegating, and so on—but the most important is respect.

▶ Check Your Knowledge

1. From what country did North America gain most of its culinary legacy?
2. Define fusion cuisine and give an example.

Developing a Restaurant

Developing a restaurant may be the ultimate entrepreneurial dream. In which other industry can you get into a business like a restaurant for only a few thousand dollars? Of course, you need to have acquired the knowledge and skills along the way by getting experience in the kind of restaurant you intend to open. Yes, independent restaurants are a rush for the owners—they are one of the few places where guests use all of their senses to enjoy the experience. Through taste, sight, smell, hearing, and touch, all employees and guests can savor the food, service, and atmosphere of the restaurant. The successful operation of a restaurant is dependent on a number of factors. Let's examine the factors that make for a successful restaurant development, from the operating philosophy to controls, and all the functions in between.

Operating Philosophy, Mission, Goals, and Objectives

At the heart of an enterprise is the philosophy of the owner. The philosophy represents the way the company does business. It is an expression of the ethics, morals, and values by which the company operates. Many companies have formal mission statements that explain their reason for being in business. Danny Meyer of Union Square Hospitality calls it "*enlightened hospitality*—meaning if your staff is happy your guests will be, too."[8] Meyer gives each of his 450 employees a voucher to dine in one of the restaurants

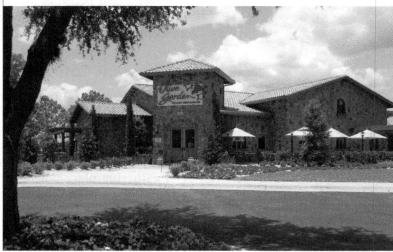

The Olive Garden, a popular Italian-themed restaurant, is part of Darden Restaurants.

every month. They have to write a report on the experience; Meyer enjoys reading them. Ever the coach and teacher, he says that it's better to have your staff tell you what's wrong than for you to have to tell them. No wonder his restaurants like Union Square Cafe, Gramercy Tavern, Eleven Madison Park, Tabla, Blue Smoke, and others are the top rated in New York.

Restaurant Market

The market is composed of those guests who will patronize the restaurant. A respective restaurant owner will analyze the market to determine whether sufficient demand exists in a particular market niche, such as Italian or Southern cuisine. A **niche** is a marketing term used to describe a specific share or slot of a certain market. A good indication of the size of the market can be ascertained by taking a radius of from one to five miles around the restaurant. The distance will vary according to the type and location of the restaurant. In Manhattan, it may only be a few blocks, whereas in rural West Virginia it may be a few miles. The area that falls within the radius is called the **catchment area**. The demographics of the population within the catchment area is analyzed to reveal age, number of people in various age brackets, sex, ethnicity, religion, income levels, and so on. This information is usually available from the chamber of commerce or data at the local library or real estate offices.

One yardstick used to determine the potential viability of a restaurant is to divide the number of restaurants in the catchment area by the total population. The average number of people per restaurant in the United States is about 500. Perhaps this kind of saturation is one of the reasons for the high failure rate of restaurants. Obviously, each area is different; one location may have several Italian restaurants but no Southern restaurant. Therefore, a Southern restaurant would be unique in the market and, if properly positioned, may have a competitive advantage. If someone in the catchment area wanted to eat Italian food, he or she would have to choose among the various Italian restaurants. In marketing terms, the number of potential guests for the Italian restaurant would be divided by the number of Italian restaurants to determine **fair market share** (the average number of guests that would, if all other things went equal, eat at any one of the Italian restaurants). Figure 1 shows a thousand potential guests. If they all decided to eat Italian in the fair market share scenario, each restaurant would receive 100 guests. In reality, we know this does not happen—for various reasons, one restaurant becomes more popular. The number of guests that this and the other restaurants receive then is called the **actual market share**. Figure 2 shows an example of the actual market share that similar restaurants might receive.

Restaurant Concept

Successful restaurant concepts are created with guests in mind. All too frequently someone thinks it would be a good idea to open up a particular kind of restaurant, only to find there are insufficient guests to make it viable.

For the winners, creating and operating a restaurant business is fun—lots of people coming and going, new faces, old friends. Restaurants provide a social gathering place where employees, guests, and management can get their adrenaline flowing in positive ways. The restaurant business is exciting and

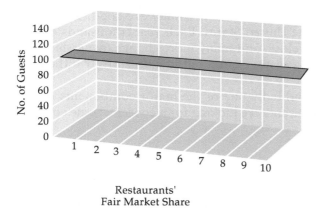

Figure 1 • Fair Market Share.

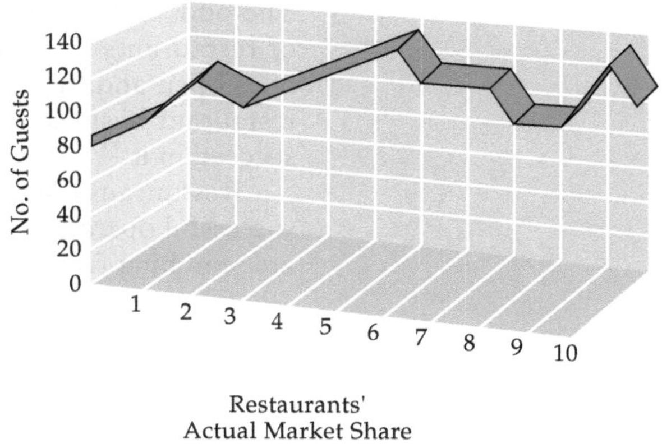

Figure 2 • Actual Market Share.

challenging; with the right location, food, atmosphere, and service it is possible to extract the market and make a good return on investment.

There are several examples of restaurant concepts that have endured over the past few decades. Applebee's, Chart House, Hard Rock Cafe, Olive Garden, Red Lobster, and T.G.I. Friday's are some of the better-known U.S. chain restaurant concepts. Naturally, there are more regional and independent concepts.

The challenge is to create a restaurant concept and bring it into being, a concept that fits a definite market, a concept better suited to its market than that presented by competing restaurants.[9] Every restaurant represents a concept and projects a total impression or an image. The image appeals to a certain market—casual, formal, children, adults, ethnic, and so on. The concept should fit the location and reach out to its target market. A restaurant's concept, location, menu, and decor should intertwine.[10]

In restaurant lingo, professionals sometimes describe restaurants by the net operating percentage that the restaurant makes. T.G.I. Friday's restaurants, for example, are usually described as 20-percent restaurants. A local restaurant may be only a 10-percent restaurant.

For the operation of a restaurant to be successful, the following factors need to be addressed:

- Mission
- Goals
- Objectives
- Market
- Concept
- Location
- Menu planning
- Ambiance
- Lease
- Other occupational costs

The odds in favor of becoming a big restaurant winner are good. Thousands of restaurants do business in the United States. Each year, thousands of new ones open and thousands more close, and many more change ownership. The restaurant business is deceptively easy to enter, but it is deceptively difficult to succeed in it.[11]

Restaurant concept is undoubtedly one of the major components of any successful operation. Some restaurants are looking for a concept; some concepts are searching for a restaurant.

Restaurant Location

The restaurant concept must fit the location, and the location must fit the concept (see Figure 3). The location should appeal to the target market (expected interests). Other things being equal, prime locations cost more, so operators must either charge more for their menu items or drive sufficient volume to keep the rent/lease costs to between 5 and 8 percent of sales.

Key location criteria include the following:

- Demographics—how many people are there in the catchment area?

- The average income of the catchment area population

- Growth or decline of the area

- Zoning, drainage, sewage, and utilities

- Convenience—how easy is it for people to get to the restaurant?

- Visibility—can passersby see the restaurant?

- Accessibility—how accessible is the restaurant?

- Parking—is parking required? If so, how many spaces are needed and what will it cost?

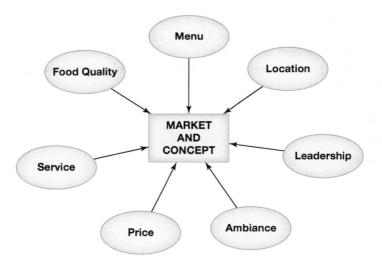

Figure 3 • Concept and Market.

(Reprinted with permission from John R. Walker and Donald E. Lundberg, *The Restaurant from Concept to Operation*, 3rd ed. [New York: John Wiley and Sons, 2001], p. 62.)

- Curbside appeal—how inviting is the restaurant?
- Location—how desirable is the neighborhood?

Several popular types of restaurant locations include the following:

- Stand-alone restaurants
- Cluster or restaurant row
- Shopping mall
- Shopping mall—freestanding
- Downtown
- Suburban

Restaurant Ambiance

The **atmosphere** that a restaurant creates has both immediate conscious and unconscious effects on guests. The immediate conscious effect is how guests react to the **ambiance** on entering the restaurant—or even more importantly as an element in the decision-making process used in selecting a restaurant. Too noisy? Are the tables too close? The subconscious is affected by mood, lighting, furnishings, and music; these play an important role in leaving a subtle impression on guests. Today, atmospherics are part of the theme and have an immediate sensory impact on customers.

Perhaps the most noticeable atmospheric restaurants are those with a theme. The theme will use color, sound, lighting, decor, texture, and visual stimulation to create special effects for patrons. Among restaurants with good atmospherics are Macaroni Grill, Panera Bread, Outback, Hard Rock Cafe, and Chart House.

▶ Check Your Knowledge

1. Imagine you are starting your own restaurant. In the process, you realize you need a mission statement. Write a mission statement for your new restaurant.
2. Define the following terms and briefly describe the role they play:
   a. Market
   b. Concept
   c. Ambiance

Sustainable Restaurants

The average American meal has a shockingly large carbon footprint, usually traveling 1,500 miles to the plate and emitting large amounts of CO_2 in the process, according to the Leopold Center for Sustainable Agriculture. Each meal created produces 275 pounds of waste a day, making restaurants the worst aggressors of greenhouse gas emissions in retail industry, says the

Boston-based Green Restaurant Association [GRA], a nonprofit organization that works to create an ecologically sustainable restaurant industry.[12]

A recent NRA [National Restaurant Association] study shows that utility costs are a big line item for restaurateurs, accounting for a median of between 2.3 percent and 3.6 percent of sales, depending on the type of operation. According to *Zagat's America's Top Restaurants*, 65 percent of surveyors said they would pay more for food that has been sustainably raised or procured. According to National Restaurant Association research, 62 percent of adults said they would likely choose a restaurant based on its environmental friendliness.[13]

Does greenings restaurant sound challenging, time-consuming, and costly? According to the Green Restaurant Association (GRA), it doesn't have to be any of those things. The GRA was founded almost 20 years ago with the mission of creating an ecologically sustainable restaurant industry, and it has the world's largest database of environmental solutions for the restaurant industry.[14] The GRA strives to simplify things because it realizes that restaurateurs have enough on their plates without worrying what kind of paper towel to order, or where they'll get next month's supply of ecofriendly dish soap.[15]

Menu Planning

The menu may be the most important ingredient in a restaurant's success. A restaurant's menu must agree with the concept; the concept must be based on what the guest in the target market expects; and the menu must exceed those expectations. The type of menu will depend on the kind of restaurant being operated.

There are six main types of menus:

A la carte menus. These menus offer items that are individually priced.

Table d'hôte menus. Table d'hôte menus offer a selection of one or more items for each course at a fixed price. This type of menu is used more frequently in hotels and in Europe. The advantage is the perception guests have of receiving good values.

Du jour menus. Du jour menus list the items "of the day."

Tourist menus. These menus are used to attract tourists' attention. They frequently stress value and food that is acceptable to tourists.

California menus. These menus are so named because, in some California restaurants, guests may order any item on the menu at any time of the day.

Cyclical menus. Cyclical menus repeat themselves over a period of time.

A menu generally consists of perhaps six to eight appetizers, two to four soups, a few salads—both as appetizers and entrées—eight to sixteen entrées, and about four to six desserts.

The many considerations in menu planning attest to the complexity of the restaurant business. Considerations include the following:

* Needs and desires of guests
* Capabilities of cooks
* Equipment capacity and layout

- Consistency and availability of menu ingredients
- Price and pricing strategy (cost and profitability)
- Nutritional value
- Accuracy in menu
- Menu analysis (contribution margin)
- Menu design
- Menu engineering
- Chain menus[16]

Needs and Desires of Guests

In planning a menu, the needs and desires of the guests are what is important—not what the owner, chef, or manager thinks. If it is determined that there is a niche in the market for a particular kind of restaurant, then the menu must harmonize with the theme of the restaurant.

The Olive Garden restaurants are a good example of a national chain that has developed rapidly during the past few years. The concept has been positioned and defined as middle of the road with a broad-based appeal. During the concept development phase, several focus groups were asked their opinions on topics from dishes to decor. The result has been extremely successful.

Several other restaurants have become successful by focusing on the needs and desires of the guest. Among them are Hard Rock Cafe, T.G.I. Friday's, Red Lobster, and Applebee's.

Capabilities of Cooks

The capabilities of the cooks must also harmonize with the menu and concept. An appropriate level of expertise must be employed to match the peak demands and culinary expertise expected by the guests. The length and complexity of the menu and the number of guests to be served are both factors in determining the extent of the cooks' capabilities.

The equipment capacity and layout affect the menu and the efficiency with which the cooks can produce the food. Some restaurants have several fried or cold items on the appetizer menu simply to avoid use of the stoves and ovens, which will be needed for the entrées. A similar situation occurs with desserts; by avoiding the use of the equipment needed for the entrées, cooks find it easier to produce the volume of meals required during peak periods.

One of the best examples of effective utilization of menu and equipment is in Chinese restaurants. At the beginning of many Chinese restaurant menus, there are combination dinners. The combination dinners include several courses for a fixed price. Operators of Chinese restaurants explain that about 60 to 70 percent of guests order those combinations. This helps the cooks because they can prepare for the orders and produce the food quickly, which pleases the guests. It would create havoc if everyone ordered à la carte items because the kitchen and the cooks could not handle the volume in this way.

Equipment Capacity and Layout

All restaurant menus should be developed with regard to the capacity and layout of the equipment. Anyone who has worked in a busy kitchen on Friday or Saturday night and been "slammed" will realize that part of the problem may have been too ambitious a menu (too many items requiring extensive preparation and the use of too much equipment).

If the restaurant is already in existence, it may be costly to alter the kitchen. Operators generally find it easier to alter the menu to fit the equipment. The important thing is to match the menu with the equipment and production scheduling. A menu can be created to use some equipment for appetizers; for this one reason, the appetizers selections on the menu often include one or two cold cuts, possibly a couple of salads, but mostly some deep-fried items or soups. This keeps the stove and grill areas free for the entrées. The desserts, if they are not brought in, are mostly made in advance and served cold or heated in the microwave. Other considerations include the projected volume of sales and the speed of service for each menu item.

Most chefs are sufficiently adaptable to be able to prepare quality meals with the equipment provided. Some may prepare a more detailed *mise en place* (everything in place to prepare a menu item), and others will go further to partially cook items so that they can be furnished to order. Of course, there is always the old standby—the daily special—that can take the pressure off the production line.

Consistency and Availability of Menu Ingredients

In the United States, most ingredients are available year-round. However, at certain times of the year, some items become more expensive. This is because they are out of season—in economic terms, the demand exceeds the supply, so the price goes up. An example of this is when a storm in the Gulf of Mexico disrupts the supply of fresh fish and shellfish and causes an increase in price. To offset this kind of situation, some operators print their menus daily. Others may purchase a quantity of frozen items when the prices are low.

FOCUS ON NUTRITION

New Frontiers in Restaurant Dining

Jim Inglis, Professor, Valencia Community College, Orlando, Florida

Over the last several years we have seen a major shift in what dishes restaurants are serving up. The cause for this change? Public interest, some of which is sparked by government legislation and some of which is driven by market or consumer demands. With laws now requiring restaurant chains in some states (soon every state) to disclose calorie counts and other nutritional information, restaurant companies have an opportunity to take advantage of and capitalize on this national movement—and many are.

Health-conscious consumers are demanding that companies change the way they do business; no longer does quantity always trump quality. Chains such as Chipotle, with the slogan "Food with Integrity,"[17] have been successful in marketing the qualities of healthy eating and serving animal products that do not contain growth hormones or antibiotics. Words like *sustainable*, *eco-friendly*, *green*, and *farm-raised* are the new catchphrases.

Some other chain concepts have also set their sights on nutrition by adding menu items with lower total calorie counts, sourcing more locally grown foods, and utilizing healthier cooking methods such as grilling or caramelizing vegetables in dishes rather than adding sugar. In fact, Seasons 52, of Darden Restaurants, "makes a promise that nothing on our menu is over 475 calories."[18] The result, they say, is "great tasting, highly satisfying food that just so happens to be good for you!"[19]

There is also the new push that came from the Obama administration to change the food pyramid, improve our public school meals, and educate children on the benefits of eating healthy and exercising. The USDA's new *My Plate* icon simplifies/replace the old food pyramid and is meant to "help consumers make healthier food choices."[20] It emphasizes the fruit, vegetable, grain, protein, and dairy food groups and clearly shows that half of what you eat every day should be fruits and vegetables. This is something that Americans as a whole are not doing, but Americans are starting to up and demand change.

So what role will the restaurant industry play in this paradigm shift through which the industry is going? This is not a fad or just a trend; I do believe the industry is going to have to embrace the concept of nutritional importance in selecting the items restaurants choose to put on their menus. On my recent visit the National Restaurant Show in Chicago, 2011, there were many examples of gluten-free products, vegan dishes, vegetarian cooking demonstrations, and so forth. We are seeing some innovative restaurant companies already incorporating many of these ideas into their menu concepts to meet the needs of today's consumer. The companies that position themselves correctly, and that can appeal to young and old alike, will be in a position to make substantial revenues, which equals substantial profits.

(Reprinted by permission of Jim Inglis.)

Price and Pricing Strategy

The target market and concept will, to a large extent, determine the menu price ranges. An example might be a neighborhood restaurant where the appetizers are priced from $3.25 and $6.95 and entrées are in the $6.95 and $11.95 price range. The selling price of each item must be acceptable to the market and profitable to the restaurateur. Factors that go into this decision include the following:

- What is the competition charging for a similar item?
- What is the item's food cost?
- What is the cost of labor that goes into the item?
- What other costs must be covered?
- What profit is expected by the operator?
- What is the contribution margin of the item?[21]

Figure 4 illustrates the factors that influence a restaurant's menu prices. There are two main ways to price menus: A comparative approach analyzes the price ranges of the competition and determines the price range for appetizers, entrées, and desserts. The second method is to cost the individual dish item on the menu and multiply it by the ratio amount necessary to achieve the desired food cost percentage. For example, to achieve a 30-percent food cost for

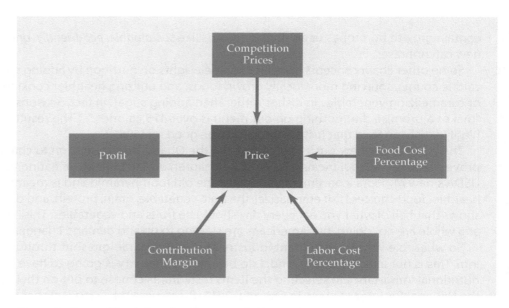

Figure 4 • Factors That Influence a Restaurant's Menu Prices.

an item priced at $6.95 on the menu, the food cost would have to be $2.09. Beverage items are priced the same way. This method will result in the same expected food cost percentage for each item. It would be great if we lived in such a perfect world. The problem is that if some items were priced out according to a 30-percent food cost, they might appear to be overpriced according to customers' perceptions. For example, some of the more expensive meat and fish would price out at $18 to $21, when the restaurant would prefer to keep entrée prices under $15. To balance this, restaurants lower the margin on the more expensive meat and fish items—as long as there are only one or two of them—and raise the price on some of the other items, such as soup, salad, chicken, and pasta. This approach is called the **weighted average**, whereby the factors of food cost percentage, contribution margin, and sales volume are weighted.

Nutritional Value

A more health-conscious customer has promoted most restaurant operators to make changes not only to the menu selections but also to the preparation methods. Restaurant operators are using more chicken, fish, seafood, and pasta items on the menus today compared with a few years ago. Beef is leaner than ever before. All of these items are being prepared in more healthful ways such as broiling, poaching, braising, casseroling, or rotisserieing instead of frying.

Increasingly, restaurants are publishing the nutritional value of their food. McDonald's has taken a leadership role in this. Other restaurants are utilizing a heart-healthy symbol to signify that the menu item is suitable for guests with concerns about heart-healthy eating. Many restaurants are changing the oil they use from oils high in saturated fat, which may be damaging to health, to 100-percent vegetable oil or canola oil, which are lower in saturated fat.

Accuracy in Menu

Laws prohibit misrepresentation of items being sold. In the case of restaurants, the so-called truth-in-menu laws refer to the fact that descriptions on the menu must be accurate. Prime beef must be prime cut, not some other grade; fresh vegetables must be fresh, not frozen; and Maine lobster had better come from Maine. Some restaurants have received sizable fines for violations of accuracy in menu.

Menu Analysis

One of the earliest approaches to menu analysis was developed by Jack Miller. He called the best-selling items *winners*; they not only sold more but were also at a lower food cost percentage. In 1982, Micheal Kasavana and Donald Smith developed menu engineering, in which the best items are called *stars*—those items that have the highest contribution margin and the highest sales. Later, David Paresic suggested that a combination of three variables—**food cost percentage** (percentage of the selling price of an item that must be spent to purchase the raw ingredients), **contribution margin**, and **sales volume**—should be used.

Another key variable in menu analysis is labor costs. A menu item may take several hours to prepare, and it may be difficult to calculate precisely the time a cook spends in preparation of the dish. Operators add the total food and labor costs together to determine prime cost, which should not exceed about 60 to 65 percent of sales. The remaining 35 to 40 percent is for overhead and profit.

Menu Engineering

Menu engineering is a sophisticated approach to setting menu prices and controlling costs. It operates on the principle that the food cost percentage of each menu item is not as important as the total contribution margin of the menu as a whole. Usually this means that the food cost percentage of a menu item could be larger than desired, yet, the total contribution margin of the menu will increase. Through menu engineering, menu items that should be repositioned, dropped, repriced, or simply left alone can be identified.

Menu Design and Layout

Basic menus can be recited by the server. Casual menus are sometimes written on a chalk or similar type board. Quick-service menus are often illuminated above the order counter. More-formal menus are generally single page, or folded with three or more pages. Some describe the restaurant and type of food offered; most have beverage suggestions and a wine selection. The more upscale American-Continental restaurants have a separate wine list.

Some menus are more distinctive than others, with pictures of the items or at least enticing descriptions of the food. Research indicates that there is a focal point at the center of the right-hand page; this is the spot in which to place the star or signature item.[22]

Like a brochure for the hotel, a menu is a sales tool and motivational device. A menu's design can affect what guests order and how much they spend.

The paper, colors, and artwork all play an important role in influencing guest decisions and help to establish a restaurant's image and ambiance.

As you can see, a number of factors make for a successful restaurant. Help is available from the U.S. Small Business Association (**www.sba.gov/category/navigation-structure/counseling-training**), which has several courses and other information for those interested in developing a business plan for a restaurant. Now, let's look at the classifications of restaurants.

Classifications of Restaurants

There is no single definition of the various classifications of restaurants, perhaps because it is an evolving business. Most experts would agree, however, that there are two main categories: **independent restaurants (indies)** and **chain restaurants**. Other categories include designations such as *fine dining, casual dining and dinner house restaurants, family,* and *quick-service restaurants.* Some restaurants may even fall into more than one category—for instance, a restaurant can be both quick service and ethnic, such as Taco Bell.

The National Restaurant Association's figures indicate that Americans are spending a lot of food dollars away from home at various foodservice operations. Americans are eating out up to five times a week—and on special occasions such as birthdays, anniversaries, Mother's Day, and Valentine's Day. The most popular meal eaten away from home is lunch, which brings in approximately 50 percent of fast-food restaurant sales.[23]

Individual restaurants (also called indies) are typically owned by one or more owners, who are usually involved in the day-to-day operation of the business. Even if the owners have more than one store (restaurant-speak for a "restaurant"), each usually functions independently. These restaurants are not affiliated with any national brand or name. They offer the owner independence, creativity, and flexibility, but are generally accompanied by more risk. For example, the restaurant may not be as popular as the owners hoped it would be, the owners lacked the knowledge and expertise necessary for success in the restaurant business, or the owners did not have the cash flow to last several months before a profit could be made. You only have to look around your neighborhood to find examples of restaurants that failed for one reason or another.

Chain restaurants are a group of restaurants, each identical in market, concept, design, service, food, and name. Part of the marketing strategy of a chain restaurant is to remove uncertainty from the dining experience. The same menu, food quality, level of service, and atmosphere can be found in any one of the restaurants, regardless of location. Large companies or entrepreneurs are likely chain restaurant owners. For example, Applebee's is a restaurant chain; some stores are company-owned, but the majority are franchised by territory.

Fine Dining

A **fine-dining restaurant** is one where a good selection of menu items is offered; generally at least fifteen or more different entrées can be cooked to order, with nearly all the food being made on the premises from scratch using raw or fresh ingredients. Full-service restaurants may be formal or casual and may be further categorized by price, decor/atmosphere, level of formality, and menu. Most fine-dining restaurants may be cross-referenced into other categories, as mentioned previously. Many of these restaurants serve **haute cuisine** (pronounced *hote*), which is a French term meaning "elegant dining," or literally "high food." Many of the fine restaurants in the United States are based on French or northern Italian cuisine, which, together with fine Chinese cuisine, are considered by many Western connoisseurs to be the finest in the world.

Most fine-dining restaurants are independently owned and operated by an entrepreneur or a partnership. These restaurants are in almost every city. In recent years, fine dining has become more fun because creative chefs offer guests fine cuisine as an art. At places like Union Square Café and Gramercy Tavern in New York, Danny Meyer is looking for guests who want spectacular meals without the fuss. Many cities have independent fine-dining restaurants that offer fine dining for an occasion—a birthday, an "expense account" (business entertaining), or other celebration.

Marco Maccioni, son of Sirio Maccioni of the famed Le Cirque, says that the sons did not want simply to clone Le Cirque. For the menu, they sought inspiration from Mama's home cooking—pizza, pasta, and comfortable, braised dishes.

Many cities have independent fine-dining restaurants that pursue those who are not content with wings and deep-fried cheese. Chefs are therefore making approachable, yet provocative food; each course is expertly prepared and may be served with wine.

Several types of restaurants are included in the fine-dining segment: various steakhouses; ethnic, celebrity, and theme restaurants. The upscale steakhouses, such as Morton's of Chicago, Ruth's Chris, and Houston's, continue to attract the expense account and "occasion" diners. Naturally, they are located near their guests and in cities with convention centers or attractions that draw big crowds.

Anthony Bourdain, owner and chef of Les Halles Restaurant, sits at one of its tables. Bourdain is the top-selling author of *Kitchen Confidential* and *A Cook's Tour*.

A DAY IN THE LIFE OF MELISSA DOAN-FIEBER

Server, Carrabba's Italian Grill

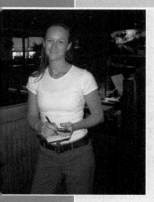

I started working in the restaurant business as a way to make money while going to school. I thought to myself, "This is a piece of cake." I soon realized that this fast-paced job is hectic and trying. Being a server is like being on center stage waiting for the next performance request. Every guest has their needs and it's up to you to figure out how they want them met. Sound scary? To some it may be; to me, I love it. Every day is something new, someone new, and never a reflection of the day before it. Over the years, I have learned that servers must obtain a few qualities: attentiveness, knowledge, hospitality, and genuine concern. Maintaining these qualities is hard during a busy shift; but in my experience, you can mess up a guest's order, and as long as you acknowledge the problem, seem concerned, and admit you're wrong, the guest will return. Restaurant goers dine out based on a number of reasons, but service is a deciding factor when choosing where to dine.

(continued)

A DAY IN THE LIFE OF MELISSA DOAN-FIEBER *(continued)*

As a server in a family-friendly fine-dining restaurant, I am never allowed to have a bad day. A typical workday starts before I even leave my house. I have to prepare a presentable uniform and gather all my tools of the trade (tie, wine key, lighter, pens, and server book). My uniform is my first impression and my instant greeting to any guest in the restaurant. Typically, I am scheduled the opening shift, and when I arrive at 3:15 P.M., it is my responsibility to start the shift with the proper amounts of lemons, butters, teas, and garnishes and to bake the bread. Every restaurant is different, but the one I work at schedules two openers and 45 minutes to set up.

Once setup is complete, I focus on making sure I have a clean section. Company policy allows a three-table maximum; this is designed to maintain consistently great service. The doors open at 4:00 P.M., and as the opener, I receive the first two tables. Each table has specific requirements, and it is part of my job to read their needs. Some guests want a quiet meal, while others are looking for entertainment and conversation. Some guests provide more specific instructions, such as allergies, food specifications, or child provisions. The restaurant I serve for is unique in two ways: first, they require their servers to know the ingredients of every item on the menu, and second, they make every item from scratch, allowing the guests to tailor items to their needs. Shortly into the shift, we are all called to the back for a "huddle-up"; here, we learn the soup, fish, and vegetable of the day, as well as the current sales contests. As the shift progresses, the chaos snowballs. Through the course of the night, I can only expect the unexpected. Steaks will be cooked improperly, guests will dislike their food, I will need manager compensations without a manager in sight, and I will always get to the ice bin right as it's emptied. The customer's perception of my service is how I get paid, and as long as I maintain my qualities, the guests will notice. My job is to run my food, meet my table's needs, and do my side work, but my service is the base of my tip.

As the evening winds down, I am cut based on the business of the restaurant. The managers cut the servers that came in first, and this time varies every night. Before I get started on my closing side work, I must finish up my tables and complete my restaurant financials. Ideally, my closing side work should be easy because everyone has running side work that maintains the tasks that need to be completed. Closing side work can consist of cleaning, restocking, and resetting for the following day. Once I am finished, I must get checked out by another server and then I can clock out, expecting a new day tomorrow.

A few ethnic restaurants are considered fine dining—most cities have a sampling of Italian, French, and other European, Latin, and Asian restaurants. Some even have fusion (a blend of two cuisines—for example, Italian and Japanese). Fusion restaurants must pay particular attention when blending two unique ethnic flavors. If successful, the dish could turn out to be the latest craze; if unsuccessful, it could be disastrous!

Celebrity chef–owned fine-dining restaurants of interest include Wolfgang Puck's Spago, in four locations; Chinois in Santa Monica, California; CUT, in four locations; and Wolfgang Puck Pizzeria & Cucina in Las Vegas and Alice Waters's Chez Panisse in Berkeley, California. Both chefs have done much to inspire a new generation of talented chefs. Alice Waters has been a role model for many female chefs and has received numerous awards and published several cookbooks, including one for children.

The level of service in fine-dining restaurants is generally high, with a hostess or host to greet and seat patrons. Captains and food servers advise guests of special items and assist with the description and selection of dishes during order taking. If there is no separate sommelier (wine waiter), the captain or food server may offer a description of the wine that will complement the meal and can assist with the order taking. Some upscale or luxury full-service restaurants have table-side cooking and French service from a gueridon cart (a wheelable cart used to add flair to tableside service; it is also used for flambé dishes). The decor of a full-service restaurant is generally compatible with the overall ambiance and theme that the restaurant is seeking to create. These elements of food, service, and decor create a memorable experience for the restaurant guest.

INTRODUCING SARAH STEGNER

Chef–Owner, Prairie Grass Café

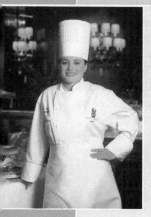

Sarah Stegner opened Prairie Grass Café in Northbrook, Illinois, with her partner, former executive chef George Bumbaris of the Ritz-Carlton Chicago, in 2004. A little history. . .

Stegner, an Evanston, Illinois, native, grew up in a family devoted to food. Her grandmother was a caterer "before women did those kinds of things," and her grandfather was an avid backyard vegetable gardener. The table was the center of the family and was where Stegner's passion for food emerged.

After a year spent studying classical guitar at Northwestern University, Stegner followed her heart and enrolled at the Dumas Pere Cooking School. She graduated with a chef's certificate one year later and was hired as an apprentice at the Ritz-Carlton Chicago.

In 1990, after six years of working in various culinary capacities (including a first job of cleaning fish for twelve hours a day), Stegner was promoted to chef of the Dining Room. She worked for years under the guiding hands of Fernand Gutierrez, former executive chef and director of food and beverage at the Ritz-Carlton Chicago, and current food and beverage director at Four Seasons Mexico City. Since then, Stegner has distinguished herself as one of America's most creative young chefs.

As a result of her talents, she has captured many national honors. Chef Stegner was named Best Chef of the Midwest in 1998 by the prestigious James Beard Foundation and the Dining Room was named one of the top five restaurants in Chicago in 1999 by *Gourmet* magazine, and it received four stars from the *Chicago Tribune*. In addition, it was rated best hotel dining room in Chicago in 1999 by the prestigious Zagat Chicago Restaurant Guide and was named Best Restaurant in Chicago in 1996 by *Gourmet*, one of the top thirteen hotel dining rooms in the United States in 1996 by *Bon Appétit*, and one of the top ten hotel restaurants in the world in 1996 by *Hotels* magazine.

Chef Stegner is recipient of the 1995 Robert Mondavi Culinary Award of Excellence and captured the national title of 1994 Rising Star Chef of the Year in America by the James Beard Foundation. She also holds the title of Prix Culinaire International Pierre Taittinger 1991 U.S. Winner, where she represented the United States in the finals in Paris and was the only female chef present at the global competition.

In recent years, Chef Stegner has enjoyed periodic training in France, under the expertise of Chef Pierre Orsi at his two-star Michelin Pierre Orsi Restaurant in Lyon, France, and with chefs Bertolli and Berard Bessin in Paris.

She also finds time to donate her talents to charitable causes. Six years ago, she founded the Women Chefs of Chicago, comprising the city's top female chefs who donate cuisine for numerous events throughout the city to raise money for charity. Under her direction, The Women Chefs of Chicago have helped raise more than $500,000 for Chicagoland charities in the past few years.

Sarah's support of her state's agriculture is reflected in her food: she uses the finest seasonal produce from Midwest vegetable farmers and cheesemakers. She works with her husband, Rohit Nambiar, who manages the front of house at Prairie Grass Café. Her mother, Elizabeth Stegner, makes the pies served at Prairie Grass Café. Sarah feels right at home in her new restaurant.

Celebrity Restaurants

Celebrity-owned restaurants have been growing in popularity. Some celebrities, such as Wolfgang Puck, come from a culinary background, whereas others, such as Naomi Campbell, Claudia Schiffer, and Elle Macpherson (owners of the Fashion Café), do not. A number of sports celebrities also have restaurants. Among them are Michael Jordan, Dan Marino, Junior Seau, and Wayne Gretzky. Television and movie stars have also gotten into the act. Oprah Winfrey was part owner of the Eccentric in Chicago for a number of years. She said she bought the restaurant because she liked a sandwich she had there, but was told that the place was closing. So she stepped in and bought it! Matt Damon and Ben Affleck once owned the Continental, and Dustin Hoffman and Henry Winkler were investors in Campanile, a popular Los Angeles restaurant. Dive, in Century City (Los Angeles), was owned by Steven Spielberg; Dan Aykroyd was one of the co-founders of the House of Blues; Robert De Niro, Christopher Walken and others own Ago; Kevin Costner, Robert Wagner, Jack Nicklaus and Fred Couples owned the Clubhouse; and musicians Kenny Rogers and Gloria Estefan are also restaurant owners.

Celebrity restaurants generally have an extra zing to them—a winning combination of design, atmosphere, food, and perhaps the thrill of an occasional visit by the owner(s).

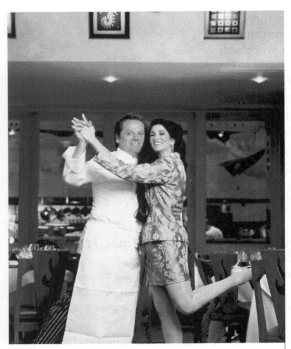

Wolfgang Puck and ex-wife Barbra Lazaroff at Spago, known for its innovative cuisine and stunning dining rooms designed by Barbra.

Steak Houses

The steak restaurant segment is quite buoyant despite nutritional concerns about red meat. The upscale steak dinner houses, such as Flemming's of Chicago, Ruth's Chris, and Houston's, continue to attract the expense account and "occasion" diners. Some restaurants are adding additional value-priced items such as chicken and fish to their menus to attract more guests. Steak restaurant operators admit that they are not expecting to see the same customer every week but hopefully every two or three weeks. The Chart House chain is careful to market its menu as including seafood and chicken, but steak is at the heart of the business, with most of its sales from red meat.

Outback Steakhouse, which is profiled in this chapter, owns and operates about a thousand Outback restaurants and about thirty Flemming's Prime Steakhouse and Wine Bars. Other restaurants in this segment include Stewart Anderson's Black Angus, Golden Corral, Western Sizzlin, which all have sales of more than $300 million each. In fact, chains have the biggest share of the segment.

Casual Dining and Dinner House Restaurants

The types of restaurants that can be included in the casual dining restaurants category are as follows:

Midscale casual restaurants. Romano's Macaroni Grill, the Olive Garden
Family restaurants. Cracker Barrel, Coco's Bakery, Bob Evans, Carrows

Ethnic restaurants. Flavor Thai, Cantina Latina, Panda Express
Theme restaurants. Hard Rock Cafe, T.G.I. Friday's, Roy's
Quick-service/fast-food restaurants. McDonald's, Burger King, Pizza Hut, Ponderosa, Popeyes, Subway, Taco Bell

CORPORATE PROFILE

Outback Steakhouse

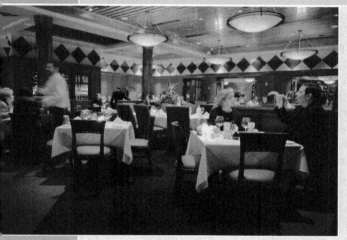

The founders of Outback Steakhouse have proved that unconventional methods can lead to profitable results. Such methods include opening solely for dinner, sacrificing dining-room seats for back-of-the-house efficiency, limiting servers to three tables each, and handing 10 percent of cash flow to the restaurants' general managers.

March 1988 saw the opening of the first Outback Steakhouse. Outback's founders, Chris Sullivan, Robert Basham, and Senior Vice President Tim Gannon, know plenty about the philosophy "No rules, just right" because they have lived it since day one. Even the timing of their venture to launch a casual steak place came when many pundits were pronouncing red meat consumption dead in the United States.

The chain went public and has since created a track record of strong earnings. It was evident that the three founders were piloting one of the country's hottest restaurant concepts. The trio found themselves with hundreds of restaurants, instead of the five they originally envisioned.

Robert Basham, cofounder, president, and chief operating officer at Outback Steakhouse, was given the Operator of the Year award at the Multi-Unit Foodservice Operators Conference (MUFSO). He helped expand the chain, a pioneer in the steak house sector of the restaurant business, to more than a thousand restaurants with some of the highest sales per unit in the industry despite the fact that they serve only dinner.

Perhaps the strongest indication of what this company is about lies in its corporate structure, or lack thereof. Despite its rapid growth, the company has no public relations department, no human resources department, and no recruiting apparatus. In addition, the Outback Steakhouse headquarters is very different from that of a typical restaurant company. There is no lavish tower—only modest office space in an average suburban complex. Instead of settling into a conservative chair and browsing through a magazine-lined coffee table (as is the case in most reception areas), at Outback you must belly up to an actual bar, brass foot rail and all, to announce your arrival.

Also, Outback's dining experience—large, highly seasoned portions of food for moderate prices—is so in tune with today's dining experience that patrons in many of its restaurants experience hour-long dinner waits seven nights a week. The friendly service is notable, from the host who opens the door and greets guests, to the well-trained servers, who casually sit down next to patrons in the booths and explain the house specialties featured on the menu.

Using such tactics and their "No rules, just right" philosophy, the founders have accomplished two main goals: discipline and solid growth. Good profits and excellent marketing potentials show just how successful the business has become. Outback also owns and operates Bonefish Grill, Flemming's Prime Steakhouse, Carabba's Italian Grill, and Roy's.

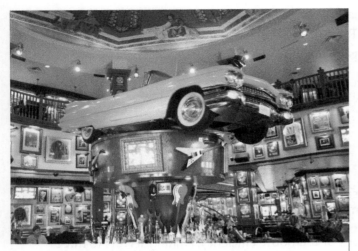

Hard Rock Cafe offers first-rate, moderately priced casual American fare with, of course, a side of rock and roll.

As implied, **casual dining** is relaxed and could include restaurants from several classifications: chain or independent, ethnic, or theme. Hard Rock Cafe, T.G.I. Friday's, the Olive Garden, Houston's, Romano's Macaroni Grill, and Red Lobster are good examples of casual dining restaurants.

Houston's is a leader in the casual restaurant segment, with about $5.5 million average per unit sales in its thirty-five restaurants. The menu is limited to about forty items and focuses on American cuisine, with a $16 average per-person ticket for lunch and a cost of $35 to $45 for dinner. While encouraging local individuality in its restaurants and maintaining exceptional executive and unit general manager stability, it succeeds with no franchising and virtually no advertising.

Over the past few years, the trend in **dinner house restaurants** has been toward more casual dining. This trend merely reflects the mode of society. Dinner house restaurants have become fun places to let off steam. A variety of restaurant chains call themselves dinner house restaurants. Some of them could even fit into the theme category.

Many dinner house restaurants have a casual, eclectic decor that may promote a theme. Chart House, for example, is a steak and seafood chain that has a nautical theme. T.G.I. Friday's is an American bistro dinner house with a full menu and a decor of bric-a-brac that contributes to the fun atmosphere. T.G.I. Friday's is a chain that has been in operation for nearly forty years, so the concept has stood the test of time.

Family Restaurants

Family restaurants evolved from the coffee shop style of restaurant. In this segment, most restaurants are individually or family operated. Family restaurants are generally located in or with easy access to the suburbs. Most offer an informal setting with a simple menu and service designed to please all the family. Some of these restaurants offer alcoholic beverages, which mostly consist of beer, wine, and perhaps a cocktail special. Usually, there is a hostess/cashier standing near the entrance to greet and seat guests while food servers take the orders and bring the plated food from the kitchen. Some family restaurants have incorporated salad and dessert bars to offer more variety and increase the average check.

The lines separating the various restaurants and chains in the family segment are blurring as operators upscale their concepts. Flagstar's acquisition of Coco's Bakery and Carrows family restaurant brands has created the high-end niche of family dining—somewhere between traditional coffee shops and the casual dining segment. The value-oriented operator in the family dining segment is Denny's. The more upscale family concepts include Perkins, Marie Callender's, and Cracker Barrel, all of which are sometimes referred to as the "relaxed" segment. These chains tend to have higher check averages than do traditional and value-oriented family chains, and compete not only with them, but also with moderately priced, casual-themed operators, such as Applebee's and T.G.I. Friday's.

Karen Brennan, Synergy Restaurant Consultants, says that people's use of restaurants is very different from five years ago. Consumers are thinking in terms of "meal solutions." The operators in this segment are seeking to capitalize on two trends affecting the industry as a whole: the tendency of families to dine out together more often, and the quest among adults for higher-quality, more flavorful food offerings.

Ethnic Restaurants

The majority of **ethnic restaurants** are independently owned and operated. The owners and their families provide something different for the adventurous diner or a taste of home for those of the same ethnic background as the restaurant. The traditional ethnic restaurants sprang up to cater to the taste of the various immigrant groups—Italian, Chinese, and so on.

Perhaps the fastest growing segment of ethnic restaurants in the United States, popularity wise, is Mexican. Mexican food has a heavy representation in the southwestern states, although, because of near-market saturation, the chains are spreading east. Taco Bell is the Mexican quick-service market leader, with a 60-percent share. This *Fortune 500* company has achieved this incredible result with a value-pricing policy that has increased traffic in all units. There are more than 7,000 units with sales of about $5 billion. Other large Mexican food chains are Del Taco, La Salsa, and El Torito. These Mexican food chains can offer a variety of items on a value menu. Our cities offer a great variety of ethnic restaurants, and their popularity is increasing.

Theme Restaurants

Many **theme restaurants** are a combination of a sophisticated specialty and several other types of restaurants. They generally serve a limited menu but aim to wow the guest by the total experience. Of the many popular theme restaurants, two stand out. The first highlights the nostalgia of the 1950s, as done in the T-Bird and Corvette Diners. These restaurants serve all-American food such as the perennial meatloaf in a fun atmosphere that is a throwback to the seemingly more carefree 1950s. The mostly female food servers appear in short polka-dot skirts with gym shoes and bobby socks.

The second popular theme restaurant is the dinner house category; among some of the better known national and regional chains are T.G.I. Friday's, Houlihan's, and Bennigan's. These are casual, American bistro-type restaurants that combine a lively atmosphere created in part by

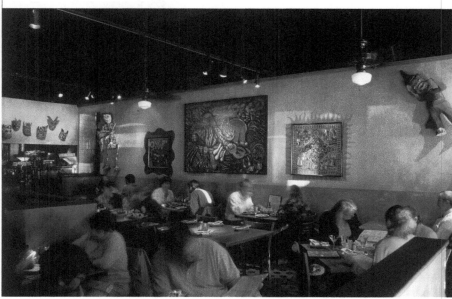

Guests being served at a Mexican restaurant.

assorted bric-a-brac that decorate the various ledges and walls. These restaurants have remained popular over the past twenty years. In a prime location, they can do extremely well.

People are attracted to theme restaurants because they offer a total experience and a social meeting place. This is achieved through decoration and atmosphere and allows the restaurant to offer a limited menu that blends with the theme. Throughout the United States and the world, numerous theme restaurants stand out for one reason or another. Among them are decors featuring airplanes, railway, dining cars, rock and roll, 1960s nostalgia, and many others.

Quick-Service/Fast-Food Restaurants

Quick-service restaurants (QSRs) consist of diverse operating facilities whose slogan is "quick food." The following types of operations are included under this category: hamburger, pizza, chicken, pancakes, sandwich shops, and delivery services.

The quick-service sector is the one that really drives the industry. Recently, the home-meal replacement and fast casual concepts have gained momentum (see Figure 5).

Quick-service or fast-food restaurants offer limited menus featuring food such as hamburgers, fries, hot dogs, chicken (in all forms), tacos, burritos, gyros, teriyaki bowls, various finger foods, and other items for the convenience of people on the go. Customers order their food at a counter under a brightly lit menu featuring color photographs of food items. Customers are even encouraged to clear their own trays, which helps reduce costs. The following are examples of the different types of quick-service/fast-food restaurants:

Hamburger. McDonald's, Burger King, Wendy's

Pizza. Pizza Hut, Domino's, Godfather's

Steak. Bonanza, Ponderosa

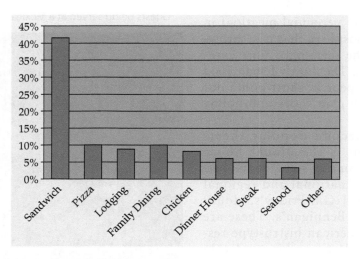

Figure 5 • Approximate Market Share of Restaurant Segments.

Seafood. Long John Silver's
Chicken. KFC, Church's, Zaxby's, Kenny Rogers Roasters, Popeyes
Sandwich. Subway
Mexican. Taco Bell, El Torito
Drive-thru/drive-in/delivery. Sonic, Domino's, Pizza Hut

Quick-service restaurants have increased in popularity because of their location strategies. They are found in very convenient locations in every possible area. Their menus are limited, which makes it easy for customers to make quick decisions on what to eat. The world equates time with money these days, and most people do not want to spend time trying to look through long menus to make an eating decision. These restaurants deliver fast service and usually include self-service facilities, too. Such restaurants also use cheaper, processed ingredients, which allow them to have extremely low, competitive prices. Quick-service restaurants also require minimum use of both skilled and unskilled labor, which increases the profit margins.

In an attempt to raise flat sales figures, more quick-service restaurant (QSR) chains are using cobranding at stores and nontraditional locations, including highway plazas and shopping centers. It is hoped that the traffic-building combos will increase sales among the separate brands, such as Carl's Jr. and Green Burrito. Many QSR chains are targeting international growth, mostly in the larger cities in a variety of countries.

Hamburgers

McDonald's is the giant of the entire quick-service/fast-food segment and serves millions of people daily. McDonald's has 32,478 stores in 117 countries with 400,000 employees and sales of $ 24 billion.[24] This total is amazing because it is more than the next three megachains combined—Burger King, KFC, and Pizza Hut. McDonald's has individual product items other than the traditional burger—for example, chicken McNuggets and burritos as well as salads and fish, which all aim to broaden customer appeal. Customer appeal has also been broadened by the introduction of breakfast and by targeting not only kids but seniors. Innovative menu introductions have helped stimulate an increase in per-store traffic.

In recent years, because traditional markets have become saturated, McDonald's has adopted a strategy of expanding overseas. It is embarking on a rapid expansion in the world's most populous nation, China, with more than 12,000 restaurants nationwide. The reason for this expansion in China is a rapidly developing middle class with a growing appetite for Western culture and food. McDonald's is now in 117 countries and has a potential audience of 3.2 billion people. Of the company's roughly 32,000 restaurants, some 8,600 are outside the United States, serving 47 million people each day.[25]

It is interesting to note that about 50 percent of total profits come from outside of the United States. More than two-thirds of new restaurants added by McDonald's are outside of the United States. McDonald's also seeks out nontraditional locations in the U.S. market, such as on military bases or smaller-sized units in the high-rent districts or gas stations.

McDonald's is taking another step toward being the most convenient food-service operation in the world by striking deals with gasoline companies Chevron, U.S. Petroleum Star Enterprise, and Mobil Oil Corporation to codevelop sites.

It is very difficult to obtain a McDonald's franchise in the United States because they have virtually saturated the primary markets. It often costs between $1 million and $2 million to open a major brand fast-food restaurant. Franchises for lesser-known chains are available for less money (about $35,000) plus the 4 percent of sales royalty fee and 4 percent fee for advertising, but an entrepreneur needs about $125,000 liquid and $400,000 net worth for an upscale, quick-service outlet, not counting land costs.

Each of the major hamburger restaurant chains has a unique positioning strategy to attract their target markets. Burger King hamburgers are flame broiled, and Wendy's uses fresh patties. Some smaller regional chains are succeeding in gaining market share from the big-three burger chains because they provide an excellent burger at a reasonable price. In-N-Out Burger, Sonic, and Rally's are good examples of this.

Pizza

The pizza segment continues to grow, with much of the growth fueled by the convenience of delivery. There are several chains: Pizza Hut, Domino's, Godfather's, Papa John's, and Little Caesar's. Pizza Hut, with 13,200 units,[26] has broken into the delivery part of the business over which, until recently, Domino's had a virtual monopoly. Pizza Hut has now developed systemwide delivery units that also offer two pizzas at a reduced price.

In response to the success of Pizza Hut's Stuffed Crust Pizza, Domino's highlighted its Ultimate Deep Dish Pizza and its Pesto Crust Pizza. It is currently advertising its new artisan pizzas, which are intended to look like bistro-style pizzas, with unusual ingredients such as spinach and feta and salami and roasted vegetables.

Chicken

Chicken has always been popular and is likely to remain so because it is relatively cheap to produce and readily available and adaptable to a variety of preparations. It also is perceived as a healthier alternative to burgers.

KFC, with a worldwide total of more than 15,000 units,[27] dominates the chicken segment. Even though KFC is a market leader, the company continues to explore new ways to get its products to consumers. More units now offer home delivery, and in many cities, KFC is teaming up with sister restaurant Taco Bell, selling products from both chains in one convenient location. KFC continues to build menu variety as it focuses on providing complete meals to families. Amazingly, there are now more than a thousand KFC restaurants in China.

Church's Chicken, with 1700 units, in 22 countries,[28] is the second largest chicken chain. It offers a simple formula consisting of a value menu featuring Southern-style chicken, spicy chicken wings, okra, corn on the cob, coleslaw, biscuits, and other items. Church's focused on becoming a low-cost provider and the fastest to market. To give customers the value they expect day in and day out, it is necessary to have unit economies in order. Systemwide, Church's now registers 34 percent in food costs and 25.9 percent labor costs.[29]

Popeyes is another large chain in the chicken segment, with 1943 units in 44 states and 27 foreign countries. It is owned by AFC, the same parent company as Church's. Popeyes is a New Orleans–inspired "spicy chicken" chain operating more than 2,000 restaurants in the United States and 25 countries.[30]

There are a number of up-and-coming regional chains, such as El Pollo Loco, of Irvine, California. It focuses on a marinated, flame-broiled chicken that is a unique, high-quality product. Kenny Rogers Roasters and Cluckers are also expanding rotisserie chains.

Sandwich Restaurants

Indicative of America's obsession with the quick and convenient, sandwiches have achieved star status. Recently, menu debuts in the sandwich segment have outpaced all others. Classics, such as melts and club sandwiches, have returned with a vengeance—but now there are also wraps and Panini.

A sandwich restaurant is a popular way for a young entrepreneur to enter the restaurant business. The leader in this segment is Subway, which operates more than 34,385 units in ninety-seven countries.[31] Cofounder Fred Deluca parlayed an initial investment of $1,000 into one of the largest and fastest-growing chains in the world. Franchise fees are $12,500, with a second store fee of $2,500.

The Subway strategy is to invest half of the chain's advertising dollars in national advertising. Franchise owners pay 2.5 percent of sales to the marketing fund. As with other chains, Subway is attempting to widen its core eighteen- to thirty-four-year-old customer base by adding Kids' Meals and Fresh Fit Choices aimed at capturing the health-conscious market. Subway has also added a breakfast menu and flatbread to its it bread offerings.

Bakery Café

The bakery café sector is headed up by Panera Bread, a 1,027-unit chain in thirty-eight states, with the mission of "a loaf in every arm" and the goal of making specialty bread broadly available to consumers across the United States. Panera focuses on the art and craft of breadmaking, with made-to-order sandwiches, tossed-to-order salads, and soup served in bread bowls.[32]

▶ Check Your Knowledge

1. Describe the different types of restaurants, and give examples of each. Highlight some of the characteristics that make up the specific restaurant types.

Trends in the Restaurant Business

- *Demographics.* As the baby boomers move into middle age and retirement, a startling statistic is emerging: forty-five- to sixty-four-year-olds (the age group with the highest income) will make up almost one-third of the U.S. population. Simply put, the largest demographic group will have the most money and will offer opportunities for restaurants that meet their needs.

- *Branding.* Restaurant operators are using the power of branding, both in terms of brand-name recognition from a franchising viewpoint and in the products utilized.

- *Alternative outlets.* Restaurants face increased competition from convenience stores ("c-stores") and home meal replacement outlets.

- *Globalization.* Corporations will continue the transnational development of restaurants.

- *Diversification.* Diversification within the various dining segments will continue.

- *Shared locations.* Restaurants will open more twin and multiple locations; restaurants such as Pizza Hut and KFC will share locations.

- *Points of service.* Restaurants will develop more points of service (for example, Taco Bell at gas stations).

- *Las Vegas.* Several restaurants and nightclubs have opened recently, such as the Strip House, CUT, and The Bank; plus, French chef Joel Robuchon at the MGM Grand was recently awarded a coveted three-star rating by the Michelin Guide.

Summary

1. Restaurants offer the possibility of excellent food and social interaction. In general, restaurants strive to surpass an operating philosophy that includes quality food, good value, and gracious service.

2. To succeed, a restaurant needs the right location, food, atmosphere, and service to attract a substantial market. The concept of a restaurant has to fit the market it is trying to attract.

3. The location of a restaurant has to match factors such as convenience, neighborhood, parking, visibility, and demographics. Typical types of locations are downtown, suburban, shopping mall, cluster, or stand-alone.

4. The menu and pricing of a restaurant must match the market the restaurant wants to attract, the capabilities of the cooks, and the existing kitchen equipment.

5. The main categories of restaurants are independent and chain. Further distinctions can be made as follows: fine dining, casual dining and dinner house, family, ethnic, and quick-service/fast-food. In general, most restaurants fall into more than one category.

Key Words and Concepts

actual market share
ambiance
atmosphere
casual dining
catchment area
celebrity-owned restaurant
chain restaurant
contribution margin
culinary arts
dinner house restaurant
ethnic restaurant
fair market share
family restaurant
fine-dining restaurant

food cost percentage
fusion
haute cuisine
independent restaurant (indie)
mother sauces
niche
nouvelle cuisine
purée
quick-service restaurant (QSR)
roux
sales volume
theme restaurant
weighted average

Review Questions

1. Describe the evolution of American culinary arts.
2. What are the five mother sauces?
3. Name some of America's finest chefs.
4. How are restaurants classified?
5. Explain why there is no single definition of the various classifications of restaurants; give examples.

Internet Exercises

1. Organization: **Charlie Trotter**
   Web site: **charlietrotters.com/restaurant**
   Summary: Charlie Trotter is regarded as one of the finest chefs in the world. Chef Trotter's restaurant has received numerous awards, yet chef Trotter is always seeking new opportunities.

   (a) What are Chef Trotter's recent activities?

2. Organization: **Olive Garden Restaurant**
   Web site: **www.olivegarden.com**
   Summary: The Olive Garden is a multiunit chain that primarily serves Italian food. It is currently operated by Darden Restaurants and has about 534 restaurants in the United States and Canada. Olive Garden strives to create a feeling of warmth and caring for every guest, which extends beyond the walls of the

restaurants into the community. Olive Garden participates in civic community service, such as delivering meals during times of crisis, sponsoring charity events, and hosting school tours of the restaurants.

(a) What kind of restaurant does the name Olive Garden represent?
(b) What is the Garden Fare? How is its menu different from the design and layout of the lunch menu?

Apply Your Knowledge

In groups, evaluate a restaurant and write out a list of weaknesses. Then, for each of the weaknesses, decide on which actions you would take to exceed guest expectations.

Suggested Activities

1. Identify a restaurant in your neighborhood and identify its catchment area. How many potential guests live and work in the catchment area?

2. Search the Web for examples of four great restaurant web sites. Compare them and share your findings in class.

Endnotes

1. National Restaurant Association, *About Us*, www.restaurant.org/aboutus/ (accessed March 22, 2011).
2. Sarah R. Labensky and Alan M. Hause, *On Cooking*, 4th ed. (Upper Saddle River, NJ: Prentice Hall, 2007), 6–7.
3. Ibid.
4. Charlie Trotter, *Charlie Trotter* (Berkeley, CA: Ten Speed Press, 1994), 11.
5. Ibid., 12.
6. "NRA Joins Healthy Dining to Promote Healthful Menu Choices," *Fast Casual*, July 18, 2006, www.fastcasual.com/article.php?id=5393 (accessed November 4, 2011).
7. This section is courtesy of Chef Michael Zema, Elgin Community College, Elgin, IL.
8. Danny Meyer, Presentation to the International hotel and Restaurant Show, New York, November 12, 2006.
9. John Walker, *The Restaurant from Concept to Operation*, 6th ed. (Hoboken, NJ: Wiley, 2011), 5.
10. Ibid., 5.
11. Ibid., 5.
12. http://www.restaurantreformer.com/, retrieved March 8, 2010.
13. Ibid.
14. http://www.dinegreen.com/restaurants/standards.asp, retrieved March 8, 2010.
15. Ibid.
16. Ibid., 208.
17. Chipotle, *What Is Food with Integrity?* www.chipotle.com/en-US/fwi/fwi.aspx (accessed November 4, 2011).
18. Seasons 52, *About Our Menu*, www.seasons52.com/menu/about_menu.asp (accessed November 4, 2011).

19. Ibid.
20. U.S. Department of Agriculture, Questions & Answers: MyPyramid Food Guidance System, www.choosemyplate.gov/global_nav/media_questions.html (accessed November 4, 2011).
21. Ibid., 211.
22. Ibid., 230.
23. Personal conversation with Jay R. Schrock, Dean, School of Hotel and Restaurant Management, University of South Florida.
24. Forbes.com, *McDonald's Corporation (NYSE: MCD): At a Glance*, http://finapps.forbes.com/finapps/jsp/finance/compinfo/CIAtAGlance.jsp?tkr=MCD (accessed April 1, 2011).
25. Ibid.
26. Yum! *Brands*, www.yum.com/company/ourbrands.asp (accessed April 1, 2011).
27. Yum! *Financial Data*, www.yum.com/investors/annualreport.asp (accessed April 1, 2011).
28. Church's Chicken, *Company History*, www.churchs.com/company-history.html (accessed April 1, 2011).
29. Ibid.
30. Popeyes Louisiana Kitchen, *Press Release: Popeyes Louisiana Kitchen Opens 2000th Restaurant Globally*, July 15, 2011, popeyes.com/article.php?articleno=MTM0 (accessed November 4, 2011).
31. Subway, *Home Page*, www.subway.com/subwayroot/index.aspx (accessed April 1, 2011).
32. Panera Bread, *Company Overview*, www.panerabread.com/about/company/mgmt.php (accessed April 1, 2011).

Glossary

Actual market share   The market share that a business actually receives; compare with the fair market share, which is an equal share of the market.

Ambiance   The combined atmosphere created by the décor, lighting, service, possible entertainment (such as background music), and other amenities, which enhances the dining or lodging experience.

Atmosphere   The combination of mood, lighting, furnishings, and music that has an immediate conscious as well as subconscious effects on guests.

Casual dining   Relaxed dining; includes restaurants from several classifications.

Catchment area   The geographical area that falls within a specific radius established to determine the size of a restaurant's market (usually one to five miles).

Celebrity-owned restaurant   A restaurant owned, or partially owned, by a celebrity.

Contribution margin   Key operating figure in menu engineering, determined by subtracting food cost from selling price as a measure of profitability.

Dinner house restaurant   A restaurant with a casual, eclectic décor that may promote a particular theme.

Ethnic restaurant   A restaurant featuring a particular cuisine such as Chinese, Mexican, or Italian.

Fair market share   A market share based on each business receiving an equal share of the market.

Fine dining   Upscale dining, usually with white tablecloths, à la carte menus, and table service.

Food cost percentage   A ratio comparing the cost of food sold to food sales, which is calculated by dividing the cost of food sold during a given period by food sales during the same period.

Fusion   The blending of two different cuisines.

Haute cuisine   Elaborate or artful cuisine; contemporary cuisine.

Independent restaurant   A nonfranchise restaurant, privately owned.

Mother sauces   One of five basic sauces that many others can be developed.

Niche   A specific share or slot of a certain market.

Nouvelle cuisine   A mid-twentieth-century movement away from classic cuisine principles. Includes shortened cooking times and innovative combinations. A lighter, healthier cuisine based on more natural flavors, including herbs.

Purée   To process food to achieve a smooth pulp.

Quick-service restaurant (QSR)   A restaurant that offers quick service.

Roux   A paste for thickening sauces, made from equal quantities of fat and flour.

Theme restaurant   A restaurant distinguished by its combination of decor, atmosphere, and menu.

Weighted average   A method of menu pricing that takes into account the food costs, percentage contribution margin, and sales volume.

Photo Credits

Credits are listed in the order of appearance.

Rade Kovac/Shutterstock
INB WENN Photos/Newscom
Hulton Archive/Getty Images
Richard Melman
Darden Restaurants
Melissa Doan-Fieber; Jim Cooper/
    AP Photo

Sarah Stegner
Alan Levenson/CORBIS
s70/ZUMA Press/Newscom
Demetrio Carrasco/DK Images
Jim Warych/DK Images

Restaurant Operations

From Chapter 7 of *Introduction to Hospitality Management,* Fourth Edition. John R. Walker. Copyright © 2013 by Pearson Education, Inc. Published by Pearson. All rights reserved.

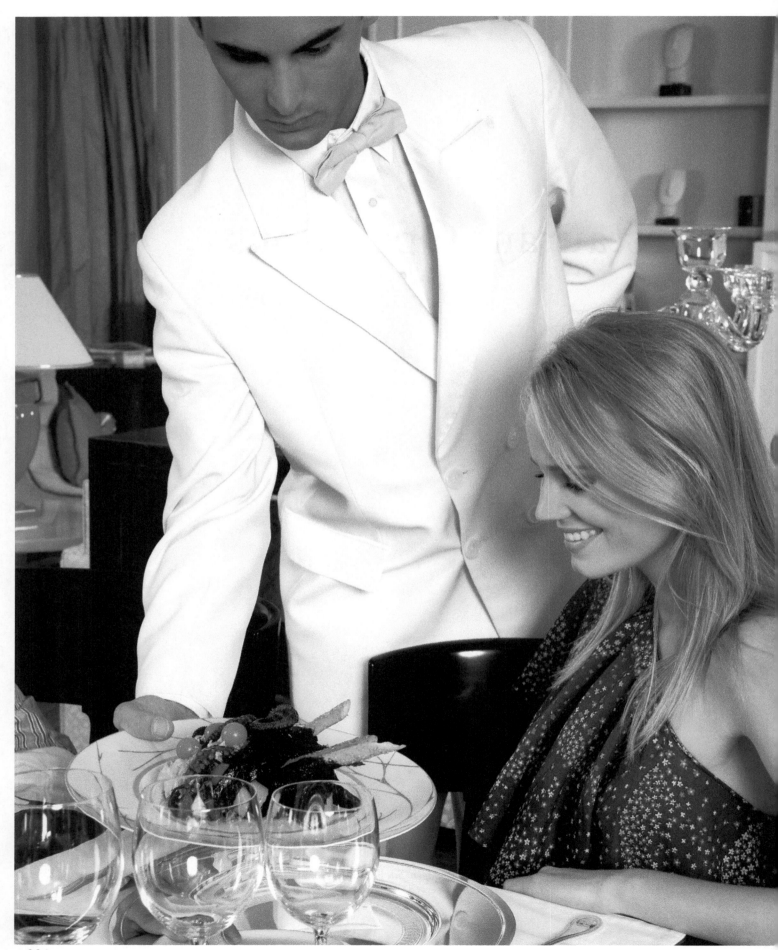

Restaurant Operations

After reading and studying this chapter, you should be able to:

- Describe restaurant operations for the front of the house.

- Explain how restaurants forecast their business.

- Outline back-of-the-house operations.

- Identify key elements of an income statement.

- Name the key restaurant operating ratios.

- Outline the functional areas and tasks of a restaurant manager's job.

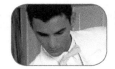
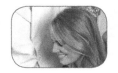
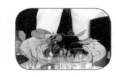
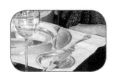

Front of the House

Restaurant operations are generally divided between what is commonly called **front of the house** and **back of the house**. The front of the house includes anyone with guest contact, from the hostess to the busser. The sample organization chart in Figure 1 shows the differences between the front- and back-of-the-house areas.

The restaurant is run by the general manager, or restaurant manager. Depending on the size and sales volume of the restaurant, there may be more managers with special responsibilities, such as kitchen manager, bar manager, and dining room manager. These managers are usually cross-trained to relieve each other.

In the front of the house, restaurant operation begins with creating and maintaining what is called **curbside appeal**, or keeping the restaurant looking attractive and welcoming. Ray Kroc of McDonald's once spent a couple of hours in a good suit with one of his restaurant managers cleaning up the parking lot of one of his restaurants. Word soon got around to the other stores that management begins in the parking lot and ends in the bathrooms. Most restaurant chains have checklists that each manager uses. In the front of the house, the parking lot, including the flower gardens, needs to be maintained in good order. As guests approach the restaurant, hostesses may hold the door open and welcome them to the restaurant. At the 15th Street Fisheries restaurant in Ft. Lauderdale, Florida, hostesses welcome the guests by assuring them that "we're glad you're here!"

Once guests are inside, the **host/hostess**, or as T.G.I. Friday's calls him or her, "smiling people greeter" (SPG), greets the guests appropriately, and, if seating is available, escorts them to a table. If there is a wait, the host/hostess will take the guests' names and ask for their table preference.

Aside from greeting the guests, one critical function of the host/hostess is to rotate arriving guests among the sections or stations. This ensures an even and timely distribution of guests—otherwise one section may get overloaded. Guests are sometimes asked to wait a few minutes even if tables are available. This is done to help spread the kitchen's workload.

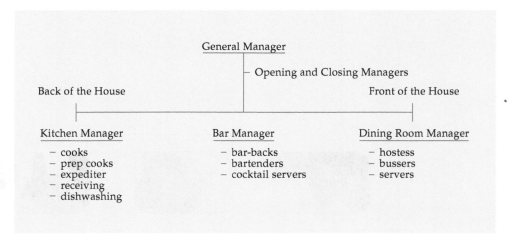

Figure 1 • Restaurant Organization Chart.

The host/hostesses maintain a book, or chart, showing the sections and tables so that they know which tables are occupied. Host/hostesses escort guests to the tables, present menus, and may explain special sales promotions. Some may also remove excess covers from the table.

In some restaurants, servers are allocated a certain number of tables, which may vary depending on the size of the tables and the volume of the restaurant. Usually, five is the maximum. In other restaurants, servers rotate within their section to cover three or four tables.

The server introduces him- or herself, offers a variety of beverages and/or specials, and invites guests to select from the menu. This is known as suggestive selling. The server then takes the entrée orders. Often, when taking orders, the server begins at a designated point and takes

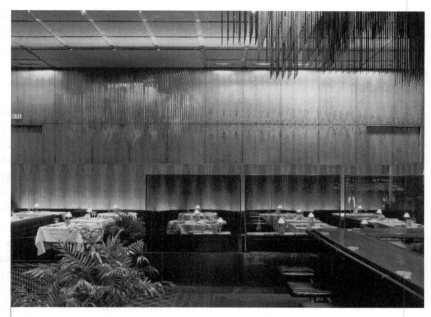

A midtown Manhattan restaurant prepares to welcome guests.

the orders clockwise from that point. In this way, the server will automatically know which person is having a particular dish. When the entrées are ready, the server brings them to the table. He or she checks a few minutes later to see if everything is to the guests' liking and perhaps asks if they would like another beverage. Good servers are also encouraged, when possible, to pre-bus tables.

Bussers and servers may clear the entrée plates, while servers suggestively sell desserts by describing, recommending, or showing the desserts. Coffee and after-dinner cocktails are also offered. Suggestions for steps to take in table service are as follows:

1. Greet the guests.
2. Introduce and suggestively sell beverages.
3. Suggest appetizers.
4. Take orders.
5. Check to see that everything is to the guests' liking within two bites of the entrées.
6. Ask if the guests would like another drink.
7. Bring out the dessert tray and suggest after-dinner drinks and coffee.

In addition to the seven steps of the table service, servers are expected to be NCO—neat, clean, and organized—and to help ensure that hot food is served hot and cold food served cold.

For example, during the lunch hour, servers may be scheduled to start at 11:00 A.M. The opening group of two or three people is joined by the closing group of the same number at around 11:45 P.M. If the restaurant is quiet, servers may be phased out early. When the closing group comes in, there is a quick shift meeting, or "alley rally." This provides an opportunity to review recent sales figures, discuss any promotions, and acknowledge any items that are "eighty-sixed"—the restaurant term for a menu item that is not available. Recognition is also given to the servers during the meetings, serving as morale boosters.

Restaurant Forecasting

Most businesses, including restaurants, operate by formulating a budget that projects sales and costs for a year on a weekly and monthly basis. Financial viability is predicted on sales, and sales budgets are forecasts of expected business.

Forecasting restaurant sales has two components: guest counts, or covers, and the average guest check. **Guest counts**, or **covers**, are the number of guests patronizing the restaurant over a given time period—a week, a month, or a year. To forecast the number of guests for a year, the year is divided into thirteen periods: twelve twenty-eight-day and one twenty-nine-day accounting periods. This ensures that accounting procedures are able to compare equal periods rather than months of unequal days. The accounting periods are then broken down into four seven-day weeks. Restaurant forecasting is done by taking into consideration meal period, day of week, special holidays, and previous forecast materializations.

In terms of number of guests, Mondays usually are quiet; business gradually builds to Friday, which is often the busiest day. Friday, Saturday, and Sunday frequently provide up to 50 percent of revenue. This, however, can vary according to type of restaurant and its location.

The **average guest check** is calculated by dividing total sales by the number of guests. Most restaurants keep such figures for each meal. The number of guests forecast for each day is multiplied by the amount of the average food and beverage check for each meal to calculate the total forecast sales. Each day, actual totals are compared with the forecasts. Four weekly forecasts are combined to form one accounting period; the thirteen accounting periods, when totaled, become the annual total.

Restaurant forecasting is used not only to calculate sales projections but also for predicting staffing levels and labor cost percentages. Much depends on the accuracy of forecasting. Once sales figures are determined, all expenditures, fixed and variable, have to be deducted to calculate profit or loss.[1]

Service

More than ever, what American diners really want when they eat out is good service. Unfortunately, all too often, that is not on the menu. With increased competition, however, bad service will not be tolerated in American restaurants. Just as American cuisine came of age in the 1970s and 1980s, service is showing signs of maturing in the twenty-first century.

A new American service has emerged. A less formal—yet professional—approach is preferred by today's restaurant guests. The restaurants' commitment to service is evidenced by the fact that most have increased training for new employees. Servers are not merely order takers; they are the salespeople of the restaurant. A server who is undereducated about the menu can seriously hurt business. One would not be likely to buy a car from a salesperson who knew nothing about the car; likewise, guests feel uneasy ordering from an unknowledgeable server.

FOCUS ON RESTAURANT OPERATIONS

The Manager's Role

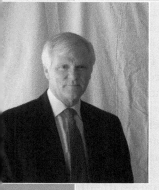

John T. Self, California State Polytechnic University, Pomona

It seems like only yesterday that I was walking into my first restaurant as a new manager trainee fresh from college. I found the restaurant industry perfect for me. It had plenty of variety, energy, and opportunity that matched my personality. I loved that I would not have to just sit behind a desk doing one thing every day. As a restaurant manager, your day will include accounting, human resources, marketing, payroll, purchasing, personal counseling, and many more functions that will challenge you.

You will be part of a management team that is the foundation of any restaurant, regardless of whether it is a chain or an independent. Managers have huge a sphere of influence, including customer service, sales, and profitability. You will be part of a management team responsible for a multimillion-dollar operation.

When you first become a manager, it is easy to be overwhelmed. You will probably feel that you will never be able to understand all the moving parts of a restaurant. However, as you grow in your management position, you will not only understand how it all works, you will also understand how you influence each part.

Being a restaurant manager offers the opportunity to grow as an individual because you will deal with so many types of people, including employees, peers, supervisors, vendors, and customers. You will learn how to get your team excited and motivated to share common goals. You will find it very rewarding to teach others about the culture of the business and will have many opportunities to make positive impacts on your staff.

The restaurant industry is the epicenter of the people business and management is at the heart of the restaurant industry. Motivating people, delegating responsibility to people, and leading people is what we are about and what we do.

Whichever company you eventually join, each will present a slightly different environment, career path, hours, days, responsibilities, and opportunities, but they all share food and people as their core.

Restaurants in the United States, Canada, and many other parts of the world all use American service, in which the food is prepared and appealingly placed onto plates in the kitchen, carried into the dining room, and served to guests. This method of service is used because it is quicker and guests receive the food hot as presented by the chef.

At Postrio in San Francisco, servers are invited to attend a one-and-a-half-hour wine class in the restaurant; about three-quarters of the forty-member staff routinely benefit from this additional training. The best employees are also rewarded with monthly prizes and with semiannual and annual prizes, which range from $100 cash, a limousine ride, dinner at Postrio, or a night's lodging at the Prescott Hotel to a week in Hawaii. Servers at other San Francisco restaurants role-play the various elements of service such as greeting and seating guests, suggestive selling, correct methods of service, and guest relations to ensure a positive dining experience. A good food server in a top restaurant in many cities can earn $50,000 or more a year.

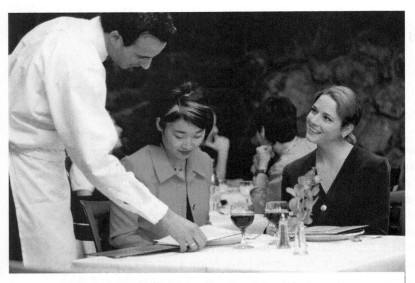
A server as a salesperson, explaining a dish on the menu to a guest.

Good servers quickly learn to gauge the guests' satisfaction levels and to be sensitive to guests' needs; for example, they check to ensure guests have everything they need as their entrée is placed before them. Even better, they anticipate guests' needs. For example, if the guest had used the entrée knife to eat the appetizer, a clean one should automatically be placed to the right side of the guest's plate. In other words, the guest should not receive the entrée and then realize he or she needs another knife.

Another example of good service is when the server does not have to ask everyone at the table who is eating what. The server should either remember or do a seating plan so that the correct dishes are automatically placed in front of guests.

Danny Meyer, owner of New York City's celebrated Union Square Cafe and recipient of both the Restaurant of the Year and Outstanding Service Awards from the James Beard Foundation, gives each of the restaurant's employees—from busser to chef—a $600 annual allowance ($50 each a month) to eat in the restaurant and critique the experience.[2]

At the critically acclaimed Inn at Little Washington in Washington, Virginia, servers are required to gauge the mood of every table and jot a number (one to ten) and sometimes a description ("elated," "grumpy," or "edgy") on each ticket. Anything below a seven requires a diagnosis. Servers and kitchen staff work together to try to elevate the number to at least a nine by the time dessert is ordered.

Suggestive Selling

Suggestive selling can be a potent weapon in the effort to increase food and beverage sales. Many restaurateurs cannot think of a better, more effective, and easier way to boost profit margins. Servers report that most guests are not offended or uncomfortable with suggestive selling techniques. In fact, customers may feel special that the server is in tune with their needs and desires. It may be that the server suggests something to the guest that he or she has never considered before. The object here is to turn servers into sellers. Guests will almost certainly be receptive to suggestions from competent servers.

On a hot day, for example, servers can suggest frozen margaritas or daiquiris before going on to describe the drink specials. Likewise, servers who suggest a bottle of fumé blanc to complement a fish dish or a pinot noir or cabernet sauvignon to go with red meat are likely to increase their restaurant's beverage sales.

Upselling takes place when a guest orders a "well" drink like a vodka and tonic. In this case, the server asks if the guests would like a Stoli and tonic. (Stoli is short for Stolichnaya, a popular brand of vodka.)

An example of the benefits of upselling is a server who describes a menu item like this: "Our special tonight is a slow-roasted aged prime Angus beef ribroast, served with roasted potatoes and a medley of fresh vegetables." Now, if this entrée costs $10 more than another beef dish on the menu, and the same thing happens with suggestions for guests to select from fish, seafood, and other meat or vegetarian items, the table's check will increase by $50 to $75. We know that a server receives about 15 percent in tips and does four or five tables that can turn twice each per night. You do the math: 15% of $50 = $7.50; if the server does four tables: $4 \times \$7.50 \times 2 =$ an additional $60 in tips.

Sustainable Restaurant Operations[3]

Sustainability is not just a philosophy about food—it's about people, attitudes, communities, and lifestyles. In the spirit of the theme of this year's International Chefs Congress—"The Responsibility of a Chef"—the ideas below come from chefs across the country. There's an idea to inspire you each day of the next month; even picking one to look into, or act on, per week is a good way to start. Almost everywhere one goes, we hear the same message: small changes and efforts can make a big difference!

1. Go local. It's not possible for everyone all the time. But when it *is* possible, support your local farmers.

2. Take your team to visit a farmer. This is good practice for remembering that each piece of food has a story and a person behind it. (And you can bring back extra produce for a special family meal.)

3. Know your seafood. The criteria for evaluating the sustainability of seafood differ from those for agriculture. Inform yourself using resources like California's Monterey Bay Aquarium's *Seafood Watch Guide*, and demand that your purveyors are informed too. If they can't tell you where a fish is from and how and when it was caught, you probably don't want to be serving it.

4. Not all bottled water is created equal. Some companies are working to reduce and offset their carbon footprint through a number of innovative measures. And some of the biggest names in the restaurant world (like *The French Laundry*) are moving away from water bottled out of house. In-house filtration systems offer a number of options—including in-house sparkling water!

5. Ditch the Styrofoam. Replace cooks' drinking cups with reusable plastic ones, and replace Styrofoam take-out containers with containers made of recycled paper. BioPac packaging is one option.

6. Support organic, biodynamic viniculture. There are incredible, top-rating biodynamic or organic wines from around the world.

7. Support organic bar products. All-natural and organic spirits, beers, and mixers are growing in popularity and availability.

8. Even your kitchen and bar mats can be responsible. Waterhog's EcoLine is made from 100 percent recycled PET postconsumer recycled fiber reclaimed from drink bottles and recycled tires.

9. Devote one morning per quarter or one morning per month to community service. Send staff to a soup kitchen, bring local kids into the kitchen, teach the kitchen staff of the local elementary school a few tricks, or spend a few hours working in the sun at a community garden.

10. The kitchen equipment of the future is green! Major equipment producers, like Hobart and Unified Brands, are developing special initiatives to investigate and develop greener, cleaner, energy-smart machines (that also save you money in the long run).

11. Shut down the computer and POS systems when you leave at night. When the computer system is on, the juice keeps flowing—shutting it down can save significant energy bill dollars over the course of a year.

12. Check the seals on your walk-in. If they're not kept clean and tight, warm air can seep in, making the fridge work harder to stay cool.

13. Compact fluorescent light bulbs (CFLs) use 75 percent less energy than incandescent bulbs. CFLs also last 10 times longer, giving them the environmental *and* economic advantage.

14. Consider wind power. Ask your energy provider about options—ConEd, for example, offers a wind power option. Though it tends to cost 10 percent more than regular energy, there's an incentive to bring the bill down by implementing other energy-saving techniques to offset the higher cost of wind power.

15. Look into solar thermal panels to heat your water. Solar Services, one of the oldest and biggest companies, will walk you through the process—from paperwork to tax credits. With the money saved on a water heater, the system will have paid for itself in two to three years.

16. Green your cleaning routine. Trade astringent, nonbiodegradable, potentially carcinogenic chemical kitchen cleaners for biodegradable, eco-safe products.

17. Use nontoxic pest control. The options are increasing, and even some of the major companies have green options.

18. Consider purchasing locally built furniture. See if there are any artisans in your state working with reclaimed wood (from trees that have fallen naturally because of storms or age).

19. Recycle your fryer oil. Biofuel companies across the country will pick it up and convert it.

20. Grow your own. Consider a roof-top garden or interior/exterior window boxes for small plants and herbs. EarthBoxes are one low-maintenance solution.

21. Cut down on shipping materials. Request that purveyors send goods with the least amount of packing materials possible. Request that Styrofoam packaging not be used.

22. Trade in white toilet paper, c-folds, and restroom paper towels. Instead, use products made of chlorine-free unbleached, recycled paper.

23. Need new toilets? There are a number of water-saving options that save anywhere from half a gallon to more than a gallon per flush. The old-fashioned brick technique is a good start too: place a brick in the tank of your toilet—the space that it takes up is water saved each time the toilet is flushed.

24. Compost garbage. Even high-volume establishments can make this happen. Keep separate cans for all food-based waste, and dump it in a compost bin out back. A common misconception about compost is that it smells bad—this is not true!

25. Recycle! Be strict about kitchen and bar staff recycling glass and plastic receptacles. Recycle cardboard and wood boxes used for produce, and any newspapers or magazines sent to the restaurant.

26. Cut down on linens. Tablecloths and napkins require a large amount of chemical cleaners, bleaches, and starches. Stay away from white, if possible. If it's not imperative, consider eliminating tablecloths all together. Go for soft cloth napkins instead of starched.

27. Ice = water + energy. Don't waste it! Don't automatically refill ice bins—wait until they truly get low, and only add as much as you need to get through the crush. Ice is expensive to produce, both in terms of money and resources.

28. If you're a small restaurant or café, without huge needs or storage space, look into joining (or forming) a local co-op for purchasing green items. Cleaning supplies, paper products, etc are all cheaper in bulk.

29. Educate yourself! From agricultural philosophy to the specifics of restaurant operations, the number of resources for green issues and practices is ever-growing. Pick up *The Omnivore's Dilemma* by Michael Pollan, the Green Restaurant Association's *Dining Green: A Guide to Creating Environmentally Sustainable Restaurants and Kitchens,* and *Sourcing Seafood, a Resource Guide for Chefs* by Seafood Choices Alliance.

30. Last but not least, educate your staff! They need to know *why* you're doing what you're doing, so that they can spread the word—to the diners, and beyond!

▶ Check Your Knowledge

1. What is considered the front of the house?

2. Define curbside appeal.

3. Suggest methods for remembering who ordered what on a table for a large party.

4. Name some of the responsibilities and duties of an assistant restaurant manager.

5. Briefly explain American service.

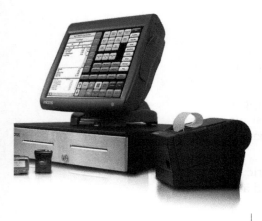

A popular point-of-sale system.

Front-of-the-House Restaurant Systems

Point-of-Sale Systems

Point-of-sale (POS) systems are very common in restaurants and other foodservice settings, such as stadiums, theme parks, airports, and cruise ships. These systems are used by hotel properties that have food and beverage and retail outlets. They are used to track food and beverage charges and other retail charges that may occur at a hotel or restaurant. A POS system is made up of a number of POS terminals that interface with a remote central processing unit. A POS terminal may be used as an electronic cash register, too.

MICROS, a leading software, hardware, and enterprise systems provider, offers Restaurant 3700, a modular suite of applications that encompasses front-of-the-house, back-of-the-house, and enterprise systems. The popular 3700 POS is a Microsoft Windows–based touchscreen system where client terminals are networked to a central POS server. Transactions are rung at the terminal and posted into the database for later analysis and reporting. The 3700 POS will support a network of kitchen printers so that orders can be presented to line cooks and chefs for food preparation. This POS system also supports use of a wireless personal digital assistant (PDA) as an order-taking device so that servers can take orders directly from the guest tableside. Mobile handheld devices can greatly speed the processing of orders to the kitchen and ultimately increase revenues as a result of faster table turns.

Kitchen Display Systems

Kitchen display systems further enhance the processing of orders to and in the kitchen. Printers in the kitchen may be replaced with video monitors and present orders to kitchen associates along with information on how long orders are taking to be prepared. Orders change color or flash on the monitor, which alerts kitchen associates to orders that are taking too long. Kitchen monitors are widely used in quick-service restaurants but are also gaining momentum in table service restaurants. Kitchen video systems also post order preparation time to a central data base for later reporting and analysis by management to determine how the kitchen is performing.

Guest Services Solutions

Guest services solutions are applications that are designed to help a restaurateur develop a dining relationship with guests. Applications include a frequent-diner management program, delivery management with caller ID interface, and guest-accounts receivable to manage home accounts and gift certificates. All these applications are accessed through the POS system and give restaurateurs the opportunity to offer their guests convenience, while allowing the restaurateurs to track who their best customers are. Guest activity is posted into the central database and management can develop targeted marketing programs based on this information.

▶ Check Your Knowledge

1. What do front-of-the-house systems entail?
2. Briefly define guest services solutions.

Back-of-the-House Restaurant Systems

Back-of-the-house systems are also known as product management systems and include inventory control and food costing, labor management, and financial reporting features. SoftCafe develops software for restaurants and foodservice operations, allowing them to create menus on personal computers. SoftCafe MenuPro creates professional menus at a fraction of the cost of print shop menus, with more than a 150 predesigned menu styles; 1500 images, watermarks, borders, and food illustrations; and more than 100 font types, and a culinary spelling checker.[4]

Restaurant Magic, based in Tampa, Florida, has several excellent restaurant management solutions: Data Central is delivered to a desktop as an enterprise-quality, secure and reliable, centralized business management solution to deliver powerful, user-friendly forms and reports to any Web-connected Windows PC in a restaurant organization. Data Central is a technological breakthrough in centralized application and database management because it is written entirely in the Visual C# language and is deployed as a Microsoft .NET Framework solution. Access to information is specified at the log-in level, and applications, reports, and important data are updated once available to all users automatically.[5] For a restaurant chain such as Outback Steakhouse, "Secure centralized management of enterprise data is more than a best practice, it is a necessity."[6] The benefits of programs such as Data Central are clear: Multistore managers can now view data for the enterprise. Store-level managers can view data for their store or for any group of stores they choose.

Restaurant Magic's Profit and Loss Reporting delivers profit and loss information on demand, consolidating information from purchasing to produce accurate cost of goods sold. All the key data is collected from the POS to track all revenues, forms of payments, and complementary activity (such as data from time clocks in order to collect labor costs) and integrate it with all other data to produce profit and loss (P&L) reporting daily, weekly, and multiperiod. The Profit and Loss Reporting allows a collaborative P&L budgeting system where the store and regional managers work together to build budgets and assess results quickly.[7]

Wireless POS Systems

Peter Perdikakis is the owner of two Skyline Chili fast-casual restaurants in Cincinnati. The restaurants are unusual in that the kitchen is open and visible to diners. Servers used to simply yell the orders across the steam table. Peter says, "You eat off china and have silverware, but it's very fast—typically you get your order about two minutes after it's ordered. Other POS systems slowed this process down because the servers had to go over to a terminal and

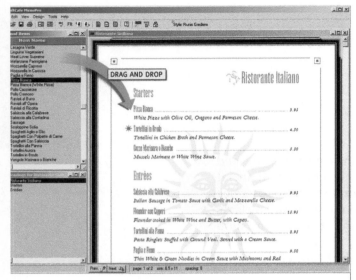

One of the menu-creation programs available from MenuPro.

write down the order," which is why Peter became interested in wireless. When he wanted to expand his operations, he selected a Pocket POS system from PixelPoint, consisting of two primary fixed terminals (one at a drive-through window and one at the check-out station), three handheld units for use on the dining floor, and another fixed unit for the back office.

The PixelPoint wireless POS system allows the servers to use a handheld PDA, which operates on the Windows CE platform, to send orders to the kitchen. Given that wireless POS systems speed up orders, their use in restaurants is likely to increase.

Labor Management

Most front-of-the-house systems have the ability to track employee working time. A back-of-the-house labor management package adds the ability to manage all of a restaurant's payroll and human resource information. A labor management system includes a human resources module to track hiring, employee personal information, vacation, I-9 status, security privileges, tax status, availability, and any other information pertinent to employees working at the restaurant. A labor management system would also include scheduling capability so that managers can create weekly schedules based on forecasted business. Schedules can then be enforced when employees check in and out so that labor costs can be managed.

The labor management package also presents actual work time and pay rates to a payroll processor so that paychecks can be cut and distributed. It also collates tips data and receipt data from the front of the house so that proper tip allocations can be reported according to IRS guidelines.

Financial Reporting

Back-of-the-house and front-of-the-house systems post data into a relational database located on the central server. The restaurant manager uses these data for reporting and decision making. P&L reports, budget variances, end-of-day reports, and other financial reports are generated from the central database. Financial management reporting needs to be flexible so that restaurant operators can manipulate it in ways that are useful to them. It is also important to get reports during the day in real time as the day unfolds so that restaurateurs can make decisions before profit is lost. Some reporting packages provide a graphical representation of the financial data displayed continuously on a monitor so that critical restaurant data is always available. This type of reporting provides restaurants with a real-time "heartbeat" for their operations.

Both back-of-the-house and front-of-the-house systems must be reliably linked so that POS food costs, labor costs, service times, and guest activity can be analyzed on the same reports. Restaurant management can then make critical business decisions armed with all necessary information. Technology is also used to collect data throughout the day for real-time budget control and "on-the-fly" management of labor effectiveness. Budgets are tight, and this is a way for management to watch, in real time, where their labor costs are at all times.

Personal Digital Assistants

Personal digital assistants (PDAs) help hospitality businesses stay effective and efficient by improving time management and helping with faster service. For example, computer systems are used today in restaurants to transmit orders to the kitchen and to retrieve and post guest payments. These actions took extra time in the past, when the computer systems were placed at a distance from the server. PDAs have been created to allow servers to control their business with their fingertips.

One leading software provider to restaurant operators is Restaurant Technology, Inc. (RTI). RTI was founded by two restaurant owners who understand the accounting applications that operate from a central platform known as the Restaurant Financial System. Working together, their accounting programs form an integrated system, with the following modules:

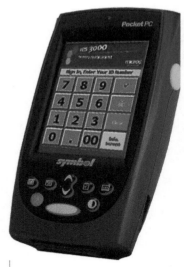

A pocket PC used in restaurants.

- Accounts payable
- Check reconciliation
- Daily store reporting
- General ledger
- Payroll
- Time keeping

PDAs can also be used in the hotel setting. Often, PDAs can be integrated with a property management system (PMS) to give housekeepers real-time information about which rooms need to be cleaned and which rooms are not occupied. In the same way, as housekeepers complete the cleaning of a room, they can send a wireless signal to the front desk to affirm that the room is ready to be occupied.

▶ Check Your Knowledge

1. Explain in what ways advances in technology aid the inventory process in restaurants.
2. What are back-of-the-house systems also known as?
3. What are the benefits of using a PDA?

Back of the House

The back of the house refers to all the areas that guests do not typically come in contact with; it is generally run by the kitchen manager. The back of the house includes purchasing, receiving, storing/issuing, food production, stewarding, budgeting, accounting, and control.

One of the most important aspects to running a successful restaurant is having a strong back-of-the-house operation, particularly in the kitchen. The kitchen is the backbone of every full-service restaurant; thus, it must be well managed and organized. Some of the main considerations in efficiently operating the back of the house include staffing, scheduling, training, food cost analysis, production, management involvement, management follow-up, and employee recognition.

Food Production

Planning, organizing, and producing food of a consistently high quality are no easy tasks. The kitchen manager, cook, or chef begins the production process by determining the expected volume of business for the next few days. The same period's sales from the previous year will give a good indication of the expected volume and the breakdown of the number of sales of each menu item. As described earlier, ordering and receiving will have already been done for the day's production schedule.

The **kitchen manager** checks the head line cook's order, which will bring the prep (preparation) area up to the par stock of prepared items. Most of the prep work is done in the early part of the morning and afternoon. Taking advantage of slower times allows the line cooks to do the final preparation just prior to and during the actual meal service.

The kitchen layout is set up according to the business projected as well as the menu design. Most full-service restaurants have similar layouts and designs for their kitchens. The layout consists of the back door area, walk-ins, the freezer, dry storage, prep line, salad bar, cooking line, expediter, dessert station, and service bar area.

The **cooking line** is the most important part of the kitchen layout. It might consist of a broiler station, window station, fry station, salad station, sauté station, and pizza station—just a few of the intricate parts that go into the setup of the back of the house. The size of the kitchen and its equipment are all designed according to the sales forecast for the restaurant.

The kitchen will also be set up according to what the customers prefer and order most frequently. For example, if guests eat more broiled or sautéed items, the size of the broiler and sauté must be larger to cope with the demand.

Teamwork, a prerequisite for success in all areas of the hospitality and tourism industry, is especially important in the kitchen. Because of the hectic pace, pressure builds, and unless each member of the team excels, the result will be food that is delayed, not up to standard, or both.

Although organization and performance standards are necessary, it is helping each other with the prepping and the cooking that makes for teamwork. "It's just like a relay race; we can't afford to drop the baton," says Amy Lu, kitchen manager of China Coast restaurant in Los Angeles. Teamwork in the back of the house is like an orchestra playing in tune, each player adding to the harmony.

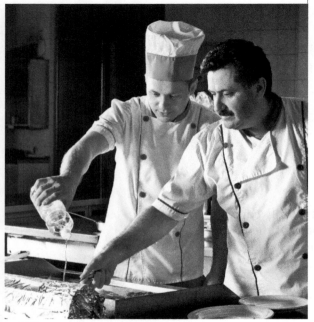

Chefs working together as a team.

Another example of organization and teamwork is T.G.I. Friday's five rules of control for running a kitchen:

1. Order it well.
2. Receive it well.
3. Store it well.
4. Make it to the recipe.
5. Don't let it die in the window.

It is amazing to see a kitchen line being overloaded, yet everyone is gratified when the team succeeds in preparing and serving quality food on time.[8]

A number of chefs are joining the green hospitality movement by encouraging the purchase of sustainable farming produce. More than 20,000 American Culinary Federation members are emphasizing organic and locally grown produce, whole-grain breads, and grass-fed meat products. Sustainable farming is making such a wave in the restaurant industry as a whole that the National Restaurant Association (NRA) began work on a multiyear plan to guide the restaurant and foodservice industry toward environmentally sound practices and to develop policy initiatives focusing on sustainability. The NRA's goal is to identify practices that can reduce costs for restaurants while encouraging the creation and use of sustainable materials and alternative energy sources.[9] As an example of a leadership role in the growth of sustainable food usage is Chipotle Mexican Grill with 1,000 restaurants that sell about 75 million pounds naturally raised meat each year. In addition, a significant portion of the chain's produce is organic. Chipotle's "Food with Integrity" mission is the cornerstone of everything they do.[10]

Kitchen/Food Production

Staffing and Scheduling

Practicing proper staffing is absolutely crucial for the successful running of a kitchen. It is important to have enough employees on the schedule to enable the restaurant, as a whole, to handle the volume on any given shift. Often it is better to overstaff the kitchen, rather than understaff it, for two reasons: First, it is much easier to send an employee home than it is to call someone in. Second, having extra employees on hand allows for cross-training and development, which is becoming a widely used method.

Problems can also be eliminated if a staffing plan is created to set needed levels. These levels should be adjusted according to sales trends on a monthly basis.

Also crucial to the smooth running of the kitchen is having a competent staff. This means putting the best cooks in the appropriate stations on the line, which will assist in the speed of service, the food quality, and the quality of the operations.

Training and Development

Implementing a comprehensive training program is vital in the kitchen because of a high turnover rate. Trainers should, of course, be qualified and experienced in the kitchen. Often, the most competent chefs are used to train new

A DAY IN THE LIFE OF JAMES LORENZ

Kitchen Manager, T.G.I. Friday's, La Jolla, California

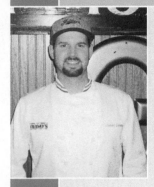

7:00 A.M. Arrive. Check the work of cleaning crew (such as clogs in burners, stoves/ovens, etc.) for total cleanliness.

7:15–7:40 A.M. Set production levels for all stations (broiler/hot sauce/expediter, cold sauce, vegetable preparation, baker preparation, line preparation: sauté/noodles, pantry, fry/seafood portioning).

8:00 A.M. The first cooks begin arriving; greet them and allocate production sheets with priority items circled.

9:00 A.M. On a good day, the produce arrives at 9:00 A.M. Check for quality, quantity, and accuracy (making sure the prices match the quotation sheet) and that the produce is stored properly.

9:30–11:00 A.M. Follow up on production. The sauté cook, who is last to come in, arrives. He or she is the closing person for the morning shift.

- Follow up on cleanliness, recipe adherence, production accuracy.
- Check the stations to ensure the storage of prepped items (for example, plastic draining inserts under poultry and seafood), the shelf life of products, and general cleanliness and that what is in the station is prepared correctly (for example, turkey diced to the right size and portioned and dated correctly).

10:45 A.M. Final check of the line and production to ensure readiness. Did everyone prepare enough?

11:00–2:30 P.M. All hands on deck. Jump on the first ticket. Pre-toast buns for burgers and hold in heated drawers. Precook some chicken breasts for salads. Monitor lunch until 2:30 P.M.

- Be responsible for cleanliness.
- Determine who needs to get off the clock.
- Decide what production is left for the remainder of the day.
- Focus on changing over the line, change the food pan inserts (BBQ sauce, etc.).

2:30–3:15 P.M. Complete changeover of the line and check the stocking for the P.M. crew:

- Complete final prep portioning.
- Check the dishwasher area and prep line for cleanliness.
- Check that the product is replaced in the store walk-in or refrigerator.
- Reorganize the produce walk-in. Check the storage of food, labels, and day dots, lids on.
- Thank the A.M. crew and send them home.

4:00–4:15 P.M. Welcome the P.M. crew.

- Place produce order (as a double check, ask the P.M. crew what they might need).

5:00 P.M. Hand over to P.M. manager.

hires. Such trainings are usually done on the job and may include study material. Some restaurants may even require new hires to complete a written test, evaluating the skills acquired through the training process.

Ensuring adequate training is necessary because the success of the business lies in the hands of the trainer and the trainee. If employees are properly trained when they begin their employment, little time and money will need to be spent on correcting errors. Thorough training also helps in retaining employees for longer periods of time.

Training, however, does not stop after the new hire passes a test. Developing the skills of all the employees is critical to the growth and success of the kitchen and, ultimately, the restaurant. A development program may consist of delegating duties or projects to the staff, allowing them to expand their horizons within the kitchen and the restaurant business. Such duties include projections of sales, inventory, ordering, schedule writing, and training.

This will help management get feedback on the running of the kitchen and on how well the development program works in their particular operation. Also, this allows for internal growth and promotion.

Production Procedures

Production in the kitchen is key to the success of a restaurant because it relates directly to the recipes on the menu and how much product is on hand to produce the menu. Thus, controlling the production process is crucial. To undertake such a task, **production control sheets** are created for each station, for example, broiler, sauté, fry, pantry, window, prep, dish, and dessert. With the control sheets, levels are set up for each day according to sales. Figure 2 shows a production sheet for a popular seafood restaurant.

The first step in creating the production sheets is to count the products on hand for each station. After the production levels are determined, the amount of product required to reach the level for each recipe is decided. After these calculations are completed, the sheets are handed to the cooks. It is important to make these calculations before the cooks arrive, considering the amount of prep time that is needed to produce before business is conducted. For instance, if a restaurant is open only for lunch and dinner, enough product should be on hand by 11:00 A.M. to ensure that the cooks are prepared to handle the lunch crowd.

When determining production, par levels should be changed weekly according to sales trends. This will help control and minimize waste levels. Waste is a large contributor to food cost; therefore, the kitchen manager should determine the product levels necessary to make it through only one day. Products have a particular shelf life, and if the kitchen overproduces and does not sell the product within its shelf life, it must be thrown away. More important, this practice allows the freshest product to reach the customers on a daily basis.

After the lunch rush, the kitchen manager checks to see how much product was sold and how much is left for the night shift. (Running out of a product is unacceptable and should not happen. If proper production procedures are followed, a restaurant will not have to eighty-six anything on the menu.) After all production is completed on all stations, the cooks may be checked out. It is essential to check out the cooks and hold them accountable for production

ITEM	PAR	ON HAND	PREP	INITIAL
FRESH CATCH				
Add Island Sauce to any fish				
BBQ Shrimp				
Casino				
Coconut Lobster				
Fried Lobster				
Ritz Crusted				
Seafood Kabob				
Stuffed Salmon				
SNAPPER				
Almondine				
Anna				
Broiled				
Fingers				
Stuffed				
FLOUNDER				
Allmondine				
Fried, Baked				
Stuffed				
GROUPER				
Baked				
Casino				
Coconut				
Coconut				
Floribean				
Fried Nutty				
Mexical				
Nuggets				
Nutty				
Potato Crusted				
Ritz				
Stuffed				
Wisconsin				
Holiday Specials				
DAILY APPETIZERS				
Oysters Maria (3 ea)				
Mozzereal Cheese Sticks (5 ea)				
Jammers, Jalapeno (4ea)				
Jammers, Seafood (10ea)				
Clam Strip Basket (6oz)				
Buffalo Shrimp (5ea)				
BBQ Shrimp (1 Skewer 5 Shrimp)				
Gator Gites (6oz)				

ITEM	PAR	ON HAND	PREP	INITIAL
WRAPS				
Ham or Turkey				
Ham & turkey				
Shrimp Salad				
Chicken Caesar				
Chicken Salad				
BLT Wrap				
DAILY SALADS				
Seafood or Chicken Salad				
Shrimp				
Chicken Mediterrarean				
PIZZA				
Shrimp or B.B.Q. Chicken				
Portabello				
SOUP & SAND				
Clamwich, Mini Grouper				
Crab Cake, Chicken Salad				
EXTRA DAILY SPECIALS				
Monday AUCE Fish				
Tues Lobster				
Wed AUCE Popcorn\Crabby Night				
Thur Prime Rib				
Beef Tips and Noodles				
Chicken Pot Pie				
Salisbury Stk				
Ham & Mac & Cheese				
Chicken Oscar				
Stone Crab Mustard Sauce				
Corn Salsa				
SPECIALS ITEMS FOR CATERING				

Pull From Freezer				
Item	Par	On Hand	Pull	Initial
				08/25/2003
				01/12/04

Figure 2 • A Production Sheet for a Popular Seafood Restaurant.

(*Source:* Anna Maria Oyster Bar, Inc.)

levels. If they are not checked out, they will slide on their production, negatively affecting the restaurant and the customer.

The use of production sheets is critical, as well, in controlling how the cooks use the products because production plays a key role in food cost. Every recipe has a particular "spec" (specification) to follow. When one deviates from the recipe, quality goes down, consistency is lost, and food cost goes up. That is why it is important to follow the recipe at all times.

Management Involvement and Follow-Up

As in any business, management involvement is vital to the success of a restaurant. Management should know firsthand what is going on in the back of the house. It is also important that they be "on the line," assisting the staff in the preparation of the menu and in the other operations of the kitchen, just as they should be helping when things are rushed. When management is visible to the staff, they are prone to do what they need to be doing at all times, and food quality is more apparent and consistent. Managers should constantly be walking and talking food cost, cleanliness, sanitation, and quality. This shows the staff how serious and committed they are to the successful running of the back of the house.

As management spends more time in the kitchen, more knowledge is gained, more confidence is acquired, and more respect is earned. Employee–management interaction produces a sense of stability and a strong work ethic among employees, resulting in higher morale and promoting a positive working environment. To ensure that policies and standards are being upheld, management follow-up should happen on a continual basis. This is especially important when cooks are held accountable to specifications and production and when other staff members are given duties to perform. Without follow-up, the restaurant may fold.

Employee Recognition

Employee recognition is an extremely important aspect of back-of-the-house management. Recognizing employees for their efforts creates a positive work environment that motivates the staff to excel and ultimately to produce consistently better-quality food for the guests.

Recognition can take many different forms, from personally commending a staff person for his or her efforts to recognizing a person in a group setting. By recognizing employees, management can make an immediate impact on the quality of operations. This can be a great tool for building sales, as well as assisting in the overall success of the restaurant.

▶ Check Your Knowledge

1. Explain the following terms: guest counts/covers, product specification, production control sheets.

2. Discuss T.G.I. Friday's five rules for running a kitchen.

TECHNOLOGY SPOTLIGHT

Reversing Restaurant Failure

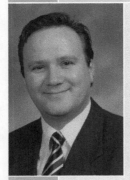

Cihan Cobanoglu, Ph.D., Dean, School of Hotel and Restaurant Management, University of South Florida, Sarasota-Manatee

In the summer of 2003, American Express aired a commercial with celebrity chef Rocco Di-Spirito purporting that "nine out of ten restaurants fail in the first year." The commercial caught the attention of an associate professor at Ohio State University's hospitality management program, H. G. Parsa. He had heard the statistic before, but, based on his thirteen years of experience in the hospitality industry, was skeptical. In fact, the statistic was somewhat of an urban legend even to American Express. After prodding the credit card company for three months as to the source of its statistic, Parsa received a written response stating that "American Express has not been able to track down a specific data source for the statistic."

In 2005, Parsa co-authored "Why Restaurants Fail," an article published in a Cornell University journal based on a study of restaurant failure. In that study, he found that the restaurant failure rate during the first year is about 30 percent—still a significant number. There are many reasons for restaurant failure: lack of cash flow, poor operational controls, high turnover, poor location, ineffective advertising and sales promotion, and so forth. In markets where net profit margins are slim, as with many quick-service operations, there's even less room for error.

In some cases, an investment in sound technology systems can help boost a restaurant's chances for success and help them avoid becoming a statistic:

- **Cost Control Software:** There are numerous cost control software options available in the market that will enable a chef and managers to make informed decisions about the cost and selling price of their menu items. For example, ChefTec (**www.cheftec.com**) will alert a manager if the cost of a menu item is over a certain price level. This allows for fluctuating inventory items to be kept under control. Additionally, cost control software allows the managers to play "what if" scenarios to determine the best price levels and contribution margins. Similarly, cost control software can alert a chef or manager if an inventory item is approaching the end of its shelf life. If it does, the chef can utilize the item in a special menu, eliminating waste and possibly even boosting sales.

- **Reverse Auction Software:** This solution can be used as a part of a menu engineering or cost control package. Eatec (**www.eatec.com**) and ChefTec both offer this feature, which allows the restaurant manager to determine a maximum price for purchase order items. The system then distributes the purchase order to suppliers electronically, allowing them to reverse bid on items. The software can even select the lowest bids for you. A manager has the freedom to purchase their products from any vendor, regardless of their bids. Of course, logic usually dictates ordering from the lowest cost provider if the qualities are equal. This system is predicted to save restaurants about 4 percent to 9 percent on food costs. In slim margin environments, this could make the difference between success and failure.

- **Point-of-Sale System:** Most restaurants have a point-of-sale system (POS); however, the majority of restaurants use only 20 percent to 30 percent of its features. Consider leveraging data from your POS system to create a menu engineering strategy: Most POS systems will report the menu mix, whereas cost control software will report contribution margins for each menu item. The result is a menu mix analysis that will allow operators to engineer their menus for higher margins. Items can then be identified as one of the four classic menu-engineering examples: "dog" items, which should be replaced; "puzzle" items, which should be repositioned on the menu; "plow horse" items, which should be re-priced; or "star" items, which should be preserved. By re-pricing plow horses and focusing on stars, restaurants can positively affect their bottom lines.

- **Computer-Based Training:** The new generation of POS systems and kitchen display systems can be used as ongoing training devices. The cost of creating these training programs is minimal, with off-the-shelf screen recorder software available from such companies as Camtasia Studio (**www.camtasia.com**) or Adobe Captivate (**www.adobe.com/captivate**). Personalized training tools will ensure high service quality and safety.

- **Other Solutions:** Opportunities for boosting the bottom line are available at nearly every juncture. Restaurants can work to make better use of their web sites (historically among the least effective in the hospitality industry) and can tap such solutions as scheduling software, table management, HACCP (hazard analysis and critical control points) alert systems, and financial management.

INTRODUCING CHRIS DELLA-CRUZ, GENERAL MANAGER OF SUSO RESTAURANT

Expectations of the General Manager

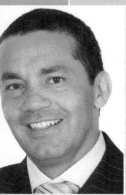

The expectations of the general manager are different in each restaurant; however, there are certain commonalities as well. Some of these commonalities are as follows:

- General managers answer directly to the owner or to regional directors of major corporations.
- General managers are expected to run good numbers for the periods. The numbers analyzed are food cost, labor cost, beverage cost. These areas are controlled to produce sufficient profit for the restaurant.
- General managers promote good morale and teamwork in the restaurant. Having a positive environment in the restaurant is of utmost importance. This will not only keep the employees happy, but it will also contribute to providing better service to the guests.

(continued)

INTRODUCING CHRIS DELLA-CRUZ, GENERAL MANAGER OF SUSO RESTAURANT (continued)

Duties and Responsibilities

The general manager of a restaurant is directly in charge of all the operations in the restaurant. General managers are also in charge of the floor managers, kitchen manager, and all the remaining employees in the restaurant.

The general manager should always check on the floor managers to ensure that all policies and regulations are being met. This will keep operations running smoothly.

Another important duty is to organize and control the staffing of the restaurant. The floor managers usually write the employee schedule; however, the general manager is still directly responsible for proper staffing for the period. This will help keep labor costs to about 20 percent of sales. The general manager is also in charge of conducting employee reviews and training.

Qualifications for a General Manager

To be hired as a general manager, the following qualifications are necessary:

- The general manager should be very knowledgeable in the restaurant business.
- He or she should have previously worked all the stations in a restaurant and be very familiar with them.
- The general manager should be able to get along with all people, be fair with all employees, and not discriminate.
- Having a degree is not the most important thing in becoming a general manager. However, a degree is very useful in moving up the ladder in a company to regional manager, regional director, and so on.

Budgeted Costs in a Restaurant

Running a good pace in the restaurant is of absolute importance. Every restaurant has different numbers to make. The following numbers came from Chris's restaurant. These numbers reflect their goals versus actual numbers run for a given week.

	Goal (%)	Actual (%)	Variance (%)
Food Cost	27.0	27.2	+0.2
Labor Cost	19.9	20.8	+0.9
Beverage Cost	19.0	18.2	−0.8

As can be seen, this restaurant did well with the beverage cost; however, the food cost and the labor cost are two areas to focus on for the upcoming week.

Making good percentages for the restaurant is the most important focus simply because this is where the restaurant makes or does not make a profit. When the general manager runs good numbers, then he or she will receive a large bonus check for contributing to the profit of the restaurant. This is why it is so important to focus on these three key areas.

Purchasing

Purchasing for restaurants involves procuring the products and services that the restaurant needs to serve its guests. Restaurant operators set up purchasing systems that determine the following:

- Standards for each item (**product specification**)
- Systems that minimize effort and maximize control of theft and losses from other sources
- The amount of each item that should be on hand (par stock and reorder point)
- Who will do the buying and keep the purchasing system in motion
- Who will do the receiving, storage, and issuing of items[11]

It is desirable for restaurants to establish standards for each product, called a product specification. When ordering meat, for example, the cut, weight, size, percentage of fat content, and number of days aged are all factors that are specified by the purchaser.

Establishing systems that minimize effort and maximize control of theft may be done by computer or manually. However, merely computerizing a system does not make it theft-proof. Instead, employing honest workers is a top priority because temptation is everywhere in the restaurant industry.

An efficient and effective system establishes a stock level that must be on hand at all times. This is called a **par stock**. If the stock on hand falls below a specified reorder point, the computer system automatically reorders a predetermined quantity of the item.

In identifying who will do the buying, it is most important to separate task and responsibility between the person placing the order and the person receiving the goods. This avoids possible theft. The best way to avoid losses is to have the chef prepare the order; the manager or the manager's designee place the order; and a third person, responsible for the stores, receive the goods together with the chef (or the chef's designee).

Commercial (for-profit) restaurant and foodservice operators who are part of a chain may have the menu items and order specifications determined at the corporate office. This saves the unit manager from having to order individually; specialists at the corporate office can not only develop the menu but also the specifications for the ingredients to ensure consistency. Both chain and independent restaurants and foodservice operators use similar prepurchase functions (see Figure 3).

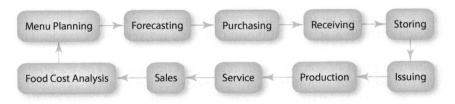

Figure 3 • Food Cost Control Process.

- Plan menus.
- Determine quality and quantity needed to produce menus.
- Determine inventory stock levels.
- Identify items to purchase by subtracting stock levels from the quantity required to produce menus.
- Write specifications and develop market orders for purchases.

Professor Stefanelli at the University of Nevada, Las Vegas, suggests a formal and an informal method of purchasing that includes the following steps[12]:

Formal	*Informal*
Develop purchase order.	Develop purchase order.
Establish bid schedule.	Quote price.
Issue invitation to bid.	Select vendor and place order.
Tabulate and evaluate bids.	
Award contract and issue delivery order.	
Inspect/receive deliveries, inventory stores, and record transactions in inventory.	Receive and inspect deliveries, store, and record transaction.
Evaluate and follow up.	Evaluate and follow up.
Issue food supplies for food production and service.	Issue food supplies for food production and service.

The formal method is generally used by chain restaurant operators and the informal one by independent restaurant operators.

A **purchase order** comes as a result of the product specification. As it sounds, a purchase order is an order to purchase a certain quantity of an item at a specific price. Many restaurants develop purchase orders for items they need on a regular basis. These are then sent to suppliers for quotations, and samples are sent in for product evaluations. For example, canned items have varying amounts of liquid. Typically, it is the drained weight of the product that matters to the restaurant operator. After comparing samples from several vendors, the operator can choose the supplier that best suits the restaurant's needs.

Receiving

When placing an order, the restaurant operator specifies the day and time (for example, Friday, 10:00 A.M. to 12:00 noon) for the delivery to be made. This prevents deliveries from being made at inconvenient times.

Receiving is a point of control in the restaurant operation. The purpose of receiving is to ensure the quantity, quality, and price are exactly as ordered. The quantity and quality relate to the order specification and the standardized recipe. Depending on the restaurant and the type of food and beverage control system, some perishable items are issued directly to the kitchen, and most of the nonperishable items go into storage.

Storing/Issuing

Control of the stores is often a problem. Records must be kept of all items going into and out of the stores. If more than one person has access to the stores, it is difficult to know where to attach responsibility in case of losses.

Items should be issued from the stores only on an authorized requisition signed by the appropriate person. One restaurateur who has been in business for many years issues stores to the kitchen on a daily basis. No inventory is kept in the production area and there is no access to the stores. To some, this may be overdoing control, but it is hard to fault the results: a good food cost percentage. All items that enter the stores should have a date stamp and be rotated using the first in–first out (FIFO) system.

First in–first out (FIFO) is a simple but effective system of ensuring stock rotation. This is achieved by placing the most recent purchases, in rotation, behind previous purchases. Failure to do this can result in spoilage.

Obviously, restaurants should maintain strict controls. Among the better-known controls are taking inventory regularly, calculating food and beverage cost percentages, having receiving done by a person other than the person who orders, using a par-stock reordering system, using one entrance/exit for employees and not permitting employees to bring bags into the restaurant with them, employing a good accountant, and, yes, checking the garbage!

Budgeting

Budgeting costs fall into two categories: fixed and variable. **Fixed costs** are constant regardless of the volume of business. Fixed costs are rent/lease payments, interest, and depreciation. **Variable costs** fluctuate with the volume of business. Variable costs include controllable expenses such as payroll, benefits, direct operating expense, music and entertainment, marketing and promotion, energy and utility, administrative, and repairs and maintenance.

Regardless of sales fluctuations, variable or controllable expenses vary in some controllable proportion to sales. For example, if a restaurant is open on a Monday, it must have a host, server, cook, dishwasher, and so on. The volume of business and sales total may be $750. However, on Friday that sales total might be $2,250 with just a few more staff. The controllable costs increased only slightly in proportion to the sales, and the fixed costs did not change.

Restaurant Accounting

To operate any business efficiently and effectively, it is necessary to determine the mission, goals, and objectives. One of the most important

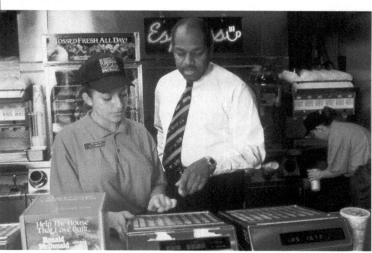

Restaurant managers also need to spend time with staff members.

goals in any enterprise is a fair return on investment, otherwise known as profit. In addition, accounting for the income and expenditures is a necessary part of any business enterprise. The restaurant industry has adopted a uniform system of accounts.

The **uniform system of accounts** for restaurants (USAR) outlines a standard classification and presentation of operating results. The system allows for easy comparison among restaurants because each expense item has the same schedule number.

Balance Sheet

A **balance sheet** for a restaurant, or any business, reflects how the assets and liabilities relate to the owner's equity at a particular moment in time. The balance sheet is mainly used by owners and investors to verify the financial health of the organization. Financial health may be defined in several ways—for example, liquidity, which means having a sufficient amount of cash available to pay bills when they are due, and debt leverage, which is the percentage of a company's assets owned by outside interests (liabilities).

CORPORATE PROFILE

T.G.I. Friday's Restaurant

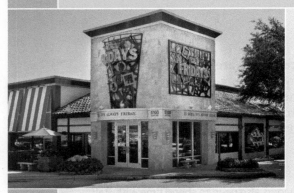

In the spring of 1965, Alan Stillman, a New York perfume salesman, opened a restaurant located at First Avenue and 63rd Street. The restaurant boasted striped awnings, a blue exterior, and yellow supergraphics reading T.G.I. Friday's. Inside were wooden floors covered with sawdust, Tiffany-style lamps, bentwood chairs, red-and-white tablecloths, and a bar area complete with brass rails and stained glass.

T.G.I. Friday's was an immediate success. The restaurant on Manhattan's Upper East Side became the meeting place for single adults.

In 1971, franchisee Dan Scoggin opened a T.G.I. Friday's in Dallas and in four other sites around the country. The success was instant; thus, began the company that is Friday's today.

By 1975, there were ten T.G.I. Friday's in eight states, but the great success that the company had seen was starting to diminish. Dan Scoggin began a countrywide tour to visit each restaurant; he talked with employees, managers, and customers to isolate the roots of successes and failures. This was the critical turning point for the company. The focus shifted from being just another restaurant chain to giving guests exactly what they wanted. The theories and philosophies Scoggin developed are the principles by which Friday's now does business.

T.G.I. Friday's goal was to create a comfortable, relaxing environment where guests could enjoy food and drink. Stained glass windows, wooden airplane propellers, racing sculls, and metal advertising signs comprised the elegant clutter that greeted guests when they entered a T.G.I. Friday's. Nothing was left to chance. Music, lights, air-conditioning, decor, and housekeeping were all designed to keep guests comfortable. Employees were encouraged to display their own personalities and to treat customers as they would guests in their own homes.

As guests demanded more, T.G.I. Friday's provided more—soon becoming the industry leader in menu and drink selection. The menu expanded from a slate chalkboard to an award-winning collection of items representing every taste and mood.

T.G.I. Friday's also became the industry leader in innovation—creating the now-famous Jack Daniel's Grill. This was the first restaurant chain to offer stone-ground whole-wheat bread, avocados, bean sprouts, and Mexican appetizers across the country. As guests' tastes continued to change, T.G.I. Friday's introduced pasta dishes, brunch items, and fettuccine.

America owes the popularization of frozen and ice cream drinks to T.G.I. Friday's, where smooth, alcoholic, and nonalcoholic drinks were made with fresh fruit, juices, ice cream, and yogurt. These recipes were so precise that T.G.I. Friday's drink glasses were scientifically designed for the correct ratio of each ingredient. These specially designed glasses have since become popular throughout the industry.

Through the years, T.G.I. Friday's success has been phenomenal. T.G.I. Friday's is privately owned by Carlson Companies, Inc., of Minneapolis—one of the largest privately held companies in the country. Today, T.G.I. Friday's has come to be known as a casual restaurant where family and friends meet for great food, fun, and conversation. Everyone looks forward to T.G.I. Friday's!

What does it take to be successful in the restaurant business, and what does it take to be a leader? The answers to these questions are crucial to success as a restaurant company. The essentials of success in business are as follows:

1. Treat everyone with respect for their dignity.
2. Treat all customers as if they are honored guests in your home.
3. Remember that all problems result from either poor hiring, lack of training, unclear performance expectations, or accepting less than excellence.
4. Remember that management tools are methods, not objectives.

As you can see, these are principles to guide decision making as opposed to step-by-step actions. However, if these principles are not followed, then actions have very short-term effects. And if you do choose to follow them, they form a base on which you can easily decide which specific actions are necessary in any given situation.

The basics of leadership are as follows:

1. Hire the right people.
2. Train everyone thoroughly and completely.
3. Be sure that everyone clearly understands the performance expectations.
4. Accept only excellence.

Here are the very basics of how to provide strong, clear leadership. However, once again these are only the minimum requirements, not all the qualities necessary to be a good leader. Individual success and that of a company such as T.G.I. Friday's are predicated on understanding and following the essentials of success in business and the basics of leadership. Whether an hourly employee or a manager, it is critical that each employee manage his or her part of the business using these philosophies.

Restaurants are one of the few, fortunate types of businesses to operate on a cash basis for income receivables. There are no outstanding accounts receivable because all sales are in cash—even credit cards are treated as cash because of their prompt payment. Typically, restaurants invest significant funds in assets, such as equipment, furniture, and building (if they own it). The balance sheet will reflect how much of the cost of these assets has been paid for, and are thus owned by the company (owner's equity), and how much is still due to outsiders (liability). Furthermore, the balance sheet will show the extent to which the company has depreciated these assets, thus providing owners and investors with an indication of potential future costs to repair or replace existing assets.

Operating or Income Statement

From an operational perspective, the most important financial document is the operating statement. Once a sales forecast has been completed, the costs of servicing those sales are budgeted on an income statement. Figure 4 shows an example of an income statement for a hypothetical restaurant.

The **income statement**, which is for a month or a year, begins with the food and beverage sales. From this total, the cost of food and beverage is deducted;

	Budgeted	Actual Amount	Percentage	Variance + (−)	Last Period	Same Period Last Year
Sales						
Food						
Beverage						
Others						
Total sales		____	100			
Cost of Sales						
Food						
Beverage						
Others						
Total cost of sales		____				
Gross profit		____				
Controllable Expenses						
Salaries and wages						
Employee benefits						
Direct operating expenses[a]						
Music and entertainment						
Marketing						
Energy and utility						
Administrative and general						
Repairs and maintenance						
Total controllable expenses		____				
Rent and other occupation costs						
Income before interest, depreciation, and taxes						
Interest						
Depreciation						
Net income before taxes						
Income taxes		____				
Net Income		____				

[a]Telephone, insurance, legal, accounting, paper, glass, china, linens, office supplies, landscaping, cleaning supplies, etc.

Figure 4 • Sample Income Statement.

the remaining total is **gross profit**. To this amount, any other income is added (for example, cigarettes, vending machines, outside catering, and telephone income). The next heading is controllable expenses, which includes salaries, wages, employee benefits, direct operating expenses (telephone, insurance, accounting and legal fees, office supplies, paper, china, glass, cutlery, menus, landscaping, and so on), music and entertainment, marketing, energy and utility, administrative and general, repairs and maintenance. The total of this group is called total controllable expenses. Rent and other occupation costs are then deducted from the total, leaving income before interest, depreciation, and taxes. Interest and depreciation are deducted leaving a total of net income before taxes. From this amount, income taxes are paid, leaving the remainder as net income.

Managing the money to the bottom line requires careful scrutiny of all key results, beginning with the big-ticket controllable items such as labor costs, food costs, and beverages, on down to related controllable items. Additionally, management may wish to compare several income statements representing operations over a number of different periods. The ideal method for comparing is to compute every component of each income statement as a percentage of its total sales. Then, compare one period's percentage to another to determine if any significant trends are developing. For example, a manager could compare labor as a percentage of total sales over several months, or years, to assess the impact of rising labor rates on the bottom line. Notice how Figure 4 has columns for budgeted, actual, percentage of sales, variance (+/−) last period, and same period last year. This really gives management good decision-making information.

Operating Ratios

Operating ratios are industry norms that are applicable to each segment of the industry. Experienced restaurant operators rely on these operating ratios to indicate the restaurant's degree of success. Several ratios are good barometers of a restaurant's degree of success. Among the better known ratios are the following:

- Food cost percentage
- Contribution margin
- Labor cost percentage
- Prime cost
- Beverage cost percentage

Food Cost Percentage

The basic **food cost percentage**, for which the formula is cost/sales × 100, is calculated on a daily, weekly, or monthly basis. The procedure works in the following manner:

1. An inventory is taken of all the food and the purchase price of that food. This is called the *opening inventory*.
2. The purchases are totaled for the period and added to the opening inventory.
3. The closing inventory (the inventory at the close of the week or period for which the food cost percentage is being calculated) and returns, spoilage,

complimentary meals, and transfers to other departments are also deducted from the opening inventory plus purchases.

4. This figure is the cost of goods sold. The cost of goods sold is divided by the total sales. The resulting figure is the food cost percentage.

The following example illustrates the procedure:

Food Sales	$3,000
Opening Inventory	1,000
Add Purchases	500
	1,500
Less Spoilage and Complimentary Meals	–100
Less Closing Inventory	–500
Cost of Goods Sold	$900

$$\frac{\text{Food Cost}(\$900)}{\text{Sales}(\$3,000)} \times 100 = 30\% \text{ Food Cost Percentage}$$

The food cost percentage calculations become slightly more complicated when the cost of staff meals, management meals and entertaining (complimentary meals), and guest food returned are all properly calculated.

Food cost percentage has long been used as a yardstick for measuring the skill of the chef, cooks, and management to achieve a predetermined food cost percentage—usually 28 to 32 percent for a full-service restaurant and a little higher for a high-volume, fast-food restaurant.

Controlling food costs begins with cost-effective purchasing systems, a controlled storage and issuing system, and strict control of the food production and sales. The best way to visualize a food cost control system is to think of the food as money. Consider a $100 bill arriving at the back door: If the wrong people get their hands on that money, it does not reach the guest or the bottom line.

Contribution Margin

More recently, attention has focused not only on the food cost percentage but also on the contribution margin. The **contribution margin** is the amount that a menu item contributes to the gross profit, or the difference between the cost of the item and its sales price. Some menu items contribute more than others; therefore, restaurant operators focus more attention on the items that produce a higher contribution margin. It works like this:

The cost of the chicken dish is $2.00, and its selling price is $9.95, which leaves a contribution margin of $7.95. The fish, which costs a little more at $3.25, sells for $12.75 and leaves a contribution of $9.50. The pasta cost price of $1.50 and selling price of $8.95 leave a contribution margin of $7.45. Under this scenario, it would be better for the restaurant to sell more fish because each plate will yield $1.55 more than if chicken were sold.

Labor Cost Percentage

Labor costs are the highest single cost factor in staffing a restaurant. Fast-food restaurants have the lowest **labor costs percentage** (about 16 to 18 percent), with family and ethnic restaurants at about 22 to 26 percent and upscale full-service restaurants at about 30 to 35 percent.

Labor costs include salaries and wages of employees, employee benefits, and their training. Foodservice is a highly labor-intensive industry, depending on the type of restaurant. Quick-service restaurants have a lower payroll cost primarily because of their limited menu and limited service. Good managers try to manage their labor costs by accurate hiring and scheduling of staff according to the restaurant's cover turnover.

The labor cost is calculated by taking the total cost of labor for a period, say $200,000, and dividing it by the total sales for the same period, $800,000, and multiplying it by 100.

$$\frac{\text{Labor Cost}}{\text{Sales}} \frac{\$200,000}{\$800,000} \times 100 = 25\%$$

Prime Cost

Combined food and labor costs are known as **prime cost**. To allow for a reasonable return on investment, prime cost should not go above 60 to 65 percent of sales.

There are various methods of control, beginning with effective scheduling based on the expected volume of business. In reality, because of the high cost of labor, today's restaurateur manages by the minute. Once a rush is over, the effective manager thanks employees for doing a great job and looks forward to seeing them again. This may appear to be micromanagement, but an analysis of restaurant operations does not leave any alternatives.[13]

$$\text{Food cost} + \text{Labor cost percentage} = \text{Prime cost}$$

Beverage Cost Percentage

The **beverage cost percentage** is calculated like the food cost percentage. The method used most often is to first determine the unit cost and then mark up by the required percentage to arrive at the selling price. This is rounded up or down to a convenient figure. The actual beverage cost percentage is then compared with the anticipated cost percentage; any discrepancy is investigated.

The NRA publishes guidelines for restaurant operations. These valuable documents help provide a guide for operators to use when comparing their restaurants with other similar establishments. If the costs go above the budgeted or expected levels, then management must investigate and take corrective action.

Beverage cost is calculated by taking the costs of beverages and dividing it by the total beverage sales and multiplying by 100.

$$\frac{\text{Cost of beverage sales}}{\text{Total beverage sales}} \times 100 \quad \text{For example} \quad \frac{4,250}{19,479} \times 100 = 21.82\%$$

Therefore, if for a casual Italian restaurant, industry comparisons would show the following:

Labor costs at 20 to 24 percent of sales

Food costs at 28 to 32 percent of food sales

Beverage costs at 18 to 24 percent of beverage sales

INTRODUCING RAY KROC

Founder of McDonald's

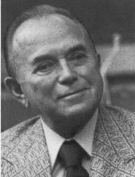

The world's greatest fast-food success story is undoubtedly McDonald's. Back in the 1950s, Ray Kroc was selling soda fountains. He received an order from Mr. McDonald for two soda fountains. Ray Kroc was so interested in finding out why the McDonald brothers' restaurant needed two machines (everyone else ordered one) that he went out to the restaurant. There he saw the now-familiar golden arches and the hamburger restaurant. Ray persuaded the McDonalds to let him franchise their operation. Billions of burgers later, the reason for the success may be summarized as follows: quality, speed, cleanliness, service, and value. This has been achieved by systemizing the production process and by staying close to the original concept—keeping a limited menu, advertising heavily, being innovative with new menu items, maintaining product quality, and being consistent.

Of all hospitality entrepreneurs, Ray Kroc has been the most successful financially. In 1982, he was senior chairman of the board of McDonald's, an organization intent on covering the earth with hamburgers. Among the remarkable things about Kroc is that it was not until age 52 that he embarked on the royal road to fame and fortune.

The original McDonald's concept was created by two brothers, Richard and Maurice, who had no interest in expanding. The McDonald brothers were content with their profitable yet singular restaurant in San Bernardino, California. However, the golden arches impressed Kroc, as did the cleanliness and simplicity of the operation.

Kroc's organizational skills, perseverance, and incredible aptitude for marketing were his genius. His talent also extended to selecting close associates who were equally dedicated and who added financial, analytical, and managerial skills to the enterprise. Kroc remained the spark plug and master merchandiser until he died in 1984, leaving a multimillion-dollar legacy.

Much of Kroc's $400 million has gone to employees, hospitals, and the Marshall Field Museum. It is distributed through Kroc's own foundation. Most important, Kroc developed several operational guidelines, including the concepts of KISS—keep it simple, stupid—and QSC&V—quality, service, cleanliness, and value. Kroc's "Never Be Idle a Moment" motto was also incorporated into the business.

Enterprises such as McDonald's are not built without ample dedication, and Ray Kroc certainly had a wealth of dedication. Today, an average McDonald's franchise can net more than $1 million annually thanks to Kroc's ingenious marketing strategies. In fact, McDonald's Corporation has become so affluent that it was named *Entrepreneur* magazine's number-one franchise.

Lease and Controllable Expenses

Lease Costs

Successful restaurant operators will ensure that the restaurant's lease does not cost more than 5 to 8 percent of sales. Some chain restaurants will search for months or even years before they find the right location at the right price. Most leases are triple net, which means that the lessee must pay for all alterations, insurance, utilities, and possible commercial fees (e.g., landscaping or parking upkeep, security).

The best lease is for the longest time period with options for renewal and a sublease clause. The sublease clause is important because if the restaurant is not successful, the owner is still liable for paying the lease. With the sublease clause, the owner may sublease the space to another restaurant operator or any other business.

Many leases are quoted at a dollar rate per square foot per month. Depending on the location, rates may range from $2.25 per square foot up to as much as $16 or more per square foot.

Some restaurants pay a combination of a flat amount based on the square footage and a percentage of sales. This helps protect the restaurant operator in the slower months and gives the landlord a bit extra during the good months.

After a lease contract is signed, it is very difficult to renegotiate even a part of it. Only in dire circumstances is it possible to renegotiate lease contracts. The governing factor in determining lease rates is the marketplace. The marketplace is the supply and demand. If there is strong demand for space, then rates will increase. However, with a high vacancy rate, rates will be driven down by the owners in an effort to rent space and gain income.

Controllable Expenses

Controllable expenses are all the expenses over which management and ownership have control. They include salaries and wages (payroll) and related benefits; direct operating expenses such as music and entertainment; marketing, including sales, advertising, public relations, and promotions; heat, light, and power; administrative and general expenses; and repairs and maintenance. The total of all controllable expenses is deducted from the gross profit. Rent and other occupation costs are then deducted to arrive at the income before interest, depreciation, and taxes. Once these are deducted, the **net profit** remains.

Successful restaurant operators are constantly monitoring their controllable expenses. The largest controllable expense is payroll. Because payroll is about 24 to 28 percent of a restaurant's sales, managers constantly monitor their employees, not by the hour but by the minute. Bobby Hays, general manager of the Chart House Restaurant in Cardiff, California, says that he feels the pulse of the restaurant and then begins to send people home. Every dollar that Bobby and managers like him can save goes directly to the bottom line and becomes profit.

The actual sales results are compared with the budgeted amounts—ideally with percentages—and variances are investigated. Most chain restaurant operators monitor the key result areas of sales and labor costs on a daily basis. Food and beverage costs are also monitored closely, generally on a weekly basis.

▶ Check Your Knowledge

1. What is the back of the house?

2. Create a recognition program that would encourage restaurant employees.

3. What is the storing/issuing process? Why is it important?

4. Briefly explain the term *contribution margin*.

Restaurant Manager Job Analysis

The NRA has formulated an analysis of the foodservice manager's job by functional areas and tasks, which follows a natural sequence of functional areas from human resources to sanitation and safety.

Human Resource Management

Recruiting/Training

1. Recruit new employees by seeking referrals.
2. Recruit new employees by advertising.
3. Recruit new employees by seeking help from district manager/supervisors.
4. Interview applicants for employment.

Orientation/Training

1. Conduct on-site orientation for new employees.
2. Explain employee benefits and compensation programs.
3. Plan training programs for employees.
4. Conduct on-site training for employees.
5. Evaluate progress of employees during training.
6. Supervise on-site training of employees that is conducted by another manager, employee leader, trainer, and so on.
7. Conduct payroll signup.
8. Complete reports or other written documentation on successful completion of training by employees.

Scheduling for Shifts

1. Review employee work schedule for shift.
2. Determine staffing needs for each shift.
3. Make work assignments for dining room, kitchen staff, and maintenance person(s).
4. Make changes to employee work schedule.
5. Assign employees to work stations to optimize employee effectiveness.
6. Call in, reassign, or send home employees in reaction to sales and other needs.
7. Approve requests for schedule changes, vacation, days off, and so on.

Supervision and Employee Development

1. Observe employees and give immediate feedback on unsatisfactory employee performance.
2. Observe employees and give immediate feedback on satisfactory employee performance.
3. Discuss unsatisfactory performance with an employee.
4. Develop and deliver incentive for above-satisfactory performance of employees.

5. Observe employee behavior for compliance with safety and security.

6. Counsel employees on work-related problems.

7. Counsel employees on non-work-related problems.

8. Talk with employees who have frequent absences.

9. Observe employees to ensure compliance with fair labor standards and equal opportunity guidelines.

10. Discipline employees by issuing oral and/or written warnings for poor performance.

11. Conduct employee and staff meetings.

12. Identify and develop candidates for management programs.

13. Put results of observation of employee performance in writing.

14. Develop action plans for employees to help them in their performance.

15. Authorize promotion and/or wage increases for staff.

16. Terminate employment of an employee for unsatisfactory performance.

Financial Management

Accounting

1. Authorize payment on vendor invoices.

2. Verify payroll.

3. Count cash drawers.

4. Prepare bank deposits.

5. Assist in establishment audits by management or outside auditors.

6. Balance cash at end of shift.

7. Analyze profit and loss reports for establishment.

Cost Control

1. Discuss factors that affect profitability with district manager/supervisor.

2. Check establishment figures for sales, labor costs, waste, inventory, and so on.

Administrative Management

Scheduling/Coordinating

1. Establish objectives for shift based on needs of establishment.

2. Coordinate work performed by different shifts—for example, cleanup, routine maintenance, and so on.

3. Complete special projects assigned by district manager/supervisor.

4. Complete shift readiness checklist.

Planning

1. Develop and implement action plans to meet financial goals.

2. Attend off-site workshops and training sessions.

Communication

1. Communicate with management team by reading and making entries in daily communication log.
2. Prepare written reports on cleanliness, food quality, personnel, inventory, sales, food waste, labor costs, and so on.
3. Review reports prepared by other establishment managers.
4. Review memos, reports, and letters from company headquarters/main office.
5. Inform district manager/supervisor of problems or developments that affect operation and performance of the establishment.
6. Initiate and answer correspondence with company, vendors, and so on.
7. File correspondence, reports, personnel records, and so on.

Marketing Management

1. Create and execute local establishment marketing activities.
2. Develop opportunities for the establishment to provide community services.
3. Carry out special product promotions.

Operations Management

Facility Maintenance

1. Conduct routine maintenance checks on facility and equipment.
2. Direct routine maintenance checks on facility and equipment.
3. Repair or supervise the repair of equipment.
4. Review establishment evaluations with district manager/supervisor.
5. Authorize the repair of equipment by outside contractor.
6. Recommend upgrades in facility and equipment.

Food and Beverage Operations Management

1. Direct activities for opening establishment.
2. Direct activities for closing establishment.
3. Talk with other managers at beginning and end of shift to relay information about ongoing problems and activities.
4. Count, verify, and report inventory.
5. Receive, inspect, and verify vendor deliveries.
6. Check stock levels and submit orders as necessary.
7. Talk with vendors concerning quality of product delivered.
8. Interview vendors who wish to sell products to establishment.
9. Check finished product quality and act to correct problems.
10. Work as expediter to get meals served effectively.

11. Inspect dining area, kitchen, rest rooms, food lockers, storage, and parking lot.
12. Check daily reports for indications of internal theft.
13. Instruct employees regarding the control of waste, portion sizes, and so on.
14. Prepare forecast for daily or shift food preparation.

Service

1. Receive and record table reservations.
2. Greet familiar customers by name.
3. Seat customers.
4. Talk with customers while they are dining.
5. Monitor service times and procedures in the dining area.
6. Observe customers being served to correct problems.
7. Ask customers about quality of service.
8. Ask customers about quality of the food product.
9. Listen to and resolve customer complaints.
10. Authorize complimentary meals or beverages.
11. Write letters in response to customer complaints.
12. Telephone customers in response to customer complaints.
13. Secure and return items left by customers.

Sanitation and Safety

1. Accompany local officials on health inspections on premise.
2. Administer first aid to employees and customers.
3. Submit accident, incident, and OSHA reports.
4. Report incidents to police.
5. Observe employee behavior and establishment conditions for compliance with safety and security procedures.

Recycling

At the end of the night at most restaurants, leftover food, paper, bottles, and cardboard typically are put in a Dumpster in the back alley, destined for a landfill. Separating garbage is dirty; it requires people and time to do it. But, several operators say making minor changes reduces trash and helps budgets. Zero waste is how Nomad Café in Berkeley, California, prefers to operate its business. It saves more than $10,000 every year by recycling and composting. Making simple changes to its daily routine of throwing out garbage also aided Scoma's in San Francisco. It color-coded the system and got staff into the habit of recycling. Scoma's saves an average of $2,000 per month.[14]

Trends in Restaurant Operations

- More flavorful food
- Increased takeout meals, especially at lunch, and more home meal replacement (for dinner)
- Increased food safety and sanitation
- Guests becoming more sophisticated and needing more things to excite them
- More food court restaurants in malls, movie theater complexes, and colleges and universities where guests line up (similar to a cafeteria), select their food (which a server places on a tray), and pay a cashier
- Steak houses becoming more popular
- With more restaurants in each segment, the segments increasingly split into upper, middle, and lower tiers
- Twin and multi-restaurant locations
- Quick-service restaurants (QSRs) in convenience stores
- The economy beginning to pick up, which is good news for many restaurants, especially fine-dining, high-end steakhouses

CASE STUDY

Short-Staffed in the Kitchen

Sally is the general manager of one of the best restaurants in town, known as The Pub. As usual, at 6:00 P.M. on a Friday night, there is a forty-five-minute wait. The kitchen is overloaded, and they are running behind in check times, the time that elapses between the kitchen getting the order and the guest receiving his or her meal. This is critical, especially if a complaint is received because a guest has waited too long for a meal to be served.

Sally is waiting for her two head line cooks to come in for the closing shift. It is now 6:15 P.M. and she receives phone calls from both of them. Unfortunately, they are both sick with the flu and are not able to come to work.

As she gets off the phone, the hostess tells Sally that a party of fifty is scheduled to arrive at 7:30 P.M. Sally is concerned, knowing that they are currently running a six-person line with only four cooks. The productivity is very high, but they are running extremely long check times. How can Sally handle the situation?

Discussion Questions

1. How would you handle the short-staffing issue?
2. What measures would you take to get the appropriate cooks in to work as soon as possible?
3. What would you do to ensure a smooth, successful transition for the party of fifty?
4. How would you manipulate your floor plan to provide great service for the party of fifty?
5. How would you immediately make an impact on the long check times?
6. What should you do to ensure that all the guests in the restaurant are happy?

CASE STUDY

Shortage in Stock

It is 9:30 Friday morning at The Pub. Product is scheduled to be delivered at 10:00. Sally specifically ordered an exceptional amount of food for the upcoming weekend because she is projecting it to be a busy holiday weekend. Sally receives a phone call at 10:30 from J&G Groceries, stating that they cannot deliver the product until 10:00 A.M. on Saturday morning. She explains to the driver that it is crucial that she receives the product as soon as possible. He apologizes; however, it is impossible to have delivery made until Saturday morning.

By 1:00 P.M., they are beginning to run out of product, including absolute necessities such as steaks, chicken, fish, and produce. The guests are getting frustrated because the staff are beginning to eighty-six a great deal of product. In addition, if they do not begin production for the P.M. shift soon, they will be in deep trouble.

On Friday nights, The Pub does in excess of $12,000 in sales. However, if the problem is not immediately alleviated, the restaurant will lose many guests and a great amount of profits.

Discussion Questions

1. What immediate measures would you take to resolve the problem?
2. How would you produce the appropriate product as soon as possible?
3. Who should you call first, if anyone, to alleviate the problem?
4. What can you do to always have enough product on hand?
5. Is it important to have a backup plan for a situation like this? If so, what would it be?

Summary

1. Most restaurants forecast on a weekly and monthly basis a budget that projects sales and costs for a year in consideration of guest counts and the average guest check.
2. To operate a restaurant, products need to be purchased, received, and properly stored.
3. Food production is determined by the expected business for the next few days. The kitchen layout is designed according to the sales forecasted.
4. Good service is very important. In addition to taking orders, servers act as salespersons for the restaurant.
5. The front of the house deals with the part of the restaurant having direct contact with guests, in other words, what the guests see—grounds maintenance, hosts/hostesses, dining and bar areas, bartenders, bussers, and so on.
6. The back of the house is generally run by the kitchen manager and refers to all areas with which guests usually do not come in contact. This includes purchasing, receiving, storing/issuing, food production, stewarding, budgeting, accounting, and control.

Key Words and Concepts

average guest check
back of the house
balance sheet
beverage cost percentage
budgeting costs
contribution margin
controllable expense
cooking line
covers
curbside appeal
employee recognition
first in–first out (FIFO)
fixed costs
food cost percentage
front of the house
gross profit
guest counts
host/hostess

income statement
kitchen manager
labor costs percentage
net profit
operating ratios
par stock
personal digital assistants (PDAs)
point-of-sale (POS) systems
prime cost
product specification
production control sheets
purchase order
receiving
restaurant forecasting
suggestive selling
uniform system of accounts
variable costs

Review Questions

1. Briefly describe the two components of restaurant forecasting.
2. Explain the key points in purchasing, receiving, and storing.
3. Why is the kitchen layout an important aspect of food production?
4. Explain the purpose of suggestive selling. What characteristics make up a good server?
5. Accounting is important to determine the profitability of a restaurant. Briefly describe the following terms:
   (a) Controllable expenses

   (b) Uniform system of accounts
   (c) Prime cost
6. What is the point-of-sales system, and why is a control system important for a restaurant operation?
7. What are the differences between the back of the house and the front of the house?
8. What steps must one take in preparing production sheets?

Internet Exercises

1. Organization: **National Restaurant Association (NRA)**
   Web site: **www.restaurant.org**
   Summary: The NRA is the business association of the food industry. It consists of 60,000 members and more than 380,000 restaurants. Member restaurants represent table service and quick-service operators,

chains, and franchises. The NRA helps international restaurants receive the benefits of the association and gives guidance for success to nonprofit members.

   (a) List the food-borne diseases listed on the NRA site. Find out about each disease and how the National Restaurant Association suggests you can prevent it.

(b) What kinds of careers are available in the restaurant and hospitality industry?

(c) What legal issues does this site advise you on if you want to start your own restaurant?

2. Organization: **Chili's Grill and Bar**
   Web site: **www.chilis.com**
   Summary: Chili's is a fun and exciting place to have burgers, fajitas, margaritas, and chili. Established in 1975 in Dallas, the chain now has more than 1,500 restaurants in the United States and twenty-nine other countries.

   (a) What requirements must you meet to open a Chili's franchise? From what you have learned about the issues involved in starting your own business, how is setting up your own business different from having a franchise?

   (b) What is a "ChiliHead"?

Apply Your Knowledge

In a casual Italian restaurant, sales for the week of September 15 are as follows:

Food sales	$10,000
Beverage sales	$2,500
Total	$12,500

1. If the food cost is 30 percent, how much did the food actually cost?
2. If the beverage cost is 25 percent of beverage sales, how much did the beverages cost?
3. If the total labor cost is 28 percent, how much money does that represent and how much is left over for other costs and profit?

Suggested Activities

1. Divide into groups of two and assign the roles of guest and server. Role-play using the concept of suggestive selling and upselling.

2. Create an income statement for an imaginary restaurant.

Endnotes

1. This section draws from John R. Walker, *The Restaurant from Concept to Operation*, 6th ed. (Hoboken, NJ: John Wiley and Sons, 2011), 86–87.
2. Personal conversation with Danny Meyer, January 14, 2004.
3. This section is adapted from http://www.starchefs.com/features/trends/30_sustainability_tips/index.shtml, retrieved March 10, 2010.
4. SoftCafé, *Make Menus on Your PC—In Minutes*, www.softcafe.com/menupro.htm. (accessed November 6, 2011).
5. Personal correspondence with Magic Software, Tampa, Florida, July 29, 2007.
6. Dusty Williams, Information Technologists," www.restaurantmagic.com/informationTech.php.
7. Data Central, "Welcome to Data Central," www.restaurantmagic.com/home.php (accessed April 2, 2011; site now discontinued).
8. Personal correspondence with James Lorenz, May 16, 2011.
9. Richard Slawsky, "Sustainable Farming Grows on Chefs," *QSR Web*, March 8, 2007, www.qsrweb.com/article.php?id=7025 (accessed November 7, 2011).
10. Chipotle, *2010 Annual Report & Proxy Statement*, http://phx.corporate-ir.net/External.File?item=UGFyZW50SUQ9NDIxMjg4fENoaWxkSUQ9NDM4OTQzfFR5cGU9MQ==&t=1 (accessed November 7, 2011).
11. This section draws from Walker, *Restaurant from Concept to Operation*, 275.
12. Walker, *Restaurant from Concept to Operation*, 275.
13. Personal conversation with Bobby Hays, general manager, Chart House Restaurant, Solana Beach, California, January 2011.
14. Jamie Popp, "Trash Talk," *Restaurants and Institutions* 116 (May 1, 2006): 75.

Glossary

Average guest check The average amount each group spends; used primarily in a restaurant setting.

Back-of-the-house The support areas behind the scenes in a hotel or motel, including housekeeping, laundry, engineering, and foodservice. Also refers to individuals who operate behind the scenes to make a guest's stay pleasant and safe.

Balance sheet Itemizes a business's assets and liabilities with regard to the owner's equity at a particular moment in time.

Beverage cost percentage Similar to food cost percentage, except that it relates to beverages.

Budgeting costs To allocate costs of operating.

Contribution margin Key operating figure in menu engineering, determined by subtracting food cost from selling price as a measure of profitability.

Controllable expenses Expenses that can be controlled by means of cost-effective purchasing systems, a controlled storage and issuing system, and strict control of food production and sales. These expenses are usually watched over by management.

Covers The guest count of a restaurant.

Curbside appeal Visual appeal and cleanliness designed to encourage people to dine in a particular restaurant.

First-in first-out (FIFO) The supplies that are ordered first are used first.

Fixed cost A cost or expense for a fixed period and range of activity that does not change in total but becomes progressively smaller per unit as volume increases.

Food cost percentage A ratio comparing the cost of food sold to food sales, which is calculated by dividing the cost of food sold during a given period by food sales during the same period.

Front-of-the-house Comprises all areas with which guests come in contact, including the lobby, corridors, elevators, guest rooms, restaurants and bars, meeting rooms, and restrooms. Also refers to employees who staff these areas.

Gross profit The amount a business earns after paying to produce or buy its products but before deducting operating expenses; the difference between sales and the cost of goods sold.

Guest counts (covers) The number of guests dining in a restaurant.

Host/hostess A greeter and "seater" at the entrance of a restaurant.

Income statement A report that lists the amount of money or its equivalent received during a period of time in exchange for labor or services, from the sale of goods or property, or as profit from financial investments.

Kitchen manager The individual who manages the kitchen department.

Labor cost percentage Similar to food cost percentage, except that it relates to labor. The formula is: Labor costs divided by net sales multiplied by 100 equals the labor cost percentage.

Net profit The amount remaining when a business makes a profit which is sales less all expenses.

Operating ratios Ratios that indicate an operation's performance.

Par stock The level of stock that must be kept on hand at all times. If the stock on hand falls below this point, a computerized reorder system automatically reorders a predetermined quantity of the stock.

Personal digital assistant (PDA) A computer system that transmits information or orders and retrieves and posts guest payments; often used in restaurants to improve time management and allow faster service.

Point-of-sale (POS) system A system used in restaurants and outlet stores that records and posts charges; consists of a number of POS terminals that interface with a remote central processing unit.

Prime cost The cost of food sold plus payroll cost (including employee benefits). This is the largest segment of a restaurant's costs.

Product specification The establishment of standards for each product, determined by the purchaser. For example, when ordering meat, the product specification includes the cut, weight, size, percentage of fat content, and so forth.

Production control sheet A checklist/sheet itemizing the production.

Receiving The back-of-the-house area devoted to receiving goods.

Restaurant forecasting The process of estimating the number of future guests, their menu preferences, and the revenue from them.

Variable cost A cost that varies according to the volume of business.

Photo Credits

Credits are listed in the order of appearance.

Fotolia
Dorling Kindersley
John Self
Doug Menuez/Getty Images, Inc. – Photodisc, RF
MICROS
SoftCafe, LLC

MICROS
T.G.I. Friday's
Michael Newman/PhotoEdit
T.G.I. Friday's
Bettmann/Corbis

Managed Services

From Chapter 8 of *Introduction to Hospitality Management,* Fourth Edition. John R. Walker. Copyright © 2013 by Pearson Education, Inc. Published by Pearson. All rights reserved.

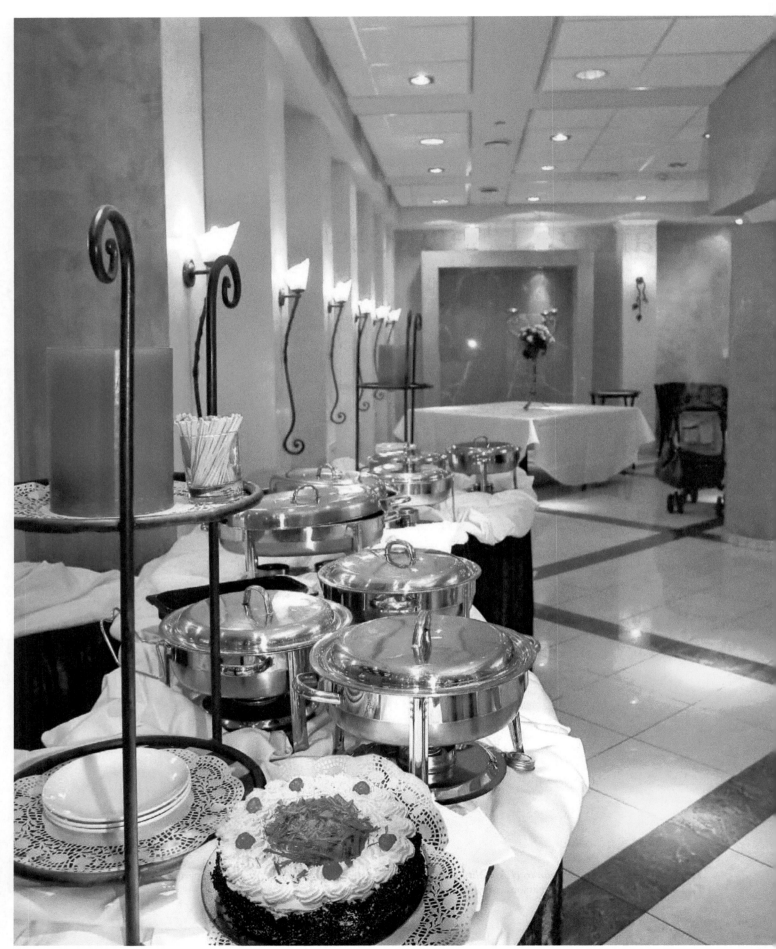

Managed Services

OBJECTIVES

After reading and studying this chapter, you should be able to:

- Outline the different managed services segments.

- Describe the five factors that distinguish managed services operations from commercial ones.

- Explain the need for and trends in elementary and secondary school foodservice.

- Describe the complexities in college and university foodservice.

- Identify characteristics and trends in health care, business and industry, and leisure and recreation foodservices.

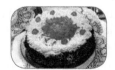
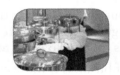
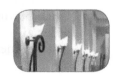
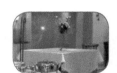

Overview

Managed services consist of foodservice and related operations, including the following:

- Airlines
- Military
- Elementary and secondary schools
- Colleges and universities
- Health care facilities
- Business and industry
- Leisure and recreation organizations
- Conference centers
- Airports
- Travel plazas

Companies and organizations such as educational or health care organizations decide if they want to operate their foodservice and related operations themselves or whether they want to contract them out to a managed services company. If they decide to operate their own foodservice, they may realize some cost savings, but if they lack the expertise, they may prefer to invite contractors to submit proposals. The company or organization can then invite contractors to make a presentation and to formally discuss and finalize all contractual details.

Several features distinguish managed services operations from **commercial foodservices** such as restaurants:

- In a restaurant, the challenge is to please the guest. In managed services, it is necessary to meet both the needs of the guest and the client (that is, the institution itself).

- In some operations, the guests may or may not have alternative dining options available to them and are a captive clientele. These guests may be eating at the foodservice operation only once or on a daily basis.

- Many managed operations are housed in host organizations that do not have foodservice as their primary business.

- Most managed services operations produce food in large-quantity batches for service and consumption within fixed time periods. For example, **batch cooking** means to produce a batch of food to serve at 11:30 A.M., another batch to serve at 12:15 P.M., and a third batch to serve at 12:45 P.M., rather than putting out all the food for the whole lunch period at 11:30 A.M. This gives the guests who come to eat later in the serving period as good a quality meal as those who came to eat earlier.

- The volume of business is more consistent and therefore easier to cater. Because it is easier to predict the number of meals and portion sizes, it is easier to plan, organize, produce, and serve meals; therefore, the atmosphere is less hurried than that of a restaurant. Weekends tend to be quieter than weekdays in managed services and, overall, the hours and benefits may be better than those of commercial restaurants.

A company or organization might contract its food- or other services for the following reasons:

- Financial
- Quality of program
- Recruitment of management and staff
- Expertise in management of service departments
- Resources available: people, programs, management systems, information systems
- Labor relations and other support
- Outsourcing of administrative functions[1]

Airlines and Airports

In-Flight and Airport Foodservice

When airlines do provide meals, foodservice either comes from their own *in-flight* business or they have the service provided by a contractor. In-flight food may be prepared in a factory mode at a facility close to but outside of the airport. In these cases, the food is prepared and packaged; then, it is transported to the departure gates for the appropriate flights. Once the food is loaded onto the aircraft, flight attendants take over serving the food and beverages to passengers.

In-flight foodservice is a complex logistical operation: The food must be able to withstand the transport conditions and the extended hot or cold holding period from the time it is prepared until the time it is served. If a food item is to be served hot, it must be able to rethermalize well on the plate. The meal should also look appetizing and taste good. Finally, all food and beverage items must be delivered on time and correctly to each departing aircraft.

Gate Gourmet is the largest in-flight food and related services provider, operating in twenty-eight countries on six continents from 122 flight kitchens and producing 250 million meals on average annually.[2] It is estimated that sales will exceed $2 billion, supported by more than 26,000 employees.

Another major player in the in-flight food service market is LSG Sky Chefs, headquartered in Neu-Isenburg, Germany. The LSG Sky Chefs group has the vision to "be the global leader in airline catering and the management of all in-flight service related processes."[3] LSG Sky Chefs consists of 130 companies with more than 200 customer service centers in 50 countries. In 2010, it produced about 460 million airline meals for more than 300 airlines worldwide.[4] The in-flight food and related services management operators plan the menus, develop the product specifications, and arrange the purchasing contracts. Each airline has a representative who oversees one or more locations and checks on the quality, quantity, and delivery times of all food and beverage items.

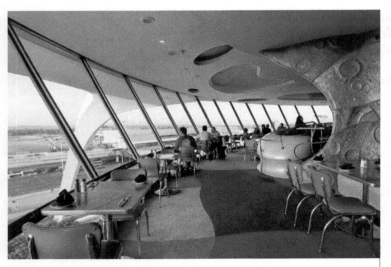

Airport restaurants from quick service to casual fine dining have seen an upswing in business as a result of the airlines cutting back on in-flight foodservice. Encounter is a restaurant at LAX (Los Angeles International Airport).

Airlines regard in-flight foodservice as an expense that needs to be controlled. To trim costs, most domestic airlines now sell snacks instead of meals on a number of short flights and even on flights that span main meal times. Both Gate Gourmet and Sky Chefs also now operate onboard retail solutions for most airlines.

International airlines try to stand out by offering superior food and beverages in hopes of attracting more passengers, especially the higher-paying business and first-class passenger. Others reduce or eliminate foodservice as a strategic decision to support lower fares. Because of the length of the flight, and the higher price paid for the ticket, international flights have better-quality food and beverage service.

On board, each aircraft has two or three categories of service, usually coach, business, and first class. First- and business-class passengers usually receive free beverages and upgraded meal items and service. These meals may consist of such items as fresh salmon or filet mignon; the rest of us get those "carry-on doggie-bags"!

A number of smaller regional and local foodservice operators contract to a variety of airlines at hundreds of airports. Most airports have caterers or foodservice contractors who compete for airline contracts. With several international and U.S. airlines all using U.S. airports, each airline must decide whether to use its own foodservice (if it has one) or to contract with one of several independent operators.

As airlines have decreased their in-flight foodservice, airport restaurants have picked up the business. Popular chain restaurants such as T.G.I. Friday's and Chili's are in several terminals, along with the quick-service restaurants such as McDonald's and Pizza Hut. These restaurants supplement airport foodservice offered by local restaurants.

▶ Check Your Knowledge

1. What are managed services?
2. Why would companies use contract management?

Military

Military foodservice is a large and important component of managed services. There are about 1.5 million soldiers, sailors, and aviators on active duty in the United States. Even with the military downsizing, foodservice sales top $6 billion per year. Base closings have prompted many military foodservice organizations to rethink services and concepts to better meet the needs of their personnel.

CORPORATE PROFILE

Sodexo

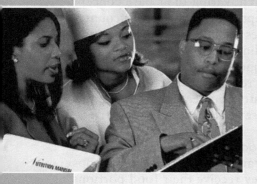

Sodexo, Inc., is a leading solutions company in North America, delivering on-site service solutions in corporate, education, health care, government, and remote site segments. Sodexo's mission is twofold: Improve the quality of daily life and contribute to the economic, social, and environmental development of the cities, regions, and countries in which it operates.

This company is also a member of the international Sodexo Alliance that was founded in 1966 by a Frenchman named Pierre Bellon with its first service provider in Marseille, France. Primarily serving schools, restaurants, and hospitals, the company soon became internationally successful by signing deals with Belgian foodservice contractors. In 1980, after considerable success in Europe, Africa, and the Middle East, Sodexo Alliance decided to expand its reach into North and South America. In 1997, the company joined with Universal Ogden Services, a leading U.S. remote-site service provider. The empire grew a year later when Sodexo Alliance and Marriott Management Services merged. The merger created a new company called Sodexo Marriott Services. Listed on the New York Stock Exchange, the new company became the market leader in food and management services in the United States. At that time, Sodexo Alliance was the biggest shareholder, holding 48.4 percent of shares on the company's capital. In 2001, however, Sodexo Alliance acquired 53 percent of the shares in Sodexo Marriott Services, which changed its name to simply Sodexo.

Today, Sodexo has more than 380,000 employees at 34,000 sites in 80 countries and serves 50 million consumers daily. In the United States, there are 120,000 employees. The goal of Sodexo is to improve the quality and life of customers and clients all over the United States and Canada. They offer outsourcing solutions to the health care, corporate, and education markets. This includes the following services: housekeeping, groundskeeping, foodservice, plant operation and maintenance, and integrated facilities management.

Sodexo's mission is to create and offer services that contribute to a more pleasant way of life for people wherever and whenever they come together. Its challenge is to continue to make its mission and values come alive through the way in which employees work together to serve the clients and customers. The values of Sodexo are service spirit, team spirit, and spirit of progress.

A leading provider of food and facilities management services in North America, Sodexo provides its services at more than 6,000 locations, including corporations, colleges and universities, health care organizations, and school districts. They are always looking to develop talent. Sodexo offers internships in foodservice and facilities management businesses as well as in staff positions such as finance, human resources, marketing, and sales. Sodexo believes that workforce diversity is essential to the company's growth and long-term success. By valuing and managing diversity at work, Sodexo can leverage the skills, knowledge, and abilities of all employees to increase employee, client, and customer satisfaction.

Sodexo has received numerous awards; among them are as follows: top ranked in the "services" category of 2010 Global Outsourcing; recognized as a Worldwise Supersector Leader for commitment to sustainable development; named one of the world's most ethical companies; number one of World's Most Admired Companies by Fortune Magazine and One of the best companies for Hourly Workers by *Working Mother* magazine.

Source: This feature draws on the following Sodexo web sites: Sodexo: *Identity & Key Figures*, http://www.sodexo.com/en/group/profile/key/figures.aspx (accessed November 8, 2011); Sodexo USA, About Us, http://www.sodexousa.com/usen/aboutus/aboutus.asp (accessed November 8, 2011).

Recent trends in military foodservice call for services such as officers' clubs to be contracted out to foodservice management companies. This change has reduced military costs because many of the officers' clubs lost money. The clubs now have moved the emphasis from fine dining to a more casual approach with family appeal. Many clubs are renovating their base concept even further, restyling according to theme concepts, such as sports or country western, for example. Other cost-saving measures include menu management, such as the use of a single menu for lunch and dinner (guests seldom eat both meals at the clubs). With proper plating techniques and portion size manipulation, a single menu (the same menu) can be created for lunch and dinner, meaning one inventory for both meals and less stock in general. To make this technique work successfully, the menu features several choices for appetizers, entrees, and desserts.

Another trend is the testing of prepared foods that can be reheated and served without much labor. Technological advances mean that field troops do not eat out of tin cans anymore; instead, they receive their food portions in plastic-and-foil pouches called meals ready-to-eat (MREs). Today, mobile field kitchens can be run by just two people, and bulk food supplies have been replaced by preportioned, precooked food packed in trays, which then are reheated in boiling water.

Feeding military personnel includes feeding troops and officers in clubs, dining halls, and military hospitals, as well as in the field. As both the budget and the numbers of personnel decrease, the military is downsizing by consolidating responsibilities. With fewer people to cook for, fewer cooks are required.

A model for such downsizing is the U.S. Marine Corps, which contracts out foodservice. With smaller numbers, they could not afford to take a marine away from training to work in the dining facilities without affecting military operations. Sodexo has the contract for the U.S. Marine Corps serves seven bases in fifty-five barracks, plus clubs and other related services. In addition, fast-food restaurants such as McDonald's and Burger King have opened on hundreds of bases; they are now installing Express Way kiosks on more bases. The fast-food restaurants on base offer further alternatives for military personnel on the move. One problem that may arise as a result of the downsizing and contracting out of military foodservice is that it is not likely that McDonald's could set up on the front line in a combat situation. The military will still have to do their own foodservice when it comes to mobilization.

Lately, military foodservice has been more innovative and creative in applying new ideas. For example, Naval Base San Diego Foodservice director Steve Hammel revaluated the base's system in terms of overall value, quality, quick service, and their packaging to enlisted personnel. He also looked at how to individualize the system for each base when each base has its own personality. Price points are also important, so the base has a $7.50 buffet and a fixed $5 lunch with different offerings every day.[5]

At another military operation in Fort Campbell, the cafeteria received a $10 million make-over and began a program of healthy eating. Out went the deep-fat fryer and in came rotisserie chicken, so now instead of selling 75 servings of fried chicken they sell 240 portions of rotisserie chicken.[6]

Smart Choices, created by VA Canteen Services, is a healthy choices menu approach that gives guests more healthy meal offerings. The campaign merges value, health, and wellness that offers a side salad, a bowl of soup, and a bottle of water totaling 235 calories or a sandwich, fruit, and a bottle of water totaling 340 calories. Interestingly, the calories, grams of fat, carbs, and protein are featured alongside the price on the receipt.[7]

Elementary and Secondary Schools

The United States government enacted the National School Lunch Act in 1946. The rationale was that if students received good meals, the military would have healthier recruits. In addition, such a program would make use of the surplus food that farmers produced.

Each day, millions of children are fed free or low-cost breakfast or lunch, or both, in approximately 101,000 schools to more than 31 million children each school day.[8] Many challenges currently face elementary and secondary school foodservice. One major challenge is to balance salability with good nutrition. Apart from cost and nutritional value, the broader social issue of the universal free meal arises. Proponents of the program maintain that better-nourished children have a better attention span, are less likely to be absent from school, and will stay in school longer. Offering free meals to all students also removes the poor-kid stigma from school lunch. Detractors from the universal program say that if we learned anything from the social programs that were implemented during the 1960s, it was that throwing money at problems is not always the best answer. Both sides agree that there is serious concern about what young students are eating. It's probably no surprise that the percentage of children who eat one serving or less of fruits and vegetables each day (excluding french fries) is as high as it is. These percentages are shown in Figure 1. One example of a school system "encouraging" a healthier meal program is in Texas, where

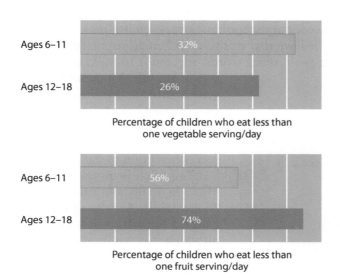

Figure 1 • Numbers of Servings of Fruit and Vegetables That Children Eat.

(*Source:* National Center Institute.)

fried chicken will no longer be a lunchtime staple and deep-fat frying is being eliminated. Instead, all potatoes, including french fries, must be oven baked and no food item can exceed 28 grams of fat. Fruits and vegetables, preferably fresh, must be offered every day for lunch and breakfast. Sodas will not be offered during the school day in middle school. The aim is to provide a healthy environment in which children can grow.[9]

The preparation and service of school foodservice meals varies. Some schools have on-site kitchens where the food is prepared and dining rooms where the food is served. Many large school districts operate a central commissary that prepares the meals and then distributes them among the schools in that district. A third option is for schools to purchase ready-to-serve meals that require only assembly at the school.

Schools may decide to participate in the **National School Lunch Program (NSLP)** or operate on their own. In reality, most schools have little choice because participating in the program means that federal funding is provided in the amount of approximately $2.72 per meal per student. Contract companies such as ARAMARK and Sodexo are introducing more flexibility in choices for students.

Meeting dietary guidelines is also an important issue. Much work has gone into establishing the nutritional requirements for children. It is difficult to achieve a balance between healthy food and costs, taking children's eating habits into account. Under the NSLP regulations, students must eat from what is commonly known as the type A menu. All the items in the type A menu must be offered to all children at every meal. The children have to select a minimum of three of the five meal components for the school to qualify for funding. However, U.S. Department of Agriculture (USDA) regulations have established limits on the amount of fat and saturated fat that can be offered: Fat should not exceed 30 percent of calories per week, and saturated fat was cut down to 10 percent of calories per week.

The government-funded NSLP, which pays in excess of $9.8 billion per year[10] for the meals given or sold at a discount to schoolchildren, is a huge potential market for fast-food chains. Chains are extremely eager to penetrate into the elementary and secondary school markets, even if it means a decrease in revenues. However, they believe that it is to their benefit to introduce Pizza Hut to young people very early—in other words, the aim is to build brand loyalty. For example, in Duluth, Minnesota, James Bruner, foodservice director for the city schools, was forced into offering branded pizza in several junior high and high schools. The local principals, hungry for new revenue, began offering Little Caesar's in direct competition to the cafeteria's frozen pizzas.

Taco Bell is in nearly 3,000 schools, Pizza Hut is in 4,500, and Subway is in 650. Domino's, McDonald's, Arby's, and others are well established in the market as well. Despite the positives, although it is not hard to convince the children, chains need to convince the adults. Much debate has arisen as to whether chains should enter the schools. Many parents feel that the school environment should provide a standard example of

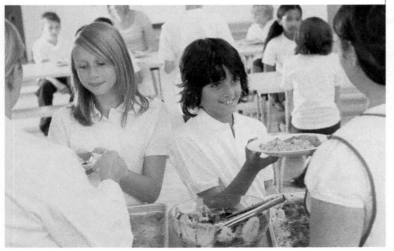
Getting kids to eat proper food is a challenge.

what sound nutrition should be, and they believe that with fast food as an option, that will not be the case.

At a school lunch challenge at the American Culinary Federation (ACF) conference, chefs from around the country developed nutritious menus geared to wean children away from junk food to healthy foods. An 80-cent limit on the cost of raw ingredients was placed on the eleven finalists. Innovation and taste, as well as healthfulness, were the main criteria used to evaluate the winning entry: turkey taco salad, sausage pizza bagel, and stuffed potatoes.

Nutrition Education Programs

Nutrition education programs are now a required part of the nation's school lunch program. As a result of this program, children are learning to improve their eating habits, which, it is hoped, will continue for the rest of their lives. To support the program, nutritional education materials are used to decorate the dining room halls and tables. Perhaps the best example of this is the food guide called MyPlate developed by the Food and Nutrition Service of the USDA. Figure 2 shows the MyPlate food guide, which illustrates what to eat each day to follow a healthy diet.

Many schools are now developing unique ways to expose children to nutrition and proper eating guidelines. Planting a garden has sparked the interest of 1,500 elementary school students at Veterans Park Academy in Florida where students were involved with the planting of a vegetable garden as a result of a $10,000 grant. Students have increased their vegetable consumption as a result of their involvement with the program and have learned firsthand the value of good nutrition by participating in after-school cooking classes to learn how to prepare the vegetables they helped grow.[11]

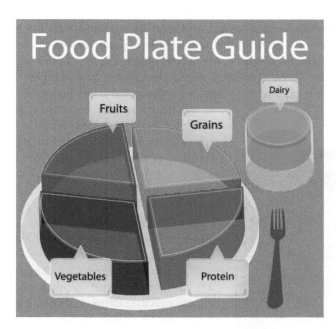

Figure 2 • The New MyPlate Healthy Eating Guide.

Colleges and Universities

College and university foodservice operations are complex and diverse. Among the various constituents of foodservice management are residence halls, sports concessions, conferences, cafeterias/student unions, faculty clubs, convenience stores, administrative catering, and outside catering.

On-campus dining is a challenge for foodservice managers because, as you well know, the clients live on campus and eat most of their meals at the campus dining facility. If the manager or contractor is not creative, students, staff, and faculty will quickly become bored with the sameness of the surroundings and menu offerings. Most campus dining is cafeteria style, offering cyclical menus that rotate every 10 or 14 days.

However, a college foodservice manager does have some advantages when compared with a restaurant manager. Budgeting is made easier because the on-campus students have already paid for their meals and their numbers are easy to forecast. When the payment is guaranteed and the guest count is predictable, planning and organizing staffing levels and food quantities are relatively easy and should ensure a reasonable profit margin. For instance, the **daily rate** is the amount of money required per day from each person to pay for the foodservice. Thus, if foodservice expenses for one semester of 98 days amount to $650,000 for an operation with 1,000 students eating, the daily rate is calculated as follows:

$$\frac{\$650,000 \div 98 \text{ days}}{1,000 \text{ students}} = \$6.63$$

College foodservice operations now offer a variety of meal plans for students. Under the old board plan, when students paid one fee for all meals each day—whether they ate them or not—the foodservice operator literally made a profit from the students who did not actually eat the meals for which they had paid. More typically now, students match their payments to the number of meals eaten: Monday through Friday, breakfast, lunch, dinner; dinner only; and prepaid credit cards that allow a student to use the card at any campus outlet and have the value of the food and beverage items deducted from his or her credit balance.

Leaders of the National Associations of College Auxiliary Services (NACAS), which represents 600 member institutes, have noticed that on-campus services and activities are undergoing continuous change.[12] The environment has become a critical part of policy and implementation that transcends parochial interests for those that best meet the needs of the institution and, ultimately, its students.

The driving forces of change on campuses are the advent and growth of branded concepts, privatization, campus cards, and computer use. A college foodservice manager today must have greater skills in retail marketing and

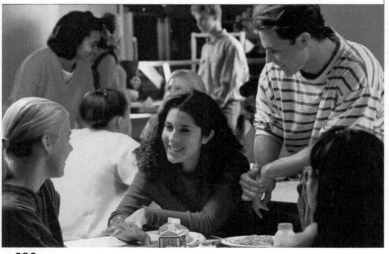

College foodservice.

INTRODUCING STEVE DOBROWOLSKI

Retail Operations Director for Dining Services, ARAMARK, University of South Florida

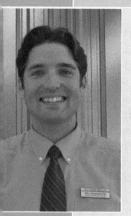

Steve began his career with ARAMARK at East Carolina University in 2000, as a shift manager for a small retail location. He quickly moved up to become the location manager of that operation and then became the assistant location manager of the largest dining hall on campus. He then became the location manager of that dining hall. In 2003, Steve transferred to New York University as the Assistant Food Service Director, managing many locations across the campus. In 2006, Steve was again promoted to Food Service Director when he transferred to the University of South Florida (USF). Most recently, in 2009, Steve was promoted to the Retail Operations Director at USF, managing all retail operations on campus.

Steve's major responsibilities are planning and managing high-volume, complex, multi-location foodservice operations at USF. Steve plans, directs, and controls all retail unit food-services and resources to meet operating and financial goals, client objectives, retail brand franchise relations, audits, and customer needs. He is also responsible for analyzing all financial reports for the retail operations, as well as reviewing all financial measurements with directors to ensure achievement of financial goals. In addition, Steve provides guidance and support in developing action plans to address areas requiring improvement and ensures compliance with ARAMARK Standard of Operations in all retail and catering operations. He interacts with USF clients daily and maintains effective client and customer relations at all levels within USF and USF dining services, including new building construction planning and renovations. He additionally regularly interfaces with ARAMARK's Regional Vice President, District Manager, Unit Directors, and their staff. Steve helps to ensure administration of human resources (HR) policies and interprets and ensures compliance with company policies such as safety, sanitation, and purchasing. Each week and month, Steve develops operational component forecasts and is able to explain any variances. Along with the Resident District Manager, Steve helps to define and hire for positions and roles for organization structure. In addition, he oversees the implementation and maintenance of new marketing and culinary concepts for retail locations.

There is no "typical" day for Steve as he oversees over 15 locations on the USF campus, in addition to the catering department for the university. A workweek usually involves meetings with various departments ranging from HR, marketing, finance, clients, catering events, customers, and his management team. In between all of these tasks, he also attends monthly meetings with students to allow them to voice their opinions and offer suggestions about the services on campus. Steve visits all of his operations often to review the notes from these meetings with the managers along with operational goals, successes, and opportunities. Steve is also the Labor Champion for the state of Florida. These duties include assisting other ARAMARK accounts with their labor management by finding efficiencies and opportunities and sharing best practices across the region. In his "spare time," on campus Steve has become known as "Mr. Fix-It," fixing equipment, lights, computers (he is also known as the IT guy) and anything else that may need his touch.

One of the most challenging responsibilities for Steve is being able to create new ideas and adapting our services daily to maintain a modern, innovative, and competitive edge in the ever-changing world of food.

Steve's favorite and most rewarding aspect of his job is that no day is ever the same. There is always something new and exciting happening. He also loves that he has opportunity to interact daily with so many great employees and customers and have the opportunity to positively influence their day!

merchandizing as students are given more discretion in how they may spend their money for food on campus.

Student Unions

As you know, the college student union offers a variety of managed services that caters to the needs of a diverse student body. Among the services offered are cafeteria foodservice, beverage services, branded quick-service restaurants, and take-out foodservice.

The cafeteria foodservice operation is often the "happening" place in the student union where students meet to socialize as well as to eat and drink. The cafeteria is generally open for breakfast, lunch, and dinner. Depending on the volume of business, the cafeteria may be closed during the nonmeal periods and weekends, and the cafeteria menu may or may not be the same as the residence foodservice facility. Offering a menu with a good price value is crucial to the successful operation of a campus cafeteria.

On campuses at which alcoholic beverage service is permitted, beverage services mainly focus on some form of a student pub where beer and perhaps wine and spirits may be offered. Not to be outdone, the faculty will undoubtedly have a lounge that also offers alcoholic beverages. Other beverages may be served at various outlets such as a food court or convenience store. Campus beverage service provides opportunities for foodservice operators to enhance profits.

In addition, many college campuses have welcomed branded, quick-service restaurants as a convenient way to satisfy the needs of a community on the go. Such an approach offers a win-win situation for colleges. The experience and brand recognition of chain restaurants such as Chick-fil-A, Moe's Southwest Grill, Au Bon Pain, Ben & Jerry's, Einstein Bros Bagels, Burger King, Smokehouse BBQ To Go, Starbucks, Beef 'O' Brady's, Pizza Hut, McDonald's, Subway, and Wendy's attract customers; the restaurants pay a fee, either to the foodservice management company or the university directly. Obviously, there is a danger that the quick-service restaurant may attract customers that the cafeteria might then lose, but competition tends to be good for all concerned. To create interest, an Iron Chef competition was held at the University of Missouri, where it gave students and chefs the opportunity to come up with innovative menu ideas, while creating a tighter knit campus community.[13]

Take-out foodservice is another convenience for the campus community. At times, students—and staff—do not want to prepare meals and are thankful for the opportunity to take meals with them. And it is not just during examination time that students, friends, and staff have a need for the take-out option. For example, tailgate parties prior to football and basketball games or concerts and other recreational/sporting events allow entrepreneurial foodservice operators to increase revenue and profits. The type of contract that a managed services operator signs varies depending on the size of the account. If the account is small, a fee generally is charged. With larger accounts, operators contract for a set percentage (usually about 5 percent) or a combination of a percentage and a bonus split. Figure 3 shows a typical college menu for the dining hall where students usually eat on campus.

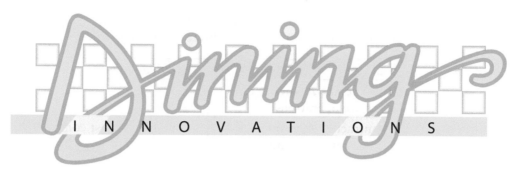

WEEK 1

	MONDAY	TUESDAY	WEDNESDAY	THURSDAY	FRIDAY
Breakfast - Cold cereal, fruit and yogurt bar, toast, juices, milks, coffee, tea, hot chocolate and fresh fruit					
Bakery:	Quick Coffee Cake	Assorted Danish	Cinnamon Coffee Cake	Sticky Top Roll	Banana Nut Muffins
Hot Cereal:	Oatmeal	Malt-O-Meal	Cream of Wheat	Grits	Oatmeal
Entrees:	Buttermilk Pancakes	Waffles	French Toast	Oatmeal Pancakes	Waffles w/Peaches
	Scrambled Eggs	Scrambled Eggs	Scrambled Eggs	Scrambled Eggs	Scrambled Eggs
	Sausage Gravy	Egg O'Muffin w/Bacon	Ham & Cheese	Chorizo & Eggs	Egg Burrito
	& Biscuits	Hearty Fried Potatoes	Omelette	Cottage Fries	Home Fries
	Cottage Fries	Bacon	Hash Browns	Sausage Links	
Lunch - Salad Bar, Rice & Chili Bar, Cereal, Build-Your-Own-Sandwich Bar & Fresh Fruit					
Soup:	Beef Barley	Italian Minestrone	Chicken Gumbo	Chicken Noodle	New England Clam Chowder
Entrees:	Baked Seafood & Rice	Chicken Tortilla	Fishwich	Cheesy Mushroom	BBQ Ham Sandwich
	Grilled Ham & Cheese	Casserole	Spanish Macaroni	Burger	Ground Beef &
	Potato Salad	Patty Melt	Ranch Beans	Hamburger	Potato Pie
	Wax Beans	French Fries	Italian Green Beans	Grilled Cheese	Whipped Potatoes
	Mixed Vegetables	Hominy	Braised Carrots &	Onion Rings	Italian Green Beans
		Spinach	Celery	Carrots	Beets
				Oriental Veg. Blend	
Dessert:	Chocolate Pudding	Applesauce Cake	Peanut Butter	Coconut Cake	Vanilla Pudding
	Soft Serve Ice Cream	Soft Serve Ice Cream	Cookies		
Dinner - Salad Bar, Cereal, & Fresh Fruit (Tortillas served at Breakfast & Dinner)					
Soup:	Beef Barley	Italian Minestrone	Chicken Gumbo	Chicken Noodle	New England Clam Chowder
Entrees:	Oven Broiled Chicken	Beef Fajitas	Roast Turkey w/Gravy	Egg Roll Over Rice	Pizza! Pizza! Pizza!
	Grilled Liver & Onions	Fried Perch	Old Fashion Beef Stew	Grilled Pork Chop	Curly Fries
	Parsley Potatoes	Spanish Rice	Whipped Potatoes	Rice	Broccoli
	Corn	Asparagus	Corn Cobbettes	Beets	Mixed Vegetables
	Zucchini	Carrots	Brussel Sprouts	Cauliflower au Gratin	
Dessert:	Chocolate Chip	Spicy Whole	Chocolate Mayo	Peach Cobbler	Best Ever Cake
	Cookies	Wheat Bar	Cake		

Figure 3 • Sample College Menu.

(Courtesy of ARAMARK.)

As with all types of contract services, there are advantages and disadvantages. Here are both from a client's (that would be your college) perspective:

Advantages	Disadvantages
Experience in size and types of foodservice operations	
Use contracted department as a model for rest of institution	Potential for lost contracts, meaning foodservice contracts are generally for a period of five years, after which bids are requested for another contract. So, the operator must maintain the service and pricing that please the client (the college/university).
Variety of services	
Resource and support available	
Hold contractor to a higher level of performance	

Managing Managed Services[14]

Operating a large $24 million university campus foodservice operation with 32 managers and 680 hourly employees is exhilarating. Each university or college campus is somewhat different, so an operator is smart to become a part of the "living and learning" campus community and align with the university's goals. Also important is to seek input into many of the decisions made so that there is more of a buy-in by the campus community.

Each year, strategic planning and marketing sessions are held with each of the key operating divisions: residential, retail, concessions, and catering; then, financial budgets are completed by month and week for every operation and category. These figures are also updated monthly throughout the year.

The managed services operating ratios vary according to the type of operation, for example, labor costs, which range from the low teens to 50 percent. For residential and retail, labor costs are high and food costs are low, whereas for concessions, labor costs are low and food costs are high. Overall, a well-run operation makes a net profit of between 5 and 15 percent.

Communications are a vital part of a successful foodservice operation. Because there is so much going on, each director and manager has regular meetings to ensure everyone is on the same page. Many day-to-day operating decisions are made by supervisors, who, along with management, all use Outlook and newsletters to communicate electronically.

Foodservice directors spend about 75 percent of their time by following up and making sure that things are still happening the way they are intended to. The fact that foodservice directors need to spend so much time controlling underlines the importance of making good hires and setting clear and concise standards.

A foodservice manager's responsibilities in a small or midsize operation are frequently more extensive than those of managers of the larger operations.

CORPORATE PROFILE

ARAMARK

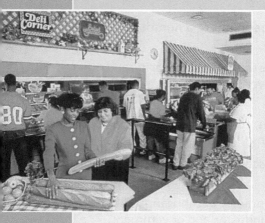

In the 1950s, Dave Davidson and Bill Fishman, both in the vending business, realized that they shared the same dreams and hopes of turning vending into a service and combining it with foodservice. And this they did—ARAMARK is the world's leading provider of quality managed services. It operates with 255,000 employees in all fifty states and in twenty-two foreign countries,[15] offering a very diversified and broad range of services to business of all sizes and to thousands of universities, hospitals, and municipal, state, and federal government facilities. Each day, they serve millions of people at more than 500,000 locations worldwide. ARAMARK's emphasis on the quality of service management was evident from the very beginning of its operations. ARAMARK entered new markets by researching the best-managed local companies, acquiring them, and persuading key managers to stay with the company.

The company's Business Purpose states that "We are a professional services organization dedicated to excellence."

- We develop and sustain our leadership position by engaging and supporting our most valuable differentiated asset: the competence, commitment and creativity of *our people*.

- We provide world-class *experiences*, *environments*, and *outcomes* for our clients and customers by developing relationships based on service excellence, partnership, and mutual understanding.

- We enable our clients to realize their *core mission*, and we will anticipate the needs and exceed the expectations of customers, by dedicating our skills in professional services—hospitality, food, facilities, and uniforms—to the goals and priorities of their institution.

- We create long-term value and capture the greatest opportunity for all ARAMARK shareholders— our people, clients, customers, communities, and shareholders—by delivering sustainable profitable growth in sales, earnings, and cash flow in a global company built on pride, integrity, and respect.

The focus on management skills at every level, especially the local one, gave ARAMARK an invaluable resource. In fact, with every acquisition, local managers were encouraged and rewarded for becoming multiskilled entrepreneurs. This approach to outsourcing is, put more simply, the ability of the company to take the best management skills and apply them to all the lines of business the company uses to diversify. Among ARAMARK operations are the following:

Parks and Destinations. ARAMARK manages food, lodging, hospitality, and support services at national parks and other recreational facilities that serve the general public.

Health Services. ARAMARK provides specialized management services for hospitals and medical services. It maintains hospital equipment valued at $5 billion and services 1,300 hospitals and senior living centers with 400,000 beds.

Colleges and Universities. A leading provider of dining facilities and conference center management to 1,000 colleges and universities. Specializing in residential dining, retail operations such as convenience stores, coffee kiosks, and late-night and branded restaurants.

(continued)

CORPORATE PROFILE *(continued)*

Conference Centers. ARAMARK manages 108 conference centers.

Convention Centers. ARAMARK offers full-service convention center operations at a number of diverse facilities across the country.

Correctional Institutions. ARAMARK Correctional Services provides a wide range of food, facility, and other customized support solutions to over 600 correctional facilities as well as over 1 million meals a day for state and municipal facilities.

Sports and Entertainment. ARAMARK offers services at recreational areas, cultural attractions, sports and entertainment venues, amphitheaters, parks, resorts, and tourists attractions.

School Districts. ARAMARK specializes in providing early-childhood and school-age education services to 4,000 schools to provide services to 7 million students.

Business and industry services. ARAMARK services millions of people annually at thousands of industry accounts, including delivering customized solutions to clients in business, industry, and government.

Uniform services. The company is America's largest provider of uniform services and work apparel for virtually all types of institutions. Millions of customers use uniform and work clothing services by ARAMARK.

ARAMARK has created an Innovation Center for corporate research, design, and product development resources. One interesting outcome is the design of a "cool" place for students to eat—it has a unique design with students in mind, different from the days of the old gym dining.

Joseph Neubauer, chairman and CEO, realizes this: "I am energized by the bright prospects for the journey ahead."

Source: Courtesy of ARAMARK.

This is because larger units have more people to whom certain functions can be delegated, such as human resources. For example, following are some of the responsibilities that the foodservice manager in a small or midsize operation might have in addition to strictly foodservice responsibilities:

Employee Relations
- Team development
- Rewards/recognition
- Drug alcohol abuse/prevention
- Positive work environment
- Coaching/facilitating versus directing

Human Resource Management
- Recruitment/training/evaluating
- Wage/salary administration
- Benefits administration

- Compliance with federal/state laws/EEOC (Equal Employment Opportunity)/Senate Bill 198
- Harassment/OSHA (Occupational Safety and Health Administration)
- Disciplinary actions/terminations
- Unemployment/wrongful disclosure

Financial/Budgeting
- Project budgets
- Actual versus projected budget monitoring (weekly)
- Controlling food cost, labor, expenses, and so on
- Record-keeping requirements/audit
- Monitoring accounts payable/receivable
- Billing/collecting
- Compliance with contracts
- Cash procedures/banking

Safety Administration
- Equipment training/orientation
- Controlling workers' compensation
- Monthly inspections/audits (federal/state/OSHA requirements/Senate Bill 198)

Safety Budget
- Work on the expensive injuries
- Reduce lost time frequency rate and injury frequency rate

Food Production/Service
- Menu/recipe development
- Menu mix versus competition
- Food waste/leftovers utilization
- Production records
- Production control
- Presentation/merchandising

Sanitation/Food-Borne Illness Prevention
- Food-borne illness (FBI) prevention
- Sanitation/cleaning schedule
- Proper food handling/storage
- Daily prevention/monitoring
- Monthly inspection
- Health department compliance

Purchasing/Recruiting

- Ordering/receiving/storage
- Food and beverage specifications/quality
- Inventory control
- Vendor relation/problems

Staff Training/Development

- On-the-job versus structured
- Safety/sanitation/food handling and so on
- Food preparation/presentation
- Guest service

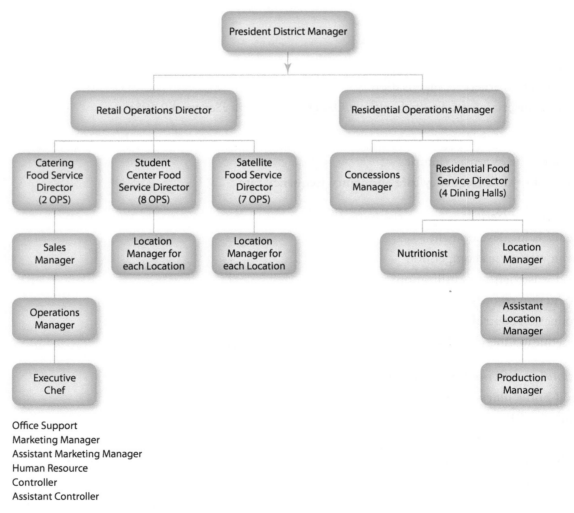

Office Support
Marketing Manager
Assistant Marketing Manager
Human Resource
Controller
Assistant Controller

Figure 3a • An Organization Chart for a Large University.

Sustainable Managed Services

Hospital foodservice directors often say that offering healthy choices in their cafeterias is a key department mission. But many operators are quick to add that they still offer the so-called unhealthy options to prevent a drop in participation and revenues. However, Raquel Frazier, food service director at La Rabida Children's Hospital in Chicago, did not have that luxury. She was mandated by the hospital's administration to make the cafeteria 100 percent healthy.[16] To meet new nutritional guidelines, food items could not exceed 450 calories, with ten grams of fat or three grams of saturated fat, and had to contain at least three grams of fiber. In addition, nutritional information for all items had to be posted on the menu and at the point of service. The outcome has been that most employees reported losing weight and keeping it off and leading a more healthy lifestyle.[17]

INTRODUCING REGYNALD G. WASHINGTON

Vice President and General Manager for Disney Regional Entertainment and Vice President of New Business Initiatives for Walt Disney Parks and Resorts

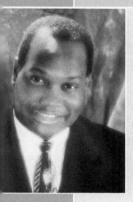

For a student majoring in hotel and restaurant management, being a general manager, president, or even chief executive officer in the food industry is a goal to be achieved. For Regynald G. Washington, not only has it been a goal reached, but a dream realized. His bright smile spells success. As a child growing up in a middle-income family in the town of Marathon in the Florida Keys, working was mandatory. At the early age of thirteen, he was introduced to the food industry. His first job consisted of waiting on and busing tables and doing other chores in the Indies Inn Resort and Yacht Club. He took this on as an exciting and new challenge.

For Regynald, attitude is everything. His positive attitude toward being the best that he can be was derived from a phrase his parents used to repeat to him: "A chip on your shoulder earns a lack of respect from colleagues, friends, and family." His great energy and pride in his work is what makes him stand out among many other leaders in the food industry. He has a quality and people-oriented mind that keeps him focused on any task he wishes to accomplish.

Regynald graduated from Florida International University with a degree in hotel and restaurant administration. He continued to work for Indies Inn Resort, but by this time he was running the food and beverage operation. This was the beginning of the long career road for Regynald G. Washington.

In the years that followed, Regynald worked as a restaurant general manager and at Concessions International, an airport food and beverage, duty free, gifts, and magazine organization in Atlanta. He was promoted to executive vice president in 1990. He then formed Washington Enterprises and developed Sylvia's Restaurant in Atlanta, which turned out to be very successful.

A few years later, though, a major entertainment company executive recruiter offered Washington an opportunity to join the new and creative food and beverage approach that the company was aiming to develop.

Regynald's secret to managing 2,500 employees and satisfying Epcot's customers is simply organization and care. Having organization and direction in your work eliminates stress and makes time for fun. Making sure that all the staff know what they are doing and that they are doing it well and serving guests hot food hot and cold food cold is all it takes. He uses a back-to-basics formula, which requires that everything go well, from making guests happy to proper staffing. Not only has his ambition and energy helped him climb

(continued)

INTRODUCING REGYNALD G. WASHINGTON *(continued)*

to the top, but he also has great concern for others and wants to help his employees learn new things and move forward in their careers. He is very well focused on quality and precision in anything and everything he does. One of his number one concerns is food safety.

To make sure everything is intact and going well, Regynald and his support team perform unannounced inspections every quarter. A specific food and beverage facility is concentrated on and fully evaluated for its table turns, guest service, food quality, and training programs. Specialists act as the guests and observe and report anything that seems less than perfect. Epcot executive chefs check the kitchen food as well as the menu. In-house sanitarians evaluate the level of sanitation at the facility. The goal of these inspections is to make sure nothing is less than perfect. Excellence is the goal for Regynald. He admires and respects the people who work with him and has ranked them as being the best food and beverage people.

Regynald is a frequent guest lecturer in educational forums and has served on the advisory boards of a number of universities for their hospitality management programs. His board service includes being a trustee of the National Restaurant Association Educational Foundation.

Regynald believes that he has achieved a lot and has had many successes during his career. His career is exciting and motivating and he has the opportunity to make a difference in people's lives every single day. This is what he always wanted and now he has it. He says, "My parents really wanted me to become a lawyer, physician, or architect. They didn't believe you could reach the top and do exciting things in the restaurant industry."

Source: This profile draws on Whit Smyth, "Regynald Washington, EPCOT's Chief of Food and Beverage, Says Pleasing Customers Is No Mickey Mouse," *Nation's Restaurant News* 33, (January 25, 1999): 28–30; personal correspondence with Regynald Washington, April 6, 2005.

A number of support staff positions offer career opportunities not only within managed services but also in all facets of hospitality operations and arrangements. They include sales, marketing, controller/audit, financial analysis, human resources, training and development, affirmative action/EEOC compliance, safety administration, procurement/distribution, technical services (recipes, menus, product testing), labor relations, and legal aspects.

A sample operating statement is shown in Figure 4. It shows a monthly statement for a college foodservice operation.

▶ Check Your Knowledge

1. In your own words, define in-flight foodservice.

2. What are some of the challenges faced by in-flight foodservice operators? What can be done to solve these problems?

3. Name the foodservice operations that constitute managed services.

4. How is each foodservice operation characterized?

5. In small groups, discuss the differences between the foodservice operations; then, share with the class.

DESCRIPTION		%	STUDENT UNION	%	TOTAL	%
SALES						
FOOD REGULAR	$ 951,178				$ 951,178	
FOOD SPECIAL FUNCTIONS	40,000				40,000	
PIZZA HUT EXPRESS			$ 100,000		100,000	
BANQUET & CATERING	200,000				200,000	
CONFERENCE	160,000				160,000	
BEER			80,000		80,000	
SNACK BAR			300,000		30,000	
A LA CARTE CAFE	60,000				60,000	
** TOTAL SALES	$ 1,411,178		$ 480,000	100.0%	$ 1,891,178	100.0%
PRODUCT COST						
BAKED GOODS	$ 9,420		$ 4,700		$ 14,120	
BEVERAGE	10,000		8,000		18,000	
MILK & ICE CREAM	11,982		2,819		14,801	
GROCERIES	131,000		49,420		180,420	
FROZEN FOOD	76,045		37,221		113,266	
MEAT, SEAFOOD, EGGS, & CHEESE	129,017		48,000		177,017	
PRODUCE	65,500		26,000		91,500	
MISCELLANEOUS					0	
COLD DRINK	0		0		0	
** TOTAL PRODUCT COST	$ 432,964		$ 176,160	36.7%	$ 609,124	32.2%
LABOR COST						
WAGES	$ 581,000		$ 154,000		$ 735,000	
LABOR—OTHER EMPLOYEES	101,500		545,000		156,000	
BENEFITS + PAYROLL TAXES	124,794		50,657		175,451	
MANAGEMENT BENEFITS	58,320		6,000		64,320	
WAGE ACCRUALS	0				0	
** TOTAL LABOR COST	$ 865,614		$ 265,157	55.2%	$ 1,130,771	59.8%
FOOD OPERATING COST- CONTROLLABLE						
CLEANING SUPPLIES	$ 24,000		$ 6,000		$ 30,000	
PAPER SUPPLIES	9,000		46,000		55,000	
EQUIPMENT RENTAL					0	
GUEST SUPPLIES					7,000	
PROMOTIONS	4,500		2,500		40,000	
SMALL EQUIPMENT	35,000		5,000		0	
BUSINESS DUES & MEMBERSHIP					3,000	
VEHICLE EXPENSE	3,000				4,300	
TELEPHONE	3,600		700		$ 22,000	
	$ 17,000		$ 5,000			

Figure 4 • An Operating Statement.

Health Care Facilities

Health care managed services operations are remarkably complex because of the necessity of meeting the diverse needs of a delicate clientele. Health care managed services are provided to hospital patients, long-term care and assisted living residents, visitors, and employees. The service is given by tray, cafeteria, dining room, coffee shop, catering, and vending.

The challenge of health care managed services is to provide many special meal components to patients with very specific dietary requirements. Determining which meals need to go to which patients and ensuring that they reach their destinations

DESCRIPTION		%	STUDENT UNION	%	TOTAL	%
LAUNDRY & UNIFORMS					0	
MAINTENANCE & REPAIRS	$ 1,200		$ 200		$ 1,400	
FLOWERS	10,000		4,000		140,000	
TRAINING					0	
SPECIAL SERVICES	18,000		3,000		21,000	
MISCELLANEOUS						
** TOTAL CONTROLLABLE SUPPLIES	$ 125,300	8.9%	$ 72,400	15.1%	$ 197,700	10.5%
OPERATING COSTS- NONCONTROLLABLE						
AMORTIZATION & DEPRECIATION	$ 13,500		$ 7,000		$ 20,500	
INSURANCE	55,717		14,768		70,485	
MISCELLANEOUS EXPENSE	12,400		4,100		16,500	
ASSET RETIREMENTS					0	
RENT/COMMISSIONS	48,000		40,000		88,000	
PIZZA HUT ROYALTIES			7,000		7,000	
PIZZA HUT — LICENSING MARKETING			7,000		7,000	
TAXES, LICENSE & FEES	5,000		500		5,500	
VEHICLE — DEPRECIATION & EXPENSE	4,000				4,000	
ADMINISTRATION & SUPERVISION						
** TOTAL NONCONTROLLABLE COST	$ 138,617	9.8%	$ 80,368	16.7%	$ 218,985	11.6%
** TOTAL COST OF OPERATIONS	$ 1,562,495	110.7%	$ 594,085	123.8%	$ 2,156,580	114.0%
EXCESS OR (DEFICIT)	(151,317)	(10.7%)	(114,085)	(23.8)	(265,402)	(14.0%)
PARTICIPATION-CONTRACTOR						
*** NET EXCESS OR (DEFICIT)						
STATISTICS						
CUSTOMER COUNT						
HOURS WORKED						
AVERAGE FOOD- SALES/CUSTOMER						

Figure 4 • An Operating Statement. *(continued)*

involve especially challenging logistics. In addition to the patients, health care employees need to enjoy a nutritious meal in pleasant surroundings in a limited time (usually thirty minutes). Because employees typically work five days in a row, managers must be creative in the development of menus and meal themes.

The main focus of hospital foodservice is the **tray line**. Once all the requirements for special meals have been prepared by a registered dietitian, the line is set up and menus color coded for the various diets. The line begins with the tray, a mat, cutlery, napkin, salt and pepper, and perhaps a flower. As the tray moves along the line, various menu items are added according to the color code for the particular patient's diet. Naturally, each tray is double- and triple-checked, first at the end of the tray line and then on the hospital floor. The line generally goes floor by floor at a rate of about five trays a minute; at this rate, a large hospital with 600 beds can be served within a couple of hours. This is time consuming for the employees because three meals a day represent up to six hours of line time. Clearly, health care foodservice is very labor intensive, with labor accounting for about 55 to 66 percent of operating dollars. In an effort to keep costs down, many operators have increased the number of help-yourself food stations, buffets, salads, desserts, and topping bars. They also focus on increasing revenues through catering and retail innovations. Operators must also contend with the fact that food costs are not totally covered by Medicare.

Hospital foodservice has evolved to the point where the need for new revenue sources has changed the traditional patient and non-patient meal-service ratios at many institutions. This situation was imposed by the federal government when it narrowed the treatment-reimbursement criteria; originally 66 percent of a typical acute-care facility's foodservice budget went toward patients' meals, with the remainder allocated for feeding the employees and visitors. In the past few years, as cash sales have become more important, the 66/33 percent ratio has reversed.

Experts agree that because economic pressures will increase foodservice managers will need to use a more high-tech approach, incorporating labor-saving sous-vide and cook–chill methods. This segment of the industry, which currently is dominated by self-operated managed services, will continue to see contract specialists, such as Sodexo, Compass, and ARAMARK Services, increase their market share at the expense of self-operated health care managed services. One reason for this is that the larger contract companies have the economy of scale and a more sophisticated approach to quantity purchasing, menu management, and operating systems that help to reduce food and labor costs. A skilled independent foodservice operator has the advantage of being able to introduce changes immediately without having to support layers of regional and corporate employees.

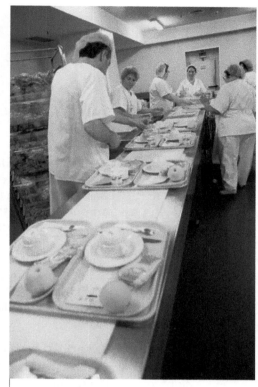

The all-important tray line in health care foodservice.

Another trend in health care managed services is the arrival of the major quick-service chains. McDonald's, Pizza Hut Express, Burger King, and Dunkin' Donuts are just a few of the large companies that have joined forces with the contract managed services operators. Using branded quick-service leaders is a win-win situation for both the contract foodservice operator and the quick-service chain.

The chains benefit from long-term leases at very attractive rates compared with a restaurant site. Chains assess the staff size and patient and visitor count to determine the size of unit to install. Thus far, they have found that weekday lunches and dinners are good, but the numbers on weekends are disappointing.

In contrast, several hospitals are entering the pizza-delivery business: They hook up phone and fax ordering lines, and they hire part-time employees to deliver pizzas made on the premises. This ties in with the increasing emphasis on customer service. Patients' meals now feature "comfort foods," based on the concept that the simpler the food is, the better—hence, the resurgence of meat loaf, pot pies, meat and potatoes, and tuna salad, which contributes to customer satisfaction and makes patients feel at home and comfortable.

Some hospitals have adopted a "room service menu" concept for patients whose diets are not restricted. Here patients are often contacted before they arrive at the hospital so that the foodservice professionals may find out the likes and requests of future patients.

TECHNOLOGY SPOTLIGHT

Management by Exception

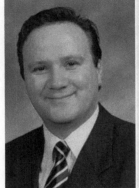

Cihan Cobanoglu, Ph.D., Dean, School of Hotel and Restaurant Management, University of South Florida, Sarasota-Manatee

While visiting industry trade shows and conferences over the past several years, I've noticed a growing number of business intelligence offerings that incorporate exception-based reporting tools into their solution. One simple reason for this trend is the large amount of data that is collected and maintained by hospitality organizations. Not only do hotels and restaurants store guest data, but they also store data related to their employees and other stakeholders, such as suppliers and vendors, blogs and bloggers, and review web sites.

For a long time, the challenge was to combine this data in a central location, mine it, and use it to predict the future. Data was often stored without any plans for further use, or it was used in isolation. Business intelligence tools have since emerged as a way to leverage this data to create a competitive advantage.

Exception-Based Approach

A traditional approach to data mining, and one that has had extreme success in bringing laser-focused insight to operations, is an enterprise-level, exception-based management and reporting solution. Exception-based reporting consolidates data from multiple end-points and systems across an enterprise and performs a rules-based analysis to provide exception reports to various stakeholders in the organization.

A key challenge in implementing a business intelligence and management-by-exception system is the integration of different systems. Following that is the importance of managing the rules that will create the exceptions. When too many noncritical exceptions are reported to management, their value will diminish, and over time those exceptions will not be taken seriously.

Solution Evolution

First-generation solutions focused on exceptions after the fact (that is, next business day). In most high-volume transaction-oriented environments like hospitality, managers receive exception-based information after the window of opportunity to affect an issue has already closed. In this scenario, the best that a manager can hope for is to view the exception report as a scorecard rather than a call to action.

Second-generation solutions focus on customized and real-time reporting. Mirus (**www.mirus.com**) offers a tool that allows users to create custom business rules based on data collected from the point of sale (POS). Another option, RealTime from Real Time Intelligence (www.jackbe.com), gathers information in the form of events and queries from property- and store-level systems, including the POS/PMS, access control, CCTV (closed-circuit TV), and facilities management, to processes this information constantly in real time against a sophisticated business-rules engine at the unit level.

The results of the analysis (the exceptions) are delivered to the appropriate person in real time. This intelligence enables management to affect a resolution before the issue becomes a statistic on tomorrow's report. Delivery may take the form of an SMS (Short Message Service) message to a cell phone, an e-mail to a PDA or standard inbox, telemetry displayed on a custom dashboard, or even a page or a phone call.

Practical Returns

Application of this technology delivers high returns in areas like labor management, compliance, loss prevention, service reparation, and information technology (IT) support. One simple advisory sent to a supervisor when any one of his or her employees is fifteen minutes away from entering overtime, coupled with metrics related to current and projected sales volume, check-ins/check-outs, or other similar information, can drastically reduce overtime and empower a manager to make informed decisions. This concept of targeted intelligence holds the promise of elevating the effectiveness of management by giving each manager, regardless of experience, the ability to perform with the experience of a seasoned colleague.

Implementing real-time exception-based reporting across the enterprise system is not easy or cheap. However, in an industry where profit margins are getting slimmer every year, an exception-based reporting system may pay for itself very quickly and help the company achieve a competitive advantage.

Business and Industry

Business and industry (B&I) managed services is one of the most dynamic segments of the managed services industry. In recent years, B&I foodservice has improved its image by becoming more colorful, with menus as interesting as commercial restaurants.

There are important terms to understand in B&I foodservice:

1. *Contractors.* **Contractors** are companies that operate foodservice for the client on a contractual basis. Most corporations contract with managed services companies because they are in manufacturing or some other service industry. Therefore, they engage professional managed services corporations to run their employee dining facilities.

2. *Self-operators.* **Self-operators** are companies that operate their own foodservice operations. In some cases, this is done because it is easier to control one's own operation; for example, it is easier to make changes to comply with special nutritional or other dietary requests.

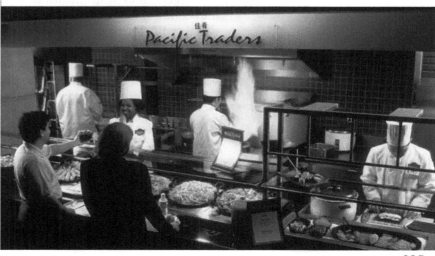

A business and industry account of Sodexo.

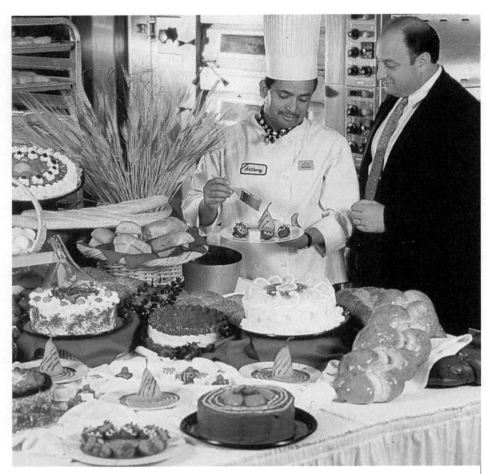

An ARAMARK business and industry foodservice account.

3. *Liaison personnel.* **Liaison personnel** are responsible for translating corporate philosophy to the contractor and for overseeing the contractor to make certain that he or she abides by the terms of the contract.[18]

Contractors have approximately 80 percent of the B&I market. The remaining 20 percent is self-operated, but the trend is for more foodservice operations to be contracted out. The size of the B&I sector is approximately 30,000 units. To adapt to corporate downsizing and relocations, the B&I segment has offered foodservice in smaller units, rather than huge full-sized cafeterias. Another trend is the necessity for B&I foodservice to break even or, in some cases, make a profit. An interesting twist is the emergence of multitenant buildings, the occupants of which may all use a central facility. However, in today's turbulent business environment, there is a high vacancy rate in commercial office space. This translates into fewer guests for B&I operators in multitenant office buildings. As a result, some office buildings have leased space to commercial branded restaurants.

B&I managed services operators have responded to requests from corporate employees to offer more than the standard fast-food items of pizza and hamburgers; they want healthier food options offered, such as make-your-own sandwiches, salad bars, fresh fruit stations, and ethnic foods.

Most B&I managed services operators offer a number of types of service. The type of service is determined by the resources available: money, space, time, and expertise. Usually these resources are quite limited, which means that most operations use some form of cafeteria service.

B&I foodservice may be characterized in the following ways:

1. Full-service cafeteria with *straight line*, *scatter*, or *mobile systems*
2. *Limited-service cafeterias* offering parts of the full-service cafeteria, fast-food service, cart and mobile service, fewer dining rooms, and executive dining rooms

FOCUS ON MANAGED SERVICES

Mega-Event Management: The Olympics—Going for the Gold

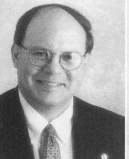

Fred J. DeMicco, Professor and ARAMARK Chair, Department of Hotel, Restaurant and Institutional Management, University of Delaware, and Penn State Walter J. Conti Professor of HRIM

ARAMARK is a world leader in providing global managed services, including food, facility, and other support services. ARAMARK has leadership positions serving the business, education, health care, sports, entertainment, and recreation management segments. Related to sports, entertainment, and food service is "serving the world" at the Olympics.

ARAMARK has a long and rich history with the Olympic Games, dating back to 1968 when it served at the Mexico City Summer Games, the largest in history at the time. Since then, the company has managed services at more Olympic Games than any other company, earning its own "gold medal" performance at both the summer and winter games over the past four decades.

ARAMARK chefs and nutritionists develop a World Menu with more than 550 recipes designed to meet the needs of athletes from 200 different countries, with different ethnic and religious backgrounds and varying nutritional needs, to help them achieve their best during their Olympic performances.

For the third time, Dr. DeMicco is taking students to the Olympic Village to work for ARAMARK. In 1996, his students worked the Summer Games in Atlanta, and they traveled to Sydney to work in the 2000 Summer Games. With 1,500 different menu items available, twenty-four hours a day, the students will have their work cut out for them. Some of the stranger dishes that appeared on athletes' plates during the 2000 Sydney Olympics included kangaroo prosciutto, smoked emu, grilled mako shark, and goat vindaloo.

"The exposure to this type of event provides more learning than any other foodservice venture," Jerome Bill, of ARAMARK, says. "Usually a small city is built, operated for approximately thirty-three days, and then is taken down just as fast. The logistics are tremendous."

ARAMARK recruits and trains more than 6,500 persons to prepare and serve more than 5 million meals during the thirty-three days the Olympics and Para-Olympics take place. The grocery list for such an event is enormous. Some of the major ingredients that ARAMARK used included 576,000 eggs, 34,000 pounds of rice, 32,800 pounds of margarine, and 9,057 pounds of shredded cheddar cheese.

"Where else can you welcome 15,000 of the best in the world into your home for dinner? It is truly the ultimate display of blending one's background, classroom experience, and human nature into an unforgettable learning environment. Students learn more than just serving and cooking; they reach the brink of fully understanding the true meaning of hospitality," said Marc Bruno, MBA, ARAMARK.

The students were able to interact with elite athletes in the world in a fast-paced and constantly changing environment. They were able to be part of providing foodservice that met the unique cultural and nutritional needs of athletes from more than 200 countries. They went in every day knowing that their jobs were critical to each athlete's peak performance.

According to a student participant, "The Olympics allowed me to get an inside view of how a mega event was run, the problems that came up, and how they were overcome. Being in the Olympic Village introduced me to working with people of many different cultures. I am currently working for NBC Olympics in the Games Services department. I am really looking forward to being part of another Olympic Games."

▶ Check Your Knowledge

1. What roles other than those strictly related to foodservice does the foodservice manager perform?

2. Briefly explain some of the tasks the foodservice manager performs. What makes each task so important?

Managed Services Other Than Food

Many companies such as Sodexo have recognized the potential to increase their market opportunities by developing service capabilities beyond food. This also offers hospitality managers the opportunity to expand their career paths as well. Typically, hospitals, colleges, schools, and businesses outsource other service departments the same as they do food. Companies on the cutting edge are able to offer clients broader packages of services. These services often come under the area of facilities management[19] and offer the following services:

- Housekeeping/custodial/environment services
- Maintenance and engineering
- Grounds and landscaping
- Procurement and materials management
- Office and mail services
- Concierge services
- Patient transportation services (hospitals)

Many colleges and universities recognize that this is an area for career opportunities and are developing courses and programs surrounding the area of facilities management. Managers who work in the managed services segment of the industry have the advantage of learning about several disciplines. In doing so, they increase their career growth potential and can find career paths similar to those available in the lodging segment of the industry.

Leisure and Recreation

The leisure and recreation[20] segment of managed services may be the most unique and the most fun part of the foodservice industry in which to work.

Leisure and recreation foodservice operations include stadiums, arenas, theme parks, national parks, state parks, zoos, aquariums, and other venues where food and beverage are provided for large numbers of people. The customers are usually in a hurry, so the big challenge of the foodservice segment is to offer the product in a very short period of time. The average professional sporting event lasts for only two to three hours of time.

What makes this segment unique and fun is the opportunity to be part of a professional sporting event, a rock concert, a circus, or other event in a stadium or arena. There is also the choice of working in a national or state park and being part of the great outdoors. The roar of the crowd and the excitement of the event make this a very stimulating place to work. Imagine *getting paid* to see the Super Bowl versus *paying* to see the Super Bowl.

Stadium Points of Service

Leisure and recreation facilities usually have several points of service where food and beverage are provided. In the typical stadium, a vendor yells, "Here, get your hot dog here!" to the fans in the stands, while on the concourse other fans get their food and beverage from concession stands. These stands offer everything from branded—meaning well-known brands—foods to hot dogs and hamburgers to local cuisine. For example, in Philadelphia the cheesesteak sandwich is popular, whereas in Baltimore, crabcake sandwiches are favored by fans. Another place for people to get food is in a restaurant, which most stadiums have as a special area. In some cases, fans must be members of the restaurant; in other cases, fans can buy special tickets that provide them with access to this facility. These restaurants are like any other except that they provide unobstructed views of the playing area.

The other major point of service is the food and beverage offered in the premium seating areas known as superboxes, suites, and skyboxes. These premium seating areas are usually leased by corporations to entertain corporate guests and customers. In each of these areas, branded and gourmet food and beverage service is provided for the guests. These facilities are capable of holding thirty to forty guests and usually have an area where the food is set up buffet style and a seating area where the guests can see the sporting or other event. In a large, outdoor stadium, there could be as many as sixty or seventy of these superbox-type facilities. For stadium foodservices, more tickets are being placed on mobile devices to enter the stadium/arena; once in the stadium, there are promotions texted to fans, and GPS locations are used in stadiums for vendor ordering.

In summary, a large stadium or arena could have vendors in the stands, concession outlets, restaurants, and superboxes all going at once and serving upward of 60,000 to 70,000 fans. Feeding all these people takes tremendous planning and organization on the part of the foodservice department. The companies that have many of the contracts for stadiums and arenas are ARAMARK, Fine Host, Sodexo, Compass Group, and Delaware North.

Other Facilities

Besides stadiums and arenas, food and beverage service is provided in several other types of facilities by the same major managed service companies that service stadiums. Most of the U.S. national parks are contracted to these companies. These parks have hotels, restaurants, snack bars, gift shops, and a myriad of other service outlets where tourists can spend their money. In addition to parks, other venues where food and beverage are offered include zoos, aquariums, tennis tournaments such as the U.S. Open in New York, and professional golf tournaments. All these events involve big numbers of people. For example, a professional golf event, which lasts a week including practice time, will have upward of 25,000 spectators per day watching the pros play. Tournament events are similar to stadium and arena foodservice operations because they also include concession stands, food and beverage areas for the fans, and "corporate tents" for special catering and company guests.

Advantages and Disadvantages

A foodservice career in this segment has several advantages, which include the unique opportunity to see professional and amateur sporting events to your heart's delight; to hear the roar of the crowd; to be in rural, scenic areas and enjoy the great outdoors; to provide a diverse set of services for the guests or fans; and to have a set work schedule.

The disadvantages of this segment include very large crowds of people to serve in a short time; a work schedule of weekends, holidays, and nights; the chance to give only impersonal service; less opportunity to be creative with food; seasonal employment; and an on-season/off-season work schedule.

Leisure and recreation foodservice is a very exciting, unique part of the hospitality industry that offers employees very different opportunities from standard hotel and restaurant jobs. With the current trend toward building new stadiums and arenas around the country, this segment offers many new career openings.

Trends in Managed Services

- College and university foodservice managers face increasing challenges. *Restaurants and Institutions* magazine asked several managers to identify some of those challenges. In general, managers mentioned trying to balance rising costs with tighter dollars. Bill Rigan, foodservice center manager at Oklahoma State University, Stillwater, points out two main challenges: the reduction of revenues from board-plan sales and increased costs such as food and utilities. He dealt with these challenges by recognizing that because he could not change the utilities or hourly rates for employees, he would have to maximize purchasing potential. He also made optimal usage of "from scratch" cooking, convenience foods, and more efficient labor scheduling.

- Martha Willis, foodservice director at Tennessee Technological University, Cookesville, sees declining enrollment and a reduction in state funding as challenges. This translates to a cutback in services and more pressure to produce a bigger bottom line. Martha intends to achieve this by filling vacant full-time positions with part-time and student employees. The savings made by not paying full-time employee benefits can amount to 30 percent of a person's wage.

- Increased use of campus cards (declining balance or debit cards)

- Increased use of grab and go—and even room service, for instance—to dorms or offices and before sporting events

- Increased use of foodservice carts at vantage points to provide service to students who may not be able to reach the main buildings in time for refreshments before the next class

- Dueling demands for foodservice managers—from students who want more freshly prepared foods in convenient locations and from administrators who want more revenue from existing sources

- Twenty-four-hour foodservice for those clients who need round-the-clock service

- Increased business in health care and nursing homes. As the population ages, there is an increased need to provide services for this important and growing segment.

- Proliferation of branded concepts in all segments of managed services, including military, school and college, business and industry, health care, and airport

- Development of home meal replacement options in each segment of the managed services sector, as a way to increase revenue

- Increasing use of fresh product. People are more health conscious and want healthy produce.

- Increased use of "social media" to promote sales and to communicate with guests

- Foodservice offering more local and sustainable menu items and practices

CASE STUDY

Gas Leak

The kitchen at a major corporation's managed services business account includes several gas and electric stoves, ovens, broilers, steamers, grills, and other appliances. On average, the kitchen serves 500 lunches. At 10:15 A.M. on a Tuesday in December, a gas leak prompts the gas company to cut off the gas supply.

Discussion Question

1. What can be done to offer the best possible lunch food and service?

CASE STUDY

Chaos in the Kitchen

Jane is the foodservice director at an on-campus dining service that feeds 800 students per meal for breakfast, lunch, and dinner. Jane arrives at her office at 7:00 A.M. (half an hour before breakfast begins) only to find many problems.

After listening to her phone messages, she finds that her breakfast cashier and one of her two breakfast dishroom employees have called in sick. The cashier position is essential, and the second dishroom person is necessary at 8:15 A.M. when the students leave to go to their 8:30 A.M. classes.

(continued)

CASE STUDY (continued)

Then, the executive chef tells Jane that one of their two walk-in refrigerators is not working properly, so some of the food is above the safe temperature of 40°F.

The lead salad person later comes to her, saying that one of the three ice machines is not working. Hence, there will not be enough ice to ice down the salad bars and to use for cold beverages at lunch.

Last, the catering supervisor tells Jane that he has just found out that there was a misunderstanding with the bakery that supplies their upscale desserts. The desserts were requested by the president of the university for a luncheon he is having that day; however, because the employee at the bakery wrote the wrong delivery date, the desserts would not be delivered. This will cause the president to be angry.

Discussion Questions

1. How should Jane handle being short a cashier and a dishroom person at breakfast?
2. What should Jane do with the food in the defective refrigerator? Should the food that is measured to be above 40°F be saved?
3. What are Jane's options concerning the ice shortage?
4. How should Jane handle the president's function, knowing that the requested desserts have not been delivered?
5. If the special dessert cannot be purchased in time, how should the catering supervisor approach this situation when speaking with the president's office?
6. What can be done to ensure that mistakes, such as the one made by the bakery employee, do not happen again?

Summary

1. Managed services operations include segments such as airlines, military, schools and colleges, health care facilities, and businesses.
2. Food has become scarce on short and medium domestic flights. Most airlines have food prepared by a contractor, such as Dobbs International or Sky Chefs.
3. Service to the military includes feeding troops and officers in clubs, dining halls, and hospitals as well as out in the field. Direct vendor delivery, menu management, prepared foods, and fast-food chains located on the base have met new trends in military foodservice.
4. Schools are either equipped with on-site kitchens and dining rooms or receive food from a central commissary. They try to balance salability with good nutrition. Today, nutrition education is a required subject in school.
5. College and university managed services operations include residence halls, cafeterias, student unions, faculty clubs, convenience stores, and catering.
6. The responsibilities of a foodservice manager are very complex. He or she is in charge of employee relations, human resource management, budgeting, safety administration, sanitation, and inventory.
7. Health care managed services operations need to provide numerous special meals to patients with very specific dietary requirements and

nutritious meals in a limited time period for employees. The main areas of concern for health care managed services operations are tray lines and help-yourself food stations.

8. Business and industry managed services operations either operate with a full-service cafeteria or limited-service cafeteria. The type of service is determined by money, space, and time available.

9. Leisure and recreation foodservice offers yet more career opportunities. It is often available at several points of service.

Key Words and Concepts

batch cooking
commercial foodservice
contractors
daily rate
liaison personnel

managed services
National School Lunch Program (NSLP)
nutrition education programs
self-operators
tray line

Review Questions

1. What are managed services operations?
2. List and explain features that distinguish managed services operations from commercial ones.
3. Describe the issues that schools are currently facing concerning school food service.
4. Explain the term *National School Lunch Program* (NSLP).

5. Identify recent trends in college foodservice management.
6. What are the pros and cons concerning fast-food chains on campus?
7. Briefly explain the complex challenges for health care managed services operations.

Internet Exercises

1. Organization: **ARAMARK**
   Web site: **www.aramark.com**
   Summary: ARAMARK is "a global leader in managed services" according to its web site. ARAMARK is an outsourcing company that provides services ranging from everyday catering to corporate apparel.
   (a) Click the "Careers" link. Go to ARAMARK's Web site and see what they are doing under the Social Responsibility heading.
   (b) What are some of the characteristics that make a star of the month?

2. Organization: **Sodexo**
   Web site: **www.sodexousa.com**
   Summary: Sodexo offers a full range of outsourcing solutions and is a leading food and facilities management services company in North America.
   (a) What corporate services does Sodexo offer?
   (b) Look at the current opportunities (at Sodexo or ARAMARK) within your area.

Apply Your Knowledge

1. From the sample operating statement (Figure 4), calculate the labor cost percentage by taking total labor cost and dividing by total sales × 100. Remember the formula:

$$\frac{\text{Cost}}{\text{Sales}} \times 100$$

2. Consider a retail operation at a local college where a grilled chicken combo, which consists of a grilled chicken breast, fries, and a 20-oz. soda, is on the menu. Find out the cost of the ingredients and write out everything needed for the combo, including its service. What is your cost price? How much would you charge customers for the item to make a reasonable profit?

Suggested Activity

Create a sample menu for a day at an elementary or high school. Then, compare your items to the MyPlate food guide and the recommended daily servings. How does your menu measure up?

Endnotes

1. Personal conversation with Susan Pillmeier, ARAMARK, and John Lee, Sodexo, July 28, 2005.
2. Gate Gourmet, *About Us*, www.gategourmet.com/gategourmet/index.php?option=com_content&view=article&id=377&Itemid=54 (accessed May 1, 2011).
3. LSG Sky Chefs, *About Us*, www.lsgskychefs.com/en/about-us.html (accessed November 8, 2011).
4. Ibid.
5. "Channeling the college environment: Viewing a military installation like a college campus can help foodservice enhance the retail experience," *Foodservice Director* (March 15, 2011): 6.
6. "Cafeteria boot camp: Fort Campbell's hospital cafeteria focuses on healthy dining after renovation," *Foodservice Director* (March 15, 2011): 8.
7. "Smart choices," *Foodservice Director* (April 15, 2011): 10.
8. United States Department of Agriculture, Food and Nutrition Service, *National School Lunch Program*, October 2011, www.fns.usda.gov/cnd/lunch/AboutLunch/NSLPFactSheet.pdf (accessed April 28, 2011).
9. Sahra Bahari, "Students can expect healthier selection," *Fort Worth Star-Telegram,* August 12, 2007.
10. United States Department of Agriculture, Food and Nutrition Service, *National School Lunch Program*, October 2011, www.fns.usda.gov/cnd/lunch/AboutLunch/NSLPFactSheet.pdf (accessed April 28, 2011).
11. "Teaching moments: School's garden spurs nutrition program for students," *Foodservice Director* (December 15, 2010): 8.
12. The National Association of College & University Food Services, *About NACUFS*, www.nacufs.org/about-nacufs-overview (accessed April 28, 2011).
13. "Smart choices," *Foodservice Director* (April 15, 2011): 1.
14. Based on an interview with Steve Dobrowolski, Retail Operations Director, ARAMARK, University of South Florida, April 27, 2011.
15. ARAMARK, *About ARAMARK*, www.aramark.com/aboutaramark/ (accessed April 28, 2010).
16. FSD Staff, "Environmental Awareness," *FoodService Director* 22(8), August 15, 2009, p. 58.
17. Ibid.
18. Personal correspondence with John Lee, director of college and external relations, Sodexho, September 13, 2005.
19. Ibid.
20. Courtesy of David Tucker.

Glossary

Contractor A company that operates a foodservice for the client on a contractual basis.

Liaison personnel Workers who are responsible for translating corporate philosophy for the contractor and for overseeing the contractor to be sure that he or she abides by the terms of the contract.

Managed services Services that can be leased to professional management companies.

National School Lunch Program The program that provides free lunches to students from a certain income level.

Nutrition education programs Programs ensuring that food served in school cafeterias follows the nutrition standards set by government programs.

Self-operator A company that manages its own foodservice operations.

Tray line The line of trays in hospital meal preparation where items are added to the tray to complete the meal order.

Photo Credits

Credits are listed in the order of appearance.

Tourism

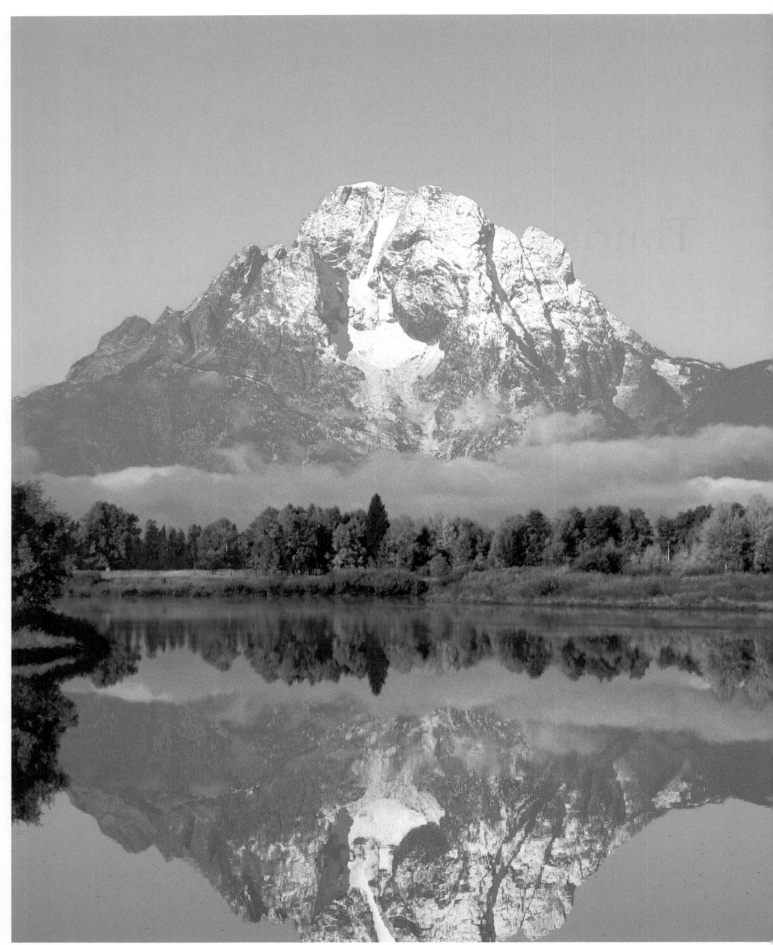

Tourism

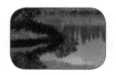
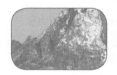
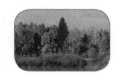
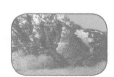

Highlights of Tourism

It is difficult to determine when tourism began because, centuries ago, very few people traveled for pleasure or business as they do today. We do know the following:

- In the fourth century B.C. (before Christ), work started on the Great Wall of China and continued for centuries until the 1600s. Although not exactly a tourist destination or attraction back then, it certainly is today.

- In 776 B.C., athletic games were held on the plain of Olympia in Greece (the modern Olympic Games were inspired by these games), and presumably people traveled there to participate or to watch.

- The Romans liked to visit the Bay of Naples, so they built a road there from Rome in 312 A.D. (*anno Domini*, after Christ). The road was 100 miles long and took four days by litter to get there (in which a nobleperson sat on a platform and was carried by some unfortunate servants).

- Religious pilgrimages to Rome and the Holy Land (now Israel) began in the 1200s, so inns sprang up to feed and accommodate the pilgrims.

- Marco Polo became the first noted European business traveler as he pioneered trade routes from Europe to China from 1275 to 1292, staying at primitive inns called *khans* along the way.

- In the 1600s, during the age of horse-drawn coach travel in England, posthouses were set up to feed and shelter travelers and change the teams of horses every few miles. The journey from London to Bristol took three days—it now takes less than three hours by rail.

- In 1841, Thomas Cook organized a group tour for 570 people to a religious meeting in England.

- Cruising began in the 1840s with the Cunard Lines crossing the Atlantic between England and North America.

- In the 1840s, the Peninsula and Oriental Steam Navigation Company (P&O) cruised the Mediterranean.

- In the 1850s, Monaco (a principality in the south of France) decided to cure its economic woes by becoming a winter haven for the rich as a health resort and a casino.

- During the age of the grand tour, from 1880 through the 1930s, wealthy Europeans toured Europe as a part of their education.

- Rail travel began in the 1800s.

- Auto travel began in the 1900s.

- Air travel began in the 1900s.

- American Airlines introduced its first transcontinental flight between New York and Los Angeles in 1959.

- In 1970, the Boeing 747 began flying 450 passengers at a time across the Atlantic and Pacific Oceans.

- In the 1970s, ecotourism and sustainable tourism became important topics.

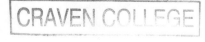

- In the 1980s, cruising became popular.

- In 1986, the United States established the Visa Waiver Program to eliminate unnecessary barriers to travel to the United States. Currently, thirty-six countries are part of the program.

- In the 2000s, tourism temporarily declined as a result of the September 11 attacks, severe acute respiratory syndrome (SARS), bird flu, and war. However, tourism is projected to grow at a rate of between 3.0 and 3.5 percent a year, according to the World Travel & Tourism Council.[1]

- In 2008, there were over 922 million international tourist arrivals, but as a result of the 2007–2010 recession, tourism was down 4 percent in 2009. However, it was expected to rise in 2010–2012.[2]

International tourism arrivals grew by almost 5 percent in the first half of 2011, consolidating the nearly 7-percent growth rate from 2010.[3]

What Is Tourism?

Tourism is a dynamic, evolving, consumer-driven force and is the world's largest industry, or collection of industries, when all its interrelated components are placed under one umbrella: tourism, travel; lodging; conventions, expositions, meetings, and events; restaurants and managed services; assembly, destination, and event management; and recreation. Tourism plays a foundational role in framing the various services that hospitality companies perform.

The leading international organization in the field of travel and tourism, the **World Tourism Organization (UNWTO)** is vested by the United Nations with a central and decisive role in promoting the development of responsible, sustainable, and universally accessible tourism, with the aim of contributing to economic development, international understanding, peace, prosperity, and universal respect for and observance of human rights and fundamental freedoms. In pursuing this aim, the organization pays particular attention to the interests of the developing countries in the field of tourism. The UNWTO's definition of tourism is, "Tourism comprises the activities of persons traveling to and staying in places outside their usual environment for not more than one consecutive year for leisure, business, and other purposes."[4]

The UNWTO plays a catalytic role in promoting technology transfers and international cooperation, stimulating and developing public–private-sector partnerships, and encouraging the implementation of the Global Code of Ethics for Tourism. The UNWTO is dedicated to ensuring that member countries, tourist destinations, and businesses maximize the positive economic, social, and cultural effects of tourism and fully reap its benefits, while minimizing its negative social and environmental impacts. Francesco Frangialli, secretary-general of the UNWTO from 1998 to 2008, writes:

The Global Code of Ethics for Tourism sets a frame of reference for the responsible and sustainable development of world tourism. It draws inspiration from many similar declarations and industry codes that have come before and it adds new thinking that reflects our changing society at the beginning of the 21st century.

With international tourism forecast to reach 1.6 billion arrivals by 2020, members of the World Tourism Organization believe that the Global Code of Ethics for Tourism is needed to help minimize the negative impacts of tourism on the environment and on cultural heritage while maximizing the benefits for residents of tourism destinations. The Global Code of Ethics for Tourism is intended to be a living document. Read it. Circulate it widely. Participate in its implementation. Only with your cooperation can we safeguard the future of the tourism industry and expand the sector's contribution to economic prosperity, peace and understanding among all the nations of the world.[5]

Through tourism, the UNWTO aims to stimulate economic growth and job creation, to provide incentives for protecting the environment and cultural heritage, and to promote peace, prosperity, and respect for human rights. Membership includes 154 countries, 7 territories, and some 400 affiliate members representing the private sector, educational institutions, tourism associations, and local tourism authorities.[6] Unfortunately, the United States is not a member, but it may soon be.

The UNWTO and the World Travel and Tourism Council (WTTC) declare the travel and tourism industry to have the following characteristics:

- A 24-hour-a-day, 7-day-week, 52-week-a-year economic driver
- Total contribution to world gross domestic product (GDP) of 9.1 percent
- Employer of 259 million people, or 8.8 percent of the global workforce, and is expected to be responsible for about 1 in 10 jobs by 2021[7]
- Leading producer of tax revenues

Given declining manufacturing and agricultural industries, and in many countries the consequent rise in unemployment, world leaders should turn to the service industries for real strategic employment gains. For many developing nations, tourism represents a large percentage of gross national product and a way of gaining a positive balance of trade with other nations.

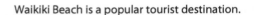

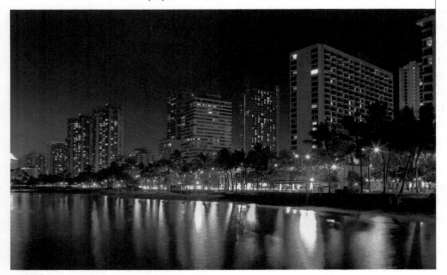

Waikiki Beach is a popular tourist destination.

▶ Check Your Knowledge

1. What role does the UNWTO play in the tourism industry?

2. Describe the characteristics of tourism.

3. How is tourism sometimes categorized?

Benefits of Tourism

Tourism is firmly established as the number-one industry in many countries and the fastest-growing economic sector in terms of foreign exchange earnings and job creation. International tourism is the world's largest export earner and an important factor in the balance of payments of most nations.

Tourism has become one of the world's most important sources of employment. It stimulates enormous investment in infrastructure, most of which helps to improve the living conditions of residents as well as tourists. It provides governments with substantial tax revenues. Most new tourism jobs and businesses are created in the developing countries, helping to equalize economic opportunities and keep rural residents from moving to overcrowded cities. Intercultural awareness and personal friendships fostered through tourism are powerful forces for improving international understanding and contributing to peace among all the nations of the world.

The UNWTO encourages governments, in partnership with the private sector, local authorities, and nongovernmental organizations, to play a vital role in tourism. The UNWTO helps countries throughout the world to maximize the positive impacts of tourism, while minimizing its possible negative consequences on the environment and societies.[8] Tourism is a collection of industries, or segments, that when combined, form the world's largest industry. Tourism offers the greatest global employment prospects. This trend is caused by the following factors:

1. The opening of borders: Despite security concerns, we can travel to more countries now than ten years ago. The United States has a Visa Waiver Program with thirty-six European countries, meaning citizens of these countries with machine-readable passports do not require a visa to visit the United States.

2. An increase in disposable income and vacation taking

3. Reasonably affordable airfares

4. An increase in the number of people with more time and money to travel

5. More people with the urge to travel

According to the WTTC—the industry's business leaders' forum—tourism and travel generate, directly and indirectly, 9.1 percent of global GDP, investment, and employment.[9] The industry is forecast to grow strongly in real terms during the next ten years. This means growth in jobs in the United States and abroad.

Long-Term Prospects: Tourism 2020 Vision[10]

Despite the terrorist attacks and a weak economic recovery, the long-term prospects for tourism appear to be good. *Tourism: 2020 Vision* is the UNWTO's long-term forecast and assessment of the development of tourism for the first twenty years of the new millennium. An essential outcome of the *Tourism: 2020 Vision* is quantitative forecasts covering a twenty-five-year period, with 1995 as the base year and forecasts for 2000, 2010, and 2020 (Figure 1).

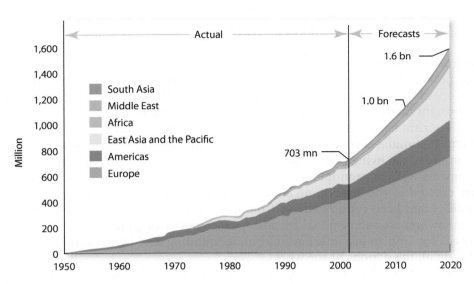

Figure 1 • Actual and Forecast Tourism Arrivals, 1950–2020.
(© UNWTO, 9284403211)

UNWTO's *Tourism Toward 2030* forecasts that international arrivals will hit 1.8 billion by the year 2030.

The total tourist arrivals by region show that by 2020 the top three receiving regions will be Europe (717 million tourists), East Asia and the Pacific (397 million), and the Americas (282 million), followed by Africa, the Middle East, and South Asia.

The fact that tourism is expected to grow rapidly presents both tremendous opportunities and challenges. The good news is the variety of exciting career prospects for today's hospitality and tourism graduates. Tourism, although a mature industry, is a young profession. Careful management of tourism and travel will be necessary to avoid repercussions and negativism toward the "pesky" tourist, which is already happening to some extent in Europe, where the sheer number of tourists overwhelms attractions and facilities.

There is an **interdependency** between the various segments of tourism, travel, lodging, foodservice, and recreation. Hotel guests need to travel to reach the hotel. They eat in nearby restaurants and visit attractions. Each segment is, to an extent, dependent on another for business.

The Five Ages of Tourism

The historical development of tourism has been divided into five distinct ages (or periods),[11] four of which paralleled the advent of a new means of transportation:

Pre–Industrial Revolution (prior to 1840)

The railway age

The automobile age

The jet aircraft age

The cruise ship age

Pre–Industrial Revolution

As early as 5,000 years ago, some ancient Egyptians sailed up and down the Nile River to visit and construct the pyramids. Probably the first journey ever made for the purposes of peace and tourism was made by Queen Hatshepsut to the Land of Punt (believed to be on the east coast of Africa) in 1480 B.C. Descriptions of this tour have been recorded on the walls of the temple of Deir el-Bahri at Luxor.[12] These texts and bas-reliefs are among the world's rarest artworks and are universally admired for their wondrous beauty and artistic qualities. The Colossi of Memnon at Thebes have on their pedestals the names of Greek tourists of the fifth century B.C.[13] The Phoenicians were among the first real travelers in any modern sense. In both the Mediterranean and the Orient (now called Southeast Asia), travel was motivated by trade. Later, the Roman Empire provided safe passage for travelers via a vast road system that stretched from Egypt to Britain. Wealthy Romans traveled to Egypt and Greece, to baths, shrines, and seaside resorts.[14] The Romans were as curious as are today's tourists. They visited the attractions of their time, trekking to Greek temples and places where Alexander the Great slept, Socrates lived, Ajax committed suicide, and Achilles was buried and to the pyramids, the Sphinx, and the Valley of the Kings—just as today's tourists do.[15] The excavated ruins of the Roman town Pompeii, which was buried by the volcanic eruption of Mount Vesuvius, revealed some twenty-plus restaurants, taverns, and inns that tourists visit even today.

The earliest Olympic Games for which we still have written records were held in 776 B.C. (though it is generally believed that the games had been going on for many years before that).[16] Thus, sports have been a motivation for tourism for a long time.

Travel in the Middle Ages was mostly for religious or trade reasons. People made pilgrimages to various shrines: Muslims to Mecca and Christians to Jerusalem and Rome. The Crusades (which began in 1095 and lasted for the next two hundred years) stimulated a cultural exchange that was in part responsible for the Renaissance.

Marco Polo (1254–1324) traveled the Silk Road, which was anything but a road as we know it, from Venice to Beijing, China. He was the first European to journey all the way across Asia to Beijing, and his journey, which lasted twenty-four years, and the tales from it became the most well-known travelogue in the Western world.[17]

Marco Polo's father and uncle had traveled extensively in Asia before Marco joined them. The journey was both difficult and dangerous (excerpts of Marco's account can be read at several Marco Polo web sites). One time, to make sure the Polo brothers

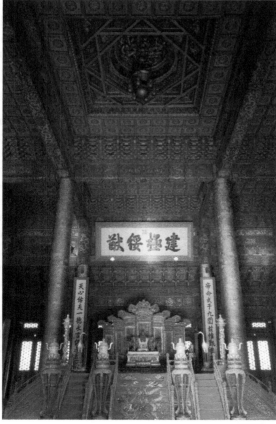

The Hall of Supreme Harmony in Beijing's Forbidden City.

would be given every assistance on their travels, Kublai Khan presented them with a golden tablet (or *paiza*, in Chinese, *gerege*, in Mongolian) a foot long and three inches wide and inscribed with the words "By the strength of the eternal Heaven, holy be the Khan's name. Let him that pays him not reverence be killed." The golden tablet was a special VIP passport, authorizing the travelers to receive throughout the Great Khan's dominions such horses, lodging, food, and guides as they required.[18] This was an early form of passport.

▶ Check Your Knowledge

1. Describe the benefits of tourism.

2. How many arrivals are forecast for 2020?

3. What are the five ages of tourism?

Rail, Automobile, and Coach Travel

Changes in the technology of travel have had widespread implications for society. In the United States, rail travel influenced the building of towns and cities, caused hotels to be built near rail depots, and opened up the West, among other things. Likewise, auto travel produced the motel and a network of highways, and the commercial jet created destination resorts in formerly remote and exotic locations, made the rental car business a necessity, and changed the way we look at geography. Although long-distance travel has always been fairly comfortable for the wealthy, it was not until the development of the railroad in the 1830s that travel became comfortable and cheap enough to be within reach of the masses.

Traveling by Train

Coast to coast, the United States has a lot of land with a fair share of mountains, canyons, forests, deserts, rivers, and other natural barriers to travel. One of the main factors that led to the development of railroads in the United States was the need to move goods and people from one region of the country to another. Farmed goods needed to be transported to industrial areas, and people wanted a quicker route to the West, especially after the discovery of gold in California. Those who already lived at the frontier wanted the same conveniences as their neighbors in the East, such as efficient postal service.

The train made mass travel possible for everyone. Long-distance travel became both cheaper and faster, making the horse and ship seem like "overpriced snails." The vast rail networks across North America, Asia, Australia, and Europe made the train station a central part of nearly every community. Naturally, entrepreneurs soon built hotels conveniently close to train stations.

Although hugely important and popular for many years, the popularity of rail travel started to decline as early as the 1920s. Why did people stop using the train? For two main reasons: the bus and the car. In addition, the Great Depression of the 1930s certainly deterred travelers. Although World War II brought a new surge in passenger numbers, people were seldom traveling for pleasure, and at the close of the war, the decline continued. Automobiles were again available, and people had the money to buy them. By 1960, airplanes had taken over much of the long-distance travel market, further reducing the importance of the train.

Facing a possible collapse of passenger rail services, the U.S. Congress passed the Rail Passenger Service Act in 1970 (amended in 2001). Shortly after, the National Railroad Passenger Corporation began operation as a semipublic corporation established to operate intercity passenger trains, a move in the direction of semi-nationalization of U.S. railroads. The corporation is known today as Amtrak.

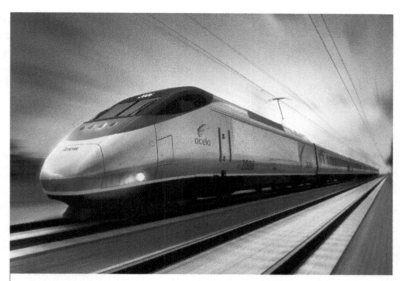

The aerodynamic Amtrak ACELA train speeding along between Washington, D.C., and New York City reaches its destination in 2 hours 45 minutes.

Rail Travel Abroad

While the United States tries to rejuvenate rail travel under the direction of Amtrak, rail service in other parts of the industrialized world is far ahead in progress. Taking the train makes good sense in densely populated areas such as those in Western Europe and parts of Asia, and high-speed networks are already well developed, often drawing most of the traffic that formerly went by air. One good example is the Eurostar, connecting the United Kingdom with mainland Europe via the thirty-one-mile-long underwater Channel Tunnel. France's TGV (Trains à Grande Vitesse) trains are perhaps the best known of them all, serving more than 150 cities in France and Europe, and traveling at about 186 mph (although they have the capacity of running at 250 mph). The TGV's most spectacular feature is the smoothness of the ride: It is like sitting in your armchair at home. Because of their importance, all trains—high speed or not—run frequently and on time. Fares are generally reasonable, and service levels are high.

Japan's Shinkansen, the bullet train system, makes the 550-mile run between Tokyo and Osaka in 3 hours and 10 minutes, down from the former rail time of 18 hours. In addition, it provides a ride so smooth that a passenger can rest a coffee cup on the windowsill and not a drop will spill, just like on the TGV.

Do you dream of exploring Europe? As a student, you have probably heard of the famous Eurail Pass. Several European nations have banded together to offer non-European visitors unlimited first-class rail service for a reduced lump-sum. However, if you want to use the Eurail Pass, be sure to purchase a pass before you leave home because not all types of passes are available in Europe and the ones that are cost on average 20 percent when bought in Europe. When visiting Europe, you can choose to travel in one country, in a few selected ones, or in all with Eurail Pass; it's up to you to choose between the different passes available. In other parts of the world, Australia offers the Austrailpass, India the Indrail Pass, Canada the Canrail Pass, and Canada and the United States the

North American Rail Pass. The new rail line in China linking Beijing to Nepal is of interest because it is one of the longest and highest rail lines in the world, and, according to some, it is going to dilute the Tibetan culture. This is one of the dilemmas of tourism: Travel and tourism can bring an economic and social development, yet it can also damage local cultures and environments.

TECHNOLOGY SPOTLIGHT

Use of the Internet for Travel

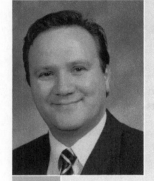

Cihan Cobanoglu, Ph.D., Dean, School of Hotel and Restaurant Management, University of South Florida, Sarasota-Manatee

Advances in information technology have made a significant impact on all parties involved in tourism industry: tourism organization, travelers, transportation companies, and travel destinations.

Development of the Internet and online booking systems has drastically changed travel agents' operations. From working with huge price catalogs, calling for seats and room availability, and faxing reservations, travel agents have moved to online reservation systems that allow convenient access to information and instant updates. All these became available due to the invention of Global Distribution Systems (GDSs). Originally, these systems were developed by airline companies to enable bookings among different airline companies. Later, they were also extended to hotels and car-rental companies. The most popular GDSs are Amadeus, Sabre, Galileo, Worldspan, and Travel Sky (a new GDS that is emerging in China). For example, more than 30,000 travel agents use Sabre and nearly 75,000 use Amadeus. GDSs provide travel agents with rapid search, booking, and confirmation facilities for airline, hotel, and car-hire products. In hospitality, GDSs are dependent on modern hotel Central Reservation Systems (CRSs), which provide full details of hotel properties, locations, room types, availability, prices, and booking conditions. If a hotel wants to make its inventory available to numerous customers and travel agents all around the world, it needs to interface its CRS to one (or several) GDSs. This interface can be done by means of a switch company, for example, Pegasus Solutions. The Internet also gave rise to online travel agencies (OTAs) such as Expedia and Travelocity. OTAs are an electronic overlay of GDSs. These sites may focus on travel reviews, online bookings, and providing relevant information to customers. There are three major OTA business models: merchant (net rate, for example, Expedia), agency (commission, for example, Booking.com), and opaque (for example, Priceline.com).

The development of information technology has greatly enhanced travelers' experience by increasing their access to information, their awareness, and the travel options available to them. Previously, travelers used to be dependent on travel agents in their search for vacation places and decision-making process. However, the extensive resources of the Internet today allow every traveler to be a travel agent on his or her own. On the Web, travelers can find information about millions of hotels, destinations, and things to do all over the world. Review web sites (for example, Tripadvisor.com) provide firsthand evaluation of hotels, destination, and attractions through the recording of people's experiences. These web sites have become one of the key forces in travel decision-making.

Airline companies have also greatly developed and improved their electronic systems in order to improve operations and customer service. As mentioned earlier, airlines were the initiators of the GDSs. Airline companies also developed comprehensive reservation systems that allow customers to create their accounts, select seating, and check in online, as well as customer relationship management (CRM) and loyalty systems. Recently, airlines introduced a new initiative by implementing electronic boarding passes. This pass is sent to a smartphone or personal digital assistant (PDA) of a traveler and does not require any printouts. This system is already available in select airports around the United States.

Traveling by Car

The internal combustion engine automobile was invented in Germany but quickly became America's obsession. In 1895, there were about 300 "horseless carriages" of one kind or another in the United States, including gasoline buggies, electric cars, and steam cars. In 1914, Henry Ford began making the Model T on the first modern assembly line, making the car available to many more Americans because of its lower cost. Even during the Great Depression, almost two-thirds of American families had automobiles. Henry Ford's development of the assembly line and construction of good, solid roads helped make the automobile the symbol of American life that it is today.

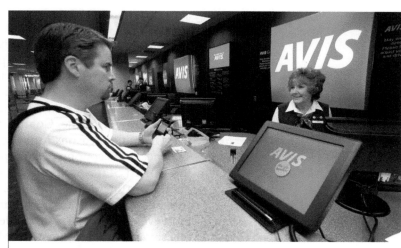

Rental cars offer business and leisure travelers the convenience of fly–drive or drive-only to facilitate tourists' needs.

The auto changed the American way of life, especially in the leisure area, creating and satisfying people's urge to travel. The automobile remains the most convenient and rapid form of transportation for short and medium distances. Without question, it has made Americans the most mobile people in history and has given them options not otherwise possible. Whereas many Europeans ride their bikes or use the bus or train to get to school or work, Americans cannot seem to function without their cars. In fact, it is not uncommon for an American to drive 20,000 miles a year.

Road trips are a must for most Americans—college students, families, and retirees alike. Travel by car is by far the largest of all segments in the ground transportation sector of the travel and tourism industry. It is no wonder, then, that the highways and byways of the United States and Canada play such important roles in tourism. The advantages of car travel are that the car brings you to places that are otherwise inaccessible. Mountain resorts, ski destinations, dude ranches, and remote beaches are just a few examples. This travel generates millions of dollars, and in certain places the local economy depends on the car tourist.

Rental Cars

Some 5,000 rental car companies operate in the United States. Waiting at nearly every sizable airport in the world are several highly competitive rental car agencies, a significant segment of the travel/tourism business. About 75 percent of their sales take place at airport counters that are leased from the airport, the cost of which is passed on to the customer. The larger companies do 50 percent or more of their business with large corporate accounts, accounts that receive sizable discounts under contract. The hurried business traveler is likely to rent a car, speed out of the airport, do his or her business in a day or two, return to the airport, and hop on a plane to return home. The pleasure traveler, however, is more likely to rent a small car for a week or more. This group constitutes about 30 percent of the rental car market. The top-five rental car companies in the United States are Hertz, Avis, Enterprise, National, and Budget. The agencies maintain approximately 625,000 rental cars that are usually new and are sold after six months to reduce maintenance costs and help avoid breakdowns.

Traveling by Bus

Although scheduled bus routes aren't as competitive as scheduled service for airlines, buses still play an important role in the travel and tourism industry, especially with regards to charter and tour services. Some bus companies even offer services such as destination management, incentive programs, and planning of meetings, events, and conferences. Some companies to check out are Gray Line Worldwide, Contiki Tours, and Canadian Tours International.

The major reasons for selecting the bus over other modes of travel are convenience and economy. Many passengers are adventurous college students from the United States and abroad or senior citizens, both with limited funds but plenty of time on their hands. Most people don't choose bus travel for long trips, however, because a flight is much quicker and often just as economical. However, in places such as the heavily populated northeast corridor, regular bus service between most sizable communities in New England and New York often makes it easier and safer for travelers to ride the bus than to drive their cars into the city. Anyone who has experienced New York City traffic will probably agree.

Another reason why buses are popular is because they allow the leisure traveler to sit back, relax, and enjoy the scenery. In addition, they are hassle free and provide an opportunity to make new friends and stop along the way. Long-distance buses offer a variety of amenities similar to an airplane, with an extra benefit of almost door-to-door service! Buses travel to small and large communities, bringing with them tourist dollars and thus a boost to the local economy.

Types of Bus Service

In addition to routes between towns and cities, bus travel includes local route service, charter service, tour service, special services, commuter service, airport service, and urban and rapid transit service. The largest and most recognized of all of the specialized travel services is Gray Line. Founded in 1910, Gray Line is a franchise operation based in Colorado. The company assembles package tours and customized tours, arranges rail and air transfers, and even provides meeting and convention services. Its major service, however, is sightseeing trips by bus. When a traveler arrives at a destination and wishes to see the town and the major tourist attractions, Gray Line is usually ready to serve. The 150-member organization carries about 28 million passengers a year at more than 200 destinations. Their trips are widely diversified, such as "around-the-town" in Paris and "around-the-country" in Thailand. In the United States, Gray Line's biggest market is Los Angeles, followed by San Francisco and then Manhattan.

▶ Check Your Knowledge

1. In what locations does rail travel make the most sense?

2. What is the future of rail travel?

3. Who are the major users of buses?

Airlines

Air travel has made it possible to build great resorts on remote islands, it has fostered multinational enterprises, and it has broadened the horizons of hundreds of millions of people. Without the airplane, most resort destinations would have been virtually impossible to build. The number of international travelers would be far fewer because of the time, money, and difficulty involved in travel. The airplane makes travel easier and more convenient because even the most remote location is just a few hours away by plane, and reasonable airfares make it possible for more people to travel by air.

Air transport has become an integral factor in the travel and tourism industry. Hotels, car rental agencies, and even cruise lines depend heavily on airplanes for profits. For instance, lower airfares result in more passengers and hence a higher occupancy at hotels. Whole towns and cities can and do benefit from this concept by receiving more taxes from tourists, which leads to better public facilities, better schools, and even lower local and property taxes.

In the United States, there are, at any one time, about 5,500 airplanes in the skies.[19] By 2012, total passenger traffic between the United States and the rest of the world is projected to reach 1 billion flights annually. In recent years, the airline has become the preferred means of travel for the long haul. The jet aircraft has made previously inaccessible places such as Bali, Boracay, and Bangkok easily accessible, for a reasonable price. Today millions of Americans travel within the United States and abroad, and millions more visit the United States because of air travel.

Over the past few years—with the exception of Southwest, AirTran, and JetBlue—major U.S. airlines have lost billions of dollars. One reason is competition from low-cost domestic and international airlines.

Since the economic recession, business travelers continue to spend less, and airlines' pension, fuel, and security costs have risen. The major airlines have laid off employees, delayed delivery of new jets, and closed some hubs, reservations, and maintenance centers in an effort to reduce costs. Several of the major U.S. airlines have been and are in financial trouble, so they are charging an additional fuel surcharge on tickets and charging for checked bags, food, beverages, and selected seats just so that they can stay in the air. Other strategies are needed to keep airlines viable.

For example, in efforts to promote passenger loyalty and operating effectiveness, the major U.S. airlines have formed strategic alliances with partner airlines to provide passengers with easier ticket purchases and transportation to destinations in countries not served by U.S. airlines. Many of the world's major airlines are grouped with either Star Alliance, Sky Team, or One World. Sky Team

American Airlines and its eleven One World partner airlines go just about anywhere. The One World partners include British Airways, Cathy Pacific Airways, and Japan Airlines.

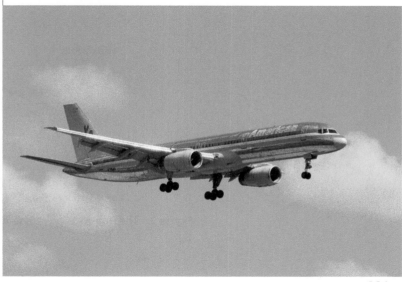

includes Delta Air Lines from the United States, Aeroflot from Russia, Aeromexico, Air Europa from Spain, Air France, Alitalia from Italy, China Airlines, China Southern, KLM from the Netherlands, Korean Air from South Korea, and others. Alliances of this nature will allow airlines access to each other's feeder markets and to resources that will enable them to compete in what will ultimately be a worldwide deregulation. A *feeder market* is a market that provides the source—in this case, passengers for the particular destination. Ultimately, any major European airline without a strategic alliance in the United States will only limit its own horizons and lose market share. Airlines have merged or taken over others to increase their scope of operations and reduce costs in an effort to stay competitive. Delta acquired Northwest Airlines and Continental was acquired by United.

Another example is Southwest Airlines. Southwest operates more efficiently than the competition does despite the fact that its workforce is unionized. Southwest gets more flight time from its pilots than does American Airlines—672 hours a year versus 371—and racks up 60 percent more passenger miles per flight attendant. These efficiencies have resulted in annual profits for thirty consecutive years as a result of Southwest's dedication to a low-cost, high-customer-satisfaction strategy.

Carriers such as Southwest, AirTran, and JetBlue have lower operating costs because they use only one type of aircraft, fly point to point, and offer a no-frills service. Their lower fares have forced many larger airlines to retreat.

To reduce losses brought about by deregulation and high labor, pension plan, and fuel costs, major carriers have eliminated unprofitable routes, often those serving smaller cities. New airlines began operating shuttle services between the smaller cities and the nearest larger or hub city. This created the hub-and-spoke system (see Figure 2).

The Hub-and-Spoke System

To remain efficient and cost effective, major U.S. airlines have adopted a **hub-and-spoke system**, which enables passengers to travel from one smaller city to another smaller city via a hub or even two hubs. Similarly, passengers may originate their

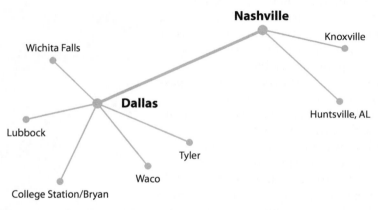

Figure 2 • The Hub-and-Spoke System.

travel from a small city and use the hub to reach connecting flights to destinations throughout the world.

The hub-and-spoke system has two main benefits: (1) Airlines can service more cities at a lower cost, and (2) airlines can maximize passenger loads from small cities, thereby saving fuel. The airlines have also used deregulation to their advantage to save money whenever possible, for instance, by cutting nonprofitable routes from some smaller cities.

New Airplanes

Boeing's first new airplane model in several years, the Dreamliner 787, takes advantage of huge advances made in aviation technology in the past decade and is capable of flying long-haul routes using up to 20 percent less fuel than today's similar-sized airplanes. Up to 50 percent of the primary structure of the plane, including the fuselage and wing, is made of components such as carbon fiber, which reduces the weight of the plane.[20]

Able to fly up to 9,700 miles without refueling, the Boeing 787 Dreamliner could easily manage a flight between New York and Moscow, Manila, or Sao Paulo or between Boston and Athens. Richard Aboulafia, chief analyst with Teal Group, comments, "If you look at it from an airline standpoint: you don't have a choice. If you don't have a 787-class aircraft and your competitor does, he can under price you and out-profit you."[21]

Boeing's competitor, Airbus, makes the Airbus A380. The giant double-decker Airbus A380 can carry up to 500 passengers for a distance of up to 8,000 miles. Singapore Airlines flew the first commercial flight of this aircraft in October 2007 between Singapore and Sydney, Australia.

Components of Airline Profit and Loss

Have you ever wondered why air travel is so expensive? You might find some answers in this section, where we look at the different costs included when you buy an air ticket. Airlines have both fixed and variable costs. *Fixed costs* are constant and do not change regardless of the amount of business. Examples are the lease of airplanes, the maintenance of airline-owned or leased terminals, interest on borrowed money, insurance, and pensions. *Variable costs* tend to rise and fall with the volume of sales or the number of flights. They include wages and salaries, advertising and promotion, fuel costs, passenger food and drink, and landing fees.

The biggest single cost for airline operations is labor, which is typically 30 to 45 percent of total operating

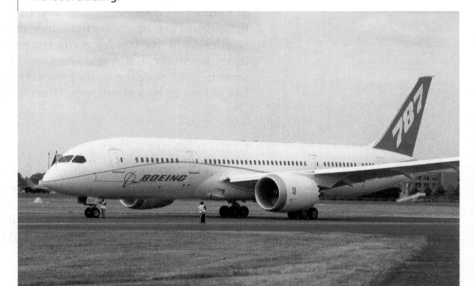

The new Boeing 787 Dreamliner is able to fly up to 9,700 miles without refueling.

costs. Senior pilots for airlines such as United and Delta can receive as much as $150,000 or more a year.[22] The median salary for a flight attendant is $56,000 or more a year, plus benefits.[23] Additionally, landing and takeoff charges charged to airlines by airports can add up to thousands of dollars per plane, depending on the airport and time of day. Passenger servicing costs such as reservations, ticketing, food, baggage handling, and an amount for additional security and fuel must also be accounted for in the ticket price. Once a schedule is set and the break-even point is reached, selling tickets to extra passengers produces large profits for airlines. Being able to offer just the right amount of discount tickets that are needed to fill a plane then becomes highly important. Capacity control is one yield-management technique for maximizing sales income by lowering the price of seats according to expected demand.

The Load Factor

A key statistic in analyzing an airline's profitability is the **load factor**, which means the percentage of seats filled on all flights, including planes being flown empty to be in position for the next day's schedule. The load factor, like the occupancy rate of a hotel, is an indicator of efficient or inefficient use. The current U.S. commercial air carrier load factor is usually around 79.74 percent. [24] The break-even point, the point at which carriers neither lose money nor make a profit, is likely to be unique on any given flight. This point is determined by the rate structure in effect, the length of the flight, the time spent on the ground, and other costs such as wages and salaries. An airline with a long-haul high-density route—for example, from New York to Los Angeles—has a decided cost advantage over another airlines' short-haul, low-density routes. The cost of flying a plane is sharply reduced once it reaches cruising altitude. A short flight thus costs more per mile than a long one does because a greater proportion of flight time and fuel is consumed in climbing to and descending from the cruising altitude.

In busy airports such as Atlanta, O'Hare, Los Angeles, and Kennedy, planes may spend much time waiting to take off or land. Every minute's wait adds dollars to personnel, fuel, and other costs. To keep costs down, the airlines have shifted to newer two-engine planes such as the Boeing 767, which enables them to reduce fuel consumption by as much as 30 percent. Aircraft have also reconfigured seat arrangements to include more seats, but this results in seats that are smaller and have less leg room for passengers. Claustrophobic? You'd better travel business class! A few years ago, American Airlines removed some rows of seats to give more leg room by spacing the remaining seats farther apart. This has proven to be a popular decision, and many others have followed.

Cruise Ships

More than 200 cruise lines offer a variety of wonderful vacations, from a Carnival cruise to freighters that carry only a few passengers. Travelers associate a certain romance with cruising to exotic locations and being pampered all day.

Being on a cruise ship is like being on a floating resort. For example, the *Diamond Princess* is a "Super Love Boat," weighing in at 116,000 tons with 18 decks and costing $400 million to build. This ship is longer than two football fields and is capable of carrying up to 2,670 passengers.[25] Cruise ship accommodations range from luxurious suites to cabins that are even smaller than most hotel rooms. Attractions and distractions range from early morning workouts to fabulous meals and nightlife consisting of dancing, cabarets, and sometimes casinos. Day life might involve relaxation, visits to the hair salon or spa, organized games, or simply reclining in a deck chair by the pool. Nonstop entertainment includes language lessons, charm classes, port-of-call briefings, cooking, dances, bridge, table tennis, shuffleboard, and more.

The cruise market has increased dramatically in recent years. About 9.0 million Americans cruise each year. Rates vary from a starting point of about $95 per person per day on Carnival Cruise Lines to $850 on the *Seabourn Yachts*. Rates typically are quoted per diem (per day) and are cruise-only figures based on double occupancy. Some 215 ships provide lake and river cruises, but most cruises are oceangoing. Casual ships cater to young couples, singles, and families with children. At the other end of the spectrum, ships that appeal to the upscale crowd draw a mature clientele that prefers a more sedate atmosphere, low-key entertainment, and dressing up for dinner. The spectacular new ships with multideck atriums and razzle-dazzle entertainment cater to the tourist market who have a median income of $50,000 a year.

Carnival Cruise Lines is the most financially successful of the cruise lines, netting about 20 percent of cruise sales. It targets adults between the ages of twenty-five and fifty-four and expects to attract millions of passengers with its spectacular atriums and round-the-clock activities. Its largest income, other than the fare itself, is from beverage service. Casino income is also high, and its casinos are the largest afloat. Carnival hopes that passengers will enjoy buying drinks and putting quarters, or preferably dollars, into the shipboard slot machines. They also hope their passengers will not mind their small cabins because the activities on the ship occupy passengers' waking hours and much of the night.

In 2009 alone, about 13.5 million passengers vacationed on a ship. As of Fall 2008, approximately 17 percent of the U.S. population target market had taken a cruise, but millions more intended to cruise in the next few years.[26] Many passengers are remarkably loyal to one particular vessel; as many as half of the passengers on a cruise may be repeat guests. Most cruise ships sail under foreign flags because they were built abroad for the following reasons:[27]

1. U.S. labor costs for ships, officers, and crew, in addition to maritime unions, are too high to compete in the world market.

2. U.S. ships are not permitted to operate casino-type gambling.

3. Many foreign shipyards are government subsidized to keep workers employed, thereby lowering construction costs.

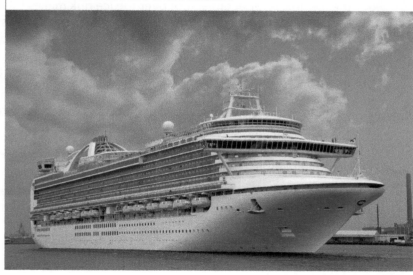

Take a Princess cruise for a dream vacation.

A DAY IN THE LIFE OF RICHARD SPACEY

Cruise Director, Royal Caribbean International

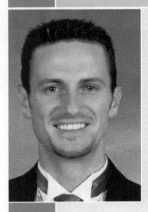

Voyager of the Seas, one of the largest and most innovative cruise ships ever built, has a total guest capacity of 3,700, with 1,200 crew members. *Voyager of the Seas* is truly a revolution in the cruising industry. A virtual city in itself, she features the world's first floating ice-skating rink, a rock-climbing wall, an inline skating track, and the largest and most technically advanced theater afloat. There is a four-story Royal Promenade shopping and entertainment boulevard spanning the length of the ship that acts as a hub for the ship's vast array of activities and entertainment. Cruise director Richard Spacey was instrumental in implementing the unique entertainment and activities program aboard with the help of a support staff of 130 people. What follows is an account of a day in the life of the cruise director of one of the largest cruise ships in the world.

Monday—First Day at Sea

7:30–8:30 A.M. Yesterday we embarked 3,650 guests in Miami and headed for our first port of call, Labadee, our own private island on the coast of Hispaniola. Before most of the guests are up for the day, I plan and submit our daily activities schedule for the rest of the voyage to our hotel director for his approval. All of the cruise director's staff management team have submitted their reports after our staff meeting at embarkation yesterday. The assistant cruise director, who also submits the payroll and overtime hours for my approval, schedules the twelve activities staff for the week. Our cruise programs administrator says that three couples were married in the wedding chapel yesterday, and they are included in the 108 couples that have chosen to spend their honeymoon with us. A special party will be held later on in the week to celebrate this happy occasion. The youth activities manager reports that there are more than 600 children aboard, ranging in age from three to seventeen. The youth activities manager and her team of thirteen are responsible for providing age-appropriate activities for our junior cruisers. We offer a special deck and pool area/arcade for children in addition to our extensive youth facilities, which include a teen disco.

A large part of our business is group and incentive business. The group coordinator appropriates lounges and facilities for these special group events under the auspices of the cruise director. There will be seminars, group meetings, presentations, and cocktail parties. We have a state-of-the-art conference center/executive boardroom/screening room in addition to a large convention facility named "Studio B," which doubles as the ice rink. A retractable floor over the ice rink makes this a great space for large conventions. The shore excursion manager reports that tour sales are good for this voyage among the fifty land-based excursions that we offer. All of this information is consolidated into a report to the hotel director that is submitted on a daily basis.

8:45–9:30 A.M. Hotel director's meeting. All of the division heads in the Hotel Department meet to discuss the daily operation of this floating hotel. Today's agenda includes a monthly safety meeting. Each division head presents his or her monthly report on safety and environmental protection. Hospitality and the safety of our guests and crew are our top priorities.

9:45 A.M. The start of my public duties. I give a daily announcement and rundown of all the activities and entertainment happenings around the ship.

10:00 A.M. Morning walk-around. Time to kick off the first session of Jackpot Bingo for the week. On my way through the promenade, I encounter our interactive performers hamming it up with our guests.

10:30 A.M. The Studio B ice rink is busy with guests skating at our first All Skate session. There are several sessions throughout the day. The ice-skating cast (ten individuals) are responsible for running the sessions as well as skating in our Ice Show.

11:00 A.M. Time to change out of my day uniform into a business suit and put on stage makeup for the taping of our onboard talk and information show, "Voyager Live." I produce this segment from the Royal Promenade. We have three video programmers and an interactive TV technician. Interactive TV allows our guests to order room service, excursions, and movies with the click of a button in the privacy of their staterooms.

12:00 noon Noon lunch with the staff in the Officers and Staff Dining Room.

1:00 P.M. Change out of the business suit into shorts and a Polo shirt to emcee the Belly Flop Competition at 1:30 P.M. poolside. This is always a popular event among our guests. It gets quite a few laughs. This is followed by horse racing, cruising style. We pick six jockeys who move six wooden horses by a roll of the dice. The betting is fierce as the guests cheer their favorite horses on. I become the track announcer for three races and the horse auctioneer. Today we auction off the six horses for our Voyager Derby later in the week. The horses go to the highest bidder, and then the "owners" run them in a race later in the week for all the money. The six horses go for $2,100. A nice pot for one lucky winner.

2:30 P.M. I stop by the Sports Court to check out the action. The sports court is full of families enjoying our Family Hour activities with the youth staff. We offer a nine-hole miniature golf course, a golf driving simulator, full-court basketball/volleyball, inline skating, table tennis, and a rock-climbing wall that rises up the smokestack 200 feet above sea level—the best view in the Caribbean. By the end of the day, 125 people will have climbed the wall.

3:00–4:30 P.M. POWER-NAP TIME. The day will not end until about 12:30 A.M. Being "on stage" and available practically twenty-four hours a day can take its toll. This nap will carry me through until the end of the evening.

6:00 P.M. Back to the office to catch up on e-mail and general administrative business. It is also time to work on budget and revenue forecasting for the upcoming year.

7:30 P.M. Off to the Royal Promenade deck to mingle with the guests at the Welcome Aboard reception. The captain gives his welcome speech, and then we send the guests off to their dinner or the show at 8:30 P.M.

8:30 P.M. Meet in the Champagne Bar with the hotel director before dinner. Tonight we will entertain guests who are on their fiftieth cruise and also a representative from an insurance company who is thinking of booking 700 guests on a future cruise with us.

9:00 P.M. On my way to the dining room, I introduce our production show in the La Scala Theater for the main-seating guests.

10:45 P.M. After dessert, I introduce the show for second-seating guests and watch the show for quality control.

11:45 P.M. After the show finishes, I do a final walk around the lounges on the ship with my assistant. Karaoke has just finished in one of the secondary lounges and we have music playing everywhere. We have thirty-five musicians comprising several bands featuring all varieties of music (string quartet, jazz ensemble, piano bar, Calypso, Latin, Top 40). The disco is lively with singles' night tonight, and there are a few couples enjoying light jazz in the Jazz Club.

12:30 A.M. A full day. Definitely a far cry from Julie on the *Love Boat*! Time for bed because I have to be on the gangway at 8:00 A.M. to welcome our guests to Labadee.

In addition, cruise ships sail under foreign flags (called flags of convenience) because registering these ships in countries such as Panama, the Bahamas, and Liberia means fewer and more lax regulations and little or no taxation.

Employment opportunities for Americans are mainly confined to sales, marketing, and other U.S. shore-based activities, such as reservations and supplies. Onboard, Americans sometimes occupy certain positions, such as cruise director and purser.

The reasons that few Americans work onboard cruise ships are because the ships are at sea for months at a time with just a few hours in port. The hours are long and the conditions for the crew are not likely to be acceptable to most Americans. No, you don't get your own cabin! Still interested? Try **www.crewunlimited.com.**

The Cruise Market

There are marked differences between the segments of the cruise industry:

Mass Market—Generally, people with incomes in the $35,000 to $74,000 range, interested in an average cost per person of between $95 and $195 per day, depending on the location and size of the cabin

Middle Market—Generally, people with incomes in the $75,000 to $99,000 range, interested in an average cost per person of $175 to $350 per day. These ships are capable of accommodating 750 to 1,000 passengers. The middle-market ships are stylish and comfortable, with each vessel having its own personality that caters to a variety of different guests. Among the cruise lines in the middle market are Princess Cruises, Norwegian Cruise Lines, Royal Caribbean, Holland America Lines, Windstar Cruises, Cunard Lines, and Celebrity Cruises.

Luxury Market—Generally, people with incomes higher than $100,000, interested in an average cost per person of more than $400 per day. In this market, the ships tend to be smaller, averaging about 700 passengers, with superior appointments and service. What constitutes a luxury cruise is partly a matter of individual judgment, partly a matter of advertising and public relations. The ships that received the top accolades from travel industry writers and others who assign such ranks cater only to the top 5 percent of North American income groups. Currently, the ships considered to be in the very top category are *Seabourn Spirit, Seabourn Legend, Seabourn Pride, Crystal Cruises Crystal Harmony, Radisson Diamond,* and *Silversea Silver Wind*. These six-star vessels have sophisticated cuisine, excellent service, far-reaching and imaginative itineraries, and highly satisfying overall cruise experiences.

The rising demand for cruising means larger ships with resort-like design, numerous activities, and amenities such as "virtual golf," pizzerias, and caviar bars. Significant growth opportunities still exist for the industry. With only about 10 percent of the cruise market tapped and with an estimated market potential of billions, the cruise industry is assured of a bright future.

► **Check Your Knowledge**

1. Why are the major U.S. airlines struggling financially?

2. Why do most cruise ships sail under foreign flags?

3. Describe the cruise market.

An Exciting Destination

Now, let's visit one of the world's most popular and exciting cities.

Think of the excitement of planning a trip to the city of Paris, which is for many the most fabulous city in the world. Known as the City of Light, it is also one of the most romantic cities. Paris is a city of beautiful buildings, boulevards, parks, markets, and restaurants and cafés. Paris has excitement. So, for tourists, what to see first is an often-asked question over morning coffee and, of course, a croissant. There are city tours, but the best way to see Paris is on foot, especially if you want to avoid the hordes of tourists hovering around the popular attractions! Take your pick from the many places of interest: You could begin with the Eiffel Tower or the Notre Dame Cathedral, the Louvre or the Musée d'Orsay, the Île de la Cité, or simply a stroll down the Champs-Elysées.

Paris began as a small village on an island called the Île de la Cité, in the middle of the river Seine. In time, Paris grew onto the Left Bank (Rive Gauche) where the University of the Sorbonne was founded, which gave instruction in Latin—thus, it became known as the Quartier Latin, or Latin Quarter. The Latin Quarter has a Bohemian intellectual character with lots of small cafés and wine bars similar to Greenwich Village and Soho in New York. Nearby is Montparnasse, an area that is popular with today's artists and painters. On the Right Bank (Rive Droit) of the river Seine are many attractions; one favorite is the area of Montmartre, with the diminutive St. Pierre Church, the domes of Sacré-Coeur, and the Place du Tertre. Just walking along the winding streets up to Sacré-Coeur gives one a feel of the special nature of Paris. Savoring the sights of the little markets with arrays of fresh fruits, vegetables, and flowers; catching the aromas wafting out from the cafés; and seeing couples walking arm in arm in a way that only lovers in Paris do add to the ambiance that captivates all who go there and provide wonderful memories.

Close-up, Sacré-Coeur is a magnificent building in gleaming white. It towers over Paris, with its five bulb-like domes resembling a Byzantine church. The view from there, one of the highest parts of Paris, is spectacular, especially at sunset.

Notre-Dame Cathedral is the most famous Gothic cathedral in the world. The thirteenth-century cathedral is adorned with

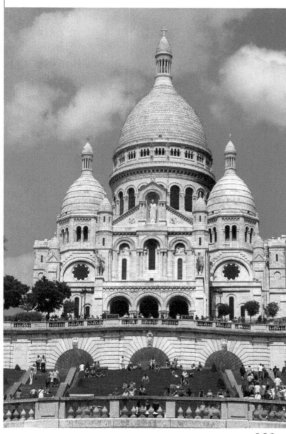

The Sacré-Coeur in Paris.

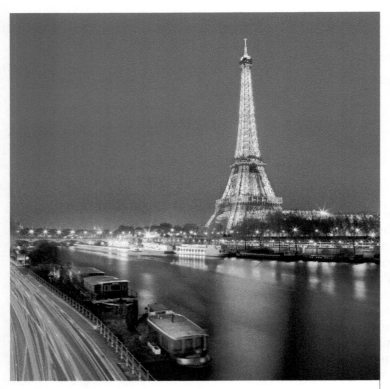

The River Seine and the Eiffel Tower at night.

ornate stone carvings depicting the Virgin Mary, signs of the Zodiac, the Last Judgment, Vices and Virtues, Christ and His Apostles, and Christ in Triumph after the Resurrection. A portal above these and other stone carvings are the gargoyles immortalized in Victor Hugo's *The Hunchback of Notre Dame* as Quasimodo's den.

The Eiffel Tower was built more than 100 years ago for a World's Fair and has become one of the most recognizable buildings in the world and a symbol of Paris. On a clear day, you can see for up to forty miles at the top of the tower.

Of the many fashionable boulevards and avenues, the Avenue des Champs-Elysées, the main boulevard of Paris, stands out as one of the most grand. The Arc de Triomphe commemorates Napoleon's victories and houses.

The Louvre, the former residence of King Louis XIV, is the world's largest palace and largest museum. It is here that priceless works of art are displayed for public view. The *Mona Lisa* and *Venus de Milo* are the star attractions of extensive collections of Chinese, Egyptian, Greek, Roman, French, and European art, sculpture, and ceramics. In the courtyard of the Louvre is the controversial Plexiglas pyramid that was built to ease overcrowding at the entrance—but perhaps in part because of its striking contrast with the palace, the lines of museum visitors are now even longer than they were before. Other museums in Paris house collections of the best works of art by the greatest painters the world has known. They represent various periods of art throughout the centuries.

The Economic Impact of Tourism

The World Travel and Tourism Council, a Brussels-based organization, suggests that the revenue from travel and tourism will be $1.850 billion (2.8 percent of GDP) in 2011 and will rise by 4.2 percent per year.[28] The total contribution of travel and tourism to GDP, including its wider economic impacts, is forecast to be $9,226.9 billion (9.6 percent) by 2021. Total contribution of travel and tourism to employment, including jobs indirectly supported by the industry, is forecasted to rise to 323,826,000 jobs (9.7 percent) by 2021.[29]

Tourism accounts for 7.72 million jobs in the United States. The United States is second to France in the number of tourists (59.7 million) but first in tourism revenues (see Figure 3).

World international arrivals, according to the UNWTO, will reach 1.8 billion by 2030, more than triple the 475 million people who traveled abroad in 1992. Nearly every state publishes its own tourism economic impact study

**International Tourism Receipts
(US $ billion)**

Rank		2009
1	United States	93.9
2	Spain	53.2
3	France	49.4
4	Italy	40.2
5	China	39.7
6	Germany	34.7
7	United Kingdom	30.0
8	Australia	25.6
9	Turkey	21.3
10	Austria	19.4

Source: World Tourism Organization (WTO)©.

Figure 3 • World's Top Ten Tourism Earners. Notice that China now features prominently as a leading tourism nation.
(© UNWTO, 9284403211)

indicating billions of dollars in tourism revenue. The Tourism Industry Association's annual *Tourism Work for America Report*[30] indicates that travel and tourism are one of the nation's leading sectors. Statistics include the following:[31]

- International travelers spend about $134.4 billion on travel-related expenses (for example, lodging, food, entertainment) in the United States annually.

- There are 7.72 million people are directly employed in the travel industry, making travel and tourism the nation's second largest employer after health services.

- Travel generates more than $100 billion a year in tax receipts. If it were not for tourism, each U.S. household would have to pay about $1,000 more per year in taxes.

- Spending by international visitors in the United States is about $31 billion more than travel-related spending by Americans outside the United States.

- Approximately 59.7 million international travelers visit the United States each year.

- Just a small percentage increase in the world market would mean millions more visitors, which would create thousands of jobs and contribute billions of dollars in new tax revenue.

By employing approximately one out of every ten workers, travel and tourism is the world's largest employer and is the world's largest industry grouping.

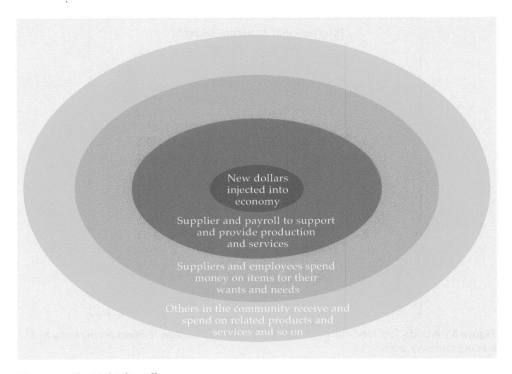

Figure 4 • The Multiplier Effect.

The Multiplier Effect

Tourists bring new money into the economy of the place they are visiting, and this has effects beyond the original expenditures. When a tourist spends money to travel, to stay in a hotel, or to eat in a restaurant, that money is recycled by those businesses to purchase more goods, thereby generating further use of the money. In addition, employees of businesses who serve tourists spend a higher proportion of their money locally on various goods and services. This chain reaction, called the **multiplier effect**, continues until there is a leakage, meaning that money is used to purchase something from outside the area. Figure 4 illustrates the multiplier effect.

In most economic impact studies to date, developed economies have a multiplier effect of between 1.5 and 2.0.[32] This means that the original money spent is used again in the community between 1.5 and 2.0 times. If tourism-related businesses spend more money on locally produced goods and services, it benefits the local economy.

Promoters of Tourism

The **Pacific Area Travel Association (PATA)** represents thirty-four countries in the Pacific and Asia that have united behind common goals: excellence in travel and tourism growth. PATA's accomplishments include shaping the future of travel in the Asia/Pacific region; it has had a remarkable record of success with research, development, education, and marketing.

Many countries have a minister of tourism, which is a cabinet-level position that can advocate tourism development, marketing, and management through the national tourism organization (NTO). Unfortunately, the United States does not have even a senior-level government official for tourism. Instead, an organization known as the Travel Industry of America (TIA) is the main body for the promotion and development of tourism in the United States. It speaks for the common interests and concerns of all components of the U.S. travel industry. Its mission is to benefit the entire U.S. travel industry by unifying its goals, coordinating private sector efforts to encourage and promote travel to and within the United States, monitoring government policies that affect travel and tourism, and supporting research and analysis in areas vital to the industry. Established in 1941, TIA's membership represents more than 2,000 travel-related businesses, associations, and local, regional, and state travel-promotion agencies.

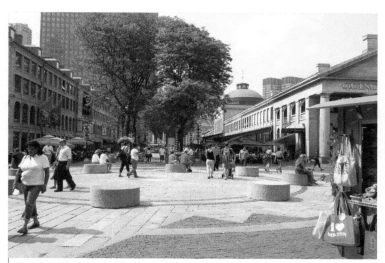

State offices of tourism promote places of interest, such as Faneuil Hall and Quincy Market in Boston.

State Offices of Tourism

In the United States, the next level of organizations concerned with tourism are the state offices of tourism. These offices are charged by their legislative bodies with the orderly growth and development of tourism within the state. They promote information programs, advertising, publicity, and research on the recreation and tourism attractions in the state.

City-Level Offices of Tourism and Convention Centers

Cities have also realized the importance of the "new money" that tourism brings. Many cities have established **convention and visitors bureaus (CVBs)**, whose main function is to attract and retain visitors to the city. The CVBs are staffed by representatives of the city's attractions, restaurants, hotels and motels, and transportation system. These bureaus are largely funded by the transient occupancy tax (TOT) that is charged to hotel guests. In most cities, the TOT ranges from 8 to 18 percent. The balance of funding comes from membership dues and promotional activities. In recent years, convention centers have sprung up in a number of large and several smaller cities. Spurred on by expectations of economic and social gain, cities operate both CVBs and convention centers.

National Offices of Tourism

National offices of tourism (NOTs) seek to improve the economy of the country they represent by increasing the number of visitors and consequently their spending in the country. Connected to this function is the responsibility to oversee and ensure that hotels, transport systems, tour operators, and tour guides maintain high standards in the care and consideration of the tourist. The main activities of NOTs are as follows:

- Publicizing the country
- Assisting and advising certain types of travelers
- Creating demand for certain destinations
- Supplying information
- Ensuring that the destination is up to expectations
- Advertising[33]

Tour Operators

Tour operators promote tours and trips that they plan and organize. A *tour* is a trip taken by an individual or group of people who travel together with a professional tour manager/escort and follow a preplanned itinerary. Most tours include travel, accommodations, meals, land transportation, and sightseeing. The tour operator negotiates discounted travel, accommodation, meals, and sightseeing and then adds a markup before advertising the package. Tour operators also offer **vacation packages** to people traveling alone. Vacation packages include a combination of two or more travel services—hotel, car rental, and air transportation—offered at a package price. Most vacation packages offer a choice of components and options, allowing the client to customize his or her package to personal interests and budget.

Travel Agencies

A *travel agent* is a middleperson who acts as a travel counselor and sells travel services on behalf of airlines, cruise lines, rail and bus transportation companies, hotels, and auto rental companies. Agents may sell individual parts of the overall system or several elements, such as air and cruise tickets. The agent acts as a broker, bringing together the client (buyer) and the supplier (seller). Agents have quick access to schedules, fares, and advice for clients about various destinations.

The American Society of Travel Agents (ASTA) is the world's largest travel trade association, with more than 20,000 members in more than 165 countries. Agents use computer reservation systems (CRSs) to access service availability and make bookings. In the United States, the main vendors of CRSs are Amadeus, Sabre, Travel Sky, Worldspan, and Galileo.

A travel agent is more than a ticket seller. Agents serve their clients in the following ways:

- Arranging transportation by air, sea, rail, bus, car rental, and so on
- Preparing individual itineraries, personally escorted tours, group tours, and prepared package tours
- Arranging for hotel, motel, and resort accommodations; meals; sightseeing tours; transfers of passengers and luggage between terminals and hotels; and

special features such as tickets for music festivals, the theater, and so forth

- Handling and advising on many details involved with travel, such as insurance, foreign currency exchange, documentary requirements, and immunizations and other inoculations needed

- Using professional know-how and experience (for example, schedules of air, train, and bus connections, rates of hotels, quality of accommodations)

- Arranging reservations for special-interest activities, such as group tours, conventions, business travel, gourmet tours, and sporting trips

However, the travel business has changed, resulting in a sharp decline in the number of travel agents, because there is less need for the traditional travel agent in the age of the Internet. Internet travel services such as Travelocity and Expedia have changed the way we book travel. As you know, it is quick and easy to go online and select travel dates, times, and fares. In fact, tourism services are among the top online purchases. As consumers, we can shop for the best price and most convenient schedule and purchase electronic tickets by entering our credit card numbers and billing information over a secure connection.

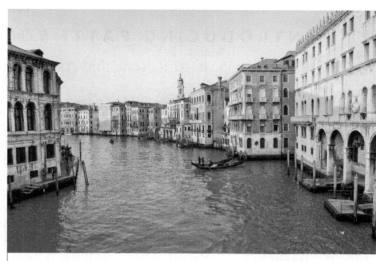

Travel agents have knowledge of destinations and can make air, ground, and hotel reservations for clients to visit popular destinations such as Venice, Italy.

Tour Wholesalers and Consolidators

Tour suppliers provide the package components for tour operators via the services of hotels, attractions, restaurants, airlines, cruise lines, railroads, and sightseeing, which are packaged into a tour that is sold through a sales channel to the public.[34] Tour wholesaling came into prominence years ago because airlines had vacant seats, which, like hotel rooms, are perishable. Airlines naturally wanted to sell as many seats as possible and found that they could sell blocks of seats to wholesalers close to departure dates. These tickets are for specific destinations around which tour wholesalers build a tour. Wholesalers then sell their tours directly through retail agents.

Consolidators work closely with airlines to purchase discounted seats that they then sell to consumers for a price that is generally about 20 percent lower than the price offered by airlines or an online service company such as Travelocity. For example, the price of a consolidator's fare for a round trip to Bali from New York is $975, but the airline or Travelocity fare can be double that. So, consolidators are the place to call or e-mail when you are interested in booking an airfare.

Destination Management Companies

A destination management company (DMC) is a service organization in the visitor industry that offers a host of programs and services to meet clients' needs. Initially, a destination management sales manager concentrates on selling the

INTRODUCING PATTI ROSCOE

Chairperson, Patti Roscoe and Associates (PRA) and Roscoe/Coltrell, Inc. (RCI)

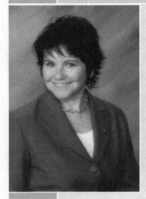

Patricia L. Roscoe landed in California in 1966, charmed by the beautiful San Diego sun compared to the cold winters in Buffalo, New York, her hometown. She was a young, brilliant middle manager who was to face the challenges of a time when women were expected to become either nurses or teachers. She became involved with the hotel industry, working for a large private resort hotel, the Vacation Village. Those were years to be remembered. She gained a very thorough knowledge of southern California tourism, as well as the inherent mechanisms of the industry. With the unforgettable help and guidance of her manager, she began to lay the foundations of her future career as a very successful leader in the field. The outstanding skills that she learned are, in fact, the very basis of her many accomplishments.

The list of her awards and honors is astounding: the prestigious CITE (Certified Incentive Travel Executive) distinction, the San Diego Woman of Accomplishment, and San Diego's Allied Member of the Year. The U.S. Small Business Administration gave her the Wonder Woman Award for her outstanding achievements in the field, and the San Diego Convention and Visitors Bureau has conferred on her the prestigious RCA Lubach Award for her contributions to the industry.

She is also extremely involved in civic and tourism organizations, including the Rotary Club, the American Lung Association of San Diego and Imperial Counties, and the San Diego Convention and Visitors Bureau.

The key to her success perhaps lies in her remarkable skill for interacting with people. It is the human resources, in fact, that represent the major strength of PRA. Its employees are experienced, dedicated, and service oriented. But what makes them so efficient is their dedication to working together as a team. Patti Roscoe guides, inspires, and motivates the teams. She is a self-admitted "softy," a creative and emotional leader who enjoys training her employees and following their growth step by step, to eventually give them the power of initiative they deserve, as a tool to encourage their creativity and originality. She constantly seeks to balance the concept of teamwork with the individual goals and private lives of her employees. It is through the achievement of such a balance that a profitable, healthy community is preserved. PRA is a bit more than a community, however: It is a family, and just like a mother, Patti's formula is discipline and love. At the same time, Patti's leading efforts are aimed at training her employees to think outside of the box, and to keep their views as broad as possible, which is the only way to rise above the commonplace, the rhetorical, and the trivial, to escape provincialism, and thus become unique individuals.

That's how the magic is done. PRA excels in creating "something that becomes exclusively yours—that has never been done before." PRA is decentralized into service teams to foster an entrepreneurial environment in which initiative and creativity can be boosted to the fullest. Therefore, PRA staff design personalized, unique events to give their customers an unforgettable time.

Since its opening in 1981, PRA has become one of the most successful destination management companies in the country, providing personal, caring service characterized by flexibility and creativity.

destination to meeting planners and performance improvement companies (incentive houses).

The needs of such groups may be as simple as an airport pickup or as involved as hosting an international sales convention with theme parties. DMCs work closely with hotels; sometimes DMCs book rooms, and other times hotels request the DMC's know-how on organizing theme parties.

Patricia Roscoe, chairperson of Patti Roscoe and Associates (PRA), says that meeting planners often have a choice of several destinations and might ask, "Why should I pick your destination?" The answer is that a DMC does everything, including providing airport greetings, transportation to the hotel, and VIP check-in; organizing theme parties; sponsoring programs; organizing competitive sports events, and so on, depending on the budget.

Sales managers associated with DMCs obtain leads, which are potential clients, from the following sources:

- Hotels
- Trade shows
- CVBs
- Cold calls
- Incentive houses
- Meeting planners

Each sales manager has a staff or team that includes people in the following positions:

- Special events manager, who has expertise in sound, lighting, staging, and so on
- Accounts manager, who is an assistant to the sales manager
- Operations manager, who coordinates everything, especially on-site arrangements, to ensure that what is sold actually happens

For example, Patti Roscoe's DMC organized meetings, accommodations, meals, beverages, and theme parties for 2,000 Ford Motor Company dealers in nine groups over three days per group.

Roscoe also works closely with incentive houses, such as Carlson Marketing or Maritz Travel. These incentive houses approach a company and offer to evaluate and set up incentive plans for the sales team, including whatever it takes to motivate them. Once approved, Carlson contacts a DMC and asks for a program.

In conclusion, thousands of companies and associations hold meetings and conventions all over the country. Many of these organizations use the services of professional meeting planners, who in turn seek out suitable destinations for the meetings and conventions. Some larger hotels and resorts now have a destination management department to handle all the arrangements for groups and conventions.

▶ Check Your Knowledge

1. Describe the economic impact of tourism.

2. Is it better to have a higher or lower multiplier effect and why?

3. Describe the promoters of tourism.

Business Travel

In recent years, business travel has declined due to[35] the general economic climate; in addition, increases in airfares, incidences in terrorism, and businesses reducing their travel budgets have negatively affected business travel.

Yet, a good percentage of the guests who check into upscale hotels around the world are traveling for business reasons. Much **business travel** is hard work, whether it is travel in one's own automobile or in the luxury of a first-class seat aboard an airplane. A good portion of business travel, however, is mixed with pleasure.

Counted as business travelers are those who travel for business purposes, such as for meetings; all kinds of sales, including corporate, regional, product, and others; conventions; trade shows and expositions; and combinations of more than one of these purposes. In the United States, meetings and conventions alone attract millions of people annually. Sometimes the distinction between business and leisure travel becomes blurred. If a convention attendee in Atlanta decides to stay on for a few days after the conference, is this person to be considered a business or leisure traveler? Business travelers, when compared to leisure travelers, tend to be younger, spend more money, travel farther, and travel in smaller groups, but they do not stay as long as leisure travelers do.

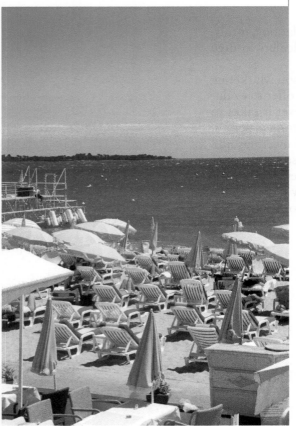

Beaches at the Cote d'Azur in southern France may be standing room only.

Social and Cultural Impact of Tourism

From a social and cultural perspective, tourism can have both positive and negative impacts on communities. Undoubtedly, tourism has made significant contributions to international understanding. World tourism organizations recognize that tourism is a means of enhancing international understanding, peace, prosperity, and universal respect for and observance of human rights and fundamental freedom for all without distinction as to race, sex, language, or religion. Tourism can be a very interesting sociocultural phenomenon. Seeing how others live is an interest of many tourists, and the exchange of sociocultural values and activities is rewarding.

Provided that the number of tourists is manageable and that they respect the host community's sociocultural norms and values, tourism provides an opportunity for a number of social interactions. A London pub or a New York café are examples of good places for social interaction. Similarly, depending on the reason for the tourist visit, myriad opportunities are available to interact both socially and culturally with local people. Even a visit to another part of the United States can be both socially and culturally stimulating. For example, New Orleans has a very diverse social and cultural heritage. Over the years, the city has been occupied by the Spanish, French, British, and Americans, so the food, music, dance, and social norms are unique to the area. The competitiveness of international destinations is based on attributes such as service quality, value for the price, safety, security, entertainment, weather, infrastructure, and natural environment.[36] Political stability is also important in determining the desirability of a destination for international tourism. Imagine the feelings of an employee in a developing country who earns perhaps $5 per day when he or she sees wealthy tourists flaunting money, jewelry, and an unobtainable lifestyle.

CORPORATE PROFILE

G Adventures

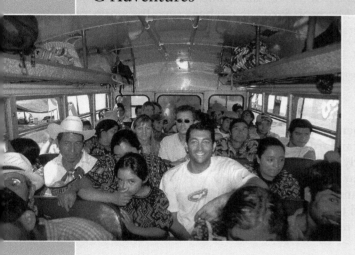

If you are tired of the one-week-in-the-Florida-sun vacation and want to do something exciting and off the beaten path, then G Adventures is the perfect company to turn to. They provide more than 1,000 small group experiences, safaris, and expeditions on all seven continents, to more than 100,000 travelers a year. This year, approximately 1.5 million more people are expected to visit their web site, some of them to change their lives forever.

G Adventure's CEO Bruce Poon Tip has been honored with the Entrepreneur of the Year Award, sponsored by NASDAQ, Ernst & Young, and the National Post. G Adventures has also been named one of Canada's 50 best managed companies and top 100 employers. Furthermore, they have greatly helped to improve the conditions in the many countries they visit.

Their philosophy, "The Freedom of Independent Travel with the Security of a Group," has been practiced since the start. They respect their travelers as individuals, and there is no requirement to be athletic to embark on one of their trips. The only thing needed is to have the spirit of adventure and the desire to experience a world totally different from what you are accustomed to.

In addition, the concept of responsible tourism is very important to G Adventures; the company employees interact with the local population, striving to leave behind only footprints. Their commitment is to support local people and communities and to protect the environment in which they travel. To that end, G Adventures developed Planeterra—the G Adventures Foundation that gives back to the people and communities that its passengers visit on their trips.

G Adventures hires people in different departments, including Operations, Product, Sales and Marketing, Finance, Human Resources, and Tour Leading. G Adventures employs more than 1,350 staff worldwide. All current postings can be found under the career section of their web site.

Maybe the most obvious choice for you is the position of G Adventures tour leader, which G Adventures calls Chief Experience Officers (CEOs). In this position, your main task is to make people's holiday dreams come true and make sure all travelers have an enjoyable time abroad.

As a CEO, most of the time the local hostel where you spend the night is your home, and your office is your backpack. On your way to work, you might have to hike the Inca Trail or canoe down the Amazon River.

(continued)

CORPORATE PROFILE (continued)

If you are interested in meeting and really interacting with people from different cultures, and like to show your passion to travelers of different backgrounds, ages, and interests, this is the perfect job for you.

Some of the requirements to work as a CEO include fluency in English and Spanish, a passion for travel, a love for Latin America (which is their main area of operations), and excellent people skills. No matter what happens and how bad your day has been, you always have to be the happy and helpful leader. Additional skills needed include awareness of, and commitment to, sustainable tourism, both environmentally and culturally, as well commitment to an eighteen-month contract. It takes time to become the perfect adventure tour leader, and once you have learned it, the company may decide to renew your contract. You also need to be resourceful, which here means being able to solve any kind of problem that might arise, expected or unexpected. Because of the nature of the work, you also need to have good health, first-aid certification, and an average level of computer literacy (Internet/e-mail/Microsoft Word/Microsoft Excel). If you have seen the world, or want to see it, in a truly interactive way, and you have leadership skills and are adventurous and brave, then this might be the perfect job for you. Why not give it a try?

Note: To apply to be a tour leader, you must complete the online application form found on the web site.

Just imagine what will happen when another 500 million people become tourists by virtue of increasing standards of living and the ability of more people to obtain passports. Currently, only about 37 percent of the U.S. population have passports, although that may increase because everyone returning to the United States from Mexico and Canada must now have a passport.[37] The population of eastern Europe and the new rich of the Pacific Rim countries will substantially add to the potential number of tourists.

Ecotourism

Ecotourism is focused more on individual values; it is "tourism with a conscience," sharing many of the same aspirations as sustainable tourism (described next). The International Ecotourism Society (TIES) defines *ecotourism* as "responsible travel to natural areas that conserves the environment and improves the well-being of local people."[38] This means that those who implement and participate in ecotourism activities should respect the following principles:

- Minimize impact.
- Build environmental and cultural awareness and respect.
- Provide positive experiences for both visitors and hosts.
- Provide direct financial benefits for conservation.
- Provide financial benefits and empowerment for local people.
- Raise sensitivity to host countries' political, environmental, and social climate.
- Support international human rights and labor agreements.[39]

Most ecotourism destinations can be found in developing countries with natural surroundings and plentiful flora and fauna. Places such as deserts, tropical rain forests, coral reefs, and ice glaciers are prime locations. Also important in ecotourism is the presence of a culture that is unique. The focus of ecotourism is to provide tourists with new knowledge about a certain natural area and the culture that is found in it, along with a little bit of adventure. As for the local inhabitants, ecotourism aims to help improve the local economy and conservation efforts. All parties are to gain a new appreciation for nature and people.

Generally, most of the more popular ecotourism destinations are located in underdeveloped and developing countries. As vacationers become more adventurous and visit remote, exotic places, they are participating in activities that should affect nature, host communities, and themselves in a positive manner. And because of the growing interests of travelers, many developed countries are following the trend and developing ecotourism programs. Ecotourism can be a main source of worldwide promotion of sustainable development geared toward tourists and communities in all countries.

Thus far, ecotourism projects tend to be developed on a small scale. It is much easier to control such sites, particularly because of limits that are normally set on the community, the local tourism business, and the tourists. Limitations may include strict control of the amount of water and electricity used, more stringent recycling measures, regulation of park and market hours, and more important, and caps on the number of visitors to a certain location at one time and the size of the business. Another reason ecotourism projects are kept small is to allow more in-depth tours and educational opportunities.

Sustainable Tourism

The increasing number of tourists visiting destinations has heightened concerns about the environment, physical resources of the place, and sociocultural degradation. The response of tourism officials has been to propose that all tourism be sustainable. The concept of **sustainable tourism** places a broad-based obligation on society, especially those involved in making tourism policy, planning for development, and harmonizing tourism and tourism development by improving the quality of a place's environment and physical and sociocultural resources. According to the UNWTO definition, sustainable tourism refers to the environmental, economic, and sociocultural aspects of tourism development, with the establishment of a suitable balance between these three dimensions to guarantee its long-term sustainability.[40]

The United Nations Environment Program (UNEP) says that sustainability principles refer to the environmental, economic, and sociocultural aspects of tourism. Sustainable

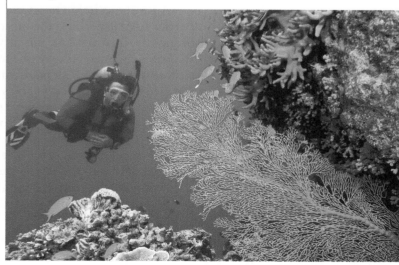

The Great Barrier Reef off the coast of Australia is one of the World Heritage sites.

tourism should (1) make optimal use of environmental resources that constitute a key element in tourism development; (2) respect the sociocultural authenticity of host communities, conserve their built and living cultural heritage and traditional values, and contribute to intercultural understanding and tolerance; and (3) ensure viable, long-term economic operations, providing socioeconomic benefits to all stakeholders that are fairly distributed, including stable employment and income-earning opportunities and social services to host communities, and contributing to poverty alleviation.

The two key factors are community-based tourism and quality tourism. Community-based tourism ensures that a majority of the benefits go to locals and not to outsiders. Quality tourism basically offers tourists "good value for their money." This also serves as a protection of local natural resources and as an attraction to the kinds of tourists who will respect the local environment and society. All tourism should be sustainable, but the problem is that all too frequently it is not.

Let's look around the world and see how the concept of sustainable tourism is applied. Europe has been criticized for lack of sustainability, but apart from the congested areas of, for example, London, Rome, and Paris, there are plenty of destinations focusing on sustainable tourism. In particular, tours to explore the ancient ruins, architecture, and cultures of Turkey and Greece are popular choices. Also, the largely untouched nature and distinctive culture of the Scandinavian countries are growing in recognition and importance.

If you want to explore Asia, join an ecotour to the snow-capped Himalayas in Nepal or the sultry jungles of Thailand. More and more places, such as Malaysia, Thailand, and the Philippines, are developing their tourism programs based on environmental conservation and protection. Looking for Shangri-la? The former hidden kingdom of the Hunza Valley in Pakistan has been opened for ecotourism, allowing a select number of tourists to see the 700-year-old Hunza Fort and village. The project has been internationally acclaimed as an outstanding example of sustainable tourism.

More adventures await you in Africa, where the tourism industry, especially ecotourism, has been growing tremendously over the past years. The most popular activity is the safari, which lets you get up close and personal with exotic wildlife such as elephants, gazelles, lions, tigers, cheetahs, and countless others. Kenya is an important destination for safaris, as are Tanzania, South Africa, Botswana, and Malawi.

Australia is home to an impressive variety of eco-friendly places. The Great Barrier Reef is perhaps the most famous spot. The "Leave No Trace" program, originally an American initiative, ensures that visitors to the reef act in a responsible manner. As a visitor to the Great Barrier Reef, you can enjoy activities such as snorkeling, fishing, diving, hiking, camping, and much more with many certified eco-friendly companies. Another area that is subject to increasing interest and attention is the massive glaciers of Antarctica.

These days, many regions of the world are designating their attractions as ecotourism sites. Vacationers are becoming more adventurous and are visiting remote, exotic places. They are participating in activities that hopefully affect nature, host communities, as well as themselves, in a positive manner.

From Yellowstone National Park in the United States to the Mayan ruins of Tikal in Guatemala, from the Amazon River in Brazil to the vast safari lands

FOCUS ON TOURISM

Ann-Marie Weldon, Johnson & Wales University, Charlotte, North Carolina

Think of the last vacation you took, or the one you are planning now. Where have you gone or where are you going? Is it somewhere exotic or is it close to home? How are you going to get there? Will you be flying, driving, or taking the train? Where are you going to stay? Are you going to a hotel, to a resort, or on a cruise ship? What will you do once you are there? Will you explore a new city, go to a museum, hang glide, visit a nature preserve, see a ball game, or visit an amusement park? What about the business traveler? Where are their business meetings? How about members of an association? Where is their convention or conference? Many people think tourism is just for the big cities or someplace they dream about visiting. As people travel, for either business or pleasure, they touch all the aspects of the hospitality industry. Tourism is what drives the need for hotels, resorts, cruise lines, restaurants, airlines, recreation, theme parks, and entertainment—in your home town or around the world.

The World Tourism Organization (UNWTO) report *Tourism: 2020 Vision*, which you learned about in this chapter, forecasts "that international arrivals are expected to reach nearly 1.6 billion by the year 2020" and "of these worldwide arrivals in 2020, 1.2 billion will be intraregional." This information may not mean anything to you right now, but each of the 1.6 billion people that are expected to travel will need a place to stay, eat, and experience something new. This indicates opportunities for new hotels, food and beverage outlets, places to hold meetings or conventions, and activities to keep guests busy. This will also provide employment potential in the traditional as well as the creative sense. We tend to forget the impact tourism has on our industry and what that means to our economy. Even in tough economic times, people still travel, though maybe not as far as they would otherwise. But they will need a way to get where they want to go and a place to stay, food to eat, and things to do once they get there.

Remember that each segment of the hospitality industry is interconnected with each other and depends on tourism—people traveling, experiencing, and exploring. Happy travels on your exciting new adventure in hospitality!

of Kenya, from the snow-capped Himalayas in Nepal to the sultry jungles of Thailand, from the Great Barrier Reef in Australia to the massive ice glaciers in Antarctica, it seems that sustainable tourism is taking place in all corners of the world. Quite frankly, some sort of ecotourism activity is happening in almost every country.

Cultural, Heritage, Nature, and Volunteer Tourism

Tourism has developed to the point that there are now several special-interest areas. *Culture* and *heritage* are "our legacies from the past, what we live with today, and what we pass on to future generations. Our cultures and natural heritages are irreplaceable sources of life and inspiration."[41] The **United Nations Educational, Scientific, and Cultural Organization** (UNESCO) has designated a number of World Heritage Sites worthy of protection and preservation because of the outstanding value to humanity of their natural and cultural heritage. There are nineteen U.S. sites on the World Heritage List, among them the Statue of Liberty and the Grand Canyon. Other places as unique and diverse as the wilds of East Africa's Serengeti, the pyramids of Egypt, the Great Barrier Reef in Australia, and the Baroque cathedrals of Latin America are also on the list. What makes the concept of world heritage exceptional is its universal application. World Heritage Sites belong to all the peoples of the world, no matter where they call home.[42]

Various examples of cultural tourism, heritage tourism, nature tourism, and volunteer tourism are as follows:

Cultural tourism. These trips are motivated by interest in cultural events such as feasts or festivals or activities such as theater, history, arts and sciences, museums, architecture, and religion. An example of **cultural tourism** is a visit to the Polynesian Center in Hawaii where you will find information on and examples of the lifestyles, songs, dance, costumes, and architecture of seven Pacific islands: Fiji, New Zealand, Marquesas, Samoa, Tahiti, Tonga, and Hawaii.

Heritage tourism. This type of tourism is motivated by historic preservation—a combination of the natural, cultural, and architectural environment. An example of heritage tourism is a visit to the Alamo in Texas, a former battlefield that attracts 3 million visitors a year.

Nature tourism. These trips are motivated by nature, such as a visit to a national park. In recent years, aging baby boomers have increasingly become interested in nature tourism and include nature attractions as a part of or a reason for their trip. (Notice that there are some similarities among these tourism areas of special interest.)

Culinary tourism. Gastronomic tours of Europe and Asia in places like Florence, Italy, and Bangkok, Thailand, have an appeal to the "foodies" among us. If not the main reason for a trip, culinary adventures are certainly a contributing reason, and the appeal is growing stronger with the advent of such programs as Anthony Bourdain's "No Reservations."

Volunteer tourism. **Volunteer tourism** provides travelers with an alternative to standard commercial vacation options. A major attraction for those who volunteer for overseas aid projects is the opportunity to travel safely and cheaply. While volunteers provide material benefits for the host community in exchange for shelter, both have the opportunity to experience each other's cultural differences. Dr. Stephen Wearing of the University of Technology in Sidney, Australia, and author of a book on volunteer tourism says:

The growth of eco-tourism, which grew out of the Green movement, proves people want an alternative, and volunteer tourism offers a similarly enriching experience.

While volunteers provide material benefits for the host community in exchange for shelter, both have the opportunity to experience each other's cultural difference.[43]

Dr. Wearing believes volunteer tourism will rival the popularity of ecotourism this decade.

Trends in Tourism and Travel

- Ecotourism, sustainable tourism, and heritage tourism will continue to grow in importance.

- Globally, the number of tourist arrivals will continue to increase by about 4 percent per year, soon topping 1 billion.

- Governments will increasingly recognize the importance of tourism not only as an economic force, but also as a sociacultural force of growing significance.

- More bilateral treaties are being signed, which will make it easier for tourists to obtain visas to visit other countries.

- The promotion and development of tourism will move even more from the public sector (government) to the private sector (involved industry segments).

- Technology will continue to advance, allowing even more information to be available more quickly to more places around the world.

- Marketing partnerships and corporate alliances will continue to increase.

- Employment prospects will continue to improve.

- Ticketless air travel will continue to increase.

- Travel and tourism bookings via the Internet will continue to increase rapidly.

- As an ever-increasing number of tourists visit destinations, managing these destinations will continue to be a challenge.

- Low-cost, no-frills airlines, such as Jet Blue, AirTran, ATA, and, of course, Southwest, will continue to gain an increased market share at the expense of the six main U.S. airlines.

- Airlines will try to entice travelers to book their trips via the airline's web site rather than through Expedia and similar sites.

- Automatic airport check-ins will become more popular.

- The cruise industry will continue to expand.

- There will be more alternative cruises.

- There will be increased concern for the health and safety of travel and tourism.

- Nature, culinary, and volunteer tourism will continue to increase.

CASE STUDY

Congratulations! You have just been appointed to your city's council. You discover that a hot topic soon to be presented to the council is the construction of a convention center. Your initial research shows that several midsized cities are considering the convention center as a way to increase economic activity, including job creation. The challenge these cities face is how to finance the convention center; projected costs are $100 million. Voters may resist a ballot to increase local taxes (either property or sales), but there is still the transient occupancy tax (TOT)—that is, taxes paid by people staying in local hotels—to consider. However, that tax is already earmarked for various local charities, and as we all know, good politicians want to get reelected, so voting against several worthy causes would not be popular. How can the center be financed and built? The city could float a bond on the market or could raise the TOT, but that might dissuade some groups from coming to your city because other cities have lower TOTs.

What would you do? What information do you need in order to decide whether to support or oppose the convention center?

Summary

1. Tourism can be defined as the idea of attracting, accommodating, and pleasing groups or individuals traveling for pleasure or business. It is categorized by geography, ownership, function, industry, and travel motive.

2. Tourism involves international interaction and, therefore, government regulation. Several organizations, such as the World Tourism Organization, promote environmental protection, tourism development, immigration, and cultural and social aspects of tourism.

3. Tourism is a collection of industries that, when combined, form the world's largest industry and employer. It affects other industry sectors, such as public transportation, foodservice, lodging, entertainment, and recreation. In addition, tourism produces secondary impacts on businesses that are affected indirectly, which is known as the multiplier effect.

4. Travel agencies, tour operators, travel managers, wholesalers, national offices of tourism, and destination management companies serve as middlepersons between a country and its visitors.

5. Physical needs, the desire to experience other cultures, and an interest in meeting new people are some of the motives of travelers. Because of flexible work hours, early retirement, and the easy accessibility of traveling, tourism is constantly growing.

6. From a social and cultural perspective, tourism can further international understanding and economically improve poorer countries. However, it can also disturb a culture by presenting it with mass tourism and the destruction of natural sites. A trend in avoiding tourism pollution is ecotourism.

7. Business travel has increased in recent years as a result of the growth of convention centers in several cities. As a result, business travelers have given a boost to hotels, restaurants, and auto rental companies. The number of female business travelers is rising as well.

8. Ecotourism is tourism with a conscience, or responsible travel to natural areas that conserves the environment and improves the well-being of the local people.

9. The concept of sustainable tourism places a broad-based obligation on society, especially those involved with tourism policy, planning, and development.

Key Words and Concepts

business travel
convention and visitors bureaus (CVBs)
cultural tourism
ecotourism
hub-and-spoke system
interdependency
load factor
multiplier effect

Pacific Area Travel Association (PATA)
sustainable tourism
tourism
United Nations Educational, Scientific, and
Cultural Organization (UNESCO)
vacation package
volunteer tourism
World Tourism Organization (UNWTO)

Review Questions

1. Give a broad definition of tourism and explain why people are motivated to travel.
2. Give a brief explanation of the economic impact of tourism. Name two organizations that influence or further the economic impact of tourism.

3. Choose a career in the tourism business and give a brief overview of what your responsibilities would be.
4. Discuss the positive and negative impacts that tourism can have on a country in relation to tourism pollution and ecotourism.

Internet Exercises

1. Organization: **World Tourism Organization (UNWTO)**
   Web site: **www.world-tourism.org/**
   Summary: The UNWTO is the only intergovernmental organization that serves in the field of travel and tourism and is a global forum for tourism policy and issues. It has about 154 member countries and 7 territories. Its mission is to promote and develop tourism as a significant means of fostering international peace and understanding, economic development, and international trade.
   (a) How much is spent on international tourism?
   (b) What does the *Tourism: 2020 Vision* predict?

2. Organization: **World Travel and Tourism Council**
   Web site: **www.wttc.org**
   Summary: The World Travel and Tourism Council is the forum for business leaders in the travel and tourism industry. With chief executives of some 100 of the world's leading travel and tourism companies as its members, the WTTC has a unique mandate and overview on all matters related to travel and tourism.
   (a) What is your opinion of the "Blueprint for New Tourism"?

Apply Your Knowledge

1. Analyze your family's and friends' recent or upcoming travel plans and compare them with the examples in the text for reasons why people travel.

2. Suggest some ecotourism activities for your community.

3. How would you promote or improve tourism in your community?

Suggested Activities

1. Go online and get prices for an airline round-trip ticket between two cities for a flight that is as follows:
   (a) More than 60 days out
   (b) 30–59 days out
   (c) 15–29 days out
   (d) 7–14 days out
   (e) for tomorrow

2. Compare the prices and share the results with your class.

Endnotes

1. World Travel & Tourism Council, *Travel & Tourism 2011*, www.wttc.org/site_media/uploads/downloads/traveltourism2011.pdf (accessed November 13, 2011).

2. World Tourism Organization (UNWTO), "In Focus: Transport," *UNTO World Tourism Barometer* 7 (June 2009), 42–46.

3. World Tourism Organization (UNWTO), *Press Release: Healthy Growth of International Tourism in First Half of 2011*, September 7, 2011, http://media.unwto.org/en/press-release/2011-09-07/healthy-growth-international-tourism-first-half-2011 (accessed November 14, 2011).

4. World Tourism Organization (UNWTO), Understanding Tourism: Basic Glossary, http://media.unwto.org/en/content/understanding-tourism-basic-glossary (accessed November 14, 2011).

5. World Tourism Organization, *Ethics and Social Dimensions or Tourism: Background*, http://ethics.unwto.org/en/content/background (accessed November 13, 2011).

6. World Tourism Organization (UNWTO), *About UNWTO*, http://unwto.org/en/about/unwto (accessed April 18, 2011).

7. World Travel & Tourism Council, *World: Key Facts at a Glance*, www.wttc.org/research/economic-impact-research/regional-reports/world/ (accessed November 14, 2011).

8. World Tourism Organization (UNWTO), *About UNWTO*, http://unwto.org/en/about/unwto (accessed November 14, 2011).

9. World Travel & Tourism Council, *World: Key Facts at a Glance*, www.wttc.org/research/economic-impact-research/regional-reports/world/ (accessed November 14, 2011).

10. World Tourism Organization (UNWTO), *Tourism: 2020 Vision* (Madrid: UNWTO, 1999).

11. Charles R. Goeldner and J. R. Brent Ritchie, *Tourism: Principles and Practices*, 9th ed. (New York: John Wiley and Sons, 2003), 42–48.

12. Goeldner and Ritchie, *Tourism: Principles and Practices*, 43.

13. Ibid.

14. Donald E. Lundberg, *The Tourist Business*, 6th ed. (New York: Van Nostrand Reinhold, 1990), 16.

15. Lundberg, *The Tourist Business*, 17.

16. N. S. Gill, "101 on the Ancient Olympic Games," *About.com*, http://ancienthistory.about.com/cs/olympics/a/aa021798.htm (accessed April 6, 2011).

17. Silk Road Foundation, *Marco Polo and His Travels*, www.silk-road.com/artl/marcopolo.shtml (accessed April 6, 2011).

18. Ibid.

19. Federal Aviation Administration, *Air Traffic: NextGen Briefing*, http://www.faa.gov/air_traffic/briefing/ (accessed November 14, 2011).

20. "Boeing Unveils Ambitious 787 Dreamliner Passenger Jet," *Philippine Star*, July 10, 2007, B8.

21. Ibid.

22. Salary.com, *Salary Wizard: Captain/Pilot in Command (Large Jet)*, http://swz.salary.com/SalaryWizard/Captain-Pilot-in-Command-Large-Jet-Salary-Details.aspx (accessed November 14, 2011).

23. Salary.com, *Salary Wizard: Flight Attendant*, http://swz.salary.com/SalaryWizard/Flight-Attendant-Salary-Details.aspx (accessed November 14, 2011).

24. Wikinvest, *Wiki Analysis: Industry-Specific Metrics*, www.wikinvest.com/industry/airlines (accessed April13, 2001).

25. Princess Cruises, *Diamond Princess*, www.princess.com/learn/ships/di/index.html (accessed November 14, 2011); and Fran Golden, *Diamond Princess Review*, Cruise Critic, www.cruisecritic.com/reviews/review.cfm?shipID=296 (accessed November 14, 2011).

26. Bob Sharak, "Cruise Vacations Are Hot Even if the Economy's Not," *Travel Marketing Decisions*, Fall 2008: 3.

27. www.cruising.org/press/overview%202006/2.cfm

28. World Travel & Tourism Council, *Economic Impact Research*, http://www.wttc.org/eng/Tourism_Research/Economic_Research/ (accessed April 13, 2011).

29. Ibid.

30. www.world_tourism.org/market_research/facts

31. World Travel & Tourism Council, *Economic Impact Research*, http://www.wttc.org/eng/Tourism_Research/Economic_Research/ (accessed April 15, 2011).

32. Personal conversation with Dr. Greg A. Dunn Vice President, Y Partnership, April 12, 2011.

33. Personal correspondence with Karen Smith and Claudia Green, June 28, 2005.

34. NTA, *Home Page*, http://ntaonline.com (accessed November 14, 2011).

35. Personal correspondence with Edward Inskeep, June 4, 2007.

36. Personal conversation with Dr. Greg A. Dunn, September 14, 2007.

37. The Expeditioner, *How Many Americans Have a Passport?* http://www.theexpeditioner.com/2010/02/17/how-many-americans-have-a-passport-2/ (accessed April 16, 2011).

38. International Ecotourism Society (TIES), *What Is Ecotourism?* http://www.ecotourism.org/site/c.orLQKXPCLmF/b.4835303/k.BEB9/What_is_Ecotourism__The_International_Ecotourism_Society.htm (accessed November 14, 2011).

39. Ibid.

40. World Tourism Organization, *Sustainable Development of Tourism: Definition*, http://sdt.unwto.org/en/content/about-us-5 (accessed November 14, 2011).

41. http://whc.unesco.org/en/about/ retrieved November 16, 2011.

42. United Nations Educational, Scientific, and Cultural Organization, *World Heritage*, whc.unesco.org/en/about (accessed November 14, 2011).

43. University of Technology, Sydney, *Volunteer Tourism Beckons*, www.uts.edu.au/new/releases/2002/January/22.html (accessed April 18, 2011).

Glossary

Business travel Travel for business purposes.

Convention and visitors bureau (CVBs) 1. An organization responsible for promoting tourism at the regional and local level. 2. A not-for-profit umbrella organization that represents a city or urban area in soliciting and servicing all types of travelers to that city or area, whether for business, pleasure, or both.

Cultural tourism Tourism related to cultural interests or pursuits.

Ecotourism Responsible travel to natural areas that conserves the environment and sustains the well-being of the local people.

Hub-and-Spoke system A system used by airlines to transport passengers from one small city to another via a larger hub.

Interdependency One hospitality entity being to some extent dependent on another; a cruise line is dependent on airlines bringing many of the passengers to the cruise ship port and to ground transportation for bringing the passengers to the ship.

Multiplier effect A concept that refers to new money that is brought into a community to pay for hotel rooms, restaurant meals, and other aspects of leisure. To some extent, that income then passes into the community when the hotel or restaurant orders supplies and services, pays employees, and so on.

Sustainable tourism Tourism that is sustainable.

Tourism Travel for recreation or the promotion and arrangement of such travel.

Vacation package A vacation that is made up of a package; that may include air and ground transportation, hotel accommodation and other goodies.

Volunteer tourism A form of tourism where people volunteer to help others or projects usually in developing countries.

World Tourism Organization (UNWTO) The leading intergovernmental tourism organization.

Photo Credits

Credits are listed in the order of appearance.

Rob/Fotolia LLC
Dhoxax/Shutterstock
Chen Chao/Dorling Kindersley
Handout Old/Reuters
ZUMA Press/Newscom
Icholakov/Dreamstime
Steven May/Alamy
E.G.Pors/Shutterstock
Royal Caribbean International

Ewa Walicka/Shutterstock
Henk Meijer/Alamy
Chuckpee54/Dreamstime
Oleg Znamenskiy/Shutterstock
Patti Roscoe
Elena Elisseeva/Shutterstock
G.A.P Aventures
Debra James/Shutterstock
Ann-Marie Weldon

Recreation, Attractions, and Clubs

From Chapter 10 of *Introduction to Hospitality Management*, Fourth Edition. John R. Walker. Copyright © 2013 by Pearson Education, Inc. Publishing as Prentice Hall. All rights reserved.

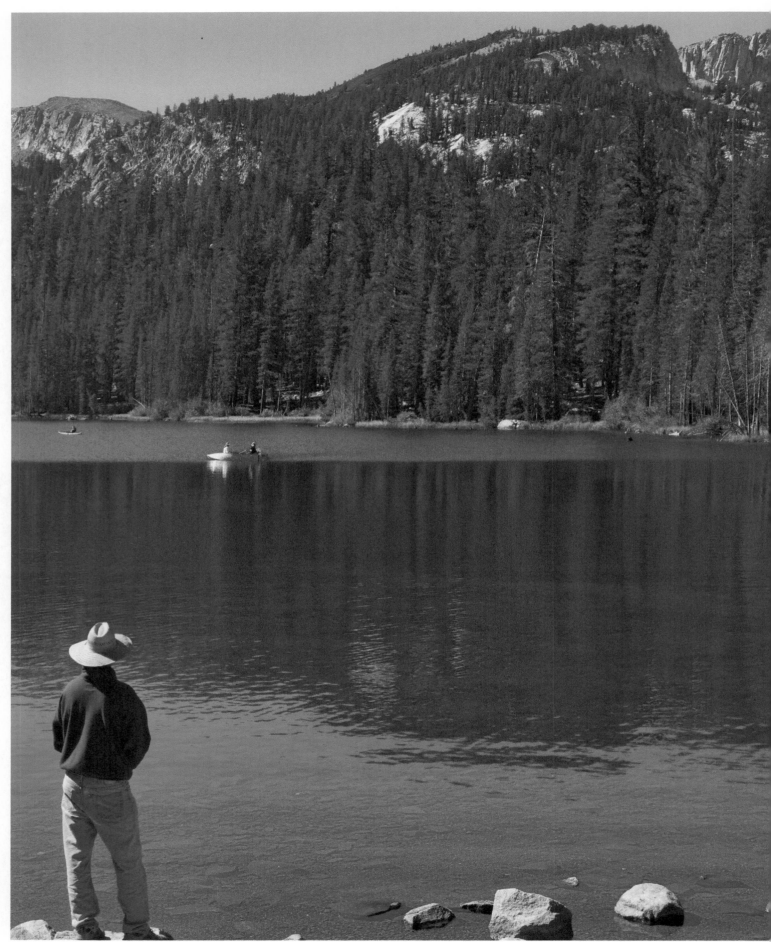

Recreation, Attractions, and Clubs

OBJECTIVES

After reading and studying this chapter, you should be able to:

- Discuss the relationship of recreation and leisure to wellness.
- Explain the origins and extent of government-sponsored recreation.
- Distinguish between commercial and noncommercial recreation.
- Name and describe various types of recreational clubs.
- Identify the major U.S. theme parks.
- Describe the operations of a country club.

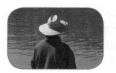
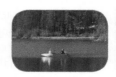
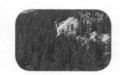
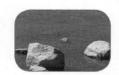

Recreational activities include both active and passive activities. Passive activities include all kinds of sports—team and individual. Baseball, softball, football, basketball, volleyball, tennis, swimming, jogging, skiing, hiking, aerobics, rock climbing, and camping are all active forms of recreation. Passive recreational activities include reading, fishing, playing and listening to music, gardening, playing computer games, and watching television or movies. **Recreation** *is an integral part of our nation's total social, economic, and natural resource environment. It is a basic component of our lives and well-being.*[1]

Recreation, Leisure, and Wellness

As postindustrial society has become more complex, life has become more stressed. The need to develop the wholeness of the person has become increasingly important. Compared to a generation ago, the stress levels of business executives are much higher. The term *burnout*—and indeed the word *stress*—has become a part of our everyday vocabulary only in recent years. Recreation is all about creating a balance, a harmony in life that will maintain wellness and wholeness.

Recreation allows people to have fun together and to form lasting relationships built on the experiences they have enjoyed together. This recreational process is called *bonding*. Bonding is hard to describe, yet the experience of increased interpersonal feeling for friends or business associates as a result of a recreational pursuit is common. These relationships result in personal growth and development.

The word *recreation* implies the use of time in a manner designed for therapeutic refreshment of one's body or mind.[2] Recreation is synonymous with lifestyle and the development of a positive attitude. An example of this is the increased feeling of well-being experienced after a recreational activity. Some people make the mistake of trying to pursue happiness as a personal goal. It is not enough for a person to say, "I want to be happy; therefore, I will recreate." Nathaniel Hawthorne wrote in the midnineteenth century: "Happiness in this world, when it comes, comes incidentally. Make it the object of pursuit, and it leads us on a wild goose chase, and it is never attained. Follow some other object, and very possibly we may find that we have caught happiness without dreaming of it."[3]

Recreation is a process that seeks to establish a milieu conducive to the discovery and development of characteristics that can lead to happiness. Happiness and well-being, therefore, are incidental outcomes of recreation. Thus, happiness may be enhanced by the pursuit of recreational activities. Personal recreational goals are equally as important as any other business or personal goals. These goals might include running a mile in under six minutes or maintaining a baseball batting average above .300. The fact that a

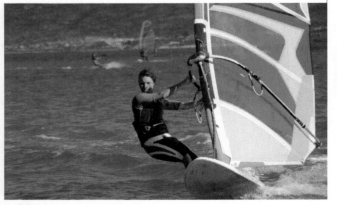

Windsurfing is definitely an active recreational activity.

person sets and strives to achieve goals requires personal organization. This helps improve the quality of life.

Leisure is best described as time free from work, or discretionary time. Some recreation professionals use the words *leisure* and *recreation* interchangeably, while others define leisure as the "productive," "creative," or "contemplative" use of free time. History shows again and again a direct link between leisure and the advancement of civilization. Hard work alone leaves no time for becoming civilized. Ironically, however, the opportunity to be at leisure is the direct result of increased technological and productivity advancements.

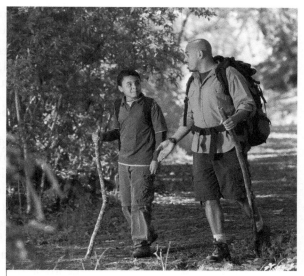

Hiking is a great exercise and an ideal way to get back to nature.

Government-Sponsored Recreation

Various levels of government that constitute **government-sponsored recreation** are intertwined, yet distinct, in the parks, recreation, and leisure services. The founding fathers of America said it best when they affirmed the right to life, liberty, and the pursuit of happiness in the Declaration of Independence. Government raises revenue from income taxes, sales taxes, and property taxes. Additionally, government raises special revenue from recreation-related activities such as automobile and recreational vehicles, boats, motor fuels, **transient occupancy taxes (TOTs)** on hotel accommodations, state lotteries, and others. The monies are distributed among the various recreation- and leisure-related organizations at the federal, state/provincial, city, and town levels. Recreation and leisure activities are extremely varied, ranging from cultural pursuits such as museums, arts and crafts, music, theater, and dance to sports (individual and team), outdoor recreation, amusement parks, theme parks, community centers, playgrounds, libraries, and gardens. People select recreational pursuits based on their interests and capabilities.

Park and recreation leaders confront daunting challenges at a time when leisure and recreational resources are highly valued community assets. Yet, securing adequate funding for staff and services can be a juggling act.[4] The following are some of the issues with which recreation professionals must deal:

- Comprehensive recreation planning
- Land classification systems
- Federal revenue sharing
- Acquisition- and development-funding programs
- Land-use planning and zoning
- State and local financing
- Off-road vehicle impacts and policy
- Use of easements for recreation

- Designation of areas (such as wilderness, wild and scenic rivers, national trails, nature preserves)
- Differences in purposes and resources (of the numerous local, state/provincial, and federal agencies that control more than one-third of the nation's land, much of which is used for recreation)

National Parks in the United States

The prevailing image of a **national park** is one of grand natural playgrounds, such as Yellowstone National Park, but there is much more to parks than that.[5] The United States has designated 397 national park units throughout the country, including a rich diversity of places and settings. The **National Parks Service** was founded in 1916 by Congress to conserve park resources and to provide for their use by the public in a way that leaves them unimpaired for the enjoyment of future generations. In addition to the better-known parks such as Yellowstone and Yosemite, the Parks Service also manages many other heritage attractions, including the Freedom Trail in Boston, Independence Hall in Philadelphia, the Antietam National Battlefield in Sharpsburg, Maryland, and the USS *Arizona* Memorial at Pearl Harbor in Hawaii. The Parks Service is also charged with caring for myriad cultural artifacts, including ancient pottery, sailing vessels, colonial-period clothing, and Civil War documents.

The ever-expanding mandate of the Parks Service also calls for understanding and preserving the environment. It monitors the ecosystem from the Arctic tundra to coral atolls, researches the air and water quality around the nation, and participates in global studies on acid rain, climate change, and biological diversity. The idea of preserving exceptional lands for public use as national parks arose after the Civil War when America's receding wilderness left unique national resources vulnerable to exploitation. Recent years have seen phenomenal growth in the system, with three new areas created in the last twenty years. These include new kinds of parks, such as urban recreational areas, free-flowing rivers, long-distance trails, and historic sites honoring our nation's social achievements. The system's current roster of 397 areas covers more than 80 million acres of land, with individual areas ranging in size from the 13-million-acre Wrangell–St. Elias National Park and Preserve in Alaska to the Thaddeus Kosciuszko National Memorial (a Philadelphia row house commemorating a hero of the American Revolution), which covers two one-hundredths of an acre.

Annual visitation to the National Park system approaches 300 million visitors, who take advantage of the full range of services and programs.[6] The focus once placed on preserving the scenery of the most natural parks has shifted as the system has grown and changed. Today, emphasis is placed on preserving the vitality of each park's ecosystem and on the protection of unique or endangered plant and animal species.

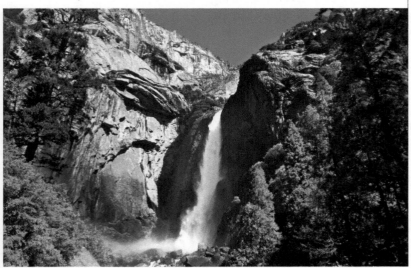

The splendor of nature awaits us in our national parks.

National Park Management

The National Park Service is in the Department of the Interior and is over-seen by a director who reports to the Secretary of the Interior. There are 397 National Parks divided into seven regions. The *Director* of the National Park Service establishes and approves service-wide natural resource policies and standards. The Director is ultimately responsible for establishing natural and cultural resource programs that conserve natural resources unimpaired for the enjoyment of future generations and for ensuring that such programs are in compliance with directives, policies, and laws.[7]

Each National Park has a superintendent, and the superintendent is responsible for understanding the park's resources and their condition. The superintendent is responsible for establishing and managing park backcountry-management programs and ensuring that they comply with directives, policies, and laws. The superintendent initiates the development of backcountry recreational use plans as necessary. The superintendent should coordinate the visitor use management plans with neighboring land managers as appropriate. Each superintendent with designated or eligible wilderness should designate a wilderness coordinator to review all activities ongoing in the wilderness.[8]

The National Park Service budget for 2011 is $3.14 billion, and it employs a staff of 21,501. Beyond these appropriated funds, the National Park Service is also authorized to collect and retain revenue from specified sources:[9]

- Recreation fees: approximately $190 million per year
- Park concessions franchise fees: approximately $60 million per year
- Filming and photography special use fees: approximately $1.2 million per year
- Additional funding comes from individual donations.

Managing a national park is a complex task that involves skilled professionals from many fields. Park management is not achieved by merely relying on experience and instincts. Whenever possible, it is based on solid scientific research, conducted not only by park staff, but by universities and independent researchers as well. Financial constraints are always an issue while managing our national parks.[10]

The Great Smoky Mountains National Park is the most visited of the National Parks, receiving about 9.5 million visitors a year. This park has the following main operating departments:

Ranger—rangers provide the chief response and visitor protection and are the sole law enforcement in the park. Rangers operate the camp grounds, perform search and rescue, and provide emergency medical services.

Resource Education—creates curriculum and delivers courses ranging from elementary students to adults and seniors. Known as "walks, talks, and tours," they cover pre-visitation to guided tours of the park.

Resource Management and Science—is responsible for the ongoing health of the natural and cultural resources.

Facility Management—responsible for a $2 billion infrastructure of roads, 350 nonhistoric buildings, and 72 bathrooms.

Administration—takes care of human resources, purchasing, contracts and property management.

Remember that the park service has the mission to conserve natural resources. This can prove very challenging, as nonnative pests and diseases threaten the biological diversity of the park, such as the case of the wolly adelgid, an aphid-like pest that kills hemlock trees. The Great Smoky Mountains National Park has about 75,000 acres of hemlock trees that are likely to be killed by these pests unless something can be found to stop the pest quickly.

Let's look at another National Park, Cape Lookout National Seashore. There are natural and cultural resources and numerous historic structures that are managed within the 56 miles of seashore. In all national parks, the need for efficient, innovative park management is especially important in order to protect the very best of this nation's rich heritage. And the law of the land dictates that, in turn, these resources, and the American public that owns them, deserve the very best that the National Park Service can give them.[11]

The National Park Service is required to maintain an up-to-date General Management Plan (GMP) for each unit of the park system. The purpose of each GMP is to ensure that the park has a clearly defined direction for asset preservation and visitor use. This foundation for decision-making is to be developed by an interdisciplinary team, in consultation with relevant offices within the Park Service, other federal and state agencies, interested parties, and the general public. The GMP should be based on use of scientific information related to existing and potential asset conditions, visitor experiences, environmental impacts, and relative costs of alternative courses of action. The GMP should take the long view, which may project many years into the future, when dealing with time frames. The plan should consider the park in its full ecological, scenic, and cultural contexts as a unit of the National Park Service and as part of a surrounding region.[12]

No two days are alike in the park service. On one day, a meth lab may be discovered; on another, a tornado may create havoc or visitors may get lost and need rescuing. Yet, every day at the Great Smoky Mountains National Park there are 8,000 visitors to take care of at the visitor center. Each visitor has questions ranging from "Where are the bathrooms?" to "Can I see a bear?"

Public Recreation and Parks Agencies

During the early part of the nineteenth century in the United States, the parks movement expanded rapidly as a responsibility of government and voluntary organizations. By the early 1900s, fourteen cities had made provisions for supervised play facilities, and the playground movement gained momentum. Private initiative and financial support were instrumental in convincing city government to provide tax dollars to build and maintain new play areas.

About the same time, municipal parks were created in a number of cities. Boston established the first metropolitan park system in 1892. In 1898, the New England Association of Park Superintendents (predecessor of the American

Institute of Park Executives) was established to bring together park superintendents and promote their professional concerns. Increasingly, the concept that city governments should provide recreation facilities, programs, and services became widely accepted. Golf courses, swimming pools, bathing beaches, picnic areas, winter sports facilities, game fields, and playgrounds were constructed.

▶ Check Your Knowledge

1. Name a few parks in the United States and in Canada. What are some characteristics that make the parks you named special?

2. Name your favorite park. Share with your classmates why it is your favorite.

Commercial Recreation—Attractions

Recreation management came of age in the 1920s and 1930s, when recreation and social programs were offered as a community service. Colleges and universities began offering degree programs in this area. Both public and private sector recreation management has grown rapidly since 1950.

Commercial recreation, often called eco- or adventure tourism, provides residents and visitors with access to an area's spectacular wilderness through a variety of guided outdoor activities. Specifically, commercial recreation is defined as outdoor recreational activities provided on a fee-for-service basis, with a focus on experiences associated with the natural environment.[13] Commercial recreation includes theme parks, attractions, and clubs.

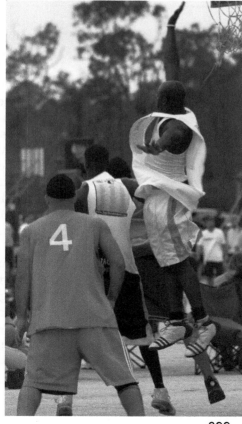

Street basketball is a great team sport.

Theme Parks

The idea of theme parks all began in the 1920s in Buena Park, California, with a small berry farm and tea room. As owner Walter Knott's restaurant business grew, different attractions were added to the site to keep waiting customers amused. After a gradual expansion, over eighty years after its humble beginnings, Knott's Berry Farm has become the largest independent theme park in the United States.

Today, Knott's Berry Farm is 150 acres of rides, attractions, live entertainment, historical exhibits, dining, and specialty shops. The park features six themes—Ghost Town, Indian Trails, Fiesta Village, the Boardwalk, Wild Water Wilderness, and Camp Snoopy, which is the official home of Snoopy and the Peanuts characters. In addition, the California Marketplace is located right outside the park, and offers fourteen unique shops and restaurants.

Knott's Berry Farm has truly been a great influence on the American theme park industry. Hundreds of parks, both independent and corporate

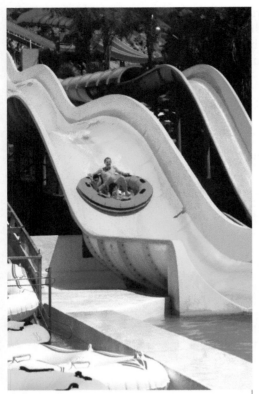

A water park is an example of a single-themed park.

owned, started to develop following the birth of Knott's. Creator Walter Knott may have figured out why amusement parks became so popular so quickly. He was quoted as saying, "The more complex the world becomes, the more people turn to the past and the simple things in life. We [the amusement park operators] try to give them some of those things."[14] Even with the ever-increasing competition, Knott's continues to attract guests with its authentic historical artifacts, relaxed atmosphere, emphasis on learning, famous food, varied entertainment, innovative rides, and specialty shopping.[15]

Knott's Berry Farm is now owned and operated by Cedar Fair Entertainment Company.

Size and Scope of the Theme Park Industry

Visiting **theme parks** has always been a favorite tourist activity. Theme parks attempt to create an atmosphere of another place and time, and they usually emphasize one dominant theme around which architecture, landscape, rides, shows, foodservices, costumed personnel, and retailing are orchestrated. In this definition, the concept of *themes* is crucial to the operation of the parks, with rides, entertainment, and food all used to create several different environments.[16]

Theme parks and attractions vary according to theme, which might be historical, cultural, geographical, and so on. Some parks and attractions focus on a single theme, such as the marine zoological Sea World parks. Other parks and attractions focus on multiple themes, such as King's Island in Ohio, a family entertainment center divided into seven theme areas: International Street, Oktoberfest, Rivertown, Planet Snoopy, Coney Mall, Boomerang Bay, and Dinosaurs Alive. Another example is Great America in California, a 100-acre family entertainment center that evokes North America's past in five themes: Home Town Square, Yukon Territory, Yankee Harbor, Country Fair, and Orleans Place.

An abundance of theme parks are located throughout the United States. These parks have a variety of attractions, from animals and sea life to thrill rides and motion simulators. There are parks with educational themes and parks where people go simply to have a good time.

Many of the country's most well known parks are located in Florida. Walt Disney World, Sea World, Water Mania, Wet 'n Wild, and Universal Studios are just a few of the many parks located in Orlando. Busch Gardens and Adventure Island are both in Tampa.

Busch Gardens, located in both Tampa, Florida, and Williamsburg, Virginia, is perhaps the most well known of the animal-themed parks. Busch Gardens is like a zoo with a twist. It features equal amounts of thrill rides and animal attractions. Guests can take a train ride through the Serengeti Plains, where zebras and antelope run wild, hop aboard a giant tube ride through the Congo River rapids, or ride on one of the parks' many world-record-holding roller coasters.

Many cities in the United States are well known for their festivals, which bring in droves of vacationers year after year. One of the most well known is Mardi Gras (Fat Tuesday) in New Orleans. Mardi Gras began more than a hundred years ago as a carnival and has evolved into a world-renowned party. Mardi Gras takes place every year in February, the day before Ash Wednesday, the beginning of Lent. The days leading up to Fat Tuesday are filled with wild parades, costume contests, concerts, and overall partying. The famous Bourbon Street is the scene for most of the party-going crowd, and it is often too crowded even to walk around. Beads are big at Mardi Gras, and thousands are given out each year. The culture of New Orleans greatly adds to the festiveness of Mardi Gras, because traditional jazz and blues can always be heard on most street corners.

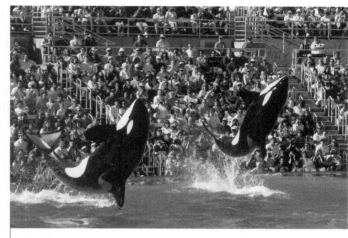

Orcas entertain the crowd at SeaWorld.

Another famous site of interest is the Grand Ole Opry in Nashville, Tennessee. The Grand Ole Opry is a live radio show in which country music guests are featured. Begun more than seventy-five years ago, the Grand Ole Opry is what made Nashville the "Music City." Since the Opry's start, Nashville created a theme park, Opryland (closed in 1997), and a hotel, the Opryland Resort. Famous musicians come from all over the world to showcase their talents, and tourists flock from everywhere to hear the sounds of the Opry and see the sites that Nashville has to offer.

Introducing Walt Disney: A Man with a Vision

In 1923, at the age of twenty-one, Walt Disney arrived in Los Angeles from Kansas City to start a new business. The first endeavor of Walt Disney and his brother Roy was a series of shorts (a brief film shown before a feature-length movie) called *Alice Comedies,* which featured a child actress playing with animated characters. Realizing that something new was needed to capture the audience, Walt Disney conjured up the concept of a mouse character. In 1927, Disney began a series called *Oswald the Lucky Rabbit.* It was well received by the public, but Disney lost the rights as a result of a dispute with his distributor.

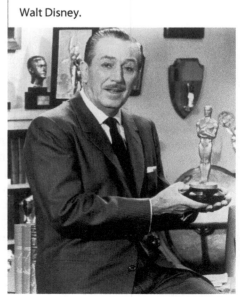

Walt Disney.

Mickey and Minnie Mouse first appeared in *Steamboat Willie,* which also incorporated music and sound, on November 18, 1928. Huge audiences were ecstatic about the work of the Disney Brothers, who became overnight successes.

During the next few years, Walt and Roy made many Mickey Mouse films, which earned them enough to develop other projects, including full-length motion pictures in Technicolor.

According to Disney, "Disneyland really began when my two daughters were very young. Saturday was always Daddy's Day, and I would take them to the merry-go-round and sit on a bench eating peanuts while they rode. And sitting there alone, I felt there should be something built, some kind of family park where parents and children could have fun together."[17]

Walt's original dream was not easy to bring to reality. During the bleak war years, not only was much of his overseas market closed, but the steady stream of income that paid for innovation dried up. However, even during the bleak years, Walt never gave up. Instead, he was excited to learn of the public's interest in movie studios and the possibility of opening the studios to allow the public to visit the birthplace of Snow White, Pinocchio, and other Disney characters.

After its creation, Disneyland had its growing pains—larger-than-expected opening day crowds, long lines at the popular rides, and a cash flow that was so tight that the cashiers had to rush the admission money to the bank to make payroll. Fortunately, since those early days, Disneyland and the Disney characters have become a part of the American dream.

By the early 1960s, Walt had turned most of his attention from film to real estate. Because he was upset when cheap motels and souvenir shops popped up around Disneyland, for his next venture, Walt Disney World, he bought 27,500 acres around the park. The center of Walt Disney World was to be the Experimental Prototype Community of Tomorrow (Epcot). Regrettably, Epcot and Walt Disney World were his dying dreams; Walt Disney succumbed to cancer in 1966.

However, Walt's legacy carries on. The ensuing years since Walt's death have included phenomenal Disney successes with Epcot, movies, a TV station, the Disney Channel, Disney stores, and Disney's Hollywood Studios theme park (formerly Disney–MGM Studios). In April 1992, EuroDisneyland, now Disneyland Paris, opened near Paris. For a variety of reasons (location, cost, climate, and culture), it was initially a failure, until his Royal Highness Prince Al Waleed Bin Talal Bin Abdula of Saudi Arabia purchased 25 percent of the Disneyland Paris Resort.

Both Walt Disney World and Disneyland have excellent college programs that enable selected students to work during the summer months in a variety of hotel, foodservice, and related park positions. Disney has also introduced a faculty internship that allows faculty to intern in a similar variety of positions.

Walt Disney World is composed of four major theme parks: Magic Kingdom, Epcot, Disney's Animal Kingdom, and Disney's Hollywood Studios (formerly Disney–MGM Studios), with more than 100 attractions, 23 resort hotels themed as faraway lands, spectacular nighttime entertainment, and vast shopping, dining, and recreation facilities that cover thousands of acres in this tropical paradise.

Walt Disney World includes tennis courts, championship golf, marinas, swimming pools, jogging and bike trails, water skiing, and motor boating. The resort also offers a unique zoological park and bird sanctuary on Discovery Island in the middle of Bay Lake that is alive with birds, monkeys, and alligators; hundreds of restaurants, lounges, and food courts; a nightclub metropolis to please nearly any musical palate; a starry-eyed tribute to 1930s Hollywood; and even bass fishing. Walt Disney World is always full of new surprises: It now features an unusual water adventure park, a "snow-covered" mountain with a ski resort theme called Blizzard Beach.

The Disney hotels are architecturally exciting and offer a number of amenities. The fun-filled Disney's All-Star Sports Resort and Disney's colorful All-Star Music Resort are categorized as value-class hotels. Disney's Wilderness Lodge is one of the park's jewels, with its impressive tall-timber atrium lobby and rooms built around a Rocky Mountain–like geyser pool. In all, the park has a cast of thousands of hosts, hostesses, and entertainers famous for their warm smiles and commitment to making every night an especially good one for Disney guests.

There is more to enjoy than ever at Walt Disney World in Mickey's PhilharMagic, which incorporated new 3D movie technology in the Fantasyland area of the Magic Kingdom; Splash Mountain, a popular flume ride in Adventureland at the Magic Kingdom; Mission: SPACE, a motion simulator ride at Epcot that mimics what an astronaut experiences; and, at Disney's Hollywood Studios, the ultimate thriller, the Twilight Zone Tower of Terror.

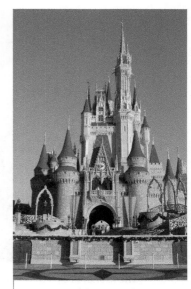

Walt Disney World.

Magic Kingdom

The heart of Walt Disney World and its first famous theme park is the Magic Kingdom. It is a giant theatrical stage where guests become part of exciting Disney adventures. It is also the home of Mickey Mouse, Snow White, Peter Pan, Tom Sawyer, Davy Crockett, and the Swiss Family Robinson.

More than forty major shows and ride-through attractions, not to mention shops and unique dining facilities, fill its seven lands of imagination. Each land carries out its theme in fascinating detail—architecture, transportation, music, costumes, dining, shopping, and entertainment are designed to create a total atmosphere where guests can leave the ordinary world behind. The seven lands are as follows:[18]

Main Street USA Experience turn-of-the-century charm with horsedrawn trolley, horseless carriages, plenty of souvenir shops, a penny arcade, and a grand-circle tour of the park on the Walt Disney World Railroad.

Adventureland Explore exotic places with the Pirates of the Caribbean, the Jungle Cruise, the Swiss Family Treehouse, the Magic Carpets of Aladdin, and the Enchanted Tiki Room.

Frontierland Experience thrills on Splash Mountain and Big Thunder Mountain Railroad, musical fun in the Country Bear Jamboree, recreation in the Shooting Gallery, and adventure in the Tom Sawyer Island caves and its raft rides.

Liberty Square Go steamboating on the Rivers of America, find mystery in the Haunted Mansion, and view the impressive Hall of Presidents with the addition of President Barack Obama in a speaking role.

Fantasyland Cinderella Castle is the gateway to Fantasyland. Fantasyland is currently undergoing a major expansion centered around the Disney Princesses, with additional emphasis on the corresponding films' villains to attract the boys. Classic Fantasyland rides include Mickey's PhilharMagic, Peter Pan's Flight, Dumbo the Flying Elephant, Mad Tea Party, It's a Small World, Prince Charming Regal Carousel, and Winnie the Pooh.

Tomorrowland Visit a sci-fi city of the future with the whirling Astro Orbiter, the shoot-em-up Buzz Lightyear's Space Ranger Spin, the interactive Monsters, Inc. Laugh Floor, the adventurous Stitch's Great Escape, the speedy Space Mountain, a new production of the Carousel of Progress, the Tomorrowland Speedway, and the elevated Tomorrowland Transit Authority.

Epcot

Epcot is a unique, permanent, and ever-changing world's fair with two major themes: Future World and World Showcase. Highlights include IllumiNations: Reflections of Earth, a nightly spectacle of fireworks, fountains, lasers, and classical music.

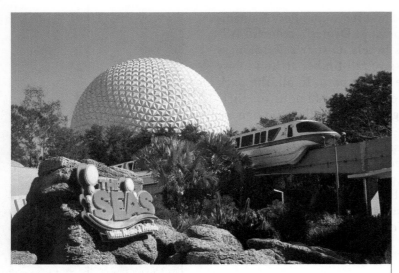

The monorail zips through Walt Disney's Epcot Center in Orlando, Florida.

Future World shows an amazing exposition of technology for the near future for home, work, and play in Innoventions. The newest consumer products are continually added. Major pavilions exploring past, present, and future are shown in the Spaceship Earth story of communications (Spaceship Earth is the geosphere symbol of Epcot). The Universe of Energy giant dinosaurs help explain the origin and future of energy. There are also Mission: Space, which launches visitors into a simulated space adventure; Test Track, a high-speed vehicle-simulation ride; Journey into Imagination; The Land, with spectacular agricultural research and environmental growing areas, and the new simulation hang-gliding ride Soarin'; and The Seas with Nemo and Friends, which houses the world's second-largest indoor ocean with thousands of tropical sea creatures.[19]

Around the World Showcase Lagoon are pavilions where guests can see replicas of world-famous landmarks and sample the native foods, entertainment, and culture of eleven nations:[20]

Mexico Mexico's fiesta plaza and boat trip on Gran Fiesta Tour Starring the Three Caballeros, plus La Hacienda de San Angel for authentic Mexican cuisine

Norway Maelstrom, a thrilling Viking boat journey, and the Akershus restaurant

China Wonders of China Circle-Vision 360 film tours from the Great Wall to the Yangtze River, plus the Nine Dragons Restaurant

Germany An authentic Biergarten restaurant

Italy St. Mark's Square street players and Tutto Italia Ristorante

United States The American Adventure's stirring historical drama

Japan Re-creation of an Imperial Palace plus the Teppan Edo restaurant

Morocco Morocco's palatial Restaurant Marrakesh

France Impressions de France film tour of the French countryside, plus the Chefs de France and Bistro de Paris restaurants

United Kingdom Shakespearean street players, plus the Rose and Crown Dining Room pub

Canada O Canada, a Halifax-to-Vancouver Circle-Vision 360° tour

Each showcase has additional snack facilities and a variety of shops featuring arts, crafts, and merchandise from each nation.

Disney's Hollywood Studios

With fifty major shows, shops, restaurants, ride-through adventures, and back-stage tours, Disney's Hollywood Studios (formerly Disney–MGM Studios) combines real working motion picture, animation, and television studios with exciting movie attractions. The newest adventure in the American Idol Experience, which puts guests center stage and under the spotlight. The famous Chinese Theater on Hollywood Boulevard houses the Great Movie Ride.

Other major attractions include the Tower of Terror, a stunning thirteen-story elevator fall; fast-paced adventure on the Rock 'n' Roller Coaster Starring Aerosmith; the Studio Backlot Tour of production facilities, Catastrophe Canyon, and New York Street; exciting shows at Indiana Jones Epic Stunt Spectacular and Muppet Vision 3D; plus a thrilling Star Wars adventure on Star Tours.

Especially entertaining for Disney fans is the Magic of Disney Animation, where guests can visit the Animation Academy and sit in on a class hosted by a Disney Animator. Favorite Disney films become entertaining stage presentations in the Voyage of the Little Mermaid theater and in Beauty and the Beast, a live, twenty-five-minute musical revue at Theater of the Stars. The best restaurants at Disney's Hollywood Studios include the Hollywood Brown Derby, 1950s Prime Time Cafe, Sci-Fi Dine-In Theater, and Mama Melrose's Ristorante Italiano.[21]

The Animal Kingdom is the newest edition to Walt Disney World. The Animal Kingdom focuses on nature and the animal world around us. Guests can go on time-traveling rides and come face to face with animals from the prehistoric past to the present. Shows are put on featuring Disney's most popular animal-based films, such as *Lion King* and *A Bug's Life*. Safari tours that bring guests up close and personal with live giraffes, elephants, and hippopotamuses are also offered at Animal Kingdom.

Walt Disney World's two water parks are Blizzard Beach and Typhoon Lagoon. Blizzard Beach has a unique ski-resort theme, while Typhoon Lagoon is based on the legend that a powerful storm swept through, leaving pools and rapids in its wake. Both parks offer a variety of slides, tube rides, pools, and moving rivers that drift throughout the parks.

All this and much more are what help make Walt Disney World the most popular destination resort in the world. Since its opening in 1971, millions of guests, including kings and celebrities from around the world and all eight U.S. presidents in office since the opening (excluding President Obama), have visited the parks. What

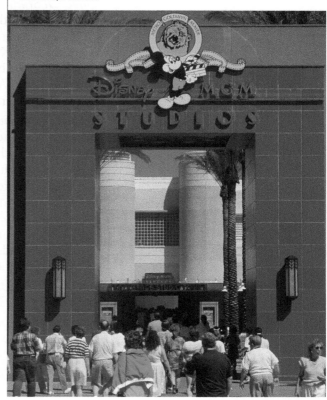

Crowds flock to the Disney's Hollywood Studios, Florida.

causes the most comments from guests is the cleanliness, the friendliness of its cast, and the unbelievable attention to detail—a blend of showmanship and imagination that provides an endless variety of adventure and enjoyment.[22]

Universal Studios

Universal Studios Hollywood has been giving guided tours on its famous movie sets for almost forty years, and tens of thousands of people visit Universal every day.[23] Since its founding, Universal Studios has become the most formidable competitor facing the Walt Disney Company.

In Orlando, Florida, Universal Studios has enjoyed huge success, despite encroaching on the "kingdom" of Disney. In addition to its Hollywood and Orlando parks, Universal has since expanded into Singapore and Japan. Future locations are planned for Dubai, United Arab Emirates and Seoul, South Korea. One reason for Universal's success is its adaptation of movies into thrill rides; another is its commitment to guest participation. Guests get to help make sound effects and can participate in "stunts," making Universal Studios more than just a "look behind the scenes."

Universal Studios is also a good example of what is predicted to occur in the future regarding amusement and theme parks. It is offering more realistic thrill rides by combining new technologies and state-of-the-art equipment. Also, the company has realized that visitors tend to go to theme parks just because they happen to be in the area. By greatly expanding the experience, NBC Universal is hoping that its improvements will make travelers want to visit Universal Studios as a one-stop destination.

Let's take a closer look at the Universal theme parks:

Universal Studios Hollywood was the first Universal park and boasts the title of the world's largest movie studio and theme park. As part of the new studio tour, visitors are taken into the tomb of the Mummy, feel the hot breath of King Kong, experience a major earthquake, and are right in the middle of a Hollywood movie shoot. Afterward, guests can "chill" at the Universal CityWalk, a street that claims to offer the best in food, nightlife, shopping, and entertainment.

Universal Orlando Resort is a destination in itself, with two theme parks, several themed resorts, and a bustling CityWalk. In Universal Studios Florida, like in the Hollywood park, you can explore the exciting world of movie making. Its newest and most exciting park, Islands of Adventure, gives you the best in roller coasters and thrill rides, whereas Wet 'n Wild gives you the opportunity to enjoy a range of cool waterslides, among other things. If you're not already exhausted by the mere thought of it, why not check out CityWalk for some food, shopping, and a taste of the hottest nightlife in town. Myriads of venues, popular with tourists and locals alike, offer an amazing variety of cool bars, hot clubs, and live music.

Universal Studios Japan features eighteen rides and shows, some brand new and others old favorites, plus great dining and shopping.

Universal Studios Singapore is the newest addition and is located within Singapore's first integrated resort.[24]

TECHNOLOGY SPOTLIGHT

Use of Technology in Recreation, Attractions, and Clubs

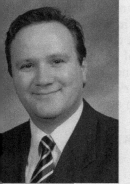

Cihan Cobanoglu, Ph.D., Dean, School of Hotel and Restaurant Management, University of South Florida, Sarasota-Manatee

Some of the technologies utilized in the recreation and clubs area are common to the rest of the hospitality industry. Depending on the size and amenities of an establishment, the following information technology systems can be used: call centers (for sales and customer service), point-of-sale systems (for retail distribution, food and beverage, rentals), and ticketing systems (for issuing tickets and passes). Besides these, there are some specific systems that can be implemented in the resorts and clubs.

Golf club property management systems would usually make the following functions available to users. The first is wide reservations options: online booking and group reservations. These systems usually can copy the guest's name on several tee times and thus help to save time on data entry. Another important function in golf clubs is tee-time management. This feature allows instant checking of tee-time availability to provide guests with a complete picture of what's available. Also, this module enables managing separate times and rates for different types of guests: public, member, twilight, and so forth. Besides this, club agents can relocate (drag and drop) one or multiple players from one tee time to another with ease. Some of the providers of club management software are Jonas Software, RTP, and CSI Software.

Radio-frequency identification (RFID) is rapidly entering the recreation and clubs niche of the hospitality industry. This is a technology that uses communication through radio waves for the purposes of tracking and identifying people or objects. RFID chips can be embedded in the guest cards or wristband. They enable authorization at the access points as well as retrieval of the guest's profile, picture, and membership privileges. The necessary components for this system are RFID chips and an antenna or "reader." The RFID antenna picks up a unique serial number from the microchip when a ticket, pass, or wristband with the RFID chip is presented. This technology helps to enhance fraud prevention on the management side and provides hands-free convenience on the guest side. RFID access systems have been widely used at European ski resorts, and now they are also spreading to the American market. In addition, RFID systems can have electronic "wallet" functionality. Often, RFID is implemented in beach resorts, where guests receive an opportunity to pay at different retail outlets without carrying an actual wallet. This provides the convenience of electronic payment to guests and encourages shopping. Moreover, RFID wristbands can be utilized at huge resorts and amusement parks in order to track children if they are lost.

Information kiosks appear often at large parks and resorts. Usually this technology allows park visitors to purchase park passes and other services on park grounds. Kiosks can be supplemented with digital displays that provide visitors with relevant information. These technologies optimize the use of parks' personnel, maximize the use of parks' resources, and ensure information is available to park visitors. These displays can digitally present pictures or event schedules of different parts of a resort or a park. This helps to attract guests to particular areas at the right time (for example, when there is an event taking place), as well as enables guests to plan a better recreation experience according to their interests.

SeaWorld Parks and Entertainment

SeaWorld Parks and Entertainment includes Busch Gardens and is a division of Blackstone Group. The animal parks not only offer guests from around the world the opportunity to see and experience the wonders of many marine and land animals, but they also have highly developed educational programs.

These programs reach millions of people a year—in the parks, on TV, and over the Internet—informing them on topics such as endangered animals, the environment, and the wonders of the ocean. In addition, SeaWorld Parks and Entertainment is active in the areas of conservation, research, and wildlife assistance worldwide.

The company is dedicated to preserving marine life. It uses innovative programs to research various wildlife dilemmas. It also participates in breeding, animal rescue, rehabilitation, and conservation efforts throughout the year. What SeaWorld Parks and Entertainment does for the preservation of animals is important to the existence of its theme parks because the research and rescue programs are subsidized through guest revenue. Also, each park offers unique shows and attractions that combine entertainment and education with a strong commitment to research and conservation.

Currently, SeaWorld Parks and Entertainment[25] runs the following parks in the United States:

SeaWorld The three SeaWorld parks are located in California (San Diego), Florida (Orlando), and Texas (San Antonio). Each park has various themes, marine and animal attractions, shows, rides, and educational exhibits. SeaWorld is based on the creatures of the sea. Guests can pet dolphins and other fish; watch shows featuring Shamu, the famous killer whale; and learn all about the mysteries of the sea. Several rides are also available at SeaWorld, and countless exhibits feature everything from stingrays to penguins.

Busch Gardens These theme parks, located in both Tampa, Florida, and Williamsburg, Virginia, feature exciting thrill rides and attractions in addition to large zoos and safari parks. The theme for the Williamsburg Park is the "Old Country." It re-creates the seventeenth-century charm of the Old World European atmosphere with a journey through nine authentically detailed European hamlets. "The Dark Continent" theme of Busch Gardens in Tampa has a distinctly African theme.

Adventure Island Also located in Tampa, Adventure Island is the only splash park in the Tampa Bay area. It is also the only water theme park on Florida's west coast featuring several unique water play areas and thrilling splash rides. The water park comprises more than twenty-five acres of fun-filled water rides, cafés, and shops.

Water Country USA Also located in Williamsburg, Water Country USA is the mid-Atlantic's largest water park, featuring state-of-the-art water rides and attractions, all set to a 1950s and 1960s surf theme, plus live entertainment, shopping, and restaurants.[26] Like Adventure Island, Water Country has an educational atmosphere to help guests, especially children, learn water safety techniques.

Aquatica Aquatica is a water park located in Orlando and operated as a companion to SeaWorld Orlando. The park is themed to the southern Pacific and features Australian- and New Zealand–based mascots. The park also features dolphins, which you ride by on one of the attractions.

Sesame Place This fourteen-acre park is located in Langhorne, Pennsylvania, and is dedicated totally to a Sesame Street theme. It was designed with the goal of stimulating children's natural curiosity to learn and explore, while building self-confidence as they interact with other children.

Discovery Cove Adjacent to Sea World in Orlando, Florida, Discovery Cove is where you can immerse yourself in adventure. It offers up-close encounters with dolphins and other exotic sea life. Guests can swim with dolphins and snorkel through a coral reef, tropical river, waterfalls, and an amazing freshwater lagoon, among other things.[27]

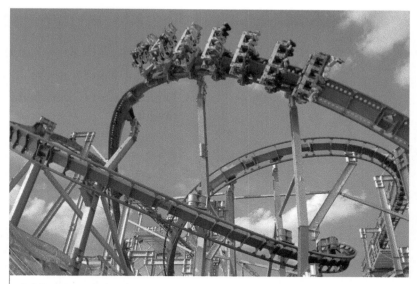

Exhilarating rides make theme parks more exciting to thrill seekers.

Hershey's

What does the name Hershey bring to mind?[28] It was at the 1893 World's Columbian Exposition in Chicago that Hershey first became fascinated with the art of chocolate. Then, Milton Hershey, a small-time candy manufacturer, decided he wanted to make chocolate to coat his caramels. He opened his new establishment in Lancaster, Pennsylvania, and named it the Hershey Chocolate Company. In the 1900s, the company started to produce mass quantities of milk chocolate, which resulted in immediate success. Soon after, Hershey decided that there was a need to increase his production facilities. He built a new factory on the farmland of south-central Pennsylvania in Derry Township. The following decades brought many product-line expansions. In 1968, the company was renamed the Hershey Foods Corporation. Today, the company is the leading manufacturer of chocolate, nonchocolate confectionery, and grocery products in North America.

In 1907, Milton Hershey opened Hershey Park as a leisure park for employees of Hershey's company. He wanted to create a place for his employees to relax and have some fun when they were not on the job. The park was small and simple, offering employees a place to picnic, canoe, and walk around the beautifully landscaped grounds. In 1908, the park started its soon-to-be huge expansion with the addition of a merry-go-round.

In the years to come, the park continued to add more rides and attractions. As the park continued to expand, the company decided to open the park's doors to the public. It became a small regional park with a pay-as-you-ride policy.

In 1971, the park underwent redevelopment to turn the small regional park into a large theme park. In addition, the company decided to add a one-time admission fee to eliminate the pay-as-you-ride policy and changed its name from Hershey Park to Hersheypark. Today, the park sits on more than 110 acres and is the home of more than sixty rides and attractions.

▶ Check Your Knowledge

1. What is Knott's Berry Farm?
2. Why did Walt Disney really create Disneyland?
3. Discuss your favorite theme park with your class. Explain why it is your favorite.

Regional Theme Parks

Just to show how varied the attractions industry is, consider the state of Florida and its attractions association. The Florida Attractions Association, founded in 1949, is a trade association representing 90-plus family-oriented attractions, including astronaut, historical, cultural, military, and scientific museums; botanical gardens; castles; collections of the unique and different; dinner entertainments; dolphin and marine parks; exhibitions of alligators, lions, monkeys, parrots, butterflies, and manatees; Native American villages; musical entertainment complexes; sightseeing trains, cruises, and boat tours; state parks; theme parks; towers; water parks; and zoological parks.

In addition to some of the larger theme parks mentioned in the preceding section, here are two others that cater to thousands of visitors each year. The Miami Seaquarium is a 38-acre tropical paradise, a place where dolphins walk on water, killer whales fly through the air, and endangered sea turtles and manatees find a safe haven.

There are eight different marine animal shows and an educational program that focuses on the mysteries of the sea even top marine scientists can't explain. In order to broaden its appeal and bring in additional revenue, the Miami Seaquarium has developed a company program for events and a schools and Scouts program to appeal to the youth market.

Marineland Dolphin Adventure in Miami began in 1938 in an effort to duplicate the variety of marine life as it exists in the wild for the purpose of making films. It was a hit with Hollywood and was used in a number of movies. Today, the park offers an array of dolphin adventures including opportunities to touch and feed the dolphins, to simulate being a trainer for the day, to make art with the dolphins, and take kayak tours in the local estuary.

Dollywood

In 1961, a small attraction with a Civil War theme called Rebel Railroad opened its doors to the public.[29] In the 1960s, the name Rebel Railroad was changed to Goldrush Junction, and the theme was changed to resemble the Wild West. This attraction is now known all across the world as Dollywood. The name came about in 1986 when Dolly Parton became a co-owner of the park. The park sits on 125 acres in the foothills of the Great Smoky Mountains in Pigeon Forge,

Tennessee. In addition to having all the rides of an amusement park, Dollywood is enriched by the culture of the Smoky Mountains. The park includes crafts such as blacksmithing, glass blowing, and wood carving. It also hosts several festivals, concerts, and musical events. Today, Dollywood brings in more than 2.5 million visitors every year and continues to be Tennessee's number one tourist attraction.[30]

Legoland

Legoland is a theme park partly owned by the Lego Group.[31] In 1968, Legoland, Billund, Denmark, opened and now has 1.6 million visitors annually. The parks are themed after—you guessed it—Legos, the brightly colored plastic bricks, gears, minifigures, and other pieces that are assembled to create models of almost anything. The parks are marketed toward young families. This is emphasized in the rides: All the parks have roller coasters that are not quite as extreme as the roller coasters found in other theme parks. Today there are five Legoland parks located in Windsor, England; Günzburg, Germany; Carlsbad, California; Billund, Denmark; and Winter Haven, Florida. Each park features a miniland, which is made up of millions of bricks that create models of landmarks and scenes from all around the world. The Windsor Legoland is one of Britain's most popular attractions, bringing 1.9 million visitors in 2010. The other parks (Californian, Danish, and German) all bring in approximately 1.4 million visitors annually. A majority interest in LegoLand's four theme parks is now owned by the Blackstore group, under its Merlin Entertainments brand.[32]

Gatorland

Gatorland is a 110-acre theme park and wildlife preserve located in Orlando, Florida.[33] It all started when Owen Godwin built an alligator pit in his backyard. After World War II, Godwin bought a sixteen-acre plot located off Florida's second-most-traveled highway. He decided that he wanted to build an attraction on his land that would provide a close-up view of Florida's animals in their native habitat. In 1949, Godwin opened the attraction's doors to the public under the name of the Florida Wildlife Institute, which he shortly after changed to the Snake Village and Alligator Farm. In 1954, Godwin once again changed the name of the attraction to its current name, Gatorland.

The 1960s brought growth to the tourism industry in Florida. As the industry grew, Gatorland continued to expand by adding a number of exhibits and attractions. Today, Gatorland features alligators, crocodiles, a breeding marsh, reptilian shows, a petting zoo, a swamp walk, educational programs, and train rides. In addition, it offers the following shows: Gator Jumparoo, which features alligators jumping four to five feet out of the water to retrieve food; Gator Wrestlin', an alligator wrestling show in which wranglers catch an alligator by hand; and Upclose Encounters, where visitors meet wildlife from around the globe. One of the oldest attractions in the area, Gatorland continues to be privately owned by Godwin's family.

Wet 'n Wild

Wet 'n Wild was founded by George Millay in Orlando, Florida, in 1977.[34] George Millay is also known as the creator of SeaWorld. Wet 'n Wild is considered the first major water park to be opened in the United States. Millay received the first Lifetime Achievement Award from the World Waterpark Association for creation of Wet 'n Wild. The association named him the official "Father of the Waterpark."

Today, Wet 'n Wild is a chain of water parks with locations in Florida and North Carolina. The Wet 'n Wild North Carolina located in Greensboro features more than thirty-six rides and attractions that are classified "from mild to wild." Wet 'n Wild Orlando also offers something for everyone. The rides fall into four categories: Thrill Rides, Multi Person Rides, Just For Kids, and Takin' It Easy. In 1998, Millay sold the Orlando Park to the Universal Studios Recreation Group.

Animal Attractions

Another sector that has been growing substantially is the one of animal attractions. Although they are usually not the main reason people visit a state or city, zoos, aquariums, and wild animal parks attract millions of visitors every year.

Zoos

Every kid's dream, and just as much fun for parents, zoos are one of those things that just don't seem to go out of style. They are forms of tourist attractions that people may visit when in a destination city such as New York, Chicago, or San Diego. Approximately 150 million people visit a U.S. zoo every year.[35] The first zoo in the United States was the Philadelphia Zoo, built in 1859. Even today, zoos are extremely popular in the United States and Canada, and almost every major city has one. In fact, the popularity of zoos was proven when the Walt Disney Company unveiled its Animal Kingdom as one way to combine the effects of visiting a zoo with the attractions of a theme park. Busch Gardens and SeaWorld also have similar parks.

Following are examples of two of the most popular and noteworthy American zoos.

San Diego Zoo, California

The San Diego Zoo attracts many tourists from across the country for a variety of reasons. It may be in part because of the favorable climate that allows the zoo to operate all year round. Also, the zoo has a large collection of animals, interactive programs, and educational programs for children.

The world-famous San Diego Zoo is located in historic Balboa Park in downtown San Diego, California. Founded in 1916 by Dr. Henry Wegeworth, the zoo's original collection totaled 50 animals. Today, it is home to over 4,000 animals of more than 800 different species. The zoo also features a prominent botanical collection with more than 700,000 exotic plants.[36] The zoo's breeding programs help not only to enhance the zoo, but also to provide hope for the survival of many endangered animals. The first baby panda ever born in captivity, Hua Mei, was born at the San Diego Zoo.[37]

The National Zoo

The National Zoological Park in Washington, D.C., is part of the respected Smithsonian Institution. More than 2,000 animals from nearly 400 species make their home in this zoo.[38] Among the rare animals featured at the National Zoo are a giant panda, komodo dragons, rare Sumatran tigers, and Asian elephants.

The National Zoo is located in a quiet residential area only minutes away from other Smithsonian museums, the Capitol, and the White House. It is not only a place to observe the behavior of certain animals, but also a place that works actively to educate visitors on conservation issues and the various interactions among living organisms. The National Zoo breeds endangered species and reintroduces the animals into their natural habitats. The zoo also participates in other visitor education programs and biological research.[39]

Aquariums

Aquariums are attractions that provide thrilling educational experiences to millions of tourists each year. They are also multi-million-dollar showpieces, displaying creatures vastly different from us who dwell on land. For example, each year, 1.6 million visitors pass through the doors of the National Aquarium in Baltimore.[40] This impressive aquarium seeks to stimulate public interest in and knowledge about the aquatic world, focusing on the beauty of these species in their natural environments. It uses only the most modern interpretative techniques to engage and get an emotional response from visitors. In fact, many visitors walk out with a desire to become more environmentally responsible.[41]

▶ Check Your Knowledge

1. What zoo is the oldest in the United States?
2. Name some rare animals you can find at the National Zoo.

Historic Places/Sites

Travelers and tourists have visited historic sites for thousands of years. The first sites visited in recorded history were the Seven Wonders of the ancient world, which included the Great Pyramid of Giza (Egypt), the Hanging Gardens of Babylon (modern-day Iraq), the Statue of Zeus at Olympia (Greece), the Temple of Artemis at Ephesus (modern-day Turkey), the Mausoleum at Halicarnassus (modern-day Turkey), the Colossus of Rhodes (Greece), and the Lighthouse of Alexandria (Egypt). Historic places, sites, and museums are a

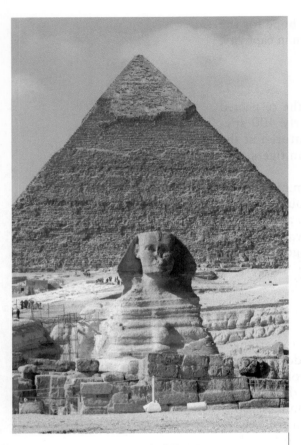

The Great Pyramid of Giza, Egypt.

part of what is now called **heritage tourism**. Heritage tourism has gained prominence in recent years, particularly with baby boomers and older adults. These groups are less likely to engage in adventure tourism and usually prefer more passive activities. Tourists visiting historic places/sites and museums are interested in the national culture. The various historic attractions appeal to a broad spectrum of the community because they are diverse and located throughout the nation.

The National Park Service maintains properties listed in the National Register of Historic Places. The **National Register of Historic Places** is the United States' official list of districts, sites, buildings, structures, and objects worthy of preservation. The more than 85,000 listings represent significant icons of American culture, history, engineering, and architecture.[42] Historic sites include buildings that have been restored and that are now being used as private houses as well as hotels, inns, churches, libraries, galleries, and museums.

Because of declining funds, galleries, museums, and heritage sites have had to become creative in raising money. They have not only had to cover operating costs, but also cater to an increasing number of visitors. To self-generate revenues, they have had to become more entrepreneurial while continuing to meet their heritage preservation and educational goals. Revenue generation has often been achieved through an increased concentration on partnerships, promotions, and packages in which the sites team up with other operators in the tourism industry, such as tour companies, hotels, restaurants, and car rental companies.

The following are a few of the most important U.S. historical attractions:

- Monticello was the home of the famous statesman Thomas Jefferson, author of the Declaration of Independence, architect of American ideals as well as noble buildings, and father of the University of Virginia. The domed mansion of Monticello is set in the beautiful Virginia countryside and is well worth a visit.

- Alamo is a small mission in San Antonio, Texas, with a rich historical background. During Texas's fight for independence from Mexico, a vicious battle took place in this town. One hundred eighty-seven Texans held out for thirteen days in a group of fortified mission buildings against General Santa Anna's army of about 2,400 soldiers. The battle resulted in a tragic Texan defeat. Not long after that, Texans everywhere united in a rallying cry: "Remember the Alamo!"[43] And people still do.

- The French Quarter in New Orleans is an original part of the city, full of life and history. Unlike historic districts in many other cities, it is still growing and evolving, regardless of the recent natural disasters.

Locals constantly wrestle with the issue of balancing evolutionary changes with the need to preserve history. Visitors can have a great time when they visit during Mardi Gras.

- The Martin Luther King Jr. National Historic Site is located in the residential section of "Sweet Auburn," Atlanta. Two blocks west of the home is Ebenezer Baptist Church, the pastorate of King's grandfather and father. It was in these surroundings of home, church, and neighborhood that "M. L." experienced his childhood. Here, he learned about family and Christian love, segregation in the days of "Jim Crow" laws, diligence, and tolerance. This important site is a reminder of King's significant contribution to the civil rights movement.

- The Grand Ole Opry in Nashville, Tennessee, is a live radio show in which country music guests are featured. Started more than 75 years ago, The Grand Ole Opry is what made Nashville "Music City." Since the Opry's start, Nashville created a theme park, Opryland (now closed), and a hotel, the Opryland Resort. Famous musicians come from all over the world to showcase their talents, and tourists flock from everywhere to hear the sounds of the Opry and see the sites that Nashville has to offer.[44]

- The Freedom Trail is a walking tour through downtown Boston that passes 16 points of interest, plus other exhibits, monuments, and shrines just off the trail, some of which are a part of the Boston National Park. This interesting walk through a part of U.S. history includes both the State House and the Old South Meeting House. The Old South Meeting House was the site of many important town meetings concerning the British colonial rule, including those that sparked the Boston Tea Party. Today, there is a multimedia exhibition depicting the area's 300-year history. The building and two other restored structures today house a bustling marketplace of more than 100 specialty shops, restaurants, and bars. Paul Revere's house is the only seventeenth-century structure left in downtown Boston. It was from this house that the silversmith left for his historic ride on April 18, 1775. Another site on the Freedom Trail is the Bunker Hill Monument.

- The Liberty Bell is housed on Market Street in Philadelphia. The bell's inscription reads, "Proclaim liberty throughout all the land unto all the inhabitants thereof," which in fact is taken from the Bible, Leviticus 25:10. For many years, it was known as the State House bell. Its popularity rose when a group of abolitionists, remembering its inscription, adopted the bell as a symbol of their cause; they nicknamed it their liberty bell. In the late 1800s, the bell went on tour around the United States. This trip was an effort to show the war-torn country that there had been a time in history when they had fought and died for a common cause. In 1915, when the tour ended, the Liberty Bell, as it was then known, went home to Philadelphia, where it remains to this day. Throughout American history, the Liberty Bell has served as a simple reminder, a symbol of freedom, independence, and liberty, not just in the United States, but also all over the world.

▶ Check Your Knowledge

1. What were the first historic sites visited in recorded history?
2. Name some important U.S. historical attractions.

Museums

Some experts have speculated that people visit museums because of some innate fascination with the past and with diverse cultures. Nobody knows for sure, but it is a fact that the number of museums in the United States has more than quadrupled since 1950. There are many types of museums, including general, art, science and technology, natural history, history, and military. Someone has to manage these operations, and the more people that travel to experience them, the more career opportunities are available in the travel, hotel, and restaurant industries. Here are a couple of the big names in the museum sector.

The Smithsonian Institution

Established in 1846 by a man who never visited the United States, this well-known institution now holds almost 140 million artifacts, works of art, and specimens. It is composed of the following museums and galleries: the Anacostia Community Museum; the Arthur M. Sackler Gallery; the Cooper-Hewitt, National Design Museum; the Freer Gallery of Art; the Hirshhorn Museum and Sculpture Garden; the National Air and Space Museum; the National Museum of African American History and Culture; the National Museum of African Art; the National Museum of American History; the National Museum of Natural History; the National Museum of the American Indian; the National Portrait Gallery; the National Postal Museum; Smithsonian American Art Museum and its Renwick Gallery, and 9 research facilities in the United States and abroad, and 169 affiliate museums, as well as the National Zoo.[45] The institution's goal is to increase and diffuse knowledge, and it is also dedicated to public education, national service, and scholarship in the arts, sciences, and history.[46] Smithsonian museums attract approximately 24.2 million visitors annually, and entrance is free. The National Zoo attracts about 2.6 million visitors annually.[47] In addition to its museums and research facilities, parts of the Smithsonian collection can be viewed online at http://www.si.edu.

The Field Museum, Chicago

The Field Museum is a "unique institution of public learning that utilizes its collections, researchers, exhibits, and educational programs to increase public knowledge . . . of the world."[48] The museum, located in Chicago, takes on two issues that it reiterates time and time again in all of its exhibits and programs. These two issues are "balancing growth with responsible environmental stewardship" and the creation of "mutual respect and understanding among cultures."[49]

The museum was founded in 1893 as a place to house biological and anthropological collections for a world exposition. These types of objects continue to form the basis of the museum's collections. In addition, the museum conducts research in the areas of geology, paleontology, archaeology, and ethnography. Furthermore, the museum houses a world-class library collection consisting of more than 20 million items.[50]

Permanent exhibits at the Field Museum range from dinosaurs to minerals and gems, plants, animals, and cultural exhibits. Temporary exhibits are also displayed from time to time. One example of this is a program entitled "The Art of the Motorcycle." This exhibit discusses the motorcycle as a cultural icon and also its technological design.

Performance Arts

Have you ever wished that you could just take off and follow your favorite band on tour? Although some people do, most of us do not have the money or time to do so. However, that does not stop us from enjoying an occasional concert, musical, theater production, comedy show, and so forth when we are at home or on the road. However, these shows and productions are usually not the primary purpose of leisure travel, although in some circumstances they might be. In Orlando or Las Vegas, for example, certain shows have taken up permanent residence. The public knows this and therefore may take a trip to Orlando or Las Vegas at their convenience so that they may see a certain production. In places like New York City and London, stopping off to see a Broadway production or a concert may be an unplanned bonus.

Theaters once were immensely important. In a time before people had access to modern inventions like radio or television, books and theater were the only entertainment available. During the industrial era of the early 1900s, the importance of theaters began to wane somewhat as people became too busy juggling work and spending time with family. In addition, many people could not afford such luxuries. In modern times, however, the theater is again gaining importance. Old theaters from the vaudeville days are now being resurrected and reopened to the public—and the public is responding. Increasing numbers of people visit the theater or opera on weekends, holidays, or just for an evening out on the town. Theater is no longer attractive only to the upper classes; affordable prices make it reasonable entertainment for almost anyone.

Concerts, musicals, and comedy shows are also becoming increasingly affordable and are included in many people's vacations schedules. As we move up the hierarchy of needs, self-actualization becomes a greater motivation, and more and more people satisfy that need with a dose of culture and performing arts.

▶ Check Your Knowledge

1. What are the goals of the Smithsonian Institution?
2. Why are theaters, concerts, musicals, and comedy shows regaining importance?

Destinations

Some destinations are major attractions in themselves. For example, a trip to Europe might include visits to cities such as London, Paris, Rome, Athens, and Madrid or just focus on one country, where visitors enjoy not only the city but also the countryside. The following sections describe some of the world's most popular destinations.

Athens, Greece

Athens, the capital city of Greece, is one of the world's oldest cities—the cradle of Western civilization and the birthplace of democracy. Classical Athens was a powerful city-state, a center for the arts, learning, and philosophy, and home of Plato's Academy and Aristotle's Lyceum.[51] History abounds in Athens, as evidenced by the Parthenon—a temple to the Greek goddess Athena built in the fifth century B.C. on the Acropolis, a flat rock above the city. Today, Athens is a bustling city of more than 3 million—all of whom seem to be on the move, hence its notorious congestion.[52]

Of the millions of tourists who go to Greece, many, after visiting Athens, take a ferry boat ride to the famed Greek Islands in the Aegean Sea. Crete, the largest island, is rugged and mountainous with beautiful beaches and a reconstruction of King Minos's Palace, which is the largest Bronze Age archeological site on Crete, dating back to between 1700 and 1400 B.C. It was probably the ceremonial and political center of Minoan civilization and culture. The strikingly beautiful island of Santorini is a remaining part of the cone of an extinct volcano that erupted some 3,500 years ago. Some of the picturesque white buildings cling to the rim of the volcano and are among the most photographed in the world. The best way up to the town on top of the hill is by donkey ride. Mikonos is a trendy island with its famed windmills and fabulous beaches, some of them nude beaches. Other often-visited islands include Rhodes, with plenty of ruins, good beaches, and nightlife, and Corfu, off the west coast of Greece, with its lush vegetation due to higher rainfall than the other islands and its excellent beaches, museum, and nightlife—including a casino—making it a favorite of package tour groups.

London

London was once the center of an empire that included approximately one-quarter of the globe. The name suggests history, pageantry, royalty, theater, shopping, museums, music, fashion, and now even food. London has several interesting areas such as Chelsea and the River Thames and Hampstead on the hill with its quaint pubs and row houses. Trafalgar Square, named after the Battle of Trafalgar in which Nelson defeated the French, is where a statue of Lord Nelson stands atop a tall column. The four large lions that guard the statue were reputedly made from the cannons of the French fleet. Nearby is Piccadilly Circus, the core of the theater and nightlife district, along with neighboring Soho, which was a former royal park and favorite hunting ground of King Henry VIII. (In Old English, the word *so* means "wild boar or pig," and *ho* means "there.") There are many other fascinating areas such as London's East End, home of the Cockneys; the impressive buildings of the Houses of Parliament, with Big Ben, the clock tower; and of course, Buckingham Palace, the queen's London residence.

Outside London's popular tourist spots are Oxford, where travelers can visit the famous university; Stratford-upon-Avon, the birthplace of William Shakespeare, where travelers can visit the house in which Shakespeare was born in 1564 and can visit Ann Hathaway's cottage, where she lived before her marriage to Shakespeare; Bath, famous for its history of therapeutic heated springs; and Stonehenge, a complex of Neolithic and Bronze Age monuments whose purpose is mysterious and unknown. Bath is England's most elegant city known for its Georgian architecture and, of course, its baths that date back to Roman times and that are reputed to ease the pain of arthritis. Many visitors enjoy the English countryside, with quaint villages and narrow winding roads and roundabouts. And visitors can always enjoy the British pubs.

Paris

Paris is a city of beautiful buildings, boulevards, parks, markets, and restaurants and cafés. Paris is exciting! So, for tourists, what to see first is an often-asked question over morning coffee and croissants. There are city tours, but the best way to see the real Paris is on foot, especially if people want to avoid the hordes of other tourists. A tour could begin at the Eiffel Tower or the Notre Dame Cathedral, the Louvre or the Musée d'Orsay, or the Île de la Cité, or with simply with a stroll down the Champs-Elysées.

Paris began as a small island called Île de la Cité, in the middle of the River Seine. In time, Paris grew onto the Left Bank (Rive Gauche), where the University of the Sorbonne was founded. The university provided instruction in Latin, so it became known as the Quartier Latin, or Latin Quarter. The Latin Quarter has a Bohemian intellectual character with lots of small cafés and wine bars similar to Greenwich Village and Soho in New York. Nearby is Montparnasse, an area that is popular with today's artists and painters. On the Right Bank (Rive Droit) of the river Seine are many attractions; one favorite is the area of Montmartre, with the domes of Sacré-Coeur and the Place du Tertre. Just walking along the winding streets up to Sacré-Coeur gives visitors a feel of the special nature of Paris. Savoring the sights of the little markets with arrays of fresh fruits, vegetables, and flowers; catching the aromas wafting from the cafés; and seeing couples walking arm in arm in a way that only lovers do in Paris add to the ambiance that captivates all who go there and provide wonderful memories.

Rome

They say, "All roads lead to Rome." Rome, the Eternal City, also called the "Cradle of Civilization," is built on seven hills beside the Tiber River, with centuries of history that seem to exude from every building. Among the most visited sites are the Colosseum, the Pantheon, the Spanish Steps, Vatican City,

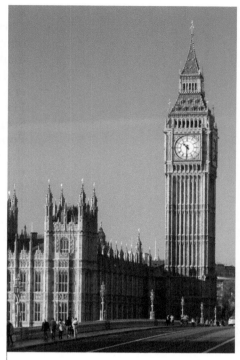

Big Ben and Westminster Abbey make London a popular destination.

419

and the Forum. The Colosseum is the ancient stadium where gladiators fought, Christians were martyred, other sports and games were played, and thousands of men fought with ferocious animals to amuse the crowds. The Pantheon, originally built in 27 B.C. as a temple to all the gods of ancient Rome, was destroyed by fire in A.D. 80, rebuilt in 126, and is likely the best preserved building of its era. The Spanish Steps, the widest steps in Europe, are situated between the Piazza di Spagna (Plaza of Spain) and the Piazza Trinità die Monti (The Holy See), the Episcopal jurisdiction of the Bishop of Rome, better known as the Pope. They are a popular hangout for tourists and residents. Vatican City is the smallest state in the world, with only 110 acres and a population of just over 800.[53] In this tiny area are St. Peter's Basilica, the Vatican Museums, and Michelangelo's *Creation*, painted on the ceiling of the Sistine Chapel, and his *Last Judgment*, on the wall behind the altar. The Roman Forum was the center of political, social, and economic life in imperial Rome, with temples, basilicas, and triumphal arches; it is the place where the Roman democratic government began. Several other interesting cities to visit in Italy include Venice, Naples, and Florence, along with the Tuscan countryside.

Managing Attractions

Managing attractions and theme parks has many similarities to managing any business. Theme park managers use the same main management functions (planning, including forecasting; organizing; decision making; and controlling).

Planning involves all types of planning that fall under two headings: strategic (long term) and tactical (short term). An example of strategic planning would be determining what kind of theme ride to build as the next major attraction or planning a new park in another country. An example of tactical planning would be forecasting the park's attendance for the next month so departments can staff correctly.

Organizing is getting everything arranged: who will do what, by whom, when, and where. For example, a theme park requires a structure to be organized for managing the process. The management team is assembled and given their assignments. Someone manages the reservations and admissions, the rides, the restaurants and foodservice, the gift shops, maintenance, marketing, human resources, and accounting and finance. Each department manager has daily, weekly, and monthly tasks that structure the organizing of the park to maximize operational efficiencies and effectiveness. Organization charts show who reports to whom and give a visual representation of the operation of the park.

Decision making can be quick and easy for the many programmed decisions—decisions that occur on a regular basis, allowing the decision to be handled with a "programmed" response. For example, when the inventory of an item falls below the reorder point, a programmed response is to order a predetermined quantity to bring the stock back up to par.

Another, more complicated type of decision making is nonprogrammed—which is nonrecurring and is caused by unusual circumstances. One example of a nonprogrammed decision is a situation with incomplete information—for example, which guest relations program or point-of-sale system to install.

The decision-making process consists of eight steps:[54]

1. Identification of the problem and definition of the problem
2. Identification of the decision criteria
3. Allocation of weights to the criteria
4. Development of alternatives
5. Analysis of alternatives
6. Selection of alternative
7. Implementation of alternative
8. Evaluation of decision effectiveness

Controlling is constantly checking to make sure that the results were what they should be. Was the actual revenue what was expected? Or, was it above or below expected, and by how much? What was the labor cost and how did it compare with the expected labor cost? Control examines performance results in all the key areas of operation.

Revenue comes from entrance ticket sales, parking, vending, retail program fees, food and beverage sales, and donations. There is a great variation among attractions. Some are for profit and others are nonprofit; however, both must operate with budgets. Many attractions obtain 70 percent of their revenue from ticket sales, approximately 15 percent income from retail, and another 15 percent from food and beverage sales. Many attractions are looking to attract new revenue by staging special events such as corporate events, Father's Day or Easter celebrations, or auto shows in the parking lot.

As managers of a business, attractions managers are also trying to stay ahead of the wave and keep on top of expenditures. They also try to retain the best employees during the slow season by cross-training them to do more than one job as the need arises. Because labor costs are the highest expense item, managers do their best to reduce labor costs by boosting the volunteer base in multiple areas.[55]

Attractions management is all about keeping the quality of product and guest service at the highest levels. It boils down to revenue minus expenses equal net profit.[56]

Clubs

Private clubs are places where members gather for social, recreational, professional, or fraternal reasons. Members enjoy bringing friends, family, and business guests to their club. Their club is like a second home, but with diverse facilities and staff to accommodate the occasion. Bringing guests to one's club can be more impressive than inviting them to one's home, and there is still a level of the same personal atmosphere as there would be if guests were invited home. Many of today's clubs are adaptations of their predecessors, mostly examples from England and Scotland. For example, the North American country club is largely patterned after the Royal and Ancient Golf Club of St. Andrews, Scotland, founded in 1758 and recognized as the birthplace of golf. Many

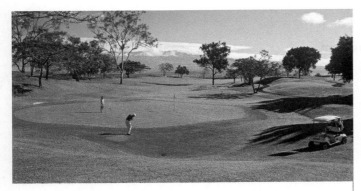

Big Island Country Club on Kona Coast of Hawaii.

business deals are negotiated on the golf course. A few years ago, country clubs were often considered to be bastions of the social elite.

Historically, the ambiance of these clubs attracted the affluent. The character of the clubs transcended generations. Member etiquette and mannerisms developed over years to a definable point by which members could recognize each other through subtleties, and those not possessing the desired qualities were not admitted.

Today there are more affluent people than ever, and their number continues to grow. The new rich are now targeted and recruited for a variety of new hybrid groups that also call themselves clubs. The newer clubs' cost of initiation and membership may be considerably less than some of the more established clubs. The stringent screening process and lengthy membership applications are now simplified, and cash is the key to admittance.

New clubs are born when a developer purchases a tract of land and builds a golf course with a clubhouse surrounded by homes or condominiums. The homes are sold and include a membership to the club. After all the homes are sold, the developer announces that the golf course and clubhouse will be sold to an investor who wishes to open it to the public. The homeowners rush to purchase the clubhouse and golf course to protect their investment. A board is formed, and the employees of the developer and all operations are usually transferred to and become the responsibility of the new owners or members.

Size and Scope of the Club Industry

There are a few thousand private clubs in North America, including both country and city clubs. When the total resources of all the clubs are considered, such as land, buildings, and equipment, along with thousands of employees and so forth, clubs have billions of dollars of economic impact.

Club Management

Club management is similar in many ways to hotel management, both of which have evolved in recent years. The general managers of clubs now assume the role of chief operating officer, and in some cases chief executive officer of the corporation. They may also have responsibility for management of the homeowners' association and all athletic facilities, including the golf courses. In addition, they are responsible for planning, forecasting and budgeting, human resources, food and beverage operations, facility management, and maintenance. The main difference between managing a club and managing a hotel is that with clubs the guests feel as if they are the owners (in many cases they are) and frequently behave as if they are the owners. Their emotional attachment to the facility is stronger than that of hotel guests who do not use hotels with the same frequency that members use clubs. Another difference is that most clubs do not offer sleeping accommodations.

CORPORATE PROFILE

ClubCorp

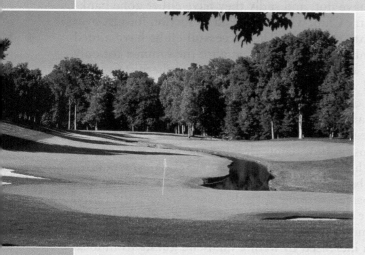

Founded in 1957, Dallas-based ClubCorp is the world leader in delivering premier golf, private club, and resort experiences. Internationally, ClubCorp owns or operates more than 150 golf and country clubs, business clubs, sports clubs, alumni clubs, and resorts in twenty-five states, the District of Columbia, and two foreign countries. ClubCorp has approximately $1.8 billion in assets. Among the company's nationally recognized golf properties are the Firestone Country Club in Akron, Ohio (site of the 2003–2005 World Golf Championships—Bridgestone Invitational) and Mission Hills Country Club in Rancho Mirage, California (home of the Kraft Nabisco Championship).

The more than forty business clubs and business and sports clubs include the Boston College Club; City Club on Bunker Hill in Los Angeles; Citrus Club in Orlando, Florida; Columbia Tower Club in Seattle; Metropolitan Club in Chicago; Tower Club in Dallas; and the City Club of Washington, D.C. The company's 14,000 employees serve the nearly 350,000 members of the ClubCorp properties.

ClubCorp is in the business of building relationships and enriching lives. The extraordinary private club environments nourish relationships old and new, as well as create a world of privacy, luxury, and relaxation where guests' every need is anticipated and every expectation exceeded. Crafting fine, private-club traditions for more than fifty years, ClubCorp has developed a signature philosophy of service that resonates with every encounter, every warm welcome, and every magic moment, joining to form the bedrock of all the clubs.

Each club has its own distinctive personality and takes pride in creating the perfect settings for casual gatherings with friends, business meetings, or formal celebrations. The clubs provide safe havens where members and their guests always are welcome. Whether looking for a country club experience or a professional retreat in which to conduct business affairs, ClubCorp's members are the beneficiaries of the ultimate in private club service and tradition.

ClubCorp clubs provide a variety of membership options and experiences for a range of lifestyle pursuits. In more than 150 private business and sports clubs, country clubs, golf courses, and resorts around the world, from Seattle to Mexico and from Boston to Beijing, ClubCorp provides for its members a haven of refuge, a home away from home, where every need is anticipated and every expectation surpassed.

Source: ClubCorp, *United States Securities and Exchange Commission Form 10-Q,* http://b2i.api.edgar-online.com/EFX_dll/EdgarPro.dll?FetchFilingHTML1?Session ID=MNp_Fy-6vHMBo-9&ID=8054747 (accessed November 15, 2011); and ClubCorp, *Company Profile,* http://www.clubcorp.com/About-ClubCorp/Company-Profile (accessed November 15, 2011).

Club members pay an initiation fee to belong to the club and annual membership dues thereafter. Some clubs also charge a set utilization fee, usually related to food and beverages, which is charged regardless of whether those services are used.

The Club Manager's Association of America (CMAA) is the professional organization to which many of the club managers belong. The association's goal is to advance the profession of club management by fulfilling the educational and related needs of the club managers. The association provides networking opportunities and fosters camaraderie among its member managers through meetings and conferences held locally and nationally. These gatherings keep managers abreast of current practices and procedures and new legislation. The general managers who join CMAA subscribe to a code of ethics.

Successful club general managers have adapted to their new and evolving environment. Some, however, have not, and sadly they have either gone bankrupt, as with Cyprus Run Country Club, which was sold at auction for just over $1 million, or gone from private to public. The successful clubs have added incentives, like becoming a member for a day or joining for the summer for only $500, to attract more members. Clubs in Florida and other southern states that attract "snowbirds"—seasonal visitors from the northern states—are offering special winter rates. For many clubs, the harsh economic climate has reduced membership, reducing revenue and making it more difficult to pay mortgages.

Most clubs have found creative ways of increasing revenue by including more items in the shops—not just golf or tennis clothing and clubs or racquets, but expanded merchandise such as jewelry, books, organic cookies, vitamins, and swim gear. In addition, clubs have expanded their offerings to include spas that offer Botox, facials, and cosmetic products. Clubs have extended their food and beverage offerings to make more money off events like weddings and social fund raisers such as the American Cancer Society and the Salvation Army. Additionally, revenue has been increased by letting high-end guests from local hotels pay handsomely for the privilege of playing the course.

Clubs are reducing expenses by paying about 40-percent-less property taxes and by trimming costly items like water for the golf course by using reclaimed water and by cutting back on the amount paid into employees' 401(k) retirement plans and by providing a fixed amount of $400 for a staff member and family per month for benefits.

Club Management Structure

The internal management structure of a club is governed by the corporation's articles of incorporation and bylaws. These establish election procedures, officer positions, a board of directors, and standing committees. Guidance and direction also are provided for each office and committee and how it will function. The general manager will usually provide an orientation for the new directors and information to help them in their new role. The members elect the officers and directors of the club. The officers represent the membership by establishing policies by which the club will operate. Many clubs and other organizations maintain continuity by having a succession of officers. The secretary becomes the vice president and the vice president becomes the president. In other cases, the person elected president is simply the person believed to be the most qualified to lead the club for that year. Regardless of who is elected president, the club's general manager must be able to work with that person and the other officers.

The president presides at all official meetings and is a leader in policymaking. The vice president is groomed for the role of president, which is usually eminent, and will in the absence of the president perform the presidential duties. If the club has more than one vice president, the titles *first*, *second*, *third*, and so on, may be used. Alternatively, vice presidents may be assigned to chair certain committees, such as membership. Board members usually chair one or more committees.

Committees play an important part in the club's activities. If the committees are effective, the operation of the club is more efficient. The term of committee

INTRODUCING EDWARD J. SHAUGHNESSY

General Manager, Belleair Country Club

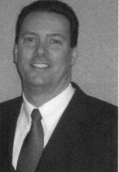

For Ed Shaughnessy, working in a country club is not just a job but a passion. Clubs feature great recreational facilities, including some fabulous golf courses, gourmet dining, the finest entertainment, and clientele who are more like family than customers. Shaughnessy has worked for three prestigious clubs in his career. He began working in clubs at the tender age of fourteen as a busser. Shortly after graduating from high school, he accepted a full-time evening bar manager position at Sleepy Hollow Country Club in New York. He worked full time at night while attending college full time until he received his A.A.S. degree. Upon graduation, he was promoted to food and beverage manager, but continued his education, taking two or three courses every semester until he earned and received his B.B.A. He was subsequently promoted to assistant general manager.

After fourteen years at the same club and on his twenty-ninth birthday, he was offered and accepted the general manager's position at Belle Haven Country Club in Alexandria, Virginia. He began an active role in the National Capital Club Managers Association and was elected president. He continued his education and earned his Certified Club Manager (CCM) designation and his Certified Hospitality Educator (CHE) designation through the Club Managers Association of America (CMAA). He stayed at Belle Haven Country Club for eight years, but wanted to live closer to sunny beaches in a warmer climate.

An opportunity at the prestigious Belleair Country Club in Belleair, Florida, was brought to Shaughnessy's attention by John Sibbald, a top recruiter in the club industry, and in 1997 Ed Shaughnessy accepted the position of general manager/chief operating officer at the Belleair Country Club. He continued his education, earning his M.B.A. in International Hotel and Tourism Management from Schiller International University, where he now teaches a variety of hospitality-related courses. Shaughnessy is still active with the CMAA and serves on the Club Foundation Allocation Committee. This committee reviews scholarship and grant applications and recommends the awarding of funds to promote education. He also serves as the ethics chair for the Florida Chapter of the CMAA.

Shaughnessy believes that there are two stages in life—growth and decay—and that we are all in one of these stages. For him, to be in the growth stage is preferred in life. He believes we are all given the choice to change our environment, and he enjoys catering to those with the highest expectations. It appears that people will always recognize and be willing to pay for great value and quality. Meticulous attention to detail and proactively providing what customers desire before they have to ask is the key to success.

No two days are the same or predictable for a general manager. One day you could be developing a strategic plan, the next you may be invited to fly on a private Lear jet to see the Super Bowl. You have to make a conscious effort to balance work and family life. A general manager should remember that although you can enjoy many of the same privileges as the elite, you are still an employee and must always set an exemplary role as a professional. A general manager's people skills are very important, as well as having a comprehensive understanding of financial statements.

The challenge for the future is finding talented and service-oriented people who are needed to exceed the constantly increasing expectations of sophisticated and discriminating club members. Shaughnessy discovered some time ago that it may be necessary to grow one's own talent among his employees, and this gives him the confidence that he will be ready to serve his customers well. Shaughnessy has a high concern for the welfare of his loyal and dedicated employees. They could lose their jobs if the club is mismanaged. These people and their families count on him to operate the club efficiently. He also recognizes that he must take proactive steps to ensure the growth and success of his club. With two waterfront golf courses, a marina, and the amenities of a full-service country club, Ed Shaughnessy is taking steps to be sure he positions the club for continued success.

membership is specified, and committee meetings are conducted in accordance with Robert's Rules of Order, which are procedural guidelines on the correct way to conduct meetings. Standing committees include the following: house, membership, finance/budget, entertainment, golf, green tennis, pool, and long-range planning. The president may appoint additional committees to serve specific functions commonly referred to as ad hoc.

The treasurer obviously must have some financial and accounting background because an integral part of his or her duties is to give advice on financial matters, such as employing external auditors, preparing budgets, and installing control systems. The general manager is responsible for all financial matters and usually signs or cosigns all checks.

It is the duty of the secretary to record the minutes of meetings and take care of club-related correspondence. In most cases, the general manager prepares the document for the secretary's signature. This position can be combined with that of treasurer, in which case the position is titled secretary–treasurer. The secretary may also serve on or chair certain committees.

The Club Managers Association of America (CMAA) has reexamined the role of club managers, and because of ever-increasing expectations, the role of the general manager has changed from the traditional managerial model to a leadership model. The new CMAA model is based on the premise that general managers or chief operating officers (COOs) are more responsible for operating assets and investments and club culture.

The basic level of competency required of a general manager or COO is management of club's operations, which includes private club management, food and beverage, accounting and financial management, human and professional resources, building and facilities management, external and governmental influences, management, marketing, and sports and recreation (see Figure 1).

The second tier of the model is mastering the skills of asset management. Today's general manager or COO must be able to manage the physical property, the financial well-being, and the human resources of the club. These facets of the manager's responsibilities are equally as important as managing the operations of the club.

The third and final tier of the new model is preserving and fostering the culture of the club, which can be defined as the club's traditions, history, governance, and vision. Many managers or COOs intrinsically perform this function; however, it is often

CMAA Code of Ethics

We believe the management of clubs is an honorable calling. It shall be incumbent upon club managers to be knowledgeable in the application of sound principles in the management of clubs, with ample opportunity to keep abreast of current practices and procedures. We are convinced that the Club Managers Association of America best represents these interests and, as members thereof subscribe to the following CODE OF ETHICS.

We will uphold the best traditions of club management through adherence to sound business principles. By our behavior and demeanor, we shall set an example for our employees and will assist our club officers to secure the utmost in efficient and successful club operations.

We will consistently promote the recognition and esteem of club management as a profession and conduct our personal and business affairs in a manner to reflect capability and integrity. We will always honor our contractual employment obligations.

We shall promote community and civic affairs by maintaining good relations with the public sector to the extent possible within the limits of our club's demands.

We will strive to advance our knowledge and abilities as club managers, and willingly share with other Association members the lessons of our experience and knowledge gained by supporting and participating in our local chapter and the National Association's educational meetings and seminars.

We will not permit ourselves to be subsidized or compromised by any interest doing business with our clubs.

We will refrain from initiating, directly or through an agent, any communications with a director, member, or employee of another club regarding its affairs without the prior knowledge of the manager thereof, if it has a manager.

We will advise the National Headquarters, whenever possible, regarding managerial openings at clubs that come to our attention. We will do all within our power to assist our fellow club managers in pursuit of their professional goals.

We shall not be deterred from compliance with the law, as it applies to our clubs. We shall provide our club officers and trustees with specifics of federal, state and local laws, statutes, and regulations to avoid punitive action and costly litigation.

We deem it our duty to report to local or national officers any willful violations of the CMAA CODE OF ETHICS.

Source: The author gratefully acknowledges the professional courtesy of the Club Managers Association of America.

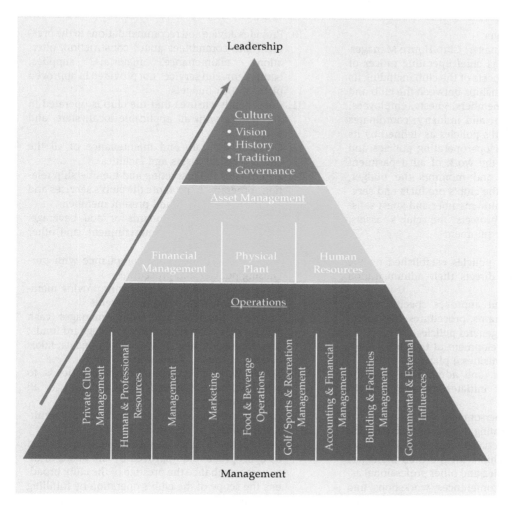

Figure 1 • Management to Leadership.

an overlooked and underdeveloped quality. A job description for club manager is given in Figure 2. The club management competencies are shown in Figure 3. Additionally, you can see an example of the overall organization of a country club in Figure 4.

Types of Clubs

Country Clubs

Nearly all **country clubs** have one or more lounges and restaurants, and most have banquet facilities. Members and their guests enjoy these services and can be billed monthly. The banquet facilities are used for formal and informal parties, dinners, dances, weddings, and so on, by members and their personal guests. Some country clubs charge what might seem to be an excessive amount for the initiation fee—as much as $250,000 in some cases—to maintain exclusivity.

I. **Position:** General Manager

II. **Related Titles:** Club Manager; Club House Manager

III. **Job Summary:** Serves as chief operating officer of the club; manages all aspects of the club including its activities and the relationships between the club and its board of directors, members, guests, employees, community, government, and industry; coordinates and administers the club's policies as defined by its board of directors. Develops operating policies and procedures and directs the work of all department managers. Implements and monitors the budget, monitors the quality of the club's products and services, and ensures maximum member and guest satisfaction. Secures and protects the club's assets, including facilities and equipment

IV. **Job Tasks (Duties):**

1. Implements general policies established by the board of directors; directs their administration and execution

2. Plans, develops, and approves specific operational policies, programs, procedures, and methods in concert with general policies

3. Coordinates the development of the club's long-range and annual (business) plans

4. Develops, maintains, and administers a sound organizational plan; initiates improvements as necessary

5. Establishes a basic personnel policy; initiates and monitors policies relating to personnel actions and training and professional development programs

6. Maintains membership with the Club Managers Association of America and other professional associations. Attends conferences, workshops, and meetings to keep abreast of current information and developments in the field

7. Coordinates development of operating and capital budgets according to the budget calendar; monitors monthly and other financial statements for the club; takes effective corrective action as required

8. Coordinates and serves as ex-officio member of appropriate club committees

9. Welcomes new club members; meets and greets all club members as practical during their visits to the club

10. Provides advice and recommendations to the president and committees about construction, alterations, maintenance, materials, supplies, equipment, and services not provided in approved plans and/or budgets

11. Consistently ensures that the club is operated in accordance with all applicable local, state, and federal laws

12. Oversees the care and maintenance of all the club's physical assets and facilities

13. Coordinates the marketing and membership relations programs to promote the club's services and facilities to potential and present members

14. Ensures the highest standards for food, beverage, sports and recreation, entertainment, and other club services

15. Establishes and monitors compliance with purchasing policies and procedures

16. Reviews and initiates programs to provide members with a variety of popular events

17. Analyzes financial statements, manages cash flow, and establishes controls to safeguard funds; reviews income and costs relative to goals; takes corrective action as necessary

18. Works with subordinate department heads to schedule, supervise, and direct the work of all club employees

19. Attends meetings of the club's executive committee and board of directors

20. Participates in outside activities that are judged as appropriate and approved by the board of directors to enhance the prestige of the club; broadens the scope of the club's operation by fulfilling the public obligations of the club as a participating member of the community

V. **Reports to:** Club President and Board of Directors

VI. **Supervises:** Assistant General Manager (Club House Manager); Food and Beverage Director; Controller; Membership Director; Director of Human Resources; Director of Purchasing; Golf Professional (Director of Golf); Golf Course Superintendent; Tennis Professional; Athletic Director; Executive Secretary

Source: Club Managers Association of America.

Figure 2 • A Job Description for a Club Manager.

Source: The author gratefully acknowledges the professional courtesy of the Club Managers Association of America.

Country clubs have two or more types of membership. Full membership enables members to use all the facilities all the time. Social membership allows members only to use the social facilities: lounges, bars, restaurants, and so on, and perhaps the pool and tennis courts. Other forms of membership can include weekday and weekend memberships.

Private Club Management
History of Private Clubs
Types of Private Clubs
Membership Types
Bylaws
Policy Formulation
Board Relations
Chief Operating Officer Concept
Committees
Club Job Descriptions
Career Development
Golf Operations Management
Golf Course Management
Tennis Operations Management
Swimming Pool Management
Yacht Facilities Management
Fitness Center Management
Locker Room Management
Other Recreational Activities

Food and Beverage Operations
Sanitation
Menu Development
Nutrition
Pricing Concepts
Ordering/Receiving/Controls/Inventory
Food and Beverage Trends
Quality Service
Creativity in Theme Functions
Design and Equipment
Food and Beverage Personnel
Wine List Development

**Accounting and Finance
  in the Private Club**
Accounting and Finance Principles
Uniform System of Accounts
Financial Analysis
Budgeting
Cash Flow Forecasting
Compensation and Benefit
  Administration
Financing Capital Projects
Audits
Internal Revenue Service
Computers
Business Office Organization
Long-Range Financial Planning

Human and Professional Resources
Employee Relations
Management Styles
Organizational Development
Balancing Job and Family
  Responsibilities
Time Management
Stress Management
Labor Issues
Leadership vs. Management

Building and Facilities Management
Preventive Maintenance
Insurance and Risk Management
Clubhouse Remodeling and
  Renovation

Contractors
Energy and Water Resource
  Management
Housekeeping
Security
Laundry
Lodging Operations

**External and Governmental
  Influences**
Legislative Influences
Regulatory Agencies
Economic Theory
Labor Law
Internal Revenue Service
Privacy
Club Law
Liquor Liability
Labor Unions

Management and Marketing
Communication Skills
Marketing Through In-House
  Publications
Professional Image and Dress
Effective Negotiation
Member Contact Skills
Working with the Media
Marketing Strategies in a Private
  Club Environment

Source: Club Managers Association of
  America.

Figure 3 • The Club Management Competences.

Source: The author gratefully acknowledges the professional courtesy of the Club Managers Association of America.

City Clubs

City clubs are predominantly business oriented, although some have rules prohibiting the discussion of business and the reviewing of business-related documents in dining rooms. They vary in size, location, type of facility, and services offered. Some of the older, established clubs own their own buildings; others lease space. Clubs exist to cater to the wants and needs of members. Clubs in the city fall into the following categories:

- Professional
- Social
- Athletic
- Dining
- University

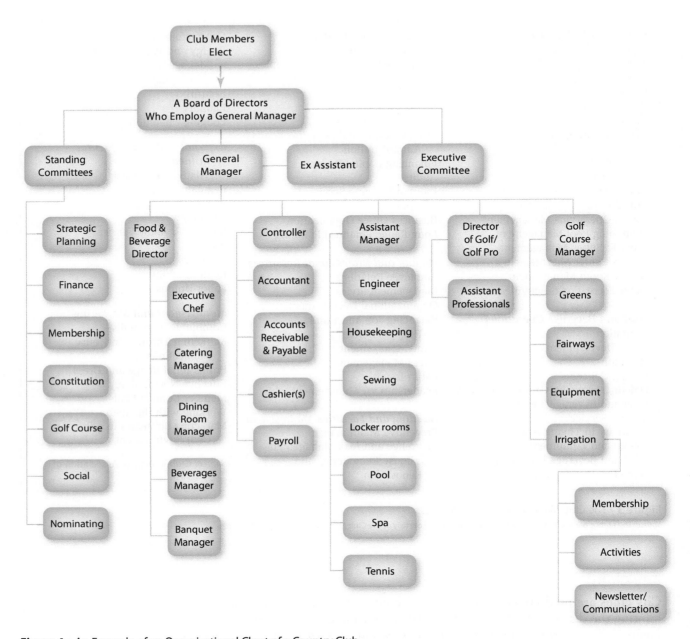

Figure 4 • An Example of an Organizational Chart of a Country Club.

- Military
- Yachting
- Fraternal
- Proprietary

Professional clubs, as the name implies, are clubs for people in the same profession. The National Press Club in Washington, D.C., the Lawyers Club in New York City, and the Friars Club for actors and other theatrical people in Manhattan are good examples.

Social clubs allow members to enjoy one another's company; members represent many different professions, yet they have similar socioeconomic backgrounds. Social clubs are modeled after the famous men's social clubs in London, such as Boodles, St. James's, and White's. At these clubs, it is considered bad form to discuss business. Therefore, conversation and social interaction focus on companionship or entertainment unrelated to business.

The oldest social club in the United States is thought to be the Fish House in Philadelphia, founded in 1832. To ensure that the Fish House would always be socially oriented rather than business oriented, it was formed as a men's cooking club, with each member taking a turn preparing meals for the membership. Other social clubs exist in several major cities. The common denominator is that they all have upscale food and beverage offerings and club managers to manage them.

Athletic clubs give city workers and residents an opportunity to work out, swim, play squash and/or racquetball, and so on. Some of the downtown athletic clubs provide tennis courts and running tracks on the roof. Athletic clubs also have lounges, bars, and restaurants at which members may relax and interact socially. Some athletic clubs also have meeting rooms and even sleeping accommodations. The newest feature is known as the executive workout. This begins with a visit to the steam room, followed by a trip to the Jacuzzi, then sauna, a massage, and nap in the resting room before showering and returning to work.

Dining clubs are generally located in large city office buildings. Memberships are often given as an inducement to tenants who lease space in the office building. These clubs are always open for lunch and occasionally for dinner.

University clubs are private clubs for alumni. University clubs are generally located in the high-rent district and offer a variety of facilities and attractions focusing on food and beverage service.

Military clubs cater to both noncommissioned officers (NCOs) and enlisted officers. Military clubs offer similar facilities as do other clubs for recreation and entertainment and food and beverage offerings. Some military clubs are located on base. The largest membership club in the country is the Army Navy Country Club in Arlington, Virginia. The club has more than 6,000 members, 54 holes of golf, 2 clubhouses, and a host of other facilities. Many of the military clubs in recent years have given over their club management to civilians.

Yacht clubs provide members with moorage slips, where their boats are kept secure. In addition to moorage facilities, yacht clubs have lounge, bar, and dining facilities similar to other clubs. Yacht clubs are based on a sailing theme and attract members with various backgrounds who have sailing as a common interest.

Fraternal clubs include many special organizations, such as the Veterans of Foreign Wars, Elks, and Shriners. These organizations foster camaraderie and often assist charitable causes. They generally are less elaborate than are other clubs, but have bars and banquet rooms that can be used for various activities.

Proprietary clubs operate on a for-profit basis. They are owned by corporations or individuals; individuals wanting to become members purchase a membership, not a share in the club. Proprietary clubs became popular with the real estate boom in the 1970s and 1980s. As new housing developments were planned, clubs were included in several of the projects. Households pay a small initiation fee and monthly dues between $30 and $50, allowing the whole family to participate in a wide variety of recreational activities.

Clearly, the opportunities for recreation and leisure abound. The goal must be to achieve a harmony between work and leisure activities and to become truly professional in both giving and receiving these services. The next few years will see a substantial increase in the leisure and recreational industries.

FOCUS ON RECREATION

Hospitality and Recreation: Inextricably Intertwined

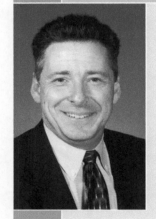

Bart Bartlett, Ph.D., Professor in Charge of Undergraduate Programs at Penn State University's School of Hospitality Management

Americans have more leisure time than ever before, and as leisure time has grown, leisure activities have evolved and grown as well. As this chapter points out, opportunities today for recreation and for careers in recreation management are vast and multifaceted. These include positions in commercial recreation (resorts, themed resorts, the ski industry), in noncommercial recreation (federal or state parks and community recreation), in clubs and sports venues, and in recreation with special populations.

Although the focus of this text is hospitality management, in many situations, recreation and hospitality go hand in hand. When a ski trip incorporates recreation on the slopes with food and beverage services in the lodge or when a hotel guest uses the hotel's business services and the spa, recreation and hospitality are both involved. When a convention center hotel provides rooms, food, and beverage; coordinates meetings and breakout sessions; and also organizes recreation and group activities during the conference, hospitality and recreation begin to merge. In fact, because our guests' total experience often involves a combination of lodging, food and beverage, and recreation, we do not want to distinguish, but instead want to ensure guest satisfaction by seamlessly integrating these different elements into the total package.

As growth in leisure travel continues to outstrip growth in business travel, the growing leisure travel market will create an increasing emphasis on recreation as an integral part of hospitality. Furthermore, though hospitality and recreation may involve different emphases, the critical customer focus and customer service skills that we love about our industry are common to all aspects of hospitality and recreation.

Resorts and resort hotels are the prototypical combination of hospitality and recreation. A mega-resort such as Walt Disney World provides an ideal example of a venue that integrates hospitality and recreation skills and services. On a Disney vacation, a family may enjoy lodging and food and beverage services provided by hotel staff and management trained in hospitality, go into the park itself to enjoy attractions and shows arranged and managed by a recreation specialist, take a break to enjoy foodservice provided by a hospitality provider, and at the end of the day enjoy dinner provided by the hospitality staff and entertainment or dancing arranged by a recreation professional.

The golf industry provides other examples. At a typical golf club, the director of golf operations is primarily involved with managing recreation activities, including scheduling and supervising play, course maintenance, and the pro shop. The clubhouse manager, meanwhile, is responsible for hospitality functions, including food and beverage operations, catering events, and membership. If either were missing, the club simply could not meet guests' and members' overall expectations.

Finally, because cruise ships are essentially floating resort hotels with many features of land-based resorts, both hospitality and recreation are required. On a cruise ship, the purser and food and beverage manager are responsible for hospitality functions, while the cruise director provides recreation programming. Both are critical parts of the cruise experience, thus providing the all-around good time guests desire and deserve.

Through this text, you are learning about hotels, restaurants, and managed services and about the knowledge and skills involved in managing these operations. This chapter talks about recreation and the opportunities to apply your hospitality skills in recreation settings. Across the spectrum, from business travelers to family vacationers, from golfing outings to business banquets, from backcountry adventures to haute cuisine dining, from white-sand Caribbean beaches to black diamond ski slopes, customer service and a focus on customer satisfaction are constants, and both hospitality and recreation skills are critical to providing a memorable guest experience. The commonalities in settings, service, and focus on guest satisfaction indicate that hospitality and recreation are indeed inextricably intertwined!

Sustainable Golf Course Management

The golf course industry recognizes sustainability as it is referenced by the Environmental Protection Agency (EPA) and the United Nations, which indicates that it is "meeting the needs of the present without compromising the ability of future generations to meet their own needs."[57] In an effort to appear sustainable, some courses call themselves "green." This is vague. However, it is not vague to say that a course engages in water-quality protection through the responsible use of all inputs, such as nutrients and pesticides.

The EPA gives a basic rundown of sustainability at http://www.epa.gov/ sustainability/basicinfo.htm#sustainability. The Environmental Institute for Golf gives information on sustainable golf management practices (www.eifg.org). Sustainable practices include the following:

- Reducing energy use especially during the peak times (a utility company's bill is much higher for consumption during peak times).

- Holding departments accountable for their energy consumption budgets by breaking down the bills by departments.

- Recycling: from aluminum cans in the clubhouse to grass clippings on the course to motor oil from the golf carts.[58]

Golf course facilities are prime candidates for reducing or reusing waste: As landfill disposal costs rise, recycling becomes even more important. Golf courses can improve their sustainability by improving grass and plant selection and by using well water and organic fertilization.

▶ Check Your Knowledge

1. Name all the types of clubs discussed here and briefly describe their functions.
2. List the important duties of a club manager.
3. Describe the operations of a country club.

Noncommercial Recreation

Noncommercial recreation includes voluntary organizations, campus, armed forces, and employee recreation, as well as recreation for special populations.

Voluntary Organizations

Voluntary organizations are nongovernmental, nonprofit agencies, serving the public at large or selected elements with multiservice programs that often include a substantial element of recreational opportunity. The best-known voluntary organizations include the Boy Scouts, Girl Scouts, YMCA, YWCA, and YM–YWHA.

In the early 1900s, YMCAs began to offer sporting facilities and programs. The Ys, though nonprofit, were pioneers in basketball, swimming, and weight

A DAY IN THE LIFE OF CHRISTIE CHAPMAN

Beverage Cart Attendant, Tampa Palms Golf and Country Club

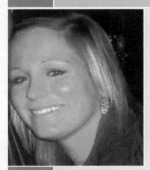

As a beverage car attendant for a golf and country club, my day starts out early at 7:30 A.M. I need to make sure I am prepared for my job, which happens to be supplying thirsty and hungry golfers on the course.

I work Tuesday through Sunday and will work additional hours or days on an as-needed basis. Organizations and other clubs often host golf tournaments at the club, and they will typically need at least one attendant for the duration of the tournament. I first start by stocking the beverage cart with beer, soda, Gatorade, liquor, and any pre-made sandwiches or snacks we offer on our menu. After I stock the cooler full of liquids and cold snacks, I have to cover everything with ice so that it will stay as cool as possible when I make my runs around the course. I also make coffee, as many golfers prefer a hot beverage during the cold mornings. This process should take no longer than an hour. I make sure I have everything I might need before I get out on the golf course, as it's often a long drive back to the clubhouse to stock up on a single item that a member or guest particularly wants.

I start the course off at Hole 18 and make my way back to Hole 1. This way, I am going against the flow of golfers, and they are more likely to need a snack or beverage a little further into their game. I stop at each group of golfers I come across to see if there is anything they need. If a member would like to purchase an item, I will either collect cash for their purchase or fill out a member ticket. The member tickets are for Tampa Palms Golf and Country Club members only, go straight to their private club account, and are billed at the end of each month. Many members golf frequently, and it is a part of my job to get to know not only the name of each member, but his or her most frequent order, member number, and so forth. If we are hosting an outside tournament, most of the golfers are not members, and therefore we require cash for all purchases made during the tournament if there are not already food and beverages provided to the golfers.

Throughout the day, especially on days with nice weather or holiday weekends, I will need to restock the cart. It's easier to restock when I'm keeping track in my head of what items are going quickest. For instance, if the last two groups of golfers each ordered Bud Lights and I haven't made a single coffee sale that morning, I'll know I don't need to make any more coffee and I'll need to stock up on Bud Lights. Even if only eight beers were purchased, the odds those two groups will be purchasing another round of Bud Lights is very likely.

At the end of my day, I unload all of my product from the cart into a fridge inside of the clubhouse. I ring in all of my member tickets, count the cash I've received, and type up an inventory sheet. The inventory sheets help me keep track of what is most popular and requested on the course, and track my sales and volume of distribution for my food and beverage director.

training. Later, commercial health clubs also began to evolve, offering men's and women's exercise. As the sports and fitness movement grew, clubs appealed to special interests. Now clubs can be classified as follows: figure salons, health clubs, bodybuilding gyms, tennis clubs, rowing clubs, swim clubs, racquetball centers, or multipurpose clubs.

A multipurpose club has more exclusive recreation programs than a health club does. Leagues, tournaments, and classes are common for racquet sports, and most clubs offer several types of fitness classes. Some innovative clubs offer automatic bank tellers, stock market quote services, computer matching for tennis competition, auto detailing, laundry and dry cleaning services, and wine-cellar storage.

Club revenue comes from membership fees, user fees, guest fees, food and beverage sales, facility rental, and so on. Human resources account for about 66 percent of expenses at most clubs.

It is amazing to realize that in the center of a city there may be several voluntary organizations, each serving a particular segment of the population. Richard Kraus writes that a study of the city of Toronto which examined various land uses and leisure programs in the city's core found the following organizations: a Boy's Club, a mission, the Center of the Metropolitan Association for the Retarded, a Catholic settlement house, a day care center, an Indian center, a YMCA and YWCA, a service center for working people, a Chinese center, a Ukrainian center, and several other organizations meeting special needs and interests. These were all in addition to public parks, recreation areas, and nineteen churches.

Campus, Armed Forces, and Employee Recreation

Campus Recreation

North America's colleges and universities provide a major setting for organized leisure and recreational programs with services involving millions of participants each year. The programs include involvement by campus recreation offices, intramural departments, student unions, residence staffs, or other sponsors. People spend much of their leisure time participating in a wide variety of organized recreational activities, such as aerobics, arts and crafts, the performing arts, camping, and sports. Recreation and fitness workers plan, organize, and direct these activities in local playgrounds and recreation areas, parks, community centers, health clubs, fitness centers, religious organizations, camps, theme parks, and tourist attractions. Increasingly, recreational and fitness workers also are found in workplaces, where they organize and direct leisure activities and athletic programs for employees of all ages.

The various recreational activities help in maintaining good morale on campus. Some use recreational activities such as sports or orchestras or theater companies as a means of gaining alumni support. Students look for an exciting and interesting social life. For this reason, colleges and universities offer a wide range of recreational and social activities that may vary from campus to campus.

Armed Forces Recreation

It is the official policy of the Department of Defense to provide a well-rounded welfare and recreational program for the physical, social, and mental well-being of its personnel. Each service sponsors recreational activities under the auspices of the Morale, Welfare, and Recreation Program (MWR), which is executed under the Installation Management Command. MWR activities are provided to all military personnel and civilian employees at all installations.

MWR programs include the following types of activities:

- Sports, including self-directed, competitive, instructional, and spectator programs
- Motion pictures
- Service clubs and entertainment
- Crafts and hobbies
- Youth activities for children of military families
- Special-interest groups such as aero, automotive, motorcycle, and power boat clubs, as well as hiking, skydiving, and rod and gun clubs
- Rest centers and recreation areas
- Open dining facilities
- Libraries

Recreation is perceived as an important part of the employee benefits package for military personnel, along with the G.I. Bill, medical services, commissaries, and exchanges.

Employee Recreation

Business and industry have realized the importance of promoting employee efficiency. Human resource experts have found that workers who spend their free time at constructive recreational activities have less absenteeism resulting from emotional tension, illness, excessive use of alcohol, and so on. Employee recreation programs may also be an incentive for a prospective employee to join a company. So, remember to ask for a signing bonus if you are a softball star and the company you are about to join wants to win the tournament!

In the United States and Canada, almost all the leading corporations have an employee recreation and wellness program. Some companies include recreation activities in their team-building and management-development programs.

Recreation for Special Populations

Recreation for special populations involves professionals and organizations who serve groups such as those with mental illness, mental retardation, or physical challenges. In recent years, there has been increased recognition of the need to provide recreational programs for special populations. These programs, developed for each of the special population groups, use therapeutic recreation as a form of treatment.

One sports program for people with disabilities that has received considerable attention in recent years is the Special Olympics, an international year-round program of physical fitness, sports training, and athletic competition for children and adults with intellectual disabilities. The program is unique because it accommodates competitors at all ability levels by assigning participants to competition divisions based on both age and actual performance.[59]

Today, the Special Olympics serves more than 1.4 million individuals in the United States and more than seventy other countries. Among the official sports are track and field events, swimming, diving, gymnastics, ice skating, basketball, volleyball, soccer, softball, floor hockey, bowling, Frisbee disk, downhill skiing, cross-country skiing, and wheelchair events. The National Parks and Recreation Association and numerous state and local agencies and societies work closely with the Special Olympics in promoting programs and sponsoring competitions.[60]

Trends in Recreation and Leisure

- An increase in all fitness activities
- A surge in travel and tourism
- In addition to a continuation of traditional recreation and leisure activities, a development of special programs targeted toward at-risk youths and latchkey children
- Several additional products in the commercial sector
- Additional learning and adventure opportunities for the elderly, such as Life Long Learning

Career Information

Theme Parks

The operation of a theme park includes countless occupations. SeaWorld Parks & Entertainment, Walt Disney Company, and others have excellent programs for employment during college. These programs provide information on career development. Upon graduation, careers may follow a number of paths. Graduates may start in any number of levels: operations management, marketing and sales, human resources, food service, planning and development, or information systems, to name but a few.

An internship is one of the best ways to get involved in the theme park industry. An internship provides valuable work experience and is a great way to learn more about various areas of the industry. Interns are very appealing to potential employers. If you are a college student who is interested in spending a summer working for one of America's premier companies, visit the Disney College Program web site at www.wdwcollegeprogram.com.

George Gonzalez, a theme park manager offers this advice:

Theme parks and attractions offer excellent career opportunities for hospitality graduates. Parks and attractions are generally organized by divisions and departments: rides, shows, animal attractions, up-close tours, special events, dining, gift shop, group events, education and classes, and animal attractions.

If you are interested in theme parks, it is a good idea to work at one during the school year and in the summer months. By gaining experience in any department, you gain an overall impression of the park and hopefully learn if a career in the theme park industry would be a good fit you. Good luck whichever career path you take.

Remember, someone has to run the Smithsonian museum and the national parks and Walt Disney World. All of these attractions have several departments, all with management ladders that can be climbed at varying speeds. Apart from the main attractions, there are careers in accounting, marketing, maintenance, and service, in addition to professional positions for entertainers, historians, and curators. Salary levels for graduates with experience is about $30,000, and for mid-level managers in the larger attractions, salary levels are about $80,000 to $120,000.[61]

Clubs

Club managers and hotel managers share many of the same responsibilities. They are in charge of preparing budgets and forecasting future sales; monitoring restaurants on the property and various internal departments, such as human resources; and making sure maintenance work is done properly. They are responsible for the overall well-being of the club. The CMAA (www.cmaa.org) gives club managers certification and other membership benefits, such as professional development and networking. Its web site is worth a visit.

Club management is different from hotel management in that guests at a club are members and feel like and sometimes behave like owners because they pay a lot of money to join the club. Because of this, many feel a stronger tie to the club and therefore expect a higher level of service.

Of the many types of clubs within the club management industry, the most predominant are golf, country, city, athletic, yacht. Country clubs are the most common. They are typically based on outdoor activities. Golf is the main draw, but other sports such as tennis and swimming are also popular. Some country clubs also offer their members a variety of classes and social activities. They typically have a lounge and/or restaurant on the property, as well. Country clubs can be private or semiprivate. If a country club is private, its facilities are only available to members; a semiprivate club offers some services to nonmembers. There is no one definite career path when it comes to club management. However, most people

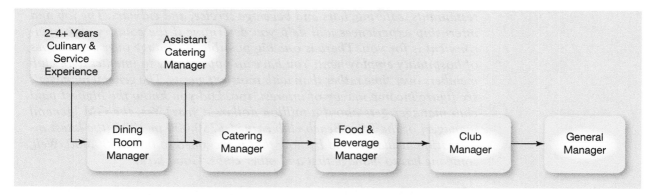

Figure 5 • A Career Path in Club Management.

make the transition to club manager from positions in kitchen or bar management (see Figure 5). It is rare that employees move from areas such as accounting to become club managers. Depending on the level of experience, one might start out as an assistant banquet or dining room manager and then progress to position as catering manager or assistant clubhouse manager. The next step occurs according to the amount of time in these positions, as well as the quality of the experience. For example, four to six years in a club that has gross income of $1.5 million in food and beverage sales would most likely lead to a club management position.

Club managers do not keep regular hours. They work long hours when the club is busy, and fewer hours when the club is slow. Club managers usually create their own schedules according to fluctuations in activity. On average, they typically work five or six days a week, 10 hours a day. Most entry-level club management positions have set salaries that range from $27,000 to $30,000. Entry-level positions are usually not subject to negotiation. Mid-level position salaries, however, can be negotiated until an agreeable sum is met. The actual salary depends on the amount of experience the employee has and the strength of his or her references. The best aspect of working as club manager is that the environment and facilities are usually top notch. Managers typically have access to the club's facilities and receive meals. ClubCorp is one of the largest corporate owners of clubs, operating more than 150 country clubs, business clubs, and golf resorts. Recent expansions in corporate ownership have made it slightly easier to enter the club management profession.

If you are serious about a career in club management, you should join the local student chapter of the CMAA. CMAA meetings are a great place for networking to find a summer job or an internship. The experience you gain during your collage tenure will provide you with the knowledge you need to begin your career in the recreation and leisure industries. Excellent opportunities for advancement come frequently. Club managers also often receive bonuses based on performance. These bonuses range from 5 to 15 percent of the manager's base salary of more than $100,000 annually. The highest paid country club manager makes about $1 million annually.

John Costello, country club general manager, offers this advice:

If you have an interest in country club management, get a job in a club, and then do an internship in one. The most likely area of initial employment is in the food and beverage department, with opportunities in dining rooms/

restaurants, catering, bars and beverage service, and culinary. The job and internship experiences will help you determine if the country club environment is for you. There is one big possible advantage over other types of hospitality employment: You have an opportunity to interact with club members over time rather than with transient guests. The general manager's six-figure income maybe of interest, too. Did you know the highest paid club manager gets about a million dollars a year? Yes, the GM [general manager] of the Palm Beach club earned $750,000 in 2006 (the latest information available) and by now that is reckoned to be $1,000,000. Well, someone has to manage that and other clubs. Good luck!"

The following are web sites where you can gather more information:

ClubCorp: www.clubcorp.com
Club Managers Association of America: www.cmaa.org
Club Management magazine: http://www.naylornetwork.com/mam-nxt/
National Parks Service: www.nps.gov
National Club Association: www.natlclub.org

CASE STUDY

Service Proposal for Guests

You recently joined the front desk of a nice resort hotel in New England, and your hotel manager has complimented you on your guest service ability. She has asked you to develop a walking/jogging trail for the guests.

Discussion Question

1. What would be some of the key elements to consider in developing a proposal for your hotel guests?

CASE STUDY

Overpopulation of National Parks

Our national parks are under serious threat from a number of sources, including congestion resulting from overvisitation, consequent environmental degradation, and pollution.

There are too many people and too many vehicles in the most popular national parks. Many visitors bring their city lifestyle, leaving garbage lying around, listening to loud music, and leaving the trails in worse shape.

Discussion Question

1. List the recommendations you have for the park superintendents to help save the parks.

Summary

1. Recreation is free time that people use to restore, rest, and relax their minds and bodies. Recreational activities can be passive or active, individual or group activities.

2. Recreational activities range from cultural pursuits such as museums or theaters, to sports or outdoor recreation such as amusement parks, community centers, playgrounds, and libraries. These services involve various levels of government.

3. National parks preserve exceptional lands for public use, emphasizing the protection of their ecosystems and endangered plant and animal species and honoring historical sites. Two of the best known of the current 397 parks in the United States include Yellowstone and Yosemite National Parks.

4. Today, city governments are increasingly expected to provide recreational facilities such as golf courses, swimming pools, picnic areas, and playgrounds as a community service.

5. Commercial recreation—for example, theme parks, clubs, and attractions—involves a profit for the supplier of the recreational activity.

6. Clubs are places where members gather for social, recreational, professional, or fraternal reasons. There are many different types of clubs such as country clubs and city clubs categorized according to the interests they represent to their members.

7. Noncommercial recreation includes governmental and nonprofit agencies, such as voluntary organization, campus, armed forces, and employee recreation, and recreation for special populations, such as the physically challenged.

Key Words and Concepts

city clubs
club management
commercial recreation
country clubs
government-sponsored recreation
heritage tourism
leisure
national park
National Parks Service

National Register of Historic Places
noncommercial recreation
recreation
recreation for special populations
recreation management
theme parks
transient occupancy tax (TOT)
voluntary organizations

Review Questions

1. Define recreation and its importance to human wellness. What factors affect an individual's decision to participate in recreational activities?

2. Describe the origin of government-sponsored recreation in consideration of the origin and purpose of national parks.

3. Briefly describe the difference between commercial and noncommercial recreation.

4. Briefly explain the purpose of a theme park and the purpose of clubs.

5. Explain the concept of recreation for special populations.

Internet Exercise

1. Organization: **Prestonwood Country Club**
Web site: **www.prestonwoodcc.com**
Summary: Prestonwood is a full-service country club that offers activities and fine food.

(a) What kinds of activities are offered at the Prestonwood Country Club?
(b) Parents may wish to take their kids on vacations. In these situations, what might this country club offer those kids?

Apply Your Knowledge

1. Create your own personal recreation goals and make a plan to reach them.

2. Describe the features of commercial versus noncommercial recreation.

Suggested Activities

1. On the Internet, research the history of Mardi Gras. Write a one-page description of the event and its cultural roots.

2. Look up your favorite theme park on the web. Think about what kind of position you would like to have at the park. If the site has job listings, tell whether any of them appeal to you.

Endnotes

1. Personal correspondence with Jay Sullivan, August 4, 2007.
2. Wikipedia, *Recreation*, http://en.wikipedia.org/wiki/recreation (November 15, 2011).
3. "Nathaniel Hawthorne," *BrainyQuote.com*, Xplore Inc. http://www.brainyquote.com/quotes/quotes/n/nathanielh163048.html (accessed November 15, 2011).
4. Peopleassets, *The PeopleAssets/California Park & Recreation Society Leadership Competency Profile*, www.peopleassets.net/cprs/reports/samplereport.htm (accessed November 15, 2011).
5. This section draws on information supplied by the National Parks Service.
6. Robert E. Manning, "Commons without Tragedy: Measuring and Managing Carrying Capacity in the National Parks," In *Natural Resource Year in Review—2006* (National Park Service, 2007): 13–14, http://www.nature.nps.gov/YearInReview/YIR2006/01_c.html (accessed November 15, 2011).
7. National Park Service, *Backcountry Recreation Management*, http://www.nature.nps.gov/Rm77/backcountry/roles.cfm (accessed May 10, 2011).
8. Ibid.
9. National Park Service, *Budget*, http://www.nps.gov/aboutus/budget.htm (accessed May 11, 2011).
10. National Park Service, *Cape Lookout National Seashore: Management*, http://www.nps.gov/calo/parkmgmt/index.htm (accessed May 10, 2011).
11. Ibid.
12. National Park Service, *General Management Planning Process: Frequently Asked Questions*, http://www.nps.gov/sero/planning/buis_gmp/buis_desc.htm (accessed May 10, 2011).
13. Wikipedia, *Recreation*, http://en.wikipedia.org/wiki/recreation (accessed November 15, 2011).
14. Personal correspondence with Knott's Berry Farm, April 2006.
15. Knott's Berry Farm, Inside the Park, http://www.knotts.com/public/park/index.cfm (accessed November 15, 2011).
16. Astrid Dorothea Ada Maria Kemperman, *Temporal Aspects of Theme Park Choice Behavior*, (Eindhoven University of Technology, 2000), http://alexandria.tue.nl/extra2/200013915.pdf (accessed November 15, 2011).
17. Todd D. MacCartney, *Excerpt from Walt Disney World Made Simple*, http://travelassist.com/mag/a12.

html (accessed November 15, 2011); Randy Bright, *Disneyland: Inside Story* (New York: Abraus, 1987), 33.

18. DIS, *Magic Kingdom*, http://www.wdwinfo.com/wdwinfo/guides/magickingdom/mkindex.htm (accessed November 15, 2011).

19. DIS, *Epcot—Future World*, http://www.wdwinfo.com/wdwinfo/guides/epcot/ep-futureworld.htm (accessed November 15, 2011).

20. DIS, *Epcot World Showcase*, http://www.wdwinfo.com/wdwinfo/guides/epcot/ep-worldshowcase.htm (accessed November 15, 2011).

21. DIS, *Disney's Hollywood Studios*, http://www.wdwinfo.com/wdwinfo/guides/mgm/st-overview.htm (accessed November 15, 2011).

22. Atlas Cruises and Tours, *Walt Disney World Vacation Packages*, www.atlastravelweb.com/waltdisneyworldpackages.shtml (site now discontinued).

23. Wikipedia, *Universal Studios Hollywood*, http://en.wikipedia.org/wiki/Universal_Studios_Hollywood (accessed November 18, 2007).

24. NBCUniversal, This Is NBCUniversal, http://www.nbcuni.com/corporate/about-us/ (accessed November 15, 2011).

25. Wikipedia, *SeaWorld Parks & Entertainment*, http://en.wikipedia.org/wiki/SeaWorld_Parks_%26_Entertainment (accessed November 15, 2011).

26. Water Country USA, *2011 Media Kit*, http://www.watercountryusa.com/AssetManagement/Assets/WIP/WC/2011%20WCUSA%20press%20kit.pdf (accessed November 15, 2011).

27. Discovery Cove, *Discover a Place beyond Words*, http://www.discoverycove.com/Explore/Discover.aspx (accessed November 15, 2011).

28. Hershey's, *Hershey's History*, http://www.thehersheycompany.com/about-hershey/our-story/hersheys-history.aspx (accessed November 15, 2011).

29. Dollywood, *About Dollywood*, http://www.dollywood.com/dollywood-q10143-c10132-About_Dollywood.aspx (accessed November 15, 2011).

30. Wikipedia, *Dollywood*, http://en.wikipedia.org/wiki/Dollywood (accessed November 15, 2011).

31. Wikipedia, *Legoland*, http://en.wikipedia.org/wiki/legoland (accessed November 15, 2011).

32. Ibid.

33. Gatorland, *History*, www.gatorland.com/history/history.html (accessed November 15, 2011).

34. Wikipedia, *Wet 'n Wild Orlando*, http://en.wikipedia.org/wiki/Wet_%27n_Wild_Orlando (accessed November 15, 2011).

35. Association of Zoos & Aquariums, *Home Page*, www.aza.org (accessed November 15, 2011).

36. San Diego Zoo, *About San Diego Zoo Global*, www.sandiegozoo.org/disclaimers/aboutus.html (accessed November 15, 2011).

37. San Diego Zoo, *Panda Baby Named in Zoo Ceremony*, www.sandiegozoo.org/news/panda_naming.html (accessed September 19, 2009).

38. Smithsonian National Zoological Park, *About Us*, http://nationalzoo.si.edu/aboutus/ (accessed September 19, 2009).

39. Ibid.

40. National Aquarium Baltimore, *Community Affairs*, www.aqua.org/communityaffairs.html (accessed September 19, 2009).

41. Ibid.

42. National Park Service, *National Register of Historic Places Program: About Us*, www.nps.gov/nr/about.htm (accessed September 19, 2009).

43. Wikipedia, *Battle of the Alamo*, http://en.wikipedia.org/wiki/Battle_of_the_Alamo (accessed November 15, 2011).

44. Opry.com, *Tour the Opry House*, http://www.opry.com/shows/TourTheOpryHouse.html (accessed November 15, 2011).

45. Smithsonian Institution, *About Us*, www.si.edu/about/ (accessed November 15, 2011).

46. Ibid.

47. Ibid.

48. Field Museum, *Mission Statement*, http://fieldmuseum.org/about/mission (accessed November 15, 2011).

49. Ibid.

50. Ibid.

51. Hellenic Ministry of Culture, *The Unification of the Archaeological Sites of Athens*, www.yppo.gr/4/e40.jsp?obj_id=90 (accessed January 20, 2009).

52. Wikipedia, *Athens*, http://en.wikipedia.org/wiki/Athens (accessed November 15, 2011).

53. Central Intelligence Agency: "Holy See (Vatican City)," *The World Factbook*, https://www.cia.gov/library/publications/the-world-factbook/geos/vt.html (accessed November 15, 2011).

54. John R. Walker, *Introduction to Hospitality Management*, 3rd ed. (Upper Saddle River, NJ: Pearson, 2010): 553–554.

55. Ibid.

56. Interview with Kurt Allen, General Manager, Marineland Dolphin Adventure, Miami, June 9, 2011.

57. Angela Nitz, "A Sustainable Term," *Club Management*, January/February 2010: 43, www.nxtbook.com/nxtbooks/naylor/MAMS0110/index.php?startpage=43&qs=sustainability#/42 (accessed November 15, 2011).

58. Angela Nitz, "Facility-wide Recycling: A Team Effort," *Club Management*, November/December 2009: 29, http://www.nxtbook.com/nxtbooks/naylor/MAMS0609/index.php?startpage=29&qs=sustainability#/28 (accessed November 15, 2004).

59. Special Olympics, *What We Do: Changing Attitudes*, http://www.specialolympics.org/changingattitudes.aspx (accessed November 15, 2011).

60. Special Olympics, "About Us," www.specialolympics.org/special+olympics+public+website/English/About_us/default.htm.

61. Interview with Bill Lupfer, CEO of the Florida Attractions Association, June 9, 2011.

Glossary

City clubs Various clubs in cities.

Club management The management of clubs.

Commercial recreation For profit recreation.

Country clubs Clubs that offer members golf and sometimes other sporting activities such as tennis and swimming along with games and social activities.

Government-sponsored recreation Recreation paid for by government taxes; includes monies sent to cities for museums, libraries, and municipal golf courses.

Heritage tourism Tourism that involves or relates to heritage.

Leisure Freedom from activities, especially time free from work or duties.

National park A park belonging to the nation.

National Parks Service The service that manages to National Parks.

Noncommercial recreation Not for profit recreation.

Recreation Refreshment of strength and spirits after work; a means of diversion.

Recreation for special populations Recreation designed to accommodate persons with disabilities, for example the Special Olympics.

Theme park A recreational park based on a particular setting or artistic interpretation; may operate with hundreds or thousands of acres of parkland and hundreds or thousands of employees.

Transient occupancy tax (TOT) Tax paid by people staying in a city's hotels.

Voluntary organization A nongovernmental, nonprofit agency serving the public.

Photo Credits

Credits are listed in the order of appearance.

Gaming Entertainment

From Chapter 11 of *Introduction to Hospitality Management,* Fourth Edition. John R. Walker. Copyright © 2013 by Pearson Education, Inc. Published by Pearson. All rights reserved.

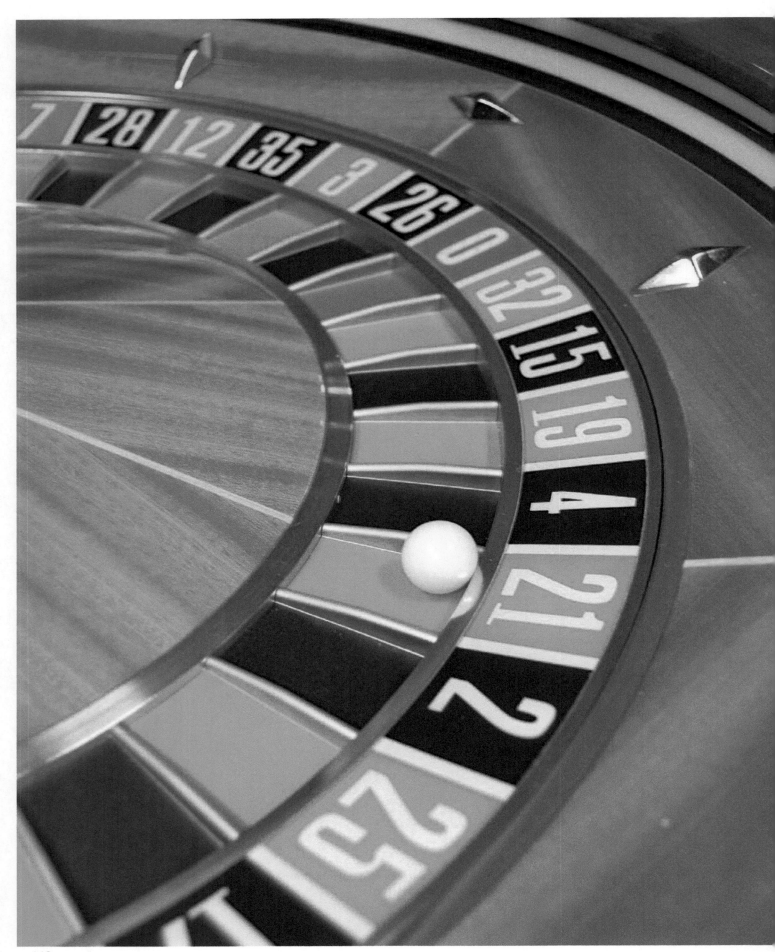

Gaming Entertainment

OBJECTIVES

After reading and studying this chapter, you should be able to:

- Outline the history of modern casinos.

- Describe the various components of modern casino hotels.

- Explain how casinos have been integrated into larger hospitality operations.

- Appreciate the spread of casino gaming across the United States and throughout the world.

- Understand the basic principles of casino operations.

- Discuss the different positions within the gaming industry.

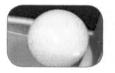
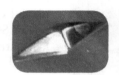
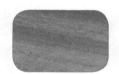

One of the most significant developments in the hospitality industry during the past three decades has been the astounding growth of the casino industry and its convergence with the lodging and hospitality industries. With its rapid expansion in North America and throughout the world, new opportunities have been created for hospitality careers within casino resorts.

The Casino Resort: A Hospitality Buffet

Today, **casino resorts** are among the most visible hospitality businesses in the world. Twenty of the thirty largest hotels in the world are casino resorts on the Las Vegas Strip.[1] Those aiming for careers in hospitality, even if they have no special interest in working on the gambling side of the operation, may find themselves considering a position in a resort that has a casino but also a full spread of lodging, food and beverage, entertainment, and retail offerings.

Even if you don't plan on working on the casino floor itself, a rudimentary understanding of the nature of gambling—and the specifics of casino gambling—is an essential tool for those who want to pursue careers in casino resorts. Today, many casino resort presidents and key executives have come up through the lodging or food and beverage side of operations; a solid understanding of what's happening in the casino—and how casino guests are different from other hospitality patrons—makes advancing through the ranks that much easier.

What Is Gambling?

In its broadest definition, **gambling** is the act of placing stakes on an unknown outcome with the possibility of securing a gain if the bettor guesses correctly.

To be considered gambling, an act must have three elements: something wagered (the bet), a randomizing event (the spin of slot reels or the flip of a card), and a payoff.

This broad definition of gambling includes many dissimilar activities: contests between animals (horse racing, cockfighting) and between humans (team and individual sports); lotteries; and games of chance played with cards, dice, and other randomizing elements. Some of the best-known games fall into the last category: Poker, blackjack, and baccarat are played with cards, and craps with dice. Slot machines, which were originally mechanical (but now electronic) devices that award prizes based on the

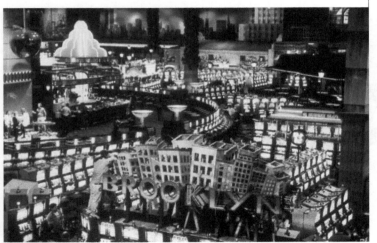

A themed gaming and slot machine area in a casino.

random stopping of reels, are also popular, and are typically the most-played games in most casinos today.

How do casinos make money from gambling? The answer lies in the kind of gambling they offer. There are two basic categories of gambling: **Social** gambling and **mercantile** (or commercial) gambling. Social gambling is conducted among individuals who bet against each other; mathematically, each player has the same chance of winning. Poker is a classic social game: Every player is drawing from the same deck and has the same opportunity to check, raise, or fold. Other social forms of gambling include dominoes and mah-jongg.

In mercantile or commercial gambling, players bet against "the house," a professional gambler or organization that accepts wagers from the general public. Mercantile games have a mathematical advantage for the casino, or a house edge that lets professionals profit from them while still offering fair games. All lotteries are mercantile games, and every game found on the casino floor is a mercantile game: There is a small guaranteed bias toward the house that, over time, ensures the casino will win more than it pays out.

The **house edge** is best explained by looking at the game of roulette, which features a wheel with thirty-eight slots numbered one to thirty-six, in addition to a single zero and a double zero. On each spin, a small ball falls into one of the thirty-eight slots. If you bet "straight up" on a number, you win thirty-five units for each one unit you bet. So if you bet one dollar straight on, you'd end up with thirty-six dollars: the one you staked, plus thirty-five more. Since the wheel has a one-in-thirty-eight chance of hitting any number, you should be paid off at a rate of 37:1, not 35:1. That extra two dollars is the house edge; it seems slight, but over time, it adds up.

The house edge is what makes casinos possible; without it, the only way to offer games of chance to the public that can generate an income would be to cheat. The house edge allows casinos to offer their customers honest games, fairly dealt, and still remain in business.

The game of poker is an interesting exception to the rule that all casino games have built-in house edges. Many casinos have poker rooms, in which players bet against each other using a table, cards, and dealer supplied by the house. The casino has no direct stake in the outcome of each hand, but instead takes a small percentage of each pot ("the rake") to defray the costs of operating the room. Though it is a popular game, poker makes little money for casinos (see Figure 1); casinos offer the game as an amenity for players who will also play straight-up mercantile games or for those who are visiting with slots or table games players.

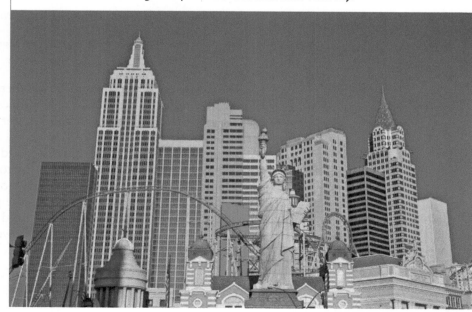

This resort on the Las Vegas Strip models itself after New York City.

Game	# of Units	n Amount	Win %	Handle
Slot Machine	49,352	2,789,753	7.22%	38,639,238
Table Games	2,802	2,904,826	11.43%	25,414,051
Total Win		5,776,570	9.02%	64,053,289

Slots detail

Game	# of Units	n Amount	Win %	Handle
1 Cent	11,674	743,101	11.55%	6,433,775
5 Cent	1,948	72,254	9.16%	788,799
25 Cent	1,948	262,773	8.33%	3,154,538
1 Dollar	5,006	298,171	6.45%	4,622,806
Multi-Denom	22,576	1,233,092	6.04%	20,415,430

Table games detail

Game	# of Units	n Amount	Win %	Handle
Twenty-one	1,404	721,822	9.98%	7,232,685
Baccarat	241	1,181,967	11.03%	10,715,929
Craps	202	267,397	11.59%	2,307,135
Roulette	274	258,886	16.80%	1,540,988
3-Card Poker	126	96,159	29.05%	331,012
Mini-Bacc	89	62,424	8.34%	748,489
Car. Stud Poker	11	6,204	26.29%	23,598
Let It Ride	59	31,225	22.31%	139,960
Pai Gow	23	17,808	14.44%	123,324
Pai Gow Poker	115	58,006	19.85%	292,222
Keno	22	6,909	28.03%	24,649
Bingo	3	1,652	7.41%	22,294
Race Book	26	26,715	16.51%	161,811
Sports Book	37	69,338	5.11%	1,356,908
Poker tables	435	81,990 (rake only; no direct win)		

Figure 1 • Las Vegas Strip 2010 Gaming Win.

Win and Handle are in thousands of dollars.

Gaming Revenue Report, Nevada Gaming Control Board, December 2010.

The house edge is a theoretical number; it describes the amount of money wagered (handle) that the casino should keep over time. For tables and slots, casinos track the hold percentage to better understand how well the casino is performing.

To understand hold percentage, we need to understand two other terms: handle (or buy-in) and win. The **handle** is the total amount of money bet at a game. The **win** is the handle minus the money paid out on winning bets—essentially, what the casino keeps. The **hold percentage** is the percentage of the total handle that is retained as win. On slot machines, the hold percentage tracks very close to the theoretical house edge. On table games, however, it is usually considerably higher than the house edge.

Though the games offered in casinos have a statistical bias toward the house, they are still games of chance. In the short run, players can get lucky and walk away with the house's money. In small-stakes games this isn't a problem, since the sheer number of bets taken tends to drive the hold percentage toward its historically expected value (see Figure 2).

Games played for high stakes, such as baccarat, are different. Because there are large amounts of money being spread over fewer decisions, these games have a great deal of volatility; in a given month, the hold percentage for a baccarat game in single casino can fluctuate wildly (see Figure 3).

Casino Win Defined

Let's say you buy into a roulette game for $100 in $1 chips. You place 100 even-money bets, winning 94 and losing 6. In this case, the following are true:

The handle is $100.
The win is $6.
The winning percentage is 6 percent.

This is very close to the theoretical house edge of 5.26 percent. But if you continued playing for another 100 bets, you might lose another 6. In this case, the handle would still be $100, but the win would be $12, and the hold percentage 12 percent.

Theoretical hold versus actual 2010 win percentage for the Las Vegas Strip

Game	House Edge	Win %
Twenty-one	Approx 1%*	9.98%
Baccarat	1.15%	11.03%
Craps	1.4% (Pass line bet)	11.59%
Roulette	5.26%	16.80%

Figure 2 ● House Edge versus Win Percentage.

Because there are several varieties of blackjack, it is difficult to provide a single 'house edge' for the game, but most games have a house edge near one percent. Gaming Revenue Report, Nevada Gaming Control Board, December 2010.

	Wheel of Fortune			Baccarat		
Month	Win	Drop	Hold	Win	Drop	Hold
Jan-07	91,717	195,126	47.00%	986,554	4,604,032	21.40%
Feb-07	92,750	188,835	49.12%	511,022	5,521,377	9.30%
Mar-07	99,949	194,208	51.46%	533,126	4,318,929	12.30%
Apr-07	88,537	182,643	48.48%	1,362,604	3,923,624	34.70%
May-07	74,434	183,663	40.53%	383,515	4,508,300	8.50%
Jun-07	85,933	176,311	48.74%	825,539	4,080,351	20.20%
Jul-07	84,886	208,992	40.62%	−406,421	4,718,282	−8.60%
Aug-07	93,739	214,358	43.73%	182,793	4,086,594	4.50%
Sep-07	55,157	155,184	35.54%	348,263	4,501,165	7.70%
Oct-07	52,935	149,538	35.40%	16,027	1,129,132	1.40%
Nov-07	77,557	173,000	44.83%	319,151	1,672,186	19.10%
Dec-07	80,646	164,742	48.95%	145,398	2,072,952	7.00%

Figure 3 ● Wheel of Fortune versus Baccarat.

Results from two Atlantic City Casinos for 2007.
Monthly gross revenue returns, New Jersey Casino Control Commission.

As a manager of a casino resort, it is important that you have an appreciation of the nature of volatility. Just because the casino department is reporting a net loss for a shift does not necessarily mean that the department is inefficient or incompetent; it may just be an expression of volatility. Over time, gaming wins will tend towards their historical average.

Managers also need to understand that, because of volatility, casinos are not like other hospitality businesses. A typical hotel, running at 95-percent occupancy for the weekend and with full restaurant bookings, will certainly make a profit. Because of volatility, even a busy casino can end up in the red for a shift or even a weekend if one high-stakes player has a run of good luck.

Comps: A Usual Part of an Unusual Business

Volatility isn't the only aspect of the casino business that makes it different from most other hospitality businesses. **Comps** are another area that set casinos apart.

Comps are complimentary goods and services offered to casino patrons in order to attract their business. Comps are found in virtually every casino, and any casino guest of consequence has expectations of receiving comps. Unlike in other hospitality operations, where comps are given primarily as part of service recovery to compensate for a customer service failure or other miscue, comps are distributed as a usual part of a casino's operation.

The value of comps varies; generally speaking, higher-producing players are given higher-value comps. For example, a small-stakes slot player might receive an offer for a discounted or free buffet; a baccarat-playing high roller, betting $10,000 a hand for several hours, might receive a full RFB (room, food, beverage) comp, with all expenses in the casino's most lavish accommodations paid for. Casino guests might also receive comps for entertainment or other gifts. Many slots players receive cash back when they reach certain play thresholds.

Comps dramatically affect casino resort operations. As shown in Figure 4, a significant percentage of nongaming services are comped.

Casinos, with thousands of guests on any given day, rely on customer **loyalty programs** to track patron play. Patrons who wish to receive comps and other offers join the casino's player loyalty club (e.g., Caesars' Total Rewards, MGM Resorts' M life, Wynn Resorts' Red Card). Slot players insert

Department	Percentage of Comps
Rooms	24.6%
Restaurants	17.0%
Beverage	34.4%

Figure 4 • Las Vegas Strip Comps.

the card they receive into the machine they are playing; the card then tracks money played and won. Table games players have a pit manager swipe their card, tracking their time of play and average bet size.

Casinos use the information they gain about a player's gambling patterns to offer him or her comps, based both on theoretical wins by the player and his or her expected levels of play. Most loyalty programs have tiered rewards structures, giving patrons an incentive to play more and unlock more rewards.

Loyalty programs are an essential part of casino marketing; many guests base the money they spend gaming around where they receive the best comps, so good casino managers know they must send out good offers to qualified players. Casinos also use sophisticated software to monitor and deliver bonuses to slot patrons as they are playing on machines. Recently, some casinos have begun tracking and rewarding nongaming spending as well, a reflection of the broadening of the casino resort revenue stream.

Types of Casino Operations

There are several different kinds of casino operations, operating on vastly different scales. At one end of the spectrum is the Nevada-style gaming tavern, which is a typical bar and restaurant that has less than sixteen electronic gaming devices, usually bar-top video poker and slot machines. At the other is a fully-developed casino resort, with (on average) a 100,000-square-foot casino featuring thousands of slot machines and dozens of table games, approximately 3,000 hotel rooms, at least a dozen bars and restaurants, meeting and convention facilities, entertainment venues, retail shopping, and pool and spa facilities.

Between these two extremes, which are both found in Las Vegas, there are several other kinds of operations. Stand-alone casinos are not very common in the United States or elsewhere in the world. Where they are found, they usually consist of only slot machines; this type operation might be called a slot parlor. In Europe, the Middle East, Africa, and South America, casinos located in hotels might be extremely small and ancillary to the general hospitality operation.

In the United States, casinos on Indian reservation can take many forms, from bingo parlors in prefabricated buildings to fully functional casino resorts with lodging, dining, and entertainment that are indistinguishable from resorts on the Las Vegas Strip. Some states allow gambling only on riverboats, which originally cruised the waterways but today are usually "boat in a moat" operations that are permanently moored and connected almost seamlessly with a hotel and resort facility. Other states allow slot machines at racetracks (called "racinos"), and in some cases these have evolved to include hotel and resort operations as well. Finally, many cruise lines have casinos as part of the amenities available to guests on their ships.

FOCUS ON CASINO RESORTS

Casino Resorts and Hospitality

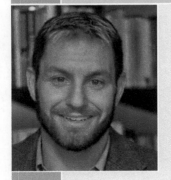

David G. Schwartz, Director, Center for Gaming Research, University of Nevada, Las Vegas

Casino resorts combine virtually every strand of the hospitality business. They've come a long way since the dusty saloons of frontier Nevada and the grimy illegal slot routes and bookmaking operations of American cities. Today, funded by mainstream capital, staffed by trained hospitality managers, and promoted globally, there is little that one can't find in a major casino resort.

It's important to note that casino resorts are so all-inclusive because it makes good economic sense. Originally, most revenues were generated on the casino floor. Yet, the nature of casino gambling—games that, over time, have a slight bias in favor of the house—demanded that casinos offer more than just gambling. To discourage spot play, in which a lucky player cashes out and leaves, casino resorts developed a number of attractions to lure and keep players near the casino. Lodging, food, beverage, and entertainment were offered as loss leaders to get players through the doors.

In the 1990s, following the opening of Steve Wynn's Mirage, the rules of the game changed. Though the old approach—offering loss leaders and focusing on gaming revenues—was profitable, there was more growth potential in a more balanced approach. Shifting the revenue center from exclusively gaming to also including rooms and particularly restaurants proved to be a lucrative decision. Guests got the chance to stay in more luxurious accommodations and sample a variety of dining experiences.

Now, major casino resorts earn most of their money from things other than gambling. But gambling is still central to their identity, and many high-value guests are primarily focused on gambling. Even if your job isn't directly on the gaming floor, it's important to remember that without gambling, the resort wouldn't exist.

At the same time, many smaller resorts still get most of their revenues from gambling, so managers of other departments may face an uphill battle for respect—and resources. If this is the case, it will be important to remind everyone that your department can help increase revenues, both by earning money itself and by contributing to an environment to which gamblers will flock.

At the end of the day, despite the sometimes obscure jargon and hard-to-figure-out gameplay, casino gambling is really no different from other hospitality operations: The idea is to help guests enjoy themselves. Guests pay for that privilege, and there are many other places where they can do so.

That's an important fact to remember: Today there are a wealth of choices for casino customers; any oversight or cut corner gives your customers an excuse to spend their money with your competition, who will gladly take it. A good casino manager, no matter what the department, will never lose sight of that fact, and will start and end each day with a single question: "What can I do to help my guests have a better time with us?" Anyone who can continue to come up with innovative but not budget-busting answers to this simple question will enjoy a long, successful career in the gaming and hospitality industry.

Components of Casino Resorts

The best example of the modern casino resort can be found on the Las Vegas Strip. These destination resorts are centered on casinos that have several types of games available:

- Slot machines
- Table games, including twenty-one (blackjack), craps, roulette, baccarat, and carnival games such as three-card poker
- Race and sports books, which accept wagers on horseracing and sporting events
- Poker rooms, where players bet against each other and where the house only keeps a portion of each pot

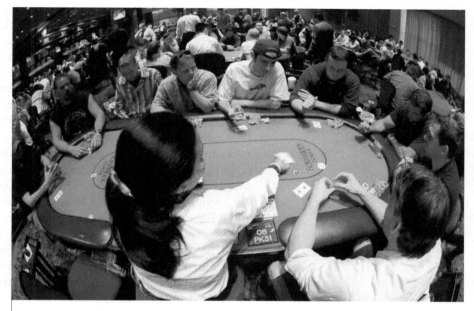

Gamblers playing poker at the Foxwoods Resort Casino in Mashantucket, Connecticut.

In most parts of the United States, slot machines produce the bulk of the revenue; on the Las Vegas Strip, due to high-stakes table play, it is closer to a 50/50 split (see Figure 1). Among table games, blackjack is most popular nationally, while on the Strip baccarat has recently become a favorite. In Macau casinos, nearly all revenue comes from high-stakes baccarat; slot machines are negligible.

Casino resorts also include the following components:

- Lodging (on average, 3,000 hotel rooms)
- Food and beverage outlets, ranging from fast food to gourmet eateries
- Entertainment venues, including lounges but also purpose-built theaters for Cirque du Soleil and similar spectaculars
- Retail shopping: Several casinos have shopping esplanades or even attached malls (Caesars Palace, Venetian, Planet Hollywood)
- Convention facilities, ranging from a few small rooms to the 1.9-million-square-foot Sands Expo Center at the Venetian/Palazzo
- Nightclubs, which are an increasingly lucrative part of the casino resort package
- Pool and spa facilities, which may be branded as "dayclubs" with DJ entertainment and bottle service available in cabanas

Casino resorts in other jurisdictions may have some, but not all, of these features. For example, outside of Nevada, sports betting is currently illegal, so those casinos will have, at most, a race book. Most casinos outside of Las Vegas, with a few notable exceptions, have smaller hotel and entertainment components.

❝ The largest casino in the world is currently the Venetian Macao, with over 800 table games and 3,400 slot machines[2]. By contrast, the typical Las Vegas Strip casino has about 90 tables and 1,200 slot machines. ❞

❝ People go to casinos and gamble for a variety of reasons, whether it's for fun, excitement, the possibility of hitting a jackpot, or just to feel challenged. ❞

Evolution of Gambling and Casinos

Gambling is among the oldest of human behaviors; archaeological evidence of gambling stretches back into prehistory, and purpose-built dice have been discovered at sites dating back to 7,000 years before the present. Gambling developed in nearly every ancient civilization of consequence and has been part of Western life since the days of Ancient Greece.

Casino resorts, as they are currently operated, are much younger, dating back only to 1941, though the casino industry has its antecedents in several earlier developments, both legal and illegal. Legal public gambling in casinos dates back to 1638, when the Grand Council of Venice awarded a franchise for a single legal casino in that city. Though that casino was closed in 1774, other European states—mostly small, resource-poor jurisdictions—also permitted gambling, usually as part of a larger spa complex; spas were Europe's first true tourist destination, and gambling was considered an essential part of many European spa communities. By 1872, however, casino-style gambling had been banned in all European countries save the tiny Mediterranean enclave of Monaco, whose Monte Carlo would grow wealthy on a decades-long monopoly.

In the United States, public gambling at cards and dice was legal intermittently during the nineteenth century in several states, including Louisiana, California, and Nevada, but by 1910 this kind of gambling—and playing at slot machines—had been outlawed everywhere in the United States. Both before and after the criminalization of all casino-style gambling, illegal gambling halls flourished in most of the major American cities.

Yet the tide soon turned toward legalization, at least in Nevada. When legislators authorized "wide open" commercial gambling there in 1931, the state was in the throes of the Great Depression. By allowing taverns and hotels to conduct games of chance, they hoped to increase tourism slightly. There was initially no state tax on gambling, and the economic impact was thought to be negligible. Reno and Las Vegas soon developed thriving downtown gambling districts, with small clubs offering slot machines and table games. These were usually simple, storefront operations with no real amenities.

The real creation of the modern casino came in 1941, with the opening of the **El Rancho Vegas**, the first casino resort on what would become the **Las Vegas Strip**. As a spa-like, self-contained destination with fine dining, entertainment, and gambling, the El Rancho Vegas appealed to casual tourists in a way that the smoky downtown gambling halls did not. Within a decade, a half-dozen other resorts joined the El Rancho Vegas, and the Las Vegas Strip was becoming a force.

These casinos were superior to gambling halls because, with rooms and a full range of amenities, they offered a diverse set of options for travelers–gamblers and nongamblers alike–and because they allowed casinos to keep visitors near the casino. Although in the short run the players might get lucky thanks to volatility, the longer they remained near the tables and slots, the more likely the casino was to end up with their money. Casinos in resorts therefore proved more profitable than stand-alone casinos, and they soon proliferated, particularly along the Strip.

By the mid-1950s, the casino resorts of the Las Vegas Strip had changed Nevada. Now numbering more than a dozen, they became an integral part of the state's economy. The legislature created a regulatory body, the Gaming Control Board, to oversee the industry, and the state began to rely on taxes extracted from casinos. With other development options failing to pan out, Nevada's casinos became the only game in town. The industry grew, and with the entrance of publicly traded corporations in the 1970s, it became more integrated into the national economic mainstream. The bulk of casinos were in Las Vegas; though Reno and Lake Tahoe remained key attractions in the north of the state, they failed to reinvent themselves, as Las Vegas did, in the face of new competition. As a result, by 2000, Las Vegas Strip casinos accounted for well over half of all state gambling revenues.

Others soon became interested in the potential of casino resorts for economic revitalization. In 1976, New Jersey voters legalized casino gambling in Atlantic City by referendum, and two years later the first legal casino on the East Coast opened. Within a few years, ten casinos were thriving in the city, helping to provide jobs, augment state revenues, and revitalize a formerly desolate resort town. Other states began exploring the possibilities of legalization, though they did so in far more restricted ways.

Riverboat gaming, which permitted games of chance only on boats, debuted in Iowa and Illinois in 1991, and soon spread throughout the Midwest and South, with a particularly robust presence in Mississippi. States like Colorado and South Dakota turned to "limited gambling" schemes, which like New Jersey confined casinos to particular towns, but also capped maximum bet sizes.

INTRODUCING STEPHEN A. WYNN

Chairman of the Board and CEO, Wynn Resorts

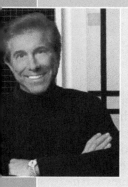

Casino developer Stephen A. Wynn is widely credited with transforming Las Vegas from a gambling venue for adults into a world-renowned resort and convention destination. As chairman of the board, president, and chief executive officer of Mirage Resorts, Mr. Wynn envisioned and built the Mirage, Treasure Island, and Bellagio—boldly conceived resorts that set progressively higher standards for quality, luxury, and entertainment. As chairman of the board and chief executive officer of Wynn Resorts, Limited, Mr. Wynn developed Wynn Las Vegas, among the world's preeminent luxury hotel resorts. Mr. Wynn also developed the Wynn Macau, a flagship Asian casino resort in Macau, where his company has been awarded a twenty-year concession by the Macau government.

Mr. Wynn began his career in 1967 as part owner, slot manager, and assistant credit manager of the Frontier Hotel. Between 1968 and 1972, he also owned and operated a wine and liquor importing company. But it was an entrepreneurial real estate deal with Howard Hughes in 1971 that produced sufficient profits for a major investment in the landmark Golden Nugget Casino. Once known only as a "gambling joint," he transformed the Golden Nugget into a Four-Diamond resort known for elegance and personal service. By 1973, at age thirty-one, Mr. Wynn controlled the property and began developing the Golden Nugget as a complete resort hotel. In 1978, Mr. Wynn used the profits from the Golden Nugget in Las Vegas to build the Golden Nugget Hotel and Casino on the Boardwalk in Atlantic City. The resort became

(continued)

INTRODUCING STEPHEN A. WYNN *(continued)*

known for its elegant facilities, television ads featuring Frank Sinatra, and its impressive lineup of superstar entertainment. From its opening in 1979 until its sale in 1986, the Atlantic City property dominated the market in revenues and profits despite its smaller size. In 1987, Mr. Wynn sold the Atlantic City Golden Nugget, which had cost $160 million, to Bally for $450 million and turned his creativity to developing the elegant Mirage Resort, which opened in 1989. With its imaginative erupting volcano and South Seas theme, the Mirage ignited a $12 billion building boom that catapulted Las Vegas to America's number-one tourist destination and fastest-growing city. In 1991, Golden Nugget Incorporated was renamed Mirage Resorts, Incorporated.

Following his staggering success at the Mirage, in 1993 Wynn opened Treasure Island, a Four-Diamond property with a romantic tropical theme indoors and a full-size pirate ship used in the daily reenactment of the Battle of Buccaneer Bay outdoors. He raised the bar again in 1998, when he opened the opulent $1.6 billion Bellagio, one of the world's most spectacular hotels. Visitors line the street in front of the hotel to watch the Dancing Waters, shooting fountains choreographed to music that "dance" on the hotel's 8.5-acre manmade lake. He then brought Mirage Resorts' standard of style to historic Biloxi, Mississippi, with the 1,835-room Beau Rivage, which blends Mediterranean beauty and Southern hospitality.

In June 2000, Mr. Wynn sold Mirage Resorts, Incorporated, to MGM for $6.6 billion and purchased Las Vegas's legendary Desert Inn Resort and Casino. The Desert Inn was closed in August 2000 and on that site Mr. Wynn began developing Wynn Las Vegas, a 2,700-room luxury destination resort that has inspired yet another wave of development on the Strip.

For every property he develops, Wynn is known for assembling a dream team of highly motivated employees who keep guestrooms and public spaces impeccable. His properties are always exceptional, drawing a commanding share of a demanding market and maintaining an exceptionally high occupancy. He is confident that both his projects and Las Vegas will continue to thrive.

Today, Mr. Wynn is active in the community and has received honorary doctorate degrees from the University of Nevada, Las Vegas, and Sierra Nevada College in northern Nevada. He is chairman of Utah's Moran Eye Institute; a trustee of his alma mater, the University of Pennsylvania; and a member of the board of the George Bush Presidential Library.

Source: Courtesy of Stephen A. Wynn.

In these years, the number of casinos in the United States has skyrocketed, as gambling halls on Indian reservations also became common. Indian gaming has its roots in the concept of tribal sovereignty, meaning that a tribe is not subject to the commercial restrictions of the state in which it is located. In the 1987 *Cabazon* decision, the Supreme Court affirmed that if a state allowed betting on bingo or card games, Indian tribes could offer these games without limits imposed by state regulators. The following year, the Indian Gaming Regulatory Act codified the rules under which Indian tribes could open "Las Vegas-style" casinos with slot machines and bank games: To do so, the tribes needed to sign a compact, or treaty, with the state in whose land the reservation sat. Frequently, these compacts specified fees that tribes would remit to state governments, often pegged to slot machine revenues, but states had no power to tax tribes; these payments were instead the result of negotiation. As of 2010, over 200 tribes in more than thirty states have some form of gambling operation, with combined annual revenues of more than $25 billion.

Casinos opened elsewhere, as well. Major cities like New Orleans and Detroit legalized a limited number of casinos within their borders, partly to spur tourism, partly to prevent the outflow of gambling dollars to neighboring jurisdictions. States like West Virginia and Delaware balked at authorizing new casino development but legalized slot machines at racetracks, businesses that came be to be known as racinos. The horseracing industry, which began to decline as track attendance fell in the 1970s, embraced the racino concept, and slot machines helped to stave off the demise of live racing in several states. In 2004, Pennsylvania authorized slot machines at racetracks, destination resorts, and urban slot parlors, signaling a further expansion of slot gaming. Gambling has proven to be a growth industry, even in areas of the country that have experienced an overall economic decline.

In addition, American-run casino operators have found that Asia is an even more lucrative market for casinos than the United States. Both Macau (concession awarded in 2002; first U.S.–owned casino opened in 2004) and Singapore (franchises awarded 2006; first U.S.–owned casino opened in 2010) have become casino powerhouses; since 2008, Macau's casino industry has become a leading gaming center with increasing revenues. See Figure 5 for a comparison of the revenues of the major gaming markets.

▶ Check Your Knowledge

1. Define the following:
   a. Handle
   b. Win
   c. House edge
   d. Hold percentage
   e. Volatility

2. Briefly describe why casino resorts are superior to stand-alone operations.

3. Explain the growth in casino gaming since the 1970s.

Year	Nevada	Las Vegas Strip	Atlantic City	Mississippi	Pennsylvania	Macau
2001	9,468,599	4,703,692	4,303,078	2,700,437	n/a	unkn
2002	9,447,660	4,654,808	4,381,406	2,717,258	n/a	2,772,500
2003	9,625,304	4,757,043	4,488,334	2,699,837	n/a	3,583,875
2004	10,562,247	5,333,508	4,806,698	2,776,970	n/a	5,172,250
2005	11,649,040	6,033,595	5,018,276	2,468,476	n/a	5,755,875
2006	12,622,044	6,688,903	5,217,613	2,570,883	31,567	7,077,875
2007	12,849,137	6,827,887	4,920,786	2,891,546	1,039,030	10,378,125
2008	11,599,124	6,126,292	4,544,961	2,721,139	1,615,565	13,596,500
2009	10,392,675	5,550,192	3,943,171	2,464,662	1,964,570	14,921,375
2010	10,404,731	5,776,570	3,565,047	2,389,779	2,486,408	23,542,875

Figure 5 • Comparative Revenues for Major Gaming Markets, 2001–2010.
All totals in thousands of dollars (U.S.)

Working in a Casino Resort

Students of the industry who understand the multidisciplinary needs of the casino business find five initial career tracks in hotel operations, food and beverage operations, casino operations, retail operations, and entertainment operations.

Hotel Operations

The career opportunities in gaming entertainment hotel operations are much like the career opportunities in the full-service hotel industry, with the exception that food and beverage can be a division of its own and not part of hotel operations. The rooms and guest services departments offer the most opportunities for students of hospitality management. Because gaming entertainment properties have hotels that are much larger than nongaming hotels, department heads have a larger number of supervisors reporting to them and more responsibilities. Reservations, front desk, housekeeping, valet parking, and guest services can all be very large departments with many employees.

Food and Beverage Operations

Gaming entertainment has a foundation of high-quality food and beverage service in a wide variety of styles and concepts. Some of the best foodservice operations in the hospitality industry are found in gaming entertainment operations. There are many career opportunities in restaurant management and the culinary arts. As with hotel operations, gaming entertainment properties are typically very large and contain numerous food and beverage outlets, including a number of restaurants, hotel room service, banquets and conventions, and retail outlets. Many establishments support gourmet, high-end signature restaurants. It is not unusual to find many more executive-level management positions in both front- and back-of-the-house food and beverage operations in gaming entertainment operations than in nongaming properties.

Casino Operations

Casino operations jobs fall into five functional areas. Gaming operations staff include slot machine technicians (approximately one technician for 40 machines), table-game dealers (approximately four dealers for each table game), and table-game supervisors. Casino service staff includes security, purchasing, and maintenance and facilities engineers. Marketing staff includes public relations, market research, and advertising professionals. Human resources staff includes employee relations, compensation, staffing, and training specialists. Finance and administration staff includes lawyers, accounts payable, audit, payroll, and income control specialists.[3]

The explosive growth of the gaming industry has increased the need for trained dealers skilled at working a variety of table games, including

blackjack, craps, roulette, poker, and **baccarat.** Through the use of textbooks and videotapes combined with hands-on training at a mock casino, future dealers learn the techniques and fine points of dealing at classes offered by both colleges and private schools.

Retail Operations

The increased emphasis on nongaming sources of revenues in gaming entertainment demands an expertise in all phases of retail operations, from store design and layout to product selection, merchandising, and sales control. Negotiating with concession subcontractors may also be a part of the overall retail activities. Retail operations often support the overall theme of the property and can often be a major source of revenue; however, retail management careers are often an overlooked career path in the gaming entertainment industry.

Entertainment Operations

Because of the increased competition, gaming entertainment companies are creating bigger and better production shows to turn their properties into destination attractions. Some production shows have climbed in the million of dollars range and require professional entertainment staffs to produce and manage them. Gaming entertainment properties often present live entertainment of all sorts, with headline acts drawing huge audiences.

Casino management is hierarchical. At the top of the management structure, a property president or general manager is in charge of day-to-day operations. Internal audit and surveillance departments report directly to the president or to the casino's board of directors, bypassing the management hierarchy because of their role in maintaining controls over cash and procedures in the casino.

Below the casino president are the vice presidents (sometimes called directors) of different divisions of the casino: the casino itself; hotel; food and beverage; entertainment; marketing (for casino guests); sales (typically directed toward business travel and group sales); retail; various support functions, including finance, which includes all casino cashiering operations; and security.

Within the casino, the vice president of gaming operations oversees a casino manager, who in turn oversees shift managers, one for each shift (day, swing, grave) of the casino's 24-hour day. The shift manager, in return, has authority over the managers on duty of each of the casino's departments, which may include slots, poker, keno, race and sports book, and casino hosts and marketing representatives, who work directly with high-value players, arranging comps and generally keeping them happy.

The slot department includes customer service representatives, who sign up players for the casino's loyalty program and technicians who keep the slot machines operational. Table games are organized into pits—clusters of about a dozen games—each run by a pit boss who reports directly to the casino shift manager. Below the pit boss, a floorperson oversees between two and four games, while one or more dealers staffs each table. The casino may have a high-limit room (also called a baccarat room) where high-stakes bets—as high as $50,000 per hand—are taken. The baccarat room frequently has its own manager who reports to the casino shift manager as well.

Other departments are managed similarly, with directors in charge of shift managers, who in turn oversee supervisors, who are then responsible for the performance of line employees.

The Mirage Effect

Since the 1990s, casino resorts on the Las Vegas Strip have seen their nongaming operations become much more central to their bottom line. In 1984, Strip casinos earned nearly 60 percent of their revenues from the casino itself; by 2008, that number had fallen below 40 percent.[4] In the 1990s, operators enlarged and upgraded their rooms. Originally merely places for gamblers to speak, rooms became attractions in and of themselves, at least partially because convention travelers were willing to pay higher premiums for better rooms. Rooms have become a major revenue center.

The rooms aren't the only part of the Strip that's become a money generator. This is because in addition to paying more for higher thread-count sheets and designer finishes, Strip visitors have eagerly opened their wallets for gourmet cuisine, delivered to them in celebrity chef eateries.

In 1992, Wolfgang Puck opened Spago in the Forum Shops at Caesars Palace. Puck, who had become famous with his restaurant of the same name on the Sunset Strip in Los Angeles, brought a different sensibility to Las Vegas eating. Spago at Caesars proved successful, and a cohort of established chefs from Paris, New York, and San Francisco followed Puck to Las Vegas, leading to an explosion of both gourmet-dining opportunities for patrons and an increase in restaurant revenues for casinos.

The cost of entertainment has gone up, too, as headliner concerts and installed shows (Cirque du Soleil alone has five) raised their production values and their prices. And with the growth of full-fledged shopping malls inside casinos, ranging from the Canal Shops at the Venetian to the Miracle Mile at Planet Hollywood, retail spending has climbed as well.

The ascendancy of nightclubs, ultra-lounges, and day clubs will further amplify the Mirage Effect. The nightclub trade, which skews to a demographic of 20- and 30-year-olds, represents a departure for Strip casinos, which traditionally considered 45-year-olds youngsters. Here, bottle service is the way of the future. Under this model, select patrons bypass the line and receive reserved tables along the dance floor in exchange for purchasing several bottles of liquor, at charges of up to $500 per bottle. By opening clubs and lounges along these lines, operators meet two objectives: They capture an extremely lucrative business, and they effectively orient new patrons to the casino.

Figure 6 shows the revenues generated by various aspects of casino resort operations.

	Daily Average	% of Total
Gaming	$557,792.48	38.70%
Rooms	$339,595.96	23.50%
Food	$222,101.89	15.40%
Beverage	$94,144.01	6.50%
Other	$228,523.55	15.80%
Total:	$1,442,157.89	100%

Casino Revenues

	Daily Average	% of Total
Tables	$252,092.10	45.20%
Slots	$282,030.71	50.60%
Poker	$11,932.21	2.10%
Race Book	$3,884.81	0.70%
Sports Book	$7,852.65	1.40%

Casino Expenses

	Daily Average	% of Revenues
Bad Debt	$14,706.78	2.60%
Comps	$156,541.94	28.10%
Gaming Taxes	$42,064.74	7.50%
Payroll	$105,581.73	18.90%
Total Expenses	$389,364.75	69.80%

Room Revenues and Occupancy

	Daily Average	% of Revenues
Sales	$256,201.04	75.40%
Comp Rooms	$83,394.91	24.60%
Available Rooms	3,089	
Rooms Occupied	2,781	
Rooms Payroll	$89,916	35.10%
Occupancy Rate	90.01%	

Number of Employees

Department	Per Casino
Casino	901
Rooms	751
Food	1,059
Beverage	291
G & A	507
Other	386
Total	3,894

In fiscal 2010, 23 casinos in the Las Vegas Strip area produced gaming revenue of more than $72 million. The averages for several key financial statistics produce a picture of the statistically "average" Strip casino and give a good snapshot of the industry standard. All of the data is excerpted from the 2010 Nevada Gaming Abstract, published by the Nevada Gaming Control Board.

Figure 6 • The Average Strip Casino: Daily Revenues.

Sustainability in Gaming Entertainment

Sustainable initiatives are constantly gaining in popularity and prestige across the gaming industry. Gaming entertainment companies continue adapting their operations and practices to fit "green" standards. Many well-known companies in gaming entertainment are leading the way to establish sustainable initiatives as the standard practice in the industry, including Harrah's Entertainment, which operates Harrah's Resort, Caesars, and Bally's in Atlantic City, along with Delaware North, and Dover Downs Hotel & Casino.

One of the leading corporations in the gaming industry, Harrah's Entertainment Inc. has undertaken a sustainable initiative in several areas of operation, including energy, waste and water conservation, as well as climate control. Harrah's executives have urged their management teams to embrace a sustainable approach to their daily practices, designated "Code Green". This sustainable initiative involves the exchange of traditional incandescent lighting to a more resourceful energy conservative lighting, as well as ventilation controls in guest rooms, and throughout hotel and casino space in some of their larger properties. Select properties feature subsidized public transportation, habitat preservation fundraisers, recycling used oil, and composting waste products. Harrah's plans to continue the future implementation of sustainable practices in select properties throughout the country.[5]

Recently, gaming entertainment companies have begun implementing sustainable initiatives into the initial construction and development of new properties. Delaware North, a well-known player in gaming industry operations has recently built a new property in Daytona Beach, Florida, which complies with all the necessary standards required to be a Leadership in Engineering and Environmental Design (LEED) certified property. LEED employs a four tier rating system for buildings, based on the level of sustainability applied during property development, and maintained upon completion. The level of certification is based on the areas of "sustainable site development, water savings, energy efficiency, materials selection, and indoor environmental quality". The Daytona property received silver certification, which is the second tier of the rating system, which followed in the footsteps of their previous sustainable site developed in West Memphis, Arkansas in 2006.[6]

Hospitality Green LLC, an environmental consulting firm has taken on the task of creating a model for "green" standards that will set precedent for which existing and future initiatives will be measured. The company directed a property-wide assessment of Dover Downs Hotel & Casino's sustainable business practices in order to collect the necessary data required to provide an appropriate model. Dover Downs Hotel & Casino is one of the most noteworthy gaming and entertainment resorts in the Mid-Atlantic region. Currently, the AAA-four diamond property is working towards the objective of becoming the first certified "green" hotel in Delaware. In addition to the assessment of Dover Down's sustainable business practices, Hospitality Green will be conducting staff training in sustainable practices that can be implemented on a daily basis. This will ensure that Dover Down's employees are knowledgeable of proper standards and procedures, in order for the property to maintain "green" status.[7]

Career Information

The growth of the gaming industry has resulted in a variety of new job openings. People choose to work in the industry because it is known to place people first, whether they are employees or customers. The industry also has many opportunities for employees to learn new skills, which lead to growth and advancement in their careers.

Employees in the gaming industry may receive many tangible benefits. Most careers include impressive benefits packages and offer many career advancement opportunities. Casinos are known to hire from within, which gives current employees a greater chance to move into better positions over time. Because the gaming industry's positions are so varied, many educational and experiential backgrounds can be adapted to a specific casino's policies.

A variety of careers are specific to the gaming industry including dealer, slot attendant, marketing director, and casino surveillance. More opportunities are becoming available every day as new technology creates more openings. For example, systems such as MindPlay's Table Management System and IGT's EZpay technology and the introduction of advanced guest service technology will surely create new and exciting technical employment opportunities within the industry.

Although it may appear as if many gaming jobs have very specific qualifications, it is important not to focus too narrowly on one sector. Knowledge of all areas of the industry is essential for advancement. For example, today's casinos now rely on entertainment as well as gaming to bring in patrons. Therefore, an employee at such a casino also needs to have knowledge of the entertainment industry and of how casinos operate such events.

To get a job in the gaming industry, one must have very thorough knowledge of the legal, regulatory, and compliance issues related to daily operations in the casino. Broken laws can result in lawsuits and cost the company large sums of money. This can be avoided if all employees have the proper background knowledge.

Even though observing daily activity in a casino provides invaluable work experience, obtaining a college or graduate degree is also crucial. It is true that much of the necessary education can take place on the job; however, applicants who have received an outside education, as well as attended gaming certification programs, have a much better chance of standing out from their competition.

A general manager in the gaming industry earns a starting average annual salary of about $82,800. A casino operator begins at about $38,000, and marketing and sales employees start out at $55,000. Positions typically include full health benefits, yearly bonuses, and other compensation, depending on the casino.

TECHNOLOGY SPOTLIGHT

Technology Use in the Casino Industry

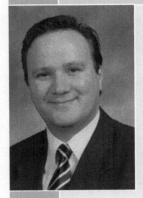

Cihan Cobanoglu, Ph.D., Dean, School of Hotel and Restaurant Management, University of South Florida, Sarasota-Manatee

Casinos are perhaps the heaviest users of technology in the hospitality industry. There are three main areas that should be considered in the casino information system: gaming technology, surveillance systems, and customer data mining.

Examples of gaming technology include slot machines and automated card shufflers. Slot machines were originally installed as an alternative to other games. They require minimal gambling knowledge and low bets (as low as one cent). Due to these factors, slot machines gained high popularity over time. The classic slot machine is configured of gears and levers. The handle mechanism that gets the system moving is connected to a metal shaft that supports the reels. A coin/bill detector identifies the payment and unlocks the brake so that the handle can move. When a game begins, the reels start moving and then are stopped by the breaking system. Special sensors built into the slot machine communicate the position of the reels to the payout system. However, technological advances have affected the way slot machines work. Most modern slot machines are computerized: The outcome of the game is being determined by a computer inside the machine. Now, the computer tells the reels where to stop. However, it does not mean that winning is impossible. Every round, the computer generates a random number (usually in the range from one to several billion), which determines where the reels will stop. All these numbers are generated in such a way that they have equal probability of hitting the jackpot.

Another important gaming technology is electronic card shufflers. This technology helps to shuffle card decks in seconds. The key point of using the technology is that it protects players from cheating. In contrast with the initial designs, modern devices are very small and convenient. Some of the main techniques of card shuffling include shelves (vertical carousels), ejectors, and mechanical fingers.

Computer surveillance systems are crucial for casino operations. Any casino can face such problems as intoxicated patrons, cheaters, thieves, and dishonest employees. Surveillance systems are necessary to ensure safety and minimize loss. Originally, surveillance systems were completely nonelectronic and were based on manager observations. However, technological advances of the previous decades enabled digital imaging technology, including facial recognition systems. Most modern versions of such systems are even capable of scanning the room in search of particular persons. Some of the vendors that provide surveillance systems are IQinVision, EZWATCH PRO, and CloseoutCCTV.com.

The casino industry is one of early adopters of data-mining techniques among all hospitality sectors. Data mining allows businesses to work with large volumes of information in order to identify unique useful patterns that can be helpful in decision making. To give an example, data mining was employed by Harrah's casinos to cluster the guests (based on demographics characteristics, preferences, loyalty points, etc.), classify them (e.g., to identify the customers with the high lifelong value), and establish association rules (e.g., if customers prefer a particular slot machine, are they all likely to be interested in any other type of a game?). The information generated by means of data mining helps to predict the value of the future guests by looking at existing ones and identifying patterns in their behavior. Having this information in hand enables managers to make important business decisions.

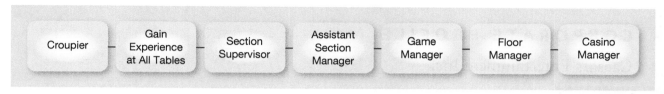

Figure 7 • A Career Path in the Gaming Industry.

Management careers can be very different, depending on your focus. If your interest is gaming management, it is important that you take courses in finance, law, human resources, management, and gambling. You also need to work in the gaming industry while in college, so that you can open doors for yourself through networking. Casinos still believe in promoting from within, and so you will have to work your way up the corporate ladder. You also need to understand that because of the continuous operation of a casino, your work schedule will vary. It is not uncommon to work several straight twelve-hour days, but the rewards for dedication and hard work can be very worthwhile: Casinos have many opportunities for advancement. Figure 7 shows an example of a career path in the gaming industry.

To see more of the types of jobs that are available in the gaming entertainment industry, go to **www.casinocareers.com/index.cfm**, where you can look up potential employers, available jobs, and areas of employment.

Trends in the Gaming Entertainment Industry

- Gaming entertainment is depending less on casino revenue and more on room, food and beverage, retail, and entertainment revenue for its profitability and growth.

- The gaming entertainment industry and lodging industry are converging as hotel room inventory is rapidly expanding in gaming entertainment properties.

- Gaming entertainment, along with the gaming industry as a whole, will continue to be scrutinized by government and public policymakers as to the net economic and social impact of its activities.

- As the gaming entertainment industry becomes more competitive, exceptional service quality will become an increasingly important competitive advantage for success.

- The gaming entertainment industry will continue to provide management opportunities for careers in the hospitality business.

CORPORATE PROFILE

Caesars Entertainment Inc.

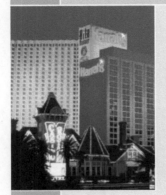

Harrah's Entertainment was founded in 1937 by William F. Harrah as a small bingo parlor in Reno, Nevada. Today, Harrah's is the largest gaming company in the world, with a portfolio of forty-eight casinos totaling 4 million square feet of gaming, which it owns or manages in three countries under the Harrah's, Caesars, and Horseshoe brand names.[1] Harrah's has twenty-eight land-based and twelve riverboat or dockside casinos, plus golf courses and combination racetrack and casinos in several states, including Nevada, Louisiana, New Jersey, Mississippi, Kansas, and Missouri. Harrah's grew by new property development, expansions, and acquisitions, and it now employs some 85,000 people, with the vision that "each of our brands will be the overwhelming first choice for casino entertainment of its targeted customers."[2] Harrah's Entertainment is focused on building loyalty and value with its customers through a unique combination of guest service, excellent products, unsurpassed distribution, operational excellence, and technology leadership.[3] The marketing strategy is designed to appeal to those who are avid players, especially those who play in more than one market.[4]

[1] Yahoo! Finance, *HET (Harrah Entertainment Inc.)*, http://finance.yahoo.com/q/pr?s=het (April 21, 2011; site now discontinued).

[2] Harrah's Entertainment, www.harras.com/harrahs-corporate/about-us.html (April 21, 2011; site now discontinued).

[3] Harrah's Entertainment, *Name of Web Site*, www.harrahs.com/harrahs-corporate/index.html (June 4, 2009; site now discontinued).

[4] www.investords.com/cgi-bin/stocksymbol.cgi?ticker=het

[5] Arnold M. Knightly, "Deal closes: Harrah's now private," *Las vegas Review-Journal*, Jan. 29, 2008, as cited by http://en.wikipedia.org/wiki/Harrah%27s_Entertainment (accessed November 18, 2011).

[6] Wikinvest, *Harrah's Entertainment*, www.wikinvest.com/Harrah's_Entertainment (accessed November 18, 2011).

CASE STUDY

Negotiating with Convention Groups

Your convention sales department receives a call from a trip director for a large convention group. The group will use many function rooms for meetings during the day and will generate a substantial amount of convention services revenue. Likewise, the group's food and beverage needs are quite elaborate, so this will be good for the food and beverage department budget. However, the group is very sensitive concerning room price and is willing to negotiate the time of week for its three-night stay.

Discussion Question

1. What are the considerations that a gaming entertainment property must take into account when determining room rates for convention groups?

CASE STUDY

VIP

A frequent guest of the casino makes a last-minute decision to travel to your property for a weekend stay. The guest enjoys gambling as a leisure activity and is one of the casino's better customers. When he arrives at the casino, he is usually met by a casino host and is treated as a VIP due to his level of wagering at the blackjack tables. This guest is worth approximately $500,000 in casino win per year to the hotel. Due to his last-minute arrangements, however, the guest cannot notify a casino host that he is on his way to the hotel. Upon arriving, he finds a very busy registration desk. He must wait in line for twenty minutes, and when he tries to check in, he is told that the hotel is full. The front-desk clerk acts impatient when the guest says that he is a frequent customer. In a fit of frustration, the would-be guest leaves the hotel and makes a mental note that all casinos have similar odds at the blackjack table and that maybe another property will give him the respect he deserves.

Discussion Question

1. What systems or procedures could you institute to make sure this type of oversight does not happen in your property?

Summary

1. The casino industry is a growing international force that includes both gambling and more traditional hospitality elements.
2. To manage a casino resort, it is necessary to understand the relationship between the casino and other departments in the operation, as well as ways that casinos are different from other businesses.
3. Casino gambling is strictly regulated by state governments, and the integrity developed over time by these regulations is necessary for the survival of the industry.
4. Nongaming revenue is increasing as a percentage of total casino resort revenue, and nongaming parts of casino resorts are gaining in prominence.

Key Words and Concepts

Baccarat
Blackjack
Casino resort
Comp
Craps
Gambling

Handle
Hold percentage
Poker
Roulette
Win

Review Questions

1. Briefly describe the history of legalized gaming in the United States.
2. What defines a gaming entertainment business?
3. Explain the attraction of gaming entertainment to the destination of a tourist.
4. Why is it necessary for strict regulations to be in force on the casino floor?
5. How are hotel operations in a gaming entertainment business different from hotel operations in a nongaming environment?

Internet Exercises

1. Organization: **Wynn Las Vegas**
   Web site: **www.wynnlasvegas.com**
   Summary: Located on the Las Vegas Strip, the Wynn Las Vegas has a lot to offer. From gaming and concerts, to hosting some of the biggest conventions, the Wynn Las Vegas will certainly keep you busy.
   (a) What are some of the gaming features that attract customers to the Wynn Las Vegas?
   (b) What are the benefits to the different packages available?

2. Pick a casino in Las Vegas and look it up on the Internet. What does it offer that sets it apart from other casinos in Las Vegas and from other casinos in the United States? In what areas is it similar to other casinos?

Apply Your Knowledge

1. Name the major gaming entertainment hotels in Las Vegas.
2. Give examples of nongaming revenue.

Suggested Activity

1. Research careers in the gaming entertainment industry. Are there more opportunities than you realized? What careers in the industry interest you the most?

Endnotes

1. Insider Viewpoint of Las Vegas, 20 *Largest Hotels in the World*, http://www.insidervlv.com/hotelslargestworld.html (accessed November 18, 2011).
2. Wikipedia, *The Venetian Macao*, http://en.wikipedia.org/wiki/The_Venetian_Macao (accessed November 18, 2011).
3. www.harrahs.com/about_us/community_relations/IPImpacts.pdf
4. University of Nevada Las Vegas, *Annual Comparison: Revenue Statistics—Las Vegas Strip Casinos with Gaming Revenue over $1,000,000*, http://gaming.unlv.edu/abstract/lv_revenues.html (accessed November 18, 2011).
5. August, 2010. http://www.leonardoacademy.org/programs/standards/gaming/news.html. Retrieved on November 16, 2011.
6. http://www.delawarenorth.com/Gaming-Entertainment-Environmental-Management.aspx Retrieved on November 16, 2011.
7. October 17, 2011. http://www.4-traders.com/DOVER-DOWNS-GAMING-ENTE-12270/news/DOVER-DOWNS-GAMING-ENTERTAINMENT-INC-Dover-Downs-Hotel-Casino-reveals-details-of-innovative-sustaina-13845599/. Retrieved on November 16, 2011.

Glossary

Baccarat   A traditional table game in which the winning hand totals closest to nine.

Blackjack   A table game in which the winning hand is determined by whether the dealer or the player gets cards that add up to a number closest to or equal to 21 without going over.

Handle   The dollars wagered, or bet; often confused with *win*. Whenever a customer places a bet, the handle increases by the amount of the bet. The handle is not affected by the outcome of the bet.

Poker   A card game in which participants play against each other instead of the casino.

Roulette   A traditional table game in which a dealer spins a wheel and players wager on which number a small ball will fall.

Win   Dollars won by the gaming operation from its customers. The net spending of customers on gaming is called the *win*, also known as *gross gaming revenue (GGR)*.

Photo Credits

Credits are listed in the order of appearance.

Andrew Moss/Fotolia
Alan Keohane/Dorling Kindersley, Ltd.
David Schwartz

Chet Gordon/The Image Works
Courtesy of the Wynn Hotel & Resort Las Vegas
Aurora Photos/Alamy

Meetings, Conventions, and Expositions

From Chapter 12 of *Introduction to Hospitality Management,* Fourth Edition. John R. Walker. Copyright © 2013 by Pearson Education, Inc. Published by Pearson. All rights reserved.

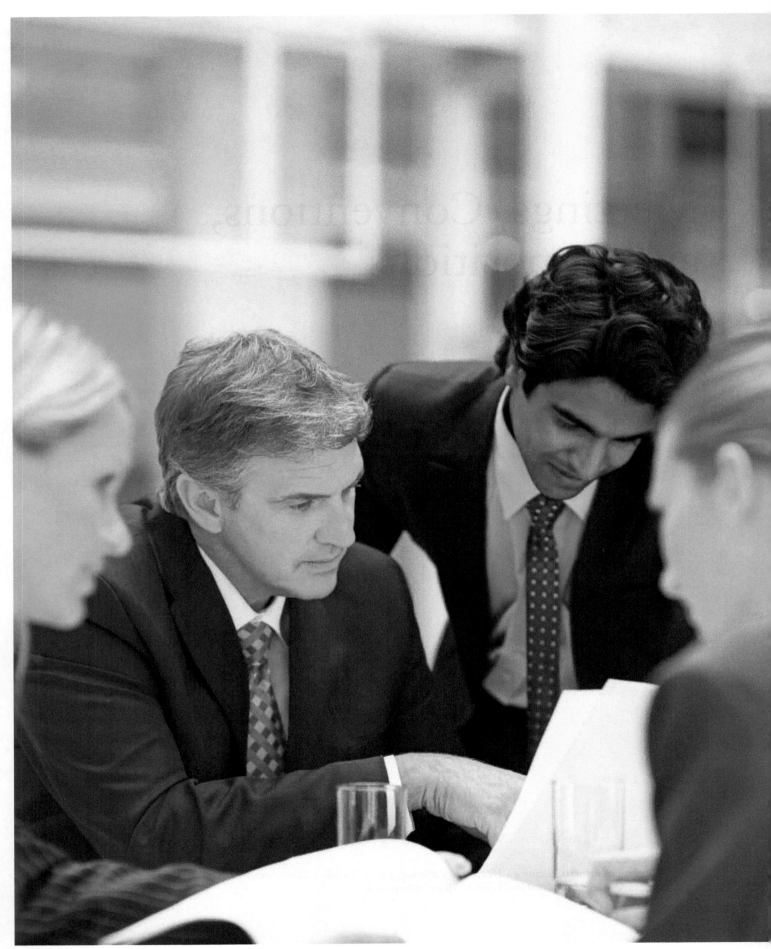

Meetings, Conventions, and Expositions

OBJECTIVES

After reading and studying this chapter, you should be able to:

- List the major players in the convention industry.

- Describe destination management companies.

- Describe the different aspects of being a meeting planner.

- Describe the different types of contractors.

- Explain the different types of meetings, conventions, and expositions.

- List the various venues for meetings, conventions, and expositions.

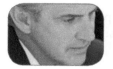
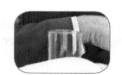
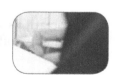
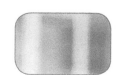

Development of the Meetings, Conventions, and Expositions Industry

People have gathered to attend **meetings, conventions,** and **expositions** since ancient times, mainly for social, sporting, political, or religious purposes. As cities became regional centers, the size and frequency of such activities increased, and various groups and associations set up regular expositions.

Associations go back many centuries to the Middle Ages and earlier. The guilds in Europe were created during the Middle Ages to secure proper wages and maintain work standards. In the United States, associations began at the beginning of the eighteenth century, when Rhode Island candle makers organized themselves.

Meetings, incentive travel, conventions, and exhibitions (MICE) represent a segment of the tourism industry that has grown in recent years. The MICE segment of the tourism industry is very profitable. Industry statistics point to the fact that the average MICE tourist spends about twice the amount of money that other tourists spend.

Size and Scope of the Industry

According to the American Society of Association Executives (ASAE), there are about 90,908 trade and professional associations[1]. The association business is big business. Associations spend billions holding thousands of meetings and conventions that attract millions of attendees.

The hospitality and tourism industries consist of a number of associations, including the following:

- American Hotel & Lodging Association (AH&LA)
- National Restaurant Association (NRA)
- American Culinary Federation
- International Association of Convention and Visitors Bureaus (IACVB)
- Hospitality Sales and Marketing Association International
- Association of Meeting Planners
- Club Managers Association of America
- Professional Convention Management Association

Associations are the main independent political force for industries such as hospitality, offering the following benefits:

- A voice in government/politics
- Marketing avenues
- Education

- Member services
- Networking

Thousands of associations hold annual conventions at various locations across North America and throughout the rest of the world. Some associations alternate their venues from east to central to west; others meet at fixed locations, such as the NRA show in Chicago or the AH&LA convention and show in New York City.

Associations have an elected board of directors and an elected president, vice president, treasurer, and secretary. Additional officers, such as a liaison person or a public relations person, may be elected according to the association's constitution.

Key Players in the Industry

The need to hold face-to-face meetings and attend conventions has grown into a multibillion-dollar industry. Many major and some smaller cities have convention centers with nearby hotels and restaurants.

The major players in the convention industry are **convention and visitors bureaus (CVBs)**, corporations, associations, meeting planners and their clients, convention centers, specialized services, and exhibitions. The wheel diagram in Figure 1 shows the types of clients that use convention centers by percentage utilization.

CVBs are major participants in the meetings, conventions, and expositions market. The IACVB describes a CVB as a not-for-profit umbrella organization

> " Meetings, conventions, and expositions provide attendees and personnel in specialized areas an opportunity to discuss important issues and new developments with their peers. "
>
> Laurel Ebert,
> The Boylston Convention Center,
> Boylston, Maryland.

> " Meetings provide managers the opportunity to give positive feedback to their employees, address employee concerns, and to emphasize projects and/or goals. "
>
> Lianne Wilhoitte,
> Wilhoitte & Associates,
> Baltimore, Maryland.

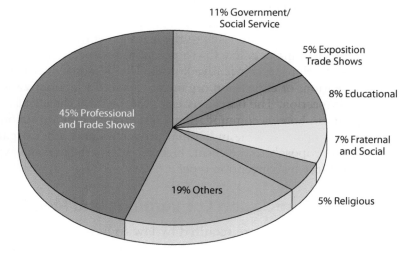

Convention Center Utilization by Market Sector

- 11% Government/Social Service
- 5% Exposition Trade Shows
- 8% Educational
- 7% Fraternal and Social
- 5% Religious
- 19% Others
- 45% Professional and Trade Shows

Figure 1 • Convention Center Clientele.

that represents an urban area and that tries to solicit business- or pleasure-seeking visitors. The CVB comprises a number of visitor industry organizations representing the various industry sectors:

- Transportation
- Hotels and motels
- Restaurants
- Attractions
- Suppliers

The bureau represents these local businesses by acting as the sales team for the city. A bureau has *five* primary responsibilities:

1. To enhance the image of tourism in the local/city area
2. To market the area and encourage people to visit and stay longer
3. To target and encourage selected associations and others to hold meetings, conventions, and expositions in the city
4. To assist associations and others with convention preparations and to give support during the convention
5. To encourage tourists to partake of the historic, cultural, and recreational opportunities the city or area has to offer

The outcome of these five responsibilities is for the city's tourist industry to increase revenues. Bureaus compete for business at trade shows, where interested visitor industry groups gather to do business. For example, a tour wholesaler who is promoting a tour will need to link up with hotels, restaurants, and attractions to package a vacation. Similarly, meeting planners are able to consider several locations and hotels by visiting a trade show. Bureaus generate leads (prospective clients) from a variety of sources. One source, associations, have national/international offices in Washington, D.C. (so that they can lobby the government), and Chicago.

A number of bureaus have offices or representatives in these cities or a sales team who will make follow-up visits to the leads generated at trade shows. Alternatively, they will make cold calls to potential prospects, such as major associations, corporations, and incentive houses. The sales manager will invite the meeting, convention, or exposition organizer to make a **familiarization (FAM) trip** for a site inspection. The bureau assesses the needs of the client and organizes transportation, hotel accommodations, restaurants, and attractions accordingly. The bureau then lets the individual properties and other organizations make their own proposals to the client. Figure 2 shows the average expenditure per delegate per stay by convention type.

Business and Association Conventions and Meetings

Publicly held corporations are required by law to have an annual shareholders' meeting. Most also have sales meetings, incentive trips (all-expenses paid trips for groups of employees that met or exceeded goals set for them), product

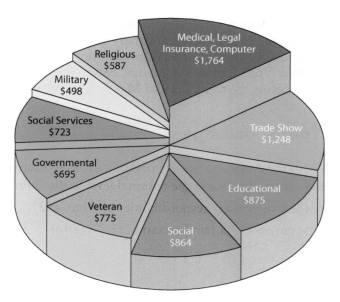

Average length of stay is 3.5 days.

Figure 2 • Average Expenditure per Delegate per Stay by Convention Type. The significance of these amounts is that given an attendance of several hundreds to thousands of guests, the economic impact quickly adds up and benefits the community in a variety of ways.

launches, focus groups, executive retreats, seminars and training sessions, and management meetings.

Corporations are big spenders, in part because they receive tax deductions on their meeting expenditures. When a corporation decides to hold a gathering, it determines what the budget will be, where the gathering will be held, and who will attend. Since the corporation typically pays for all expenses associated with attending the meeting, hotels, resorts, and convention centers compete for this lucrative business.[2] In the United States, almost 1.1 million corporate events are held annually, with a total attendance of 84 million. The total direct spending on these events is over $30 billion per year, with the average corporate event generating almost $550,000.[3] Corporations also arrange incentive trips—paying all expenses for a special vacation for the employee or customer and a significant other at a hotel, at a resort, or on a cruise ship.

Associations represent the interests of their members and gather at the state, regional, national, and international levels for professional industry–related reasons; for annual congresses, conventions, and conferences; and for scientific, educational, and training meetings.

Conventions are a major source of income for associations, as they charge attendees a registration fee and charge vendors for booth space (this gives vendors a chance to sell their products to attendees). Association conventions and meetings attract crowds ranging from hundreds to over 100,000, which only the larger convention facilities like New York, Orlando, Las Vegas, San Francisco, and Chicago can handle. The next level of convention facilities includes cities like Washington, D.C., San Diego, Dallas/Fort Worth, Miami, Boston, and Phoenix/Scottsdale.

The larger associations book their dates several years ahead, some in the same place at the same time of year; others move around the country. For example, the AH&LA holds its annual convention during the second week of November in New York City at the Javits Center, and the NRA holds its annual convention during the third week of May in Chicago at McCormick Place.

► Check Your Knowledge

1. According to the American Society of Association Executives (ASAE), how many associations operate at the national level in the United States?
2. What are the five primary responsibilities of a bureau?
3. What is the purpose of a familiarization (FAM) trip?

Destination Management Companies

A destination management company (DMC) is a service organization within the visitor industry that offers a host of programs and services to meet clients' needs. Initially, a destination management sales manager concentrates on selling the destination to meeting planners and performance improvement companies (incentive houses).

The needs of such groups may be as simple as an airport pickup or as involved as an international sales convention with theme parties. DMCs work closely with hotels; sometimes a DMC books rooms, and another time a hotel might request the DMC's expertise on organizing theme parties. Patricia Roscoe, chairperson of Patti Roscoe and Associates (PRA), says that meeting planners often have a choice of several destinations and might ask, "Why should I pick your destination?" The answer is that a DMC does everything, including airport greetings, transportation to the hotel, VIP check-in, arranging theme parties, sponsoring programs, organizing competitive sports events, and so on, depending on budget. Sales managers associated with DMCs obtain leads, which are potential clients, from the following sources:

- Hotels
- Trade shows
- CVBs
- Cold calls
- Incentive houses
- Meeting planners

Each sales manager has a staff or team, which can include the following:

- A special events manager, who will have expertise in sound, lighting, staging, and so on
- An accounts manager, who is an assistant to the sales manager

- A theme-events creative director
- An audiovisual specialist
- An operations manager, who coordinates everything, especially on-site arrangements, to ensure that what is sold actually happens

For example, Patti Roscoe's DMC organized meetings, accommodations, meals, beverages, and theme parties for 2,000 Ford Motor Company dealers in nine groups over three days for each group.

Roscoe also works closely with incentive houses, such as Carlson Marketing and Maritz Travel. These incentive houses approach a company and offer to set up incentive plans for companies' employees, including whatever it takes to motivate them. Once approved, Carlson contacts a DMC and asks for a program.

Meeting Planners

Meeting planners may be independent contractors who contract out their services to both associations and corporations as the need arises or they may be full-time employees of corporations or associations. In either case, meeting planners have interesting careers. According to the International Convention Management Association (ICMA), about 212,000 full- and part-time meeting planners work in the United States.

The professional meeting planner not only makes hotel and meeting bookings but also plans the meeting down to the last minute, always remembering to check to ensure that the services that have been contracted have been delivered. In recent years, the technical aspects of audiovisual and simultaneous translation equipment have added to the complexity of meeting planning. The meeting planner's role varies from meeting to meeting, but may include some or all of the following activities:

Premeeting Activities

- Estimate attendance
- Plan meeting agenda
- Establish meeting objectives
- Set meeting budget
- Select city location and hotel/ convention site
- Negotiate contracts
- Plan exhibition
- Prepare exhibitor correspondence and packet
- Create marketing plan
- Plan travel to and from site

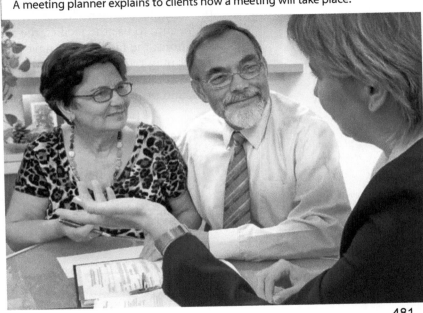

A meeting planner explains to clients how a meeting will take place.

- Arrange ground transportation
- Organize shipping
- Organize audiovisual needs

On-Site Activities

- Conduct pre-event briefings
- Prepare VIP plan
- Facilitate people movement
- Approve expenditures

Postmeeting Activities

- Debrief
- Evaluate
- Give recognition and appreciation
- Plan for next year

As you can see, this is quite a long list of activities that meeting planners handle for clients.

Service Contractors

Service contractors, *exposition service contractors*, *general contractors*, and *decorators* are all terms that have at one time or another referred to the individual responsible for providing all of the services needed to run the facilities for a trade show. Just as a meeting planner is able to multitask and satisfy all the demands in meeting planning, a general exposition contractor must be multitalented and equipped to serve all exhibit requirements and creative ideas.

The service contractor is hired by the exposition show manager or association meeting planner. The service contractor is a part of the facilities management team, and, to use the facility, the sponsor must use its service contractor. In other situations, the facility may have an exclusive contract with an outside contractor, and it may require all conventions and expositions to deal with this contractor. Today, there are Internet service companies that can take reservations, prepare lists, and provide all kinds of services via the Internet for meeting planners.

▶ Check Your Knowledge

1. What is a destination management company?
2. What are the primary responsibilities of professional meeting planners?

CORPORATE PROFILE

Hawai's Convention Center

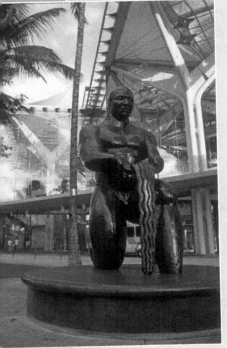

The Hawai'i Convention Center (HCC) on the island of Oahu, Hawaii, is consistently recognized by meeting planners and conventioneers as the world's most desirable convention and meeting destination and has built its reputation around being a facility where business and *aloha* meet.

Hawaiian hospitality values are recognized as the most sophisticated and genuine in the world. To take advantage of this, the HCC offers each employee training in the Hawaii Institute of Hospitality, a program of the Native Hawaiian Hospitality Association (NaHHA). The seminar, headed by the Hawaii Institute of Hospitality, is just one element of a series of *Na Mea Ho'okipa* (Hawaiian hospitality) training for the staff at the center. More than teaching hospitality, *ho'okipa* advocates a personal behavior system based on Hawaiian values and a heightened "sense of place." "*Ho'okipa* is about understanding who we are and how we fit into this place, and the HCC has always had a fundamental sense of how it, as a viable economic powerhouse and ultimate host, fits successfully within Hawaii's cultural environment," says Peter Apo, director of the NaHHA.

Ho'okipa training also includes a novel approach to orienting staff to the concept of place, the most integral element of the visitor experience. A walking tour through historic Waikiki reiterates that it is not merely high rises and hotels, but one of the most sacred, culturally important places in Hawaii. The "Hawai'i Advantage" is a strategy to position the Convention Center and Hawaii as the world's most desirable convention and meeting destination. This advantage is channeled through various facets, each one an instrumental consideration for meeting planners. The premise is that Hawaii as a destination expounds on aspects including, but not exclusive to, location, productivity, competitive shipping, value of facility, destination appeal, industry support, and customer service in a way that no other destination can. And, of course, no other destination offers "business with aloha."

"The Hawai'i Advantage is a powerful concept that works on several levels; it distinguishes the HCC from other venues and is an initiative rooted in testimonials of past convention attendees," says Joe Davis, general manager of the HCC. "The Convention Center and Hawaii offers conventioneers an unmatched experience. Once we get them here for the first time, we know they will rebook," says Davis.

HCC highlights include the following:

- One million square feet of meeting facilities, including an exhibit hall, theaters, and expansive conference rooms
- Convention Television (CTV)—an exclusive service with the capability to broadcast convention information in 28,000 hotel rooms in Waikiki, as well as on screens within the convention center. CTV is an expedient way for organizations to reach out to conventioneers with its message, as well as to showcase sponsors, VIPs, and trade show participants.
- Designed with a "Hawaiian Sense of Place"—the Center captures the essence of the Hawaiian environment with a soaring, glass-front entry; a 70-foot misting waterfall; and mature palm trees

(continued)

CORPORATE PROFILE *(continued)*

- A $2 million Hawaiian art collection of unique pieces commissioned for specific locations within the building, and a rooftop outdoor function space complete with a tropical garden of native flora
- The center's state-of-the-art technical features include fiber-optic cabling, multilingual translation stations, satellite and microwave broadcast capability, and videoconferencing

The HCC's recent list of awards includes the following:

- Prime Site Award from *Facilities & Destinations* magazine
- Planners' Choice Award—Recognition for Excellence in the Hospitality Industry—*Meeting News* magazine
- Ranked as North America's most attractive convention center in the METROPOLL X study, Gerard Murphy & Associates

The HCC's web site (**http://www.hawaiiconvention.com/**) offers the following information:

The Las Vegas Convention and Visitors Authority (LVCVA) hosts hundreds of conventions attended by more than a million delegates. The LVCVA is organized in the followed way: State law establishes the number, appointment, and terms of the authority's board of directors. A twelve-member board provides guidance and establishes policies to accomplish the LVCVA mission.

Seven members are elected officials of the county, and each represents one of the incorporated cities therein; the remaining five members are nominated by the Las Vegas Chamber of Commerce, and each represents a different segment of the industry. The board is one of the most successful public/private partnerships in the country. Under the presidency of Manuel J. Cortez, the LVCVA and its board of directors have received numerous awards.

The LVCVA's organizational structure is shown in the accompanying diagram. The board of directors employs a president (executive) to serve as chief executive officer. Other members of the executive staff are vice president of marketing, vice president of operations, and vice president of facilities. The marketing division's first priority is to increase the number of visitors to Las Vegas and southern Nevada. The marketing division is composed of eight teams that specialize in various market segments to increase the number of visitors and convention attendance: marketing services, convention sales, tour and travel, corporate and incentive, international, wholesalers/special events, consumer advertising, and news bureau.

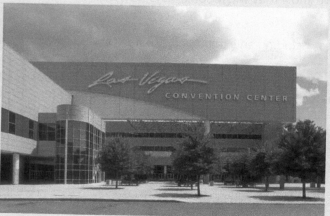

The marketing services team is responsible for providing visitor services including research, registration, convention housing, hotel/motel reservations, and visitor information. The research team tracks the dynamics of the Las Vegas and Clark Country tourism marketplace, along with the competitive gaming and tourism environment. The registration department coordinates and provides temporary help for conventions and trade shows being held in Las Vegas.

The housing division receives and processes hotel and motel housing forms from convention and trade show delegates, forwarding the reservations to participating hotels daily. The reservations department operates toll-free telephone lines, transferring the calls of travel agents, tourists, conventioneers, and special event attendees to hotel and motels within a requested location and price range.

The convention sales team coordinates convention sales efforts at the authority and contributes to the success of convention sales citywide by providing sales leads to the hotels. Sales managers travel throughout the United States and the world, meeting with association meeting planners to sell the benefits of holding conventions in Las Vegas. Members of the team also attend numerous conventions and trade shows, where they host or sponsor special events and functions to entice conventions and trade shows to Las Vegas.

Familiarization trips for travel agents are conducted by team members to generate enthusiasm and excitement around Las Vegas bookings. Travel agent presentations are also scheduled in both primary and selected secondary airline market cities. Similar events are also scheduled for Laughlin, which also advertises a 1-800 number for tourism information.

The corporate and incentive markets are traditionally considered the high end of the travel industry. These buyers are extremely sophisticated and value-conscious and are looking for the highest-quality facilities and amenities. Corporate and incentive team members attend various trade shows throughout the United States and Canada, as well as selected cities in Europe and Asia, promoting Las Vegas as a complete, value-oriented, flexible, and accessible resort destination for corporate meetings.

The operations division is divided into teams that are discussed in the following sections.

Finance

The finance division maintains a general accounting system for the authority to ensure accountability in compliance with legal provisions and in accordance with generally accepted accounting principles. Finance is composed of financial services, accounting, and payroll activities. Additional responsibilities include the preparation of the authority's annual financial report (CAFR) and the annual budget. The CAFR has received the Government Finance Officers Association (GFOA) Excellence in Financial Reporting Award a number of times in recent years.

Materials Management

Materials management supports the marketing, operations, and facilities divisions by providing for purchasing of materials, services, and goods needed to meet its goals and objectives. Materials management is responsible for the storage and distribution of various supply items through an extensive warehousing program, as well as through printing and mail distribution.

Security

The security division provides protection of the authority's property, equipment, employees, and convention attendees 24 hours a day, 365 days a year, and also oversees paid parking and fire safety functions. The team patrols both the convention center and Cashman Field properties and is trained in first-aid assistance. Several officers have been recognized by the authority board and convention organizations for providing life-saving measures to convention attendees.

Information Technology

The information technology division (ITD) is responsible for efficiently and effectively meeting the automation and information needs of the authority. The ITD sustains a staff of technically competent professionals to design, maintain, implement, and operate the systems necessary to support the goals of the authority.

The author gratefully acknowledges that this section draws on information given by the Las Vegas Convention and Visitors Authority.

TECHNOLOGY SPOTLIGHT

Meeting, Convention, and Exposition Technology

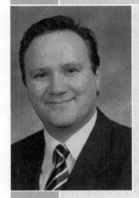

Cihan Cobanoglu, Ph.D., Dean, School of Hotel and Restaurant Management, University of South Florida, Sarasota-Manatee

Managing meetings, conventions, and expositions may be a challenging task. Technology comes to the rescue! There is software available in the market to help manage meetings, conventions, and expositions. One of the market leaders of this segment is Delphi by Newmarket International (**www.newmarketinc.com/products/delphi.aspx**). Some of the features of this software include the following:

- Providing forecast values that better estimate guestroom pickup, ensuring the desired mix between group and transient business
- Responding to Requests for Proposal (RFPs) from the software
- The ability to flag and determine which accounts should track transient production from the Property Management System
- Enhanced suite logic that enables guestroom configurations of suites for more accurate inventory reporting
- Customized guestroom security that lets you move guestrooms in and out of inventory for a specified period of time
- Configurable security settings that limit changes on key booking information
- Guestroom overblock controls that allow for specific room types to be overblocked while restricting other room types
- Simplified guestroom rate fields that drastically reduce time-consuming data entry

Similarly, there are online solutions for managing meetings. RegOnline (**http://www.regonline.com/**) offers online event management, registration, and planning software. This software allows anyone to create an event web site and allows registrants to self-register to the event. Additionally, it generates nametags and attendee lists.

With the advance of smartphones, a lot of conference and event-management applications were introduced for mobile phones such as iPhone and Droid. Some examples of these are as follows:

QuickMobile (www.quickmobile.com)—Features include full conference schedule, personal agenda building, area guide, search capabilities for attendees/speakers/exhibitors, integration with social media including Twitter/Facebook/Pathable, and messaging. QuickMobile builds apps for the iPhone, iPad, Blackberry, Android and mobile web, providing greater ease of use than companies that provide only mobile web versions.

Follow Me (www.core-apps.com)—Follow Me was the mobile app for the 2010 Consumer Electronic Show, one of the largest shows in the tradeshow industry. Features include a full conference schedule, personal agenda builder, maps, exhibit hall way-finding (you are a dot on the map), course notes/literature pickup, session alerts, Twitter integration, and sponsorship revenue sharing. Core-Apps also build native apps for the major smartphones (iPhone, Android, Blackberry) and mobile web for the rest.

SNIPP (www.snipp.com)—This application allows meeting planners to send text messages (SMS) to attendees. It is a low-cost, fast communication channel.

NearPod (www.nearpod.com)—NearPod creates iPod and iPad applications for surveys, data collection, prize giveaways, presentation tools, and metric tools with applications for meetings and trade shows.

Foursquare (www.foursquare.com) and Gowalla (www.gowalla.com)—These location-aware mobile applications allow people to check in at a location to network with others and to share with friends. Although originally used in restaurants, bars, and so forth, these applications are starting to be used for events.

Types of Meetings, Conventions, and Expositions

Meetings

Meetings are conferences, workshops, seminars, or other events designed to bring people together for the purpose of exchanging information. Meetings can take any one of the following forms:

- *Clinic.* A workshop-type educational experience in which attendees learn by doing. A clinic usually involves small groups interacting with each other on an individual basis.

- *Forum.* An assembly for the discussion of common concerns. Usually, experts in a given field take opposite sides of an issue in a panel discussion, with liberal opportunity for audience participation.

- *Seminar.* A lecture and a dialogue that allow participants to share experiences in a particular field. A seminar is guided by an expert discussion leader, and usually thirty or fewer persons participate.

- *Symposium.* An event at which a particular subject is discussed by experts and opinions are gathered.

- *Workshop.* A small group led by a facilitator or trainer. It generally includes exercises to enhance skills or develop knowledge in a specific topic.

The reason for having a meeting can range from the presentation of a new sales plan to a total quality management workshop. The purpose of meetings is to affect behavior. For example, as a result of attending a meeting, a person should know or be able to do certain things. Some outcomes are very specific; others may be less so. For instance, if a meeting were called to brainstorm new ideas, the outcome might be less concrete than for other types of meetings. The number of people attending a meeting can vary. Successful meetings require a great deal of careful planning and organization. Figure 3 shows convention delegates' spending in a convention city.

Meetings are set up according to the wishes of the client. The three main types of meeting setups are theater style, classroom style, and boardroom style:

- Theater style generally is intended for a large audience that does not need to make a lot of notes or refer to documents. This style usually consists of a raised platform and a lectern from which a presenter addresses the audience.

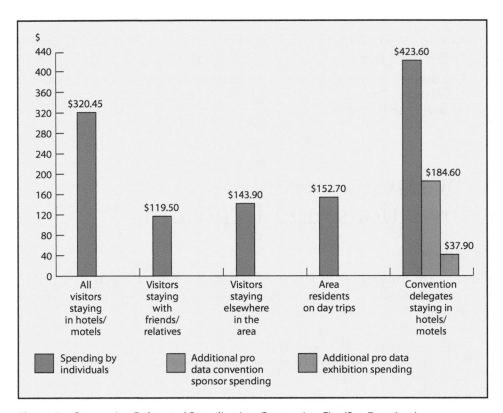

Figure 3 • Convention Delegates' Spending in a Convention City (San Francisco).
Source: J.R. Schrock.

- Classroom setups are used when the meeting format is more instructional and participants need to take detailed notes or refer to documents. A workshop-type meeting often uses this format.
- Boardroom setups are made for small numbers of people. The meeting takes place around one rectangular table.

Association Meetings

Every year there are thousands of association meetings that spend millions of dollars sponsoring many types of meetings, including regional, special interest, education, and board meetings. The things that top the list of what an association meeting planner looks for when choosing a meeting destination include the availability of hotels and facilities, ease of transportation, distance from attendees, transportation costs, and food and beverage. Members attend association meetings voluntarily, so the hotel should work with meeting planners to make the destination seem as appealing as possible.

Associations used to be viewed as groups that held annual meetings and conventions with speeches,

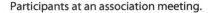
Participants at an association meeting.

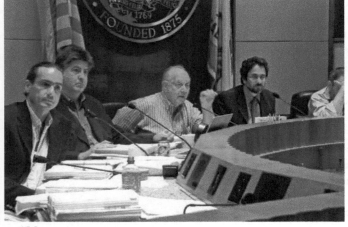

entertainment, an educational program, and social events. They have changed in activity and perception.

Conventions and Expositions

Conventions are generally larger meetings with some form of exposition or trade show included. A number of associations have one or more conventions per year. These conventions raise a large part of the association's budget. A typical convention follows a format like the following:

1. Welcome/registration
2. Introduction of the president
3. President's welcome speech, opening the convention
4. First keynote address by a featured speaker
5. Exposition booths open (equipment manufacturers and trade suppliers)
6. Several workshops or presentations on specific topics
7. Luncheon
8. More workshops and presentations
9. Demonstrations of special topics (e.g., culinary arts for a hospitality convention)
10. Vendors' private receptions
11. Dinner
12. Convention center closes

Figure 4 shows a convention event profile for a trade show.

Conventions are not always held in convention centers; in fact, the majority are held in large hotels over a three- to five-day period. The headquarters hotel is usually the one in which most of the activity takes place. Function space is allocated for registration, the convention, expositions, meals, and so on.

Expositions are events that bring together sellers of products and services at a location (usually a convention center) where they can show their products and services to a group of attendees at a convention or trade show. Exhibitors are an essential component of the industry because they pay to exhibit their products to the attendees. Exhibitors interact with attendees with the intention of making sales or establishing contacts and leads for follow-up. Expositions can take up several hundred thousand square feet of space, divided into booths for individual manufacturers or their representatives. In the hospitality industry, the two largest expositions are the AH&LA's conference, held in conjunction with the International Hotel/Motel & Restaurant Show (IHMRS; held annually in November at the Javits Center in New York), and the NRA's annual exposition held every May in Chicago. Both events are well worth attending.

Types of Associations

An association is an organized body that exhibits some variety of volunteer leadership structure, which may employ an activity or purpose that the leadership shares in common. The association is generally organized to promote and

16:15:28

San Diego
Convention Center Corporation
EVENT PROFILE

EVENT STATISTICS

Event Name:	San Diego Apartment Association Trade Show	ID:	9506059
Sales Person:	Joy Peacock	Initial Contact:	8/3/2005
Event Manager:	Trish A. Stiles	Move In Date:	6/22/2009
ConVis Contact:		Move In Day:	Wednesday
Food Person:		Move In Time:	6:01 am
Event Tech.:		First Event Date:	6/23/2009
Event Attend.:		First Event Day:	Thursday
Nature of Event:	LT Local Trade Show	Start Show Time:	6:01 am
Event Parameter:	60 San Diego Convention Center	End Show Time:	11:59 pm
Business Type 1:	41 Association	# of Event Days:	1
Business Type 2:	91 LOCAL	Move Out Date:	6/23/2009
Booking Status:	D Definite	Move Out Day:	Thursday
Rate Schedule:	III Public Show, Meetings and Location	Out Time:	11:59 pm
Open to Public:	No	Date Confirmed:	8/3/2005
Number of Sessions:	1	Attend per Sesn:	3000
Event Sold By:	F Facility (SDCCC)	Tot Room Nights:	15
Abbrev. Name:	/6/Apartment Assn	Public Release:	Yes
Est Bill Amount:	Rent - 6,060.00 Equip –	0.00 Food –	0.00
Last Changed On:	8/20/05 in: Comment Maintenance	By – Joy Peacock	

This Event has been in the facility before

CLIENT INFORMATION

Company: San Diego Apartment Assn, a non-profit Corporation
Contact Name: Ms. Leslie Cloud, Sales and Marketing Coord.
1011 Camino Del Rio South, Suite 200, San Diego, CA 92108   ID: SDAA
Telephone Number: (619) 297-1000
Fax Number: (619) 294-4510
Alternate Number: (619) 294-4510

Company: San Diego Apartment Assn, a non-profit Corporation
Alt Contact Name: Ms. Pamela A. Trimble, Finance & Operations Director
1011 Camino Del Rio South, Suite 200, San Diego, 92108
Telephone Number: (619) 297-1000
Fax Number: (619) 297-4510

EVENT LOCATIONS

ROOM	MOVE IN	IN USE	ED	MOVE OUT	BS	SEAT	RATE	EST. RENT	ATTEND
A	6/22/09 6:01 am	6/23/09	1	6/23/09 11:59 pm	D	E	III	6,060.00	5,000
AS	6/22/09 6:01 am	6/23/09	1	6/23/09 11:59 pm	D	E	III	0.00	10
R01	6/22/09 6:01 am	6/23/09	1	6/23/09 11:59 pm	D	T	III	0.00	450
R02	6/22/09 6:01 am	6/23/09	1	6/23/09 11:59 pm	D	T	III	0.00	350
R03	6/22/09 6:01 am	6/23/09	1	6/23/09 11:59 pm	D	T	III	0.00	280
R04	6/22/09 6:01 am	6/23/09	1	6/23/09 11:59 pm	D	T	III	0.00	280
R05	6/22/09 6:01 am	6/23/09	1	6/23/09 11:59 pm	D	T	III	0.00	460

FOOD SERVICES

ROOM	DATE	TIME	BS ATTEND	EST. COST FOOD SERVICE
There are No Food Services booked for this event

Figure 4 • Convention Event Profile for a Trade Show.

(Courtesy San Diego Convention Center.)

INTRODUCING JILL MORAN, CSEP

Principal and Owner, JS Moran, Special Event Planning & Management

In my life, there is no typical day. As the owner of a special event company, I provide a variety of services to corporate, nonprofit, and social clients. I must be able to communicate successfully with a client at one moment, a vendor at the next, and a prospect at another. My job also involves managing the growth of my company, hiring the right staff and vendors for projects, and getting each job done from start to finish in a professional and timely manner.

As a business owner, I am required to keep my eye on many facets of the company almost daily. Some areas are a must to attend to such as billing, scheduling, and marketing. The squeakiest wheel that gets the most grease, though, is the actual ongoing projects. Once a project is secured, the contracting, planning, and execution stages quickly follow after the initial handshake. These components of meeting and event planning can be time and energy consuming as the details are planned out and put into motion. Event details may involve researching, attending meetings, generating event documents, developing creative concepts and themes, securing vendors to satisfy event details, or executing an event. In the planning of any given event or conference, I may be required to attend off-site visits with vendors, venues, or clients as well as use the computer or telephone to facilitate the planning process. Visits to art supply, furniture, fabric stores, or storerooms of linen or décor vendors are also key elements as theme and design elements are worked on. Review of entertainment or speakers, planning of room layouts or trade show and exhibition space, or discussion with graphic artists also fits into the necessary details covered during the planning phase of an event.

A typical day may involve early computer time to work on production schedules, time lines, e-mails to vendors or clients, follow-up on contracts, or focused time spent on a new proposal. I find early morning (before 9 A.M.) or evening (after 8 P.M.) to be the best time for these activities. This is when I get the least telephone interruptions, and it is before or after scheduled appointments that would require my time out of the office. During the typical business day, phone calls, planning activities, and appointments occupy most of the day. If I am working on an international project, there is more flexibility with this because of the time differences.

While the execution phase of projects and events keeps me busy moment to moment, the strategic planning and business management of my company also demand attention. The challenge for me as the owner of a small business is to carve out time for the marketing and sales arm of the business—to take time to prospect for new business at the same time that I am in the execution phase of events, so that when one project comes to an end, another will be waiting in the wings. I do this by developing fresh marketing materials using photos or components of recent meetings and events; creating video or DVD–style materials to post on my web site or to send to clients; making calls to colleagues, prospects, or venues to say "hello" or touch base; and attending luncheons or visits with past clients to keep in touch. I also try to spend time getting a pulse on new markets to explore or niche areas to develop in my business. I typically subscribe to a wide variety of industry and professional magazines and try to end my day flipping through and tearing out articles that may be useful.

Sometimes I feel I eat, sleep, and live special events, and in many ways, I do. But work doesn't take up every moment of my life. As a mother and wife, I still try to create a fun, loving home for my family by cooking dinner almost every night and by walking daily with my husband and two dogs. These breaks during the day give me downtime and a chance to regroup. I am also active in the music ministry at my local church as a youth choir director, which offers me spiritual and community involvement. I also belong to a book group, which I often attend without finishing the book. There are only so many hours in the day, and I seem to use them up very quickly. But at the end of each day, I am always looking forward to the next!

Source: Courtesy of Jill Moran.

enhance that common interest, activity, or purpose. The association industry is significant in many respects—total employees, payroll, and membership—but in one area, it is the undisputed leader: It's the big spender when it comes to conventions and meetings. The following sections discuss different types of associations that participate in meetings, conventions, and expositions.

Historical Associations

Today's associations find their roots in historical times. Ancient Roman and Asian craftsmen formed associations for the betterment of their trade. The Middle Ages found associations in the form of guilds, which were created to ensure proper wages were received and to maintain work standards.

Types of Historical Associations

Trade Associations

A trade association is an industry trade group that is generally a public relations organization founded and funded by corporations that operate in a specific industry. Its purpose is generally to promote that industry through public relations (PR) activities such as advertising, education, political donation, political pressure, publishing, and astroturfing.[4]

Professional Association

A professional association is a professional body or organization, usually nonprofit, that exists to further a particular profession and to protect both the public interest and the interests of professionals.[5]

Medical and Scientific Associations

These associations are professional organizations for medical and scientific professionals. They are often based on their specific specialties and are usually national, often with subnational or regional affiliates. These associations usually offer conferences and continuing education. They often serve in capacities similar to trade unions and often take public policy stances on these issues.

Religious Organizations

Religious organizations include those groups of individuals who are part of churches, mosques, synagogues, and other spiritual or religious congregations. Religion has taken many forms in various cultures and individuals. These groups may come together in meeting places to further develop their faith, to become more aware of others who have the same faith, to organize and plan activities, to recognize their leaders, for fund-raising, and for a number of other reasons.

Government Organizations

There are thousands of government organizations in the United States made up of numerous public bodies and agencies. These types of organizations can range from federal, state, and local organizations. There are five basic types of local governments. Three of these are general-purpose governments; the remaining two include special-purpose local governments that fall into the category of school district governments and special district governments.

Types of Meetings

There are different types of meetings and purposes for having a meeting. Some of the types of meetings are annual meetings that are held by private or public companies, board and committee meetings, fund-raisers, and professional and technical meetings. The following sections describe some of the more popular types of meetings.

Annual Meetings

Annual meetings are meetings that are generally held every year by corporations or associations to inform their members of previous and future activities. In organizations run by volunteers or a paid committee, the annual meeting is generally the forum for the election of officers or representatives for the organization.

Board Meetings, Committee Meetings, Seminars and Workshops, Professional and Technical Meetings

Board meetings for corporations must be held annually, and most corporations hold meetings monthly or four times a year. Of course, not all are held in hotels, but some are, and that brings in additional revenue at the hotel. Committee meetings are generally held at the place of business and only occasionally are held in hotels. Seminars are frequently held in hotels, as are workshops and technical meetings. To meet these needs, hotels and convention centers have convention and meeting managers who go over the requirements and prepare proposals and event orders and budgets.

Corporate Meetings, Conventions, and Expositions

Meetings are mostly held by either the corporate or nonprofit industries. Both association and corporate meeting expenditures are in the billions of dollars each year. Corporations in various industries hold lots of meetings mostly for reasons of educating, training, decision making, research, sales, team building, the introduction of a new product, organization or reorganization, problem solving, and strategic planning. Corporate meetings may be held for the employees or for the general public. For employees of a company, a corporate meeting is a command performance. The major objective of corporate meeting planners is to ensure that the meetings are successful.

SMERF

Many participants in meetings are organized by either an association, a corporation, or **social, military, educational, religious, and fraternal groups (SMERF)**. Often, these groups are price conscious, because of the fact that the majority of the functions sponsored by these organizations are paid for by the individual, and sometimes the fees are not tax deductible. However, SMERF groups are flexible to ensure that their spending falls within the limits of their budgets; they are a good filler business during off-peak times.

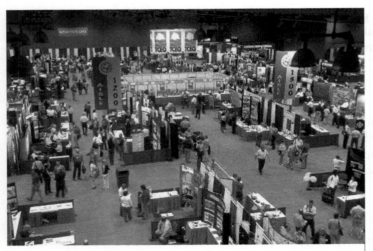

The show floor of the Environmental Quality Trade Fair and Conference.

Incentive Meetings

The **incentive market** of MICE continues to experience rapid growth as meeting planners and travel agents organize incentive travel programs for corporate employees to reward them for reaching specific targets. Incentive trips generally vary from three to six days in length and can range from a moderate trip to an extremely lavish vacation for the employee and his or her partner. The most popular destination for incentive trips is Europe, followed closely by the Caribbean, Hawaii, Florida, and California. Because incentive travel serves as the reward for a unique subset of corporate group business, participants must perceive the destination and the hotel as something special. Climate, recreational facilities, and sightseeing opportunities are high on an incentive meeting planner's list of attributes for which to look.

▶ Check Your Knowledge

1. What are three different types of meetings described in this chapter and what is their purpose?
2. What is SMERF?

Meeting Planning

Meeting planning includes not only the planning but also the successful holding of the meeting and the postmeeting evaluations. As the following sections discuss, there are a number of topics and lots of details to consider. (See Figure 5.)

Needs Analysis

Before a meeting planner can start planning a meeting, a *needs analysis* is done to determine the purpose and desired outcome of a meeting. Once the necessity of the meeting has been established, the meeting planner can then work with the party to maximize the productivity of the meeting. The key to a productive meeting is a meeting agenda. The meeting agenda may not always fall under the responsibility of the meeting planner, but it is essential for the meeting planner to be closely involved with the written agenda and also with the core purpose of the agenda, which may be different from what is stated. For example, a nonprofit organization may hold a function to promote awareness of its objectives through a fun activity, but its hidden agenda is to raise funds for the organization.

The meeting agenda provides the framework for making *meeting objectives*. The meeting planner must know what the organization is trying to accomplish so as to be successful in the management of the meeting or conference. It is helpful for the meeting planner, regardless of what role he or she plays, to plan the meeting with the meeting objectives in mind. The meeting's objectives provide

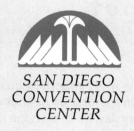

SAN DIEGO CONVENTION CENTER

EVENT MANAGER

DEFINITION

Under moderate direction from the services manager, plans, directs, and supervises assigned events and represents services manager on assigned shifts.

KEY RESPONSIBILITIES

- Plans, coordinates, and supervises all phases of the events to include set ups, move ins and outs, and the activities themselves
- Prepares and disseminates set-up information to the proper departments well in advance of the activity, and ensures complete readiness of the facilities
- Responsible for arranging for all services needed by the tenant
- Coordinates facility staffing needs with appropriate departments
- Acts as a consultant to tenants and the liaison between in-house contractors and tenants
- Preserves facility's physical plant and ensures a safe environment by reviewing tenants plans; requests and makes certain they comply with facility, state, county, and city rules and regulations
- Prepares accounting paperwork of tenant charges, approves final billings, and assists with collection of same
- Resolves complaints, including operational problems and difficulties
- Assists in conducting surveys, gathering statistical information, and working on special projects as assigned by services manager
- Conducts tours of the facilities

MINIMUM REQUIREMENTS

- Bachelor's degree in hospitality management, business, or recreational management from a fully accredited university or college, plus two (2) years of experience in coordinating major conventions and trade shows
- Combination of related education/training and additional experience may substitute for bachelor's degree
- An excellent ability to manage both fiscal and human resources
- Knowledge in public relations; oral and written communications
- Experienced with audiovisual equipment

225 Broadway, Suite 710 • San Diego, CA 92102 • (619) 239-1989
FAX (619) 239-2030
Operated by the San Diego Convention Center Corporation

Figure 5 • An Event Manager's Job Description.

A DAY IN THE LIFE OF ALEXANDRA STOUT

Professional Meeting Planner

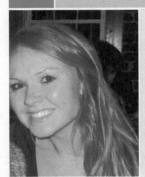

In most careers, organization and communication are two of the most important qualities to have. As a professional meeting planner, organization and communication defines what needs to be done on a daily basis. I work with different clients every day. No client is the same, and no client will have the same request as another, so being able to listen effectively to the wants and needs of an individual or group of individuals is what I focus on first. The second step is understanding the purpose the client has for their meeting or conference and organizing the details to carry out that purpose.

When I initially meet with a client, some know exactly what they need, and others only have an idea of what they need, which is often a challenge. For the clients who only have an idea, I must cover all aspects of their meeting by asking them what message they want to send. Once I reveal that message, I can ask additional questions that will assist in creating a successful meeting. For example, will there be guest speakers, food and/or beverages, accommodations, printed material, or special audiovisual equipment?

Company A is hosting three guest speakers at its annual conference. Who will be greeting the guests on the day of the meeting? Where will they be staying? How will they be arriving at the venue?

Clients that host larger meetings or conferences often have more detailed requests, as it is not a reoccurring event. Organizations like Company A that will have guest speakers attend will also have larger requests such as catered meals, blocked hotel rooms in the area or at the venue for the duration of the conference, and transportation to and from the airport and the venue location. Other organizations have monthly or bimonthly meetings, and their needs are the same from week to week. Company B plans on presenting a PowerPoint presentation during its monthly regional sales meeting, it will need a projector, screen, and appropriate audio and visual elements, as well as coffee and pitchers of water for its employees. Company B also asks for an assortment of fruit and breakfast pastries to be displayed by the coffee and water. Since Company B has its sales meeting on a monthly basis, its requests from month to month rarely change.

More recently, virtual meetings have been increasing in popularity. This option not only makes travel less demanding for members of an organization but is also more cost effective. "Go to" meetings allow a high volume of individuals to join a virtual conference through their computers. With a telephone, computer microphone, and speakers, everyone can communicate with one another, share ideas, and present information just the same as a conventional meeting.

By first listening and determining the purpose and impression the client wants to communicate to another organization, its own, or a group of individuals, I am then able to organize that message into a plan. Clients always have a message they want to get across; whether it be motivation to boost employee morale within a company or to make a lasting impression on a group of potential customers for a given product for sale, a meeting always has a purpose, and my job is to create and fulfill that request from start to finish.

the framework from which the meeting planner will set the budget, select the site and facility, and plan the overall meeting or convention.

Budget

Understanding clients and knowing their needs are both extremely important; however, the budget carries the most weight. Setting the *budget* for the meeting is more successful if the meeting planner is involved in the budget planning throughout and before making a finalized decision on how much to spend in each area. Setting the budget for the meeting is not a simple task. Knowing how much there is available to spend will help the meeting planner to better guide clients with parameters by which the event is designed. Budgets are planned for various activities and the amount of the budget needed fluctuates for different sites. Therefore, a working budget is necessary to be used as a guideline for making decisions for necessary changes. When changes in the budget are made, it is wise to communicate with the meeting planner these decisions so that the planning of activities is within budgetary constraints. Revenue and expenditure estimates must be accurate and be as thorough as possible to make certain that all possible expenditures are included in the budget prior to the event.

Income for a meeting, convention, or exposition comes from grants or contributions, event sponsor contributions, registration fees, exhibitor fees, company or organization sponsoring, advertising, and the sale of educational materials.

Expenses for a meeting, a convention, or an exposition could include, but are not limited to, rental fees; meeting planner fees; marketing expenses; printing and copying expenses; support supplies, such as office supplies and mailing; on-site and support staff; audiovisual equipment; speakers; signage; entertainment and recreational expenses; mementos for guests and attendees; tours; ground transportation; spousal programs; food and beverage; and on-site personnel.

Request for Proposal and Site Inspection and Selection

No matter how large or small a meeting, it is essential that clear meeting specifications are developed in the form of a written *request for proposal/quote (RFQ)*, rather than contacting hotels by telephone to get a quote. Many larger hotels and convention centers now have online submission forms available.

Several factors are evaluated when selecting a meeting site, including location and level of service, accessibility, hotel room availability, conference room availability, price, city, restaurant service and quality, personal safety, and local attractions. Convention centers and hotels provide meeting space and accommodations as well as food and beverage facilities and service. The convention center and a hotel team from each hotel capable of handling the meeting will attempt to impress the meeting planner. The hotel sales executive will send particulars of the hotel's meeting space and a selection of banquet menus and invite the meeting planner for a site inspection. During the site inspection, the meeting planner is shown all facets of the hotel, including the meeting rooms, guest sleeping rooms, the food and beverage outlets, and any special facility that may interest the planner or the client.

Negotiation with the Convention Center or Hotel

The meeting planner has several critical interactions with hotels, including negotiating the room blocks and rates. Escorting clients on site inspections gives the hotel an opportunity to show its level of facilities and service. The most important interaction is typically with the catering/banquet/conference department associates, especially the services manager, maître d', and captains; these frontline associates can make or break a meeting. For example, meeting planners often send boxes of meeting materials to hotels expecting the hotel to automatically know for which meeting they are intended. On more than one occasion, they have ended up in the hotel's main storeroom, much to the consternation of the meeting planner. Fortunately for most meeting planners, once they have taken care of a meeting one year, subsequent years typically are very similar.

Contracts

Once the meeting planner and the hotel or conference facility have agreed on all the requirements and costs, a contract is prepared and signed by the planner, the organization, and the hotel or convention center. The *contract* is a legal document that binds two or more parties. In the case of meetings, conventions, and expositions, a contract binds an association or organization and the hotel or convention center. The components that make up an enforceable contract include the following:

1. *An offer:* The offer simply states, in as precise a manner as possible, exactly what the offering party is willing to do, and what he or she expects in return. The offer may include specific instructions for how, where, when, and to whom the offer is made.

2. *Consideration:* The payment exchanged for the promise(s) contained in a contract. For a contract to be valid, consideration must flow both ways. For example, the consideration is for a convention center to provide services and use of its facilities in exchange for a consideration of a stated amount to be paid by the organization or host.

3. *Acceptance:* The unconditional agreement to the precise terms and conditions of an offer. The acceptance must mirror exactly the terms of the offer for the acceptance to make the contract valid. The best way to indicate acceptance of an offer is by agreeing to the offer in writing.[6]

Most important to be considered legally enforceable, a contract must be made by parties who are legally able to contract, and the activities specified in the contract must not be in violation of the law. Contracts should include clauses on "attrition and performance," meaning that the contract has a clause to protect the hotel or convention facility in the event that the organizer's numbers drop below an acceptable level. Because the space reserved is supposed to produce a certain amount of money, if the numbers drop, so does the money; unless there is a clause that says something like "there will be a guaranteed revenue of $$$ for the use of the room/space." The performance part of the clause means that a certain amount of food and beverage revenue will be charged for regardless of whether it is consumed.

Organizing and Preconference Meetings

The average lead time required for organizing a small meeting is about three to six months; larger meetings and conferences take much longer and are booked years in advance. Some meetings and conventions choose the same location each year and others move from city to city, usually from the East Coast to the Midwest or West Coast.

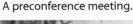
A preconference meeting.

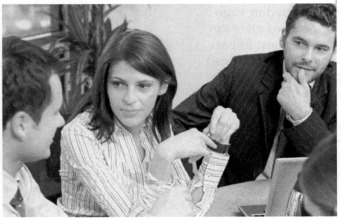

Conference Event Order

A conference event order has all the information necessary for all department employees to be able to refer to for details of the setup (times and layout) and the conference itself (arrival, meal times and what food and beverages are to be served, and the cost of items so that the billing can be done). An example of a conference event order is given in Figure 6.

EVENT DOCUMENT
REVISED COPY
/6/SAN DIEGO INTERNATIONAL BOAT SHOW
Tuesday, January 4, 2005–Tuesday, January 11, 2005

SPACE: Combined Exhibit Halls AB, Hall A - How Manager's Office, Box Office by Hall A, Hall B – Show Manager's Office, Mezzanine Room 12, Mezzanine Room 13, Mezzanine Rooms 14 A&B, AND Mezzanine Rooms 15 A&B

CONTACT: Mr. Jeff Hancock
National Marine Manufacturers Association, Inc.
4901 Morena Blvd.
Suite 901
San Diego, CA 92117
Telephone Number: (619) 274-9924
Fax Number: (619) 274-6760
Decorator Co.:   Greyhound Exposition Services
Sales Person: Denise Simenstad
Event Manager: Jane Krause
Event Tech.:   Sylvia A. Harrison

SCHEDULE OF EVENTS:

Monday, January 3, 2005   5:00 am–6:00 pm   Combined Exhibit Halls AB
Service contractor move in GES,
Andy Quintena

Tuesday, January 4, 2005   8:00 am–6:00 pm   Combined Exhibit Halls AB
Service contractor move in GES,
Andy Quintena
12:00 pm–6:00 pm
Combined Exhibit Halls AB
Exhibitor move in

Wednesday, January 5, 2005   8:00 am–6:00 pm   Combined Exhibit Halls AB
Exhibitor move in
Est. attendance: 300

Thursday, January 6, 2005   8:00 am–12:00 pm   Combined Exhibit Halls AB
Exhibitor final move in
11:30 am–8:30 pm   Box Office by Hall A
OPEN: Ticket prices, Adults $6, Children 12 & under $3

Figure 6 • Conference Event Document.
(Courtesy of the San Diego Convention Center Corporation.)

FOCUS ON MARKETING

Meetings and Conventions Information Search

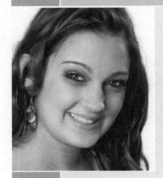

Amanda Alexander, M.S., Ph.D., Student

The meeting and conventions industry is one of the fastest growing sectors of the tourism and hospitality field, with expenditures in the billions of dollars and annual revenue growth. An event planner is responsible for organizing convention personnel and securing accommodations, transportation, guest speakers, food service, or equipment needs for the organization and production of an event. An event planner can act as a gatekeeper of information to his or her client, and therefore it is important that information is disseminated to the event planner and then the client. Understanding how event planners obtain their information is vital for the meeting and convention businesses.

Event planners can obtain information through various mediums including print, TV, radio, Internet, and word of mouth. The continuing advancement of Internet capabilities has allowed businesses to showcase their product or services in a way that hasn't been possible before, for example, through virtual tours of a property. Social media sites have changed how information is presented and how users can interact with other users to get personal experiences (virtual word of mouth) and reviews of a business. Applications on phones have allowed individuals to "check in" when they arrive at locations and then post this information on social media sites; this can create awareness of a business that otherwise may have not occurred. While many social media sites are driven by consumers, a business should monitor the site to ensure that negative comments are handled from a customer service perspective.

Even though the Internet offers many strategic opportunities, the medium that has been shown to be trusted and deemed most reliable by event planners is word of mouth. Word of mouth occurs when information is passed from one person to another. An individual will give attention to a source (another person) if the source is considered to be significant in making a decision. So how does a business ensure that event planners are receiving information via word of mouth? The following are a few tactics that will encourage word-of-mouth marketing to reach event planners:

- Making convention and visitors bureaus and destination management companies aware of your services and products through site visits and trials
- Having a sales member make cold calls to event planners and be available to meet one on one with event planners
- Creating a presence within organizations/associations such as the International Special Event Society (ISES) during meetings and annual conventions
- Following up after an event planner has used your business to find out what could have made the experience more positive (this will be an indication of what event planners are saying to others about your business)

Working in the meeting and conventions industry can be very exciting and rewarding, but to achieve success, whether an event planner or a business that offers services or products, knowing where and how to present information that leads to a decision is vital. As with all marketing tactics and strategies, the goal is to gain attention by the target market and create awareness of a product/service that is needed by the target market.

Postevent Meeting

A postevent meeting is held to evaluate the event—what went well and what should be improved for next time. Larger conferences have staff from the hotel or convention center where the event will be held the following year so that they can better prepare for the event when it is held at their facility.

Venues for Meetings, Conventions, and Expositions

Most of the time, meetings and functions are held in hotels, convention centers, city centers, conference centers, universities, corporate offices, or resorts, but more and more, meetings are housed in unique venues such as cruise ships and historical sites.

City Centers

City centers are good venues for some conferences because they are convenient to reach by air and ground transportation. There is plenty of action in a major city center; attractions range from cultural to scenic beauty. Most cities have a convention center and several hotels to accommodate guests.

Convention Centers

Convention centers throughout the world compete to host the largest exhibitions, which can be responsible for adding several million dollars in revenue to the local economy. Convention centers are huge facilities with parking, information services, business centers, and food and beverage facilities included.

Usually, convention centers are corporations owned by county, city, or state governments and are operated by a board of appointed representatives from the various groups having a vested interest in the successful operation of the center. The board appoints a president or general manager to run the center according to a predetermined mission, goals, and objectives.

Convention centers have a variety of expositions and meeting rooms to accommodate both large and small events. The centers generate revenue from the rental of space, which frequently is divided into booths (one booth is about 100 square feet). Large exhibits may take several booths' space. Additional revenue is generated by the sale of food and beverages, concession stand rentals, and vending machines. Many centers also have their own subcontractors to handle staging, construction, lighting, audiovisual, electrical, and communications.

In addition to the megaconvention centers, a number of prominent centers also contribute to the local, state, and national economies. One good example is the Rhode Island Convention Center. The $82 million center, representing the second largest public works project in the state's history, is located in the heart of downtown Providence, adjacent to the 14,500-seat Providence Civic Center. The 365,000-square-foot center offers a 100,000-square-foot main exhibit hall, a 20,000-square-foot ballroom, eighteen meeting rooms, and a full-service kitchen that can produce 5,000 meals per day. The exhibit hall divides into four separate halls, and the facility features its own telephone system, allowing individualized billing. A special rotunda function room at the front of the building features glass walls that offer a panoramic view of downtown Providence for receptions of up to 365 people. Extensive use of glass on the façade of the center provides ample natural light throughout the entrance and prefunction areas.

Conference Centers

A conference center is a specially designed learning environment dedicated to hosting and supporting small- to medium-sized meetings, typically between twenty and

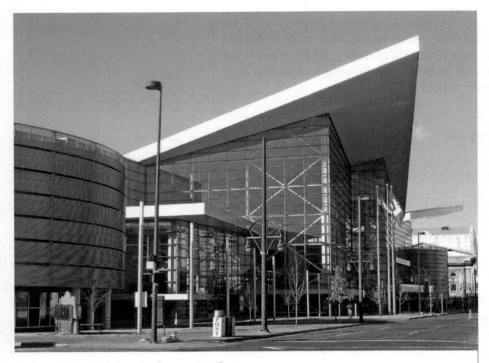
Denver, Colorado, Convention Center.

fifty people.[7] The nature of a conference meeting is to promote a distraction-free learning environment. Conference centers are designed to encourage sharing of information in an inviting, comfortable atmosphere, and to focus sharply on meetings and what makes them effective. Although the groups that hold meetings in conference centers are typically small in terms of attendees, there are thousands of small meetings held every month. Increasingly, hotels are now going after executive meetings where expense is not a major issue.

Hotels and Resorts

Hotels and resorts offer a variety of locations from city center to destination resorts. Many hotels have ballrooms and other meeting rooms designed to accommodate groups of various sizes. Today, they all have web sites and offer meeting planners to help with the planning and organizing of conferences and meetings. Once the word gets out that a meeting planner is seeking a venue for a conference, there is plenty of competition among the hotels to get the business.

Cruise Ships

Meeting in a nontraditional facility can provide a unique and memorable experience for the meeting attendee. However, many of the challenges faced in traditional venues such as hotels and convention centers are also applicable to these facilities. In some cases, planning must begin much earlier for alternative meeting environments than with traditional facilities. A thorough understanding of goals and objectives, budget, and attendee profile of the meeting is essential to negotiate the best package possible. A cruise ship meeting is a uniquely different meeting setting and offers a number of advantages to the attendees such as discounts, complimentary meals, less outside distraction while at sea, entertainment, and visiting more than one destination while unpacking only once![8]

Colleges and Universities

More and more, alternative venues for meeting places include facilities such as colleges, universities, and their campuses. The paramount consideration in contemplating use of campus-based facilities is to know the nature of the target audience.[9] A certain knowledge and evaluation of the participants are inevitable and invaluable because, most of the time, the relative cost of campus-based meetings is less expensive than a medium-priced hotel.

Sustainable Meetings, Conventions, and Expositions

The meetings industry is becoming more responsible in its environmental stewardship, and it makes economic sense to do so. Companies that choose to do so are reporting higher gross margins, higher return on sales, higher return on assets, and a stronger cash flow within its own organization. Although there are some upfront costs with going green, the end result is generally a significant savings.[10]

Taking small steps to go green can make an enormous difference in a company's bottom line, as well as in the environment. Simply switching from bottled water to pitchers of water for attendees saved Oracle $1.5 million at its Open World event in San Francisco. Reusing name-badge holders saved another $500 in just one year. In addition to monetary savings to these groups, the amount of waste deposited into a landfill was dramatically reduced, just by making these small changes.

Convention centers are going green by reducing the heat, light, and power consumption. LEED (Leadership in Energy and Environmental Design) buildings require far less energy to air-condition the building, less electric lighting due to increased natural lighting, and less water consumption because of low-flow toilets and faucets that supply water when a sensor is triggered.

In an effort to encourage and support sustainability, various industry certifications have been introduced, including the Green Meeting Guide and the Certification in Green Meetings and Events (CGME). CGME is designed to help meeting planners organize meetings in a sustainable and socially responsible way. Additionally, there are carbon footprint calculators.

Career Information

Meetings, incentive travel, conventions, and expositions (the MICE segment) offer a broad range of career paths. Successful meeting planners are detail-oriented, organized people who not only plan and arrange meetings, but also negotiate hotel rooms and meeting space in hotels and convention centers.

Incentive travel careers include aspects of organizing high-end travel, hotels, restaurants, attractions, and entertainment. With big budgets, this can be an exciting career for those interested in a combination of travel and hotels in exotic locations.

Conventions and convention centers offer several career paths, from assistants to event managers to sales managers for a special type of account (e.g., associations) or territory. Senior sales managers are expected to book large conventions and expositions—yes, everyone has their quota. Event managers plan and organize the function/event with the client once the contract has been signed. Salaries range from $35,000 to $70,000 for both assistants on rise to sales or event managers. Careers are also possible in the companies that service the MICE segment.

Someone has to equip the convention center, get it ready for an exposition, and supply all the food and beverage items. Off-premise catering for special events also offers careers for creative people who like to come up with concepts and themes around which an event or function may be planned.

For all career paths, it is critical to gain experience in the areas of your interest. Ask people you respect to be your mentor. Ask questions! When you show enthusiasm, people will respond with more help and advice. Figure 7 illustrates a career path to becoming a meeting planner; Figure 8 shows an event manager's job description at a convention center.

John Moors, former administrator of the Tampa Convention Centre, offers the following advice: "The convention and meeting industry needs qualified candidates. Many come into the convention side of the industry with transferable skills from hotels and resorts with basic business principles. We hire personalities, not résumés. It does not take long to learn how to set up a meeting room. It does, however, take experience to learn how to lead people—this leadership aspect is very important. Get your degree! But remember, it's not only what you learn in the classroom, but also your demonstrated ability to stick to something and achieve it. So get into the industry and find a mentor. Good luck!"

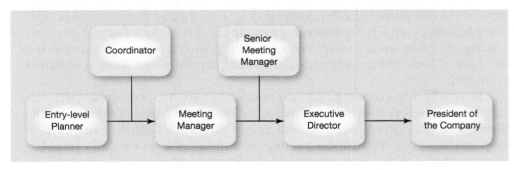

Figure 7 • A Career Path to Becoming a Top-Level Event Manager.

SAN DIEGO
CONVENTION
CENTER

EVENT MANAGER

DEFINITION

Under moderate direction from the services manager, plans, directs, and supervises assigned events and represents services manager on assigned shifts.

KEY RESPONSIBILITIES

- Plans, coordinates, and supervises all phases of the events to include set-ups, move ins and outs, and the activities themselves
- Prepares and disseminates set-up information to the proper departments well in advance of the activity, and ensures complete readiness of the facilities
- Responsible for arranging for all services needed by the tenant
- Coordinates facility staffing needs with appropriate departments
- Acts as a consultant to tenants and the liaison between in-house contractors and tenants
- Preserves facility's physical plant and ensures a safe environment by reviewing tenants' plans; requests and makes certain they comply with facility, state, county, and city rules and regulations
- Prepares accounting paperwork of tenant charges, approves final billings, and assists with collection of same
- Resolves complaints, including operational problems and difficulties
- Assists in conducting surveys, gathering statistical information, and working on special projects as assigned by services manager
- Conducts tours of the facilities

MINIMUM REQUIREMENTS

- Bachelor's degree in hospitality management, business, or recreational management from a fully accredited university or college, plus two (2) years of experience in coordinating major conventions and trade shows
- Combination of related education/training and additional experience may substitute for bachelor's degree
- An excellent ability to manage both fiscal and human resources
- Knowledge in public relations; oral and written communications
- Experienced with audiovisual equipment

225 Broadway, Suite 710 • San Diego, CA 92102 • (619) 239-1989
FAX (619) 239-2030
Operated by the San Diego Convention Center Corporation

Figure 8 • Event Manager's Job Description.

Trends in Meetings, Conventions, and Expositions

- More people are going abroad to attend meetings.
- Some international shows do not travel very well (i.e., agricultural machinery). Thus, organizations such as Bleinheim and Reed Exposition Group airlift components and create shows in other countries.
- Competitiveness has increased among all destinations. Convention centers will expand and new centers will come online.

- The industry needs to be more sophisticated. The need for fiber optics is present everywhere.
- Compared to a few years ago, large conventions are not as well attended, and regional conventions have more attendees.

CASE STUDY

Double-Booked

The convention bureau in a large and popular convention destination has jurisdiction over the convention center. A seasoned convention sales manager, who has worked for the bureau for seven years and produces more sales than any other sales manager, has rebooked a 2,000-person group for a three-day exposition in the convention center. The exposition is to take place two years from the booking date.

The client has a fifteen-year history of holding conventions, meetings, and expositions in this convention center and has always used the bureau to contract all space and services. In fact, the sales manager handling the account has worked with the client for seven of the fifteen years. The bureau considers this client a "preferred customer."

The convention group meeting planner also appears in a magazine ad giving a testimony of praise for the convention bureau, this particular sales manager, and the city as a destination for conventions.

Shortly after the meeting planner rebooks this convention with the bureau, the bureau changes sales administration personnel, not once, but three times. This creates a challenge for the sales manager in terms of producing contracts, client files, and event profiles, and in the recording and distribution of information. The preferred customer who rebooked has a contract, purchase orders for vendor services, a move-in and setup agenda, and an event profile, all supplied by the sales manager. The sales manager has copies of these documents as well. The two hotels where the group will be staying also have contracts for the VIP group.

As is the nature of this particular bureau, other sales managers have been booking and contracting space for the same time period as the group that rebooked. In fact, the exhibit hall has been double-booked, as have the breakout rooms for seminars, workshops, and food and beverage service. The groups that were contracted later are all first-time users of the facility.

This situation remains undetected until ten days prior to the groups' arrival. It is brought to the attention of the bureau and convention center only when the sales manager distributes a memo to schedule a precconvention meeting with the meeting planner and all convention center staff.

Because of the administrative personnel changes, necessary information was not disseminated to key departments and key personnel. The convention center was never notified that space has been contracted for the preferred customer. The preferred customer has been told about this potentially catastrophic situation. Now there is a major problem to rectify.

Discussion Questions

1. Ultimately, who is responsible for decision making with regard to this situation?
2. What steps should be taken to remedy this situation?
3. Are there fair and ethical procedures to follow to provide space for the preferred customer? If so, what are they?
4. What measures, if any, should be taken in handling the seasoned sales manager?
5. What leverage does the meeting planner have to secure this and future business with the bureau?
6. What might the preferred customer do if it is denied space and usage of the convention center?
7. How can this situation be avoided in the future?

Summary

1. Conventions, meetings, and expositions serve social, political, sporting, or religious purposes. Associations offer benefits such as a political voice, education, marketing avenues, member services, and networking.
2. Meetings are events designed to bring people together for the purpose of exchanging information. Typical forms of meetings are conferences, workshops, seminars, forums, and symposiums.
3. Expositions bring together purveyors of products, equipment, and services in an environment in which they can demonstrate their products. Conventions are meetings that include some form of exposition or trade show.
4. Meeting planners contract out their services to associations and corporations. Their responsibilities include premeeting, on-site, and postmeeting activities.
5. The convention and visitors bureaus are nonprofit organizations that assess the needs of the client and organize transportation, hotel accommodations, restaurants, and attractions.
6. Convention centers are huge facilities, usually owned by the government, where meetings and expositions are held. Events at convention centers require a lot of up-front planning and careful event management. A contract that is based on the event profile and an event document is part of effective management.

Key Words and Concepts

associations
convention
convention and visitors bureaus (CVBs)
convention center
exposition
familiarization (FAM) trip
incentive market

meeting
meeting planner
meetings, incentive travel, conventions, and exhibitions (MICE)
social, military, educational, religious, and fraternal groups (SMERF)

Review Questions

1. What are associations and what is their purpose?
2. List the number of different people and organizations involved with meetings, conventions, and expositions.
3. List the primary sources of revenue and expenses involved in holding a meeting, a convention, and an exposition.
4. Describe the main types of meeting setups.
5. Explain the difference between an exposition and a convention.
6. List the duties of CVBs.
7. Describe the topics a meeting planner needs to deal with before, during, and after a meeting.

Internet Exercises

1. Organization: **Best of Boston**
   Web site: **www.bestboston.com**
   Summary: Best of Boston is an event-planning company that specializes in putting together packages for different events, such as conventions, corporate events, private parties, and weddings.
   > (a) Explore this web site for events and list the different kinds of events this organization can organize.
   > (b) After browsing the web site, discuss the importance of networking in the meetings, conventions, and expositions industry.

2. Organization: **M & C Online**
   Web site: **www.meetings-conventions.com**
   Summary: This excellent web site offers in-depth information on meetings and conventions from different perspectives, ranging from legal issues to unique themes and concepts.
   > (a) Click the "Latest News" heading (it's on the left side of the page). What is the latest news?
   > (b) Click "Current Issue" (at the top of the page), then "On the Cover" (on the left side near the top). See what the cover stories are, and then share your findings with your class.

Apply Your Knowledge

Make a master plan with all the steps necessary for holding a meeting or seminar on careers in hospitality management.

Suggested Activity

Contact meeting planners in your area, and, with permission of your professor, invite them to speak to the class about their work and how they do it.

Prepare questions in advance so that they may be given to the speaker ahead of time.

Endnotes

1. http://www.asaecenter.org/advocacy/contentASAEOnly.cfm?ItemNumber=16341
2. George G. Fenich, *Meetings, Expositions, and Conventions: An Introduction to the Industry*, 3rd ed. (Upper Saddle River, NJ: Pearson, 2012), 23.
3. George G. Fenich, *Meetings, Expositions, and Conventions: An Introduction to the Industry*, 25.
4. Wikipedia, *Trade Association*, http://en.wikipedia.org/wiki/Trade_association (accessed November 21, 2011).
5. Wikipedia, *Professional Association*, http://en.wikipedia.org/wiki/Professional_association (accessed November 21, 2011).

6. Steven Barth, *Hospitality Law: Managing Issues in the Hospitality Industry* (Hoboken, NJ: John Wiley and Sons, 2006), 26–29.
7. Professional Convention Management Association, *Professional Meeting Management*, 4th ed. (Dubuque, IA: Kendall/Hunt, 2004), 557–561.
8. Professional Convention Management Association, *Professional Meeting Management*, 564–565.
9. Professional Convention Management Association, *Professional Meeting Management*, 552.
10. George G. Fenich, *Meetings, Expositions, and Conventions: An Introduction to the Industry*, 249.

Glossary

Convention   A generic term referring to any size business or professional meeting held in one specific location, which usually includes some form of trade show or exposition. Also refers to a group of delegates or members who assemble to accomplish a specific goal.
Convention center   A large meeting place.
Exposition   An event held mainly to promote informational exchanges among trade people. A large exhibition in which the presentation is the main attraction, as well as being a source of revenue for an exhibitor.
Familiarization (FAM) trip   A free or reduced-price trip given to travel agents, travel writers, or other intermediaries to promote destinations.
Meeting   A gathering of people for a common purpose.
Meeting planner   An individual who coordinates every detail of meetings and conventions.

Photo Credits

Credits are listed in the order of appearance.

Yuri Arcurs/Shutterstock
Alexander Raths/Fotolia
Dorling Kindersley/Nigel Hicks/DK Images
Alan Keohane/Dorling Kindersley, Ltd
Dana White/PhotoEdit
Jill Moran

Bob Daemmrich/PhotoEdit
Alexandra Stout
Marcin Balcerzak/Shutterstock
Dr. Amanda Alexander, University of Missouri
Dean Allen Caron/Shutterstock

Special Events

From Chapter 13 of *Introduction to Hospitality Management*, Fourth Edition. John R. Walker. Copyright © 2013 by Pearson Education, Inc. Published by Pearson. All rights reserved.

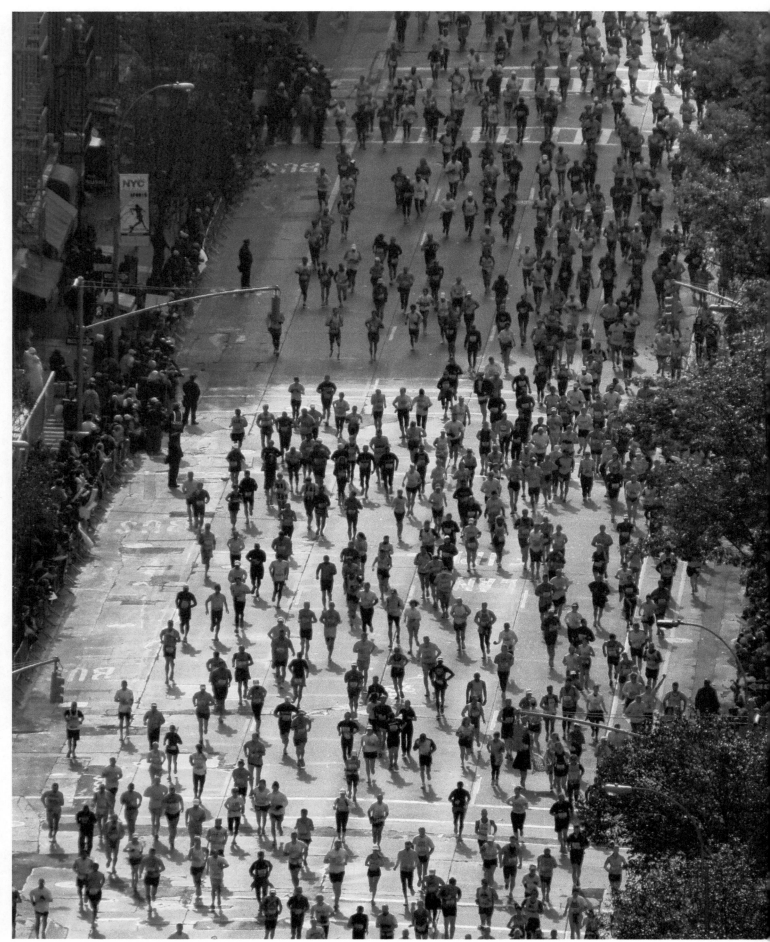

Special Events

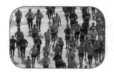
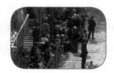
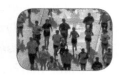
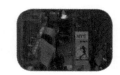

*The **special events industry** is a dynamic, diverse field that has seen considerable growth and change over the past forty years. Today, the industry employs professionals who work together to provide a broad range of services to create what is termed a special event. But what is a special event? Dr. Joe J. Goldblatt, a leading academic and author in the special events field, distinguishes between daily events and special events in the following manner:*

Daily Events	Special Events	Examples of Special Events
Occur spontaneously	Are always planned	A convention
Do not arouse expectations	Always arouse expectations	A meeting
Usually occur without a reason	Are usually motivated by a reason for a celebration	A festival or wedding

*He uses these contributing factors to shape a definition of a special event: "A special event recognizes a unique moment in time with ceremony and ritual to satisfy specific needs."[1] The scope of this definition is very broad and encompasses many "moments." Special events include countless functions, such as **corporate seminars** and **workshops**, **conventions** and **trade shows**, **charity balls** and **fundraisers**, **fairs** and **festivals**, and **social functions** such as **weddings** and **holiday parties**. It is for this reason that the industry has seen such growth and presents so much potential for future careers and management opportunities.*

Food, clothing, and shelter are the accepted basic physical needs that humans require. Following those needs is an emotional need to celebrate, which has a direct impact on the human spirit. All societies celebrate—whether publicly or privately, as individuals or in groups. The need to celebrate has been recognized by corporations, public and government officials, associations, and individuals. This has contributed to the rapid growth of the special events industry with a wide range of possible employment opportunities. When you consider all of the planners, caterers, producers, event sites, and others that become part of the special event, you can imagine the potential for future careers and employment possibilities.

Event management is a newcomer in the hospitality industry compared with the hotel and restaurant industries. Yet as you will soon learn, special events is a field that doesn't have rigid boundaries. Closely related fields that may overlap include marketing, sales, catering, and entertainment. Future growth trends in special events management provide plenty of career opportunities in all hospitality sectors.

This chapter gives you an overview of the special events industry. You will learn about the various classifications of special events and where future career opportunities can be found. You will find information on the skills and abilities required to be successful in the field. Information on special events organizations, strategic event planning, and the future outlook of the industry will allow you to take a glimpse into this exciting, rewarding, and evolving field. As Frank Supovitz, Vice President of Special Events for the National Hockey League in New York, says, "The stakes have never been higher. Sponsors are savvier. Audiences are more demanding. And, event producers and managers are held accountable by their clients to meet their financial and marketing goals more than ever before. . . . So before the lights go down and the curtain rises, reach out for the experience and expertise in these pages . . . and explore the opportunities in special events management."[2]

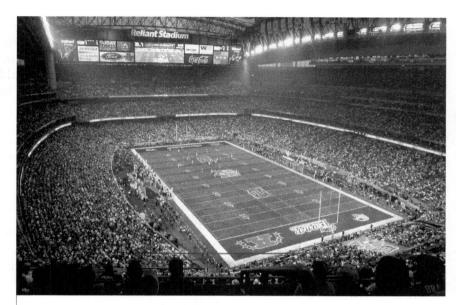

Someone has to manage this incredible event, the Super Bowl.

What Event Planners Do

Event planning is a general term that refers to a career path in the growing field of special events. Its forecast includes a growing demand for current and future employment opportunities. Like several other professions, event planning came about to fill a gap—someone needed to be in charge of all the gatherings, meetings, conferences, and so on that were increasing in size, number, and spectacle among the business and leisure sectors. Corporate managers had to step away from their assignments to take on the additional challenges of planning conventions and conferences. Government officials and employees were displaced from their assignments to arrange recruitment fairs and military events. Consequently, whenever a special event was to be held, the planner became a person whose job description did not include "planning."

The title **event planner** was first introduced at hotels and convention centers. Event planners are responsible for planning an event, from start to finish. This includes setting the date and location, advertising the event, and providing refreshments or arranging catering services, speakers, or entertainment. Please keep in mind that this is a general list and will vary depending on the type, location, and nature of the event.

" Associations can be a valuable resource for students interested in a career in event management. Many offer scholarships and provide a great networking opportunity. "

Karen Harris

A VGM Career Book, *Opportunities in Event Planning Careers*, has the following to say about a good candidate: "In addition to good organizational skills, someone with a creative spirit, a flair for the dramatic, a sense of adventure, and a love of spectacle could expect to flourish in this field." Highlighted skills and characteristics of a future professional in this field include the following:

Computer skills

Willingness to travel

Willingness to work a flexible schedule

Experience in delegating

Willingness to work long hours

Negotiating skills

Verbal and written communication skills

Enthusiasm

Project management skills

Follow-through skills

Ability to work with high-level executives

Budgeting skills

Ability to initiate and close sales

Lots of patience

Ability to handle multiple tasks simultaneously

Ability to be a self-starter

Ability to interact with other departments[3]

Event Management

Event management can be as small as planning an office outing, to something larger like organizing a music festival and as large as planning the Super Bowl or even the Olympics. Events can be one-off, annual (happening each year), or every four years, as for the Olympics. Things do not just happen by themselves; it takes a great deal of preparation to stage a successful event. To hold a successful event, the organizer should have a vision and leader/manager skills in the following key result areas: marketing, financial, operational, and legal. Getting good sponsorship is a big help. Sponsors provide money or in-kind contributions and receive recognition as sponsors of the event, including use or display of their logos in the event's promotion. Sponsors expect to get something in return for their sponsorship, so give them something tangible that will help their corporation or organization. Each year, thousands go to festivals and events of all kinds, and most, if not close to all, events receive some sponsorship, because it is too costly to stage an event without sponsorship.

Event management requires special skills in marketing and sales (to attract the business in the first place), planning (to ensure all details are covered and that everything will be ready on time), organization (to make sure all key staff know what to do, why, when, where, and how), financial (a budget needs to be made and kept to), human resources and motivation (the best people need to be selected and recruited, trained, and motivated), lots of patience, and attention to detail and endless checking on them. To gain business, event managers prepare a proposal for the client's approval and contract signature. There are some important how-tos in preparing an event proposal: Find out as much information as possible about the event (if it has been previously held) or what

> The art of networking will allow you to build a contact base that will help you succeed in the event industry.
>
> Karen Harris

516

the client really has in mind. Ask organizers, attendees, providers, and others what went right and what went wrong or what could be improved on next time the event is organized. Write the proposal in business English, no elaborate or florid language. Finally, do the numbers—nobody wants a surprise—do a proforma invoice so that the client will know the costs, and surprise the client by being on time and on budget.

An event can be costly to put on; in addition to advertising, there is a location charge, security costs, labor costs, and production costs (this may be food, beverage, and service, but also staging and decor). Usually, the event manager has a good estimate of the number of ticket sales expected. He or she then budgets the costs to include the entertainment and all other costs, leaving a reasonable profit.

Event management also takes place at convention centers and hotels, where event managers handle all the arrangements after the sales manager has completed the contract. The larger convention center events are planned years in advance. As stated earlier, the convention and visitors bureau is usually responsible for the booking of conventions more than eighteen months ahead. Obviously, both the convention and visitors bureau and the convention center marketing and sales teams work closely with each other. Once the booking becomes definite, the senior event manager assigns an event manager to work with the client throughout the sequence of pre-event, event, and postevent activities.

The booking manager is critical to the success of the event by booking the correct space and working with the organizers to help them save money by allocating only the space really needed and allowing the client to begin setting up on time. A contract is written based on the event profile. The event profile stipulates in writing all the client's requirements and gives all of the relevant information, such as which company will act as decorator/subcontractor to install carpets and set up the booths.

The contract requires careful preparation because it is a legal document and will guarantee certain provisions. For example, the contract may specify that the booths may only be cleaned by center personnel or that food may be prepared for samples only, not for retail. After the contract has been signed and returned by the client, the event manager will from time to time make follow-up calls until about six months before the event, when arrangements such as security, business services, and catering will be finalized. The event manager is the key contact between the center and the client. He or she will help the client by introducing approved subcontractors who are able to provide essential services.

Two weeks prior to the event, an event document is distributed to department heads. The event document contains all the detailed information that each department needs to know for the event to run smoothly. About ten days before the event, a WAG (week at a glance) meeting is held. The WAG meeting is one of the most important meetings at the convention center because it provides an opportunity to avoid problems—like two event groups arriving at the same time or additional security for concerts or politicians. About this same time, a preconvention or pre-expo meeting is held with expo managers and their contractors— shuttle bus managers, registration operators, exhibit floor managers, and so on. Once the setup begins, service contractors marshal the eighteen-wheeler trucks to unload the exhibits by using radio phones to call the trucks from a nearby depot. When the exhibits are in place, the exposition opens and the public is admitted.

The following sections discuss the stages in the event-planning process.

Research

The first stage of event planning is to answer the following simple questions:

1. Why should a special event be held?
2. Who should hold it?
3. Where should it be held?
4. What should the focus of the event be?
5. What outcomes are expected?

Once answers to these questions are available, you can move to the second stage of event planning.

Design

The second stage in the event-planning process can be both the most exciting and the most challenging. This stage allows freedom in creativity and the implementation of new ideas that support the objectives of the special event. The design process is a time when an event manager or team can brainstorm new innovative ideas or develop adaptations to previous events to make them better, grander, and more exciting for the attendees. The design process seeks to obtain original and fresh ideas that will create an event in which it's worth investing. The event may be a corporate meeting or it may be a beachside wedding, yet the design of the event will have a lasting impression on those who attend it.

Planning

Planning, the third stage in the event-planning process, is often led by the budget determined for the event. The planning process includes contracting out services and arranging all other activities that will become part of the event. The planning process may include the following tasks:

- Determine event budget
- Select the event site
- Select hotel accommodations
- Arrange transportation
- Negotiate contracts
- Arrange catering
- Arrange speaker, entertainment, music
- Organize audiovisual needs

- Create marketing plan for the event
- Prepare invitations or event packets

The type and size of the event will ultimately determine the steps required for the planning process. The information you learn about planning from your other courses and studies will help you if you choose to pursue a career in event management.

Coordination

The process of **coordination** can be compared to a director leading a band. The band may have rehearsed a piece of music countless times, and yet during a concert the director still has the ability to "direct" or control the performance. Similarly, the event manager engages in the process of coordinating the event as it unfolds. This may be a stressful time because of unforeseen problems that occur, or it may be a truly rewarding time with a flawless execution. Regardless, coordination of the event may involve decision-making skills and abilities as the event progresses.

Coordination also relates to the human resource aspect of the special event. Event managers are leaders who, through example, motivate others. As an event manager, you will engage in coordinating staff and/or volunteers to carry out the special event's planned objectives and goals. As mentioned earlier, empowering your staff will create a positive environment and will make your job of coordinating their efforts that much easier.

Evaluation

Evaluation should take place during each of the stages of the event-planning process and is a final step that can measure the success of the event in meeting the goals and objectives. If you take a look at the event-planning process diagram in Figure 1, you will notice that it is a continuous process. Outcomes are compared to expectations and variances investigated and corrected.

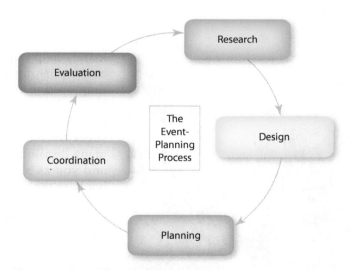

Figure 1 • Event-Planning Process Diagram.

Challenges and Tools for Event Planners and Managers

If you are at this point considering a professional career in event management, there are event-planning tools that you can use to your advantage as you pursue a career in this field. There are four primary challenges professional event managers face: time, finance, technology, and human resources.

Time management plays an important role in event planning, and it is an element that can be used effectively by budgeting your time the same way that you would your finances. Delegating tasks to the appropriate people, keeping accurate records and lists, preparing agendas before meetings, and focusing on what items deserve top priority are all examples of how to use time management effectively.

Financial management becomes important for an event planner when it becomes necessary for you to evaluate financial data, management fees, vendor fees, and so forth. This does not mean that you have to be a financial wizard; however, knowledge in this area will greatly enhance your opportunity to make profitable and sound decisions. There are resources that can be used in this area such as obtaining help or counsel from a financial professional and using technology that will help with event accounting.

Utilizing technology as a tool in event management can be a great opportunity to assist in the previous two areas. Software programs for word processing, financial management, and database management can help in daily tasks and event planning. Other technology products that are used by event professionals include laptop computers, cell phones, handheld devices, event management software, and the Internet.

The final tool relates to the effective management of your human resources. Empowering your employees is the key to success. As a manager and leader, you must train your employees and/or volunteers and give them the necessary information to perform their jobs. It is critical to select the right people, empower them, and develop their skills. This will ultimately help you succeed in accomplishing your goals. Empowering event staff can be used to allow them to make important decisions—successful events require many decisions to be made, and you as a manager will not have the time to make all of them. Empowering your team is the greatest tool you can use to become an effective leader and improve the performance of your staff.

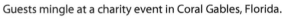
Guests mingle at a charity event in Coral Gables, Florida.

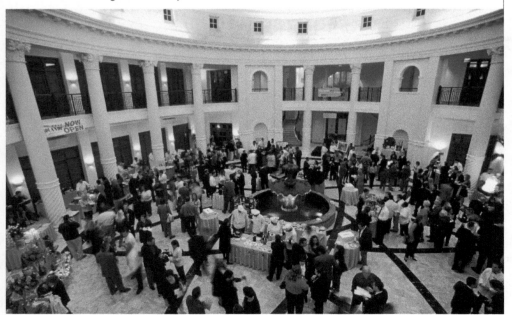

► Check Your Knowledge

1. Give some examples to distinguish the differences between a daily event and a special event.
2. What are event planners responsible for?
3. Name the stages in the event-planning process.

Classifications of Special Events

The special events industry has been divided up into the following classifications:

- Corporate events (seminars, workshops, meetings, conferences)
- Association events (conventions, trade shows, meetings)
- Charity balls and fund-raising events
- Social functions (weddings, engagement parties, holiday functions)
- Fairs and festivals
- Concerts and sporting events

A poll taken from a wide variety of event professionals in the industry, *Event Solutions Black Book*, lists the following as the most popular types of event sites:

Hotel/resort	62.0 percent
Convention center	32.5 percent
Tent/structure	32.6 percent
Banquet hall	29.0 percent
Outdoors	21.8 percent
Corporate facility	28.4 percent
Museum/zoo/gardens	12.4 percent
Arena/stadium/theater	18.0 percent
Restaurant	16.1 percent
Private residence	22.8 percent
Club	16.7 percent[4]

With those figures in mind, take a closer look at the various classifications that make up this exciting industry. Each category has its own unique characteristics, rewards, and challenges. As a human resource specialist would say, "It's important to put the right person in the right position." This statement also holds true for special events. Any career selection, especially for a person seeking the management level, should look for the correct "fit." With such a vast array of options, you may find one that ignites your passion for the field, you may find several that are the wrong size before finding the right one, or you may decide that this is not the right match for your personality and goals. The following may help you to decide whether your future holds a professional career in the special events industry.

Corporate Events

Corporate events continue to lead the industry in terms of event business. About 80 percent of the event market is corporate events.

Corporate event managers are employed by the company to plan and execute the details of meetings for the corporation's employees, management, and owners. The growing use of special events in the corporate arena created the need for positions dedicated to the planning and management of them. The corporate event planners engage in the following management activities: They are involved in the planning and organizing of events, and they play a key leadership role. Additionally, the planner must possess the following skills: effective communication, ability to coordinate various activities, and attention to detail.

Corporate events include the following: annual meetings, sales meetings, new product launches, training meetings and workshops, management meetings, press meetings, incentive meetings, and awards ceremonies.

Corporate events benefit several sectors of the hospitality industry. For example, a client may hold an event at a major attraction like Sea World or a resort like The Breakers. Each corporate client can provide the hotel, restaurants, airlines, and other businesses in the destination's economy with tens of thousands of dollars. Corporate event planners will consider the factors most important to the attendees when using a hotel as part of the event, including corporate account rates for lodging, amenities such as fitness centers and business centers, airport transportation, and quick check-in and check-out at the hotel. Therefore, corporate event planners should have strong negotiating skills to book lodging and convention services as needed.

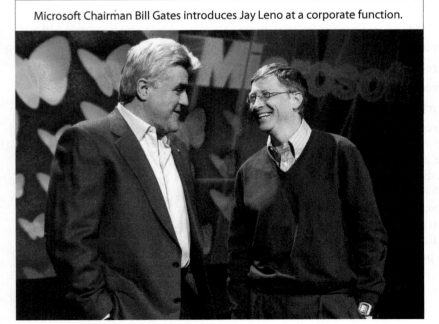

Microsoft Chairman Bill Gates introduces Jay Leno at a corporate function.

Association Events

There are more than 6,500 associations in the United States alone. The majority of the large association conventions are planned two to five years ahead of time, and the destination is a determining factor in the planning process. The American Medical Association and the American Dental Association are two of the most recognized examples of associations that hold large conventions. In the hospitality industry, the National Restaurant Association (NRA), the American Hotel & Lodging Association (AH&LA), and, at a global level, the International Association of Convention and Visitors Bureaus are a few of the many associations that hold conventions. Associations account for millions in generated revenue. This stems from the millions of people who attend thousands of meetings and conventions. For example, the American Marketing Association holds more than twenty conferences annually, which generates approximately a million for each hotel.

Events relating to associations can range from a monthly luncheon at a private club or hotel to a yearly convention that may comprise an educational seminar(s) with an opportunity to network with other association members. Associations generally hire full-time paid planners to manage the yearly national membership meeting that is a requirement for most associations as part of their bylaws. Larger associations with greater financial resources often hire full-time meeting and convention management professionals who are involved in the large association events as well as other association events, including board meetings, educational seminars, membership meetings, professional meetings, and regional meetings.

Other opportunities for employment are widespread. They may include a position as a convention manager, a special events manager in a hotel, a conference manager, or a special events manager at a private club for the events held by local associations.

In the event-planning industry, professional associations have a great impact in contributing to the development of their members. Professional associations provide training, certification, networking, and assistance with business plans and other consulting services for their members.

Charity Balls and Fund-Raising Events

Charity balls and fund-raising events provide a unique opportunity for the event manager to work with the particular group or charity, and a theme is usually chosen for the event. The event manager is then responsible for selecting the location and coordinating all of the details that will determine the success of the event, which may include catering, entertainment, décor, lighting, floral arrangements, invitations, rentals, public relations, transportation, security, and technical support.

One of the key skills that a person entering this category must possess is the ability to plan the event on a set and often limited budget. Why is this skill so critical? These events are used to raise funds toward a set group or charity, and every dollar that is spent on the event is thereby one less dollar that could go toward the cause. Nevertheless, these events are expected to be extravagant—so a little creativity can go a long way in the planning and implementing of the theme. The event manager should also have strong negotiating skills to bargain with vendors on reduced rates or in some cases donated services or products. A smart planner will know how to market and sell the positive public relations that the event could provide to the vendors.

The demand for fund-raising event planners/managers is one that holds solid ground. To prove this point, *Opportunities in Event Planning Careers* quoted an in-house event planner as stating, "One of the major advantages of working for a nonprofit as an in-house planner for almost six years was that I never had to look for work. There were always new events to take on."[5]

"Associations can be a valuable resource for students. Many offer scholarships and provide a great networking opportunity. I received a scholarship from the American Association of University Women and was therefore prompted to join as a student affiliate. Students interested in a career in event management can gain valuable experience by attending the meetings and, more importantly, becoming involved. Volunteering is rarely turned down!"

Karen Harris

"Volunteering is one of the best ways to gain experience in the event industry, and charity/fund-raising events provide a great opportunity. I recently had the opportunity to volunteer as a banquet server for the "Star Night Gala." More importantly, however, I was provided the opportunity to meet various people involved in the planning and to ask questions! Check your local paper for "upcoming events." In addition, I found a local Charity Register that provides a calendar of events for the upcoming year.

Volunteers are not paid. Not because they are worthless, but because they are priceless."

University of South Florida, Circle K International motto.

"The ability to learn as a volunteer truly is priceless!"

Karen Harris

Social Events

Social function planners or managers work on a broad variety of events. This category of special events includes the traditional wedding and party planners with which most of us are already familiar. This category of event planning includes weddings, engagement parties, birthday parties, anniversary parties, holiday parties, graduation parties, military events, and all other social gatherings or events. A social event planner/manager is usually responsible for selecting the venue, determining any themes and/or design schemes, ordering or planning decorations, arranging for catering and entertainment, and having invitations printed and mailed.

SMERF, which stands for social, military, educational, religious, and fraternal organizations, is a category of organizations that also falls into the category of social events. Individuals of these organizations often pay for the events, meaning the events are price sensitive. Needless to say, budgeting skills are important for those working with these groups.

Weddings are the most widely recognized social event. Wedding planners are a key player in the social event category. The title seems glamorous and has a certain perception that most of us will hold; yet the management involved in planning a wedding involves strict attention to detail. Don't forget that the planner is responsible for creating what is considered to be the most important day of a couple's life. "Realize this is a business," says Gerard J. Monaghan, president of the Association of Bridal Consultants. "A fun business to be sure, but a business nonetheless." Effective wedding planners will have contacts formed for a variety of services, such as venues like hotels, wedding locations, decorating, catering, bridal shops, musicians, photographers, florists, and so forth.

Today's weddings are more expensive than those of the past, and they are often longer. Weddings have become true "special events" because of the willingness of family and friends to travel longer distances to celebrate with the bride and groom. Many weddings today have become minivacations for those attending.

▶ Check Your Knowledge

1. What events continue to lead the industry in terms of event business?
2. When are the majority of large association conventions planned?
3. What are the key skills that a person entering the charity event category must possess?
4. What is SMERF?

Fairs and Festivals

The word *fair* is likely to evoke memories of cotton candy, funnel cakes, Ferris wheels, and other games. These memories are very important to why a fair is considered a special event, but the purpose of most fairs in the United

States is usually related to the agriculture industry. A professional staff chosen by an elected committee usually produces them. Fairs are generally held at the local, county, or state level.

Festivals are planned events that are often themed to the celebration's purpose. Cultures, anniversaries, holy days, and special occasions are commonly celebrated as a festival. Mardi Gras, for example, celebrates the beginning of Lent. Food and entertainment are greatly emphasized when planning a festival. **Festivals.com** is a site that allows you to search for festivals held throughout the world. The variety of festivals is astounding—art, music, sporting, literary, performing arts, air shows, science, and even children's festivals. The web site describes cultural festivals as "Magical parades. Fabulous feasts. Dizzying dancing. The spirit of celebration crosses languages, oceans, continents and cultures, as people revel in their heritages and communities."[6]

The following is a small sampling of festivals—some are commonly known, and others are surprising:

Oktoberfest

Mardi Gras

Biketoberfest

Hispanic Heritage Festival

Street Music Festival

American Dance Festival

Polar Bear Jumpoff Festival

Gilroy Garlic Festival

Bagelfest

One of the key strategies in planning special events for fairs and festivals is to determine the purpose of the event early on. It is important to analyze the "available manpower" in the form of both professionals and volunteers who will assist in staging the event. The **International Festival & Events Association (IFEA)** provides an opportunity for event managers from around the world to network and exchange ideas on how other festivals excel in sponsorship, marketing, fund-raising, operations, volunteer coordination, and management. The IFEA is highlighted later in the chapter.

Concerts and Sporting Events

Concert promoters are an alternative career choice relating to special events. For the purpose of this text, smaller concert and music events will be the focus. Woodstock, in 1969, was a large music festival that has been labeled as a transformational event—it transformed the participants and society. Many concerts are planned as fund-raisers, such as Live Aid, which raised millions of dollars to benefit starving people of Africa through a concert that included major rock performers. On a smaller scale, universities may provide a concert as a special event.

Opening ceremonies, halftime shows, and postgame shows for sporting events provide another "arena" an event manager can select as a career path. Shows such as these are highly visible because of the large number of sporting events that are televised. This provides a unique challenge for the event manager—to satisfy the millions of television viewers as well as those watching in the stadium (or whatever the venue may be).

Sporting events have historically been more popular than other forms of entertainment. This is probably because of our competitive nature and a desire to watch those who compete—a kind of flashback to the gladiator days of old. It is important to remember when planning special events in the sports environment that the primary attention should remain on the athletes and the competition. Therefore, the special event should be staged to add to and not subtract from the sport itself. Special events may even attract additional viewers and fans to the sport. The role of special events in the sports category has plenty of room for growth and expansion as professional sports become more and more competitive.

Sports entertainment is a field that will likely see considerable growth in the future. Just think, someone has to plan, organize, and run the halftime shows and the events before and after the game. A large audience awaits your Super Bowl–sized imagination, which can ensure that every sporting event is a winning experience for the most important player of all—the fan.

Mega Sporting Events

Mega sporting events are some of the biggest moneymakers in the industry. Both large and small communities embrace mega sporting events because of the positive economic impact. Activities in sports have brought forth tremendous economic impacts.

INTRODUCING SUZANNE BAILEY

Event Director

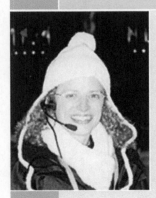

Suzanne graduated from Southern Utah University with a B.A. in Business Administration, Marketing, in 1996. Eager to get her career started, she accepted an entry-level position at Bowl Games of America (BGA), a student travel/special events production company that produces several NCAA bowl game halftime shows including the Orange Bowl (Miami, FL), Sugar Bowl (New Orleans, LA), Liberty Bowl (Memphis, TN), Alamo Bowl (San Antonio, TX), and the Gator Bowl (Jacksonville, FL). BGA recruits high school marching bands and dance groups to perform in the field shows along with guest stars. The students earn an opportunity to perform by excelling in competitions and working fund-raisers to pay for their three- to five-day trip. Within a year, Suzanne settled into the division of the company that interested her most—the tiny but growing dance division of BGA, BGA Performance, as an executive assistant.

Suzanne worked with the director of BGA Performance to create an entirely new marketing strategy, which eventually led to great success within the dance division. Rather than working with small high school dance groups exclusively, BGA Performance set up a commission system with large private dance competition companies, which would market the bowl game performance opportunities to their competition winners. This marketing strategy led to 300-percent growth in the first year.

Suzanne worked her way up the ladder to associate director and eventually director of BGA Performance. Her work changed dramatically with the seasons. During dance competition season, the marketing effort was immense—that was the time to make the big sales push. Every day, Suzanne created and sent hundreds of invitation packets to private dance competition companies and made as many sales phone calls as possible. She also reviewed audition tapes and selected dancers for the bowl game halftime shows. Once most of the dancers signed up for the bowl game they would perform in, Suzanne's work shifted to customer service and show production. A few months prior to each event, Suzanne traveled to each city with the dance directors and/or chaperones to give them a preview of what would happen during the event with their dancers.

Finally, the events took place. Suzanne became an event director during the actual events. Suzanne traveled to the destination city a few days before the dancers arrived to confirm with hotel group sales managers, caterers, rehearsal site workers, and bowl game executives. She met and directed her on-site staff (choreography team and event staff). The workdays of the events could be long and exhausting, full of excitement and anticipation. Much of the time was devoted to rehearsals, with some fun activities also included. Catered lunches, beach parties, and evening dinner/dance parties for the group at famous spots like Mardi Gras World in New Orleans are a few examples of some activities. The dancers enjoyed every minute of their week, including the long, hard rehearsals in the sun (or rain, or even snow, depending on the city). Game day (or show day) was always the most exciting of the days. After much hard work and preparation, the dancers went out on the field for their five minutes of fame. They performed, along with famous guest stars and the BGA–recruited marching bands, to a live stadium audience in the tens of thousands and often to a national television audience. This was when the position as director of BGA Performance really pays off. The excitement of the show outweighed all the frustrations and challenges of actually putting it all together. It was extremely rewarding to watch the young people have the time of their lives! For Suzanne, the next day was usually spent traveling to the next bowl game city and starting the process all over again.

After working on bowl game halftime shows for about six years, the 2002 Olympics came to Salt Lake City, Suzanne's hometown. Having worked with the dance choreographer and other directors of the Olympic Opening and Closing Ceremonies team for bowl game shows, she was offered a position as Senior Production Coordinator, Volunteer Cast, with the Ceremonies Production Team. She left her position at BGA Performance to work on the Olympic Ceremonies. The Olympic Opening Ceremony is truly the pinnacle of live productions. Suzanne helped manage a team of fifteen cast coordinators, who worked with more than 4,000 volunteer cast members and 200 production staff volunteers. Suzanne facilitated communication between choreographers, stage managers, the producers, and the cast. She managed all aspects of casting for the ceremonies, from recruitment to auditions to performer selection to the actual live performance. This was truly an opportunity of a lifetime for Suzanne. She enjoyed every minute of her work with the Ceremonies Production Team.

After the Olympics, Suzanne started her family and now accepts work as a subcontractor for specific events and shows. She enjoys tackling one project at a time according to her own schedule. The special events world is an exciting, exhausting, and fun place to work.

The *Olympic Games* is the hallmark of all sporting events, attracting more than 6 million people to the host city. That is a lot of people traveling, staying in hotels, eating in restaurants, and possibly looking at the host city's attractions. The Olympics is an international sporting event that takes place every two years, and it consists of both summer and winter games. The Olympics attract more people than any other sporting event, making it easy to see why the Olympics play an important role in the industry.

The *World Cup* features the best soccer teams in the world. It is an international competition that takes place every four years. However, the World Cup is an ongoing competition, as the qualifying rounds take place over the three years before the final rounds in which the championship is awarded. Close to one million people actually attend the World Cup, and millions more tune in via television or the Internet.

The *Super Bowl* is an annual competition between the two best American football teams. It is a tradition that the game is held on "Super Bowl Sunday," typically occurring in late January or early February. Over the years, this day has become a holiday to many Americans. Super Bowl is one of the most-watched U.S. TV broadcasts of the year and not just for the game. People also tune in to see the much-discussed commercials, on which millions of advertising dollars are spent. People also tune in to watch the halftime show, during which some of the most popular musical artists perform.

The *World Series* is the fight for the title of best baseball team in the United States. The series is played every year starting in October between the champions of the American League and National League and caps off the Major League Baseball (MLB) postseason. Today, the series winner is determined through a best-of-seven playoff. The winning team is awarded the World Series Trophy, and each player receives a World Series ring.

There are four major men's golf championships known as the *Majors*. The *Masters Tournament* is an annual gathering of the world's best golf players on the Augusta Golf Course. Champions of the Masters are automatically invited to play in the other three majors for the following five years, and earn a lifetime invitation to the Masters. The *U.S. Open Championship* is a men's open championship held in June of each year. The U.S. Open Championship is on the official schedule of the PGA Tour and the European Tour. The U.S. Open takes place on a variety of golf courses. The *British Open* is the oldest of the four major championships in men's golf. It is played annually on a links course (located in coastal areas causing frequent wind, on sandy soil, often amid dunes, with few water hazards and few if any trees). The *U.S. PGA Championship* is the final championship of the year, held in August. Champions of the PGA are also automatically invited to play in the other three majors for the next five years and are exempt from qualifying for the PGA Championship for life.

There are a number of boat races held on an annual basis. The *America's Cup* is perhaps the most famous of yachting races. In addition to the yacht races, it is also a test of boat design, sail design, fund-raising, and managing people. The races are held in a series that currently involves a best-of-nine series of match racing (a duel between two boats).

Cruise lines are also creating specialized sports cruises, enabling spectators and participants to enhance their skills, to meet professional athletes, to attend major events, and simply to immerse themselves in their favorite sports.

Where Do Event Planners Work?

- Hotels/resorts
- Private corporations
- Associations

- Caterers
- The government
- Private clubs
- Convention centers
- Bridal businesses
- Event production companies
- Nonprofit organizations
- Advertising agencies
- Self-employed

Required Skills and Abilities for Event Management

Special events management, like any other form of management, requires certain skills and abilities. The act of carrying out a successful event takes more than just an idea—it takes leadership, communication, project management, effective negotiating and delegating skills, the ability to work within a budget, the ability to multitask, enthusiasm, social skills, and even the ability to make contacts. The following sections will provide an overview of skills critical to effective event management.

Leadership Skills

As a leader, the event manager will wear many hats. The first is to inspire the staff and volunteers by providing valid reasons as to why they should want to assist in achieving the established goals for the event. In this role, the event manager will also act as a salesperson. The second hat represents the event manager's responsibility to provide tools for the staff and volunteers to achieve the goals. This includes training and coordination. The third hat the event manager will wear will be that of a coach. The event manager as a leader will act as mentor and provide a support system to build a team. Staff and volunteer motivation is an important factor for effective event management. Leadership ability is the number-one skill for successful event managers. The goal of an event manager is to become a leader who can direct a team of employees and/or volunteers who will respect, admire, and follow your direction to accomplish the established goals.

Effective event leadership can transform the people on your team. Empowering your event team to find their own solutions will benefit both the people and the event. It will allow the team members to create new opportunities for themselves and stimulate personal growth. For the event, empowerment will enable goals and objectives to be achieved quickly. Following are suggestions given by Dr. Joe Jeff Goldblatt, CSEP, for event leadership:

- Event leadership enables your team members to find the motivation to continue achieving the event goals and objectives.

- You cannot motivate others; they must motivate themselves by identifying clear personal goals and objectives.

- Volunteers are the lifeblood of most events. Recruiting, training, coordinating, and rewarding are critical to the success of this activity.

- The three styles of event leadership are democratic, autocratic, and laissez-faire. Each style may be used during the course of the event.

- Policies, procedures, and practices serve as the blueprint for event decision making.[7]

Ability to Communicate with Other Departments

The success of an event manager greatly depends on the ability of involved individuals to communicate effectively with one another. Communication can take different forms: oral, written, and electronic. It is very important for event managers to become effective communicators in order to maintain clear communications with all staff, volunteers, stakeholders, and other departments.

Written communications are an essential tool for record keeping and providing information to be mass distributed. Another way to communicate with other departments is through a meeting.

Delegating

One person cannot do everything, but managers seldom delegate enough. This contradiction is typical in the events business. The secret is to plan ahead of time and allow time for tasks to be delegated to others to help facilitate the smooth operation of an event. For successful delegation, a climate of trust and a positive working environment are needed. Also required is a committed associate who will complete the delegated task and who will communicate effectively throughout the process.

Project Management Skills

Event planning and management can be time consuming. Therefore, a good planner should have effective project management skills to be equipped to balance all of the elements of one event (or more if there are other events going on at the same time). Project management is the act of completing the project(s) on time and within budget. Project management is a perfect fit for the special events industry, where the entire event or components of an event can be managed as projects. Following are management tools by George G. Fenich that may be used to assist in event project management:

- Flow charts and graphs used for scheduling certain programs that will happen at the event. Look at any program of a meeting, and you will see start times and end times of a particular seminar, when the coffee break is to occur, when and where the lunch will be held, followed by the resumption of the meeting. A charting of the scheduling of the activities helps to guide your attendees and guests.

- Clearly defined work setup and breakdown schedules for the event. These provide the event manager with an opportunity to determine tasks that may have been overlooked in the initial planning process for the event.

- Policy statements will need to be developed to help guide in the decision-making process and the fulfilling of commitments. Some of the commitments would be to human resources, sponsorships, security, ticketing, volunteers, and even to paid personnel for the event.[8]

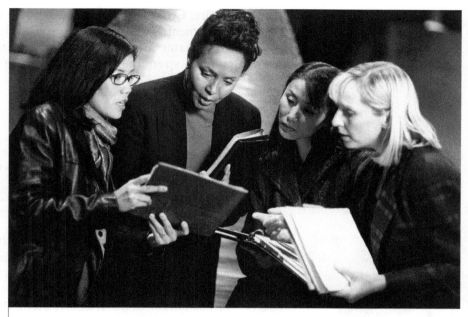

Meeting planners coordinating events during a meeting.

Negotiating Skills

Negotiation is the process by which a meeting planner and supplier (hotel representative, for example) reach an agreement on the terms and conditions that will govern their relationship before, during, and after a meeting, convention, exposition, or event. Effective negotiators will enter the negotiation with a good idea of what they want.

A seasoned negotiator gives the following tips:

- Do your homework. Develop a "game plan" of the outcomes sought, and prioritize your needs and wants. Learn as much about the other side's position as you can.

- Keep your eyes on the prize. Do not forget the outcome sought.

- Leave something on the table. It may provide an opportunity to come back later and renew the negotiations.

- Do not be the first one to make an offer. Letting the other person make the first move sets the outside parameters for the negotiation.

- Bluff, but do not lie.

- When there is a roadblock, find a more creative path. Thinking "outside the box" often leads to a solution.

- Timing is everything. Remember that time always works against the person who does not have it and that 90 percent of negotiation usually occurs in the last 10 percent of the time allocated.

- Listen, listen, listen . . . and do not get emotional. Letting emotions rule a negotiation will cause one to lose sight of what result is important.[9]

The planning and execution of a special event may involve the negotiation of several contracts. The most important is generally the one with the facility or event site. Contracts with other services may include destination management, entertainment, catering, temporary employees, security, and audiovisual equipment, to name a few. Event managers should keep the following two words in mind to strengthen their negotiating skills and position: information and flexibility.

A DAY IN THE LIFE OF TINA FORDE

Events Assistant at the Waldorf Astoria Orlando and Hilton Bonnet Creek

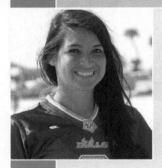

A day in the life of an events assistant is never the same. While I might be doing similar tasks on a day-to-day basis, everything is very different as you encounter each client. Each day is certainly an adventure, always leaving you thinking what will come next. This is an adventure I love.

As an events assistant at the Waldorf Astoria Orlando and Hilton Bonnet Creek, my first and most important task is to assist the events managers with anything they need. There are four managers whom I assist on a daily basis: Those managers are the Assistant Director of Events, two Senior Event Managers, and an Event Manager. I report to the Event Manager on a daily basis.

Through our meetings, my job is to help pre-plan any event that will be taking place at one of our sites. Once I understand what the event entails, I place all of the specifications, or "specs," the client has requested onto Banquet Event Orders, or BEOs. BEOs are like the road map for any event. The BEO will take you from point A to point B while ensuring the client's every request is fulfilled.

There are two types of BEOs: Food and Beverage, and Meeting. If I put together a food and beverage BEO, it would consist of every food item for each meeting, reception, break, or event that will be taking place. The banquet department will use this BEO information to know when, where, and what to set up for each event. Meeting BEOs will include information regarding the setup of the room, audio visual equipment, electric services, and any other specific needs the client has requested.

While working closely with the logistics of events, I also assist with transporting VIP clients that will be staying at one of our hotels. This includes arranging appropriate modes of transportation to and from airports and our hotels, fulfilling client requests, ensuring amenities provided meet the client's expectations, and other duties such as screening the client's telephone calls.

On a monthly basis, I also set up in-house meetings for both properties. Each department has monthly meetings, and it is my job to block times, block rooms, create the space, organize BEOs, and so forth. This also includes orientation for new employees; if Human Resource needs a space to introduce employees to the property and begin the training process, I must ensure that their needs are met for the space.

Because each event is never the same, communication and organization are the most important qualities to have when working as an events assistant. Clients may change their mind, something may not go as originally planned, and being able to adapt to situations while satisfying the client is the core of my job. If you can multitask, react quickly to situations that may become problematic, and balance working well with others and communicating effectively, you can become successful in this line of work.

I truly enjoy every aspect of being an events assistant. No day of work is the same, and being dedicated to what I love to do has helped me succeed with this job. My efforts as an assistant and the love for my career ensure that each event is as successful as the next.

Coordinating and Delegating Skills

The management of staff and volunteers involves coordinating their duties and job performance to enable you to accomplish the goals of the event. As the manager, you are responsible for assigning supervisors or group leaders to oversee the performance of the employees and/or volunteers. It is important to provide coaching and mentoring when working with staff and volunteers to arrive at the event's goals and objectives. When employees can see the purpose and value of their work as well as the outcomes of their work, they usually become more excited about achieving the goals and objectives.

Budgeting Skills

Budgeting is an activity that allows managers to plan the use of their financial resources. In the event industry, the event planner may be working with a fixed budget determined by an association, a SMERF group, or an individual (a wedding or an engagement). In other cases, the budget may be more flexible—a large corporation, for example, that has greater financial resources. Budgeting is a required skill in all hospitality fields, including the special events industry.

The financial history of previous identical or similar events, the general economy and your forecast of the future, and the income expenses you reasonably believe you can expect with the resources available are all factors to be considered in creating an event budget. Even though most event managers will view the budgeting aspect as the least interesting in their job, it is an area that should be carefully managed and is critical for success. The better you become in your budgeting skills, the more you will be able to use resources for other, "more creative" activities.

Ability to Multitask

Because of the nature of the business, an effective event manager should have the ability to multitask. During the planning and staging of the event, your ability to administrate, coordinate, market, and manage will be put to the test. Your job is ultimately to conduct and take control of whatever needs to be done to carry out your goals and objectives. You may encounter several problems arising at the same time, and an effective solution would be to delegate tasks accordingly.

Enthusiasm

As you've probably heard time and time again by now, in any hospitality field the risk of burnout is high and the work is demanding. At the same time, however, the rewards are great and so is the satisfaction when the event is a complete success. As perfectly stated by Norman Brinker, chairman of the board of Brinker International, "Find out what you love to do and you'll never work a day in your life. . . . Make work like play and play like hell!"[10] Enthusiasm and passion. Drive and determination. These are all qualities that will contribute to the success of an event manager/planner. As shown in the profile of Suzanne Bailey, the special events industry is an "exciting, exhausting, and fun place to work." For those with the right enthusiasm and passion, it can be a truly rewarding career path.

Effective Social Skills

Social skills are an important trait for any management position, including one in the special events industry. Social skills are critical in making those you do business with feel comfortable, in handling situations appropriately, and in eliminating barriers that get in the way of accomplishing your goals. Communication is a critical social skill as is another social skill—listening. Social etiquette is another skill that can make or break a career, and it is a practiced skill that can be acquired. Social etiquette is defined as exhibiting good manners established as acceptable to society and showing consideration for others. Professionals in the hospitality industry, including the special events field, must be proficient in proper social etiquette. Service is one of the largest products offered; therefore, social skills and etiquette are required to be successful. Proper social etiquette is required in planning special events, and correct social manners are key to business success.[11] Effective social skills are also critical to leading a motivated group of staff and/or volunteers. How well you communicate, coach, instruct, lead, and listen is a reflection of how well you will succeed as a manager.

Ability to Form Contacts

Many of us have heard the phrase, "It's not what you know, but who you know." Does this statement hold any value in the special events industry? It certainly does. An event may require various services, vendors, suppliers, or products. Here's how it works: An event planner prepares a specification of what is required and requests potential suppliers to submit their prices. The event planner then goes over this information with the client, and they make a decision as to who will provide the services. Over time, event planners quickly find out who is the best provider and therefore the one with whom they prefer to work.

> We've all heard the term "networking" before. It is a practice worth the time and effort. Networking is one of the benefits of joining an association (explained in the next section). The art of networking will allow you to build a contact base that will help you succeed in the event industry. What would happen if your caterer backed out of a contract at the last minute? First of all, make sure you have a contract. Beyond that, having a strong contact base will allow you to plan for those "unexpected" occurrences that are bound to happen at some point in your career.
>
> Karen Harris

► Check Your Knowledge

1. What does the International Festival & Events Association (IFEA) provide?
2. What is project management?
3. Define the process of negotiation.

Special Event Organizations

Like other hospitality industries, professional associations are a key contributor to the professional development of the special events field. Professional associations provide training and prestigious certification to their members, and membership provides an opportunity to network with other professionals in the field. Furthermore, associations can help members connect with vendors that provide products and services relating to special events.

CORPORATE PROFILE

International Special Events Society

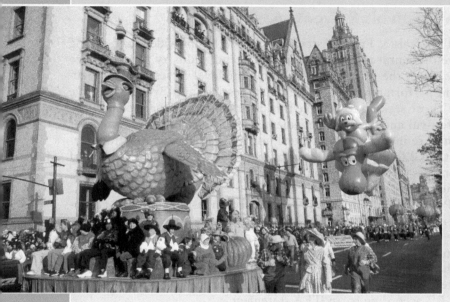

Members of the International Special Events Society organize events like the Macy's Thanksgiving Day Parade

The **International Special Events Society (ISES)** was founded in 1987 and has grown to involve nearly 7,200 members who are active in forty-nine chapters around the world.[12] The organization includes professionals representing special events producers (from festivals to trade shows), caterers, decorators, florists, destination management companies, rental companies, special effects experts, audiovisual technicians, party and convention coordinators, hotel sales managers, specialty entertainers, and many others.

The ISES was founded with the objective to "foster enlightened performance through education while promoting ethical conduct. ISES works to join professionals to focus on the 'event as a whole' rather than its individual parts."[13] The organization has formed a solid network of peers that allows its members to produce quality events for their clients while benefiting from positive working relationships with other ISES members.

The ISES awards a designation of Certified Special Events Professional (CSEP), which is considered to be the benchmark of professional achievement in the special events industry. "It is earned through education, performance, experience, service to the industry, portfolio presentation and examination, and reflects a commitment to professional conduct and ethics,"[14] as stated by ISES. The program includes a self or group study program, point assessment of experience and service, application form, and exam.[15] Visit the ISES web site at **www.ises.com** for further information.

ISES Mission Statement

The mission of ISES is to educate, advance and promote the special events industry and its network of professionals along with related industries.

To that end, we strive to . . .

- Uphold the integrity of the special events profession to the general public through our "Principles of Professional Conduct and Ethics"
- Acquire and disseminate useful business information
- Foster a spirit of cooperation among members and other special events professionals
- Cultivate high standards of business practices[16]

Professional associations also provide their members with help in creating a business plan and other forms of consultation. Job banks and referral services are even provided by some associations. The following sections provide a brief overview of the key associations relating to the special events industry.

International Festivals & Events Association

The International Festivals & Events Association (IFEA) has provided fund-raising and modern developmental ideas to the special events industry for forty-five years. The IFEA began the program to enhance the level of festival management training and performance with a Certified Festival and Event Executive (CFEE) in 1983. Those seeking to achieve this distinguished title are committed to excellence in festival and event management, are using it as a tool for career advancement, and are in search of further knowledge. The organization currently has more than 2,000 plus professional members,[17] who are informed of industry developments through IFEA publications, seminars, an annual convention and trade show, and ongoing networking.[18]

"The CFEE Program is a four-part process based on festival and event management experience, achievements and knowledge. Enrolling in the program and fulfilling the requirements . . . is the first step. Completing the application is next. Successfully completing an oral interview with member(s) of the CFEE Commission is the third. After achieving the CFEE designation, the fourth step is to maintain the designation through continuing education and participation in the profession,"[19] according to an IFEA statement.

The benefits of joining this association and meeting the CFEE requirements include the ability to negotiate a better income or financial package, recognition by other industry professionals, and the inside knowledge that it provides for the festival industry. Visit the IFEA web site at **www.ifea.com** for further information.

Meeting Professionals International

Meeting Professionals International (MPI) is a Dallas-based association with nearly 19,000 members.[20] MPI believes that "as the global authority and resource for the $102.3 billion meeting and event industry, MPI empowers meeting professionals to increase their strategic value through education, clearly defined career pathways, and business growth opportunities." MPI offers professional development in two certification programs:

- Certified Meeting Professional (CMP)
- Certification in Meeting Management (CMM)

The CMP program is based on professional experience and academic examination. After gaining certification, the professional may use the CMP designation after his or her name on business cards, letterheads, and other printed items. Additionally, studies show that CMPs earn up to $10,000 more annually than non–CMPs.[21]

The CMM program is directed toward senior-level meeting professionals and provides an opportunity for continuing education, global certification and recognition, potential career advancement, and a networking base.[22] Visit the MPI web site at **www.mpiweb.org** for more information.

Hospitality Sales and Marketing Association International

Hospitality Sales and Marketing Association International (HSMAI) is the largest and most active travel industry sales and marketing membership organization in the world, with over 7,000 members in 47 chapters from 12 countries,[23] representing hotels and resorts, airlines, cruise lines, car rental agencies, theme parks and attractions, convention and visitors bureaus, destination management companies, reservations sales organizations, restaurants, golf and recreation sites, and much more. Membership is open to anyone involved in one of the sales, marketing, management, educational, planning, or reporting disciplines within the hospitality industry, including those involved in promoting, producing, or delivering support services to the travel, tourism, hospitality, convention, and meeting industries.[24]

HSMAI's mission is to be the leading source for sales and marketing information, knowledge, business development, and networking for professionals in tourism, travel, and hospitality.[25] HSMAI offers certification courses in Hospitality Sales Executive, Revenue Management, Sales Competencies, Hospitality Marketing Executive, and Hospitality Business Acumen.

Local Convention and Visitors Bureaus

A convention and visitors bureau (CVB) is a not-for-profit organization that is located in almost every city in the United States and Canada. Many other cities throughout the world also have a CVB or convention and visitors association (CVA). Simply stated, the CVB is an organization with the purpose of promoting tourism, meetings, and related business for its city. The CVB has three primary functions:

1. Encourage groups to hold meetings, conventions, and trade shows in the city or area it represents
2. Assist those groups with event preparations and during the event
3. Encourage tourists to visit the historic, cultural, and recreational opportunities the destination offers

The CVB does not engage in the actual planning or organizing of meetings, conventions, and other events. However, the CVB assists meeting planners and managers in several ways. First, it will provide information about the destination, area attractions, services, and facilities. Second, it provides an unbiased source of information to the planner. Finally, most of the services offered by the CVB are at no charge because they are funded through other sources, including hotel occupancy taxes and membership dues. Therefore, it can provide an array of services to event planners and managers. A sample of general services provided by a CVB include the following:

- CVBs act as a liaison between the planner and the community.
- CVBs can help meeting attendees maximize their free time through the creation of pre- and postconference activities, spouse tours, and special evening events.

- CVBs can provide hotel room counts and meeting space statistics.
- CVBs can help with event facility availability.
- CVBs are a network for transportation—shuttle service, ground transportation, and airline information.
- CVBs can assist with site inspections and familiarization tours.
- CVBs can provide speakers and local educational opportunities.
- CVBs can provide help in securing auxiliary services, production companies, catering, security, and so forth.

TECHNOLOGY SPOTLIGHT

GPS Drives Customers to Your Door

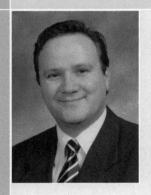

Cihan Cobanoglu, Ph.D., Dean, School of Hotel and Restaurant Management, University of South Florida, Sarasota-Manatee

On a trip to San Francisco, I had a meeting with a client that finished just before lunch time. Needless to say, I was hungry, and being in San Francisco, I knew I could find some interesting eateries. Instead of asking for recommendations at the front desk, I did something that I have been doing since the first day I bought my Garmin Nuvi 660 Global Positioning System (GPS). I left my hotel, turned it on, and was able to browse through a list of nearby restaurants, some of which I would never have found otherwise.

As the GPS guided me to a Turkish restaurant called Alaturka, a thought crossed my mind, one that I shared with the owner when I arrived: "Did you know that I found your restaurant using my GPS?" The owner had no idea.

But should he? My thoughts and the owner's inexperience with GPS led me to pursue a research study on the topic of U.S. consumer use of GPS with Dr. Silvia Ciccarelli of the University of Rome. Preliminary results are very promising for the hospitality industry.

Dashboard Results

As evidenced by the presence of GPS on the list of hot holiday items for 2007, a growing number of U.S. consumers are using GPS in their everyday lives. This is further supported by the study's findings: Only 33 percent of the U.S. consumers we polled had not used a GPS within the last 12 months, and only 4 percent did not know what a GPS was. Among those who had used a GPS within the last year (63 percent), 14 percent had rented or borrowed a GPS, 7 percent had a built-in GPS in their vehicle, 28 percent owned a portable/dashboard GPS, and 5 percent had a phone with GPS capabilities.

The vast majority of consumers (94 percent) agree that a GPS makes life easier, and 84 percent indicate that they feel safer with a GPS. What's more, 11 percent even indicate that they cannot travel without a GPS. For many consumers, a GPS is a personal thing—approximately 30 percent name their GPS (e.g., Jack, Jill), while 34 percent talk to their GPS (e.g., "Good job, Jack!" or "OK, Jill, take me there!").

However, the most important and relevant finding for the hospitality industry is that 30 percent of respondents said that they travel more because of their GPS. More than half (55 percent) of consumers would like their GPS to suggest tourist attractions to them, and 42 percent think that a GPS could help them plan their vacation. Furthermore, 65 percent of consumers who used a GPS in the past 12 months found and ate in restaurants that they did not previously know of because of their GPS. When it comes to lodging, 51 percent found hotels this way, and 47 percent were able to find tourist attractions with the help of their GPS.

Marketing Opportunities

The increasing use of the GPS has not gone unnoticed. Recognizing the powerful marketing opportunity that a GPS offers, Dunkin' Brands inked a first-of-its-kind licensing agreement with GPS manufacturer Tom-Tom (**www.tomtom.com**). Under the terms of the agreement, users could download the Dunkin' Donuts and Baskin Robbins logos onto their devices as points of interest. The systems could also be programmed so that drivers were alerted as they approach a local Dunkin' Donuts or Baskin Robbins location.

GPS maker Garmin (**http://www.garmin.com/us/**) announced a partnership with MAD MAPS that will provide scenic reminders that traveling by car or motorcycle is more than simply reaching a destination.[26]

GPS: Here to Stay

If you haven't already noticed, the one take-away from this study should be that a GPS is a powerful marketing tool. These systems drive business to hospitality operations. Accordingly, hotels and restaurants need to contact GPS manufacturers to ensure that they are listed in GPS databases and that their listing provides the correct information for GPS users. Hospitality operators should also offer downloadable point-of-interest information on their web site so customers can input location information into their GPS. GPS is a tool that's here to stay, so don't get left behind.

Sustainability in Special Events

What drives hospitality and tourism companies to incorporate sustainability standards into their business practices and daily operations? What do these companies gain from employing Sustainability standards?

The recent increase in special event tourism has triggered the emergence of sustainable event standards. Britain has recently developed a system of standards for event management, which highlights policies and procedures necessary to implement sustainability. Event managers can use these standards as a benchmark for how to train employees on proper sustainable practices before, during, and after events. Currently in the U.S., ASTM International is creating a guide for sustainable event management called, "the New Guide for Standard Practice for the Evaluation and Selection of Destinations for Meetings, Events, Trade Show, and Conferences," which credits much of its content to the British system of standards.[27]

Sustainable event tourism refers to the implementation of practices and procedures which help conserve both the natural environment and the special event space. Special event tourism is one of the most lucrative and fastest growing segments of the tourism industry.[28] Special events are provided for a variety of reasons, which range from creating market demand for the host location as a desirable destination, generating publicity for the event's sponsors, achieving a specific purpose or goal, developing awareness of a particular cause or idea, etc.[29] Whatever the reason may be, special events play an important role in consumer's images, attitudes and perceptions of host destinations.[30] Because special events bring tourism to certain locations, it is the responsibility of the event host to employ sustainable practices, in order to preserve local resources and cultural interests.[31]

Sustainable event tourism not only provides environmental advantages, but financial returns as well. The organizations who are dedicated to incorporating sustainable programs into their business plans can expect to see the greatest return on investment as a result of cost reduction, revenue increase, etc.[32] Some practices that can result in financial gain include, conserving energy such as light spill from event and security lighting, turning off lights whenever they are not in use, utilizing low carbon fuels and renewable energy, ensuring appropriate waste and cleaning procedures are followed, utilizing low emission vehicles, reducing vehicle usage and increasing shared transportation.[33] Ultimately, the implementation of sustainable practices can increase the benefits of being in the special events business, as well as the excitement of actually hosting an event.

The Special Events Job Market

Becoming a special events consultant or an off-premise catering/event specialist requires a delicate balance of many skills. Experience gained from several avenues will propel you to the heights of success. As with any career, an "experience ladder" must be climbed.

First, allow yourself to gain all the experience you can in the food and beverage aspect of the hospitality industry. If time and resources permit, it is highly recommended that you gain knowledge from a culinary arts program. Second, experience gained as a banquet food server in a high-volume convention or resort hotel property is invaluable. Also, paying your dues as a guest service agent at a hotel front desk or as a concierge provides you with the opportunity to hone your customer service skills. Promote yourself to a banquet manager or a CSM (convention service coordinator), which provides the opportunity to learn and perfect organizational skills—to which end is the ability to multitask and deal with hundreds of details simultaneously. After all, the business of special events is the business of managing details.

The next step is obtaining a sales position. An excellent appointment to aspire to is an executive meeting manager, sometimes called a small meeting manager, in a convention or conference hotel. Here, you are responsible for booking small room blocks (usually twenty rooms or less), making meeting room arrangements, creating meal plans, and setting audiovisual requirements. On a small scale, hundreds of details are coordinated for several groups at any one time. From this position, you may laterally move to a catering sales position within a hotel.

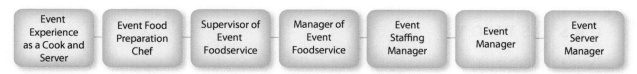

Figure 2 • A Career Path for an Event Manager.

The catering sales position in a hotel will expose you to many different kinds of events: weddings, reunions, corporate events, holiday events, and social galas and balls. In this position, one either coordinates or has the opportunity to work with various vendors. This is where the florists, prop companies, lighting experts, entertainment agencies, rental companies, and audiovisual wizards come into play. Two to three years in this capacity grooms you for the next rung on the ladder.

Now, you can pursue several different angles: being promoted to a convention service manager within a hotel, moving into off-premise catering as a sales consultant, joining a production company, or perhaps affiliating yourself with a destination management company (DMC). Typically, without sales experience within a DMC, your first experience with them will be as an operations manager. Once proficient in this capacity, you then join the sales team.

After another two years creating and selling your heart out, you will be ready for the big leagues. The palette is now yours to paint your future. How about aspiring to be the next Super Bowl halftime creator and producer? Or perhaps creating the theme and schematics for the Olympics is in your future. Many avenues are available for exploring. Call on your marketing ideas, your business sense, your accounting skills, your aptitude for design, and your discriminating palette for creating unique entertaining and dining concepts. Continually educating yourself and discovering fresh ideas through adventurous experiences are essential to designing and selling special events. Don't forget to embark on as many internships as you can in the name of gaining knowledge and experience. Show your enthusiasm for what is different and unconventional. Know that creativity has no boundaries. Visualize the big picture and go for it! Figure 2 shows a career path for an event manager.

Trends in the Special Events Industry

- The special events industry is forecast to grow because clients want ever more spectacular events.

- Events are increasingly more complex, involving multimedia presentations, elaborate staging, and frequently upscale food and beverage service.

- Technology presents both an opportunity and a challenge—an opportunity in that it can facilitate event planning and management, and a challenge in that new software programs must be mastered.

CASE STUDY

Not Enough Space

Jessica is the event planner for a large convention center. A client has requested an exhibition that would not only bring excellent revenue but that is an annual event that several other convention centers would like to host.

Exhibitions typically take one or two days to set up, three or four days of exhibition, and one day to break down. Professional organizations handle each part of the setup and breakdown.

When Jessica checks the space available on the days requested for the exhibition, she notices that another exhibition is blocking part of the space needed by her client.

Discussion Question

1. What can Jessica do to get this exhibition to use the conventon center without inconveniencing either exhibition too much?

Summary

1. Special events differ from daily events, which occur spontaneously, do not arouse expectations, and usually occur without reason, in that they recognize a unique moment in time with ceremony and ritual to satisfy specific needs and are always planned.
2. The special events industry is a growing field that will provide many professional career opportunities in event management and planning.
3. Special events planners and managers have filled a need that was first introduced at hotels and convention centers. They are responsible for planning the event from start to finish.
4. The special events industry can be grouped into several smaller classifications, including corporate events, association events, charity balls and fund-raising events, social functions, fairs and festivals, and concert and sporting events.
5. The event-planning process includes the following steps: research, design, planning, coordination, and evaluation.
6. Special events planners can work in a variety of settings. They range from hotels/resorts, convention centers, and private clubs to self-employment.
7. Critical skills and abilities required for a career in special events management include leadership skills, effective communication, project management skills, negotiating skills, coordinating and delegating skills, budgeting skills, multitasking abilities, enthusiasm, effective social skills, and the ability to form contacts.
8. The special events industry has its own selection of professional associations that offer certification, continuing education, and networking to their members. The International Special Events Society (ISES), International Festivals & Events Association (IFEA), and Meeting Professionals International (MPI) are three of the largest and most recognized professional associations in the field. Local convention and visitors bureaus (CVBs) are organizations that can be valuable

resources to the special events industry. A CVB has the purpose of promoting tourism, meetings, and related business for its city.

9. The management of time and finances, along with technology and human resources are event-planning tools that can be utilized to your advantage as you pursue a career in this field.

10. The special events industry does not have rigid boundaries. Closely related fields that may overlap include catering, marketing, sales, and entertainment.

Key Words and Concepts

charity balls
conventions
coordination
corporate events
corporate seminars
event planner
event planning
fairs and festivals

International Festival & Events Association (IFEA)
International Special Events Society (ISES)
Meeting Professionals International (MPI)
social functions
special events industry
trade shows
weddings and holiday parties
workshops

Review Questions

1. What do event planners do?
2. What are the challenges for event planners and managers?
3. Describe three of the classifications of special events.

4. Explain the skills and abilities required for event management.

Internet Exercises

1. Organization: **International Special Events Society (ISES)**
   Web site: **www.ises.com**
   Click on "Learn." Look for ISES Eventworld under "Education & Programs" and see what an ISES Eventworld can do for professional development and who should attend.

2. Organization: Meeting Professionals International
   www.mpiweb.org/resources/jobs/default.asp
   Go to "Career Development," click on "Career Connections," and check out a couple of good jobs.

Apply Your Knowledge

Make a plan for a local event in your area. List all the headings and formulate a budget.

Suggested Activity

Attend a special event and write a brief report on the event and its planning and organization.

Endnotes

1. Joe J. Goldblatt, *Special Events: Best Practices in Modern Event Management*, 2nd ed. (New York: John Wiley and Sons, 1997), 2; Joe J. Goldblatt, *Special Events: The Art and Science of Celebration* (New York: Von Nostrand Reinhold, 1990), 1–2.
2. Frank Supovitz, "Foreword," in Joe J. Goldblatt, *Special Events: Best Practices in Modern Event Management*, 2nd ed. (New York: John Wiley and Sons, 1997), iv.
3. Blythe Cameson, *Opportunities in Event Planning Careers* (New York: McGraw-Hill, 2002), 4–7.
4. Event Solutions, *2004 Black Book* (Tempe, AZ: Event Publishing, 2004), 22
5. Blythe Cameson, *Opportunities in Event Planning Careers*, 115.
6. Festivals.com, *Culture*, www.festivals.com/culture/ (accessed November 27, 2011).
7. Goldblatt, *Special Events: Best Practices in Modern Event Management*, 129–139.
8. George G. Fenich, *Meetings, Expositions, Events, and Conventions: An Introduction to the Industry* (Upper Saddle River, NJ: Pearson Education, 2005), 181–182.
9. Fenich, *Meetings, Expositions, Events, and Conventions*, 366.
10. Norman Brinker, presentation to the National Restaurant Association, May 14, 1994.
11. Judy Allen, *Event Planning Ethics and Etiquette: A Principled Approach to the Business of Special Event Management* (Etobicoke, Ontario, Canada: John Wiley and Sons, 2003), 79.
12. International Special Events Society (ISES), *ISES 2010–2011 Fact Sheet*, www.ises.com/portals/0/About_ISES.pdf (accessed November 27, 2011).
13. Ibid.
14. International Special Events Society, *Learn*, http://www.ises.com/Learn/tabid/78/Default.aspx (accessed November 27, 2011).
15. International Special Events Society (ISES), *Certified Special Events Professional (CSEP)*, http://isesew.vtcus.com/CSEP/index.aspx (November 27, 2011)
16. International Special Events Society (ISES), *ISES Vision and Mission*, www.ises.com/MediaCenter/ISESVisionandMission/tabid/92/Default.aspx (accessed November 27, 2011).
17. http://www.ifea.com/joomla1_5/index.php
18. International Festivals & Events Association (IFEA), *About the IFEA*, www.ifea.com/about_ifea_main.htm (accessed November 30, 2011).
19. http://www.ifea.com/joomla1_5/index.php
20. http://www.mpiweb.org/Portal/Research/BusinessBarometer/download (retrieved November 30, 2001).
21. Cameson, *Opportunities in Event Planning Careers*, 36–41.
22. Meeting Professionals International, *CMM: Certification in Meeting Management*, www.mpiweb.org/Education/CMM (accessed November 27, 2011).
23. Hospitality Sales and Marketing Association International (HSMAI), *About HSMAI*, www.hsmai.org/GlobalAbout.cfm (accessed November 27, 2011).
24. Hospitality Sales and Marketing Association International (HSMAI), *HSMAI Information*, www.hsmai.org/Mission.cfm (accessed June 8, 2011).
25. Hospitality Sales and Marketing Association International (HSMAI), *About HSMAI*, www.hsmai.org/GlobalAbout.cfm (accessed November 27, 2011).
26. http://www8.garmin.com/pressroom/corporate/102907.html

27. O'Connor, M.C. (July 8, 2010). On the Agenda: Sustainable Event Standards. http://www.triplepundit.com/2010/07/on-the-agenda-sustainable-event-standards/. Retrieved on November 17, 2011.

28. Reid, S., & Arcodia, C. (2002). Understanding the role of stakeholders in event management.

29. Turney, Michael. (2009). Special events generate publicity but are they effective public relations. http://www.nku.edu/~turney/prclass/sections/special_events.html. Retrieved on November 17, 2011.

30. Chalip, L., Green, C., & Hill, B. (2003). Effects of sport media on destination image and intentions to visit. *Journal of Sport Management*, 17, 214–234.

31. Okech, Roselyne N. (2011). Promoting sustainable festival events tourism: a case study of Lamu Kenya. *Worldwide Hospitality and Tourism Themes*. Vol. 3 No. 3.

32. Beer, Mitchell. (November 14, 2011). Commentary: New Green Standards Help Make Sustainability Sustainable. http://meetingsnet.com/green_meetings/commentary_beer_new_green_standards_1114/?YM_MID=1272883&YM_RID=operations@meetingstrategiesworldwide.com. Retrieved on November 17, 2011.

33. http://www.london2012.com/documents/locog-publications/london-2012-sustainability-events-guidelines.pdf. Retrieved on November 17, 2011.

Glossary

Charity ball   A gala dinner-dance event whose purpose is to raise funds toward a group or charity.

Convention   A generic term referring to any size business or professional meeting held in one specific location, which usually includes some form of trade show or exposition. Also refers to a group of delegates or members who assemble to accomplish a specific goal.

Corporate events   Annual meetings, sales meetings, new product launches, training meetings, workshops, management meetings, press meetings, incentive meetings, and awards ceremonies.

Corporate seminar   A corporate meeting whose purpose is to exchange ideas; a conference.

Event planner   An individual who is responsible for planning an event from start to finish. Duties include setting the date and location; advertising the event; and providing refreshments or arranging catering services; and arranging speakers and/or entertainment.

Event planning   A general term that refers to a career path in the growing field of special events.

Fairs and festivals   Planned events that are often themed to the celebration's purpose.

Fund-raiser   An event whose purpose is to raise funds for a group or charity.

International Festivals & Events Association   An organization that provides an opportunity for event managers from around the world to network and exchange ideas on how other festivals excel in sponsorship, marketing, fund-raising, operations, volunteer coordination, and management.

Social functions   Events that include weddings, engagement parties, and holiday functions.

Special events industry   An industry that employs professionals who work together to provide a broad range of services to create what is termed a *special event*.

Trade show   Generally, a large display of products and services available for purchase, promoting information exchange among trade people. Trade shows frequently take place in convention centers where space is rented in blocks of 10 square feet. Also called *exposition*.

Weddings and holiday parties   Of all social gatherings, weddings are the most widely recognized social event.

Workshop   A usually brief, intensive educational program conducted by a facilitator or a trainer, designed for a relatively small group of people, that focuses especially on techniques and skills in a particular field. Emphasizes interaction and exchange of information among a relatively small number of participants.

Photo Credits

Credits are listed in the order of appearance.

Leadership and Management

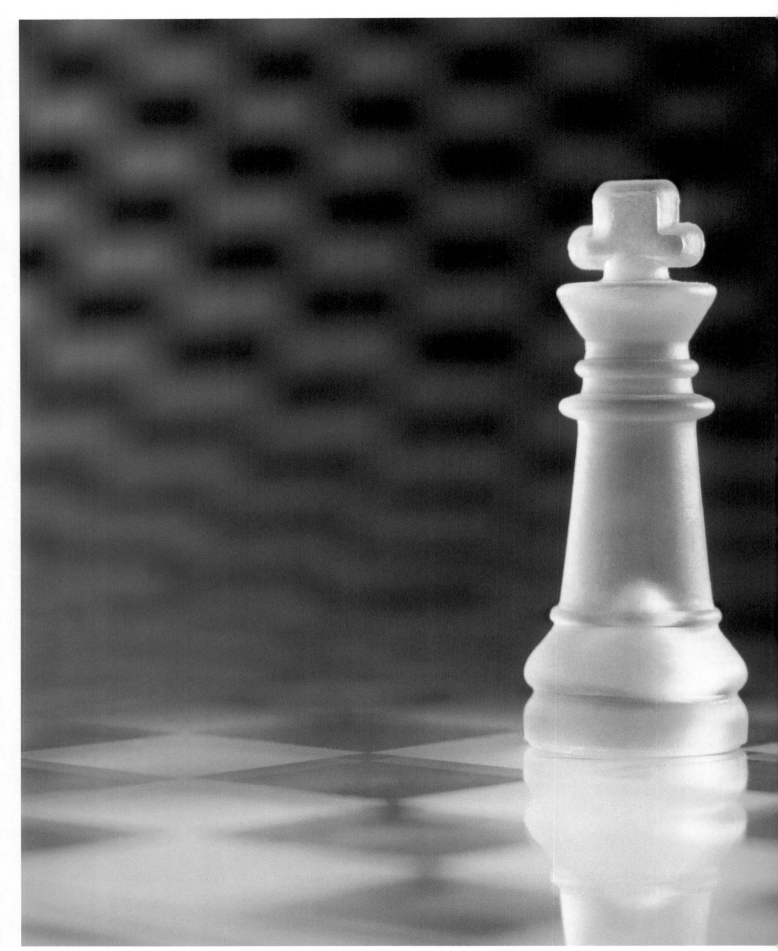

Leadership and Management

OBJECTIVES

After reading and studying this chapter, you should be able to:

- Identify the characteristics and practices of leaders and managers.

- Define *leadership* and *management*.

- Differentiate between leadership and management.

- Describe the key management functions.

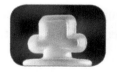
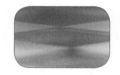
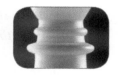
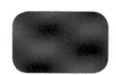

Leadership

Our fascination with **leadership** goes back many centuries. Lately, however, it has come into prominence in the hospitality, tourism, and other industries as these industries strive for perfection in the delivery of services and products in an increasingly competitive environment. Leaders can and do make a difference when measuring a company's success.

One person working alone can accomplish few tasks or goals. You have probably already experienced being part of a group that had good leadership. It might have been with a school, social, sporting, church, or other group in which the leader made a difference. The reverse might also be true: You may have been in a group with ineffective leadership. Few groups can accomplish much without an individual who acts as an effective leader. The leader can and often does have a significant influence on the group and its direction.

Characteristics and Practices of Leaders

So, what are the ingredients that result in leadership excellence? If you look at the military for examples of leadership excellence, you see that leaders can be identified by certain characteristics. For example, the U.S. *Guidebook for Marines* lists the following leadership traits:

- Courage
- Decisiveness
- Dependability
- Endurance
- Enthusiasm
- Initiative
- Unselfishness

- Integrity
- Judgment
- Justice
- Knowledge
- Loyalty
- Tact

A Marine officer would likely choose integrity as the most important trait. Integrity has been defined as "doing something right even though no one may be aware of it."

In addition to these leadership traits, the following identifiable practices are common to leaders:

1. *Challenge the process.* Be active, not passive; search for opportunities; experiment and take risks.
2. *Inspire a shared vision.* Create a vision; envision the future; enlist others.
3. *Enable others to act.* Do not act alone; foster collaboration; strengthen others.
4. *Model the way.* Plan; set examples; strive for small wins.
5. *Encourage the heart.* Share the passion; recognize individual contributions; celebrate accomplishments.

Definitions of Leadership

Because of the complexities of leadership, the different types of leadership, and individual perceptions of leaders, *leadership* has several definitions. Many definitions share commonalities, but there are also differences. In terms of hospitality leadership, the definition "Leading is the process by which a person with vision is able to influence the activities and outcomes of others in a desired way" is appropriate.

Leaders know what they want and why they want it—and they are able to communicate those desires to others to gain their cooperation and support. Leadership theory and practice has evolved over time to a point where current industry practitioners may be identified as transactional or transformational leaders.[1]

INTRODUCING HORST SCHULZE

West Paces Hotel Group

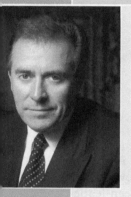

Horst Schulze is a legendary leader in the hospitality industry and one of the most influential hospitality industry leaders of our time. His vision helped reshape concepts of guest service throughout the hospitality and service industries.

Mr. Schulze grew up in a small village in Germany, and he was eleven years old when he told his parents that he wanted to work in a hotel. When he was fourteen, his parents took him to the finest hotel in the region, where they had an "audience" with the general manager—it lasted ten minutes, and he didn't speak to him again for the next two years! Everyone, including young Schulze's mother, the general manager, and the restaurant maître d', told him how important the guests were, so with knees shaking, young Schulze found himself in the restaurant working as a busser. The maître d' made a favorable impression on the young man because he was respected by both guests and staff alike. So, when Horst had to do an essay for his hotel school (he attended hotel school on Wednesdays), he chose the title, "We Are Ladies and Gentlemen Serving Ladies and Gentlemen." He kept the essay because it was the only A he received, but that A also became the foundation of his philosophy to create service excellence.

Mr. Schulze now speaks on guest service to thousands every year, graciously sharing with others his knowledge and experience. He says that there are three aspects of service[2]:

1. Service should be defect free.
2. Service should be timely.
3. People should care.

It is the caring piece that is service. The guest relationship begins when a guest perceives that he or she has contacted you, and the human contact should begin with a warm welcome. Mr. Schulze adds that all hospitality businesses should be doing four things[3]:

1. Keeping guests equals loyalty, meaning guests trust you and are happy to form a relationship with you.
2. Find new guests.

(continued)

INTRODUCING HORST SCHULZE *(continued)*

3. Get as much money as you can from the guest without losing him or her.
4. Create efficiencies.

Mr. Schulze also worked with Hyatt Hotels and Hilton Hotels. After joining the Ritz-Carlton as a charter member and vice president of operations in 1983, Mr. Schulze was instrumental in creating the operating and service standards that have become world famous. He was appointed executive vice president in 1987, and president and chief operating officer (COO) in 1988. Under his leadership, the group was awarded the Malcolm Baldrige National Quality Award in both 1992 and 1999; it was the first and only hotel company to win even one such award. In 2002, Mr. Schulze, along with several former Ritz-Carlton executives, formed the West Paces Hotel Group to create and operate branded hotels in several distinctive market segments. The canon of the company is as follows: "The West Paces Hotel Group is in business to create value and unparalleled results for our owners by creating products which fulfill individual customer expectations."[4]

They offer significant opportunities within three profiles[5]:

1. Ultra-luxury hotel properties in gateway cities and spectacular resort destinations
2. Luxury hotel accommodations for frequent travelers
3. Management of select independent hotel properties

West Paces has hotels and resorts under two brands: Solis and Capella. They can be viewed at **http://www.westpaceshotels.com**.

Transactional Leadership

Transactional leadership is viewed as a process by which a leader is able to bring about desired actions from others by using certain behaviors, rewards, or incentives. In essence, an exchange or transaction takes place between leader and follower. Figure 1 shows the transactional leadership model. This figure illustrates the coming together of the leader, the situation, and the followers. A hotel general manager who pressures the food and beverage director to achieve certain goals in exchange for a bonus is an example of someone practicing transactional leadership.

Transformational Leadership

Leadership involves looking for ways to bring about longer-term, higher-order changes in follower behavior. This brings us to transformational leadership. The term **transformational leadership** is used to describe the process of eliciting performance above and beyond normal expectations. A transformational leader

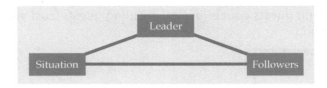

Figure 1 • Transactional Leadership Model.

is one who inspires others to reach beyond themselves and do more than they originally thought possible; this is accomplished by raising their commitment to a shared vision of the future.

Transformational leaders practice a hands-on philosophy, not in terms of performing the day-to-day tasks of subordinates, but in developing and encouraging their followers individually. Transformational leadership involves three important factors:

1. Charisma
2. Individual consideration
3. Intellectual stimulation

Of course, it is also possible to be a charismatic transformational leader as well as a transactional leader. Although this does involve a measurable amount of effort, these leaders are guaranteed to rake in success throughout their careers.

Examples of Excellence in Leadership

Dr. Martin Luther King Jr. was one of the most charismatic transformational leaders in history. King dedicated his life to achieving rights for all citizens through nonviolent methods. His dream of how society could be was shared by millions of Americans. In 1964, Dr. King won the Nobel Peace Prize.

Another transformational leader is Herb Kelleher, the co-founder, Chairman Emeritus, and former CEO of Southwest Airlines. He was able to inspire his followers to pursue his corporate vision and reach beyond themselves to give Southwest Airlines that something extra that set it apart from its competitors.

Kelleher recognizes that the company does not exist merely for the gratification of its employees. He knows that Southwest Airlines must perform and must be profitable. However, he believes strongly that valuing individuals for themselves is the best way to attain exceptional performance. Passengers who fly Southwest Airlines may have seen Herb Kelleher because he travels frequently and previously was likely to be found serving drinks, fluffing pillows, or just wandering up and down the aisle, talking to passengers. The success of Southwest and the enthusiasm of its employees indicate that Herb Kelleher achieved his goal of weaving together individual and corporate interests so that all members of the Southwest family benefit. Kelleher is a great transformational leader who is able to lead by visioning, inspiring, empowering, and communicating.[6]

In their fascinating book *Lessons in Leadership: Perspectives for Hospitality Industry Success*, Bill Fisher, former president and CEO of the American Hotel & Lodging Association and current Darden Eminent Scholar in Restaurant Management at the University of Central Florida,

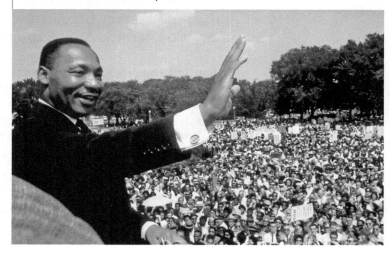

Martin Luther King Jr., one of the most charismatic transformational leaders of the twentieth century, giving his famous "I Have a Dream" speech.

and Charles Bernstein, an editor of *Nation's Restaurant News*, interviewed more than 100 industry leaders and asked each to give advice in an up-close-and-personal manner. Here is an example of the leaders' answers: "Experience is a hard teacher. It gives the test first, and then you learn the lesson[7]."

Richard P. Mayer, former chairman and CEO of Kentucky Fried Chicken and president of General Foods Corporation, says that the key traits and factors he looks for in assessing talent include the following:

- Established personal goals
- The drive and ambition to attain those goals, tempered and strengthened with integrity
- Proven analytical and communications skills
- Superior interpersonal capabilities
- A sense of humor
- An awareness and appreciation of the world beyond his or her business specialty
- Receptivity to ideas (no matter the source)
- A genuine, deep commitment to the growth and profitability of the business

Success has as many meanings as there are people to ponder it. One concept of success is to couple one's personal and family interests, dreams, and aspirations with a business or professional career such that they complement and fortify each other. Another aspect of leadership is the ability to motivate others in a hospitality working environment; decision making is also essential. These are discussed later in the chapter.

FOCUS ON LEADERSHIP

Leadership—The Basis for Management

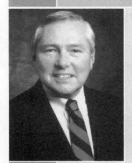

William Fisher, Darden Eminent Scholar in Restaurant Management, Author and Former Executive Vice President of the National Restaurant Association and the American Hotel & Lodging Association

The concept and practice of leadership as it applies to management carries a fascination and attraction for most people. We all like to think we have some leadership qualities, and we strive to develop them. We look at leaders in all walks of life, seeking to identify which qualities, traits, and skills they possess so that we can emulate them. A fundamental question remains: What is the essence of leadership that results in successful management as opposed to failed management? At least part of the answer can be found within the word itself:

1. *Loyalty*. Leadership starts with a loyalty quadrant: Loyalty to one's organization and its mission, loyalty to organizational superiors, loyalty to subordinates, and loyalty to oneself. Loyalty is multidirectional, running up and down in the organization. When everyone practices it, loyalty bonds occur, which drives high morale.

Loyalty to oneself is based on maintaining a sound body, mind, and spirit so that one is always "riding the top of the wave" in service to others.

2. *Excellence.* Leaders know that excellence is a value, not an object. They strive for both excellence and success. Excellence is the measurement you make of yourself in assessing what you do and how well you do it; success is an external perception that others have of you.

3. *Assertiveness.* Leaders possess a mental and physical intensity that causes them to seek control, take command, assume the mantle of responsibility, and focus on the objective(s). Leaders do not evidence self-doubt, as they are comfortable within themselves that what they are doing is right, which, in turn, gives them the courage to take action.

4. *Dedication.* Leaders are dedicated in mind, body, and spirit to their organization and to achievement. They are action oriented, not passive, and prefer purposeful activity to the status quo. They possess an aura or charisma that sets them apart from others with whom they interact, always working in the best interest of their organization.

5. *Enthusiasm.* Leaders are their own best cheerleaders on behalf of their organization and people. They exude enthusiasm and instill it in others to the point of contagion. Their style may be one of poise, stability, clear vision, and articulate speech, but their bristling enthusiasm undergirds their every waking moment.

6. *Risk management.* Leaders realize that risk taking is part of their management position. They manage risk, rather than letting it manage them, knowing full well that there are no guaranteed outcomes, no foregone conclusions, no preordained results when one is dealing with the future. Nonetheless, they measure risk, adapt to it, control it, and surmount it.

7. *Strength.* Leaders possess an inner fiber of stamina, fortitude, and vibrancy that gives them a mental toughness, causing them to withstand interruption, crises, and unforeseen circumstances that would slow down or immobilize most people. Leaders become all the more energized in the face of surprises.

8. *Honor.* Leaders understand they will leave a legacy, be it good, bad, or indifferent. True leaders recognize that all their relationships and actions are based on the highest standard of honor and integrity. They do the right things correctly, shun short-term, improper expediency, and set the example for others with high-mindedness, professional bearing, and unassailable character.

9. *Inspiration.* Leaders don't exist without followers. People will follow leaders who inspire them to reach beyond the normal and ordinary to new levels of accomplishment, new heights of well-being, and new platforms for individual, organizational, and societal good. Inspiration is what distinguishes a leader from a mere position holder, as the leader can touch the hearts, minds, and souls of others.

10. *Performance.* At the end of the day, leader/managers rise or fall on the most critical of all measurements: their performance. Results come first, but the ways in which results are achieved are also crucial to sustaining a leader's role. Many dictators don't last despite results, and many charismatics don't last despite personal charm.

These ten elements together spell LEADERSHIP! Always remember, if you want to develop a leadership quality, act as though you already possess it!

Demands Placed on Leaders

Demands on a leader in the hospitality industry include those made by owners, the corporate office, guests, employees, regulatory agencies, and competitors (Figure 2). In response to many demands, the leader must balance two additional forces: how much energy to expend on getting results and how much to expend on relationships (Figure 3).

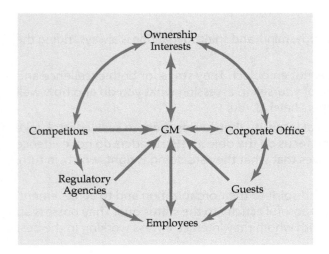

Figure 2 • Dynamics of Demands on Leaders in the Hospitality Industry.

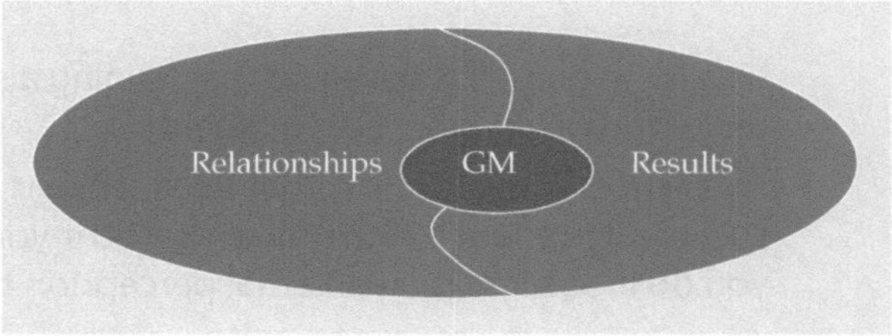

Figure 3 • Amount of Energy the Leader Needs to Spend on Getting Results and Maintaining Relationships.

Applied social scientists such as Peter Drucker, powerful industry leaders such as Bill Marriott, and public service leaders such as former New York mayor Rudolph Giuliani all seem to have common traits, among which are the following:

1. High ego strength
2. Ability to think strategically
3. Orietation toward the future
4. A belief in certain fundamental principles of human behavior
5. Strong connections that they do not hesitate to display
6. Political astuteness
7. Ability to use power both for efficiency and for the larger good of the organization

Leaders vary in their values, managerial styles, and priorities. Peter Drucker, the renowned management scholar, author, and consultant of many years, has discussed with hundreds of leaders their roles, goals, and performance. These discussions took place with leaders of large and small organizations, with for-profit and volunteer organizations. Interestingly, Drucker observes the following:

All the leaders I have encountered—both those I worked with and those I watched—realized:

1. The only definition of a leader is someone who has followers. Some people are thinkers. Some are prophets. Both roles are important and badly needed. But without followers, there can be no leaders.
2. An effective leader is not someone who is loved or admired. She or he is someone whose followers do the right things. Popularity is not leadership. Results are.

3. Leaders are highly visible. They therefore set examples.

4. Leadership is not about rank, privileges, titles, or money. It is about responsibility.[8]

Drucker adds that regardless of their enormous diversity with respect to personality, style, abilities, and interests, effective leaders all behave in much the same way:

1. They did not start out with the question "What do I want?" They started out asking, "What needs to be done?"

2. Then they asked, "What can and should I do to make a difference?" This has to be something that both needs to be done and fits the leader's strengths and the way he or she is most effective.

3. They constantly asked, "What are the organization's mission and goals? What constitutes performance and results in this organization?"

4. They were extremely tolerant of diversity in people and did not look for carbon copies of themselves. It rarely even occurred to them to ask, "Do I like or dislike this person?" But they were totally—fiendishly—intolerant when it came to a person's performance, standards, and values.

5. They were not afraid of strength in their associates. They gloried in it. Whether they had heard of it or not, their motto was the one Andrew Carnegie wanted to have put on his tombstone: "Here lies a man who attracted better people into his service than he was himself."[9]

6. One way or another, they submitted themselves to the mirror test—that is, they made sure the person they saw in the mirror in the morning was the kind of person they wanted to be, respect, and believe in. This way they fortified themselves against the leader's greatest temptations—to do things that are popular rather than right and to do petty, mean, sleazy things.[10]

Finally, these leaders were not preachers; they were doers.

The most effective leaders share a number of skills, and these skills are always related to dealing with employees. The following suggestions outline an approach to becoming a hospitality industry leader rather than just a manager:

- *Be decisive.* Hospitality industry leaders are confronted with dozens of decisions every day. Obviously, you should use your best judgment to resolve the decisions that come to roost at your doorstep. As a boss, make the decisions that best meet both your objectives and your ethics, and then make your decisions known.

- *Follow through.* Never promise what you can't deliver, and never build false hopes among your employees. Once expectations are dashed, respect for and the reputation of the boss are shot.

- *Select the best.* A boss, good or bad, is carried forward by the work of his or her subordinates. One key to being a good boss is to hire the people who have the best potential to do what you need them to do. Take the time and effort to screen, interview, and assess the people who have not only the skills that you require, but also the needed values.

- *Empower employees.* Give people the authority to interact with the customer. The more important people feel, the better they work.

- *Enhance career development.* Good bosses recognize that most of their people want to improve themselves. However, career development is a two-edged sword: If we take the initiative to train and develop our people properly, then the competition is likely to hire them. The only way a boss can prevent the loss of productive workers looking for career development is to provide opportunities for growth within the organization and to maintain an empowering work environment.

CORPORATE PROFILE

The Ritz-Carlton Hotel Company: A Commitment to Excellence and Quality Service Worldwide

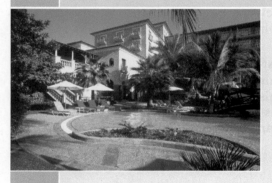

The Ritz-Carlton Hotel Company was officially organized in the summer of 1983, although the Ritz-Carlton history and tradition long precede that date. Indeed, this tradition has entered our language: To be "ritzy" or "putting on the ritz" denotes doing something with class. With the purchase of the Ritz-Carlton Boston and the acquisition of the exclusive rights to use the name came a rich heritage.

The legacy of the Ritz-Carlton begins with the celebrated hotelier Cesar Ritz, the "king of hoteliers and hotelier to kings." Cesar Ritz's philosophy of service and innovations redefined the luxury hotel experience in Europe through his management of the Ritz Paris and the Carlton in London. The Ritz-Carlton Boston revolutionized hospitality in the United States by creating luxury in a hotel setting.

Cesar Ritz died in 1918, but his wife Marie continued the expansion of hotels bearing his name. In the United States, the Ritz-Carlton Investing Company was established by Albert Keller, who bought and franchised the name. In 1927, the Ritz-Carlton Boston was opened by Edward N. Wyner, a Boston real estate developer, with room rates of $15 per night. Because of the reputation of Ritz in Europe and the cosmopolitan society in Boston, Wyner knew the Ritz-Carlton name would secure immediate success.

Fast-forward to 1983, when William B. Johnson acquired the rights to establish the Ritz-Carlton Hotel Company. The company now operates seventy-seven hotels worldwide.[1] Further expansion plans are included for Africa, Asia, the Caribbean, the Middle East, and the Americas.[2]

The Ritz-Carlton Hotel Company was named the winner of the prestigious Malcolm Baldrige National Quality Award in 1992 and again in 1999. The Ritz-Carlton is the only hospitality organization ever to have

[1]The Ritz-Carlton, *Fact Sheet*, http://corporate.ritzcarlton.com/en/Press/FactSheet.htm (accessed November 28, 2011).
[2]The Ritz-Carlton, *Future Opening*, http://www.ritzcarlton.com/en/Locations/Upcoming.htm (accessed November 28, 2011).

won this coveted honor for quality management, given by the U.S. Department of Commerce. Seven categories make up the award criteria: leadership, strategic planning, customer and market focus, information and analysis, human resources focus, process management, and business results. At the Ritz-Carlton, a focus on these criteria has resulted in higher employee and customer satisfaction, and increased productivity and market share. Perhaps most significant is increased profitability.

Horst Schultze, founding president and CEO, whose vision and leadership was the driving force behind the success in obtaining the Malcolm Baldrige Awards. Since joining the company, Herve Humler has been responsible for the successful opening of several hotels. This expansion continues with seven hotels and resorts slated for opening over the next decade. The Ritz-Carlton Residences and the Ritz-Carlton Club were also successfully developed and launched under Cooper's tenure.

Committed employees rank as the most essential element to Ritz-Carlton's success. All employees are schooled and carry a pocket-sized card stating the company's Gold Standards, which include a credo, motto, three steps of service, and twenty Ritz-Carlton basics. Each employee is expected to understand and adhere to these standards, which describe processes for solving problems that guests may have as well as detailed grooming, housekeeping, and safety and efficiency standards. "We are Ladies and Gentlemen serving Ladies and Gentlemen" is the motto of the Ritz-Carlton, exemplifying anticipatory service provided by all staff members. "Every employee has the business plan of the Ritz-Carlton—constantly reinforcing that guest satisfaction is our highest mission," says Hulmer.

The company has quickly grown a collection of the finest hotels around the world. Several of these hotels are historic landmarks, following a commitment of the company to preserving architecturally important buildings. Some examples are the Ritz-Carlton New York, Central Park; the Ritz-Carlton, San Francisco; the Ritz-Carlton, Philadelphia; the Ritz-Carlton, New Orleans; and the Ritz-Carlton, Huntington Hotel & Spa. Each property is designed to be a comfortable haven for travelers and a social center for the community. The architecture and artwork are carefully selected to complement the hotel's environment. "We go to great lengths to capture the spirit of a hotel and its locale," says Cooper. "This creates a subtle balance and celebrates a gracious, relaxed lifestyle. The Ritz-Carlton is warm, relaxed yet refined; a most comfortable home away from home." The Ritz-Carlton Hotel Company is now owned and operated by Marriott International.

In recent years, the role of the hotel general manager (GM) has changed from that of being a congenial host, knowledgeable about the niceties of hotelmanship, to that of a multigroup pleaser. Guests, employees, owners, and community should all not only be satisfied but be delighted with the operation's performance.

Many GMs are so bogged down with meetings, reports, and "putting out fires" that they hardly have any time to spend with guests. One GM who makes time for guests is Richard Riley, GM of the fabulous Shangri-La Hotel Makati in Manila, the Philippines. Richard extends an invitation for guests to visit with him in the hotel lobby between 5:00 and 7:00 P.M. every Thursday. As GM of a luxury Caribbean resort in Barbados, West Indies, the author of this text personally greeted every guest to the property. Obviously, there is a difference between a small resort and a large city hotel. Resort guests stay for at least two, sometimes four, weeks in high season, so they need individual attention.

TECHNOLOGY SPOTLIGHT

Use of Social Networking Tools in the Hospitality Industry

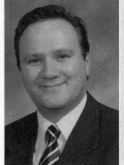

Cihan Cobanoglu, Ph.D., Dean, School of Hotel and Restaurant Management, University of South Florida, Sarasota-Manatee

One of the most significant recent advances in consumer-based information technology is the introduction, and extremely fast adoption, of social networking tools. Today there are more than 800 million active users on Facebook, according to the site, with its popular "friending" approach to making connections. On any given day, 50 percent of these users log into their accounts. More than 250 million photos are uploaded daily; more than 350 million active users access Facebook through a mobile device; and more than 70 languages are used on the site.[1]

In the business arena, thousands, if not millions, local businesses have active pages on Facebook and those pages have created billions of fans combined. Twitter, with its 140-character "tweeting" approach to getting the word out, is powerful in its own right, with an estimated 32.1 million users in 2009, a growth of nearly 2,000 percent over the 1.6 million users in 2008.

Marketing rules used to dictate that a happy customer would tell three friends about your establishment and an angry customer would tell eleven friends. This is no longer the case; in both instances, whether happy or displeased, customers can easily reach tens if not hundreds of contacts. Given the vastness of social media connections and networks, this can quickly multiply into thousands or more potential customers with word-of-mouth insight into your products and service.

Hotels and Restaurants in the Fray

Many hotel and restaurant operators are aware that social media tools can and should be leveraged for their businesses, but they struggle to identify specific return on investment. In fact, according to Hospitality Technology's 12th annual Restaurant Technology Study, although nearly one-half of restaurants recognize that there is value in Twitter as a marketing tool, only one-third of restaurant operators use it. There exist, however, many successful examples of hotels using social networking sites to generate awareness and additional revenue opportunities. As of press time, Seattle's Hotel 1000, as a single property, has about 3,083 Facebook fans, and Excalibur Hotel and Casino in Las Vegas has more than 60,397. Hilton Hotels has more than 128,436, and Sheraton Hotels has more than 108,173 fans, while Olive Garden Restaurants has more than 1,891,748 fans.

While the size of the fan base is important, the true value is in the interaction. A quick scan of these Facebook pages shows two factors for success: First, they have personality and build emotional connections, and second, people respond and interact on these pages.

Strategies for Success

Social networking tools can be used for more than connecting to external customers. Companies also use these tools to find employees and to solicit feedback from current and potential customers on menu items, decorations, room design, and more. They can even be used as a venue to prompt customers to suggest new menu items. If encouraged properly, employees can be ambassadors of your company in their own social networks.

[1]Facebook, *Statistics*, http://www.facebook.com/press/info.php?statistics (accessed November 28, 2011).

One creative example of a hotel's use of social networking to boost guest participation is demonstrated by Pod Hotel New York's own social networking site, The Pod Culture message board. When guests make reservations online, they are invited to become a member of the Pod Community. There, they can choose a log-in and password and participate in an array of forums: Drink with Me, Eat with Me, Shop with Me, Go Out with Me, and so forth.

Though social networking tools are powerful, they must be well planned and carefully implemented to avoid pitfalls. If you ask for customers' opinions, listen to them. What's more, managing social networking tools will take time. For this reason, each company should assign personnel to the task of monitoring and regularly updating its social networks. Some hotel companies are recruiting managers dedicated to online services and e-commerce initiatives. Many are combining this responsibility with a revenue, marketing, or front office manager.

My recommendation to all hotels and restaurants would be to connect to their guests, employees, families, and vendors through different social networking tools. If you are not doing this already, you are behind the curve.

▶ Check Your Knowledge

1. What three factors does transformational leadership involve?
2. Define *leadership*.
3. Describe some examples of leadership.
4. Explain the demands placed on leaders.

Hospitality Management

Managers plan, organize, make decisions, communicate, motivate, and control the efforts of a group to accomplish predetermined goals. Management also establishes the direction the organization will take. Sometimes this is done with the help of employees or outside consultants, such as marketing research specialists. Managers obtain the necessary resources for the goals to be accomplished, and then they supervise and monitor group and individual progress toward goal accomplishment.

Managers, such as presidents and CEOs, who are responsible for the entire company, tend to focus most of their time on strategic planning and the organization's mission. They also spend time organizing and controlling the activities of the corporation. Most top managers do not get involved in the day-to-day aspects of the operation. These duties and responsibilities fall to the middle and supervisory management. In hospitality lingo, one would not expect Bill Marriott to pull a shift behind the bar at the local Marriott hotel. Although capable, his time and expertise are better used in shaping the company's future. Thus, although the head bartender and Bill Marriott may both be considered management, they require slightly different skills to be effective and efficient managers.

What Is Management?

Management is simply what managers do: plan, organize, make decisions, communicate, motivate, and control. *Management* is defined as "coordinating and overseeing the activities of others so that their activities are completed efficiently and effectively."[11] In looking at this statement, you can see that the functions of management and working with and through the work of others are ongoing. Additionally, management involves getting efficient and effective results.

Efficiency is getting the most done with the fewest number of inputs. Managers work with scarce resources: money, people, time, and equipment. You can imagine the rush in the kitchen to be ready for a meal service. But it's not enough

A DAY IN THE LIFE OF STEPHANIE SUMMERALL

Director of Sales and Marketing, Intercontinental Hotels Group

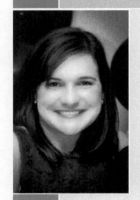

"Choose a job you love and you will never have to work a day in your life." Well, this quote could not be further from the truth, yet those of us who have chosen to work in the amazing field of hospitality would never consider making a move! There is something indescribable about being invited into the lives of a family planning a 50th wedding anniversary, a young bride obsessing over every last detail, a Fortune 500 company organizing its annual investors conference, and a political campaign trying to capture the perfect setting to deliver its message. It's a wonderfully infectious environment and one worth every ounce of hard work.

I began my career working as Director of Member Relations at Mission Hills Country Club in Palm Springs, California, a position that I was nowhere near ready to take on. Thankfully, I had the wonderful fortune of working with a fantastically talented team of professionals and from them I learned the skill needed to cultivate strong business relationships, I learned how to get creative when things didn't go as planned, and I became as resilient, as this field requires you to be in order to achieve success. Four years later in December 2004, I moved to London and, with a great deal of luck, managed to receive the most glamorous position imaginable, Senior Sales Manager for Claridge's, The Berkeley, and The Connaught, three of the most prestigious hotels in the world.

Being in sales is the most rewarding, but can also be the most illusory, of hospitality jobs. To many, being in the sales department means having a very cushy job. After all, we do enter through the front doors and are seen entertaining over lunches and cocktail receptions, but what isn't so obvious are the hours of researching new businesses, countless hours of telephone calls to qualify possible leads, and the pressure of exceeding revenue numbers that are set each month, each quarter, each year. I believe a close comparison can be made between sales and childbirth: Once it all comes together and you are holding a beautifully signed deal in your hands and your client is happy and smiling at you, you quickly forget about the heartache that came along the way . . . what a blessing it is! Although most of us chose this field because we have a desire to serve people and work creatively, it is a business like any other. I feel Mr. Henry Ford said it best, "A business absolutely devoted to service will have only one worry about profits. They will be embarrassingly large."[12] During these recent economic times, it is amazing the swing of successful hotels and those in financial struggle. They aren't located in different cities, they aren't vastly different in size, they are evenly matched in product, but they are indescribably different in their service delivery.

to just be efficient; management is also about being effective. **Effectiveness** is "doing the right thing." As an example, cooks do the right thing when they cook the food correctly according to the recipe and have it ready when needed.

Who Are Managers?

The changing nature of organizations and work has, in many hospitality organizations, blurred the lines of distinction between managers and nonmanagerial employees. Many traditional jobs now include managerial activities, especially when teams are used. For instance, team members often develop plans, make decisions, and monitor their own performance. This is the case with total quality management.

So, how do we define who managers are? A manager is someone who works with and manages others' activities to accomplish organizational goals in an efficient and effective way. Managers are often classified into three levels: **frontline managers** are the lowest-level managers; they manage the work of line employees. They may also be called supervisors. A front-office supervisor, for example, takes charge of a shift and supervises the guest service agents on the shift.

Middle managers are akin to department heads; they fall between frontline managers and top management. They are responsible for short- to medium-range plans, and they establish goals and objectives to meet these goals. They manage the work of frontline managers.

Top managers are responsible for making medium- to long-range plans and for establishing goals and strategies to meet those goals. Figure 4 shows the three levels of management plus nonmanagerial employees.

Key Management Functions

The key management functions are planning, organizing, decision making, communicating, human resources and motivating, and controlling. These management functions are not conducted in isolation; rather, they are interdependent and frequently happen simultaneously or at least overlap. Figure 5 shows the key management functions leading to goal accomplishment.

Hospitality companies exist to serve a particular purpose, and someone has to determine the vision, mission, and strategies to reach or exceed the goals. That someone is management. The **planning** function involves setting the company's goals and developing plans to meet or exceed those goals. Once plans are complete, **organizing** is undertaken to decide what needs to be done, who will

Top Managers
Middle Managers
Front-line Managers
Nonmanagerial Associates

Figure 4 • Three Levels of Management Plus Nonmanagerial Associates.

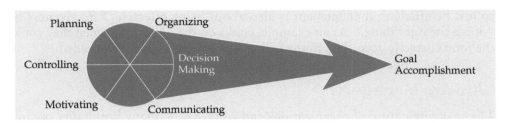

Figure 5 • Key Management Functions Leading to Goal Accomplishment.

do it, how the tasks will be grouped, who reports to whom, and who makes decisions.

Decision making is a key management function. The success of all hospitality companies, whether large, multinational corporations or sole proprietorships, depends on the quality of the decision making. Decision making includes determining the vision, mission, goals, and objectives of the company. Decision making also includes scheduling employees, determining what to put on the menu, and responding to guest needs.

Communication with and motivation of individuals and groups are required to get the job done. **Human resources and motivating** involves attracting and retaining the best employees and keeping morale high.

Controlling is the final management function that brings everything full circle. After the goals are set and the plans formulated, management then organizes, communicates, and motivates the resources required to complete the job. Controlling includes the setting of standards and comparing actual results with these standards. If significant deviations are seen, they are investigated and corrective action is taken to get performance back on target. This scientific process of monitoring, comparing, and correcting is the controlling function and is necessary to ensure that there are no surprises and that no one is guessing what should be done.

Managerial Skills

In addition to the management functions of forecasting, planning, organizing, communicating, motivating, and controlling, managers also need other major skills: conceptual, interpersonal, and technical.

Conceptual skills enable top managers to view the corporation as a complete entity and yet understand how it is split into departments to achieve specific goals. Conceptual skills allow a top manager to view the entire corporation, especially the interdependence of the various departments.

Managers need to lead, influence, communicate, supervise, coach, and evaluate employees' performances. This necessitates a high level of interpersonal human skills. The abilities to build teams and work with others are human skills that successful managers need to cultivate.

Managers need to have the technical skills required to understand and use modern techniques, methods, equipment, and procedures. These skills are more important for lower levels of management. As a manager rises through the

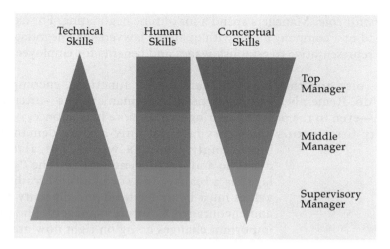

Figure 6 • Management Skill Areas Required by Management Level.

ranks, the need for technical skills decreases and the need for conceptual skills increases.

You next need to realize the critical importance of the corporate philosophy, culture, and values, and of a corporation's mission, goals, and objectives. Figure 6 shows the degree of managerial skills required by top managers, middle managers, and supervisory managers.

The Manager's Changing Role

Managers may still have subordinates, but today's successful manager takes more of a team leader/coach approach. There are, of course, other ways to "slice and dice" what managers do. For example, managers don't just plan, organize, make decisions, communicate, motivate, and control. They wear a variety of hats, including the following:

- *Figurehead role.* Every manager spends some time performing ceremonial duties. For example, the president of a corporation might have to greet important business guests or clients or represent the corporation by attending dinners.

- *Leader role.* Every manager should be a leader, coaching, motivating, and encouraging employees.

- *Liaison role.* Managers spend a lot of time in contact with people in other departments both within the organization and externally. An example would be the sales manager liaising with the rooms division director.

- *Spokesperson role.* The manager is often the spokesperson for the organization. For example, a manager may host a college class visit to the property.

- *Negotiator role.* Managers spend a lot of time negotiating. For example, the head of a company along with qualified lawyers may negotiate with a union representative to establish wages and benefits for employees.

These roles, together with the management functions, encompass what managers do. Remember, managers need to be many things—often in quick succession—even to the point of wearing two or more hats at once.

Twenty-first-century managers face not only a more demanding and increasingly complex world, but also a more dynamic and interdependent one. The "global village" is a reality, and sociocultural traditions and values must be understood and diversity respected and encouraged by future managers. The two most important changes going on right now are the technological advances and the internationalization of hospitality and tourism. The extent to which you as a future **leader/manager** can master these events and functions will determine your future.

The manager's role is not only internal but also external. For instance, a manager must be responsive to market needs and income generation. Managers must continually strive to be innovative by realizing efficiencies in their respective areas of responsibility through process improvement—for example, by determining how to reduce long check-in lines at airports and hotels. Some companies use innovative and creative ways to streamline the check-in procedures to make the process a more worthwhile experience for the guests. Disney, for instance, uses the creative approach of sending Mickey and the gang to entertain the guests while they stand in line.

A General Manager's Survival Kit

Ali Kasiki is a top-level manager at the Peninsula Beverly Hills, California. He holds the title of managing director and is involved in creating and implementing broad and comprehensive changes that affect the entire organization. Ali offers his list of tips:

- Know yourself, your own core competencies, and your values.
- Hire a seasoned management team.
- Build barriers of entry; that is, make yourself indispensable.
- Be very flexible.

You, Too, Are a Manager

Your classmates have just voted you to be the leader/manager of the summer study-abroad trip to France. None of you knows much about France or how to get there, what to do when you get there, and so on. Where would you start? (Resist the temptation to delegate the whole trip to a travel agent, please.)

You might start by thinking through what you need to do in terms of planning, organizing, deciding, communicating, motivating, and controlling. What sort of plans will you need? Among other things, you'll need to plan the dates your group will be leaving and returning, the cities and towns you'll visit, the airline you'll take there and back, how the group will get around France, and where you'll stay when you're there. As you can imagine, plans like these are very important: You would not want to arrive at Orly Airport with a group of friends who are depending on you and not know what to do next.

Realizing how much work is involved—and that you cannot do it all and still maintain good grades—you get help. You divide up the work and create an organization by asking someone to check airline schedules and prices, another person to check hotel prices, and someone else to research the sights to see and the transportation needs. However, the job won't get done with the group members simply working by themselves. Each person requires guidance and coordination from you: The person making the airline bookings can't confirm the bookings unless she knows in what city and airport the trip will originate. Similarly, the person making the hotel arrangements can't make any firm bookings until he knows what cities are being visited. To improve communications, you could set up regular meetings, with e-mail updates between meetings. Leadership and motivation could be a challenge because two of the group members do not get along well. So, ensuring that everyone stays focused and positive will be a challenge.

Of course, you'll have to make sure the whole project remains in control. If something can go wrong, it often will, and that's certainly the case when groups of people are traveling together. Everything needs to be double-checked. In other words, managing is something managers do almost every day, often without even knowing it.

Source: Adapted from Gary Dessler, *A Framework for Management* (Upper Saddle River, NJ: Prentice Hall, 2002) 8.

- Get close to your guests and owners to define reality versus perception.
- Show leadership, from both the top and the bottom.
- Delegate. There is no way you can survive without delegation.
- Appeal to trends.
- Trust your instincts.
- Take risks and change the ground rules.
- Don't become overconfident.
- Look successful, or people will think you're not.
- Manage the future—it is the best thing you can do. Bring the future to the present.[13]

Sustainable Leadership

Sustainable leadership is individual leadership that benefits the long-term good of society by positively influencing people, creating change, and demonstrating values that support the highest principles of society.[14]

The United Nations has developed a blueprint for Corporate Sustainability Leadership. The blueprint has four parts under the following headings:[15]

1. Global Compact
   a. Full coverage and Integration across principals
   b. Robust management policies and procedures
   c. Mainstreaming into corporate functions and business units
   d. Value chain implementation

2. Tracking action in support of broader UN goals and issues
   a. Core business contributions to UN goals and issues
   b. Strategic social investments and philanthropy
   c. Advocacy and public policy engagement
   d. Partnership and collective action

3. Engaging with UN global compact
   a. Local network and subsidiary engagement
   b. Global and local networking groups
   c. Issue-based and sector indicatives
   d. Promotion and support of the UN global compact

4. The cross-cutting components
   a. CEO commitment and leadership
   b. Broad adoption and oversight
   c. Stakeholder engagement
   d. Transparency and disclosure

Many business leaders, including hospitality ones, are becoming increasingly more concerned about sustainability. Not only are they concerned about the environment but also social responsibility. Leaders and managers need to steer the organization on a path of sustainability for all associates to follow.

If leaders stress the importance of sustainability then others will follow. Sustainability does not happen by itself; it needs leaders to promote it. From cities that do not allow styrofoam food containers to reducing water, paper, and electric consumption it all comes together when leaders focus on sustainability in all the key result areas of their operations.

Distinction Between Leadership and Management

Managing is the formal process in which organizational objectives are achieved through the efforts of subordinates. *Leading* is the process by which a person with vision is able to influence the behavior of others in some desired way. Although managers have power by virtue of the positions they hold, organizations seek managers who are leaders by virtue of their personalities, their experience, and so on. The differences between management and leadership can be illustrated as follows:

Managers
- Work in the system
- React
- Control risks
- Enforce organizational rules
- Seek and then follow direction
- Control people by pushing them in the right direction
- Coordinate effort

Leaders
- Work on the system
- Create opportunities
- Seek opportunities
- Change organizational rules
- Provide a vision to believe in and strategic alignment
- Motivate people by satisfying basic human needs
- Inspire achievement and energize people[16]

▶ Check Your Knowledge

1. What is management and what are the three management skill areas?
2. Explain levels of management.
3. Describe the key management functions.
4. What is the distinction between leadership and management?

Ethics

Ethics is a set of moral principles and values that people use to answer questions about right and wrong. Because ethics is also about our personal value system, there are people with value systems different from ours. Where did the value system originate? What happens if one value system is different from another? Fortunately, certain universal guiding principles are agreed on by virtually all religions, cultures, and societies. The foundation of all principles is that all people's rights are important and should not be violated. This belief is central to civilized societies; without it, chaos would reign.

Today, people have few moral absolutes; they decide situationally whether it is acceptable to steal, lie, or drink and drive. They seem to think that whatever is right is what works best for the individual. In a country blessed with so many diverse cultures, you might think it is impossible to identify common standards of ethical behavior. However, among sources from many different times and places, such as the Bible, Aristotle's *Ethics*, William Shakespeare's *King Lear*, the Koran, and the *Analects* of Confucius, you'll find the following basic moral values: integrity, respect for human life, self-control, honesty, and courage. Cruelty is wrong. All the world's major religions support a version of the Golden Rule: Do unto others as you would have them do unto you.[17]

In the foreword to *Ethics in Hospitality Management*, edited by Stephen S. J. Hall,[18] Dean Emeritus of Cornell University, Robert A. Beck poses this question: "Is overbooking hotel rooms and airline seats ethical? How does one compare the legal responsibilities of the innkeeper and the airline manager to the moral obligation?" He also asks, What is a fair or reasonable wage? A fair or reasonable return on investment? Is it fair or ethical to underpay employees for the benefit of investors?

English Common Law, on which American law is based, left such decisions to the "reasonable man." A judge would ask the jury, "Was this the act of a reasonable man?" Interestingly, what is considered ethical in one country may not be in another. For instance, in some countries, it is considered normal to bargain for room rates; in others, bargaining would be considered bad form.

Ethics and morals have become an integral part of hospitality decisions, from employment (equal opportunity and affirmative action) to truth in menus. Many corporations and businesses have developed a code of ethics that all employees use to make decisions. This became necessary because too many managers were making decisions without regard for the impact of such decisions on others. Stephen Hall is one of the pioneers of ethics in hospitality; he has developed a code of ethics for the hospitality and tourism industry, as follows:

1. We acknowledge ethics and morality as inseparable elements of doing business and will test every decision against the highest standards of honesty, legality, fairness, impunity, and conscience.
2. We will conduct ourselves personally and collectively at all times so as to bring credit to the hospitality and tourism industry.
3. We will concentrate our time, energy, and resources on the improvement of our own products and services and we will not denigrate our competition in the pursuit of our success.
4. We will treat all guests equally regardless of race, religion, nationality, creed, or sex.
5. We will deliver all standards of service and product with total consistency to every guest.
6. We will provide a totally safe and sanitary environment at all times for every guest and employee.
7. We will strive constantly, in words, actions, and deeds, to develop and maintain the highest level of trust, honesty, and understanding among guests, clients, employees, employers, and the public at large.
8. We will provide every employee at every level all the knowledge, training, equipment, and motivation required to perform his or her tasks according to our published standards.
9. We will guarantee that every employee at every level will have the same opportunity to perform, advance, and be evaluated against the same standard as all employees engaged in the same or similar tasks.
10. We will actively and consciously work to protect and preserve our natural environment and natural resources in all that we do.
11. We will seek a fair and honest profit, no more, no less.[19]

As you can see, it is vitally important for future hospitality and tourism professionals to abide by this code. The following sections present some ethical dilemmas in hospitality. What do you think about them?

Ethical Dilemmas in Hospitality

Previously, certain actions may not have been considered ethical, but management often looked the other way. A few scenarios follow that are not seen as ethical today and are against most companies' ethical policies:

1. As catering manager of a large banquet operation, the flowers for the hotel are booked through your office. The account is worth $15,000 per month.

A florist offers you a 10-percent kickback to book the account with him. Given that your colleague at a sister hotel in the same company receives a good bonus and you do not, despite having a better financial result, do you accept the kickback? If so, with whom do you share it?

2. As purchasing agent for a major hospitality organization, you are responsible for purchasing $5 million worth of perishable and nonperishable items. To get your business, a supplier, whose quality and price are similar to others, offers you a new automobile. Do you accept?

3. An order has come from the corporate office that guests from a certain part of the world may only be accepted if the reservation is taken from the embassy of the countries. One Sunday afternoon, you are duty manager and several limos with people from "that part of the world" request rooms for several weeks. You decline, even though there are available rooms. They even offer you a personal envelope, which they say contains $1,000. How do you feel about declining their request?

Trends in Leadership and Management

- Many leaders will be leading a more diverse group of associates.
- Many entry-level employees will not have basic job skills.
- There will be an increasing need for training.
- There will be a need to create leaders out of line managers.
- Leaders will need to manage sales revenue all the way to the bottom line.
- Independent business units will be established to make their own profit, or that department will be subcontracted out.
- Instead of keeping a person on payroll for a function that is only needed occasionally, that service will be outsourced to specialists.
- The amount of full-time employees will be cut and more part-time employees will be hired to avoid paying benefits.
- Keeping up with technological advances and their benefits will be an increasing challenge.
- Social and environmental issues will continue to increase in importance.
- A greater emphasis will be placed on ethics.

CASE STUDY

Performance Standards

Charles and Nancy both apply for the assistant front-office manager position at a 300-room upscale hotel. Charles has worked for a total of eight years in three different hotels and has been with this hotel for three months as a front-office associate. Initially, he had a lot of enthusiasm. Lately, however, he has been dressing a bit sloppily and his figures, cash, and reports have been inaccurate. In addition, he is occasionally rattled by demanding guests.

Nancy recently graduated from college with honors, with a degree in hospitality management. While attending college, she worked part-time as a front desk associate at a budget motel. Nancy does not have a lot of experience working in a hotel or in customer service in general, but she is quite knowledgeable as a result of her studies and is eager to begin her career.

It appears that Charles would be considered a prime candidate for the office manager position because of his extensive experience in other hotels and his knowledge of the hotel's culture. In view of his recent performance, however, the rooms division manager will need to sit down with Charles to review his future career development track.

Discussion Questions

1. What are the qualifications for the job that should be considered for both applicants?
2. How should the discussion between the rooms division manager and Charles be handled? Make specific recommendations for the rooms division manager.
3. Who would be the better person for the job? Why?

CASE STUDY

Reluctant to Change

You have just been appointed assistant manager at an old, established, but busy, New York restaurant. Your employees respond to your suggested changes with "We have always done it this way." The employees really do not know any other way of doing things.

Discussion Question

1. How should you handle this situation?

Summary

1. Leadership is defined as the process by which a person is able to influence the activities and outcomes of others in a desired way.
2. Contemporary leadership includes transactional and transformational types of leadership.
3. Increased demands placed on hospitality leaders include ownership, corporate, regulatory, employee, environmental, and social interests. Leaders must balance results and relationships.
4. Managing is the process of coordinating work activities so that they are completed efficiently and effectively with and through other people.
5. Leaders, according to Peter Drucker, realize four things and behave in much the same way.
   a. A leader is someone who has followers—some people are thinkers, and some are prophets.
   b. An effective leader is not someone who is loved or admired, but rather someone whose followers do the right things. Popularity is not leadership; results are.
   c. Leaders are highly visible. Leaders set examples.
   d. Leadership is not about rank, privileges, titles, or money. It is about responsibility.
6. There are six key management functions: planning, organizing, decision making, communicating, motivating, and controlling. However, in addition to these functions, managers occasionally have to fill roles such as figurehead, leader, spokesperson, and negotiator.
7. The difference between management and leadership is that the former is the formal process in which organization objectives are achieved through the efforts of subordinates, and the latter is the process by which a person with vision is able to influence the behavior of others in some desired way.

Key Words and Concepts

communication
controlling
decision making
effectiveness
efficiency
ethics
frontline managers
human resources and motivating
leader/manager

leadership
management
managing
middle managers
organizing
planning
top managers
transactional leadership
transformational leadership

Review Questions

1. What kind of leader/manager will you be?
2. Give examples of the management functions as they apply to the hospitality industry.
3. Discuss the changing role of managers.
4. Define leadership and name the essential qualities of a good leader.
5. Distinguish between transactional and transformational leadership.

Internet Exercises

1. Organization: **WetFeet.com**
   Web site: **www.wetfeet.com**
   Summary: WetFeet.com is an organization dedicated to helping you make smarter career decisions. WetFeet.com provides inside understanding of jobs and careers for both job seekers and recruiters. By all means, take the time to check this one out! Click on "Careers & Industries" at the bottom of the page and scroll down to "General Management" under "Careers." Answer the following questions.

   (a) What are the requirements for becoming a GM, and what tips does WetFeet.com have to offer?
   (b) The "General Management" section illustrates several attributes that managers have in common. In groups, list these attributes and discuss their significance.

2. Organization: **American Management Association**
   Web site: **www.amanet.org**
   Summary: The American Management Association (AMA), a practitioner-based organization, offers a wide range of

management development programs for managers and organizations.
Find the section titled "Articles and White Papers." Choose two current reports on leadership. Read through these and make a bullet list of the key information. Then, write a description of how this information might affect the way a hospitality manager plans, organizes, makes decisions, communicates, motivates, and controls.

3. Organization: **Ritz-Carlton Hotel Company**
   Web site: **http://corporate.ritzcarlton.com/en/Default.htm**
   Summary: Ritz-Carlton hotels are known for their superior luxury and service in the hospitality industry. This particular Web exercise illustrates how Ritz-Carlton maintains its culture of service excellence. Take a look at the Ritz-Carlton Leadership Center. Click on "Leadership Center." Now answer the following questions:

   (a) What kinds of courses does the Leadership Center offer?
   (b) **What are the seven habits of highly effective people?**

Apply Your Knowledge

Your resort has management vacancies for the following positions: executive chef, executive housekeeper, and front-office manager.

List the traits and characteristics that you consider essential and desirable for these positions.

Suggested Activity

Think of someone you admire as a leader. Make a list of the qualities that make him or her a good leader.

Endnotes

1. For a more detailed review of the many leadership theories, consult one of the many texts on the topic.
2. Horst Schultz, Presentation to the University of South Florida School of Hotel and Restaurant Management, March 26, 2005.
3. Ibid.
4. West Paces Hotel Group, *Philosophy*, http://www.westpaceshotels.com/mission.htm (accessed November 26, 2011).
5. West Paces Hotel Group, *Home Page*, http://www.westpaceshotels.com/home.htm (accessed November 26, 2011).
6. Jay R. Schrock, Presentation to University of South Florida students and faculty, May 2, 2005.
7. Vernon Saunders Law, Major League Baseball player. http://assets.teamusa.org/assets/documents/attached_file/filename/23291/Sports_Quotes_p._27–76_ver_3.16.10.pdf retrieved Jaunary 1, 2012.
8. Adapted from Peter F. Drucker, "Foreword," in *The Leader of the Future*, ed. F. Hesselbein, et al., xii–xiii (San Francisco: Josey-Bass, 1996).
9. George Ambler, "Peter Drucker on Effective Leadership," *The Practice of Leadership*, Aug. 6, 2006, http://www.thepracticeofleadership.net/peter-drucker-on-effective-leadership (accessed November 27, 2011).
10. Drucker, "Foreword," ix.
11. Stephen P. Robbins and Mary Coulter, Management 9th ed., Pearson, Upper Saddle River, NJ: 2007. P. 7.
12. BrainyQuote, *Henry Ford Quotes*, http://www.brainyquote.com/quotes/quotes/h/henryford151873.html (accessed November 28, 2011).
13. Personal correspondence with Ali Kasiki, August 4, 2005.
14. http://www.highlandconsultinggroupinc.com/programs/sustainable.html retrieved November 17, 2001.
15. http://www.unglobalcompact.org/docs/news_events/8.1/Blueprint.pdf retrieved on November 19, 2011.
16. Vadim Kotelnikov, *Ten3 Business e-Coach*, version 2005a, http://www.1000ventures.com/business_guide/crosscuttings/e_coach.html.
17. Religious Tolerance, *Shared Belief in the "Golden Rule" (a/k.a. Ethics of Reciprocity)*, http://www.religioustolerance.org/reciproc.htm (accessed November 28, 2011).
18. Stephen S. Hall, ed., *Ethics in Hospitality Management: A Book of Readings* (East Lansing, MI: Educational Institute, American Hotel & Lodging Association, 1992), 75.
19. Hall, *Ethics in Hospitality Management*, 108.

Glossary

Control   The provision of information to management for decision-making purposes. The process of monitoring activities to ensure that they are being accomplished as planned and of correcting any significant deviations.

Effectiveness   Completing activities so that organizational goals are attained; also referred to as "doing the right things" or "getting things done."

Efficiency   Getting the most output from the smallest amount of inputs; also referred to as "doing things right" or "getting things done well."

Ethics   The study of standards of conduct and moral judgment; also, the standards of correct conduct.

Frontline manager/supervisor   A low-level manager who manages the work of line employees and has guest contact.

Leader-manager An individual whose duties combine the functions of leadership and management.

Leadership The influence of one person over another to work willingly toward a predetermined objective.

Management The process of coordinating work activities so that an organization's objectives are achieved efficiently and effectively with and through other people.

Middle manager A manager between the first-line level and the top level of the organization who manages the work of first-line managers.

Planning The process of defining the organization's goals, establishing an overall strategy for achieving those goals, and developing a comprehensive set of plans to integrate and coordinate organizational work.

Top manager A manager at or near the top level of the organization who is responsible for making organization-wide decisions and establishing the goals and plans that affect the entire organization.

Transactional leadership A type of leadership that focuses on accomplishing the tasks at hand and on maintaining good working relationships by exchanging promises of rewards for performance.

Transformational leadership A type of leadership that involves influencing major changes in the attitudes and assumptions of organization members and building commitment for the organization's mission, objectives, and strategies.

Photo Credits

Credits are listed in the order of appearance.

Control

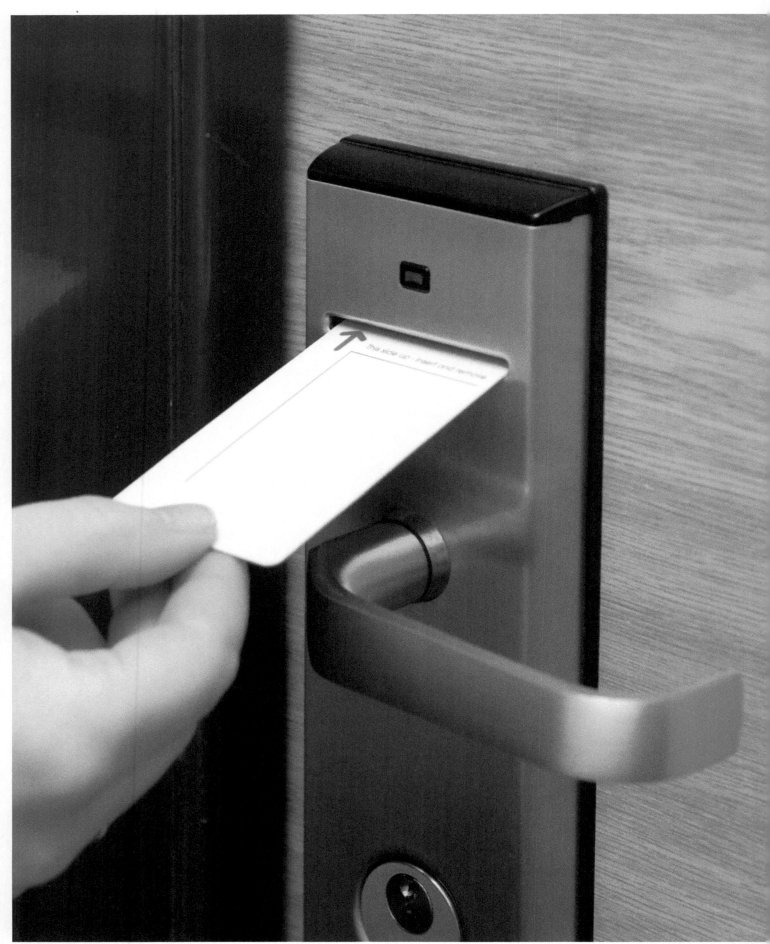

Control

OBJECTIVES

After reading and studying this chapter, you should be able to:

- Define control.
- Give reasons why control is important.
- Describe the four-step control process.
- Distinguish among the three types of control.
- Explain the important financial controls.
- Describe the qualities of an effective control system.
- Outline the contemporary issues in control.

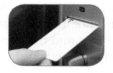
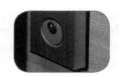
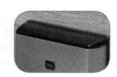
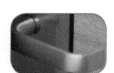

Did you ever get to the end of the week or the month and discover that you'd run out of money? Well, at one time or another, we all have, and yes, it's because we didn't exercise proper control. But control is not only about keeping our finances in order—it has a much broader and more important role to play in hospitality management. All hospitality managers need to use a variety of control measures to check whether the results they achieve are in line with expectations and, if not, to take corrective actions. The control process even sets the parameters for managerial action by setting up control by exception, meaning that managers take action only if the results are outside the acceptable range. Control is often used in conjunction with techniques such as total quality management by allowing associates and management to establish guest service levels.

Control is about keeping score and setting up ways to give us feedback on how we are doing. The feedback leads to corrective action, if necessary. For instance, if a chef and restaurant manager forecast 250 covers and 320 actually come, then they will have to "prep" more food items in a hurry and guide servers to recommend certain dishes in order to avoid running out of too many menu items. These and the many other examples we will read about in this chapter are all control related.

Control has close links to each of the other management functions, especially planning, which, as we know, includes setting goals and making plans on how to reach the goals.

What Is Control?

Control provides a way to check actual results against expected results. Action can then be taken to correct the situation if the results are too far from the expected outcome. If labor costs are 26 percent and they were expected to be 23 percent, the difference is only 3 percent, but that 3 percent could add up to thousands of dollars.

Control is the management function that provides information on the degree to which goals and objectives are being accomplished. Management engages in controlling by monitoring activities and taking corrective actions whenever the goals are not being met. An effective control system ensures that activities that lead to the attainment of the organization's goals are completed.

Control is far broader than you might think. It's not just about checking on outcomes; it is also about providing guidelines and mechanisms to keep things on track by making sure there are no surprises when the results are known. Control is also about keeping your eyes and ears open. Every place seems to have someone who steals, so as a Swiss hotel manager mentor once said to me in his heavy accent, "John, before you can stop someone else stealing the chicken, you must first know how to steal the chicken." The best way to avoid these losses is to have a tight control system.

Why Is Control Important?

Why is control so important? Control is important because it's the final link in the management functions. It's the only way managers know whether organizational goals are being met and, if not, why not. Controlling is involved with planning, organizing, and leading. Figure 1 shows the relationship between controlling and the other management functions.

Goals give specific direction to managers. Effective hospitality managers need to follow up constantly to ensure that what others are supposed to do is being done and that goals are being met. Managers need to develop an effective control system—one that can provide information and feedback on employee performance. An effective control system is important because managers need to delegate duties and empower employees to make decisions. But managers are responsible for performance results, so they also need a feedback mechanism—which control provides.

Given that management involves leading, planning, organizing, communicating, motivating, and controlling, you might easily get the impression that maintaining control is just something managers do after they are finished planning, organizing, and leading. For example, controlling always requires that

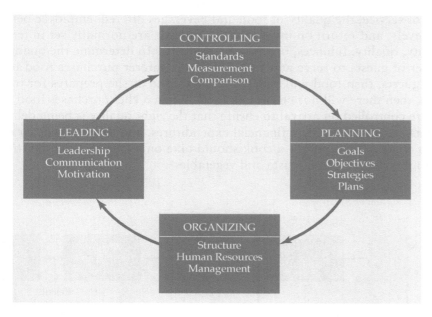

Figure 1 • Relationship between Controlling and the Other Management Functions.

Source: Modified from Stephen P. Robbins and Mary Coulter, *Management*, 8th ed. (Upper Saddle River, NJ: Prentice Hall, 2005), 460.

some desirable outcomes, such as targets, standards, or goals, be set. Similarly, much of what managers do when they have their leadership hats on involves making sure that employees are doing and will do the things they are supposed to do. However, the sort of self-motivation that derives from empowering teams and putting them in charge is often the better alternative.

▶ Check Your Knowledge

1. Define control.
2. Why is control important?

The Control Process

The **control process** is a five-step process of determining goals, setting standards, measuring actual performance, comparing actual performance against those standards, and taking managerial action to correct deviations or inadequate performances (Figure 2). These standards are the specific goals created during the planning process against which performance progress can be measured.

Setting Standards

In the hospitality industry, setting standards generally means establishing the levels of service, the quality of food and beverages offered, employee performance levels, and return on investment. Standards are normally set in terms of quantity, quality, finances, or time. A caterer has to determine the quantity or number of guests to serve at a function. If the caterer purchases food for too many guests, then food will be left over, but if he or she prepares for too few guests, then there will not be enough food. When a chef purchases food items, they are controlled on arrival to ensure that the right quality is being delivered. Budgets are used to control financial expenditures, and time is used, for example, to control labor costs—a cook should take only a certain number of minutes to prepare a batch of pasta and vegetables.

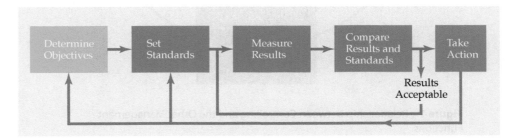

Figure 2 • The Control Process.

A word of caution: When developing a method of measurement, one must be absolutely sure that the goals are indeed measurable. Now, as convoluted as that may sound, let's illustrate the point.

Suppose after careful planning, with input from staff, all agree that labor costs are too high at 28 percent. So the decision is made to reduce labor costs, and that becomes a stated goal—one to which it is hard to object. At the end of the month, the kitchen still has a labor cost of 28 percent, so it has not achieved the goal. During your discussion with the personnel responsible, they claim that their plan to reduce labor costs will not be effective until two months hence. You remind them that the goal was to reduce labor costs, they agree that it was, and you point out that last month's labor cost and this month's are the same. Who is correct here? The answer: neither. The goal of reducing labor costs is inadequate and it is not measurable or attainable on your part. The kitchen staff has put a plan into effect that they feel will reduce labor costs by the end of the following month; they feel they are doing all that you asked. The dilemma is that the goal lacks specificity. Had the goal been to decrease labor costs to 24 percent by the end of February, it would be measurable and attainable. Then we could say to the kitchen staff that they hadn't met the stated goal, but because we didn't quantify the goal, they are correct.

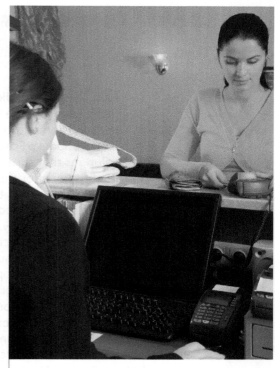

Information for control purposes can be acquired by a variety of methods, including checklists.

Measuring

Managers must first know what they are measuring and how they are measuring it before they can measure expected performance. Personal observation—by monitoring subordinates to make sure things are done right—is the simplest and most common way of comparing actual performance to standards. So, for example, the chef can see whether the cook is cutting, slicing, and dicing correctly and whether the right amount is being prepared according to the standardized recipe.

Direct Supervision

The purpose of direct supervision is to detect problems of associate-specific actions as they occur and to make corrections immediately in order to keep associates' actions in line with management's expectations.

How We Measure

Four common sources of information frequently used by managers to measure actual performance are personal observation, statistical reports, oral reports, and written reports.

Management by walking around (MBWA) is the best way to make personal observations. MBWA is a phrase used to describe when a manager is out in the work area, interacting directly with associates and exchanging information about what is happening. MBWA can pick up factual omissions, facial expressions, and tones of voice that may be missed by other sources. Front-office managers will not be aware of how guests are being checked in during the busy early evening check-in period if they are in their offices at that time.

A DAY IN THE LIFE OF CHERRY CERMINARA

Dietitian and General Manager, Sodexo, Gibsonia, Pennsylvania

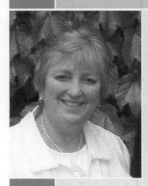

I am a registered dietitian and general manager operating a K–12 school foodservice program. I work for the management company Sodexo. Sodexo has been contracted to manage the food and nutrition program for the school I serve. It is a five-building, 4,000-student operation. Sodexo School Services leads the nation in providing food and facilities management solutions that support the educational process. From nutrition education to monitoring air quality, our efforts enable students and faculty to perform at a high level consistently. Every day, Sodexo serves the needs of more than 400 school districts. Our expertise allows school administrators to focus on education leadership activities. Best of all, our partnering approach always saves money. Our programs have been tested, and the results are conclusive: Sodexo's food service and facilities management solutions improve the quality of life for students, faculty, and the communities we serve.

As the general manager for this operation, a day in my life includes hiring, training, and managing employees; ordering foods; taking inventory; budget management; financial reporting; menu preparation; production; and nutrition. School meals operations are regulated by the U.S. Department of Agriculture for nutrition according to age-specific needs. Both breakfast and lunch are served. We even provide nutrition education both in the classroom and in the lunchroom.

Other areas of concentration include food safety following HACCP (hazard analysis and critical control points) and physical safety for the employees and our customers. We are audited every year by NSF and at least twice per year by the county health department. As a manager, I focus my day-to-day operations on customer service. Although the audience is captive, they are still our customers. We look at the students, staff, parents, and administration as our customers. If I cannot train my employees to respect this aspect of their performance, we will lose revenue and perhaps lose the business to someone perceived to provide a better service. Providing management services to Pine-Richland School District in Gibsonia, Pennsylvania, is really a pleasure. Students are interested in what they eat. They enjoy their meal periods and expect great service. Well-managed, trained, and enthusiastic employees work at Pine-Richland. All of these elements contribute to the company's success.

Statistical reports provide information in the form of data that measures results and can be used for comparative purposes. They also use charts, graphs, and other displays that are easy to visualize. Some managers keep charts on the key result areas and plot the department's progress. Others place safety charts on the associate notice board. These charts visually display the importance of safety and the number of accident-free days, which is another type of goal often sought.

Control information can be acquired through oral reports, conferences, meetings, one-on-one conversations, or telephone calls. The advantage of oral control reports is that they can be quick and allow instant feedback in the form of a two-way conversation. A manager can inquire about the status of a function and get immediate feedback from the banquet captain. In the often fast-paced hospitality industry, oral control communication is often more effective than other forms of communication. For example, every time a restaurant service team has an "alley rally" (a quick huddle/meeting), they are, in part, using oral control communication to let servers know what to sell, what the specials are—so guests can be encouraged to order them—instead of "slamming" the kitchen with multiple à la carte orders.

Written reports are also used to measure performance. Like statistical reports, these are slower yet more formal than personal observation or oral reports. Written reports generally have more information than oral ones and are usually easy to file and retrieve. General managers usually expect to see the "daily report," which gives details of the performance results from the day before, on their desks as they walk into their offices. However, they also want a verbal report from any department they may visit on the way to the office, such as, "Did we sell out last night?"

Given the varied advantages of each of these measurement approaches, comprehensive control efforts by managers should use all four sources of information.

What We Measure

We measure results to see how they compare with expectations. What we measure is more critical than how we measure—what if we are measuring the wrong thing? The results we measure include guest satisfaction, labor costs, food and beverage costs, employee satisfaction, rooms and room rates, bed sheets, energy costs, insurance, and labor turnover.

In simple terms, we measure labor costs because they are the highest of the variable costs. Did we meet our goal of a 24-percent labor cost reduction? Next, did we meet our goal of a 28-percent food cost? To find out if we met our goals, we would need to set up control measuring procedures regarding the daily monitoring of labor costs. Estimates of sales are given to department heads, who then plan and organize their labor costs accordingly. In other words, if we know our sales we can then keep our labor costs at 24 percent. For example, for food and beverage cost control, we would scrutinize ordering, purchasing, storing, issuing, preparing, and serving of the various food items. We would take inventory, calculate the actual cost of the food, and express the cost as a percentage of sales. Remember, it's the cost over sales times 100.

Whenever performance results can be measured, it is desirable to consider a results-accountability system. Some control criteria are applicable to any management situation. For instance, because all managers, by definition, coordinate the work of others, criteria such as employee satisfaction or turnover and absenteeism rates can be measured.

Most managers have budgets set in dollar costs for their areas of responsibility. Keeping costs within budget is, therefore, a fairly common control measure. However, one of the main purposes of control is to influence behavior. Therefore, a results-accountability control system must be able to detect deviations from desired results quickly enough to allow for timely corrective management action.

Effective Managers

Effective managers first control the "big ticket" items that will be costly if not controlled. Once the more costly items are under control, they can move on to other, less costly items.

Having timely information and acting on that information is crucial in avoiding the following situation: Why is it that at some hospitality operations each month's income statement results take almost a month to complete? Because of the delay in producing the results, thousands of dollars are lost before any problems can be fixed.

Comparing Results

Comparing results with expectations shows the amount of variation between actual performance and the standard or expected results. Some variation is generally seen between the expected and the actual results—but how big is the variation? The range of variation is the acceptable difference between the actual and expected results.

Managers are concerned with the size and direction of the variance. Let's look at an example: If guest surveys show that one department is not performing up to expectations, then management would make decisions to have the problem fixed. But what if that didn't work? Then more drastic action would be necessary. Meanwhile, the survey scores would continue to drop. Management would quickly find out in which direction and how fast the barometer of guest satisfaction was moving.

Taking Managerial Action

The final step in the control process is taking managerial action. **Correcting actual performance** is used by managers if the source of the performance variation is unsatisfactory. For instance, **corrective action** may include changing the way the job tasks are done, changing strategy (doing different tasks), changing structure (changing supervisors'/managers' compensation practices), changing training programs, redesigning jobs, or firing employees.

A manager who decides to correct actual performance then has to make another decision: Does he or she use **immediate corrective action**, which corrects problems at once to get performance back on track, or **basic corrective action,** which looks at how and why performance has deviated and then proceeds to correct the source of deviation? Many managers say they don't have time to take corrective action, yet they are the ones perpetually "putting out fires."

Effective managers analyze deviations and, when the benefits justify it, take the time to pinpoint and correct the causes of variance. This kind of control begins with effective associate selection and training. Hiring the right person for the job and ensuring that associates are properly trained increase the chance that associates can be trusted to do the right thing.

Good communication is critical to associate control for a number of reasons. The most important reason is that good communication helps associates understand what is expected of them. Employee performance reviews take on added significance when viewed from the control perspective. Rather than a method of reviewing past performance, they become a control technique. By rewarding and praising desired behavior, management can use performance reviews

Whom Do We Bill?

A funny lack-of-control story happened at a five-star hotel restaurant close to Christmas, when a guest signed the check for his table's extravagant business lunch as "S. Claus." The server, thinking that the guest had signing privileges, gave the check to the restaurant cashier, who in turn sent it up to the billing office so that it would go out to the client at the end of the month. Three days later, the check came back to the restaurant with the question "Which company is he with?"

to shape future behavior. The opposite will be true of undesirable behavior. Performance reviews are also a good time to consider training, reassignment, raises, and promotion decisions.

It is important to note the motivating influences of raises and promotions and how they act as a form of control. Granting raises and awarding promotions based solely on operating results criteria and desired behavior send an important message to all associates. Those actions say that performance and behavior are being monitored and are the basis for personnel decisions. In this way employee actions are controlled.

▶ Check Your Knowledge

1. What are the elements of the control process?
2. Briefly describe the four common sources of information managers use to measure employee performance.
3. Explain the difference between immediate corrective action and basic corrective action.

Types of Control

Managers can use controls *in advance* of an activity (feedforward control), *during* the activity (concurrent control), and *after* the activity has been completed (feedback control). Figure 3 shows the three types of control.

Feedforward control focuses on preventing anticipated problems because it takes place in advance of the work activity. For example, by carefully explaining

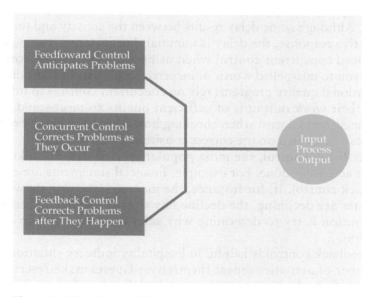

Figure 3 • Three Types of Control.

the policy on billing for catering functions, a catering manager uses feedforward control to explain to the client that an accurate number of people attending the function must be given in order for the correct space to be allocated for the function. A follow-up number is to be given three months, one month, and two weeks before the event, and final guaranteed numbers are required forty-eight hours before a function. This is the number for which food is purchased, prepared, and charged accordingly. By working closely with the client, the catering manager ensures that there are no surprises.

In the kitchen, recipes are an example of feedforward control; they prescribe the quantity of each ingredient necessary to make a particular dish. Recipes also help with consistency by making each dish look and taste the same. (That could be good or bad!) Without recipes, we know the result is going to be a disaster.

Another example of feedforward control occurred when McDonald's opened in Moscow. McDonald's sent quality control experts to help Russian farmers learn techniques for growing high-quality potatoes and bakers to teach processes for baking high-quality breads. Why? Because McDonald's strongly emphasizes product quality no matter the geographic location. It wants a McDonald's cheeseburger in Moscow to taste like one in New York.[1]

Airlines do preventive maintenance on their aircraft; restaurants do the same on their kitchen equipment to prevent any breakdowns during operation. Resorts and hotels also conduct preventive maintenance on the building, the air conditioning system, and so on. These are all examples of feedforward controls.

Feedforward controls are helpful in that they encourage managers to *prevent* problems rather than *react* to them. The challenge is that feedforward controls take more time to organize than the other types of control; however, they save time in the long run.

Concurrent control is a type of control that takes place while a work activity is in progress. When control is enacted while the work is being performed, management can correct problems before they become too costly. The best form of concurrent control is direct supervision, when a manager can concurrently monitor the actions of associates and correct problems as they occur. Although some delay results between the activity and the manager's corrective response, the delay is minimal. For instance, you may have experienced concurrent control when using word-processing software that alerts you to misspelled words or incorrect grammar. In addition, many organizational quality programs rely on concurrent controls to inform workers if their work output is of sufficient quality to meet standards. Chefs use concurrent control when checking how a recipe is being prepared; the cook can be guided on the correct consistency of a product.

Feedback control, the most popular type of control, takes place after the activity is done. For example, financial statements are examples of feedback control. If, for instance, the income statement shows that sales revenues are declining, the decline has already occurred. The manager's only option is try to determine why sales decreased and to correct the situation.

Feedback control is helpful in hospitality industry situations in which a number of activities repeat themselves: Guests make reservations, are welcomed, checked in, roomed, wined and dined, and so on, so resorts and hotels have developed several controls that help measure and report on

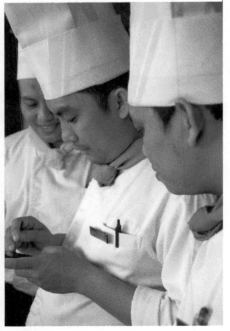

Chefs frequently use concurrent control.

these activities. These controls include guest surveys, comment cards, and outside checkers who stay at a property and give a detailed report to management on their findings.

Feedback control has two advantages over feedforward and concurrent control. First, feedback provides managers with meaningful information on how effective their planning efforts were. Feedback that indicates little variance between standard and actual performance is evidence that the planning was generally on target. If the deviation is significant, a manager can use the information when formulating new plans to make them more effective. Second, feedback control can enhance employee motivation. Associates generally want information on how well they have performed.

T.G.I. Friday's food cost percentage was expected to be 27 percent and the actual was 27.2 percent, meaning the variance was 0.2 of a percentage point. That is feedback control. When a theme park forecasts an attendance of 30,000 on a particular day and the actual comes in at 32,000, that's feedback control.

Other Types of Control

Corporate Control

The catering manager of a large convention and banqueting department received a memo stating that no overtime could be worked unless the food and beverage (F&B) director authorized it in advance. For a busy department that did thousands of dollars in business every day and was responsible for most of the F&B division's profit, that memo from the corporate office was not well received—how can we prevent clients from changing their minds at the last minute, and how dare the corporate office impose on our operation in this way? In retrospect, the department was caught up in a blanket policy to reduce labor costs by using feedforward control, and it worked because many of the not-so-profitable departments were abusing overtime payments to their associates. The convention and banqueting department services manager planned and scheduled the work more effectively, and the catering managers were able to persuade clients to avoid last-minute room changes by explaining that it would involve additional charges at overtime rates. Incentives were also given to clients to select room setups that would involve fewer complete room changes (from a dinner to a classroom setup when a cabaret might be equally as suitable). Substantial company-wide savings were made, and the convention and banqueting department reacted positively to the change (after a brief period of complaining). They also saved several thousand dollars, which, of course, went straight to the bottom line.

Food and Beverage Controls

Ask any food and beverage operator about controls and you are likely to get a serious look followed by a comment about how important control is to the operation. Lots of money can be made or lost depending on how tight the control is. Most operations take inventory and calculate the food and beverage costs expressed as a percentage of sales at least once, sometimes twice, a month.

When you become a manager and assume responsibility for controlling food and beverage items, the first thing to do is to get the locks changed because you have no idea who has access to what. The second thing is to review all control procedures. If you really want to exercise tight control, insist that all orders have your signature or approval—that way, you know what should be received. Next, the stores need to be under the authority and responsibility of one person who is held accountable for all items under his or her control.

▶ Check Your Knowledge

1. When is feedforward control used?
2. What is the difference between concurrent control and feedback control?

Operational Financial Controls

At the operational level in the hospitality industry, the financial controls mainly consist of **budgets** and **income statements**. Budgets "guesstimate" the sales figure for the month/year and allow for up to a specific dollar amount to be spent on any cost of goods sold or controllable-costs item. Just preparing the budget has a control-like effect on managers. They are responsible for the financial outcome of their departments and rely heavily on budgets. Instead of just allowing departments to budget the same amount year in and year out, **zero-based budgeting** has managers begin with a budget of zero dollars and justify all the cost of goods sold, controllable costs, and capital expenditures (such as equipment) they plan on making so that there will be an appropriate amount of profit.

Income statements show the actual sales and expenditures for a month or year. They are used extensively in the hospitality industry as a means of control because they are results driven. Managers use the results for controlling the next period's performance. For example, if the results of the beverage department come in below expectations, then corrective action in the form of increased spot-checks would immediately be instigated, along with more frequent inventory checks. Figure 4 shows a hotel income statement.

As stated earlier, but worth repeating, good managers first control the "big ticket" items that will be most costly if not controlled. Once the most costly items are under control, managers can move on to controlling other items. Looking at the labor costs in a hospitality operation, is the largest of the controllable costs. Labor costs, like any other, need to be controlled in line with sales. Each department will have its own desired labor cost expressed as a percentage of sales. If sales go up, it is easier to control labor costs. However, if sales go down, then management must "control" labor costs in order to avoid losing more than absolutely necessary. Management also needs to be fair with associates. After the September 11, 2001, tragedy, Marriott set an example at

INCOME STATEMENT
APRIL 2012

	CURRENT MONTH						YEAR TO DATE					
	CURRENT	%	BUDGET	%	LAST YR	%	CURRENT	%	BUDGET	%	LAST YR	%
REVENUE												
ROOMS	291,371	61.5%	310,270	66.3%	312,768	66.5%	1,106,897	63.5%	1,150,835	66.1%	1,167,731	64.3%
FOOD	136,868	28.9%	111,503	23.8%	108,176	23.0%	453,192	26.0%	414,868	23.8%	449,848	24.8%
BEVERAGE	22,830	4.8%	23,717	5.1%	26,470	5.6%	90,041	5.2%	84,787	4.9%	100,355	5.5%
TELEPHONE	5,473	1.2%	4,593	1.0%	6,686	1.4%	18,634	1.1%	17,390	1.0%	28,852	1.6%
SUNDRIES	367	0.1%	651	0.1%	798	0.2%	2,020	0.1%	2,368	0.1%	2,868	0.2%
OTHER INCOME	16,605	3.5%	17,270	3.7%	15,109	3.2%	72,914	4.2%	71,108	4.1%	66,559	3.7%
TOTAL REVENUE	473,514	100.0%	468,004	100.0%	470,007	100.0%	1,743,698	100.0%	1,741,356	100.0%	1,816,213	100.0%
DEPT EXPENSES												
ROOMS	68,874	23.6%	68,671	22.1%	63,403	20.3%	272,356	24.6%	273,771	23.8%	246,979	21.2%
FOOD	138,332	101.1%	115,108	103.2%	96,580	89.3%	468,515	103.4%	427,109	103.0%	398,509	88.6%
BEVERAGE	12,809	56.1%	11,080	46.7%	11,464	43.3%	46,567	51.7%	41,676	49.2%	49,675	49.5%
TELEPHONE	4,636	84.7%	4,867	106.0%	5,628	84.2%	20,543	110.2%	19,793	113.8%	21,234	73.6%
SUNDRIES	213	58.0%	418	64.2%	990	124.1%	1,957	96.9%	1,578	66.6%	2,744	95.7%
OTHER INCOME	10,531	63.4%	12,741	73.8%	12,956	85.8%	43,047	59.0%	56,513	79.5%	44,364	66.7%
TOT DEPT EXPENSES	235,395	49.7%	212,885	45.5%	191,021	40.6%	852,985	48.9%	820,440	47.1%	763,505	42.0%
DEPT PROFIT	238,119	50.3%	255,119	54.5%	278,986	59.4%	890,713	51.1%	920,916	52.9%	1,052,708	58.0%
UNDIST EXPENSES												
ADMIN & GENL	47,054	9.9%	38,531	8.2%	43,762	9.3%	206,582	11.8%	168,784	9.7%	184,744	10.2%
MARKETING	26,619	5.6%	30,139	6.4%	15,458	3.3%	91,079	5.2%	88,953	5.1%	57,023	3.1%
REPAIR & MAINT	26,767	5.7%	39,621	8.5%	37,668	8.0%	142,323	8.2%	165,966	9.5%	130,646	7.2%
GROUNDS	22,662	4.8%	26,650	5.7%	29,897	6.4%	108,114	6.2%	107,024	6.1%	95,284	5.2%
UTILITIES	20,494	4.3%	26,785	5.7%	19,010	4.0%	85,988	4.9%	99,652	5.7%	83,380	4.6%
TOT UNDIST EXP	143,596	30.3%	161,726	34.6%	145,795	31.0%	634,086	36.4%	630,379	36.2%	551,077	30.3%
GROSS OPER PROFIT	94,523	20.0%	93,393	20.0%	133,191	28.3%	256,627	14.7%	290,537	16.7%	501,631	27.6%
FIXED EXPENSES												
PROP TAXES	5,734	1.2%	5,734	1.2%	5,099	1.1%	27,015	1.5%	26,983	1.5%	24,443	1.3%
INSURANCE	2,622	0.6%	2,622	0.6%	1,700	0.4%	10,488	0.6%	10,488	0.6%	6,800	0.4%
INTEREST	1,220	0.3%	1,252	0.3%	1,345	0.3%	4,944	0.3%	5,008	0.3%	5,442	0.3%
INCOME TAXES	0	0.0%	0	0.0%	0	0.0%	0	0.0%	0	0.0%	0	0.0%
DEPREC	26,000	5.5%	26,000	5.6%	26,000	5.5%	104,000	6.0%	104,000	6.0%	100,000	5.5%
TOT FIXED EXP	35,576	7.5%	35,608	7.6%	34,144	7.3%	146,447	8.4%	146,479	8.4%	136,685	7.5%
NET INCOME	58,947	12.4%	57,785	12.3%	99,047	21.1%	110,180	6.3%	144,058	8.3%	364,946	20.1%

	CURRENT	BUDGET	LAST YR	CURRENT	BUDGET	LAST YR
ROOMS AVAIL	2,580	2,580	2,670	10,320	10,320	10,680
ROOMS OCCUPIED	1,495	1,670	1,797	5,747	6,078	6,529
OCCUPANCY %	57.9%	64.7%	67.3%	55.7%	58.9%	61.1%
AVG RATE	$151.63	$147.30	$141.56	$147.84	$147.09	$142.50

Figure 4 • Hotel Income Statement. (Courtesy of Hospitality Concepts, San Diego.)

many of its hotels and resorts by not laying off any associates—it instead reduced everyone's hours, which did a lot to keep associates loyal.

In managerial accounting, food and beverage costs are the next largest to be controlled after labor costs. Attractions such as Sea World, clubs, resorts, hotels, and restaurants all offer food and beverages to their guests. All food and beverage items need to be costed and priced in advance to yield a certain percentage—let's say 24 percent. We all know that these percentages will vary from one organization to another; the point is both that food and beverage departments need to be controlled to produce the expected results and that income statements provide written feedback control.

Things such as recipes, portion control, proper purchasing, storage, issuing, and preparation of all food and beverage items help ensure that items reach the guest correctly. Next, we need to ensure that all monies reach the bank—no fingers in the cash register! No bags in the kitchen, no internal trades between departments. A proper system must be in place for recording all sales and ensuring that the correct amount is received from guests. Hospitality operators can choose from several point-of-sale systems and front- and back-of-the-house systems to assist the control process in making the job easier.

Qualities of an Effective Control System

Effective control systems tend to have certain characteristics in common.[2] The importance of these qualities varies with the situation; however, all effective control systems exhibit the following ten characteristics:

1. *Accuracy.* An effective control system is reliable and produces valid data.
2. *Timeliness.* An effective control system provides timely information.
3. *Economy.* An effective control system is economical to operate.
4. *Flexibility.* An effective control system is flexible enough to adjust to changes and opportunities.
5. *Understandability.* The users can understand an effective control system.
6. *Reasonable criteria.* Control standards are reasonable and attainable.
7. *Strategic placement.* Because managers can't control everything, they must choose to control factors that are strategic to the organization's performance.
8. *Emphasis on exceptions.* Managers can't control all activities; control devices call attention only to the exceptions.
9. *Multiple criteria.* Measures decrease tendencies toward a narrow focus.
10. *Corrective action.* The control system not only indicates significant deviations, but also suggests appropriate corrective action.

Experienced managers use effective controls by exception, meaning that if the results are outside the acceptable predetermined limits, then they take action; otherwise they concentrate on something else.

Contingency Plans and Control

The most important contingency plan factor that affects the design of an organization's control system is the size of the organization. The control system should vary according to the organization's size. A small organization relies more on informal and personal control approaches. Here, concurrent control (direct supervision) is probably the most cost effective. However, as organizations increase in size, direct supervision is likely to be supplemented by an expanding formal control system of reports, regulations, and rules. Very large organizations typically have highly formalized and impersonal feedforward and feedback controls. Contingency plans and control cover the *what-ifs*—what if our sales dip 8 percent? What will we do? Reduce associate hours, reduce expenditures, and attempt to boost sales.

As you move up in the organization's hierarchy, there is a greater need for several different types of control; this reflects increased operational complexities. Additionally, the greater the degree of decentralization, the more managers will need feedback on employees' decisions and performance results. Managers who delegate authority for making decisions and performing work are still ultimately responsible for the actions of those to whom the authority was delegated.

The importance of an activity influences whether and how it will be controlled. However, if a particular error can be highly damaging to the organization, extensive controls to prevent that error are likely to be implemented. It simply makes sense to control the big-ticket items.

Adjusting Controls for Cultural Differences

Control is used quite differently in other countries.[3] The differences in organizational control systems of global organizations are seen primarily in the measurement and corrective-action steps of the control process. In a global hospitality corporation, managers of foreign operations tend to be controlled less directly by the home office, for no other reason than the distance keeps managers from being able to observe work directly. Because distance creates a tendency to formalize controls, the home office of a global company often relies on extensive formal reports for control. Global companies rely on the power of information technology to provide speedy control reports of results.

Technology's impact on control also can be seen when comparing technologically advanced nations with less technologically advanced countries. In countries such as the United States, Japan, Canada, the United Kingdom, France, Germany, and Australia, managers of global companies use indirect control devices, particularly computer-related reports and analyses, in addition to standardized rules and direct supervision, to ensure that work activities are going as planned.

In less technologically advanced countries, managers tend to rely more on direct supervision and highly centralized decision making for control. Also, constraints on what corrective actions managers can take may affect managers in foreign countries because laws in some countries do not allow managers the option of choosing the facilities, laying off employees, taking money out of the country, or bringing in a new management team from outside the country.

Contemporary Issues in Control

One issue that can arise from control systems involves information technology: Technological advances in computer hardware and software have made the process of controlling much easier, but these advances have brought with them difficult questions regarding what managers have the right to know about employee behavior.[4] Another issue is workplace privacy.

Workplace Privacy

If you work, do you think you have a right to privacy at your workplace? What can your employer find out about you and your work? You may be surprised by the answer. Why do managers feel they must monitor what employees are doing? One reason is that employees are hired to work, not to surf the Web checking stock prices, placing bets at online casinos, or shopping for presents for family or friends.

Personal on-the-job Web surfing costs millions of dollars a year in wasted computer resources and billions of dollars in lost work productivity. Another reason why managers monitor employee e-mail and computer usage is that they don't want to risk being sued for creating a hostile workplace environment because of offensive messages or an inappropriate image displayed on a coworker's computer screen. Concern about sexual harassment is one of the reasons why companies may want to monitor or keep backup copies of all e-mail. This can help establish what actually happened if an incident arises and can help managers react instantly. Managers also need to be certain that employees are not inadvertently passing information on to others who could use that information to harm the company.

A Prepay Restaurant

There is a great hole-in-the-wall restaurant in New York City where arguably the best front-end control system is in place. Servers have to pay the cooks for the guest's food—so they will definitely get the money from the guests.

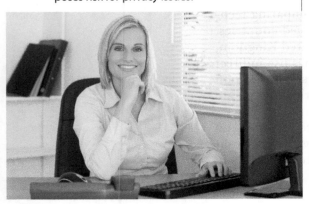

Increased use of computers at the workplace poses risk for privacy issues.

Employee Theft

Would it surprise you to know that a high percentage of all organizational theft and fraud is committed by employees, not outsiders? Any unauthorized taking of company property by employees for their personal use constitutes employee theft, including fraudulent filing of expense reports and removing equipment, software, and office supplies from the company premises. Hospitality businesses have long faced serious losses from employee theft caused by loose financial controls, especially at the start-up of a business.

Why do employees steal? There are several perspectives. Industrial loss-prevention professionals suggest that people steal because the opportunity presents itself through lax controls and favorable circumstances. Some people have different financial problems or pressures such as gambling debts. People steal because they can rationalize whatever they're doing as being correct and appropriate behavior. Hospitality associates also steal because they often feel underpaid, so whether it's a phone call here or a knife, fork, and spoon there, if the opportunity arises, they may take advantage of it. Notice how the concepts of feedforward, concurrent, and feedback control to identify measures for deterring or reducing employee theft apply.

Workplace Violence

Factors contributing to workplace violence include employee stress caused by long working hours, information overload, daily interruptions, unrealistic deadlines, and uncaring managers.

You may not think that these factors apply to where you work, but some of these factors appear in a good many corporations, especially with the pressure of making a profit in the increasingly competitive 24/7/365 environment.

Control is critical in the hospitality industry because we need to know how we are doing all the time. We need to know whether goals are being met and standards reached or exceeded. According to the situation, well-managed hospitality businesses use a variety of controls to provide the necessary information to management for decision-making purposes.

INTRODUCING MICHAEL R. THORPE

The Leader of the Future Will Be a Holistic One

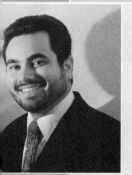

Michael R. Thorpe, who has earned a bachelor of science degree in hotel and restaurant management, is an outstanding example of the leadership skills that can be acquired throughout the school and college career.

Mike's leadership abilities developed from an early age, with his involvement in the Boy Scouts of America. Looking back at that memorable time, Mike recognizes how important it is for a leader to be a good role model. He emphasizes the fact that it is necessary to make a sharp distinction between "good" leaders and "bad" leaders, thus establishing a learning process that is based on the identification of both "shoulds" (positive examples, experiences, activities, skills) and "should nots" (mistakes, negative attitudes). Mike's experience with the Boy Scouts provided him with fundamental values and skills, which were acknowledged when he achieved the rank of Eagle Scout.

In high school as well as in college, Mike progressively developed and used his leadership skills. He believes that the key to learning is involvement. In fact, he always took part in school activities, also emphasizing the importance of maintaining a broad horizon of interests. In particular, Mike chose to actively participate in a variety of extracurricular activities, including academic, service-oriented, and sports organizations. He stressed the belief that there is a strict correlation among such fields, which shapes the overall personality of the leader. "The leader of the future will be a holistic one," Mike says.

Mike's involvement in academic organizations, such as the student body government council, in sports (as captain of the football team and vice president of the football club), and in service-oriented enterprises

INTRODUCING MICHAEL R. THORPE

(such as the Hosteur's Society HRTM Club, to which he was elected president), helped him develop the necessary skills for high-quality interaction with people. He learned that a good leader is someone who can gather a group of individuals and coordinate each single talent, skill, propensity, and personality into a successful team, joining forces in the pursuit of one common goal. Each member of the team must be fulfilled in his or her need for belonging, personal satisfaction, recognition, and so on. To accomplish this task, Mike understood that a leader must also be extremely respectful of each individual's personal life, needs, problems, cultural background, and diversity, setting aside personal likes and dislikes. Diversity also provides an opportunity for the leader to learn from the people he or she guides, an opportunity that every leader must have the humility and willingness to pursue.

In Mike's words, the leader must act as the "glue" that unites people and the organizer who finds the right place for each individual, a place in which he or she will be able to excel and perform at his or her full potential.

Work experience throughout his college career also taught Mike that workers will function at their best in a work environment that is appealing and challenging and that provides them with the right tools—in terms of knowledge, motivation, rewards, and climate—to produce the optimal outcome.

To achieve such results, Mike excludes, as much as possible, the carrot-on-a-stick approach. He feels that such a method is a superficial remedy that doesn't get to the root of the problem—and thus doesn't solve it—and doesn't consider that a leader deals with human beings intrinsically characterized by a distinct intelligence and personality. Furthermore, when dealing with subordinates' failures or mistakes, Mike prefers to approach the person(s) in question from his or her point of view, trying to understand the cause of the inefficiency and establish whether that person's poor performance is determined by his own possible leadership mistake.

Mike greatly respects a leader who creates a sense of cooperation, community, and teamwork. Just as in a family, the leader should step down from an ivory tower and be open to each member of the team, listen, and be willing to help with possible personal problems, emphasizing the importance of open communication. And as in a family, the leader must be a caring parent who can also progressively impose discipline and obtain the results expected depending on the members' potential.

Mike understands the role of a father because he has a six-year-old who represents, among other things, the ultimate challenge for leadership. "Workers' livelihoods do depend on the employer/leader."

▶ Check Your Knowledge

1. Briefly explain zero-based budgeting.
2. List the qualities of an effective control system.
3. What are some contributors to workplace violence?

Controlling Sustainability

One of the most important aspects of implementing sustainable practices in hospitality and tourism is the management of sustainable controls. Hotels and restaurants as well as other businesses and organizations must constantly monitor and manage the different aspects of sustainable practices, such as energy, waste, lighting, water, heating and cooling, temperature and other sources that consume energy. More recently, focus is being placed on integrating sustainability into the planning and development of businesses in the industry. New technologies, such as management control systems are at the forefront of sustainable practices, which provide necessary controls to monitor and conserve resources and decrease unnecessary waste production resulting in an establishment's enhanced environmental performance.[5]

Energy Management

One of the biggest trends of sustainability in hospitality establishments is energy management through temperature and lighting controls in guestrooms, and throughout hotels. There are a variety of solutions to lighting controls, including occupancy sensors, time switches, energy efficient bulbs, etc. Panasonic Home & Environment recently released the WhisperWelcome ventilation system to a number of lodging establishments to install in their guest bathrooms. This new innovative technology includes both motion and humidity sensors that control the lighting and fans in the bathroom. Hotel owners can efficiently save energy resulting in an increase of money and guest satisfaction. Another feature of the product is the option to include a wall-mounted condensation sensor that controls the fan's activity by determining the level of humidity and air temperature in the room.[6]

The Westin Alexandria Hotel has recently announced their plans to install Telkonet Inc.'s new suite energy management system, EcoSmart. The EcoSmart system will be in charge of controlling the water source heat pumps in each of the hotel's guestrooms. The system will monitor the thermostat based on motion sensors and adjust the temperature when the rooms are unoccupied. The ultimate benefit of this new system is projected energy savings of 34% annually, which translates to approximately $42,000. Telekonet's CEO claims "Clients have been very generous with their positive feedback on the aesthetics and ease of use of our in-room thermostats. Perhaps most exciting is feedback we've received on EcoCentral, which is Telkonet's cloud-based platform for management and reporting, and is one of the most comprehensive occupancy-based management platforms available."[7]

Waste Reduction

The tourism industry serves many millions of visitors annually. The waste generated by tourists constitutes a large portion of a destination's commercial waste stream. There are many reasons lodging establishments are placing more focus on sustainable practices promoting waste reduction which include "complying with state waste management laws and regulations, improving their image among customers, saving money, and protecting the environment."[8] The increase in sustainable practices throughout the hospitality and tourism industry has resulted from an increase in the public's interest. Restaurants, lodging establishments, and other businesses are finding that promoting a "green" image provides innumerous benefits, resulting in more long-term cost-savings. Recycling waste materials has allowed many establishments to save money by decreasing garbage collection fees. "Reducing the amount and/or toxicity of materials entering the solid waste stream prior to recycling, treatment, or disposal is waste reduction."[9]

There are several steps to planning and organizing a waste reduction and recycling program, which begins by arranging a team of employees dedicated to the cause. Next, your team should conduct an audit that determines what is thrown away on a consistent basis in order to evaluate the production of average weekly waste. Then your team can develop a plan with a mission and waste reduction goals to accomplish. The plan should include a system of collecting and storing recyclables. Then you should contact a facility that will collect your recycled materials and make arrangements for recyclables to be collected on a weekly basis. Your team should not only implement this program, but they should encourage all employees to implement the program as well. Finally, you should establish a way to monitor and control the waste reduction and the benefits provided by implementing the program.

Trends in Control

Increasing use of technology for control helps make the job of control not only easier but also much quicker. Quicker results mean decisions to make necessary changes are made sooner, thus avoiding further losses. Handheld devices that take inventory are an example of how technology can assist management with inventory taking.

CASE STUDY

The Ritz-Carlton

The Ritz-Carlton is an outstanding hotel providing luxury service to its guests. In contrast with the standard goals of typical business hotels—to provide a home away from home—the Ritz-Carlton decided to take it a step further and provide luxury accommodation to industry executives, meeting and corporate travel planners, and other affluent travelers. The chain is based in Atlanta and runs twenty-five luxury hotels that pursue excellence in each market.

Recently, the hotel company was awarded the U.S. government's Malcolm Baldrige National Quality Award. The award praised Ritz-Carlton for its participatory leadership, thorough information gathering, coordinated planning and execution, and trained workforce that was ready "to move heaven and earth" to satisfy its customers. Thinking about control, what types of control mechanisms did Ritz-Carlton need to achieve excellence?

Ritz-Carlton's corporate motto is "Ladies and gentlemen serving ladies and gentlemen." All employees are expected to practice the company's "Gold Standards." These standards are made up of a service credo and the basics of premium service, including processes for solving any problem guests may have.

The difference between this luxury chain and other hotel companies is that its employees are "certified" after the common basic orientation followed by an on-the-job training. This certification to work for Ritz-Carlton is reinforced daily by frequent recognition for achievement, performance appraisal, and daily "lineups." Annual surveys are given to make sure the employees know the quality standards the hotel company expects of them as well as to determine their level of satisfaction with the company. One year, 96 percent of the employees surveyed ranked excellence in guest services as their primary duty. Workers are empowered by the company to do whatever it takes to solve any sort of problem a customer may encounter. Employees are required to assist their coworkers in dealing with a guest satisfaction issue, leaving no room for any excuse as to why a customer problem was not solved on the spot. In this way, the guest is truly treated as a king; guest satisfaction comes first—always.[1]

Discussion Questions

1. In what ways does Ritz-Carlton use control to ensure high-quality service?
2. How does the company maintain and foster its employees' high level of commitment?

[1] Adapted from Gary Dessler, A Framework for Management (Upper Saddle River, NJ: Prentice Hall, 2002), 376–377.

Summary

1. Control is the management function that provides information on the degree to which goals and objectives are being accomplished.
2. Control is important because it's the final link in the management function. An effective control system is important because managers need to delegate duties and empower employees to make decisions.
3. The control process can be described as setting standards, measuring actual performance, comparing actual performance against those standards, and taking managerial action to correct deviations or inadequate performances.
4. Managers can use controls *in advance of* an activity, which is called feedforward control; *during* the activity, which is called concurrent control; and *after* the activity, which is called feedback control.
5. Budgets and income statements are primarily used for financial control. Budgets

"guesstimate" the sales figure for the month or year and allow for up to a specific dollar amount to be spent on any cost of goods sold or controllable costs item. Income statements show the actual sales and expenditures for a month or year.

6. Effective control systems have ten characteristics: accuracy, timeliness, economy, flexibility, understandability, reasonable criteria, strategic placement, emphasis on exceptions, multiple criteria, and corrective action.
7. Contemporary issues in control include the increasing use of technological advances, which raise the issue of workplace privacy. Additionally, workplace violence and employee theft are issues in the control process.

Key Words and Concepts

basic corrective action
budget
concurrent control

control
control process
correcting actual performance

corrective action
feedback control
feedforward control
immediate corrective action

income statement
management by walking around (MBWA)
measurement
zero-based budgeting

Review Questions

1. Imagine a restaurant that is lacking any kind of control. Describe the negative and positive aspects of this environment and then answer the following question: Why is control necessary?

2. If you were a manager of a Hilton resort in the Bahamas, what way of measuring actual employee performance would you use and why? What are the pros and cons of your chosen method?

3. Explain the three different types of control. Think of a situation in which you have been controlled. Which type of control works best for you?

4. Describe how you envision an effective control system. What types of control would you use? How would you measure employee performance? How would you keep employee theft under control? What about workplace violence? Which operational financial control would you implement?

Internet Exercise

Organization: **The ePolicy Institute**
Web site: **www.epolicyinstitute.com/disaster/ stories.asp**
Summary: This site summarizes e-disaster stories.

(a) Do you think that it's fair for employers to monitor their employees' e-mails?
(b) What would you do if you caught your boss reading your e-mails?

Apply Your Knowledge

You are a restaurant manager. The month-end food cost percentage has just arrived on your desk, and it shows that the actual food cost percentage is 12 percent above budget. What will you do?

Endnotes

1. Stephen P. Robbins and Mary Coulter, *Management*, 8th ed. (Upper Saddle River, NJ: Prentice Hall, 2005), 486.
2. W. H. Newman, *Constructive Control Design and Use of Control Systems* (Upper Saddle River, NJ: Prentice Hall, 1975), 33.
3. Robbins and Coulter, *Management*, 475.
4. Ibid.
5. Muhammad Jamil, Che Zuriana, and Hodgkinson, Lynn, and Thomas Lane, Eifiona. (2009). The Effect of Management Control System on Hotel Environmental Performance. http://ijs.cgpublisher.com/product/pub.41/prod.582. Retrieved December 15, 2011.
6. Hasek, Glenn. (6/20/2011). New Bathroom Ventilation Systems Make Saving Money, Energy Easy. http://www.greenlodgingnews.com/new-bathroom-ventilation-systems-make-saving-money. Retrieved December 15, 2011.
7. www.greenlodgingnews.com. (8/24/2011). Alexandria Hotel Selects Telekonet EcoSmart Energy Management. http://www.greenlodgingnews.com/alexandria-hotel-selects-telkonet-ecosmart-energy. Retrieved December 15, 2011.
8. Sherman, Rhonda. (1996). Waste Reduction and Recycling for the Lodging Industry. http://www.bae.ncsu.edu/programs/extension/publicat/wqwm/ag473_17.html. Retrieved December 15, 2011.
9. Florida Department of Environmental Protection. Waste Best Management Practices: Guidelines for All Hotel Areas. http://www.treeo.ufl.edu/greenlodging/content/_wst.htm. Retrieved on December, 15, 2011.

Glossary

Basic corrective action   An action that examines how and why performance deviated and then proceeds to correct the source of deviation.

Budget   An itemized listing, usually prepared annually, of anticipated revenue and projected expenses.

Control   The provision of information to management for decision-making purposes. The process of monitoring activities to ensure that they are being accomplished as planned and of correcting any significant deviations.

Income statement   A report that lists the amount of money or its equivalent received during a period of time in exchange for labor or services, from the sale of goods or property, or as profit from financial investments.

Measurement   An evaluation or basis of comparison in order to ascertain the dimensions, quantity, or capacity of something.

Zero-based budgeting   Managers begin with a budget of zero dollars and justify all the costs of goods sold, controllable costs, and planned capital expenditures in order to ensure an appropriate profit after the deduction of all expenses.

Photo Credits

Credits are listed in the order of appearance.

Planning

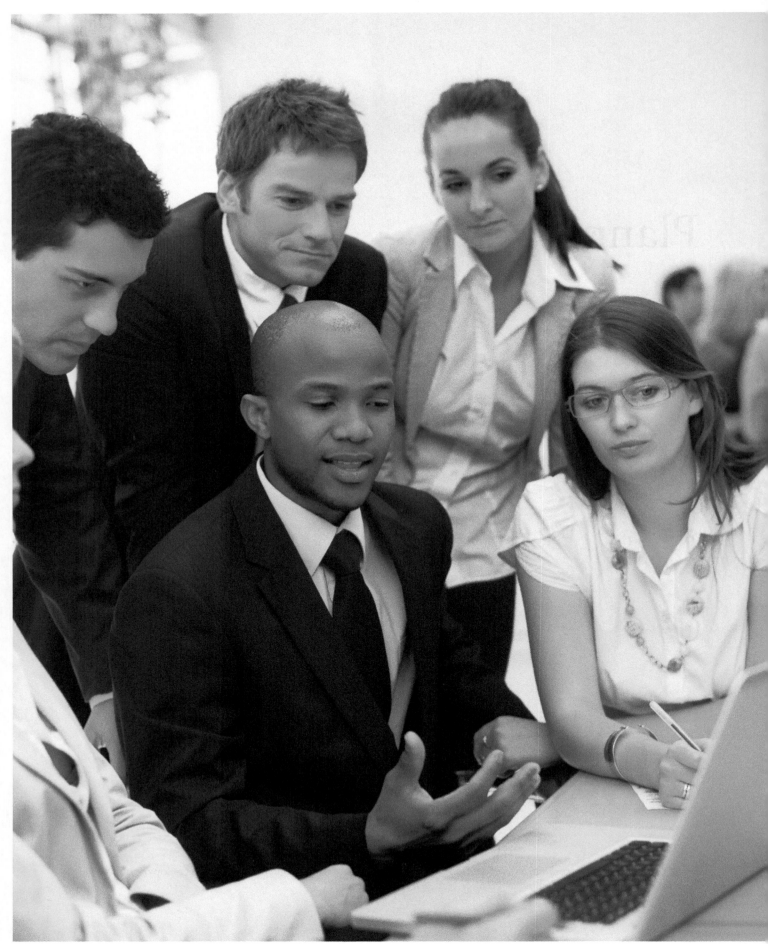

Planning

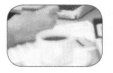
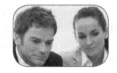
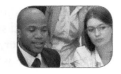
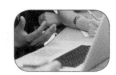

What Is Planning?

Things don't just happen by themselves—well, at least not the way we'd like them to. Remember the time, on a hot day, when you walked into an ice cream store and ordered your favorite flavor, only to be told they were out if it. You were expecting to be delighted but instead were disappointed. A lack of planning was likely the root cause of this negative experience. Someone forgot to order the flavor of ice cream in time for you to enjoy it. This is an example of simple but important planning. There are, as we shall see, more complex forms of planning.

Planning involves selecting the various **goals** that the organization wants to achieve and the **strategies** (actions) to be taken to ensure that those goals are accomplished. In organizations, executives determine where the organization is and where it wants to go. Goals are established for each of the **key operating areas**. In the hospitality industry these would include, but not be limited to, the following key operating areas:

> *Guest satisfaction:* The goal is 100-percent guest satisfaction. The current score may be 89 percent, so the planning element would be to plan strategies as to how to reach 100 percent.
>
> *Employee satisfaction:* The goal is 100-percent employee satisfaction. Let us assume it is currently 87 percent; a plan is then made to create strategies to bring it up to 100 percent.
>
> *Productivity:* Productivity is measured in many different ways across departments. For example, the kitchen of a hotel would look at the number of meals served, and the front desk would look at the number of guests checked in and out. Another way is to divide the total revenue by the number of full-time equivalent employees or person-hours worked. A goal might be set to increase the earnings per employee by 10 percent, and the plan would call for strategies to meet or exceed the goal. Similar examples would apply to the following key result areas: food and beverage preparation, foodservice, guest services, marketing and sales, rooms division, operating ratios, human resources, physical property, security, and finances. Strategies are then developed to ensure that the goals are met or exceeded.

All managers do some form of planning, whether informal or formal. Informal planning is often done at the last minute, and there is little or no sharing of goals and strategies with others in the organization. The owner has a vision of what he or she wants to accomplish and just goes ahead and does it. This is frequently the situation in small businesses; however, informal planning also occurs even in larger organizations. One weakness of informal planning is that it lacks continuity.

Formal planning occurs when specific goals covering a period of up to several years are identified and shared with all associates and when strategies are developed stating how each goal will be reached. When planning is discussed in this chapter, we are referring to formal planning. Several types of planning exist, but we will examine the main ones used in the hospitality industry.

Think of a summer trip to France. Your plans might include the following: how you plan to get to the airport, your airline and flight times, the airport of arrival, how you'll get into Paris, your hotel, and the itinerary of what to do each day in each city visited. Think for a moment: What if you didn't plan? The group would not know what flight to take or, on arrival in France, how to get into central Paris and then how and where to find a place to stay. This would be chaotic and stressful, to say the least. Now think of your career plans. Perhaps your goal is to have a successful career in one of the many areas of hospitality management. Successfully completing your degree, along with work experience, would facilitate accomplishing your goal. So, we can see that planning provides direction and a sense of purpose.[1] Remember the wonderful line in *Alice's Adventures in Wonderland* when Alice is lost and asks the Cheshire Cat which way to go? The Cat asks her where she wants to go. Alice replies, "I don't much care—." The Cat replies, "Then it doesn't matter which way you go."

Planning can also help identify potential opportunities and threats. Planning helps facilitate the other functions of management—organization, decision making, communication, motivation, and especially control—because planning establishes what needs to be done and how it is to be done, and control looks at how well we have done compared to how well we expected to do.[2]

The Purpose of Planning

Planning gives direction not only to top management but also to all associates as they focus on goal accomplishment. The purpose of planning is to determine the best goals and strategies to achieve organizational goals. Figure 1 shows the hierarchy of planning in organizations. Notice that top executives do most of the strategic planning and first-line managers do most of the operational planning.

Planning provides the road map of where the organization is going. Planning also helps coordinate the efforts of associates toward goal accomplishment. Planning assists in risk reduction by forcing managers to look ahead and anticipate change so that they can plan scenarios to react to those potential changes.

Strategic Planning and Strategic Management

The two main categories of plans are strategic (long-term) plans and operational (short-term) plans. Associated with strategic plans are business plans and feasibility studies, which deal with the structure of the plan and provide the details necessary for obtaining finance or other approvals for the operation.

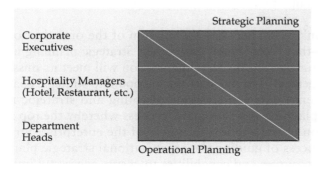

Figure 1 • The Hierarchy of Planning in Organizations.

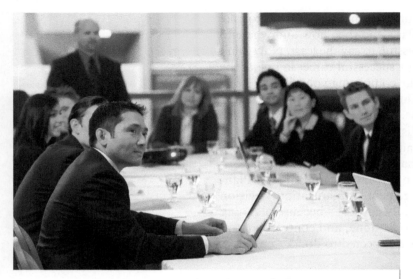

Executive committee members planning the future direction and performance of their property.

Strategic planning creates the long-range plans that steer an organization toward its goals in the accomplishment of its mission and vision. The strategic planning process involves top management, who, in simple terms, identify where the organization is and where it wants to go. There is a strong link between strategic planning and strategic management. The planners figure out what to do, and management implements the plan.

How does a large hospitality company with the mission of being a global entity determine which markets to focus on? Should it focus on expansion in Canada, Europe, Latin America, or Asia? Which market would be more beneficial? And can it enter more than one market at a time? What will the method of entry into these markets be? Will a strategy appropriate for one country work in another? Pick up a copy of the *Wall Street Journal*, *Business Week*, a hospitality trade magazine, or a major newspaper, and you are bound to find articles on or references to business strategy. In the hospitality industry, strategies are devised that become the road map of how to succeed in increasing guest satisfaction, gaining market share, increasing profits, and so on.

Strategic management develops the mission, goals, and strategies of the organization by identifying the business of the corporation today and the business it wants for the future, and then by identifying the course of action it will pursue, given its strengths, weaknesses, opportunities, and threats (internal and external environments).

Strategic management is a critical part of planning and the management process. There are three main strategic management tasks: (1) developing a vision and mission statement, (2) translating the mission into strategic goals, and (3) crafting a strategy (course of action) to move the organization from where it is today to where it wants to be.

Given the frequency of change in the environment, managers must conduct effective strategic planning in order to respond to the challenges of managing in a highly competitive environment. In other words, a good strategic plan should include detailed prescriptions of how a business wishes to implement its mission in the highly competitive environment, coupled with allowances for responding to extraordinary events.

A direct link exists between the mission of the organization and strategic management—they complement each other. Strategic planning involves creating a long-term strategy for how the organization will meet its mission. The job of strategic management is to translate the mission into strategic goals.

The difference between strategic planning and strategic management is that strategic planning is a systematic process whereby the top management of an organization charts the future course of the enterprise. Strategic management is the process of guiding the organizational strategic plan and acquiring the necessary resources and capabilities to ensure successful implementation of the plan in the context of emergent situations caused by the level of environmental turbulence.[3]

A strategy is the "how to" action necessary to accomplish goals and missions. In the hospitality industry, for instance, there are six steps to strategic planning:

1. Create a vision.

2. Find out what your guests want.

3. Do an environmental scan.

4. Identify critical issues.

5. Formulate strategies for the future.

6. Create your action plan and act on it, then monitor results.

Strategic Planning/Management Process

Most of the strategic planning that takes place at the top management level is called *corporate-level strategy*. Figure 2 shows the strategic management process. Notice that it begins with identifying the organization's mission, goals, and objectives. The process then involves analyzing the organization's environment and resources and identifying its strengths, weaknesses, opportunities, and threats. The strategic management process then entails the organization formulating strategies, implementing them, and evaluating the results.

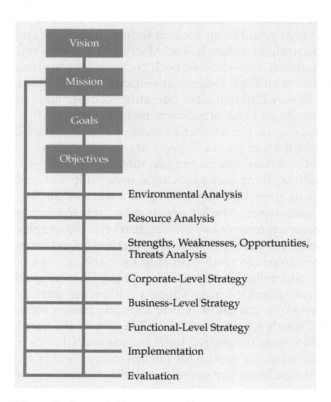

Figure 2 • Strategic Management Process.

▶ Check Your Knowledge

1. Name four purposes of planning.

2. What are the two main categories of planning?

3. What are the three main strategic management tasks?

Corporate-Level Strategies

There are three corporate strategies:

1. Growth: (a) market penetration, (b) geographic expansion, (c) product development, (d) horizontal integration
2. Strategic alliance/joint venture
3. Diversification

At the highest corporate level, many organizations consist of a portfolio of several businesses or divisions. For instance, Disney's portfolio includes movies, theme parks, and the ABC network. Hilton Worldwide's portfolio includes Conrad Hotels & Resorts, Doubletree by Hilton, Embassy Suites Hotels, Hampton Hotels, Hilton Hotels & Resorts, Hilton Garden Inn, and Homewood Suites by Hilton. These and other companies need a corporate-level strategy to plan how best to meet the mission of the company. For example, a few years ago, after careful strategic planning, Hilton decided to form a separate company made up of its gaming entertainment hotels, and Marriott decided to sell its foodservice operations to Sodexo. This allowed both corporations to focus on best meeting their missions with their lodging operations. Hilton found that operating casino hotels was very different from operating its other hotel brands. Marriott decided that growing its hotel brands was its best strategy.

Corporations choose the number of areas of business in which they want to operate. McDonald's and Panda Express are focused in one area, but Hilton, Marriott, and others have several brands, ranging from full-service hotels and extended-stay hotels all the way to vacation ownership and senior living. Most companies want to grow, and they must plan a strategy for that growth. There are four growth strategies: **Market penetration** aims to increase market share by promoting sales aggressively in existing markets. **Geographic expansion** is a strategy in which a company expands its operations by entering new markets—this is in addition to concentrating on existing markets. An example would be Hilton entering and enhancing its position in the Chinese market by entering into an agreement with Air China, China's leading air carrier. The agreement allows for cross-participation in Hilton Honors, Hilton's guest reward program, and Air China's Companion Club. The aim of the partnership between one of the world's most recognized hotel brands and China's leading airline is to provide enhanced global service for the increasing number of business travelers in China and to address the strong competitive situation with international airlines in the local business travel market after China's entry into the World Trade Organization.[4]

A DAY IN THE LIFE OF JESSICA LEIBOVICH

Chef/Owner, Entree Nous, San Diego, California; "Best Personal Chef," *San Diego Magazine*

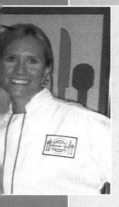

I begin planning my day as a personal chef the night before I cook for a client. Using a program called Mastercook, a recipe database software, I begin menu planning and customizing a menu for the clients that I will be cooking for the following day. I usually choose five entrées and side dishes, trying to keep a variety of one seafood, two chickens, one beef or pork, and one vegetarian selection. The side dishes are combinations of fresh vegetables, whole grains, and starches. This combination of meals may change based on the likes and dislikes of each client along with any special diets they may be on. After the menu planning, I use Mastercook to create a shopping list. This is all done the night before a cook date.

The day I am going to cook, I start my workday at approximately 8:30 A.M. I begin at my computer by printing out the shopping list for the day, along with each of the recipes I will be preparing for my client. I also type up heating instructions for the client. Before I leave the house, I go through the shopping list for the day and place all of the nonperishable items I already have into my rolling cooler. Then I go through the list and identify which stores I will need to shop at for each of the items.

Before leaving, I load my car with my cooler and my portable kitchen kit. I make sure to bring my shopping list, recipes, and heating instructions. I am in my car, ready to leave, around 9:15 A.M.

I usually need to go to at least three stores: one for my dry goods, one for my meat and produce, and one for seafood. Occasionally, I may need to visit a store if I cannot locate something I need at the others. As I shop, I check off my shopping list as I go.

I am finished shopping around 10:00 A.M. and begin to drive to my client's home. Each day, I go to a different client's house. Some of my clients I cook for every week, and others may only be once a month. Once I arrive, I bring in all of the groceries, my cooler from home, my portable kitchen kit, and the recipes and heating instructions.

Once everything is in from the car, I remove it from the bags and place it on the counters. I put all perishable items such as meat and dairy in the refrigerator. I then set up a cutting board and knife and wash my hands. I quickly go over my recipes and decide which ones need the longest cooking time and need to be started first. I also need to decide on the rotation of the items in the oven so I will not have more than two things in the oven at any given time. Eventually, I get in a rhythm and cook for about four to five hours, preparing each entrée and side dish. My day cooking is spent washing, cutting, and trimming vegetables and meat. Then I may sauté, braise, roast, bake, or stew any particular dish, depending on what the menu selections are for that day. Sometimes I am preparing desserts and need to bake as well. Fresh salads are also often requested, so the blender may be buzzing with homemade salad dressings. At one time, there may be items on three burners while two different items are in the oven. One thing I always make sure to do is to clean as I go. Otherwise, I would have quite a mess at the end of the day. As I am finished with an item, I clean it up and set it aside to dry.

As I finish preparing items, I place them in ovenproof Pyrex and Corningware containers to store them in the refrigerator or freezer, depending on the client. As each item cools, I place a label identifying each item along with the date and number of servings on a sealable lid. I leave the items to cool briefly and then place them in the refrigerator. If the client will not be eating them within the next two days, they place them in the freezer to enjoy at a later date.

At the end of the day, it all comes together, and the full menu is completed. As I am finished with an item, I place it back in my cooler. That way, when I am done, there will be no more items left on the counters. Once all the cooking is complete, I carefully clean the kitchen and leave it exactly the way it was when I arrived. I then load up my car with my portable kitchen and rolling cooler. This is usually at about 3:00 P.M.

When I arrive back home, about 4:00 P.M., I bring in my things and unload my cooler. I place everything back in its place in the cabinets. That evening I will prepare the menu and shopping list and begin again for the next day.

For more information, including menus and background information, please visit my web site at **www.chefjessica.com**.

The third form of growth strategy is **product development**, such as Hilton Garden Inn or a new restaurant menu item. The fourth type of growth strategy is **horizontal integration**, which is the process of acquiring ownership or control of competitors with similar products in the same or similar markets. Hilton's purchase of Promus Corporation (Embassy Suites) was an example of horizontal integration.

Strategic alliances or **joint ventures** are yet other methods for a corporation to fulfill its mission. It wanted to expand operations into Asia and Europe—the two main air travel growth areas—but lacked the resources necessary for opening up routes to several additional countries, and it was not allowed to do so by foreign governments because of the competition it would bring to national airlines. So American Airlines formed a "One World" alliance with several other airlines including Aer Lingus, British Airways, Cathay Pacific, Finnair, Iberia Airlines, LAN Chile, Qantas, and more than 20 affiliate carriers to feed each other passengers, code share some flights, and share resources, thus saving money and offering the consumer a better deal with the economy of scale.

Another strategy is diversification, in which companies expand into other types of business—related or unrelated. Celebrity chef Emeril "Bam!" Lagasse's expansion into TV dinners is an example of diversification.

Strengths, Weaknesses, Opportunities, and Threats Analysis

A major strategic planning technique that is widely used in the hospitality and tourism industry is a **SWOT analysis**: an analysis of *s*trengths, *w*eaknesses, *o*pportunities, and *t*hreats. A SWOT analysis is used to assess the company's internal and external strengths and weaknesses, to seek out opportunities, and to be aware of and avoid threats. A SWOT analysis is conducted in comparison with a company's main competitors. This makes it easier to see the competitors' strengths, weaknesses, opportunities, and threats. It also makes it easier to plan a successful strategy. Each operator can decide what the key points are for inclusion in the SWOT analysis. The eleven P's of hospitality marketing include the traditional four P's of marketing—place (or location), product, price, promotion—but add three other P's (people, process, physical evidence) and four new P's (personalization, participation, peer-to-peer, and predictive modeling). All plans need to be implemented; Figure 3 shows how plans follow goals and strategies. Notice that strategic plans are implemented through action plans, operating plans, and standing plans.

Environmental Scanning and Forecasting

Environmental scanning is the process of screening large amounts of information to anticipate and interpret changes in the environment. Environmental scanning creates the basis for forecasts. **Forecasting** is the prediction of future outcomes. Information gained through scanning is used to form scenarios. These, in turn, establish premises for forecasts, which are predictions of future

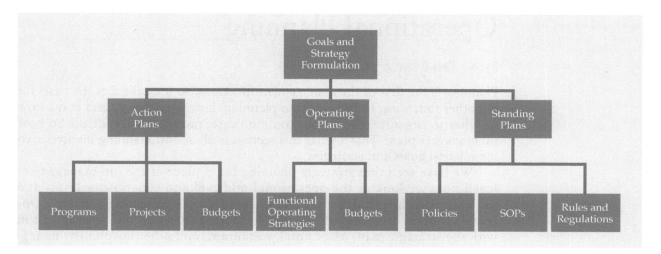

Figure 3 • How Plans Follow Goals and Strategies.

outcomes. The two main types of outcomes that managers seek to forecast are future revenues and new technology breakthroughs. However, any component in the organization's general or specific environment may receive further attention. Both Marriott International and Disney's Magic Mountain's sales levels drive purchasing requirements, production goals, employment needs, inventories, and numerous other decisions. Similarly, your university's income from tuition and state appropriations will determine course offerings, staffing needs, salaries, and so forth. These examples illustrate that predicting future revenue is a crucial first step in planning for success.

As you can imagine, the forecasting done by the president of Hilton Worldwide is very different from the forecasting done by a restaurant manager or department head. The president of Hilton needs to assess the broad economic, political, social, cultural, technological, and financial implications that may impact any forecast. For instance, should Hilton open a hotel in Providence, Rhode Island, or a different city? The desire of Hilton to have a presence in these markets must be considered along with the economic and other environmental factors in each market location. The president must also consider the probability of success of the new property. Another scenario is that of the president of a major chain restaurant corporation trying to forecast in a changing business environment. What if minimum wage is increased? What if health care is mandated? How would these changes affect the corporation?

▶ Check Your Knowledge

1. Briefly explain the four growth strategies of corporations: (a) market penetration, (b) geographic expansion, (c) product development, and (d) horizontal integration.

2. What does SWOT analysis stand for?

3. What is environmental scanning?

Operational Planning

How Do Managers Plan?

Planning is the first of the management functions, so it establishes the basis for the other functions. In fact, without planning, how would managers know how or what to organize, decide on, communicate, motivate, or control? So how do managers plan? That's what this section is all about. Planning involves two main parts: goals and strategies.

We have seen that strategic planning takes place at the top management level; now we look at the operational midlevel and supervisory levels and see that most hospitality managers have a shorter planning horizon. **Operational plans** are generally created for periods of up to one year and fit in with the strategic plan. Most hotel, restaurant, and other hospitality managers plan for periods ranging from hourly, daily, weekly, monthly, to up to 90 days.

Operational plans provide managers with a step-by-step approach to accomplish goals. The overall purpose of planning is to have the entire organization moving harmoniously toward the goals. The following are the seven steps in operational planning:

1. *Setting goals.* The first step in planning is identifying expected outcomes—that is, the goals. The goals should be specific, measurable, and achievable, and should reflect the vision and mission of the organization.

2. *Analyzing and evaluating the environment.* This involves analyzing political, economic, social, and other trends that may affect the operation. The level of turbulence is evaluated in relation to the organization's present position and the resources available to achieve the goals.

3. *Determining alternatives.* This involves developing courses of action that are available to a manager to reach a goal. Input may be requested from all levels of the organization. Group work is normally better than individual input.

4. *Evaluating alternatives.* This calls for making a list of the advantages and disadvantages of each alternative. Among the factors to be considered are resources and effects on the organization.

5. *Selecting the best solution.* This analysis of the various alternatives should result in determining one course of action that is better than the others. It may, however, involve combining two or more alternatives.

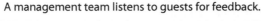

A management team listens to guests for feedback.

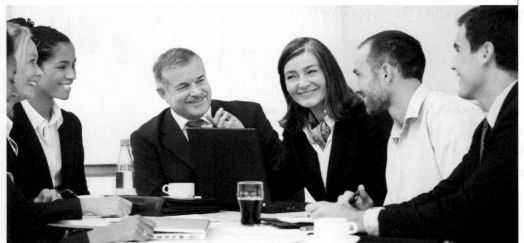

6. *Implementing the plan.* Once the best solution is chosen, the manager needs to decide the following:

   a. Who will do what?

   b. By when?

   c. What resources are required?

   d. At what benefit?

   e. At what cost?

   f. What reporting procedures will there be?

   g. What authority will be granted to achieve the goals?

7. *Controlling and evaluating results.* Once the plan is implemented, it is necessary to monitor progress toward goal accomplishment.

Operational Goal Setting

Goal setting is the process of determining outcomes for each area and associate. Once the vision and mission have been determined, organizations set goals in order to meet the mission. The goals are set for each of the key operating areas mentioned earlier. No one can work as effectively without specific goals and daily, weekly, monthly, quarterly, semiannual, and annual evaluation reports to assess progress toward goal accomplishment; if progress is lacking, adjustments must be made to change course.[5] Examples of the goals and information a sales department should record and analyze each month follow.

Group Room Nights

- Booked this month and year to date by market segment and salesperson
- Actual consumed room nights this month, year to date by month, by market segment, and "on the books" for months to come
- Actual average group room rates by month, year to date, and on the books for months to come

Individual Room Nights

- Actual room nights booked by month and year to date by market segment
- Local corporate clients—actual individual and group room nights booked by month and year to date
- Occupancy—actual by month, year to date, and same time last year
- Revenue per available room (REV PAR)—actual by month, year to date, and same time last year
- Packages—number sold for each type by month, year to date, and zip code origin[6]

Another example would be setting productivity goals. Productivity refers to the amount of labor (input) it takes to do a particular task (output). Productivity is measured in labor costs, which are expressed as a percentage of sales, for each department. Because labor costs are the highest of the operational costs, it is critical to keep them in line with budget. Productivity and labor costs can be compared across similar operations to determine which is more efficient. Suppose the goal for a family restaurant's labor costs is 23 percent of sales. If sales go up, then so too can the labor cost—but proportionately. But what if sales go down? Then so will labor costs—again, proportionately. The skill of management is to operate efficiently and effectively. It is easy to operate a hospitality business when it is busy; the skill comes in running a hospitality business that is operating at only 50 to 60 percent capacity, or worse still, even less.

Expressing goals in specific, measurable terms is important because it allows us to measure our progress toward goal accomplishment. Goals are set for each of the key result areas (departments or elements of a business that determine its success; for example, in a restaurant, guest satisfaction scores, sales, food costs, labor costs, and beverage costs are all key result areas).

An example would be a restaurant where guest satisfaction scores are currently 87 percent. The goal is a score of 95 percent. A time by which the goal is to be met is also identified, as is the individual who is to be responsible for its accomplishment.

Planning expert George Morrisey presents a four-point model for use in formulating goals.[7] Here is an example using Morrisey's model:

1. Increase guest satisfaction scores
2. From 87 to 95 percent
3. By December 31, 20XX
4. At a cost of $500 for training

Operational Objectives

Objectives state how the goals will be met. Objectives are operational statements of activities that should be quantifiable and attainable within a stated time. If the goal is to achieve a food cost percentage of 28.5 percent by October 15 and maintain it until further notice at a cost not to exceed $100 or 10 working hours, the food and beverage director and executive chef must do the following:

- Achieve the desired food cost percentage by having the menu items priced and their costs calculated.

- Control portion sizes by establishing an exact portion for each menu item and watching to see that it is maintained.

- Ensure that regular and spot checks are done on inventory and that the food cost is calculated correctly. Take a physical count of all food items accurately, including all items in the freezers, the kitchen, the storeroom, the banquet kitchen, and so on, and calculate their costs accurately.

- Ensure that all sales and food costs are included in the calculations. Check that all guest food charges are included in the calculations—especially any functions for the day of the inventory if the food is included—and that the sales are also included.

- Use any leftover food within 48 hours.

- Maintain a vigilant loss prevention program with security. Check bags leaving the property and do not allow any bags in the kitchen.

- Ensure that all food sales are recorded and paid for.

Collectively, these objectives ensure that the goal will be met. Each goal needs to have written step-by-step objectives that state how they will be met.

Management Concepts and Approaches

We can see from the preceding examples that it makes sense if the associates who are going to be responsible for achieving the goals are also the ones involved in setting them. Some years ago this concept lead to **management by objectives (MBO)**, a managerial process that determines the goals of the organization and then plans the objectives, that is, the how-tos of reaching the goals. With MBO, associates usually establish the goals and objectives and review them with management. MBO works because associates have been involved with setting goals and objectives and are likely to be motivated to see them successfully achieved. The MBO process consists of six steps:

1. *Set organizational goals.* Top management sets goals for the company in each key result area.

2. *Set departmental goals.* Department heads and their team members jointly set supporting goals for their departments' key result areas.

3. *Present goals.* Department heads present goals and gain approval from senior management.

4. *Discuss department goals.* Department heads present department goals and ask all team members to develop their own individual goals.

5. *Set individual goals.* Team members set their own goals with their supervisor, and timetables are assigned for accomplishing those goals.

6. *Give feedback.* The supervisor and team members meet periodically to review performance and to assess progress toward goals.

MBO goals need to be specific, measurable, and challenging but attainable, just like any other goals. The main purpose of an MBO program is to integrate the goals of the organization and the goals of the associates so that they are in focus. Over the years, MBO has proved very successful and has, in some organizations, been superseded by **total quality management (TQM)**. TQM not only involves planning but also touches on the other functions of management. The idea of improving efficiency and increasing productivity while placing a larger emphasis on quality has caught on fast. Originally designed by Japanese businesses to help

INTRODUCING TIM MULLIGAN

Area Director of Human Resources, Sheraton Hotels, San Diego

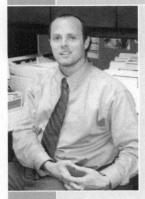

Meet Tim Mulligan, area director of human resources for Sheraton Hotels, San Diego, California. Tim feels that the important elements in planning are knowing what the desired outcome will be, having the instructions followed by the organization, and being a good time manager to help ensure goal attainment.

Goal setting can be divided into two types: annual goals for managers, which have to be in line with career growth, annual bonuses, and so forth, and annual goals for employees, which need to be stated in terms of individual development. According to Tim, the objectives need to be in line with company objectives, individual hotel objectives, and personal growth objectives.

Operational plans are important to meet financial goals (profit), guest satisfaction goals, and employee satisfaction goals.

Specific plans are important to reach day-to-day success with goals and objectives (e.g., check-in, recruiting, hiring process, room cleaning).

Single-use plans are used only for special events, such as holiday parties or Human Resources (HR) receptions.

Standing plans are annual plans, such as benefit enrollment and management screening plans. They are also used for company policies, such as tuition reimbursement or training programs.

Tim gave these examples for contingency factors in planning. If the occupancy of the hotel decreases, the HR department has a plan for layoffs. On the other hand, if a need to hire a significant amount of new staff exists, then the HR department has a plan in place for a mass-hiring action.

Forecasting in the HR department differs from forecasting in other departments, according to the HR director. In the HR field, there is a need for more accurate information on a business level, to determine needs on a staffing level, and the need for dollar amounts for advertising, recruiting, background checks, drug tests, training, and so forth.

In response to a question about which benchmarking practices he believes are the most successful, Tim named turnover rates, employee retention, the employee satisfaction index, and the guest satisfaction index.

In the field of technology, a new trend in planning is the optimal business model. This model works with drivers and is based on the business practice. As an example, this model can determine the amount of hours available for scheduling and the maximum amount of money you can spend to stay within a budget. Two more trends are an online employee evaluation model and a goal-setting process called the performance management process.

reconstruct the economy after World War II, today TQM is widely applied in most industrialized countries. The hospitality industry has embraced quality management with open arms, asking for input from all levels of employees and calling for teamwork. Ultimately, the customer rates the team on quality, value, and product—and the customer does not lie. An example of TQM is asking a group of associates to suggest ways to improve the guest experience by addressing specific challenges (actually problems, but industry professionals prefer to be positive and use the term *challenges*) that the hospitality operation has in delivering exceptional service.

Take guest check-in as an example. The TQM team would include members from the front office and guest services (bellpersons, etc.) who identify lineups for check-in from 4:00 to 7:00 P.M. The group writes a challenge or problem statement, and various ways of improving the situations are presented. They may include the following:

- Using a special desk for airport check-ins
- Handling convention and group guest check-ins in another location (the rooming list is made up in advance and rooms allocated with keys encoded and ready for distribution to guests)
- Cross-training and using associates from other departments to assist with the check-ins
- Adopting an "all hands on deck" approach to have members of management available to assist with check-ins in various ways
- Having additional help available for housekeeping to get the rooms ready more quickly

An example of TQM in the restaurant industry is asking servers in a restaurant for help solving the challenge of reducing the guests' waiting time for tables during rush periods. Once the problem or challenge statement is written, the TQM team can focus on ways to improve the guest experience by suggesting ideas to turn tables more quickly. The head chef might automatically take on the role of coach, as opposed to that of supervisor. Implementing TQM will have the natural outcome of teamwork because one employee cannot improve quality on his or her own. The chef uses motivation and inspiration to keep the team in high spirits, and each employee is important in his or her own way. Emphasis is placed on recruiting, training, and keeping quality employees to ensure that the TQM approach will be a success.

Benchmarking is a concept that identifies the best way of doing something and the companies that excel in that area (*best-practices companies*). The best practice is noted and emulated or even improved on by other companies. In the spirit of cooperation, companies are expected to share information, so you need to give as well as receive.

The history of benchmarking begins in the 1970s.[8] Japanese companies would take trips to industrialized nations to study their large, successful industrial companies and take that knowledge home to apply to their local companies. By aggressively emulating others, they were able to supersede the company being imitated by improving on the success strategy. Meanwhile, benchmarking has become a global trait. Some companies are even benchmarking companies outside their own industry. For example, IBM carefully studied Las Vegas casinos to apply their strategy of reducing employee theft at IBM.

How do you benchmark? First of all, a team is formed. The duty of this team is to identify companies to be benchmarked. Next, the team must determine the best possible way of collecting the data, which can be collected internally as well as externally. Once collected, the data must be analyzed to determine

CORPORATE PROFILE

Choice Hotels International

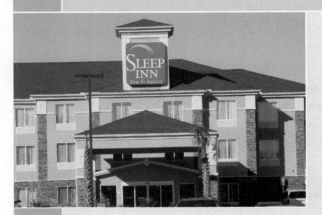

The story of Choice Hotels began in 1968 when Gerald (Jerry) Petitt, a Dartmouth engineering and business student, was seeking summer employment with IBM.[1] He blew the roof off the company's pre-employment test scores. The test scores were brought to the attention of Robert (Bob) C. Hazard Jr., who was in charge of the Coors Brewery account. This had an appeal for the ski bum in Petitt, who was originally from Denver. Bob Hazard says that Jerry Petitt did more in one summer for IBM's efforts to design a production system for the brewery than a team of five engineers did in two years.

Bob Hazard decided then, more than twenty-five years ago, to keep this talented person. They progressed in their careers with spells at American Express and Best Western; they eventually went on to Silver Spring, Maryland, where they took a sleepy, stagnating lodging company called Quality Inns from 300 properties to more than 6,000 hotels in 30 countries and territories.[2] Because they had been so successful at Best Western, they were enticed to join Quality in 1980 for equity plus $500,000 annual salaries.

Bob and Jerry brought to Quality (now Choice Hotels) a combination of engineer-builders and entrepreneur-marketers. They quickly set about changing the mausoleum management style—"Where you don't get creative thinking, where you try to pit good minds against each other." Instead, you get, "What will the chairman think?" and, "We can all go along with it—or look for another job."[3]

To illustrate the change of management style, Bob Hazard draws the upside-down management organization, where the bosses are the millions of guests at 6,000 hotels worldwide. He and Jerry Petitt, of course, were on the bottom.[4]

The strategy of changing the corporate culture, of taking advantage of emerging technological and management trends with emphasis on marketing-driven management over operations, has worked for Choice Hotels. The development of brand segmentation was perhaps its best move. Choice Hotels International is now an international hotel franchisor consisting of the following brands: Comfort Inn, Comfort Suites, Quality, Sleep Inn, Clarion, Cambria Suites, MainStay Suites, Suburban, Econo Lodge, Rodeway Inn, and Ascend Collection.

More recently, Choice has reorganized, creating market area management teams strategically placed so that licensees can be closer to support staff. Each field staff manager has 45 properties and helps with sales, training, quality assurance reviews, and operations consolidations.

[1] This draws on Philip Hazard, "The Bob and Jerry Show," *Lodging* 19 (December 1993): 37–41.

[2] Choice Hotels, *Investor Information,* http://investor.choicehotels.com/phoenix.zhtml?c=99348&p=IROL-irhome (accessed October 1, 2011).

[3] Ibid., 58.

[4] Choice Hotels, *Investor Information,* http://investor.choicehotels.com/phoenix.zhtml?c=99348&p=IROL-irhome (accessed October 1, 2011).

where the success lies and where the differences lie. The last step is to create an action plan on how to improve on the newly gained data—that is, what steps need to be taken to implement it.

The question to be answered is, "How do these companies obtain internal information on other companies they are benchmarking?" An initial team is formed, the members of which may have contacts among customers, suppliers, or employees of the company they are planning on benchmarking. Companies often are glad to swap success stories and information with others, not only informing about themselves but being informed about others as well. Successful companies can often be identified by the number of quality awards they have won. In addition, trade associations typically know who the successful companies are, and you can analyze financial data to help determine which companies to benchmark. Having employees who will implement the benchmarked changes helps ensure their commitment to service or product improvement.

Benchmarking is an operational tool that can be used to guide corporate strategy as well as operations strategies.[9] The process in an ideal setting is to compare company operations with those of other companies that exhibit best practices. Note that best practices are often found outside the company's industry grouping. For example, the Federal Aviation Administration has contracted with Disney to help reduce the long lines at airports occasioned by more severe security measures due to the threat of terrorism. In many instances, best practices adopted from outside the hospitality industry sometimes must be modified to fit the context.

Policies, Procedures, and Rules

Policies, procedures, and rules are examples of standing plans. **Policies** set broad guidelines for associates to use when making decisions. For example, it is the policy of most hotels to pay the room and tax at another hotel and provide a taxi or hotel limo when "walking" a guest.

Procedures specify what to do in given situations. An example would be when a former classmate calls you to request a room for the next weekend. However, the hotel is forecasting 94-percent occupancy, and company procedures, unfortunately for your friend, state that no employees or their friends may stay at complimentary or discounted rates if the hotel is forecast to be more than 90-percent occupied. Policy and procedures often go together.

A **rule** is a specific action guide that associates must follow. Consider this example: Under no circumstances shall an employee serve alcoholic beverages to minors or intoxicated guests.

Budgeting

Most of us are familiar with budgets; we learned about them when we received our first allowance as a child. Remember how often we had it spent before the week was up? That's why organizations plan the use of their financial resources. A **budget** is a plan allocating money to specific activities. There are budgets for revenues (sales) and costs (expenses) for capital equipment—equipment that has an expected life of several years.

Budgets are popular because they force managers to anticipate expected sales and to budget expenses accordingly—that is, not to spend it all before the week is up! Budgets are used extensively in all levels of hospitality organizations, from the corporate level to the smallest departments. Once an estimate of a particular department's revenues is determined, the costs are then budgeted, leaving a portion for profit. This is also called the bottom line. Here's an example of a budget: A restaurant expects 750 guests in a given week; at an average check of $15, this means sales will be $11,250 for the week. This allows management to budget labor costs, usually to a predetermined percentage of sales (normally between 18 and 24 percent, depending on the type of restaurant). Food, beverage, and other costs are budgeted in the same way. Figure 4 shows a detailed restaurant budget listing all the items of

Restaurant Operational Budget	Budget ($ Thousands)	%	Actual Variance +(–)
Sales			
Food	750.0	75	
Beverage	250.0	25	
Other	0.0		
Total Sales	1,000.0	100	
Cost of Sales			
Food	225.0	30.0	
Beverage	55.0	22.0	
Other	0.0		
Total Cost of Sales	280.0	28.0	
Gross Profit	720.0	72.0	
Controllable Expenses			
Salaries and wages	240.0	24.0	
Employee benefits	40.0	4.0	
Direct operating expenses	60.0	6.0	
Music and entertainment	10.0	1.0	
Marketing	40.0	4.0	
Energy and utility	30.0	3.0	
Administrative and general	40.0	4.0	
Repairs and maintenance	20.0	2.0	
Total Controllable Expenses	480.0	48.0	
Rent and other occupation costs	70.0	7.0	
Income before interest, depreciation, and taxes	170.0	17.0	
Interest	10.0	1.0	
Depreciation	20.0	2.0	
Net Income before Taxes	140.0	14.0	

Figure 4 • Restaurant Operational Budget.

expenditure. Note that the column on the right-hand side is for the percentage of sales to which the dollar amount refers. This percentage is helpful in that it can be easily compared with other similar restaurant operations. In fact, restaurant companies use percentages to check on a manager's performance. If one restaurant manager gets a food cost percentage of 28.5 and another gets 33 percent, then the corporate office will be asking the latter manager questions!

Budgets are popular because they can be used with a variety of applications, all over the world. Budgets are planning techniques that force managers to be fiscally responsible. Notice that the "Actual" and "Variance" columns in Figure 4 have no entries in them yet. As soon as the period (usually a month) is over, the results can be totaled and any variances recorded.

Budgets are created by department heads once a year and are revised monthly or as necessary. First, the projected revenue is forecasted, and then all fixed and variable costs are allocated to ensure that the required profit is attained. Forecasting revenues is not easy—there are so many variables—but it has to be done. If the business was operating the previous year(s), there is a history. For a new business, the operator's experience, information from similar operations, environmental factors, forecasting models, and calculated guesswork equal a "guesstimate" of sales.

Budgets intertwine with (1) scheduling, because scheduling equals labor costs, the largest controllable budget item; (2) purchasing, because that contributes to food, beverage, and other costs; and (3) controlling, because we want to compare budget to actual revenue and expenditure results.

▶ Check Your Knowledge

1. What is the difference between operational planning and strategic planning?
2. Define benchmarking.
3. Why is it important to have a budget?
4. Give an example of goal setting.
5. Briefly describe the six steps of the MBO process.

Scheduling

Scheduling of associates is a planning activity that involves taking the business forecast and allocating an appropriate number of staff to give the necessary level of service. Because of the increasing cost of wages and benefits, schedules must be planned very carefully to avoid being overstaffed or understaffed. Because the hospitality industry mostly operates 24/7, we need to staff all departments with appropriate coverage day and night.

Staffing each area or department with an adequate number of associates costs money and is necessary just to open the doors. For example, a restaurant needs a host to greet and seat guests, a server or two, a prep cook or two, a cook or two, a dishwasher, a bartender, and a manager. This is the minimum acceptable staffing level regardless of the number of guests. The same holds true for all areas of the hospitality industry. The problem is that we never know exactly how many guests we will have, and one day can be busy and the next quiet. That's why accurate forecasting, as discussed earlier, is so important.

Obviously, the level of service will vary from one lodging operation to another. A full-service hotel may have 24-hour bell service, whereas a limited-service hotel will not offer it. An amusement park may be open up to 12 hours a day and may need at least two shifts. A restaurant may be open for up to 12 hours a day and may need two shifts, depending on whether it serves breakfast, lunch, or dinner. The hospitality industry, in order to keep costs down and remain competitive, uses a large number of part-time employees. Many hospitality departments have a skeleton staff of full-time employees augmented by several part-time ones as the business needs them.

Project Management

Project management means exactly that—managing a project. Project management is the task of completing the project on time and within budget. In the hospitality industry, we have a variety of projects at each level of the corporation. At the corporate level, for instance, there is the construction of a new hotel or restaurant. At the unit level, there is the alteration or renovation of an existing building; at the department level, there is the installation of a new piece of equipment or a new point-of-sale system. But project management is broader than these examples. What about the senior prom? That's a project, too. So are most of the catering functions that take place at convention centers and hotels.

Hospitality companies are increasingly using project management because the approach fits well with the need for flexibility and rapid response to perceived market opportunities. Sometimes an organization has a specific need for a project that does not fit into a regular planning schedule, so it uses project management. Project management works like this: Say the project is for the organization to become more environmentally friendly. A hospitality organization will create a team of associates from various departments and challenge them to come up with a plan to accomplish the goal of becoming more environmentally friendly. Figure 5 shows the steps in the project planning process.

The process begins with clearly defining the project's goals. This step is necessary because the manager and team need to know exactly what's expected. All activities and the resources needed to do them must then be identified. What labor and materials are needed to complete the project? Once the activities have been identified, the sequence of completion needs to be determined. What

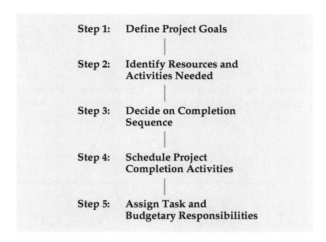

Figure 5 • Steps in the Project Planning Process.

Activity	Week						
	1	**2**	**3**	**4**	**5**	**6**	**7**
Consult with beverage staff	✓						
Establish goals and determine wines to be tasted		✓					
Arrange tasting			✓				
Taste wines				✓			
Make selection and determine pricing					✓		
Prepare and print wine list						✓	✓

Figure 6 • A Gantt Chart for a Restaurant Owner Planning a New Wine List.

activities must be completed before others can begin? Which can be done simultaneously? This step is actually done using flowchart-type diagrams such as a Gantt chart or a PERT network (see Figures 6 and 7). Next, the project activities need to be scheduled.

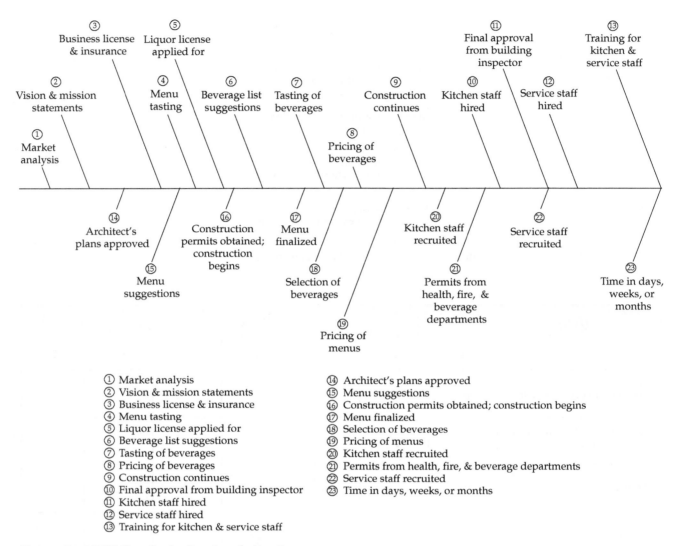

① Market analysis
② Vision & mission statements
③ Business license & insurance
④ Menu tasting
⑤ Liquor license applied for
⑥ Beverage list suggestions
⑦ Tasting of beverages
⑧ Pricing of beverages
⑨ Construction continues
⑩ Final approval from building inspector
⑪ Kitchen staff hired
⑫ Service staff hired
⑬ Training for kitchen & service staff

⑭ Architect's plans approved
⑮ Menu suggestions
⑯ Construction permits obtained; construction begins
⑰ Menu finalized
⑱ Selection of beverages
⑲ Pricing of menus
⑳ Kitchen staff recruited
㉑ Permits from health, fire, & beverage departments
㉒ Service staff recruited
㉓ Time in days, weeks, or months

Figure +7 ● A PERT Chart for the Opening of a New Restaurant.

Time estimates for each activity are done, and these estimates are used to develop an overall project schedule and completion date.[10] Tasks and budgetary responsibilities for each step are then assigned.

▶ Check Your Knowledge

1. Describe the minimum acceptable staffing level for a restaurant as it relates to scheduling.

2. What are the steps in project management?

Sustainable Planning

Tourism is the largest growing segment of the hospitality industry throughout the world. The increase in tourism can be seen as having both negative and positive effects on locations, depending on what they can and choose to offer the tourist market. Tourism can provide many economic, social, cultural and environmental benefits to a destination, but it can also incur certain costs as well. Planning for sustainable tourism requires identifying opportunities in a particular area and balancing them with possible limitations placed on tourism development, in order to capitalize on the strengths and diminish the negative effects that can befall on the environment. At the heart of sustainable planning is a focus on protecting the community and their environment from being misused.

Sustainable planning should be initiated with certain intentions in mind, such as using resources responsibly with an environmentally conscious approach, maintaining respect for local heritage and different cultures living in the community, improving the quality of life in the community, and encouraging the preservation of the various ways of life. Decision making should be structured by the local government, with objectives focused on long-term strategies to solve current problems and prevent future problems that might occur. Decisions should involve a strong collaboration between public and private sectors of the community. They should affect different sectors of the community, while demonstrating the impact various segments have on one another as a result of tourist development.

There is a strong need for planning in sustainable tourism by way of setting goals and objectives, and ensuring that they are successfully achieved. In order to prevent plans from failing, it is important for the plans to be readily adaptable to changes in the environment, community, or other factors involved in tourism development. Plans should include a strong "strategic vision," and decision making should occur from a top-down hierarchy of executives and others invested in the planning and development of the destination. Finally, plans must be well-defined and properly communicated in order to ensure a smooth implementation that corresponds with the overall philosophy.

The proper structure for constructing a plan includes:

1. Philosophy, or vision, and a mission statement
2. Situational analysis of environmental factors
3. Strategic goals and objectives
4. Ways you plan to achieve and implement these goals and objectives
5. How you will measure success

Based on the level of tourism planning, the goals and objectives may be smaller scale, and narrower in focus, such as for an individual site or destination property within a community, or larger in scale, and generally long-term, such as a region, a nation, or several countries. While the majority of tourism planning involves local community involvement, larger scale planning more often requires collaboration with political and legal entities, as well as different levels of government and various business organizations. Policies and procedures must be established and implemented in structured plans before they are approved for further development. The outline of the plan must highlight a number of elements depending on the size of the plan, generally including primary organizations involved, infrastructure, goods, services and facilities, financing, marketing and promotion, human resources, additional programs offered, etc. Finally, it is necessary to provide a blueprint that physically defines the step-by-step breakdown of the plan in action. Once the plan is initiated, it is the goal of the public sector and the private sector to effectively manage the operation from start to finish.[11]

Trends in Planning

Given the environment of rapid change in today's hospitality business, planning needs to be done on time, yet methodically, to keep pace with rapid environmental/global changes. Technology, especially the Internet, can be used to overcome time and distance, allowing for more people to have input into the planning process. Associates can contribute to the planning process online instead of going to meetings.

CASE STUDY

Shell's Seafood Restaurant

Shell's Seafood Restaurant caters weddings and other events in a small New England town. The following is an overview of the planning—or lack of planning—that took place last summer. Jason, the restaurant's general manager, together with the wedding couple, planned a garden wedding and reception in a town park near the restaurant. At first, it seemed as if there were too many choices and decisions to be made, but as they went through the lists they had prepared, they were all pleased with the arrangements.

They chose a wedding ceremony time of 2:00 P.M., followed by a reception at 2:30 P.M. The wedding couple and their families wanted it to be a special occasion but did not want to spend a fortune, so they decided to use Shell's Seafood Restaurant because they had enjoyed meals there in the past. Jason prepared a menu that the couple liked: cream of asparagus soup, chicken fricassee, potatoes au gratin, cauliflower Mornay, and for dessert, crème brûlée. Jason also suggested white and red house wines with an allocation of $3/4$ bottle per person. The wedding couple's aunt made the cake, and it was delivered to the park, but when Jason's staff assembled it, the weight of the top two tiers caused the cake to sink into the thin layer of icing and fall over.

The wedding ceremony was a success, but as you can imagine, the reception was not.

Discussion Question

1. List the planning errors that were made.

Summary

1. Planning involves selecting the various goals that the organization wants to achieve and the actions (objectives) that will ensure that the organization accomplishes the goals.
2. Goals are set for each of the key operating areas.
3. Planning gives direction, not only to top managers, but also to all associates as they focus on goal accomplishment.
4. Strategic (long-term) planning and strategic management involve identifying the business of the corporation and the business it wants for the future, and then identifying the course of action it will pursue, given its strengths, weaknesses, opportunities, and threats.
5. There are three main strategic management tasks: developing a vision and mission statement, translating the mission into strategic goals, and creating a strategy or course of action to move the organization from where it is today to where it wants to be.
6. Strategic planning and management take place at the higher levels of management. This is known as corporate-level strategy.
7. There are four growth strategies: market penetration, geographic expansion, product development, and horizontal integration.
8. A strengths, weaknesses, opportunities, and threats (SWOT) analysis is a key strategic management technique.
9. Environmental scanning is the process of assessing information about the economic, social, political, and technological environment to anticipate and interpret changes in the environment.
10. Operational plans are generally for periods of up to one year and dovetail with the strategic plan.
11. There are seven steps in operational planning: setting goals, analyzing and evaluating the environment, determining alternatives, evaluating alternatives, selecting the best solution, implementing the plan, and controlling and evaluating results.
12. Benchmarking is a concept that identifies the best way of doing something and the companies that excel in the area under study.
13. Policies, procedures, and rules are examples of standing plans. Policies set broad guidelines, procedures specify what to do in given situations, and rules are specific action guides that associates must follow.
14. Budgets are plans allocating money for specific activities. They are popular because they force managers to anticipate expected sales and to budget expenses accordingly.
15. Goal setting is determining the outcomes for the organization and associates.
16. Objectives state how goals will be met. Management by objectives is a managerial process that determines the goals of the organization then plans the objectives.
17. Project management is the task of completing a project on time and within budget.

Key Words and Concepts

benchmarking
budget
environmental scanning
forecasting
geographic expansion
goal
goal setting
horizontal integration
joint venture
key operating areas

management by objectives (MBO)
market penetration
objective
operational plans
policy
procedure
product development
project management
rule

scheduling
strategic alliance
strategic management
strategic planning
strategy
SWOT analysis
total quality management (TQM)

Review Questions

1. What does planning involve?
2. How are goals and objectives different?
3. What is strategic planning?
4. What is the distinction between SWOT analysis and environmental screening analysis?

5. Why do companies use policies, procedures, and rules?

Internet Exercise

Organization: Your restaurant chain
Web site: The company's URL
Summary: Fast-food chains need to know what their competitors are doing or going to do. In this exercise, you will select fast-food company web sites and see what you can find out about your competitors.

Apply Your Knowledge

1. Benchmarking can be an important tool and source of information for managers. It can also be useful to students, as you'll see in this team-based exercise. In your small group, discuss study habits that each of you has found to be effective from your years of being in school. As a group, come up with a bulleted list of at least eight effective study habits in the time allowed by your professor. When the professor calls time, each group should combine with one other group and share ideas, again in the time allowed by the professor. In this larger group, be sure to ask questions about suggestions that each small group had. Each small group should make sure it understands the suggestions of the other group with which it is working. When the professor calls time, each small group will then present and explain the study habit suggestions of the other group with which it was working. After all groups have presented their suggestions, the class will come up with what it feels are the "best" study habits of all the ideas presented.

2. In groups of four, develop a plan for your formal class graduation dinner with a prominent guest speaker.

Endnotes

1. Draws on Gary Dessler, *A Framework for Management,* 2nd ed. (Upper Saddle River, NJ: Prentice Hall, 2002), 99.
2. Ibid., 100.
3. Personal conversation with Kenneth E. Crocker, Ph.D., professor, Francis Marion University College of Business, May 15, 2008.
4. Odyssey Media Group, "Hilton Joins Air China Companion Card Frequent Flyer Program," *Asia Pacific News,* January 9, 2002, http://www .odysseymediagroup.com/apn/Editorial-Hotels-And-Resorts.asp?ReportID=31401 (accessed December 16, 2011).

5. Personal conversation with Stephen Deuker, director of marketing, Ritz-Carlton, Sarasota, Florida, April 18, 2008.
6. Ibid.
7. Dessler, *A Framework for Management*, 108.
8. Stephen P. Robbins and Mary Coulter, *Management*, 8th ed. (Upper Saddle River, NJ: Prentice Hall, 2005), 228–230.
9. Personal conversation with Kenneth E. Crocker, June 15, 2010.
10. Robbins and Coulter, *Management*, 240.
11. www.unescap.org. Sustainable Integrated Tourism Planning. http://www.unescap.org/ttdw/Publications/TPTS_pubs/Pub_2019/pub_2019_ch1.pdf. Retrieved on December 2, 2011.

Glossary

Benchmarking Searching for the best practices among competitors or no competitors that lead to their superior performance.

Budget An itemized listing, usually prepared annually, of anticipated revenue and projected expenses.

Forecasting Predicting future outcomes.

Geographic expansion A strategic growth alternative of aggressively expanding into a new domestic and/or overseas markets.

Goal A specific result to be achieved; the end result of a plan.

Goal setting Traditionally, goals are set at the top level of an organization and then broken down into subgoals for each level of the organization so that the levels work together toward the achievement of the ultimate goals.

Horizontal integration The acquisition of ownership or control of competitors that are competing in the same or similar markets with the same or similar products.

Joint venture An approach to going global that involves a specific type of strategic alliance in which the partners agree to form a specific, independent organization for some business purpose.

Key operating areas The most important functional areas of an organization that work and interact toward the achievement of the organization's goals.

Management by objectives (MBO) A managerial process that determines the goals of the organization and then plans the objectives and the method to be used to reach the goals.

Market penetration A strategy to boost sales of current products by more aggressively permeating the organization's current markets.

Objective A specific result toward which effort is directed.

Operational plans Plans for operations and organization.

Policy A guideline that establishes parameters for making decisions.

Procedure A series interrelated sequential steps that can be to respond to a well structured problem.

Product development The strategy of improving products for current markets to maintain or boost growth.

Project management The process of completing a project's activities on time, within budget, and according to specifications.

Rule A very specific action guide that associates must follow.

Scheduling Detailing what activities have to be done, the order in which they are to be completed, who is to do each, and when they are to be completed.

Strategic alliance An approach to the expansion of a business's activities (entering new markets) that involves a partnership with another organization(s) in which both share resources, guests and knowledge in serving existing clients and in the development of new products and services.

Strategic management The process of identifying and pursuing the organization's strategic plan by aligning internal capabilities with the external demands of its environment, and then ensuring that the plan is being executed properly.

Strategic planning Identifying the current business of a firm, the business it wants for the future, and the course of action it will pursue.

Strategy/tactics Actions taken to achieve goals.

SWOT analysis A strategic planning tool for analyzing a company's strengths, weaknesses, opportunities and threats.

Total quality management (TQM) A managerial approach that integrates all of the functions and related processes of a business such that they are all aimed at maximizing guest satisfaction through ongoing improvement.

Photo Credits

Organizing

From Chapter 16 of *Introduction to Hospitality Management*, Fourth Edition. John R. Walker. Copyright © 2013 by Pearson Education, Inc. Publishing as Prentice Hall. All rights reserved.

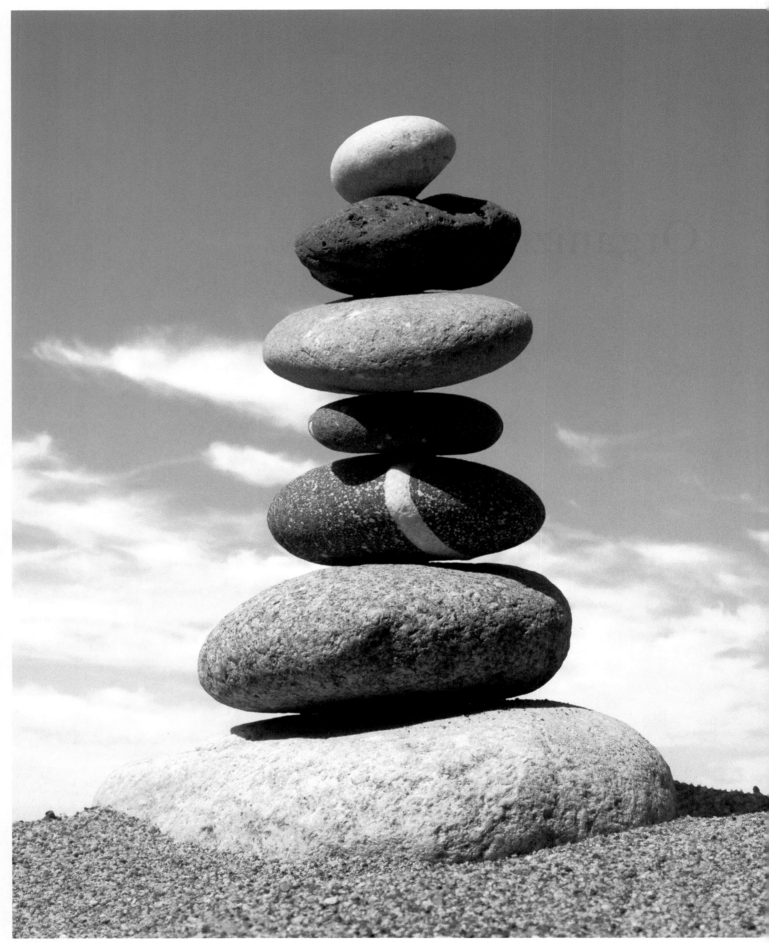

Organizing

OBJECTIVES

After reading and studying this chapter, you should be able to:

- Describe organizational structure and organizational design.

- Explain why structure and design are important to an organization.

- Identify the key elements of organizational structure.

- Explain team-based structures and why organizations use them.

- Describe matrix structures, project structures, independent business units, and boundaryless organizations.

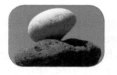
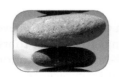
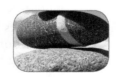
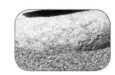

From Planning to Organizing

Howard Schultz, head of Starbucks Corporation, knows that with more than 17,000 Starbucks stores worldwide, organizing the company is no easy task.[1] Such an organization needs training departments to turn college students into café managers (who know, for example, that every espresso must be pulled within 23 seconds or be thrown away), departments that sell coffee to United Airlines and supermarkets, and a way to manage stores in locations as far away as the Philippines and China. How to organize is, therefore, not an academic issue to Schultz. He has discovered that planning and organizing are inseparable. When his company was small, its strategy focused on high-quality coffee drinks provided by small neighborhood coffeehouses. This strategy in turn suggested the main jobs for which Schultz had to hire lieutenants—for example, store management, purchasing, and finance and accounting. Departments then grew up around these jobs.

As Schultz's strategy evolved to include geographic expansion across the United States and abroad, his organization also had to evolve. Regional store management divisions were established to oversee the stores in each region. Today, with Starbucks coffee also being sold to airlines, bookstores, and supermarkets, the company's structure is evolving again, with new departments organized to sell to and serve the needs of these new markets. What Schultz discovered is that the organization is determined by the plan; that is, strategy determines structure.

Schultz has talked about making sure growth doesn't dilute the company's culture. Analysts (who watch companies for investment purposes) believe that Starbucks must determine how to contend with higher materials prices and enhanced competition from lower-priced fast-food chains, including McDonald's and Dunkin' Donuts.[2] Schultz announced his five-point plan on March 19, 2008, to reaffirm the chain's place as the world's coffee authority. "By embracing our heritage, returning to our core—all things coffee—and our relentless commitment to innovation, we will reignite the emotional connection we have with our customers and transform the Starbucks Experience."[3] Chris Muller, writing in *Restaurants and Institutions* magazine, says that Starbucks is a mature product offering in a significantly different marketplace. Upmarket coffee is not as relevant to every portion of the consuming public as it was ten years ago. Energy drinks, healthy menus, and online music delivery are all factors that were not present in the market when Starbucks caught the growth wave. Muller suggests the following[4]:

1. Starbucks should loosen its "centralized command and control" organization model and move to franchising in a "federalist" model. Franchises should be offered only to current store managers and long-term employees.

2. Starbucks is in the "lifestyle" beverage business and needs to reestablish its product offerings to connect to its core customer base, but unfortunately, the aging baby-boomer generation, which made Starbucks so successful, now wants healthy choices (e.g., lower calories, smaller portions).

3. Many members of the millennial generation (born after 1982), do not drink coffee on a regular basis, but do like high-energy drinks and possibly

adult chocolate beverages. According to Muller, this demographic group is less focused on an "individual" moment spent in the "Third Place" (the place between home and work) and more on doing team-based activities with a social message for their community (e-mail is out; Facebook is in).

4. Starbucks should lower its prices, offer less bitterness and faster service across the system, and realize that coffee aroma is not as meaningful as convenience of purchase. Starbucks needs to offer food—healthy, good-tasting, authentic, and made-for-you menu items with low carbon footprints.

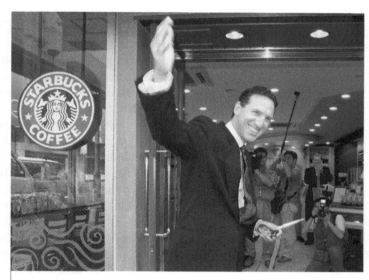

Howard Schultz inviting guests into one of the new Starbucks outlets.

Muller also suggests that Starbucks needs to remember that 50 years ago McDonald's had only one protein and five total items. Focus is great for efficiency and rapid growth, but it will not sustain a business model as a business reaches maturity and needs billions of dollars in sales.[5] In 2008, Starbucks announced that it was realigning and reducing its nonretail workforce by almost 1,000 and closing 600 stores in an effort to strengthen its focus on customers. Of course, skeptics would ask how such a reduction would actually improve the focus on its customers.

The Purpose of Organizing

The purpose of **organizing** is to get a job done efficiently and effectively by completing the following tasks:

- Divide work to be done into specific jobs and departments.
- Assign tasks and responsibilities associated with individual jobs.
- Coordinate diverse organizational tasks.
- Cluster jobs into units.
- Establish relationships among individuals, groups, and departments.
- Establish formal lines of authority.
- Allocate and deploy organizational resources.

This chapter covers these important aspects of organization, but first we need to know what organization is. *Organization* refers to the arrangement of activities so that they systematically contribute to goal accomplishment. No one person can do all the things necessary for a hospitality organization to be successful. Imagine just one person trying to do all the different tasks that make a restaurant meal memorable.

Defining Organizational Structure

In the past few years, organizational structures have changed quite a bit. Traditional approaches were questioned and reevaluated as managers searched for structures that would best support and facilitate employees doing the organization's work. The structure needs to be efficient but also have the flexibility needed in today's dynamic environment. The challenge for managers is to design an organizational structure that allows employees to efficiently and effectively do their work.

An **organizational structure** is like a skeleton in that it supports the various departments in an organization. It provides the total framework by which job tasks are divided, grouped, and coordinated. In today's leaner and meaner hospitality business environment, organizations are flatter—meaning they have fewer levels of managers. They are also structured to better fulfill the needs of the guests. A typical example is the change of mind-set that turned the traditional organizational chart upside down, as shown in Figure 1. The general manager used to be at the top of the organizational chart and the frontline associates at the bottom—the guests never appeared on the chart! Now we have the guests at the top of the inverted pyramid and the general manager near the

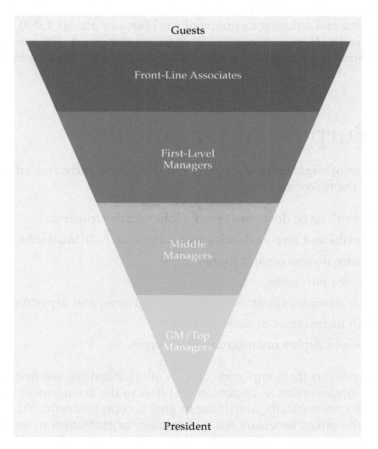

Figure 1 • The New "Upside-Down" Organizational Chart.

bottom (the president of the organization is at the very bottom of the pyramid). Given higher labor costs, there are also fewer associates to do the same amount of work. Organizations have had to become more flexible in their desire to delight the guest. Some hotels have created rapid-reaction teams of associates who respond to urgent guest needs. These teams are composed of members from several different departments who come together in an effort to please the guest. More information about this and other types of teams is discussed later in this chapter.

Work Specialization and Division of Labor

Marriott International had humble beginnings as the Hot Shoppes restaurant chain. Mr. and Mrs. Marriott probably decided what was going to be on the menu, then purchased the food, cooked it, and served it. They also collected the money and made sure everything was to their guests' liking. It's fun and stimulating to have your own business, to see the results of food well prepared and served, and to see gratified guests returning. Now consider the organizational structure of Marriott International today.

Presently, **work specialization** is used to describe the extent to which jobs in an organization are divided into separate tasks. One person does not do the entire job. Instead, a job is broken down into steps, and a different person completes each step. In the hospitality industry, we use work specialization in various departments, but not to the extent that heavy industry does. The reason is that, in the hospitality industry, we are not producing a commodity, so the line cook is likely to continue to prepare a variety of different dishes. However, the concept does apply to a banquet kitchen when a line is created to plate the food. In such a situation, each person adds a particular part of the meal to the plate, and someone checks it and places it in the heated rolling cart. In other departments, such as housekeeping, work specialization has some application: In making up guest rooms, housekeepers may work in pairs, with each specializing in a particular task. However, because the tasks are very repetitive, housekeepers prefer to do more than one task to avoid boredom.

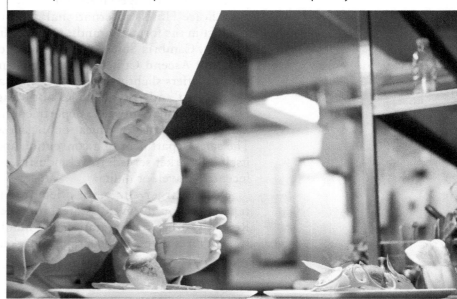

Work specialization allows professionals to focus on their specialty.

Departmentalization

We are all familiar with government departments such as the Department of Motor Vehicles and the Department of Labor, and your college probably has departments of admissions, financial aid, and student affairs, to name just a few. Once jobs have been divided up by work specialization, they have to be grouped back together

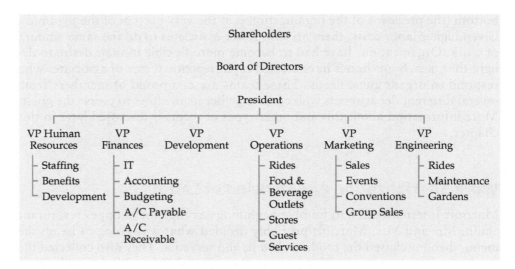

Figure 2 • Organization Chart for a Theme Park.

so that the common tasks can be coordinated. This is called **departmentalization**. Every organization has its own form of departmentalization according to its needs. The organization's structure is shown in its **organization chart** (Figure 2).

Departments are created to coordinate the work of several associates in a given area. An example is housekeeping in a hotel or marketing and sales for a convention center. The main question facing company presidents is, "What form of organization will best meet the company's goals?" Should the company be organized by function, product, service, guest, or territory, or by a combination of these?

The simplest form of departmentalization is by **function**. A large hotel rooms division has a reservations department, uniformed service department, front desk, communications department, concierge, housekeeping, and so on—each with its own specialized function.

Choice Hotels International departmentalizes its lodging properties by **product** in the form of brands: Comfort Inn, Comfort Suites, Quality, Sleep Inn, Clarion, Cambria Suites, MainStay Suites, Suburban, Econo Lodge, Rodeway Inn, and Ascend Collection. Each brand attracts a slightly different target market, offers slightly different services, and is managed independently.

Sodexo and ARAMARK, both huge multinational corporations with billions of dollars in sales, departmentalize by **guest** needs. They have departments or divisions for education, business and industry, health care, and so on. The sales department of a convention and visitors bureau may departmentalize itself by market served: travel industry, medical, legal, insurance, leisure travel, incentive travel, or military.

Many larger companies departmentalize by **territory** when they have representation in several states, provinces, and countries. For example, Avis Rent A Car has representation in a number of states, provinces, and countries. It recognizes that each geographic market has its own nuances.

Authority and Responsibility

Authority is closely associated with chain of command (see next section) because it gives managers the right to exercise their power in a given situation. Authority should be commensurate with responsibility. In other words, managers should exercise power only in accordance with their position. In recent years, managers have increasingly empowered associates to make more decisions—particularly in the hospitality industry. We have to ensure that our guests are delighted. Some companies have empowered their employees to do whatever it takes to please the guest, even to the extent of **comping** (providing free of charge) a room if necessary.

In the hospitality industry it is very important to have not only formal authority but also respect. Associates are quick to gauge the credibility of new supervisors or managers to see how much they know and to determine whether they can help out by getting their hands dirty in an emergency. Someone who has "been there" is likely to gain the associates' respect if he or she can step in and help out during a crisis. Managers are often given authority but lack the in-depth knowledge of the department to really be able to lead by example. Simply put, "You've got to know your onions." When managers lack credibility and there-fore respect, it is much more difficult for associates to work with them to get the job done. Thus, many companies require that a newly appointed manager have experience in the area or at least an accelerated apprenticeship in the area for which he or she will be responsible, thus building up his or her credibility.

When authority is delegated, so should commensurate **responsibility**. That means that you are responsible for the performance of your operation and the associates who work with you. That can sometimes be a big responsibility. What if an associate serves an alcoholic drink to a guest who is intoxicated and that guest later drives off and has an accident, injuring not only himself but also another innocent party? Are you responsible? Yes! As manager of the department or restaurant, you are not only responsible but liable, as well.

▶ Check Your Knowledge

1. Why is organizing important?
2. What are the drawbacks of work specialization?
3. Describe ways managers can departmentalize work activities.

Chain of Command

Organization charts show not only the structure and size of the organization but also the **chain of command** (Figure 3). Departments are clearly indicated, and titles may be used to show each associate's position. The chain of command begins at the top of the organization—in the case of a large, publicly traded company such as Marriott International, with the board of directors, who are elected by the shareholders. The board of directors selects a president or chief

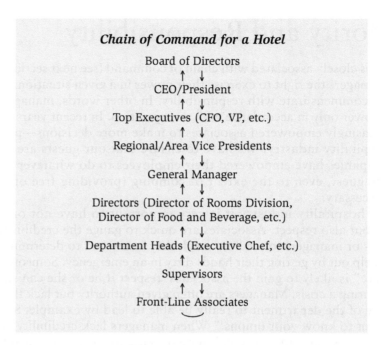

Figure 3 • An Example of a Hotel's Chain of Command.

executive officer (CEO), and the president selects the top executives such as the chief financial officer (CFO) and vice president of marketing. The president and the executive team develop plans that are presented to the board for approval, and then they implement those plans. The chain of command is helpful for associates who have questions or need advice because they will know whom to ask. Similarly, they know to whom they are responsible for their work performance. The chain of command should flow from the top to the bottom of the organization and up from the bottom to the top. This is usually illustrated by lines of authority that indicate who is responsible for what or over whom.

Increasing Span of Control

How many associates can a manager supervise? The answer used to be between 8 and 12. Now, however, the answer is likely to be 12 to 18. The reason for this increase in span of control is that organizations need to be more competitive with not only other U.S. companies but foreign ones, too. Consider the cost savings realized by eliminating levels of management: If there are two organizations, both with 4,000 employees, and one organization has a span of control of 10 and the other 15, the organization with the wider span of control will have fewer levels of management and lower costs because there will be fewer managers. But how much will this save? Well, if the average manager makes $65,000 a year, then the total savings

The Guest Is God

An industry consultant was once in Japan giving a seminar with another colleague. The colleague began by saying that in business today the guest is king, and as he was saying that a gentleman rushed down from the back row and grabbed the microphone and told the audience that the guest is not king but God! The gentleman was the company president. Reflecting on this unusual happening, the consultant realized just how much the Japanese revere their guests.

would be $9.36 million. Having said that, many hospitality corporations have increased their span of control, it is also fair to say that they realize that there is a point when the number of people reporting to managers overburdens associates. At that point, managers don't have the time to give advice, nor do they have time to properly supervise their associates, so standards decline. So what factors determine the appropriate span of control? It depends on the type of work being done. Is it straightforward or complex? Are the associates highly skilled and well trained, or is training needed? Other factors include the degree to which standardized procedures are in place, the information technology available, the leadership style of the manager, and how experienced the manager is in the area of concern.

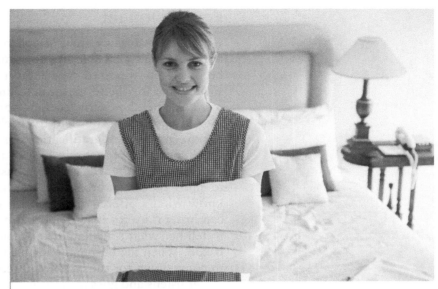

Empowerment allows associates to own the guest request and check to see that it has been fulfilled.

A DAY IN THE LIFE OF ANDREA KAZANJIAN

Ritz-Carlton Members Club, Sarasota, Florida

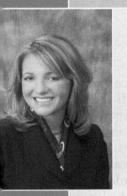

Andrea Kazanjian serves as director of membership for the Ritz-Carlton Members Club in Sarasota, Florida. In her role, Kazanjian is charged with developing and implementing strategies that shape the membership experience for this unique and exclusive luxury-tier brand extension.

A day in the life of Andrea Kazanjian consists of conducting membership training workshops, developing professional and successful Membership Sales Executive and Members Services teams, designing all membership collateral and messaging, and managing a number of marketing campaigns. These are just a few of the techniques she will use to help the organization meet the aggressive membership recruitment and sales goals outlined by the ownership.

Kazanjian earned a Bachelor of Science degree in Hotel, Restaurant, and Travel Administration from the University of Massachusetts, Amherst, on a swimming scholarship as a Division I swimmer and team captain. A native of Albany, New York, she is a board member of the Sarasota Chamber of Commerce Young Professionals Group and a volunteer for the community outreach subcommittee, a member of the Junior League of Sarasota, a representative of the Sarasota Chamber of Commerce Leadership Luncheon Series, a member of the United Way of Sarasota, and a leader of the Ritz-Carlton, Sarasota, campaign.

An extension of the Ritz-Carlton Hotel Company, LLC, the Ritz-Carlton Members Club is a luxury-tier, nonequity membership that combines the benefits of a private social club with the tradition of personalized Ritz-Carlton services and world-class amenities designed to complement the Sarasota lifestyle. Members have the opportunity to access the Members Beach Club on Lido Key, the Members Spa Club, and the Tom Fazio–designed Members Golf Club.

Empowerment

Given the increasing span of control, **empowerment** has become an industry norm. As managers delegate more authority and responsibility, associates have become empowered to do whatever it takes to delight the guest. Frontline associates are in a better position to know guests' wants and needs than management, so it makes sense to empower them to take care of satisfying guests. In the old days, associates had to check with management before making a decision to ensure guest gratification. Let's look at an example: A husband and wife check into a hotel that advertises a room rate that includes a buffet breakfast. Unfortunately, the wife catches a nasty virus and is not well enough to go down to enjoy the buffet breakfast. Her husband says that he will call her to let her know what's offered at the buffet so that she can choose something and he can bring it up for her. He goes down to the restaurant and dutifully calls her to tell her what's available. She tells him what she wants: scrambled eggs and bacon. When the husband explains to a server that his wife is sick and not able to come down for the buffet and requests a tray to carry up her breakfast, the server listens and goes to consult a more senior server, but not the manager. The husband then explains all over again and once more asks for a tray. This time he is told that food cannot be taken upstairs. The husband then says, "My wife is sick and needs something to eat and drink. We've already paid for it. . . . Get the manager here now!" The server later comes over to say that the duty manager says the husband can choose anything from the cold section of the buffet but not the hot part. That does it. The guest demands that the general manager, not the duty manager, be summoned. You get the picture. All of this could have been avoided if only the associates had been empowered to use their discretion in order to satisfy the guest's request.

Centralization and Decentralization

Some organizations make most of the decisions at the corporate office and inform unit managers of them. This process is called **centralization**. If the top managers make the organization's key decisions with little or no input from subordinates, then the organization is centralized. Other organizations make most of the decisions at the unit level or with input from associates. This is **decentralization**. In reality, organizations are never completely centralized or decentralized because they could not function if all decisions were made by the CEO, nor could they function properly if all decisions were made at the lowest level. Figure 4 illustrates the difference between a centralized and a decentralized organization.

Many companies become more centralized in an effort to save costs and improve service to associates. A good example is Choice Hotels' restructuring of its franchise services. However, because of rapid changes in the hospitality business, many organizations are becoming more flexible and responsive; this means the organizations are becoming more decentralized. In large companies especially, lower-level managers who are "closer to the action" and typically have more detailed knowledge about problems and how best to solve them are empowered to delight the guest.

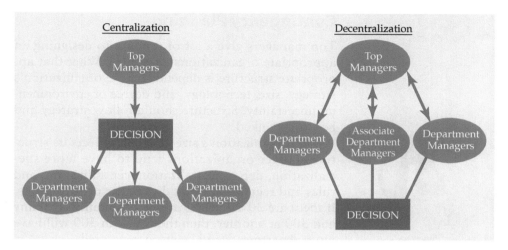

Figure 4 • Centralization versus Decentralization in an Organization.

▶ Check Your Knowledge

1. How are the chain of command and span of control used in organizing?
2. Describe the factors that influence greater centralization and the factors that influence greater decentralization.

Organizational Design Decisions

Organizations are structured in different ways, depending on which structure best suits their needs. A company with 20 associates will look very different from one with 10,000 associates. However, even organizations of comparable size don't necessarily have similar structures. What works for one organization may not work for another. How do managers decide which structure is best for them? That decision depends on certain contingency factors that we are about to discuss.

Coordination of Activities

When there are only a few associates in an operation, everyone can catch up quickly, but as a business expands, problems can and do occur unless there is good **coordination of activities**. The hospitality business is fast paced—guests want something now or even sooner! Departments need to communicate quickly and often in order to keep up with guest requests. You may have experienced an occasion when something did not go as planned—perhaps a check-out delay at your hotel or charges on your bill that were not yours, but now you're in a rush to get to the airport. You get the picture—someone made a mistake!

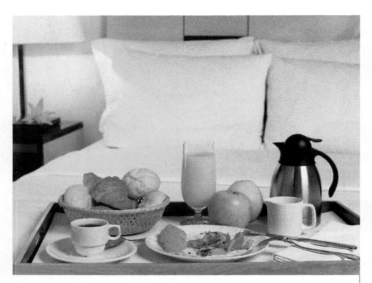

Coordination of various functions and areas is critical in exceeding guest expectations. Room service requires the coordination of a variety of people, including those who take the order from the guest, kitchen personnel who cook the food, and, of course, those who deliver the meal and later retrieve the tray and dishes.

Contingency Planning

Top managers give a lot of thought to designing an appropriate organizational structure. What that appropriate structure is depends on the organization's strategy, size, technology, and degree of environmental uncertainty. Structure should follow strategy and be closely linked.

An organization's size generally affects its structure. Larger organizations tend to have more specialization, departmentalization, centralization, and rules and regulations than do smaller organizations. If there are 30 associates at one hospitality company and 300 at another, then the one with 300 will have more departments and be more structured.

Every organization has some form of technology that relates to structure. Consider a hotel company that has a central reservations center. The central reservations center can hold the inventory of all the hotels in the chain, be far more efficient in offering available rates and rooms to callers than individual hotels, and also make the inventory available to travel agents and Internet travel organizations. A central reservations center can also do a better job of controlling and maximizing revenue for the available rooms than many decentralized centers.

Technology has enabled restaurant chains to transfer data and store menus and operations and training manuals via the Internet. In some cases, this has led to a change in organizational structure. In the hospitality industry, technology has tended to help the existing structure perform better—sometimes with fewer associates. A convention center may have the latest software program for reserving and allocating space, but it will not significantly change the organization's structure; someone must take the guest requests and enter them into the program.

Contingency factors deal with what hospitality organizations refer to as the *what-ifs*. What if such-and-such happens? The company plans and organizes for several possible outcomes. After the terrorist attacks on September 11, 2001, many hospitality companies immediately planned and organized for a drastic drop in business. Departments were greatly reduced, reorganized, or even closed in an effort to reduce losses.

Contemporary Organizational Designs

Team-Based Structures

In response to competitive market demands for organizations that are lean, flexible, and innovative, managers are finding creative ways to structure and organize work and to make their organizations more responsive to guest needs. The first of the contemporary designs is a **work team structure**; either the complete organization or a part of it is made up of teams that perform the duties necessary to delight the guest (Figure 5). This concept is, like many, borrowed from business but has relevance for hospitality managers. Perhaps the best use of this concept for

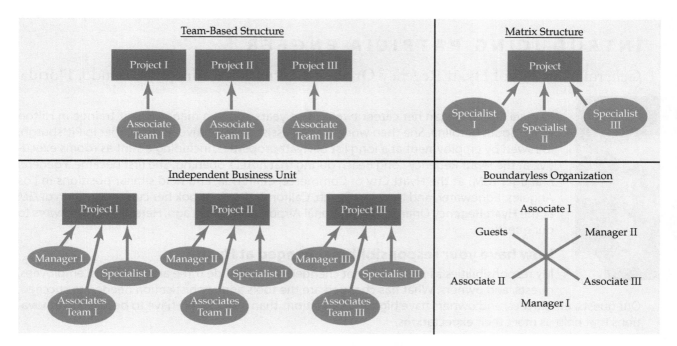

Figure 5 • The Four Types of Contemporary Organizational Designs.

hospitality managers is with total quality management (TQM). Basically, teams of mostly frontline associates take on the challenge of improving guest services and products. At first, these teams are often made up of associates from one department but later can be made up of associates from different departments. This actually improves coordination between departments. Sales departments can work well in teams, as can the banquet kitchen, and for that matter most departments in a hospitality operation. However, the team is more likely to consist of associates from one department as opposed to associates from several departments. In any event, teams tend to be more productive. There are two main types of work teams: integrated and self-managed. *Integrated work teams* are given a number of tasks by the manager, and the team gives specific assignments to members. *Self-managed work teams* are assigned a goal, and the team plans, organizes, leads, and controls to achieve the goal.[6]

Matrix and Project Structures

The matrix structure is an organizational structure that assigns specialists from different departments to work on a project—for example, a new attraction, restaurant, or hotel opening. The specialists come together to pool their knowledge and experience to work on the project. During this time, they may have two bosses: their department head plus the project manager. To work effectively, project managers and department heads need to communicate on a regular basis. Matrix structures are appealing to organizations that want to speed up the decision-making process or get projects accomplished more quickly.

A matrix structure, however, does not work for everyone. It can be disruptive because the participants must take leave from their current positions, and then, once the project is completed, they need to return to their original

INTRODUCING PATRICIA ENGFER

General Manager of Hyatt Regency Orlando International Airport, Orlando, Florida

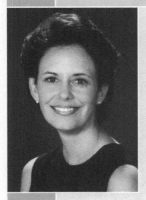

Patricia Engfer began her career twenty-five years ago as a management trainee in Hilton Head, South Carolina. She then worked as an assistant executive housekeeper in Pittsburgh, followed by employment at a long list of Hyatt properties, including a stint as rooms executive at the Hyatt Regency Long Beach during that hotel's opening. She first became a general manager (GM) at the Hyatt City of Commerce, California, and held similar positions in Los Angeles, Edgewater, and Newport Beach, California. Patricia took her current position of GM at the Hyatt Regency Orlando International Airport a few years ago. Here are Pat's answers to our questions.

How have your responsibilities changed at Hyatt?

My responsibilities as a GM have not changed. They include three areas of focus: employees, guests, and owners. What has changed are the tools and sophistication needed to succeed. Our guests, employees, and owners have higher expectations than ever. So, we have to be open to innovations that help us meet their expectations.

How did you grow into your position as a GM?

Hyatt does a great job of developing careers one position at a time. That gives each of us the opportunity to develop skills while preparing for the next step. Coming up through the rooms division and working in convention, resort, airport, and city-center hotels prepared me to manage hotels in different markets. The common thread is how you interact with people in each location.

What is the biggest challenge of your job?

We all know that the current business climate is challenging and requires focus and dedication from every member of the team to look at opportunities to drive sales and manage costs.

Do women and minorities have equal opportunities at Hyatt?

Yes. But you must have drive and determination and be willing to give 100 percent. Being a woman has never been a disadvantage. To the contrary, Hyatt has provided an environment that makes it possible to have the best of both worlds, a career and a fabulous family.

Do you have a mentor at Hyatt?

Over the years I have looked to several mentors who have helped me develop in several ways. Steve Trent hired me, and we have kept in close contact through the years. Locally, I have developed friendships with women who are true leaders, including Glenda Hood, former mayor of Orlando and former Secretary of State of Florida. Another is Linda Chaplin, our past county chairperson, who runs an economic think tank at the University of Central Florida. These women started out raising families, began volunteering time, and today are driving the vision of central Florida. That is truly inspirational.

How do you welcome new employees to your property?

I tell employees the only limits they face are the ones they put on themselves. Hyatt offers training to be successful, but only the employees can bring the personality and commitment. How many other companies offer a great work environment and the opportunity to live almost anywhere and to grow rapidly, while never having to hop from one company to another? If you put forth the effort, Hyatt provides a platform for success where employees of all races and genders are embraced.

positions. Additionally, having more than one manager can be frustrating. **Project structures** are similar to matrix structures, but employees in a project structure continuously work on projects; members of a project do not return to their departments after project completion. An example of a project structure in the hospitality industry would be a preopening team for attractions, hotels, resorts, and restaurants. Teams of employees become part of the project team because they have specific knowledge and expertise. Once the project is complete, the members go on to the next project.

Independent Business Units

Some hospitality companies have adopted the concept of **independent business units (IBUs)** to encourage departments not only to delight the guest but also to watch the money all the way to the bottom line. In other words, the IBU becomes its own independent business and makes decisions accordingly, with little or no need to get approval for routine operational decisions. The unit can implement strategies that will improve guest satisfaction or reduce costs by finding a quicker or better way of doing something. Forming IBUs is an excellent strategy to get associates to realize the total picture of revenue and expenses for a department. It forces associates to engage in all elements of management in order to make a profit. IBUs also enable management to look seriously at departments not making a sufficient profit contribution, with a view toward making changes and improvements or eliminating the department. Departments that once had a loss are now making a profit as a result of the company installing an IBU system of organizational design.

Boundaryless Organizations

Another contemporary approach to organizational design is the **boundaryless organization,** an organization whose design is not defined by, or limited to, the horizontal, vertical, or external boundaries imposed by a predefined structure.[7] The term *boundaryless organization* was coined by Jack Welch, former chairman of General Electric, who wanted to eliminate vertical and horizontal boundaries within GE and break down external barriers between the company and its customers and suppliers. This idea may sound odd, yet many of today's most successful organizations are finding that they can most effectively operate in today's environment by remaining close to the guest and being flexible and unstructured. The boundaryless organization seeks to eliminate the chain of command, to have appropriate spans of control, and to replace departments with empowered teams. Hospitality organizations are moving in this direction but are not there yet. Some may feel that this is not a concept that will work for hospitality organizations, whereas others may think it's a great idea. Hospitality companies recognize that it is important to stay close to the guest but are challenged to create a boundaryless organization.

Teams and Employee Involvement

Teams are task-oriented work groups; they either can be formally appointed or can evolve informally. We all work with others, to a greater or lesser extent, in order to meet or exceed goals. Both formal and informal teams make important contributions to the company and to satisfaction of associates' needs. For example, an informal team from one hotel saved the company more than $250,000 a year after the team made a proposal about energy savings. Not only did the team members receive a sizable bonus, but their employee satisfaction scores were significantly higher than those of associates who did not participate in the team.

Teams are great for doing work that is complex, interrelated, or more than one person can handle. Harold Geneen, while chairman of ITT, said, "If I had enough arms and legs, I'd do it all myself." We all know that associates cannot do everything themselves because of limitations of arms and legs, time, expertise, knowledge, and other resources. There is a certain "buzz" in a restaurant on a busy Friday night; when the kitchen is getting "slammed," you know what teamwork is or isn't!

The funny thing about teams, as you have probably experienced by now, is that you don't always get to choose who you work with—just as when you do term papers and projects in teams. And even when you do get to choose classmates, it sometimes doesn't work out. Your teammates don't do their fair share, or something else doesn't work. Yet in the hospitality industry, we are constantly working in teams to exceed guest expectations. So how can we make teams more effective?

Group Dynamics

Why are some groups more successful than others? Why does a team of mediocre players sometimes beat a team of superior players? You've probably experienced a situation in which, seemingly against all odds, a team excels. Remember the survival programs on television. A group of people was dropped off in some remote place, and over a period of time the group members had to survive as teams, *but* they could vote people "off the island." Imagine if we did that in the hospitality industry!

Why and how some teams succeed and others don't is called *group dynamics* and includes variables such as the abilities of the group's members, the size of the group, the level of conflict, and the internal pressures on members to conform to the group's norms. Sometimes external influences inhibit the group's performance. Corporate may dictate policies that make it more difficult for the group to succeed, or there may be a shortage of resources. One of the fascinating aspects of group dynamics is the members of the group. You may have experienced a group project at college. Sometimes you had to choose with whom you worked, and sometimes your group members were selected randomly. Which worked best?

How Companies Use Teams at Work

Hospitality companies use teams at work in a variety of ways. One way is to structure the organization into teams from the start. Instead of departments, they are called teams. This implies, of course, that employees must be **team players**, which is vital in the fast-paced hospitality industry. Another way management can use teams is through TQM programs that involve associates working in teams to constantly improve the guest experience. Teams are formed from either individual departments or several different departments. They choose an area of the operation that needs improvement, usually one of guest concern, and proceed to make changes that will benefit the guest. TQM teams have made important contributions to the industry and continue to do so.

CORPORATE PROFILE

Darden Restaurants

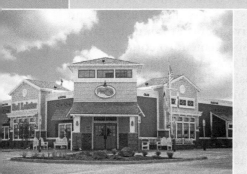

Bill Darden was just 19 when he opened his first restaurant in 1938. It was a twenty-five-seat luncheonette in Waycross, Georgia, called the Green Frog that promised "service with a hop."[1] Fast-forward to 1968, when the first Red Lobster opened in Lakeland, Florida. Today, Red Lobster is the largest full-service seafood dining company in the world, serving nearly 3 million meals a week.

The vision of Darden restaurants "is to be a company that positively affects meaningfully more guests, employees, communities and business partners—a company that matters even more than we do today."[2] Darden has nearly 180,000 employees working together in 1,900 restaurants serving 400 million meals a year, making it a global leader in hospitality by creating many lasting memories for its guests.[3]

Darden brands include Red Lobster, Olive Garden, Longhorn Steakhouse, The Capital Grille, Bahama Breeze, and Seasons 52. Darden has a commitment to quality that is unsurpassed in the industry. At Olive Garden, they are committed to Hospitaliano! and providing 100-percent guest delight through a genuine Italian dining experience. This passion for Italy led to the establishment of Olive Garden's Culinary Institute of Tuscany, where managers and team members go for cultural immersion designed to inspire, motivate, and educate.[4] Longhorn Steakhouse creates a relaxing atmosphere reminiscent of a Western rancher's home, where guests can unwind and savor a great steakhouse meal. The Capital Grille is a fine dining restaurant known for its dry-aged steaks, fresh seafood, award-winning wine list, and personalized professional service. The Capital Grille has received numerous awards, including many "Best of Awards of Excellence" from *Wine Spectator* magazine and the "Achievement of Excellence Award" from the American Culinary Federation.[5]

Bahama Breeze is a Caribbean-themed restaurant offering food and drinks popular in the islands. The Bahama Breeze menu features familiar favorites, including seafood, chicken, and steak, accented with the flavorful and colorful ingredients of the Caribbean. Seasons 52 is a grill and wine bar concept with the addition of private dining rooms and a Chef's table.

Careers at Darden can be viewed at **www.darden.com/careers/** along with examples of Darden's culture, stories, and Darden university relations.

[1] Darden, Our History, www.darden.com/about/photo_history.asp (accessed October 1, 2011).

[2] Darden, Our Company, www.darden.com/about/ (accessed October 1, 2011).

[3] Ibid.

[4] Darden, Olive Garden, www.darden.com/restaurants/olivegarden/ (October 1, 2011).

[5] Darden, The Capital Grille, www.darden.com/restaurants/capitalgrille/ (accessed October 1, 2011).

Self-managed teams make decisions that were once made by managers. This saves managers time, allowing them to concentrate on more important things. For example; hotel housekeepers who score highly on room inspections no longer need to have their rooms checked by a floor housekeeper. These teams of housekeepers actually receive a bonus for superior performance, and the hotel saves the salary of the floor housekeepers. Self-managed teams work successfully in several types of hospitality organizations such as theme parks and convention centers.

How to Build Productive Teams

Building productive teams is critical to the success of any organization, especially in the service-oriented hospitality industry. In recent years, the introduction of TQM processes has significantly increased the number of teams in the hospitality industry. At the heart of TQM is process improvement, and associate participation is the heartbeat. **Productive teams** are built by giving associates the authority, responsibility, and encouragement to come together to work on guest-related improvements that will not only enhance the guest experience but also make the associates' jobs easier. Teams need leadership, which is either appointed by management or chosen by the team. As with any other endeavor, goals and objectives need to be set, and the team must be given the resources it needs to accomplish those goals. It is amazing to see the enthusiasm that teams can generate as they work on improving the guest experience. Associates come up with great ideas that can save money and provide guests with better service. Team building happens when members interact to learn how each member thinks and works. Through close interaction, team members learn to develop increased trust and openness. When a team focuses on setting goals, determining who will plan on accomplishing what by when, and so on, the team should be on its way to becoming a high-achieving team.

Job Rotation

Job rotation is an excellent way to relieve the possible boredom and monotony that can be a disadvantage of work specialization because it gives associates a broader range of experiences. Once associates have mastered the jobs they were hired to do, boredom tends to set in. Job rotation creates interest and helps develop associates to take on additional responsibilities. The management training programs of some of the major hospitality corporations are good examples of job rotation; graduates spend a few months in several departments before selecting an area of specialization. Even then, frontline managers are likely to move through a few departments to build up their knowledge and experience. Job rotation does create some additional costs, mostly in the areas of training and reduced productivity, because as associates move into new positions, they need time to become proficient in their new roles. A major benefit of job rotation is that associates become well rounded in the operation of the corporation, and many associates are promoted as a result of gaining the additional knowledge and experience.

Job Enlargement and Job Enrichment

Job enlargement increases the scope of the associates' work. Originally, it was intended as a way of maintaining interest in the work; more recently, it has become an economic necessity. Today, hospitality management professionals have more work and responsibilities than ever before—that's why workplace stress has become an issue. However, no one in the hospitality industry can say that his or her job is uneventful. In our business, no two days are alike, and for many that's one of the fascinations of the hospitality business, despite the increased workload. **Job enrichment** adds some planning and evaluating responsibilities to a position. It gives associates greater control over their work by allowing them to assume some tasks typically done by their supervisors.

Organizing for Sustainability

Sustainability in the hospitality and tourism industry is on the rise now more than ever before. Today's pioneers are faced with decisions that not only affect their business currently, but they must also prepare for challenges ahead in an unpredictable future. The task of implementing effective sustainable practices in hospitality and tourism is the responsibility of all entities that are affected by this industry, both large and small. Organizational leadership befalls on corporations, local governments and agencies, city convention and visitors' bureaus, as well as citizens, employees, and consumers of individual communities. Organizing for sustainability requires structured planning and actions in which individuals are contributing to, operating within, or cooperating in a larger environmentally active system. The necessity of a business or organization to adapt to sustainable practices is contingent on specific markets, their competition, and the degree of social consciousness within the market.[8]

Sustainable initiatives are established for different purposes, namely in providing value to those invested in an organization. In a hotel or restaurant company, this could include stakeholders, employees, consumers, and community members who are affected by tourism that is created as a result of the organizations existence. The increase in technology over the past decade has provided an outlet for expansion into sustainable initiatives that make sense from a firm's financial perspective. The increase in hotels and restaurant's installation of sustainable practices and technology in their daily business operations has encouraged advanced competition between firms, causing a heightened degree of focus on organizational effectiveness in implementing sustainable planning. It is common to see both competition and collaboration between organizations in the same market.

Organizing resources for hospitality and tourism development can be thought of as an integrated system of supply and demand factors. The demand is created by international and domestic use of attractions, facilities, and services. The supply factors include transportation and other infrastructure (airports, roads, rail, cruise terminals, etc.), water, electric, sewage disposal, attractions, accommodations and foodservice, other hospitality and tourist services.[9] Organizing a sustainable effort must take place at many levels of an organization. Beginning with a top to bottom approach, from the boardroom to the lowest level on the organization chart a commitment by all is required to optimize sustainability. The top level of management can make policy, plans, and procedures for the organization to follow. Middle and lower levels of management can put the plans into actions resulting in greater sustainability.

Trends in Organizing

- Computerized scheduling programs save the organizer time and limit the error margin for being overstaffed or understaffed.

- The fact that recipes are just a click away on the Internet helps speed the organizational process tremendously.

- The new dynamic of multitasking has caused a drastic change in the organizational chart. For example, today, front-desk workers are responsible for much more than just checking guests in and out. Through multitasking, they simultaneously act as phone operators, customer service agents, tour guides, and, occasionally, concierges.

- A new trend following the September 11, 2001, tragedy is to decentralize organizations.

- Reduced occupancies at most hotels have led to a reduction in staff and managerial positions. This in turn has led to more decentralized organizations with fewer levels of management.

- Another trend is the outsourcing of some hospitality jobs like accounting, which can be done in India and the Philippines for a much lower cost than in the United States.

- There is a trend of utilizing outsourced employees for some departments such as housekeeping. This reduces payroll, and benefits are not offered as these workers are not actually hotel employees.

CASE STUDY

The Organization of Outback Steakhouse

Chris Sullivan, Bob Basham, Trudy Cooper, and Tim Gannon—cofounders of the Outback Steakhouse concept—began their restaurant careers as a busser, dishwasher, server, and chef's assistant, respectively. So how did they manage to build one of the all-time most successful restaurant concepts? Their careers may have had humble beginnings, but they had the money to excel. Chris and Bob met at Bennigan's (part of Steak and Ale). They honed their management skills under the mentorship of industry legend Norman Brinker, who later financed Chris and Bob's franchised chain of Chili's restaurants in Georgia and Florida. They later sold the Chili's restaurants back to Brinker for $3 million. This seed money allowed them to develop a restaurant concept with which they had been toying.

The concept was for a casual-themed steakhouse. Because the partners did not want to do a western theme (it had already been done by others) and because at the time there was a lot of hype about Australia, they opted for an Australian theme. Australia had just won the America's Cup (a major yacht race held every four years), and the movie *"Crocodile" Dundee* was popular. As with all new restaurant concepts, they searched for a suitable name. Beth Basham came up with the idea of "Outback" for the name of the

CASE STUDY

steakhouse—she wrote it on a mirror in lipstick. The Outback-themed concept was just what the partners wanted—a casual, fun, family atmosphere and the highest-quality food, which is reflected in Outback's 40-percent food cost (the industry norm for steakhouses is about 36 percent). Chris and Bob asked Tim Gannon, who at the time hardly had enough money to buy the gas to drive to Tampa, to join them. Organizationally, each of the partners brought something to the table. Chris was the visionary, Bob the operations person, Tim the chef, and Trudy the trainer. Later, they realized they needed a numbers guy, and in 1990, Bob Merritt became CFO.

Instead of fancy marketing research, the partners did lots of talking and observation on what people were eating—remember, this was a time when eating red meat was almost taboo. The partners figured that people were not eating as much red meat at home, but when they dined out, they were ready for a good steak.

Initially, the partners thought of setting up one restaurant and then a few more, which would allow them to spend more time on the golf course and with their families. So the success of Outback surprised the partners as well as the Wall Street pundits. The organization grew quickly, and by the mid-1990s, more than 200 stores were open; the partners also signed a joint venture partnership with Carrabba's Italian Grill, giving them access to the high-end Italian restaurant segment.

Same-store sales increased year after year, and the partners looked forward to 500 or even 600 units. Financial analysts were amazed at the rise in Outback's stock. So, to what can we attribute Outback's success? It's a well-defined and popular concept, has a great organizational mantra of "No Rules—Just Right," and has the best-quality food and service in a casually themed Australian outback–decor restaurant. The typical Outback is a little more than 6,000 square feet, with about 35 tables seating about 160 guests and a bar area that has 8 tables and 32 seats. Outback's target market is "A" demographics and a "B" location, which is often a strip mall. Another aspect of Outback's organization is that servers handle only 3 tables at a time; this increases their guest contact time and allows for more attention to be paid to each table. Outback also offers an Australian-themed menu with a higher flavor profile than comparable steakhouses. The design of the kitchen takes up about 45 percent of the restaurant's floor space—12 percent more than other similar restaurants. This extra space represents a potential loss of revenue, but this is the way Outback wanted it done because they realized the kitchen does not run well when it's being "slammed" on a Friday or Saturday night.

There is no organization chart at Outback Steakhouse; everyone at the unpretentious corporate headquarters in Tampa is there to serve the restaurants. There is no corporate human resources department; applicants are interviewed by two managers and must pass a psychological profile test that gives an indication of the applicant's personality. Outback provides ownership opportunities at three levels in the organization: individual restaurant level, multistore joint venture and franchises, and an employee stock ownership plan. Because there is no middle management, franchisees report directly to the president. Outback's founders had fun setting up the concept and want everyone to have fun, too—they sometimes drop in on a store and ask employees if they are having fun. Not only are they doing that—they are laughing all the way to the bank!

Discussion Questions

1. From an organizational perspective, can Outback continue to grow with so little organizational structure?

2. What kind of organizational structure would you suggest for Outback Steakhouse?

Summary

1. The purpose of organizing is to get jobs done efficiently and effectively.
2. Goals are accomplished by organizing the work to be done into specific jobs and departments; assigning tasks and responsibilities associated with individual jobs; coordinating diverse organizational tasks; clustering jobs into units; establishing relationships among individuals, groups, and departments; establishing formal lines of authority; and allocating and deploying organizational resources.
3. Organizational structure is the total framework through which job tasks are divided, grouped, and coordinated.
4. Organizational structure is divided into work specialization, departmentalization, authority and responsibility, chain of command, delegation, increasing span of control and empowerment, and centralization and decentralization.
5. Organizational designs and decisions consist of coordination, contingency factors, common organizational design, contemporary organizational design, IBUs, and the boundaryless organization.
6. Teams are task-oriented work groups; they either can be formally appointed or can evolve informally.

Key Words and Concepts

authority
boundaryless organization
centralization
chain of command
comping
contingency factors
coordination of activities
decentralization
departmentalization
empowerment
function
guest
independent business unit (IBU)
job enlargement
job enrichment

job rotation
organizational structure
organization chart
organizing
product
productive teams
project structure
responsibility
self-managed teams
team
team player
territory
work specialization
work team structure

Review Questions

1. Looking to the future, which is the best organization structure for a theme park? A 50-room resort? A midpriced Italian restaurant? An economy 100-room hotel? A 3,000-room casino hotel?
2. Describe a work team structure.
3. Compare and contrast a matrix structure and a project structure.
4. When might an organization design its structure around independent business units?

Internet Exercise

Organization: Your choice of company
Web site: The company's URL
Summary: Pick a major corporation, such as one mentioned in the text, and go to its web site to look for answers to the following questions:

(a) What different types of product offerings does the company have?

(b) In how many countries or regions is the company represented?
(c) What kind of divisions does the company have?
(d) Have different types of guest groups been identified?

Apply Your Knowledge

1. Mini Project: This project is based on a real-life experience of the executive chef at the Sheraton Hotel in San Diego. The project is to organize an off-site event, which is an event that is planned and organized by the Sheraton staff but does not take place at the hotel itself.

2. The Sheraton typically caters the annual San Diego Zoo fund-raiser every year. The attendance for this event is roughly 1,000 people. The caterers organize and cater a reception followed by dinner. Your challenge is to plan this off-site event using the planning techniques and organizational skills you have learned so far.

Endnotes

1. Starbucks, *Starbucks Company Profile*, www.starbucks.com/assets/aboutuscompanyprofileq42011121411final.pdf (accessed December 19, 2011).
2. www.rimag.com/blog-starters/2008-03-28.asp.
3. Ibid.
4. *An Alternate Plan for Starbuck's Renewal*, www.rimeg.com/blog/910000491/post/1500025350.html
5. Ibid.
6. Robert N. Lussier, *Management Fundamentals* (Cincinnati, OH: South-Western, 2003), 198.
7. See, for example, G. G. Dess, et al., "The New Corporate Architecture," *Academy of Management Executive*, August 1995, 7–20.
8. Mohrman, Susan A. (2011). "Organizing for Sustainable Effectiveness: Taking Stock and Moving Forward." http://www.hbs.edu/units/ob/pdf/Mohrman-Organizing for Sustainable Effectiveness.pdf (retrieved December 15, 2011).
9. John R. Walker and Josielyn T. Walker, *Tourism: Concepts and Practices*, Pearson, Upper Saddle River, N.J. 2011. P. 201.

Glossary

Authority   The rights inherent in a managerial position to tell people what to do and to expect them to do it.

Boundaryless organizations   Organizations not limited to or bound by vertical or horizontal boundaries.

Centralization   The degree to which decision making is concentrated at a single point in the organization.

Chain of command   The continuous line of authority that extends from upper organizational levels to the lowest levels in the organization and clarifies who reports to whom.

Comping   Offering a complimentary service without charge.

Contingency factors   Factors contingent upon various circumstances occurring; planning for the what ifs.

Decentralization   The degree to which lower level employees provide input or actually make decisions.

Departmentalization   Organizing resources into departments.

Empowerment   The act of giving employees the authority, tools, and information they need to do their jobs with greater autonomy.

Function   An assigned duty or activity.

Guest   A person who is the recipient of hospitality in the form of entertainment—at someone's home, as a visiting participant in a program, or as a customer of an establishment such as a hotel or restaurant.

Independent business unit (IBU)   A business that makes decisions with little or no need to obtain approval for routine operational decisions from higher up in the organization.

Job enlargement   A horizontal increase in the number of similar tasks assigned to a job.

Job enrichment   A vertical expansion of planning and evaluating responsibilities which act as motivators and make the job more challenging.

Job rotation   The systematic movement of workers from job to job to improve job satisfaction, reduce boredom, and enable employees to gain a broad perspective over the work process within the entire organization.

Organizational structure   Formal arrangement of jobs and tasks in an organization.

Organization chart   A chart that illustrates the organization-wide division of work by charting who is accountable to whom and who is in charge of what department.

Product   A tangible good or intangible service produced by human or mechanical effort or by a natural process.

Productive teams   Workplace teams built by giving associates the authority, responsibility, and encouragement to come together to work on guest-related improvements that will enhance the guest experience and make the associates' jobs easier.

Project structure   An organizational structure in which employees work continuously on projects.

Responsibility   The obligation to perform any assigned duties.

Self-managed team   A type of work team that operates without a manager and is responsible for a complete work process or a segment of it.

Team   A task-oriented work group that either evolves informally or is appointed formally.

Team player   An employee who is committed to the team's objectives, members, and goals.

Territory   The area for which a person is responsible as a representative or agent; a sphere of action or interest.

Work specialization   The degree to which tasks in an organization are divided into individual jobs; also called division of labor.

Work team structure   Work structure into teams of employees to delight the guest.

Photo Credits

Credits are listed in the order of appearance.

Communication and Decision Making

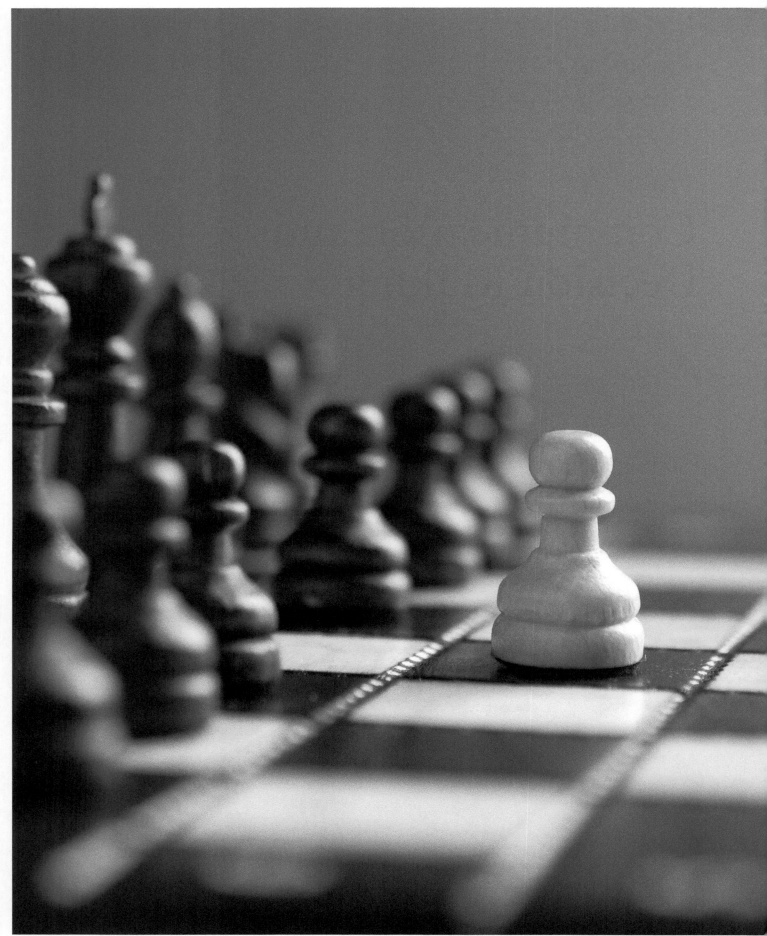

Communication and Decision Making

After reading and studying this chapter, you should be able to

- Define communication.

- List barriers to effective interpersonal communication and how to overcome them.

- Differentiate between formal and informal communication.

- Explain communication flows and networks.

- Outline the eight steps in the decision-making process.

- Know the difference between rational, bounded rational, and intuitive decisions.

- Identify situations in which a programmed decision is a better solution than a nonprogrammed decision.

- Differentiate the decision conditions of certainty, risk, and uncertainty.

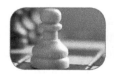 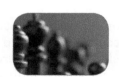 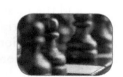 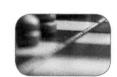

Managerial Communication

Communication is the oil that lubricates all of the other management functions of forecasting, planning, organizing, motivating, and controlling. Additionally, because managers spend a high percentage of their time communicating, the communication function becomes doubly important. Managers interact with others throughout the day by the following means:

- Personal face-to-face meetings
- Telephone
- Mail/fax
- Memos, reports, logbooks, and other internal/external written communication
- E-mail, web sites

The simplest method of communication involves a sender, a message, and a receiver. However, merely sending a message does not ensure that the message will be received and understood correctly. Several factors can lead to distortion of the message, such as noise interference, poor listening skills, and inappropriate tuning. The middle of a busy lunch service is not the right time to be asking the chef a question about the company's policy on sick-pay benefits. In this chapter, we explore various barriers to effective communication and the importance of good communication to a manager.

What Is Communication?

Communication is the exchange of information and meaning. The essence of communication is the exchange of information. Another important aspect of communication is understanding the meaning. The sole transfer of information is not enough to ensure successful communication; the actual meaning of the information must be understood, as well. An employee receiving information from a manager in Spanish will find that information of little use if the employee does not understand Spanish. Perfect communication results when a sender communicates a thought or idea and the receiver perceives it exactly as envisioned by the sender. Just because the receiver does not agree with the message does not mean that the communication process has failed. You can disagree with something even though you fully understand the message.

Managerial communication includes two different types: **Interpersonal communication** occurs between two or more individuals, and **organizational communication** includes all the different forms, networks, and systems of communication that occur among individuals, groups, or departments within an organization.

The Interpersonal Communication Process

Communication between two or more people is described as interpersonal communication.[1] The **interpersonal communication process** is made up of seven elements: the sender, encoding, the message, the channel, the receiver, decoding, and feedback (Figure 1). Before communication can take place, a *message* must exist and be conveyed. This message is sent from the sender and is passed to the receiver. The message is *encoded* and then passed by way of a medium, a *channel*, from the sender to the receiver; because of this, the message travels in a converted form. The message is then retranslated by means of *decoding*. When successful communication has taken place, the receiver gives *feedback* to the sender indicating that he or she has correctly understood the message being conveyed.

Noise is often a part of the interpersonal communication process. Noise can consist of various activities going on in the background, such as sounds of machinery or coworkers, or it can be as simple as static in the telephone line or illegible print. Therefore, noise is considered a somewhat constant disturbance in the communications process and the cause of distortions of the message. Each element in the process can be influenced and distorted by disturbances (see Figure 1). The sender conveys a message by encoding it. During this process, major things could go wrong and distort the message. The sender can have too little or too much knowledge. He or she can't communicate what he or she does not know.

However, if the proper explanations aren't given, the receiver could falsely interpret the message. Too much knowledge may cause the message not to be understood at all. Preexisting attitudes and the cultural system of the sender can influence the encoding of the message as well. Attitudes and beliefs about

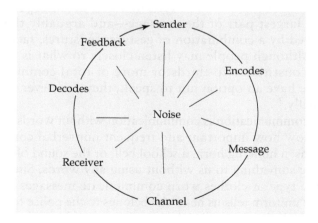

Figure 1 • Interpersonal Communication Process.
Source: Derived from Stephen P. Robbins and Mary Coulter, *Management,* 8th ed. (Upper Saddle River, NJ: Prentice Hall, 2005), 258.

subject matters will leave their traces in the message and may be picked up by the receiver.

The message itself, such as a written document, an oral speech, or gestures and facial expressions, can be influenced by disturbances. Noise will influence listening skills during an oral speech. Faulty equipment can lead to disruption of the message if it is conveyed through e-mail or fax. Symbols such as pictures, words, and numbers that are selected by the sender to convey his or her message can be influenced by noise.

The channel used to convey the message is important to the entire communications process. If you choose to use speech to communicate with a person who has a hearing impairment, the message may not be understood as the sender intended it to be. Whether the sender chooses to use an office memorandum, a phone call, e-mail, gestures, or pictures to convey the message will play a large role in how accurately the receiver will understand it. Using two channels can sometimes eliminate distortion—for example, oral speech followed by a written summary.

The receiver is limited by the same factors as the sender. If he or she has too little knowledge of the subject, distortions will take place. Likewise, if he or she has too much knowledge, too much can be read into a simple message. The preexisting attitudes and beliefs of the individual also play a role in how distorted the message will be after the decoding has taken place.

Communicating Interpersonally

Managers can communicate in various ways. Examples include face-to-face, telephone, e-mail, fax, group discussions and meetings, memos, formal presentations, bulletin boards, mail, employee publications, and teleconferencing. Communication experts generally agree that when two people are engaged in a face-to-face conversation, only a small fraction of the total message they share is contained in the words they use. A large portion of the message is contained in vocal elements such as tone of voice, accent, speed, volume, and inflection. The largest part of the message—and arguably the most important—is conveyed by a combination of gestures, postures, facial expressions, and clothing. Although people may listen closely to what is said, nonverbal behavior may constitute two-thirds or more of total communication. And although people have an option not to speak, they can never be uncommunicative nonverbally.[2]

Nonverbal communication is communication without words. Examples from everyday life show how important and frequent nonverbal communication is. Ambulance sirens, a honking horn, a school bell, or the sound of a ringing phone all communicate something to us without using any words. Similarly, gestures, actions, and the type of clothes worn communicate messages to us. A person wearing a police uniform tells us he or she belongs to the police force. In the same manner, the type of car a person drives or the size of his or her house conveys to others a message about that person. All of these forms of communication are nonverbal.

Body language consists of facial expressions, gestures, and any other ways of communicating a message with your body. For example, when you smile or laugh, you convey a message of joy or friendliness. In the same manner, rolling your eyes indicates disbelief or even annoyance. Emotions are typically conveyed purely by body language.

Verbal intonation is using your voice to emphasize certain parts of a phrase or certain words. For example, consider the phrase, "What are you doing?" An abrasive, loud intonation of the voice will indicate that the person is upset, angry, and even defensive. However, if the same sentence is said in a calm, soft voice, it will be perceived as genuine interest or concern or a friendly inquiry. Verbal intonation is almost more important than the words themselves. A common saying is that it is not *what* you say but *how* you say it. Managers should keep this very important fact in mind.

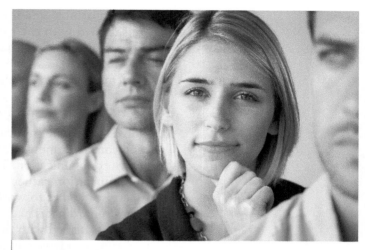

Facial expressions, a part of body language, convey different meanings.

▶ Check Your Knowledge

1. What is the difference between interpersonal and organizational communication?

2. What are three ways of communicating interpersonally?

3. Describe the interpersonal communication process.

Barriers to Effective Interpersonal Communication

Many elements can influence interpersonal communication.[3] The following sections discuss some of the major barriers.

Perception

Everybody perceives things differently. This is due to people having different backgrounds, upbringings, personal experiences, and major influences in their lives. No two people are alike, and neither are their perceptions. Whereas one person may be optimistic and perceive a message in a positive light, another may be a pessimist and see only negative aspects of the message. Unwanted news is easily screened out and forgotten, whereas things we want to hear are remembered for a longer period of time.

Semantics

The actual meaning of words, or **semantics**, is the cause of many failed communication efforts. The literal meaning of words and the actual meaning can be two different things, but they can be expressed in the same way. For instance, if a restaurant manager tells a server to make guests feel comfortable, she doesn't necessarily mean that the server will bring pillows, blankets, or even beds into the dining area. The manager may have meant to make customers feel comfortable in a nonphysical way, by attending to them, making sure they are satisfied with their order, and making sure their water glasses are refilled promptly. Employing jargon, specialized terminology, or technical language that may be used widely within an organization may be ineffective if used with new employees or people who are not familiar with it.

Nonverbal Communication

Nonverbal communication—communication through body language—is a typical means of communication. However, it can also be considered a barrier to effective communication. The weight of decoding a message lies with the nonverbal communication rather than on the actual encoded message. For example, if a supervisor comes to work in the morning disgruntled about morning traffic, his or her subordinates may misinterpret the angry facial expression as the supervisor being dissatisfied with their work, although he or she never actually said so. The next time you have a conversation with someone, be aware of your own nonverbal communication: what you are expressing with gestures and facial expressions.

Misinterpretations of nonverbal communication are especially dominant in cross-cultural communication. Gestures and expressions mean different things in different cultures. For example, in most Asian and African countries, it is considered impolite to make direct eye contact with the person you are speaking to, whereas it is considered courteous to look the speaker in the eye in most Western cultures.

Ambiguity

Ambiguity, vagueness, or uncertainty can occur in a message being conveyed. A message may be ambiguous, meaning the person receiving the message is uncertain about the actual meaning. If a manager asks an employee to come to her office as soon as possible, it could mean immediately or next week when the employee has some free time. When the words of a message are clear, but the intentions of the sender aren't, ambiguity occurs. The employee may be unclear as to why the manager wants to see him in the office now. Ambiguity may also be described as the receiver's uncertainty about the consequences of the message. The employee may think or ask, "What will happen if I don't go to her office immediately?"

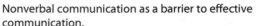

Nonverbal communication as a barrier to effective communication.

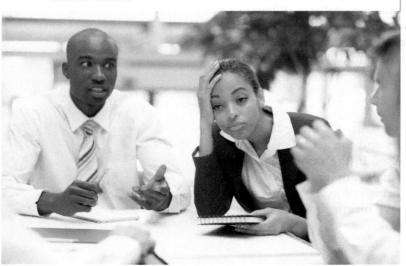

Defensiveness

When people feel that they are being verbally attacked or criticized, they tend to react defensively. The reaction could be making sarcastic remarks, being overly judgmental, or simply screening out the unpleasant parts of the conversation. This often happens when employees refuse to realize personal flaws. Using defense mechanisms helps them screen out the negative image of themselves, so they can keep their self-esteem. However, acting defensively is a barrier to effective communication.

Overcoming Barriers to Effective Interpersonal Communication

Because barriers to effective interpersonal communication do exist, there are ways to improve on communication to largely overcome them. An essential part of a manager's job is to be an effective communicator. The suggestions discussed in the following sections should help make interpersonal communication more effective.

Use Feedback

Offering feedback,[4] the last step in the communication process, will eliminate misunderstandings and inaccuracies regarding the message being conveyed. The feedback can be verbal or nonverbal. After the receiver has decoded the message, the sender should make sure the message has been understood. It can be as simple as asking the employee, "Did you understand what I said?" The ideal response to this question will be more than a yes or no answer. The best form of verbal feedback is a quick restatement and summary of the message that has been conveyed: "You said you switched my shift tomorrow to the night shift." This way the sender can be sure that the message has been correctly understood.

The nonverbal form of feedback consists of various reactions to a message. First, the sender can watch for nonverbal cues as to whether the message has been understood. Eye contact, facial expression, scratching the head, or shrugging the shoulders all can indicate how accurately the message has been received and understood. Furthermore, the actions following the message can be used as feedback. A manager who is explaining a new serving procedure to the staff will know how accurately the message has been understood by observing the staff to see whether they follow the new procedure. If some servers do not follow the new procedure, the manager will have to clarify or restate the message.

Active Listening

There is a difference between hearing and actually listening.[5] You may hear what your manager is saying, but did you *really* listen? Hearing is passive, and listening is a deliberate act of understanding and responding to the words being heard. The first step to **active listening** is listening for the total meaning. For example, if a manager tells an employee that the room occupancy is down this quarter, instead of responding, "Don't worry, it'll be fine," the employee can recognize that a problem exists. The second step is to reflect the feelings. This is an important step for the sender of the message because it helps him or her communicate the emotional part of the message. The receiver would reflect it by saying something like, "This situation must be stressful for you." The last step is to note all nonverbal cues and respond to them. These cues might include hand gestures or facial expressions.

Avoid Triggering Defensiveness

Defensiveness is one of the main barriers to effective communication. By avoiding the tendency to criticize, argue, or give advice, senders can avoid triggering defensive behavior. People don't like being criticized because it diminishes their self-image. Phrases that convey blame or finger-pointing are typically useless.

The receiver will respond by arguing or storming off, and the communication will have largely failed. A solution to this is to allow a cooling-off period so that both parties can regain their composure. Generally, managers should avoid overly negative statements.

Interpersonal Dynamics

Leaders will get the best results with and through their associates if they adopt these simple suggestions: You must have a great attitude toward your associates, meaning you accept them as colleagues and treat them fairly, with respect; you establish a climate of trust; and you include your associates in as much decision making as possible. Be sensitive to cultural differences and learn more about the cultures of your associates. Learn the best ways to communicate with your associates. Make sure that your associates know what is expected of them. Actively listen to associates. Involve your associates. Train associates and develop them so they can reach their full potential. Above all, have fun!

► Check Your Knowledge

1. Define semantics.
2. Explain ambiguity as it relates to communication barriers.
3. What are three ways of overcoming communication barriers?

Organizational Communication

Organizational communication is necessary in managerial communication. The fundamentals include formal communication vs. informal communication, communication flow patterns, and formal and informal communication networks.

Formal and Informal Communication

The two major forms of organizational communication are formal and informal communication. Formal communication is used by managers to communicate job requirements to their employees. It follows the official chain of command. **Formal communication** occurs when, for instance, a manager tells an employee his or her schedule for the following week. The subject matter is always job related and is seen as essential to the employment.

Informal communication does not follow a company's chain of command or structural hierarchy. The subject matter may be job related but may not be essential to performing job duties. Examples of informal communication are employees talking at the water fountain, in the lunchroom, or at company gatherings. In every organization, employees form relationships with each other, whether as acquaintances or as friends. Employees use informal communication to satisfy their need for social interaction, and it can also improve an organization's performance by fostering better employee relationships and providing a faster, more efficient communication channel.[6] The "grapevine" is a form of informal communication.

Communication Flows and Networks

Communication flows in various directions: upward, downward, laterally, diagonally, and so on, as we will discuss in the following sections.

Upward Communication

Upward communication takes place when managers or superiors rely on their subordinates for receiving information. Information flows upward from employees to managers. This type of communication is important to managers because it helps them determine the satisfaction level of their employees, how employees feel about their jobs and the organization in general, and if employees have problems with coworkers or even with the manager. Some managers even encourage their subordinates to give them ideas about how to make improvements in the organization. Some examples of upward communication include manager performance reports, employee surveys, suggestion boxes, and informal group sessions with other coworkers.

Downward Communication

Communication flowing down from supervisor to employee is considered **downward communication**. Managers use this type of communication for various purposes: to inform employees of company policies, procedures, employee evaluations, or job descriptions and to discuss the future of the employee. Downward communication is often used to inform, direct, coordinate, and evaluate employees.

Lateral Communication

Communication that takes place between the employees of a company who are on the same hierarchical level in the organization is called *lateral communication*. This type of communication is used by employees to discuss their environment and the organization in general. Lateral communication is also used by cross-functional teams to facilitate communication. The important thing to remember is always to let the supervisor know about decisions made through lateral communication.

Diagonal Communication

Communication that takes place between employees who are on different hierarchical levels and in different departments of the organization is called *diagonal communication*. An example of this type of communication is that of a chef communicating with a front-desk receptionist. The two employees are not on the same level, nor are they in the same department of a hotel. Through e-mail, almost every employee is able to communicate efficiently with any other employee in the same organization. However, as with lateral communication,

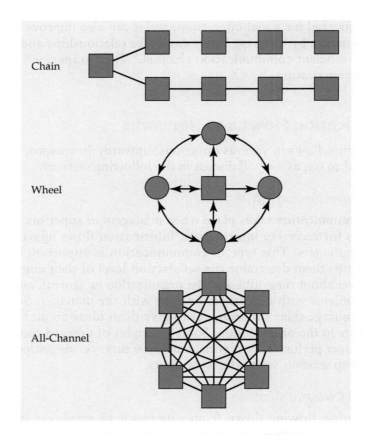

Figure 2 • Three Organizational Communication Networks.
(*Source:* Derived from Stephen P. Robbins and Mary Coulter, *Management*, 7th ed. Upper Saddle River, NJ: Prentice Hall, 2002), 295.)

the employees must make a point to update their managers on decisions made during this type of communication.

Two of the forms of communication flow, vertical and lateral, can be combined in various forms. These new forms are called **communication networks**. The most common are chain, wheel, and all-channel (Figure 2) networks, as well as the grapevine.[7]

Chain, Wheel, and All-Channel Communication Networks

Communication in a chain network flows according to the existing chain of command in an organization. This includes downward as well as upward communication flows. This type of network is highly accurate; no information can be lost, and the path the message travels is precise. On the downside, the chain network is only moderately fast and moderately popular with employees.

The wheel network is a network in which communication flows between a strong leader and each individual in a group or team. In this network, the coworkers do not need to communicate with each other; they communicate solely with their leader. The advantage to this type of communication is that it is relatively speedy and accurate. However, this type of communication is usually not very popular with employees.

The all-channel communication network is differentiated from others by its freely flowing communication between all members of a group or team. This means that the leader communicates with employees, and employees all communicate with each other. This type of network is very popular with employees, and messages travel very fast. However, the accuracy of the message is not always at 100 percent.

One thing to remember is that every unique situation will require a different communication network. No one network is perfect for every situation.

The Grapevine

The grapevine may be the most popular and important communication network in an organization. One survey reported that 75 percent of employees hear about matters first through rumors on the grapevine.[8] The grapevine is an informal organizational communication network and an important source of communication for the managers of an organization. Through the local informal grapevine, issues that employees consider a reason for stress and anxiety are made known. This network acts as a very effective feedback mechanism and as a filter that sorts out only the issues that employees find important. The negative aspect of this communication network is the occasional rumor that travels through it. This is pretty much unavoidable; however, successful managers can eliminate the negative impact of rumors. This can be done by speaking openly and honestly with employees about any negative feelings or important decisions that are made.

► Check Your Knowledge

1. Define informal communication.

2. What is the difference between lateral and diagonal communication?

3. Elaborate on the wheel communication network.

The Decision-Making Process

All individuals in organizations, small or large, are faced with the task of decision making. This can involve decisions as simple as where to have lunch or as complex as the best place to locate a new franchise. A comprehensive, detailed **decision-making process** is used to make a complex decision. However, the same model can also be used for simple decisions.

The decision-making process consists of eight major steps (Figure 3):

1. **Identification and definition of problem**
2. **Identification of decision criteria**
3. **Allocation of weights to criteria**

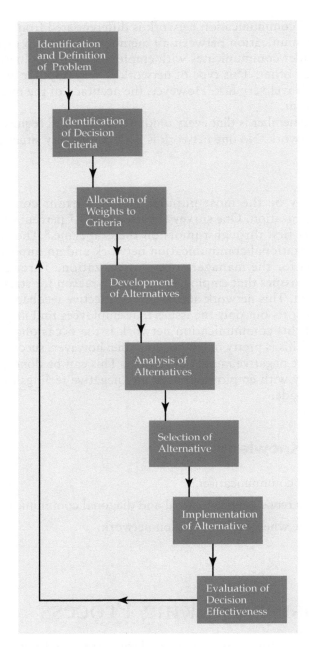

Figure 3 • Eight-Step Decision-Making Process.

4. Development of alternatives
5. Analysis of alternatives
6. Selection of alternative
7. Implementation of alternative
8. Evaluation of decision effectiveness

This model can be used for most decisions, from simple ones such as what to buy for dinner to complex corporate decisions about new marketing strategies. So let's take a closer look at each step of the decision-making process.

Step 1: Identification and Definition of Problem

Let's say that we are experiencing a discrepancy between current and desired results. In this case, the decision-making process begins with identifying and defining the problem(s). It is not always easy to identify the problem because other issues may muddy the waters. In a hotel setting, problem situations can be identified with respect to, say, guest check-in. In some of the larger city-center, convention-oriented hotels, long lines of guests are frequently waiting to check into the hotel. Defining this problem is best done by writing a problem statement: "The problem is that it takes too long for guests to register." Once the problem has been accurately stated, it becomes easier to move to the next step in the decision-making process.

Another example comes to us from Herb Kelleher, former president of Southwest Airlines, when he decided to remove the closets at the front of Southwest planes. This was in response to a problem: It was taking too long to turn around the planes. To be competitive and successful, it is necessary to reduce the turnaround time in order to squeeze more flights into each day. The situation that caused or contributed to the turnaround problem was that the first people on the plane typically went to the closets first and then grabbed the nearest seats. On landing, the departing passengers were held up while the people in the front rows rummaged through the closets for their bags. The airline now turns around about 85 percent of its flights in twenty minutes or less and is one of the most profitable airlines.

Step 2: Identification of Decision Criteria

Once the problem has been identified and defined, we need to determine the criteria relevant to the decision. Suppose the problem is that we are hungry; the decision criteria might then be the following:

1. What type of food would we prefer?
2. How much time do we have to eat?
3. How much do we want to spend?
4. How convenient is parking?
5. What is the restaurant's reputation?
6. How is the food quality?
7. How is the service?
8. How is the atmosphere?

These criteria must have been developed by a group that wants to eat out at a restaurant. Criteria that are not identified are usually treated as unimportant.

INTRODUCING PATRICIA TAM

Vice President of Standards and Corporate Relations, Halekulani Corp., Waikiki, Hawaii

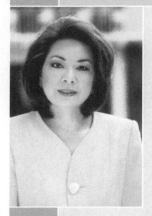

Patricia Tam is a role model to everyone who wants to pursue a career in the hospitality industry. It is not hard to see why. Patricia is a woman of great ambition and ability. She has proved herself capable of succeeding at almost anything she attempts to do.[1] Patricia is of Chinese heritage and was brought up in Hawaii. During her childhood years, her ambition was to become an English teacher. Joining the hospitality industry never entered her mind. In fact, she didn't stay in a hotel until she was a young adult: "I was going along with some friends to the mainland for one of the first times I'd been off the island."

When she finished college at age 23, she became proprietor of a bakery. She was then recruited by Amfac Corp. to open a bakeshop at its Royal Lahaina Hotel on Maui in 1975. She says, "When I opened the bakeshop there, I liked the whole aura of resort life, not just because of the guests' experience, but because of the beach and the large infrastructure." She enrolled in the resort's management training program, which would be the start of a long and successful career journey in the lodging industry. Patricia started working at Halekulani in 1983. Halekulani was first constructed in 1907 as a beachfront home accompanied by five bungalows. In 1983, it reopened as a 466-room low-rise complex. It is Waikiki's premier five-diamond resort.

When Patricia became general manager of Halekulani, the situation was less than desirable. She was promoted in the post–Gulf War period, and the once-glorious Pacific destinations had stagnated. Because most of Hawaii's visitors were Asian, Japan's ongoing recession added to the difficult times. In the 1960s, Hawaii experienced its tourist boom years. But during the early 1990s, Hawaii had to fight for every bit of the global destination market it could capture. Patricia says, "We're sitting in an arena right now where the first one to the finish line is the winner. And I think that it's more exciting to be working in this business now than it would have been in the boom years, when all you had to worry about was how many people you couldn't accommodate tonight."

Patricia realizes that the hotel business can make either a profit or a loss. "I think for a lot of us who get into the business, we see the fun part of it: the bartending, the wait help, the restaurant excitement, the chance to meet really fabulous people from around the world. We see one side of the vision of what luxury properties are all about," she explains. "But there's the other side of it, which is that it is a business, and what do businesses do? They've got to make money."

Patricia believes that outstanding guest services make a good hotel and maintain guest loyalty. She pays careful attention to detail and perfection and lets nothing pass her by. Even guest complaints are discussed one by one. She says, "You can get so worked up about the attention to detail that unless you're communicating with staff, it can be pretty challenging for them in terms of how to keep this hotel perfect. Not everybody knows how. But everybody tries to keep it that way." Maintaining her great reputation as a general manager as well as the hotel's reputation as a superior destination is reflected by her drive for perfection. John Sharpe, president of the Toronto-based Four Seasons hotel, nominated Patricia to be hotelier of the year. Halekulani, meaning "house befitting heaven," was voted best hotel in the world by *Gourmet* magazine. It has held its AAA five-diamond rating for years. It was a finalist for *Condé Nast Traveler*'s Reader's Choice Best Tropical Resorts award and ranked in the top three hotels in the country in Zagat's U.S. hotel, resort, and spa survey. Its well-known restaurant, La Mer, is Hawaii's only AAA-rated five-diamond restaurant, and it has been known as such for years.

[1] This profile draws on Tony De la Cruz, "Independent Hotelier of the World, Patricia Tam, Reaching for Resort Perfection," *Hotels*, November 1999, 64; and "Tam takes broader role at Halekulani Corp.," *Pacific Business News*, August 6, 2004, www.bizjournals.com/pacific/stories/2004/08/02/daily56.html (accessed December 21, 2011).

Courtesy Patricia Tam

Patricia has served as a hotel assistant manager, rooms division director, and acting general manager, and also as general manager of Halekulani's adjacent sister property, the four-diamond Waikiki Parc hotel. In 1993, she became the general manager of Halekulani. Through it all, she always wanted more. She says, "I could work the operations in a very good management way, but I never had to be the person responsible for the final decision making on a lot of things. The challenge, the intimidation of that process, coming back over as the general manager, was quite overwhelming to me. But that was also my proudest moment because that's when I realized that I really had to buckle down." The readers of *Hotels* magazine have named Patricia Hotelier of the World.

As for her personality, Patricia is a genuine person who doesn't credit only herself. She doesn't forget that her success depends on an ongoing and mutually beneficial relationship between Halekulani's owner, Halekulani Corp., and herself. She says, "I look at it as a kind of management proposition where you can always learn every day." She adds, "Every day you can learn something new, not only about how to maintain a luxury property, but how to develop it and take it to the next level, because that's what it's all about."

Step 3: Allocation of Weights to Criteria

To decision makers, decision criteria all have different levels of importance. For instance, is the expected cost of the meal more important than the atmosphere? If so, a higher weight should be attached to that criterion.

One method used to weigh the criteria is to give the most important criterion a weight of 10 and then score the others according to their relative importance. In the meal example, the cost of the meal may receive a weight of 10, whereas the atmosphere may be awarded a weight of 6. Figure 4 lists a sample of criteria and weights for restaurant selection.

Step 4: Development of Alternatives

In developing alternatives, decision makers list the viable alternatives that could resolve the problem. No attempt is made to evaluate these alternatives—only to list them. The alternatives for the restaurant scenario are shown in Figure 5.

How much do we want to spend?	10
What type of food would we prefer?	8
How much time do we have?	6
How is the food quality?	9
How is the atmosphere?	6
How is the service?	7
How convenient is parking?	6
What is the restaurant's reputation?	6
How far do we want to go to a restaurant?	7

Figure 4 • Criteria and Weights in Restaurant Selection.

KFC

Taco Bell

Pizza Hut

McDonald's

Applebee's

The Olive Garden

Wendy's

Figure 5 • Restaurant Alternatives.

Step 5: Analysis of Alternatives

The alternatives are analyzed using the criteria and weights established in Steps 2 and 3. Figure 6 shows the values placed on each of the alternatives by the group for the restaurant scenario (it does not show the weighted values). The weighted values of the group's decision about which restaurant to go to are shown in Figure 7.

	KFC	Taco Bell	Pizza Hut	McDonald's	Applebee's	Olive Garden	Wendy's
Price	9	10	10	10	7	7	9
Type of food	7	8	9	8	8	9	9
How much time	9	9	7	10	7	6	10
Quality of food	7	7	8	7	8	8	8
Atmosphere	7	7	8	7	9	9	7
Service	6	6	7	7	8	9	7
Convenient parking	10	10	10	9	10	10	10
Restaurant reputation	8	8	8	7	8	9	8
How far away	8	8	8	10	7	7	8
Total	71	73	75	76	72	74	75

Figure 6 • Analysis of Alternatives.

	KFC	Taco Bell	Pizza Hut	McDonald's	Applebee's	Olive Garden	Wendy's
Price	90	100	100	100	70	70	90
Type of food	56	64	72	64	64	72	72
How much time	54	54	42	60	42	36	60
Quality of food	63	63	72	63	72	72	72
Atmosphere	42	42	48	42	54	54	42
Service	42	42	49	49	56	63	49
Convenient parking	60	60	60	56	60	60	60
Restaurant reputation	48	48	48	42	48	54	48
How far away	56	56	56	70	49	49	56
Total	511	529	547	546	515	530	549

Figure 7 • Weighted Values Analysis.

Once the weighted values are totaled, we can see that Pizza Hut and Wendy's are the restaurants with the highest scores. Notice how these are not the restaurants with the highest scores before the weighted values were included.

Step 6: Selection of Alternative

The sixth step is to select the best alternative. Once the weighted scores for each alternative have been totaled, it will become obvious which is the best alternative.

Step 7: Implementation of Alternative

We next need to ensure that the alternative is implemented so that the decision is put into action. Sometimes good decisions fail because they are not put into action.

Step 8: Evaluation of Decision Effectiveness

The final step in the decision loop is to evaluate the effectiveness of the decision. As a result of the decision, did we achieve the goals we set? If the decision was not effective, then we must find out why the desired results were not attained. This would mean going back to Step 1. If the decision was effective, then no action, other than recording the outcome, needs to be taken.

How Managers Make Decisions

Managers are the main decision makers in any organization. Although all employees face daily decisions, the choices a manager makes impact the future of the organization. Decision making is an integral part of all four primary managerial functions: planning, organizing, leading, and controlling.

Making Decisions: Rationality, Bounded Rationality, and Intuition

The first criterion for making a decision is that it must be rational. Several assumptions are made to define what a rational decision really is. First, the decision itself would have to maximize value and be consistent within natural constraining limits. This means that the choice made must maximize the organization's profitability. Tying in with this is the natural assumption that the manager making the decision is pursuing the organization's values and profitability, not his or her own interest.

One assumption of **rationality** as it relates to the decision maker is that he or she is fully objective and logical. When making the decision, a clearly stated goal must always be kept in mind. This goes hand in hand with starting with a problem statement.

Bounded rationality means that managers make decisions based on the decision-making process that is bounded, or limited, by an individual's ability to gain information and make decisions. Managers know that their decision-making skills are based on their own competency, intelligence, and, last but not least, rationality. They are also expected to follow the decision-making process model. However, certain aspects of this model are not realistic with respect to true-life managerial decisions, which are made with respect to bounded reality. This comes into play, for example, when decision makers cannot find all of the necessary information to analyze a problem and all of its possible alternatives. Therefore, they find themselves **satisficing**, a term used by management scholar and author Peter Drucker that means accepting a solution that is just good enough, rather than maximizing. Consider this example: A chef for a major hotel chain has to prepare a banquet for fifty people. On the menu is half a chicken for every guest, which means that the chef needs twenty-five whole chickens for this banquet. He purchases the chickens at a market twenty-five miles away, where he has made the same purchase before for $60. Because he has made purchases from this market before, he knows the quality of the food they sell. What the chef does not know is that there is a free-range chicken farm only ten miles away that would have sold him the twenty-five chickens for the same price. Instead of researching his alternatives, the chef satisfices himself with the first option that comes to mind and settles on it, assuming it is probably not the best but is good enough. This behavior is rationally bounded because the best solution to be found is bounded by the chef's ability to research all alternatives instead of settling on the first acceptable one that comes to mind.

Most decisions that managers make are not based on perfect rationality because of various factors, such as time constraints on researching all possible solutions or lack of resources to do the research. Therefore, decisions are typically based on bounded rationality. In other words, managers make decisions based on alternatives that are just satisfactory. At the same time, though, the decision maker will be strongly influenced by an organization's culture, power considerations, internal politics, and an **escalation of commitment**. An escalation of commitment happens when the commitment to a prior decision is increased despite evidence to the contrary. For example, consider the decline of the Planet Hollywood restaurant chain. At the launch of the chain, the team of marketing professionals deemed it economically sensible to set a high price on burgers and other food items. The restaurant set out to be a novelty establishment, although the target customers were middle-class citizens. Although it was evident that the decision to have high-priced products in a middle-class establishment was doomed for failure from the beginning, the decision makers stuck with it. The inevitable took place, and Planet Hollywood went belly up and was forced to close locations all around the world. The negative consumer reaction was predictable, but the decision makers escalated their commitment to the set prices even though it was a bad decision. Rather than search for new alternatives, they did not want to admit to making a bad decision and simply increased their commitment to the original one.[9]

Using rationality and common sense to influence decision making is very important—we must not forget the role of plain and simple human intuition. Intuition is used in everyday life, such as knowing not to grab a hot baking pan with your bare hands. It ranges all the way to the corporate level, where managers often use their own intuition when making corporate decisions. **Intuitive decision**

making is a subconscious process of making decisions on the basis of experience and accumulated judgment. Five different identified aspects of intuition comply with the different types of decisions made. The first is a *values-* or an *ethics-based decision*. Managers will recall the ethics system they were raised with and base their decisions on personal morals. The second is an *experience-based decision*.

A DAY IN THE LIFE OF DENISE SIMENSTAD

National Sales Manager, San Diego Convention Center, San Diego, California

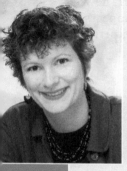

Denise Simenstad is the national sales manager at the San Diego Convention Center. Her work here starts early and usually ends when the timing is good. What she does in those hours, though, is good customer service and remarkable work.

Denise comes in to work at about 8:00 A.M. When she arrives at her office, she checks her voice mail, e-mail, and inbox messages. From then on, the day is not her own. She's working and attending to customer activity.

Her day-to-day activities keep her busy throughout the day. First, Denise responds to customer inquiries. These inquiries consist of prospective customers calling her to inquire about date and space availability at the convention center, the cost of renting meeting rooms or exhibit halls, and checking whether other, similar shows are booked in the facility.

She then usually leads a tour or, as it is better known, a "site inspection" of the facility to show customers the available physical space, including the lobby, exhibit halls, ballroom, meeting space, and outdoor space. Then she shows them the ancillary services that the convention center provides, such as the audiovisual facilities, food and beverage, telecommunications, security services, business services center, and so on. All of this makes for a complete tour.

Denise then prepares proposals (dates, rates, and space letter) for prospective customers. This ranges from a group of 100 people for one day to a trade show for 15,000 people to 250,000 guests for five days. She includes a package of information concerning the floor plans, rates, regulations, and other pertinent information.

After all of that, Denise answers customers' questions about the facilities available and capabilities. She fields questions on the sizes of rooms, capacities of the facilities, rates, distance between pillars on the exhibit floor, floor loads, dimensions of freight doors, number of committable hotel rooms in the downtown area, number of packages available, and more.

Then comes the duty of issuing and negotiating license agreements (contracts) with outlines, dates, space and rates, insurance requirements, indemnification issues, cancellation clauses, guarantees, and so on.

To start wrapping up, Denise attends meetings with other sales managers in the office to discuss business strategy concerning who is considering them for a meeting, how they can close the deal, what other managers are working on, what type of business seems to be prevalent right now, and so on. The sessions continue with yet another meeting with event managers, the people responsible for the operational aspect of an event once it is contracted. In this meeting, they all go over any operational concerns and check to ensure that promised sales are delivered. If a client is in-house, they send a gift to his or her hotel room (just prior to arrival) and then go on the floor to check the show and ensure that clients are satisfied with service received.

The day usually ends at about 5:30 P.M. for Denise. The day can go on even longer if a customer is in town. In this case, she makes sure that her customers are wined and dined and well attended to by entertaining them; providing breakfast, lunch, and/or dinner; and basically showing them what San Diego is all about.

Courtesy of Denise Simenstad.

Through trial and error, the manager has gained experience and will base a decision on past learning. *Affect-initiated decisions* are those that are based on a manager's emotions and feelings. The fourth type is a *cognitive-based decision*. The manager's previous training, learned skills, and gained knowledge influence the decision-making process. Last, the manager may use his or her subconscious mind to retain data and process it in such a way that it will influence the type of decision he or she will make.

Intuition and rationality are separate but are often used in combination in most decision making. The two complement each other to offer the manager an ideal solution for the decision-making process. As an example, consider a manager who has to make a decision on a situation that is similar to one he has come across in the past. Instead of using careful analytical rationality, he will make a decision based on a "gut feeling" and act quickly with what appears to be limited information. The decision is ultimately made based on his experience and accumulated judgment.

▶ Check Your Knowledge

1. List criteria for making a rational decision.

2. Give an example of satisficing.

3. What are the five aspects of intuition?

Types of Problems and Decisions

Several different types of decisions match different types of problems. They are applied as solutions, depending on the various situations that arise. Managers who are aware of these differences can use them to their advantage.

The two major types of decisions are programmed decisions and nonprogrammed decisions. A **programmed decision** involves situations that recur on a regular basis, allowing the response to be handled with a "programmed" response. In a programmed decision, the response will occur on a repetitive basis; for example, when the number of New York steaks goes below a specified number, an order for more is automatically placed. Programmed decisions generally become a standard operating procedure. Alternatives are not necessary most of the time because the problem statement is familiar, and therefore the solution is in close reach because of past successful decisions made. The response to a shortage of New York steaks is simply a reorder; the alternatives are truly limited. A programmed decision is made in response to a recurring problem; the approach to dealing with it has become repetitive and therefore does not require a careful analysis.

A **nonprogrammed decision** is nonrecurring and is made necessary by unusual circumstances. The type of problem that induces a nonprogrammed decision is a poorly structured problem. These types of problems are usually new or unusual to the decision maker. More often than not, the information on the problem is incomplete or unavailable. This generally increases the difficulty gradient of finding an appropriate solution. Most important, though, the problem is unique and nonrecurring, such as which computer hardware and software a restaurant

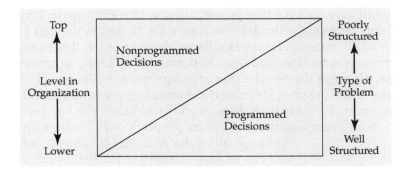

Figure 8 • Nonprogrammed and Programmed Decisions.

Source: Derived from Stephen P. Robbins and Mary Coulter, *Management*, 7th ed. (Upper Saddle River, NJ: Prentice Hall, 2002), 161.

should install or whether to expand through franchising or company-owned restaurants. These distinctive decision situations are not likely to recur for several years and require a custom-made decision.

The more sophisticated a company is, the more programmed decisions are made. Many large corporations have policy and procedure manuals to guide managerial and supervisory decision making. Nonprogrammed decisions call for greater analysis, innovation, and problem-solving skills. Figure 8 diagrams programmed and nonprogrammed decisions according to the level in the organization and type of problem.

Decision-Making Conditions

In a perfect world, we would have all the information necessary for making decisions. However, in reality, some things are unknowable. This leads us to decision-making conditions. Decision making includes three major conditions: certainty, risk, and uncertainty. These three conditions each have individual characteristics.

The ideal situation for making a decision is one of **certainty**. A decision of certainty includes knowing all of the alternatives and therefore having no risk involved when making a decision, because the outcome is known. A good example for this condition is a hotel investment specialist who is allotted a share of the hotel's profit. The investor's options are clear and defined. He knows exactly how much interest is earned on bonds and how much interest is offered by various banks, the security issues, and how many years it will take for them to mature.

Making a decision that involves **risk** is one of the most common situations. Here the decision maker is not certain of the outcome of the situation. However, through personal experience, or a simple "gut feeling," she can estimate the probability of the outcome. Although not all alternatives are properly researched, by using historical data, probabilities can be assigned to various alternatives and the best probable outcome can ultimately be chosen. This is called a *risk condition* as it relates to decision making and is characterized by having some knowledge of the outcome of the various alternatives, combined with the element of unpredictability.

For example, a popular hotel is thinking about adding on family apartments to its property. So far, the largest room it has is a double; the family rooms would need to have beds for four people, along with a kitchenette. Perusing past historical data helps make the decision somewhat clearer. In the past year alone, 40 percent of all customers were families of three or more. Reviewing the customer comments, managers find that the demand for a family apartment is relatively large. Although the construction of an apartment building will cut into the revenue, the rental profit made from these more expensive apartments is likely to outweigh costs in fewer than three years. In addition, the hotel is hoping to attract an even larger family crowd to its property once it offers apartments.

Although all of the past data is valuable information and can to some extent predict the future, a factor of risk is involved because there is always some level of unpredictability about the future.

Uncertainty situations are characterized by having to make a decision when the outcome is not certain and when reasonable outcome estimates can't be made either. These situations often arise when alternatives to the decision are limited because of lack of adequate information. Although conditions of uncertainty are not as common as situations of risk, managers still find themselves confronted with uncertainty in decision-making situations.

Rational Decision Making

Professional managers at the Sheraton Hotel and Resort in San Diego provided us with a real-life problem that deals with making rational decisions: How much space should we reserve for large parties? For example, if a group of 500 reserves a room and only 300 show up, the other 200 spaces are basically "dead space," which could have been rented out to another party of 200 people. To protect itself from this kind of dilemma, the hotel has attached a food and beverage price to each room. If you reserve the room, the food and beverage price is charged automatically, even if the guests don't show up.

Decision-Making Styles

Decision makers differ in their way of thinking; some are rational and logical, whereas others are intuitive and creative. Rational decision makers look at the information in order. They organize the information and make sure it is logical and consistent. Only after carefully studying all of the given options do they finally make the decision. Intuitive thinkers, on the other hand, can look at information that is not necessarily in order. They can make quick decisions based on their spontaneous creativity and intuition. Although a careful analysis is still required, these types of people are comfortable looking at all solutions as a whole as opposed to studying each option separately.

The second dimension in which people differ is each individual's **tolerance for ambiguity**. Managers who have a high tolerance for ambiguity are lucky in that they save a lot of time while making a decision. These individuals can process many thoughts at the same time. Unfortunately, some managers have a low tolerance for ambiguity. These individuals must have order and consistency in the way they organize and must process the information so as to minimize ambiguity.

Upon review of the two dimensions of decision making—way of thinking and tolerance for ambiguity—and their subdivisions, four major decision-making styles become evident[10]:

1. The **directive style** entails having a low tolerance for ambiguity as well as being a rational thinker.

"No ... I mean yes."

A former CEO always said "no" first because he could always change his mind to "yes" later. Today it may be better to say, "Let me get back to you on that request," or, "Let's discuss this—can you meet with me on Monday at 10:00 A.M.?"

CORPORATE PROFILE

Starwood Hotels

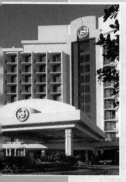

Starwood is one of the world's largest hotel and leisure companies. Its brand names include St. Regis, the Luxury Collection, Sheraton, Westin, W, Four Points by Sheraton, Le Méridien, Aloft, and Element by Westin. Through these brands, Starwood is well represented in most major markets around the world. Operations are grouped into two business segments: hotels and vacation ownership operations. Revenue and earnings are derived primarily from hotel operations, which include the operation of owned hotels, management and other fees earned from hotels managed pursuant to management contracts, and the receipt of franchise and other fees.

Starwood's hotel business emphasizes global operation of hotels and resorts primarily in the luxury and upscale segment of the lodging industry. It seeks to acquire interests in, management of, or franchise rights for properties in this segment. The hotel portfolio includes owned, leased, managed, and franchised hotels totaling 1,027 hotels, with approximately 302,000 rooms in approximately 100 countries.

Starwood's revenues and earnings are also derived from development, ownership, and operation of vacation ownership resorts, marketing and selling vacation ownerships in the resorts, and providing financing to customers who purchase such interests. Generally, these resorts are marketed under the preceding brand names. There are 23 vacation ownership resorts in the United States and the Bahamas.[1]

Starwood has assumed a leadership position in markets worldwide based on superior global distribution, coupled with strong brands and brand recognition. The upscale and luxury brands continue to capture market share from competitors by aggressively cultivating new customers while maintaining loyalty among the world's most active travelers. The strength of Starwood's brands is evidenced, in part, by the superior ratings received from hotel guests and from industry publications. The November 2004 edition of *Condé Nast Traveler* magazine named four Starwood properties in the top 100 Best in the World, with more than 30 properties listed in the Readers' Choice Awards list. In addition, the January 2005 issue included 51 Starwood properties among its prestigious Gold List and Gold List Reserve—more than any other hotel company. For the third year in a row, Starwood was named the World's Leading Hotel Group at the World Travel Awards.

Starwood has distinguished and diversified hotel properties throughout the world, including the St. Regis in New York City; the Phoenician in Scottsdale, Arizona; the Hotel Gritti Palace in Venice, Italy; the St. Regis in Beijing, China; and the Westin Palace in Madrid. These are among the leading hotels in the industry and are at the forefront of providing the highest quality and service.

Starwood's primary business goal is to maximize earnings and cash flow by increasing the profitability of its existing portfolio, selectively acquiring interests in additional assets, increasing the number of hotel management contracts and franchise agreements, acquiring and developing vacation ownership resorts and selling VOIs, and maximizing the value of owned real estate properties, including selectively disposing of noncore hotels and "trophy" assets that may be sold at significant premiums. Starwood plans to meet these goals by leveraging its global assets, broad customer base, and other resources and by taking advantage of scale to reduce costs. The uncertainty relating to political and economic environments around the world and consequent impact on travel in their respective regions and the rest of the world make financial planning and implementation of Starwood's strategy more challenging.

For more information, go to www.starwood.com.

[1] Starwood Hotels and Resorts, *Company Overview*, www.starwoodhotels.com/corporate/company_info.html (accessed December 21, 2011).

Individuals who fall into the category of having a directive decision-making style are usually logical and very efficient. They also have a primary focus on the short run and are relatively quick decision makers. Directive decision makers value speed and efficiency, which can cause them to be remiss in assessing all alternatives, such that decisions are often made with minimal information.

2. Decision makers who have an **analytic style** of decision making have a large tolerance for ambiguity. Compared to directive decision makers, these individuals require more information before making their decisions and, consequently, they consider more alternatives. Individuals with an analytic style are careful decision makers, which gives them leeway to adapt or cope to unique situations.

3. Decision makers who have a **conceptual style** of decision making look at numerous alternatives and are typically very broad in their outlook. Their focus is on the long run of the decision made. These individuals are typically creative and often find creative solutions to the problem with which they are dealing.

4. Decision makers who work well with others are said to have a **behavioral style** of decision making. This entails being receptive to suggestions and ideas from others as well as being concerned about the achievements of their employees. They commonly communicate with their coworkers through meetings. These individuals try to avoid conflict as often as possible, because acceptance by others is very important to them.

At least one of these decision-making styles is always used by managers. However, decision makers often combine two or more styles to make a decision. Most often, a manager will have one dominant decision-making style and will use one or more other styles as alternates. Flexible individuals vary their decision-making styles according to each unique situation. If the style is to consider riskier options (analytic style) or if the decision is made based on suggestions from subordinates (behavioral style), each style will eventually bring the decision maker to the optimal solution for the unique problem he or she is facing.

▶ Check Your Knowledge

1. Name the two dimensions of decision-making styles.
2. Briefly describe the conceptual style of decision making.

Sustainable Communication and Decision Making

Sustainability in the hospitality industry is a trend that is constantly gaining in popularity. There is a steady increase in environmental consciousness, which has resulted in a higher demand for eco-friendly initiatives. More often we are seeing hoteliers build sustainable practices and policies into their daily operations. In order to successfully implement sustainable initiatives, it is important to effectively communicate sustainable goals internally to employees and investors, as well as to guests. Sustainable initiatives are driven from within an organization through employee encouragement and involvement. The decision to employ sustainable practices is generally made from the top of an organization; however, it must be supported by everyone in order to prevail.[11]

In communicating sustainable practices to guests, hoteliers can use a variety of informational approaches either directly or indirectly. Some hotels post their information in guestroom compendiums, while others tell guests directly upon check-in. Many hotels attempt to establish guest involvement by surveying guests to gain feedback on the effectiveness of communicating their sustainable practices. The goal is to inform guests of what the hotel advocates without being overly aggressive. Guests should feel a sense of care and commitment to their well-being, and the surrounding environment. The decision to adapt to sustainable practices is made because of the increase in interest and attractiveness from a guest perspective.[12]

The stakeholders of a company are involved in much of the decision making, which gives them the responsibility of determining the role of sustainability within their operation. It is often necessary to establish a communication strategy, "which should identify how information, awareness creation, advocacy, network building, conflict migration, and communication platforms should be supported." In determining the level of sustainability implemented, different forms of communication are needed, which can range from meetings and conventions to emails, the internet, advertisements, and forms of telecommunications. Depending on the size of the organization, "there is a need for effective communication from the central to the regional and local levels."

Because tourism heavily impacts local communities, it is important to effectively communicate sustainable initiatives by fostering a degree of participation from the local population. Some strategies to involve the local population in tourism development include training, meetings, workshops, special events, projects, etc. It is beneficial to harbor trust by creating relationships with local communities, and considering their needs and concerns. There are also various barriers to communication with different communities, which can include differences in culture, language, perceptions, priorities, and forms of communication. These barriers can be overcome by "awareness-raising activities, and dialogue between businessmen and communities to aid in understanding different points of views, opinions and interests."[13]

Trends in Communication and Decision Making

- Trends such as improving technology to aid with communication are likely to continue. Voice mail, e-mail, and the Internet will increasingly assist hospitality managers and associates with speedier communications. All-way radio connectivity, which allows associates to communicate live, enables them to better serve the needs of discriminating guests.

- An integral part of management's decision-making process is the management support system (MSS). The MSS has two distinctive elements: the management information system (MIS) and the decision support system (DSS). The MIS provides managers with all information needed to run the business, so it is valuable for making routine decisions. Usually included in the information flow are daily or monthly sales data, daily inventory, and employee hours and salaries, to name a few. The DSS, unlike the MIS, which deals with structured, routine business information, is designed to offer the manager information to help solve nonroutine problems. The DSS processes both internal and external data.

CASE STUDY

Guests Complaining about Waiting Too Long for Elevators

Guests at a busy eight-story four-star hotel are constantly complaining about having to wait too long for the elevator. At 8:00 A.M., some of the elevators are in use by the housekeeping department, whose associates are going up to begin work on the guest rooms. At the same time, room service has an elevator blocked off to serve in-room breakfasts because the kitchen and the banqueting departments are using the service elevators. Then, at about 10:30 A.M., the housekeepers use the elevators to go down for their morning break. The general manager recognizes your potential and asks you to come up with suggestions to take care of the problem/challenge.

Discussion Question

1. What suggestions do you have to remedy the situation described?

Summary

1. The definition of communication is the transfer and understanding of meaning. Managerial communication is divided into two categories: interpersonal communication and organizational communication. Interpersonal communication takes place between two or more people, and organizational communication consists of all the networks and systems of communication that exist in an organization.

2. The interpersonal communication process can be disrupted or can fail based on several factors. To improve your interpersonal communication skills, you need to eliminate as much noise during the communication process as possible; that is, close the door to your office or move to a quiet space in the building. Inform yourself about how knowledgeable the receiver is on the subject. Be sure to provide adequate explanations if the receiver's knowledge is limited. Lastly, pick the appropriate channel of communication to ensure successful conveyance of the message.

3. Barriers to effective interpersonal communication include misunderstood perception, misuse of semantics, misguided use of nonverbal communication, ambiguous messages, and defensiveness. Ways to overcome these barriers are through use of feedback, active listening, and avoiding defensiveness.

4. Managers use formal communication to communicate job requirements to their employees. It follows the official chain of command. Informal communication does not follow a company's chain of command or structural hierarchy. The subject matter is typically not job related and is not essential to performing job duties.

5. Communication flows are part of the organizational communication process. Upward communication flows from the employees to the manager. Downward communication flows from manager to employees. Lateral communication takes place among employees who are on the same organizational level. Diagonal communication cuts across organizational levels as well as work areas. The four different types of communication networks are the chain, the wheel, the all-channel, and the grapevine.

6. The decision-making process consists of eight steps: (1) identification and definition of problem, (2) identification of decision criteria, (3) allocation of weights to criteria, (4) development of alternatives, (5) analysis of alternatives, (6) selection of alternative, (7) implementation of alternative, and (8) evaluation of decision effectiveness.

7. Although all employees in a company make decisions on a regular basis, in the end it is the manager's decisions that count. His or her decisions usually represent the final word and are valued as "the right decision." Decision making is a large part of all four primary managerial functions: planning, organizing, leading, and controlling. Hence, *managing* is a synonym for *decision making*.

8. A rational decision is based on the following assumptions: The decision is value maximizing and within natural limits, and the manager making the decision is fully objective and logical and has the organization's economic interest in mind. As a result, the rational decision-making is simple and has a clearly defined goal, limited alternatives, minimal time pressure, low cost for seeking and evaluating alternatives, an organizational culture that supports risk taking and innovation, and measurable and concrete outcomes. Bounded rationality suggests that managers make decisions that are bounded by an individual's ability to process information. Managers often cannot possibly analyze all available information and all alternatives, so they satisfice instead of maximize. Finally, intuitive decision making is a subconscious process of making decisions on the basis of experience and accumulated judgment, including ethics learned.

9. Programmed decisions require a problem situation that is a frequent occurrence, allowing the response to be handled with a routine approach. Programmed decisions generally become standard operating procedures. A nonprogrammed decision is nonrecurring and made necessary by unusual circumstances. These types of problems are usually new or unusual to the decision maker. More often than not, the information on the problem is incomplete or unavailable.

10. The decision condition of certainty includes knowing all of the alternatives and therefore having no risk involved when making a decision, because the outcome is pretty much known. Uncertainty situations are characterized by having to make a decision when the outcome is not certain and reasonable outcome estimates can't be made because of lack of adequate information. In risk situations, the decision maker is not certain of the outcome of the situation. However, through personal experience, historical data, or a simple "gut feeling," he or she can estimate the probability of the outcome.

11. Decision-making styles vary depending on a person's way of thinking—rational or intuitive—and a person's tolerance for ambiguity, which can be low or high. Combinations of these differences give us the directive style (low tolerance for ambiguity and rational way of thinking), the analytic style (high tolerance for ambiguity and rational way of thinking), the conceptual style (high tolerance for ambiguity and intuitive way of thinking), and the behavioral style (low tolerance for ambiguity and intuitive way of thinking).

Key Words and Concepts

active listening
allocation of weights to criteria
analysis of alternatives
analytic style
behavioral style
body language
bounded rationality
certainty
communication
communication networks
conceptual style
decision-making process
development of alternatives
directive style

downward communication
escalation of commitment
evaluation of decision
  effectiveness
formal communication
identification and definition of
  problem
identification of decision criteria
implementation of alternative
informal communication
interpersonal communication
interpersonal communication
  process
intuitive decision making

nonprogrammed decision
nonverbal communication
organizational communication
programmed decision
rationality
risk
satisficing
selection of alternative
semantics
tolerance for ambiguity
uncertainty
upward communication
verbal intonation

Review Questions

1. The most important aspect of a manager's job is typically described as decision making. Do you believe this is so? Explain.
2. When reviewing some important decisions you have made, would you describe them as mostly rational or intuitive decisions? What are the characteristics of each? How does intuition affect the decision-making process?
3. During the communications process, if the receiver disagrees with the sender, does this always mean that the message has not been properly understood? Or could it mean something else? Explain.
4. How can the grapevine be used to a company's advantage?
5. When communication is not effective, is it always the fault of the receiver? Discuss all options.

Internet Exercise

Organization: **Starbucks**
Web site: **www.starbucks.com**
Summary: Starbucks founder Howard Schultz has resumed his role of CEO and made plans for the reorganization of Starbucks to restore what he calls the "distinctive Starbucks experience" and to focus on the guest. He has made several decisions, including focusing on espresso standards and other important tenets of coffee education, and all Starbucks locations were closed for a three-hour training session one day. Schultz continues to communicate via his messages on the company web site.

(a) Read about Starbucks and see if you agree with Schultz's decisions.
(b) What do you think about his communications? How could communications be improved?

Apply Your Knowledge

1. Select a hospitality-related problem and write a problem statement. Then, using the decision-making steps, show how you would solve the problem.

Endnotes

1. Draws on Stephen P. Robbins and Mary Coulter, *Management,* 8th ed. (Upper Saddle River, NJ: Prentice Hall, 2005), 282.
2. Paul Preston, "Nonverbal communication: Do you really say what you mean?" *Journal of Healthcare Management*, March/April 2005, 83.
3. Anne E. Beall, "Body language speaks," *Communication World*, March/April 2004, 18.
4. Draws on Gary Dessler, *A Framework for Management,* 3rd ed. (Upper Saddle River, NJ: Prentice Hall, 2004), 282.
5. Draws on Robbins and Coulter, *Management*, 265.
6. Ibid., 293–296.
7. Ibid., 294–295.
8. "Heard it through the grapevine," cited in *Forbes*, February 10, 1997, 22.
9. Personal conversation with John Horne, president, Anna Maria Oyster Bar restaurants, April 14, 2008.
10. Adapted from Robbins and Coulter, *Management,* 147.
11. Greenhotelier. (December 2010). Communicating Sustainability to Your Employees. http://www.responsibletravelreport.com/trade-news/spotlight/trade-news/2300-communicating-sustainability-to-your-employees. Retrieved on December 4, 2011.
12. Tixier, Maud. (November 4, 2008). The Hospitality Business Communication and Encouragement of Guest's Responsible Behavior and Their Diverse Responses. http://www.esade.edu/cedit/pdfs/papers/pdf7.pdf.
13. World Tourism Organization. (2006). Communication and Sustainable Tourism. http://www.usaid.gov/our_work/agriculture/landmanagement/pubs/commun_sust_tourism.pdf.

Glossary

Active listing Listening for full meaning without making premature judgments or interpretations.

Allocation of weights to criteria Allocating different levels of importance to decision criteria according to a weighting method.

Analysis of Alternatives Analyzing alternatives according to the "weights to criteria" method.

Analytic style A style of decision making marked by great tolerance for ambiguity and consideration of several alternatives, fostering adaptability to various situations.

Behavioral style A decision-making style characterized by a low tolerance for ambiguity and an intuitive way of thinking.

Body language Gestures, facial expressions, body postures, and other movements of the body that convey meaning, such as the emotional state and attitude of the person.

Bounded rationality Decision making based on or limited by an individual's ability to gain information.

Certainty The condition of knowing in advance the outcome of a decision.

Communication The exchange of information and the transfer of meaning.

Communication networks Networks that enable and facilitate the communications process.

Conceptual style A decision-making style that involves considering numerous alternatives in order to find creative solutions to the problem.

Decision-making process The process of developing and analyzing alternatives and choosing from among them.

Development of alternatives Listing possible alternatives that could resolve a problem.

Directive style A decision-making style characterized by a rational way of thinking and low tolerance for ambiguity.

Downward communication Communication flow within the organization from supervisor or manager to employees.

Escalation of commitment Increased commitment to a previous decision despite evidence that it may have been wrong.

Evaluation of decision effectiveness Determination of whether specified goals have been achieved.

Formal communication Communication that takes place within a prescribed organizational work agreement.

Identification of decision criteria Identifying criteria important for making decisions.

Implementation of alternative Implementing the selected alternative.

Informal communication Does not follow a company's chain of command or structural hierarchy, and the subject matter is typically not job related or essential to performing job duties.

Interpersonal communication Communication between two or more people.

Intuitive decision-making A subconscious process of making decisions on the basis of experience and accumulated judgment.

Nonprogrammed decision A unique decision that requires a custom made solution.

Nonverbal communication Communication transmitted without words through body posture, gestures, and mimics.

Organizational communication All the patterns, networks, and systems of communication within an organization.

Programmed decision A repetitive decision that can be handled by routine approach.

Rationality Consistent with or based on reason; logical. A rational decision needs to be value maximizing and consistent within natural restraining limits.

Risk The conditions under which the decision maker is able to estimate the likelihood of certain outcomes.

Selection of alternative Choosing the alternative with the highest weighted score.

Semantics The study of the actual meaning of words.

Tolerance for ambiguity Individuals with a high tolerance for ambiguity are very time efficient in making decisions because they are able to process many thoughts at the same time. Those with a low tolerance for ambiguity need more time to make a decision because they process information in a consistent and ordered way in order to minimize ambiguity.

Uncertainty A situation in which a decision maker has neither certainty nor reasonable probability estimates available.

Upward communication Upward information flow within the organization from employees to supervisors or managers.

Verbal intonation Use of the voice to emphasize certain parts of a phrase or certain words.

Photo Credits

Credits are listed in the order of appearance.

Index